Mayo Clinic Gastrointestinal Surgery

MAYO CLINIC GASTROINTESTINAL SURGERY

EDITED BY

KEITH A. KELLY, M.D.
MICHAEL G. SARR, M.D.
RONALD A. HINDER, M.D.

Illustrated by
Stephen P. Graepel

SAUNDERS

An Imprint of Elsevier

SAUNDERS

An Imprint of Elsevier

The Curtis Center
Independence Square West
Philadelphia, Pennsylvania 19106

NOTICE

Care has been taken to confirm the accuracy of the information presented and to describe generally accepted practices. However, the authors, editors, and publisher are not responsible for errors or omissions or for
any consequences from application of the information in this book and make no warranty, express or
implied, with respect to the contents of the publication. This book should not be used apart from the
advice of a qualified health care provider.

The authors, editors, and publisher have exerted efforts to ensure that drug selection and dosage set forth
in this text are in accordance with current recommendations and practice at the time of publication. However,
in view of ongoing research, changes in government regulations, and the constant flow of information relating
to drug therapy and drug reactions, the reader is urged to check the package insert for each drug for any change
in indications and dosage and for added warnings and precautions. This is particularly important when the recommended agent is a new or infrequently used drug.

Some drugs and medical devices presented in this publication have U.S. Food and Drug Administration
(FDA) clearance for limited use in restricted research settings. It is the responsibility of health care providers to
ascertain the FDA status of each drug or device planned for use in their clinical practice.

Printed in the United States of America

Last digit is the print number: 9 8 7 6 5 4 3 2 1

DEDICATION

This book is dedicated to the Mayo Clinic surgeons of the past, upon whose shoulders we stand, and to the Mayo Clinic surgeons of the future, who will carry on the work after us.

FOREWORD

Mayo Clinic Gastrointestinal Surgery is the first Mayo Clinic book to cover the broad field of gastrointestinal surgery, a field in which Mayo Clinic surgeons have had a long and extensive experience. This book brings that experience to others.

The book exemplifies the cooperative individualism, the continuity of experience, and the innovations in gastrointestinal surgery as practiced at Mayo Clinic today. It outlines the development of gastrointestinal operations at Mayo Clinic through the years. Surgeons from all three Mayo Clinic practices—Rochester, Jacksonville, and Scottsdale—participated in writing the book. Such a cooperative endeavor is a Mayo Clinic tradition that dates back to our founders, William (Will) J. Mayo, M.D., and Charles (Charlie) H. Mayo, M.D.

In surgical practice at Mayo Clinic, cooperative endeavors are ultimately dependent on the individual surgeon, especially on his or her honesty. To quote from Dr. Will, "...be honest. I mean honesty in every conception of the word: let it enter into all the details of your work; in the treatment of your patients and in your association with your brother practitioners."

Did the Mayo brothers demonstrate such honesty in their surgical practice? Helen Clapesattle, author of the book *The Doctors Mayo*, provides the answer. By 1905, Drs. Will and Charlie were recognized and celebrated as the originators of the no-loop method of gastroenterostomy. U.S. surgeons began referring to it as the "Mayo operation." Dr. Will put a stop to that. According to Clapesattle, Dr. Will said that "all he and Charlie had done was gather up good ideas from many men, assemble them as a whole, and tie a string around them, so that all they could claim credit for was the string." The importance was improved patient care and not the individual surgeon's or physician's career or reputation.

The phrases "cooperative individualism," "honesty in every conception of the word," "continuity of experience," and "building on the knowledge of others" embody the "Mayo way," a distinctive expression of the spirit that binds Mayo Clinic surgeons to their patients and to each other. That spirit is captured in this book.

Oliver H. Beahrs, M.D.

PREFACE

The Mayo Clinic was founded about 100 years ago, at which time gastrointestinal surgery was a key part of the practice. In fact, the spectacular results that the Mayo brothers achieved with cholecystectomy and gastroenterostomy did much to put Mayo Clinic on the map.

Many changes have occurred in gastrointestinal surgery since the Mayos' early efforts. We are now at the beginning of a new century, just over 100 years later. It seems the right time for a book about gastrointestinal surgery as practiced at Mayo Clinic today. Some of the operations we do now were done by the Mayo brothers in the early 1900s (such as inguinal hernia repair and cholecystectomy), but others they perhaps only dreamed of (such as hepatic transplantation and proctocolectomy with ileal pouch-anal canal anastomosis to restore fecal continence). The techniques of operating also have changed markedly, especially with the recent emergence of laparoscopic and minimally invasive technology.

This book is written entirely by current staff at all three Mayo Clinic sites—Rochester, Jacksonville, and Scottsdale. It is intended for surgeons who practice gastrointestinal surgery, gastroenterologists, and others interested in gastrointestinal disease in the United States and abroad and for their fellows, residents, and students.

The book is not an encyclopedia of surgery but focuses instead on the major diseases we treat as gastrointestinal surgeons, from the esophagus to the anal canal. The presentation has a definite clinical orientation and a major emphasis on "how we do it" at Mayo Clinic: the indications for operation, the operations done, and the outcomes of the procedures. Sections on etiology, pathophysiology, pathology, and diagnosis are also included but are purposely not the emphasis of the chapters. We hope that what we do at Mayo Clinic will be of use to those who practice elsewhere.

The editors thank everyone who made this book possible: the authors, their secretaries, the members of Mayo Clinic's superb Section of Scientific Publications, the staff at WB Saunders, and especially our families, who supported us during this effort. This book is the product of the spirit of "cooperative individualism" that pervades Mayo Clinic.

Keith A. Kelly, M.D.
Michael G. Sarr, M.D.
Ronald A. Hinder, M.D.

ACKNOWLEDGMENTS

The editors greatly appreciate the encouragement for this project given to us by Joseph G. Murphy, M.D., Chair of the Section of Scientific Publications at Mayo Clinic. The superb work done by LeAnn Stee, Head of the Section of Scientific Publications at Mayo Clinic, Mary Ann Clifft, Editor at Mayo Clinic in Scottsdale, Arizona, and their editorial colleagues, Roberta J. Schwartz and Sharon L. Wadleigh, strengthened the project immensely by turning our rough texts into polished outcomes. The masterful drawings and art work of Stephen P. Graepel, our medical illustrator, lent a clarity to the operative procedures beyond that which our words could describe. Jeffrey A. Satre, who did the design and layout of the book, assembled our typewritten pages and tables and our illustrations into the attractive format found throughout the book, and John P. Hedlund, proofreader, made sure that the aberrations that always creep in were taken out. Lastly, we recognize with heartfelt appreciation the contribution of our wives, Ann Kelly, Barbara Sarr, and Philla Hinder, who supported us with love, patience, and tolerance throughout the many hours devoted to this enterprise.

LIST OF CONTRIBUTORS

Maher A. Abbas, M.D.
Chief Resident Associate in Surgery, Mayo Graduate School of Medicine; Instructor in Medicine, Mayo Medical School; Rochester, Minnesota

Mark S. Allen, M.D.
Chair, Division of General Thoracic Surgery, Mayo Clinic; Associate Professor of Surgery, Mayo Medical School; Rochester, Minnesota

Yvonne Baerga-Varela, M.D.
Consultant, Division of Trauma, Critical Care and General Surgery, Mayo Clinic; Assistant Professor of Surgery, Mayo Medical School; Rochester, Minnesota

Michael P. Bannon, M.D.
Consultant, Division of Trauma, Critical Care and General Surgery, Mayo Clinic; Assistant Professor of Surgery, Mayo Medical School; Rochester, Minnesota

Oliver H. Beahrs, M.D.
Emeritus Member, Department of Surgery, Mayo Clinic; Emeritus Roberts Professor of Surgery, Mayo Medical School; Rochester, Minnesota

Carolyn Stickney Beck, Ph.D.
Mayo Center for Humanities in Medicine; Assistant Professor of History of Medicine; Rochester, Minnesota

Thomas C. Bower, M.D.
Consultant, Division of Vascular Surgery, Mayo Clinic; Professor of Surgery, Mayo Medical School; Rochester, Minnesota

Kenneth J. Cherry, Jr., M.D.
Consultant, Division of Vascular Surgery, Mayo Clinic; Professor of Surgery, Mayo Medical School; Rochester, Minnesota

Daniel C. Cullinane, M.D.
Consultant, Division of Trauma, Critical Care and General Surgery, Mayo Clinic; Assistant Professor of Surgery, Mayo Medical School; Rochester, Minnesota

Claude Deschamps, M.D.
Consultant, Division of General Thoracic Surgery, Mayo Clinic; Professor of Surgery, Mayo Medical School; Rochester, Minnesota

Richard M. Devine, M.D.
Consultant, Division of Colon and Rectal Surgery, Mayo Clinic; Associate Professor of Surgery, Mayo Medical School; Rochester, Minnesota

Jessica S. Donington, M.D.
Chief Resident in Thoracic Surgery, Mayo Graduate School of Medicine, Rochester, Minnesota

John H. Donohue, M.D.
Consultant, Division of Gastroenterologic and General Surgery, Mayo Clinic; Professor of Surgery, Mayo Medical School; Rochester, Minnesota

Eric J. Dozois, M.D.
Senior Associate Consultant, Division of Colon and Rectal Surgery, Mayo Clinic; Instructor in Surgery, Mayo Medical School; Rochester, Minnesota

Roger R. Dozois, M.D.
Former Chair, Division of Colon and Rectal Surgery, Mayo Clinic; Emeritus Professor of Surgery, Mayo Medical School; Rochester, Minnesota

Hope J. Edmonds, M.D.
Fellow in Family Medicine, Mayo Graduate School of Medicine, Rochester, Minnesota

David R. Farley, M.D.
Consultant, Division of Gastroenterologic and General Surgery, Mayo Clinic; Associate Professor of Surgery, Mayo Medical School; Rochester, Minnesota

Michael B. Farnell, M.D.
Chair, Division of Gastroenterologic and General Surgery, Mayo Clinic; Professor of Surgery, Mayo Medical School; Rochester, Minnesota

Richard J. Fowl, M.D.
Chair, Department of Surgery, Mayo Clinic, Scottsdale, Arizona; Associate Professor of Surgery, Mayo Medical School, Rochester, Minnesota

Debora J. Fox, M.D.
Fellow in Colon and Rectal Surgery, Mayo Graduate School of Medicine, Rochester, Minnesota

Mark E. Freeman, M.D.
Resident in Surgery, Mayo Graduate School of Medicine, Rochester, Minnesota

Jeffrey M. Gauvin, M.D.
Gastrointestinal Surgical Scholar, Division of Gastroenterologic and General Surgery, Mayo Clinic, Rochester, Minnesota

Peter Gloviczki, M.D.
Chair, Division of Vascular Surgery, Mayo Clinic; Professor of Surgery, Mayo Medical School; Rochester, Minnesota

Clive S. Grant, M.D.
Consultant, Division of Gastroenterologic and General Surgery, Mayo Clinic; Professor of Surgery, Mayo Medical School; Rochester, Minnesota

Richard J. Gray, M.D.
Senior Associate Consultant, Division of General Surgery, Mayo Clinic, Scottsdale, Arizona; Assistant Professor of Surgery, Mayo Medical School, Rochester, Minnesota

Leonard L. Gunderson, M.D.
Chair, Department of Radiation Oncology, Mayo Clinic, Scottsdale, Arizona; Getz Family Professor and Professor of Oncology, Mayo Medical School, Rochester, Minnesota

Thomas M. Habermann, M.D.
Consultant, Division of Hematology and Internal Medicine, Mayo Clinic; Professor of Medicine, Mayo Medical School; Rochester, Minnesota

Jacques P. Heppell, M.D.
Head, Section of Colon and Rectal Surgery, Mayo Clinic, Scottsdale, Arizona; Professor of Surgery, Mayo Medical School, Rochester, Minnesota

Glenroy Heywood, M.D.
Gastrointestinal Surgical Scholar, Division of Gastroenterologic and General Surgery, Mayo Clinic, Rochester, Minnesota

Ronald A. Hinder, M.D.
Chair, Department of Surgery, Mayo Clinic, Jacksonville, Florida; Professor of Surgery, Mayo Medical School, Rochester, Minnesota

Dawn E. Jaroszewski, M.D.
Chief Resident Associate, Division of General Surgery, Mayo Clinic, Scottsdale, Arizona; Instructor in Surgery, Mayo Medical School, Rochester, Minnesota

Daniel J. Johnson, M.D.
Chair, Division of General Surgery, Mayo Clinic, Scottsdale, Arizona; Associate Professor of Surgery, Mayo Medical School, Rochester, Minnesota

Corey J. Jost, M.D.
Fellow in Vascular Surgery, Mayo Graduate School of Medicine; Instructor in Surgery, Mayo Medical School; Rochester, Minnesota

Keith A. Kelly, M.D.
Former Chair, Department of Surgery, Mayo Clinic, Scottsdale, Arizona; Former Chair, Department of Surgery, Mayo Clinic, Rochester, Minnesota; Emeritus Roberts Professor of Surgery, Mayo Medical School, Rochester, Minnesota; Consultant in Research, Mayo Clinic, Scottsdale, Arizona

Michael L. Kendrick, M.D.
Resident in Surgery, Mayo Graduate School of Medicine, Rochester, Minnesota

Alexander Klaus, M.D.
Research Fellow in Surgery, Mayo Graduate School of Medicine, Rochester, Minnesota

Louis A. Lanza, M.D.
Chair, Division of Cardiovascular and Thoracic Surgery, Mayo Clinic, Scottsdale, Arizona; Assistant Professor of Surgery, Mayo Medical School, Rochester, Minnesota

J. Kirk Martin, Jr., M.D.
Consultant, Section of General Surgery, Mayo Clinic, Jacksonville, Florida; Professor of Surgery, Mayo Medical School, Rochester, Minnesota

Elizabeth J. McConnell, M.D.
Senior Associate Consultant, Section of Colon and Rectal Surgery, Mayo Clinic, Scottsdale, Arizona; Assistant Professor of Surgery, Mayo Medical School, Rochester, Minnesota

Donald C. McIlrath, M.D.
Former Chair, Department of Surgery, Mayo Clinic; Emeritus Professor of Surgery, Mayo Medical School; Rochester, Minnesota

Christopher R. Moir, M.D.
Chair, Division of Pediatric Surgery, Mayo Clinic; Associate Professor of Surgery, Mayo Medical School; Rochester, Minnesota

David M. Nagorney, M.D.
Consultant, Division of Gastroenterologic and General Surgery, Mayo Clinic; Professor of Surgery, Mayo Medical School; Rochester, Minnesota

Heidi Nelson, M.D.
Chair, Division of Colon and Rectal Surgery, Mayo Clinic; Professor of Surgery, Mayo Medical School; Rochester, Minnesota

Santhat Nivatvongs, M.D.
Consultant, Division of Colon and Rectal Surgery, Mayo Clinic; Professor of Surgery, Mayo Medical School; Rochester, Minnesota

Scott L. Nyberg, M.D.
Consultant, Division of Transplantation Surgery, Mayo Clinic; Associate Professor of Surgery, Mayo Medical School; Rochester, Minnesota

W. Andrew Oldenburg, M.D.
Head, Section of Vascular Surgery, Mayo Clinic, Jacksonville, Florida; Assistant Professor of Surgery, Mayo Medical School, Rochester, Minnesota

Daniel J. Ostlie, M.D.
Chief Resident in Surgery, Mayo Graduate School of Medicine; Instructor in Surgery, Mayo Medical School; Rochester, Minnesota

Peter C. Pairolero, M.D.
Chair, Department of Surgery, Mayo Clinic; Professor of Surgery, Mayo Medical School; Rochester, Minnesota

John H. Pemberton, M.D.
Consultant, Division of Colon and Rectal Surgery, Mayo Clinic; Professor of Surgery, Mayo Medical School; Rochester, Minnesota

Barbara A. Pockaj, M.D.
Consultant, Division of General Surgery, Mayo Clinic, Scottsdale, Arizona; Assistant Professor of Surgery, Mayo Medical School, Rochester, Minnesota

Mikel Prieto, M.D.
Consultant, Division of Transplantation Surgery, Mayo Clinic; Assistant Professor of Surgery, Mayo Medical School; Rochester, Minnesota

Florencia G. Que, M.D.
Consultant, Division of Gastroenterologic and General Surgery, Mayo Clinic; Assistant Professor of Surgery, Mayo Medical School; Rochester, Minnesota

David A. Rodeberg, M.D.
Consultant, Division of Pediatric Surgery, Mayo Clinic; Assistant Professor of Surgery, Mayo Medical School; Rochester, Minnesota

Joaquin A. Rodriguez, M.D.
Fellow in Surgery, Mayo Graduate School of Medicine, Rochester, Minnesota

Charles B. Rosen, M.D.
Consultant, Division of Transplantation Surgery, Mayo Clinic; Associate Professor of Surgery, Mayo Medical School; Rochester, Minnesota

Juan M. Sarmiento, M.D.
Senior Associate Consultant, Division of Gastroenterologic and General Surgery, Mayo Clinic; Assistant Professor of Surgery, Mayo Medical School; Rochester, Minnesota

Michael G. Sarr, M.D.
Consultant, Division of Gastroenterologic and General Surgery, Mayo Clinic; Professor of Surgery, Mayo Medical School; Rochester, Minnesota

Mark D. Sawyer, M.D.
Consultant, Division of Trauma, Critical Care and General Surgery, Mayo Clinic; Assistant Professor of Surgery, Mayo Medical School; Rochester, Minnesota

Steven E. Schild, M.D.
Consultant, Department of Radiation Oncology, Mayo Clinic, Scottsdale, Arizona; Associate Professor of Oncology, Mayo Medical School, Rochester, Minnesota

Richard T. Schlinkert, M.D.
Consultant, Division of General Surgery, Mayo Clinic, Scottsdale, Arizona; Professor of Surgery, Mayo Medical School, Rochester, Minnesota

Stephen L. Smith, M.D.
Consultant, Section of General Surgery, Mayo Clinic, Jacksonville, Florida; Assistant Professor of Surgery, Mayo Medical School, Rochester, Minnesota

Mark D. Stegall, M.D.
Chair, Division of Transplantation Surgery, Mayo Clinic; Associate Professor of Surgery, Mayo Medical School; Rochester, Minnesota

Luca Stocchi, M.D.
Resident in Colon and Rectal Surgery, Mayo Clinic, Rochester, Minnesota

William M. Stone, M.D.
Chair, Division of Vascular Surgery, Mayo Clinic, Scottsdale, Arizona; Associate Professor of Surgery, Mayo Medical School, Rochester, Minnesota

James M. Swain, M.D.
Senior Associate Consultant, Division of General Surgery, Mayo Clinic, Scottsdale, Arizona; Assistant Professor of Surgery, Mayo Medical School, Rochester, Minnesota

Geoffrey B. Thompson, M.D.
Consultant, Division of Gastroenterologic and General Surgery, Mayo Clinic; Professor of Surgery, Mayo Medical School; Rochester, Minnesota

Victor F. Trastek, M.D.
Consultant, Division of Cardiovascular and Thoracic Surgery, Mayo Clinic, Scottsdale, Arizona; Professor of Surgery, Mayo Medical School, Rochester, Minnesota

Jon A. van Heerden, M.D.
Consultant, Division of Gastroenterologic and General Surgery, Mayo Clinic; Fred C. Andersen Professor and Professor of Surgery, Mayo Medical School; Rochester, Minnesota

Grettel K. Wentling, M.D.
Resident in Surgery, Mayo Graduate School of Medicine, Rochester, Minnesota

Bruce G. Wolff, M.D.
Consultant, Division of Colon and Rectal Surgery, Mayo Clinic; Professor of Surgery, Mayo Medical School; Rochester, Minnesota

Tonia M. Young-Fadok, M.D.
Consultant, Section of Colon and Rectal Surgery, Mayo Clinic, Scottsdale, Arizona; Associate Professor of Surgery, Mayo Medical School, Rochester, Minnesota

Salman Zaheer, M.D.
Fellow in Thoracic Surgery, Mayo Graduate School of Medicine, Rochester, Minnesota

Shaheen Zakaria, M.D.
Resident in Surgery, Mayo Graduate School of Medicine, Rochester, Minnesota

Nicholas J. Zyromski, M.D.
Research Fellow in Surgery, Mayo Graduate School of Medicine, Rochester, Minnesota

TABLE OF CONTENTS

1. **On Being a Mayo Clinic Surgeon**   *Keith A. Kelly, M.D.; Jon A. van Heerden, M.D.; Carolyn Stickney Beck, Ph.D.* 1

2. **Gastroesophageal Reflux and Esophageal Hiatal Hernia**
   Alexander Klaus, M.D.; Ronald A. Hinder, M.D. 23

3. **Achalasia and Other Esophageal Motility Disorders**
   Jessica S. Donington, M.D.; Mark S. Allen, M.D. 37

4. **Epiphrenic Esophageal Diverticula**   *Ronald A. Hinder, M.D.; Joaquin A. Rodriguez, M.D.* 49

5. **Cancer of the Esophagus**   *Dawn E. Jaroszewski, M.D.; Claude Deschamps, M.D.; Leonard L. Gunderson, M.D.; Louis A. Lanza, M.D.; Victor F. Trastek, M.D.; Peter C. Pairolero, M.D.* 57

6. **Gastric Adenocarcinoma**   *Barbara A. Pockaj, M.D.* 75

7. **Primary Gastric Lymphoma**   *Clive S. Grant, M.D.; Thomas M. Habermann, M.D.* 91

8. **Peptic Ulcer**   *Richard J. Gray, M.D.; Keith A. Kelly, M.D.* .103

9. **Disorders of Gastrointestinal Motility and Emptying After Gastric Operations**
   Keith A. Kelly, M.D.; Michael G. Sarr, M.D.; Ronald A. Hinder, M.D. 127

10. **Morbid Obesity**   *Michael G. Sarr, M.D.; Keith A. Kelly, M.D.; Geoffrey B. Thompson, M.D.; Florencia G. Que, M.D.* 139

11. **Hepatocellular Carcinoma and Intrahepatic Cholangiocarcinoma**
    Juan M. Sarmiento, M.D.; David M. Nagorney, M.D. 159

12. **Hepatic Metastases From Extrahepatic Cancers**   *Florencia G. Que, M.D.; John H. Donohue, M.D.; David M. Nagorney, M.D.* 177

13. **Benign Tumors and Cysts of the Liver**   *Glenroy Heywood, M.D.; Florencia G. Que, M.D.* 191

14. **Liver Diseases Necessitating Liver Transplantation**   *Charles B. Rosen, M.D.* 209

15. **Biliary Stone Disease**   *Shaheen Zakaria, M.D.; Salman Zaheer, M.D.; John H. Donohue, M.D.* 225

16. **Benign Biliary Strictures**   *Grettel K. Wentling, M.D.; Juan M. Sarmiento, M.D.; J. Kirk Martin, Jr., M.D.; David M. Nagorney, M.D.* 247

17. **Cancer of the Gallbladder**   *John H. Donohue, M.D.* 261

18. **Pancreatic and Periampullary Carcinoma**   *Glenroy Heywood, M.D.; Michael B. Farnell, M.D.* 271

19. **Islet Cell Tumors**   *Geoffrey B. Thompson, M.D.* 299

20. **Acute and Chronic Pancreatitis**   *Nicholas J. Zyromski, M.D.; Michael L. Kendrick, M.D.; Michael G. Sarr, M.D.* 321

21. **Pancreas Transplantation After Complications of Diabetes Mellitus**   *Mikel Prieto, M.D.; Scott L. Nyberg, M.D.; Mark D. Stegall, M.D.* 341

22. **Cystic Tumors of the Pancreas**   *Glenroy Heywood, M.D.; Jon A. van Heerden, M.D.* 351

23. **Thrombocytopenia and Other Hematologic Disorders**
    James M. Swain, M.D.; Richard T. Schlinkert, M.D. 365

24. **Malignant Tumors of the Small Intestine** *Hope J. Edmonds, M.D.;*
    J. Kirk Martin, Jr., M.D.; Keith A. Kelly, M.D. 375

25. **Villous Tumors of the Duodenum** *Jeffrey M. Gauvin, M.D.; Michael B. Farnell, M.D.* 387

26. **Small Intestinal Diverticula** *Daniel J. Ostlie, M.D.; Keith A. Kelly, M.D.* 397

27. **Crohn's Disease** *Debora J. Fox, M.D.; Bruce G. Wolff, M.D.* 409

28. **Small Bowel Obstruction** *Yvonne Baerga-Varela, M.D.* 421

29. **Acute Mesenteric Ischemia** *Richard J. Fowl, M.D.* 441

30. **Acute Mesenteric Venous Thrombosis** *Peter Gloviczki, M.D.; Kenneth J. Cherry, Jr., M.D.;*
    Thomas C. Bower, M.D.; Corey J. Jost, M.D. 447

31. **Chronic Mesenteric Ischemia** *W. Andrew Oldenburg, M.D.* 457

32. **Visceral Artery Aneurysms** *William M. Stone, M.D.; Maher A. Abbas, M.D.* 467

33. **Colonic Motor Disorders: Constipation** *Luca Stocchi, M.D.; John H. Pemberton, M.D.* 475

34. **Diverticular Disease of the Colon** *Tonia M. Young-Fadok, M.D.* .489

35. **Colon Cancer** *Debora J. Fox, M.D.; Heidi Nelson, M.D.* 507

36. **Ischemic Colitis** *Mark D. Sawyer, M.D.* 519

37. **Appendicitis** *Michael P. Bannon, M.D.* 525

38. **Chronic Ulcerative Colitis** *Keith A. Kelly, M.D.; Roger R. Dozois, M.D.* 533

39. **Colonic Volvulus** *Richard M. Devine, M.D.* 553

40. **Familial Adenomatous Polyposis** *Eric J. Dozois, M.D.; Roger R. Dozois, M.D.* 559

41. **Cancer of the Rectum** *Jacques P. Heppell, M.D.; Elizabeth J. McConnell, M.D.;*
    Steven E. Schild, M.D. 569

42. **Common Anorectal Problems** *Santhat Nivatvongs, M.D.* 589

43. **Rectal Prolapse and Solitary Rectal Ulcer Syndrome** *Santhat Nivatvongs, M.D.* 627

44. **Abdominal Trauma** *Daniel J. Johnson, M.D.; Daniel C. Cullinane, M.D.* 637

45. **The Unclosable Abdomen and the Dehisced Wound**
    Daniel C. Cullinane, M.D.; Michael P. Bannon, M.D. 653

46. **Ventral and Incisional Hernias** *David R. Farley, M.D.; Mark D. Sawyer, M.D.;*
    Michael G. Sarr, M.D. 665

47. **Inguinal Hernia: Open Repair** *Mark E. Freeman, M.D.; Stephen L. Smith, M.D.* 679

48. **Endoscopic Inguinal Hernia Repair** *David R. Farley, M.D.; John H. Donohue, M.D.* 691

49. **Common Pediatric Gastrointestinal Disorders**
    David A. Rodeberg, M.D.; Christopher R. Moir, M.D. 699

Index 723

On Being a Mayo Clinic Surgeon

Keith A. Kelly, M.D.
Jon A. van Heerden, M.D.
Carolyn Stickney Beck, Ph.D.

AN EXPERIMENT IN COOPERATIVE INDIVIDUALISM[1,2]

Shortly after joining the Mayo Clinic staff in 1967, one of the authors (K.A.K.) began attending the annual Mayo Clinic staff dinner. According to a long-standing tradition at this event, retiring surgeons and physicians are honored with an encomium and gift. Retirees approaching the stage to receive these items had been past presidents of the American College of Surgeons, the American Neurosurgical Association, the American Orthopaedic Association, and the American College of Physicians. The list went on. As a new person on the staff, Dr. Kelly wondered, "Where did the Mayo Clinic get all these great people who added so much to Mayo and to American surgery and medicine during their careers?" Before long, the answer was clear. Mayo Clinic had placed into the hands of its staff the tools they needed to develop spectacular careers, which in turn brought honor to the individuals and to the clinic. What is it about Mayo Clinic that allows this kind of personal and institutional growth?

This insight and continuing search for understanding about Mayo Clinic echo the observations and curiosity of many others. The educational potential in this curiosity is summarized in Helen Clapesattle's seminal pronouncement on the Mayo brothers' ideals: "Whether (such) attitudes and qualities can be perpetuated in an organization beyond the generation of the founders is a social question of the first magnitude. As an experiment in cooperative individualism, the Mayo Clinic deserves watching—and not by doctors alone."[1]

MAYO CLINIC HISTORY AND CULTURE

Beginning as a Family

There are many important dates in the history of Mayo Clinic, but there is no founding date. The Mayo family did not preconceive the group practice of medicine. It grew from their focus on, and broad understanding of, the needs of the patient, a yearning to discover through education and research, and, most fundamentally, their relationships with each other.

William Worrall Mayo immigrated to the United States in 1846 from Manchester, England, and worked his way west from New York City, earning his M.D. degree from Indiana Medical College in La Porte in 1850 (Fig. 1). He settled in Rochester, Minnesota, in 1863 as a Civil War examining surgeon for the Union enrollment board, first Minnesota district. Fiercely self-reliant, resourceful, and full of pioneering spirit, Dr. Mayo was nonetheless guided by his prevailing wisdom, "No man is big enough to be independent of others." Dr. Mayo's axiom is most likely the seed that developed into the integrated group practice of Mayo Clinic.

Dr. Mayo's prevailing wisdom was akin to the guiding principle of his wife, Louise Abigail Wright Mayo, whom their son Charles (Charlie) Horace described as "a real good doctor herself"[3] (Fig. 2). In his senior years, their son William (Will) James recalled this principle: "We should not over stress the duty other people owe to us but should bear in mind what our duty is to other people; the moral obligation is essentially mutual."[4] Honoring their parents'

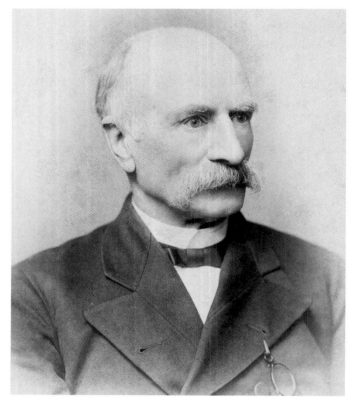

Fig. 1. William Worrall Mayo, M.D.

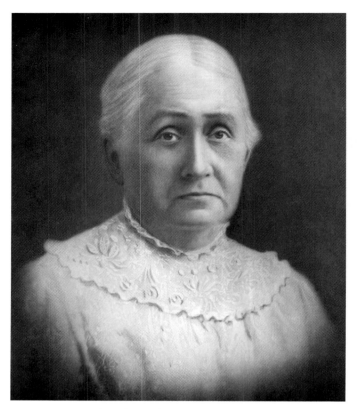

Fig. 2. Louise Abigail Wright Mayo.

wisdom and principles, Will and Charlie often said, "We grew up to be physicians" (Fig. 3 and 4). When Will received his M.D. degree from the University of Michigan in 1883, he returned home to join his father's practice. Charlie followed in 1888 after graduating from Chicago Medical College of Northwestern University.

In 1910, 5 years after his election as president of the American Medical Association, Dr. Will delivered the commencement address entitled "The Necessity of Cooperation in the Practice of Medicine" at Rush Medical College. The Mayo family philosophy rings clearly in his words: "The best interest of the patient is the only interest to be considered and in order that the sick may have the benefit of advancing knowledge, union of forces is necessary..."

> *I would admonish you, above all other considerations, to be honest. I mean honest in every conception of the word: let it enter into all the details of your work; in the treatment of your patients and in your association with your brother practitioners. Should you have no stronger incentive, be assured that, to be other than fair, generous, and sincere, will ultimately spell ruin and not success. Jealousy in the medical profession is proverbial and it has done more to retard development than all other restricting influences combined.*[5]

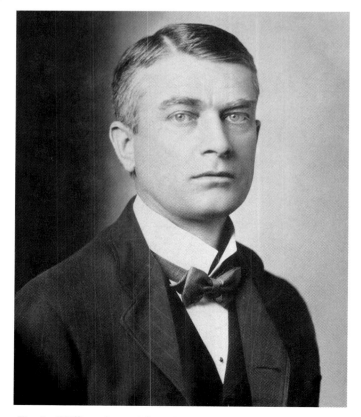

Fig. 3. William James Mayo, M.D.

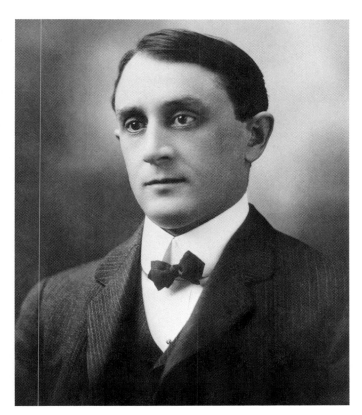

Fig. 4. Charles Horace Mayo, M.D.

The Mayo brothers believed that individual talent, energy, and imagination should always be in service as a shared resource to meet the needs of the patient. Their unwillingness to compromise this fundamental principle is expressed in Dr. Will's firing of Fred W. Rankin, M.D., a masterful surgeon who was married to Dr. Charlie's daughter Edith. Not even an exceptionally skilled surgeon who was a member of the Mayo family was excused from the responsibility for collegial effort and collective commitment expected of Mayo Clinic staff members.

Seventy years after Dr. Will's address at Rush Medical College, Mayo Clinic surgeon Oscar T. (Jim) Clagett, M.D. (Fig. 5), described the Mayo brothers' capacity to express this philosophy in dealing with the staff:

> *A particular attribute in the genius of the Mayo brothers was their ability to recognize qualities of leadership and talents in younger colleagues. They then provided opportunities and an environment and freedom to grow and develop as fast and as far as each individual's talents, energy, and imagination would allow. Age and experience were respected by the staff of the Mayo Clinic, but there was no hierarchy of position or power that ever inhibited or deterred the advancement of an enthusiastic, capable younger individual. The Mayo brothers were never afraid that others might grow to overshadow them and their own accomplishments. Instead, they encouraged*

and took pride in the innovations, advances, and contributions that came from their younger colleagues.[6]

Integrating the Group Practice

The Mayos knew that working as a team offered the best possibilities for patient care. As their ideas were implemented in their practice, pooling of resources in the care of patients resulted in efficiency in practice management. Currently, this integrated group practice system allows a patient to see a surgeon, a physician, and a host of other consultants in the same building on a single day. Consultations are centralized and diagnostic facilities are readily available. The broad nature of the approach has encouraged innovation, bringing wide-ranging ideas and knowledge to bear on the patient's problem in order to provide better care than one person alone could provide.

Pooling of resources has long been a hallmark of research, education, and patient care at Mayo Clinic. Dr. Clagett attributed the origins of this approach to weekly staff meetings, pathology conferences, and informal seminars. Staff members have an unusual opportunity to consider a large number and wide range of medical and surgical problems. Dr. Clagett noted that during his 40 years of experience, beginning in 1935, Mayo Clinic physicians and surgeons took seriously their responsibility for sharing their knowledge with all their professional colleagues. As a result,

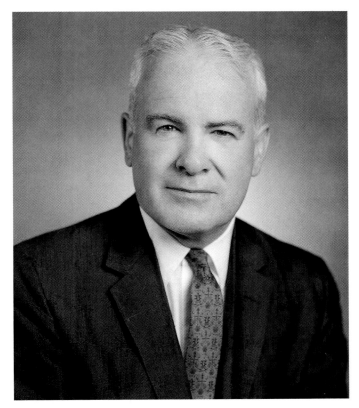

Fig. 5. Oscar T. (Jim) Clagett, M.D.

they devoted considerable effort to presenting papers at professional meetings. This research and education effort was directed toward serving the needs of patients, no matter where they might receive their medical care. According to Dr. Clagett, the ongoing peer review system that has prevailed at Mayo Clinic since its inception has helped to prevent unnecessary surgical procedures. Accordingly, this system has fostered conservation of financial resources available for health care.[7]

Conserving financial resources to serve patients was always a central concern of the Mayo brothers. In 1919, they founded Mayo Properties Association, known today as Mayo Foundation. This legal and financial structure meant that the Mayos, their partners, and all future Mayo Clinic physicians and surgeons would receive a salary and not profit personally from the proceeds of the practice. In 1926, the Mayo brothers explained their intentions:

> Because it was believed that the possibilities for good of the institution should in no way be hampered by individual ownership it was early determined that the future should be made as secure as possible by placing the Clinic and all its properties, both personal and real, without reservation, in the hands of trustees to be used for the benefit of this and future generations.[8]

The Mayo brothers' generosity and sweeping sense of responsibility also are reflected in their attention to a wide range of patient needs. For example, they insisted that the clinic's responsibility for patients extended beyond the door of the examining room to include their entire stay in Rochester.[9]

Since the earliest days of Mayo Clinic, the integrated group practice has involved not only surgeons and physicians but also the entire health care team, including physicians' assistants, nurses, paramedical personnel, secretaries, chaplains, custodians, and all other staff members. Mayo Clinic has demonstrated that an integrated group practice can provide excellent, compassionate, and cost-effective medical care. This "experiment in cooperative individualism" has stimulated the development of other such practices, both nationally and internationally. In the year 2000, there were approximately 7,000 group practices in the United States.

Mayo Clinic has continued to expand its practice during the past 40 years. Today, approximately 500,000 patients are seen within the Mayo Clinic system each year. As a result, surgeons at the clinic have a vast experience in treating a wide variety of surgical problems. This expansive practice also allows individual Mayo Clinic surgeons to focus on particular areas. Large series of operations in specific areas, including uncommon diseases, are accomplished in such a system.

Mayo Clinic provides surgeons with superb clinical facilities in both the outpatient and the hospital setting. State-of-the-art diagnostic equipment and laboratories are always available to facilitate patient care.

Focusing on the Patient
The Mayo Clinic medical records system enhances the ability of the staff to work as a team focusing on the individual patient. Each new patient coming to Mayo Clinic is given a unique identification number. A personal medical record follows each patient throughout the clinic. The record is sent from the outpatient area to the diagnostic laboratories and to the hospitals and operating rooms, depending on the location of the patient at any time. All data regarding the patient, including clinical evaluation, diagnostic tests, and operative and pathologic reports, are included in the record and kept in a single patient history packet.

The Mayo Clinic medical records system was initiated in 1907. It was developed by Henry S. Plummer, M.D. (Fig. 6), and Miss Mabel C. Root (Fig. 7), a Rochester native who was not formally educated beyond high school. William F. Braasch, M.D., who joined the staff of Mayo Clinic in the same year and helped to establish the Section of Urology, observed the impact of this system on the organization of Mayo Clinic (Fig. 8):

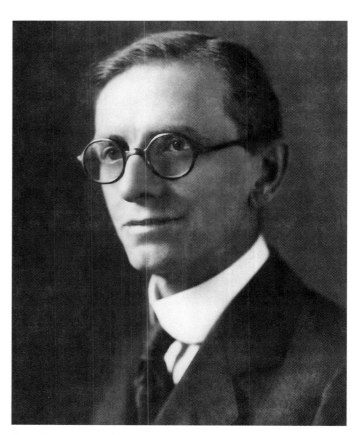

Fig. 6. Henry S. Plummer, M.D.

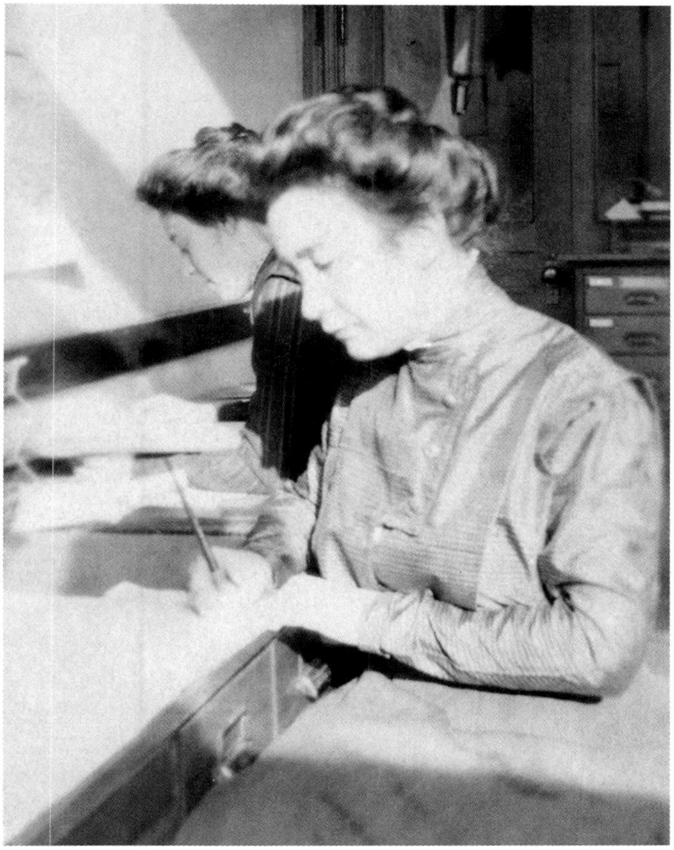

Fig. 7. Miss Mabel C. Root.

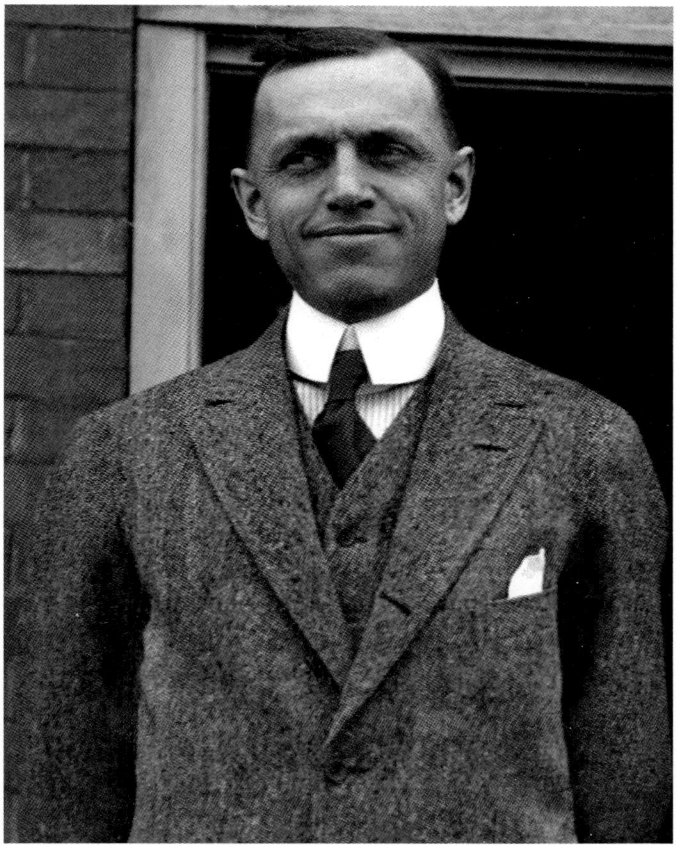

Fig. 8. William F. Braasch, M.D.

The organization of the diagnostic staff according to special fields having been established with benefit in expediting patient care, other essential factors involved the patient's course while undergoing diagnosis and appropriate care. Dr. Plummer held that fundamental to the success of a system involving the patient's examination and treatment was the concept that the patient must be regarded as a unit by members of the staff and that the one serial number given the patient on registration ought to be used in all divisions of the Clinic. Dr. Will also held similar ideas; he believed that the patient must be regarded as a whole and not be divided clinically, so to speak, to represent several fields. He emphasized the point, moreover, that the patient should continue to have the personal interest of the clinician in the section to which he had been assigned at the time he registered. The fundamental principle, according to which any member of the entire staff is available for consultation when examination of the patient indicates such a need, was firmly established at this time.[10]

As Dr. Braasch recalled, from that point on, consultation among various clinical specialties was routine at Mayo Clinic. This system automatically keeps specialists in touch with problems in other medical fields. Dr. Will insisted that specialist members of the staff stay current in other fields of medicine by examining patients who were likely to require a more routine diagnosis. This insistence was based on one of the Mayos' strongest convictions: "the combined wisdom of a man's peers is greater than that of any individual."[11]

How strongly did the Mayo brothers believe that the examining physician and the consulting surgeon should be scrupulously collegial in leading the team caring for the patient? Dr. Braasch's remembrance of the Mayos suggests the depth of their commitment to this principle: "When either Dr. Will or Dr. Charlie saw a patient who had a serious or complicated lesion he would ask the examining physician to call the other Mayo brother in consultation."[12]

The Mayo brothers envisioned and implemented collective wisdom based on consensus generated through an extensive committee system. In their view, this was the most trustworthy and efficient approach to pooling resources. They also had the wisdom and courage to proclaim that this "union of forces" could ultimately benefit the patient only if it was conveyed through a unique relationship jointly created by the physician and the patient.

The Mayo Clinic medical record system was designed to support such relationships. This system, now nearly a century old, was recently computerized. The patient history is now in electronic form, but the principles of organization remain the same as they were in 1907. A careful record is made of all the major diagnoses for the patient and of all the operations that the patient has undergone. The system currently contains the records of more than 6 million patients. Virtually all are immediately available for review and analysis. This database provides an enormous clinical resource for the study of particular diseases or operations.

In fact, one of the major strengths of Mayo Clinic is the continuous evaluation and analysis of the system, with the production of reports regarding treatment outcomes of large groups of patients with the same disease and the same operation. Conclusions regarding efficacy of procedures and suggestions for changes in patient management are drawn from these reports. Mayo Clinic considers these records to belong to Mayo Foundation and not to specific individuals. In accordance with the integrated group practice system, Mayo Clinic papers are written on the basis of the collective experience of Mayo Clinic staff, not on the basis of the experience of any particular surgeon.

Mayo Clinic continues to recognize that the strengths of the integrated group practice ultimately depend on the time-honored physician-patient relationship. Accordingly, Mayo Clinic identifies an individual physician for each patient. Each physician caring for a patient has autonomy to treat that patient as he or she best sees fit. It is clear that patients cannot be cared for by a committee. An individual physician, developing the physician-patient relationship, is in the best position to direct the care of each patient. Surrounded and advised by other Mayo Clinic consultants and allied health staff, the physician tailors the system in a unique way to meet the needs of the patient. With this approach, each patient-physician encounter is an expression of "cooperative individualism."

Focusing on Relationships

Over the years, many Mayo Clinic physicians and surgeons have become legendary because of their gifts for creating relationships with both patients and colleagues. Dr. Clagett described Donald C. Balfour, M.D., a surgeon at Mayo Clinic from 1907 to 1947 (Fig. 9):

> He had all the attributes of an ideal surgeon. He immediately won the confidence of his patients and in every way exemplified the art of physician-patient relationships to such a degree as to make an imperishable impression on patients, colleagues, and assistants.
>
> He carried the qualities of heart and mind into the operating room and created an atmosphere of dignity, confidence, and coordination. He was a superb craftsman and operated with dexterity and speed. His unfailing kindness, understanding, and encouragement won the affection and respect of everyone.[13]

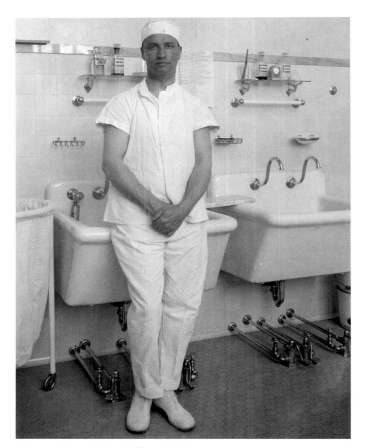

Fig. 9. Donald C. Balfour, M.D.

Continuity of experience through the kind of collegial relationships exemplified by Dr. Balfour and others is a key element of Mayo Clinic, according to John W. Kirklin, M.D., pioneer cardiovascular surgeon at Mayo Clinic from 1944 to 1966 (Fig. 10). In his 1985 Reynolds Historical Lecture at the University of Alabama, "Lessons Learned From the History of the Mayo Clinic," Dr. Kirklin reflected on his 22 years at Mayo Clinic:

> In the first five years of my career as a surgeon at the Mayo Clinic during about 10% of my time I did what little cardiac surgery there was to do and 90% of my time I did what I had been trained to do: abdominal, breast, general thoracic and neck surgery. We were still doing some gastrojejunostomies at that time. I learned to do that operation and many others from Dr. W. J. Mayo. Dr. Donald Balfour, who married Dr. Will's daughter, Carrie, became a world famous gastric surgeon and he learned to do this operation from Dr. Will Mayo. Dr. Waltman Walters, subsequently himself a famous surgeon (whose wife was Dr. Will Mayo's other daughter, Phoebe), learned to do this operation from Dr. Will and Dr. Balfour. It was my great good fortune to learn to do this operation from Dr. Walters and from a surgeon that Dr. Walters trained, Dr. Jim Clagett. I have always felt that one of the most unique parts of my surgical

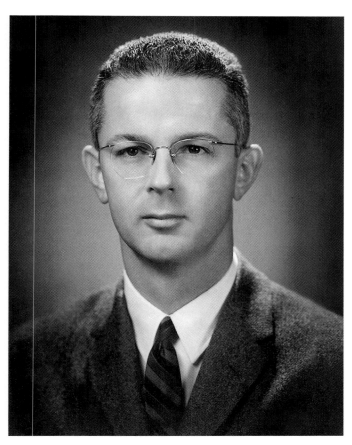

Fig. 10. John W. Kirklin, M.D.

training was that I learned from the accumulated wisdom of Dr. W. J. Mayo and his brother and that I inherited the results of a continuous surgical experience of over 50 years from my teachers. Thus I have always felt that one of the great lessons from the surgical successes of Dr. Mayo and his great clinic is that continuity of experience enhances patient care, research and education.

The academic world is often characterized by frequent changes in the location of the principal players. Many of my friends in academic life through the years have worked in one institution for 5 to 8 years and then in another for a similar period of time, and finally in a third. There is no way they could have had a continuous experience in patient care or education or research or even in administration. Their own personal experiences have limited value without this continuity.[14]

Mayo Clinic develops surgeons who aspire to be like Dr. Balfour, Dr. Kirklin, and other leaders, because the incentives for work are professional and not economic. Each staff member is paid a salary, which is independent of productivity. This arrangement allows the surgeon to advise an operation for a patient based solely on what is best for the patient. The decision to operate does not place any extra money in the pocket of a surgeon at Mayo Clinic.

A focus on professional rather than economic incentives is a distinguishing feature of Mayo Clinic surgeons. Unaware of this focus, visiting surgeons often direct their questions toward the business dimension of surgery at Mayo Clinic. One of the authors (J.v.H.) responds to such questions by saying, "We have no idea. We honestly do not concern ourselves with the financial aspects of patient care. In our day-to-day work, money does not raise its head." This response is typical of Mayo Clinic surgeons' answers to such questions. Mr. Harry J. Harwick, chief administrative officer at Mayo Clinic from 1908 to 1952, explained the administrative foundation for such responses (Fig. 11): "...non-medical sections developed to serve physicians, to the end that physicians might more effectively serve patients."[15]

Although their incentives are not primarily economic, Mayo Clinic surgeons and physicians do work hard. The professional incentives that motivate them are based in part on peer recognition. Members of the team want to keep up their end of the work and are eager to do their part. Recognition, by themselves and others, that they are doing their part is an important incentive. It is noteworthy that the volume of procedures done by each Mayo Clinic surgeon is surprisingly uniform throughout each division within the Department of Surgery.

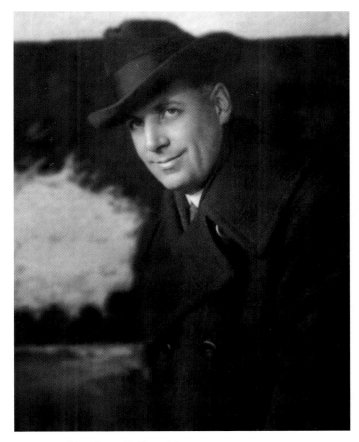

Fig. 11. Mr. Harry J. Harwick.

Serving Patients Through Research and Education

Mayo Clinic recognized early on that providing the best possible care for patients necessitates a professional environment that supports and encourages both research and education. This interdependence is symbolized clearly in the Mayo Clinic logo, which shows three interlocking shields (Fig. 12). The largest shield represents practice and the primary principle that "the needs of the patient come first." The two smaller, but interlocking, shields represent research and education: the development of new knowledge and the teaching of others integrated with, and dedicated to, patient care.

In the educational programs at Mayo Clinic, physicians-in-training and medical students are assigned to surgical services and integrated into the health care team. Mayo Clinic surgeons teach in the clinic, in the hospital, in the operating rooms, and in conferences, seminars, and lectures. Teaching is an important part of the professional life of a Mayo Clinic surgeon. As in most other U.S. medical centers, Mayo Clinic physicians who are in residency training programs are referred to as "residents." Before the 1970s, they were called "fellows," a term chosen because of its Middle English meaning, "companions in studies." Today, there are more than 1,200 Mayo Clinic residents. More than 80 of these residents serve in general surgical training programs. Mayo Clinic still has fellows; they usually serve as advanced trainees in special programs outside the residency programs.

Research has been an important part of Mayo Clinic from the inception of the practice. A 1912 report documents the presence of an experimental laboratory at Mayo Clinic and a designated director of research. Research has expanded since then to include more than 200 full-time researchers. In addition, about a third of clinicians at

Mayo Clinic have ongoing projects in clinical or basic research. The Mayo Clinic annual research budget totals about $120 million, two-thirds of which comes from external, non-Mayo sources.

The integrated group practice concept also extends to the interaction between the practicing clinical surgeon and the research team. Advances made in the basic science laboratories and in the clinical study units can be readily implemented in the clinic and on the hospital wards because of the close working relationships between the research and the clinical teams. Some Mayo Clinic surgeons straddle the fence between research and practice and work in both areas. Almost all surgeons have some interaction with the researchers, forming the needed teams that bring new advances from the bench to the bedside. Perhaps Mayo Clinic's most distinguished example of this type of collaboration was between Edward C. Kendall, Ph.D., and Philip S. Hench, M.D. (Fig. 13). Dr. Kendall isolated the adrenal hormone cortisone and Dr. Hench applied this discovery to patient care. They received the Nobel Prize for their efforts in 1950.

Serving the Public Good

Mayo Clinic evolved from a partnership of physicians and surgeons to a private foundation for the public good. There are no stockholders and no private owners or other individuals who personally profit from the activities of Mayo Clinic. Mayo Foundation and its staff serve the public as a nonprofit organization. In accordance with the Mayos' conviction that physicians, not administrators, should direct the practice, the Mayo Clinic Board of Governors is led by a physician, and all major committees are led by physicians. A physician-led clinic is more likely to be anchored in the principle that "the needs of the

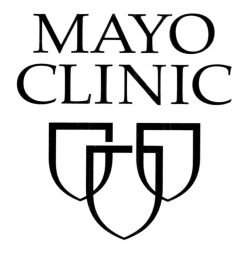

Fig. 12. Mayo Clinic logo.

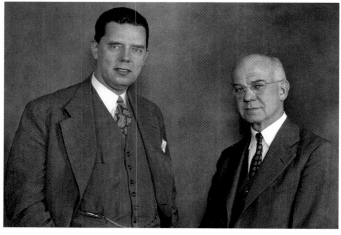

Fig. 13. Philip S. Hench, M.D. (left), *and Edward C. Kendall, Ph.D.* (right).

patient come first" than a clinic led by individuals who are not directly responsible for patient care.

In recent years, Mayo Foundation has benefited from the inclusion of distinguished public members in leadership roles. The Mayo Foundation Board of Trustees, on which public members serve, advises the Mayo Clinic Board of Governors about the long-term directions of the clinic. The Board of Governors, all Mayo Clinic employees, carry out the day-to-day operations.

According to Mr. Harwick, the board must set policy based on the best interest of the patient, the institution, and the individual staff member. Each Mayo Clinic committee and department is responsible for finding the most beneficial balance of these interests.[16]

Mayo Clinic surgeons contribute to the governance of the clinic. Many have served as chair of the Board of Governors, members of the Board of Governors, and chairs of important committees. James T. Priestley, M.D., Ph.D. (Fig. 14), served on the Board of Governors as a member from 1947-1956 and was chair from 1956-1964. Dr. Clagett described Dr. Priestley's consummate surgical and administrative skills in humanistic service to his patients and colleagues:

> He was a superb technical surgeon who made even the most difficult operation look easy. He was always calm and unruffled and operated with efficiency and dispatch and with a minimum of wasted motion.
>
> Dr. Priestley exerted his leadership in a quiet, subtle, but very effective manner. He would sit and listen attentively to opinions of all members of a decision-making body without entering into the discussion himself to any significant degree. At the end of the discussion, in a few carefully chosen words he would summarize the problem and suggest a solution that would be effective and that everyone could accept even though their previously expressed viewpoints may have diverged considerably from the final solution. He never used his own position to try to force others to follow his own judgments but by his personality, integrity, wisdom, and tact accomplished results that satisfied everyone.[17]

Dr. Priestley exemplified the leadership that has given surgeons a major role in shaping Mayo Clinic. Many Mayo Clinic surgeons have dedicated their expertise to meeting the new challenges that seem to appear constantly. These surgeons have led the clinic in new directions only when consensus has been reached among peers on committees.

Under the tutelage of Dr. William J. Mayo, Mr. Harwick pioneered a system for lay medical administration that supported leadership by groups of medical and surgical peers. His reflections on administrators' partnerships with physicians and surgeons at Mayo Clinic began with his

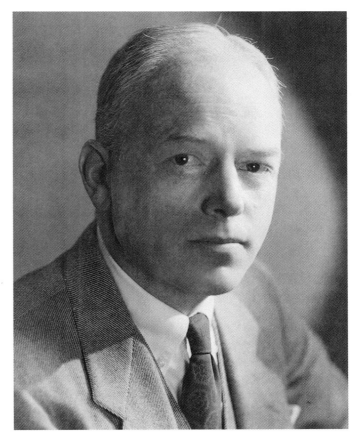

Fig. 14. James T. Priestley, M.D., Ph.D.

considerable skepticism of the committee system when it was first established by the Mayo brothers in the 1920s. He eventually arrived at an enthusiastic approval of this key Mayo Clinic element:

> Through the Committee System a great reservoir of talent, combining the experience of the older men and the fire of the younger, is brought to bear on a variety of problems facing the Clinic...our committees do a spectacularly good job in finding, within the framework of Clinic traditions and principles, the best solution to any given situation...Within their jurisdictions, Clinic committees have a real and significant authority...the vast majority of Board members came up through the hard apprenticeship of the Committee System.[18]

The effectiveness of the committee system depends on collegiality between physicians and administrators. Mr. Harwick was insightful about the necessary complementarity of administrative work at Mayo Clinic. He observed that individualism characterizes the temperament and training of most physicians. Because administrators are not competitive with physicians in regard to medical and surgical skill and training, they can function as catalysts to foster consensus among differing physicians and surgeons.[19]

Reaching Out to Other Regions

Mayo Clinic is distinguished from other tertiary care centers of excellence by its small-town origins and development. The Mayo Clinic experience supports the contention that people in small towns are friendly and open and often know one another by first name. A feeling of family and mutual support and respect among individuals is usually expected and experienced. Among Mayo Clinic surgeons, these tendencies manifest as a dedication to support and further their colleagues' careers equal to their concern with their own interests.

Mayo Foundation opened a Mayo Clinic in Jacksonville, Florida, in 1986 and in Scottsdale, Arizona, in 1987. Each of these Mayo Clinic group practices is led by a physician who is chair of the site's Board of Governors, just as at Mayo Clinic in Rochester. The overall direction of Mayo Clinic policy, however, is set by Mayo Foundation. Mayo Clinic considers itself as one foundation in three locations. Considerable effort is devoted to maintaining a small-town atmosphere at all three sites, even though Jacksonville and Scottsdale are in large metropolitan areas.

DAILY LIFE OF MAYO CLINIC SURGEONS

Following the Calendar

Each surgeon at Mayo Clinic is assigned to either an orange or a blue schedule. Orange days and blue days alternate sequentially. Surgeons on the orange schedule operate on orange days and consult on blue days, whereas surgeons on the blue schedule operate on blue days and consult on orange days. Thus, each surgeon operates every other day. On nonoperating days, surgeons are in the clinic seeing preoperative and postoperative patients. The entire surgical service, staff and residents, goes to the clinic to see the patients. This approach ensures that the residents participate with the staff in the continuity of care and follow-up of patients. This system likely was initially devised by the Mayo brothers to ensure that one brother was in the clinic and one in the operating room on a daily basis.

Surgeons usually start the day at 7 a.m. They meet their residents and colleagues for an educational conference from 7 a.m. to 7:45 a.m. or for an administrative meeting. After the meetings, half the surgeons proceed to the operating room with their residents. The other half of the surgeons and their residents who are not operating that day make rounds in the hospital, seeing patients on their own services and seeing new patients on other services who might need operation the next day.

As surgeons make rounds in the hospital at Mayo Clinic in Rochester, their patients are identified by a card with an emblem on it, chosen by the surgeon as a symbol of his or her service (Fig. 15).[20] Each card is attached to the wall next to the doorway to the patient's room. The surgeon can walk down the hall and quickly identify his or her patients by the presence of this card. These cards reflect some aspect of the surgeon's personality or career. For example, the card for Oliver H. Beahrs, M.D., depicted a magic wand. Performing magic tricks is one of Dr. Beahrs' major interests. After rounds, the surgeon and the resident staff proceed to the clinic for patient consultations.

Patient Consultations

Most patients who come to Mayo Clinic are seen by an internist or a family practitioner before they meet with a surgeon. These medical practitioners do a thorough medical evaluation of the patient. This allows the surgeon, when he or she comes for consultation, to focus specifically on the surgical problem, being aware of the comorbid conditions that could modify surgical decisions. This collaboration between physicians and surgeons for the benefit of patients is a keystone to integrated group practice.

When a patient's physician contacts the surgical desk to request a surgical consultation, the name and location (within the clinic) of the patient are written on a card, which is given to the surgeon when he or she arrives to begin consulting. The surgeon and the residents then go to the patient's location, usually in the departments of internal medicine, general medicine, or family practice within the outpatient area of Mayo Clinic. The location of the surgeons in these medical outpatient areas is carefully tracked by a system of colored lights at the entrance to each consultation room, so that the surgeon can always be located.

Each surgeon is identified by a particular light color. When the surgeon goes into the consultation room, this color is illuminated on a light panel at the door so that the secretaries and desk personnel in that area can identify the room in which the surgeon is consulting. After the surgeon's arrival, the primary physician and surgeon discuss the case, review the data, and consider the results of diagnostic tests before the surgeon's visit with the patient. Often the internist or family practitioner will give an opinion about the diagnosis and the need for operation. The surgeon then enters the patient's room and meets the patient. The patient is examined, the test results are reviewed again, the diagnosis is confirmed or disputed, and the factors for or against an operation are discussed. A decision is made with the patient's full participation. The surgical team then moves to the next patient on the list and a similar sequence follows. At the end of the consulting day, patients evaluated in the clinic and the hospital who need an operation on the following day have been identified, and the entire list is forwarded to the operating room suite for scheduling.

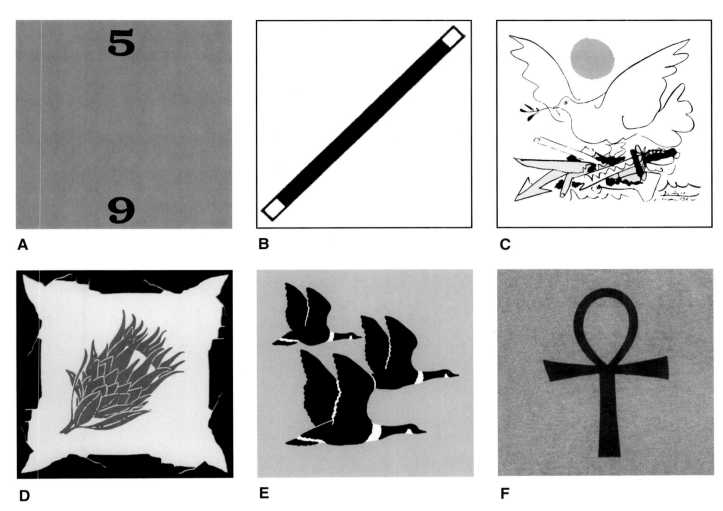

Fig. 15. Door cards of Mayo Clinic surgeons. (A), Early door card, like that of Dr. Charles H. Mayo. "When a diagnostician had a patient for one of the (Mayo) brothers to see he stepped into the hall and stuck a piece of colored cardboard above the doorframe, a red card for Dr. Charlie, a green card for Dr. Will. The earliest door cards were austerely simple. Numbers on these cards might identify a particular surgeon in a service, the number of post-operative days for a patient, or they might indicate a patient's condition."[20] (B), The card of Oliver H. Beahrs, M.D., was the first to depart from tradition by depicting a magic wand, a symbol of Dr. Beahrs' hobby. (C), The card of Martin A. Adson, M.D., is a reproduction of a famous Picasso lithograph of a peace dove flying over the broken tools of war. According to Dr. Adson, the picture expresses better than any words the essence of his profession—the triumph of hope. (D), The card of Jon A. van Heerden, M.D., features a protea, the national flower of South Africa—his native country. The border motif represents the outline of Table Mountain in the port of Cape Town, South Africa. (E), Canada geese, found year-round in Rochester, Minnesota, are depicted on the card of Roger R. Dozois, M.D., a native of Canada. The three birds flying in unison represent the consultant along with his two residents, and the blue sky is a symbol of a happy patient and a happy service. (F), The card of Keith A. Kelly, M.D., depicts an ankh, the ancient Egyptian medical symbol representing good health, life, longevity, and immortality. The ankh is green, the color used by the Greeks to represent medicine. The light brown background portrays the Nile River, whose eternal flow evokes the endless stream of sick patients seeking the surgeon's aid.

Many surgeons have two operating rooms. The two-room arrangement allows the surgeon to move back and forth between rooms. While the surgeon is performing and directing the critical portion of an operation in one room, the resident staff completes the noncritical portion of another operation in the other room. This sequence continues until all operations scheduled for that day are completed. The two-room approach maximizes use of the surgeon's time, energy, and ability and allows the team to do a series of complex cases efficiently.

Various operating techniques have been developed at Mayo Clinic. For example, when gowning, the Mayo Clinic surgeon usually puts on the left glove first and then the right. The Balfour retractor, the Mayo stand, the Mayo scissors, the Adson pickups, and the Harrington, Behrens, and Adson-Beckman retractors are some of the instruments designed by Mayo Clinic surgeons which are still in common use at Mayo Clinic. Certain operative techniques are also common to Mayo Clinic surgeons. For example, the gallbladder is usually removed by dissecting bluntly from the gallbladder toward the common bile duct, as opposed to dissecting sharply from the common bile duct toward the gallbladder.

Over the years, Mayo Clinic has generated a sustainable balance between standardization and individuality. Striving to achieve and sustain this balance is the process Helen Clapesattle identified as "an experiment in cooperative individualism." The Doctors Mayo demonstrated an innate ability to seek and hold this balance. As early as 1926, observers of Mayo Clinic recognized this achievement:

> As their surgical work increased it became necessary for the Doctors Mayo to associate with themselves other surgeons to take over part of the operative work. From the first, however, they followed the policy of training their own associate surgeons, a policy which has resulted in a surgical corps with a perhaps unparalleled unity of ideals and standards, but in which personal initiative has been fostered to a remarkable degree. The beginning of this policy was in 1905.[21]

Supporting the Surgeon

Dr. Beahrs (Fig. 16), a surgeon at Mayo Clinic from 1950 to 1979, confirms this observation in his Commentary that follows this chapter:

> The surgeon not only participates in establishing the clinical diagnosis but also has to make the decision, alone, whether to operate. Each surgeon decides how best to perform an operation on the basis of his or her training and experience and the disease process presented...For this reason, no single "Mayo way" has evolved as the only way to perform an operation at Mayo Clinic...Congenial reasoning among Mayo Clinic surgeons results in universal judgment regarding surgical problems and their management.

Dr. Beahrs' insight reveals how the surgeon's distinctive approach blends imperceptibly with collective wisdom in the examination and treatment of the patient. In this way, he deepens our understanding of Mayo Clinic as "an experiment in cooperative individualism."

Dr. Braasch enhanced this understanding by providing an example of cooperative individualism in the integrated group practice approach to surgery:

> At the request of Dr. Will, a member of the diagnostic staff often was present at the time of an operation; he would read the clinical data in the case and show the roentgenograms to the "gallery" of visiting surgeons. I was frequently present

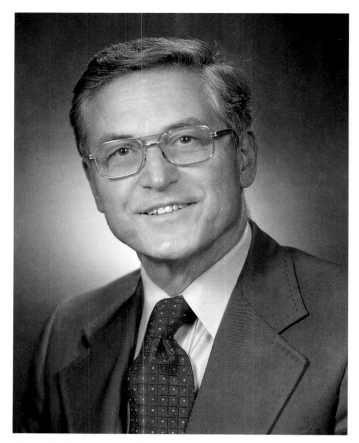

Fig. 16. Oliver H. Beahrs, M.D.

when renal operations were performed, and I discussed the diagnosis. One reason I was asked to be in the operating room was to demonstrate the value of close cooperation between surgeon and diagnostician.

> Dr. Will, in addressing the audience prior to the beginning of an operation upon a patient with a renal lesion, often would say, "Gentlemen, as far as this case is concerned, Dr. Braasch is the architect and tells me what to do. I am only the carpenter."[22]

Mayo Clinic surgeons frequently consult with each other before and during operations. It is not unusual for a Mayo Clinic surgeon to call a colleague during an operation to discuss a potential solution to a difficult problem. Advice can be given and a decision made to effect the best possible outcome for the patient. Occasionally, a colleague joins the operating surgeon at the operating table when additional expertise is required.

When specific skills are required for specific portions of an operation, Mayo Clinic surgeons operate as a multidisciplinary team. For example, an operation for recurrent carcinoma of the rectum invading the sacrum, during which a resection of the bony sacrum, removal of a portion of the spinal canal, and excision of a portion of the rectum are needed, will combine the skills of an orthopedic surgeon, a neurosurgeon, and a colorectal surgeon, each contributing his or her own skills to the effort. Another example is the use of intraoperative radiotherapy, which requires the efforts of a surgeon and a radiation oncologist.

Mayo Clinic operating rooms are characterized by a unique integrated practice between surgeons and surgical pathologists. Every specimen removed in the operating room is taken to the surgical pathology laboratory, where a pathologist is present for immediate examination of the specimen and consultation with the surgeon. Most specimens are tested by gross examination and histologic examination with the frozen section technique. The results of these tests are immediately conveyed by intercom or in person to the surgeon in the operating room. The pathologist often brings the specimen to the operating room to demonstrate the pathologic findings to the surgical team. This interaction allows the surgeon to adjust the operation accordingly.

Cooperation during the operation also may extend outside the departments of surgery. Other specialists may enter the operating room to perform specific functions. For example, a gastroenterologist may perform upper or lower gastrointestinal endoscopy during an operation to direct the surgeon to a particular area within the gastrointestinal tract.

Another interesting and unique Mayo Clinic practice is radiologic evaluation of the operative site. After each operation, radiography of the operative site is done before the patient is transferred to the recovery room. This is done to ensure that no foreign materials, sponges, or instruments remain.

For many years at Mayo Clinic in Rochester, surgeons followed a distinctive tradition on the completion of each operation. The surgeon stepped into the corridor outside the operating room to be met in person by a surgical recorder. The recorder transcribed in shorthand the surgeon's dictation of the operative report. Because the surgeon had just completed the operation, he or she was able to identify clearly and accurately all aspects of the procedure. This prompt dictation ensured the accuracy of the operative report. The surgical recorder just as promptly processed the report in his or her office, which was in the operating suite. The series of reports completed that day were available at the end of the operative day for the surgeon to proofread, correct, and sign. The report was then entered into the patient's record and was immediately available for use throughout Mayo Clinic. Today, surgeons at all Mayo Clinic locations dictate operative reports by telephone immediately after each operation. Each transcribed report is then immediately entered into the patient's medical record, becoming available to all Mayo Clinic staff members responsible for the patient's care.

At the completion of the operative day, the surgeon and staff make rounds as indicated. Surgeons remain on call during the evenings and weekends for management of their particular services. The residents stay in touch with the staff during these times. There is cross-coverage of surgical services when surgeons are not available, are out of town, or are ill; this allows for continuing care in the absence of a particular surgeon. In general, when surgeons are in town, they cover their own surgical services.

Continuing Education and Research

Mayo Clinic provides the staff with adequate time for vacation, study, and professional travel. Each surgeon is allowed 18 trip days for professional purposes and is encouraged to travel widely in the United States and abroad to learn from others, to present Mayo Clinic data, to take part in seminars, and to serve in medical and surgical organizations. The Mayos themselves traveled extensively, and their absences were made possible by the integrated group practice. When one of the Mayo brothers was out of town, the other was at home carrying on the practice, teaching, and doing research. The traveler brought back to the group new ideas and new directions, which could then be implemented to better serve the overall goal of caring for patients. Mayo Clinic surgeons have served in many major, prominent national organizations. In doing so, they have contributed much to the development of American surgery.

Vacation time is generous and increases with the person's age and length of service at Mayo Clinic, from 22 days for persons younger than 40 years and less than 5 years of service on staff to 35 days for persons 60 years or older or with 25 years of service on staff. The combination of 35 vacation days and 18 professional trip days means that senior surgeons may be away from their home base for almost 11 work weeks each year.

Some Mayo Clinic surgeons have designated time for research, called "category I" time. This time is used during the working day to conduct clinical or basic science research. All surgeons are encouraged to be innovative in their practice, to study their patients, and to evaluate the outcomes of the practice in their clinical series. Academic activities lead to academic promotion in Mayo Medical School. Surgeons usually climb the academic ladder steadily, reaching associate professor from assistant professor in 5 to 8 years and full professor after another 5 to 8 years.

MAYO CLINIC CONTRIBUTIONS TO GASTROINTESTINAL SURGERY

The development of an integrated group practice has allowed Mayo Clinic surgeons to make many contributions to gastrointestinal surgery. The reputation of Mayo

Clinic probably was built initially on the excellent results achieved by early Mayo Clinic surgeons with two emerging operations of the time: cholecystectomy for gallstones and gastroenterostomy for ulcers (Fig. 17). The Mayos reported large series of these operations in association with low morbidity and mortality rates and rapid recovery at a time when operations were not always followed by favorable outcomes. Other early Mayo Clinic contributions included development of the low anterior resection for cancer of the proximal rectum and distal sigmoid colon by Doctors Claude F. Dickson, John M. Waugh, and others, endoscopic injection of esophageal varices by Dr. Braasch, and advances in resection of the stomach for cancer by Doctors Balfour and H. Waltman Walters (Fig. 18).

Other examples are use of anterior resection for rectal prolapse by Dr. Beahrs and the development of a unique type of pyloroplasty by E. Starr Judd, M.D. (Fig. 19). Louis A. Buie, M.D., perfected an operation for hemorrhoids. A clamp he devised is still used today. Martin A. Adson, M.D., developed hepatic resection for metastatic colon cancer and determined the scientific basis for the procedure (Fig. 20). F. Henry (Bunky) Ellis, M.D. (Fig. 21), perfected the extended Heller myotomy for esophageal achalasia. James T. Priestley, M.D., performed the first total pancreatectomy for islet cell disease. Early colonic pull-through operations for rectal cancer were pioneered by B. Marden Black, M.D. (Fig. 22). Stuart W. (Tack) Harrington, M.D. (Fig. 23), developed operations for repair of esophageal hiatal hernia and devised a special retractor to facilitate exposure of the esophageal hiatus through the transabdominal route. Dr. Clagett and Dr. Walters perfected

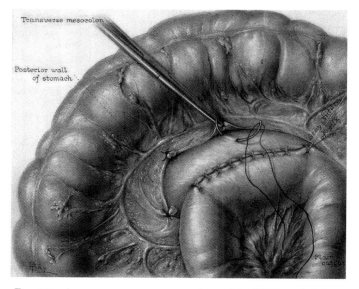

Fig. 17. A gastroenterostomy as performed by William J. Mayo, M.D., in 1915. (From Mayo WJ: Chronic duodenal ulcer. JAMA 64:2036-2040, 1915.)

gastrectomy in the treatment of peptic ulcer, and Dr. Oliver H. Beahrs was one of the early pioneers in the development of the continent ileostomy for patients who required proctocolectomy for ulcerative colitis.

CURRENT FORCES OF CHANGE

Striving for Cost-Effectiveness

Surgery and medicine are constantly changing, a phenomenon as true today as in the past. Mayo Clinic continues to evolve in response to these current forces of change. A major challenge of current practice is to continue to deliver outstanding care while maintaining cost-effectiveness. This has meant a careful review of all the steps of patient management and use of buildings, equipment, and other resources. The standard remains that "the needs of the patient come first." However, if cost-effective means can be found to maintain this standard without compromising patient care, they are pursued.

The growth of Mayo Clinic has resulted in a shortage of space. As a result, pressures are working against the system of consultations by surgeons on the medical floors. Surgeons' use of examining rooms on medical floors has resulted in pressure in some areas to send patients to a surgical "clinic" for their consultations. In such cases, the patient may have to return to the clinic on another day for the surgical consultation. This process has been particularly apparent in the newer practices at Mayo Clinic in Scottsdale and Mayo Clinic in Jacksonville. Managing surgical consultations in this manner has a negative impact on the integrated group practice, because it often precludes a face-to-face discussion between the surgeon and the physician. When this occurs, the surgeon must rely on the written record and on the patient interview. Although this approach works well for most patients, occasionally it needs to be supplemented by a telephone call to the internist or a face-to-face meeting. The belief is that surgeons are most cost-effective when they are in the operating room. There is thus pressure for the medical work-up to be almost totally completed by nonsurgical staff and for the surgeon to have only very brief visits before operation. Mayo Clinic has resisted this process and has deemed it important for the surgeon to spend adequate time preoperatively in consultation with the physicians and with the patients to ensure that the correct decisions are made and appropriate operations are planned. Nonetheless, there are constant pressures to change this system.

Patients today are at times reluctant to have an operation the day after a consultation. They need time to discuss their plans with their families, to have families travel from distant sites to Mayo Clinic, and to arrange

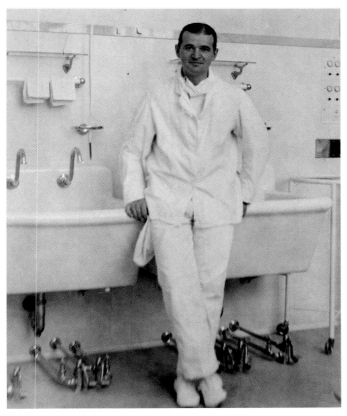

Fig. 18. H. Waltman Walters, M.D.

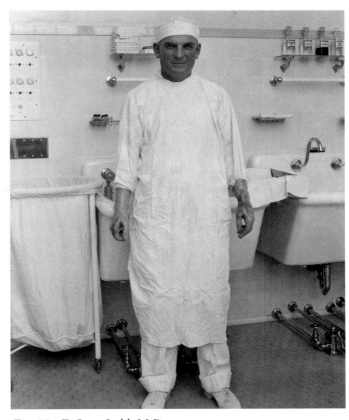

Fig. 19. E. Starr Judd, M.D.

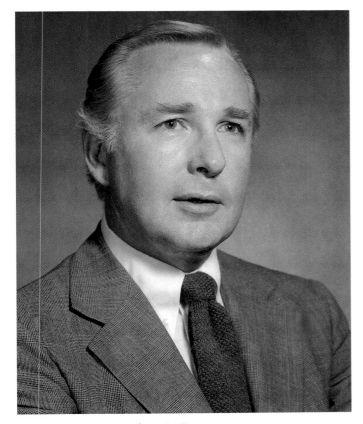

Fig. 20. Martin A. Adson, M.D.

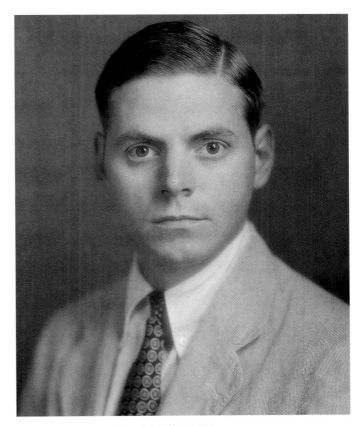

Fig. 21. F. Henry (Bunky) Ellis, M.D.

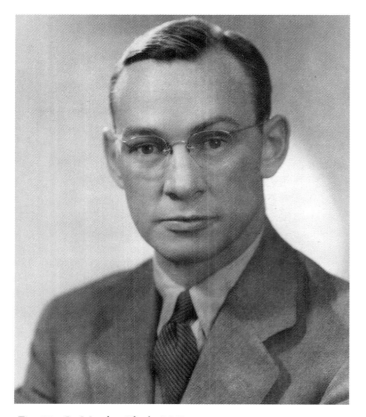

Fig. 22. B. Marden Black, M.D.

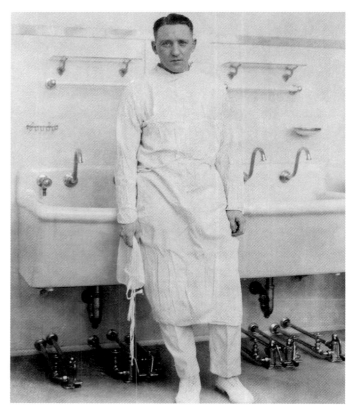

Fig. 23. Stuart W. (Tack) Harrington, M.D.

their personal affairs. As in the past, this has a negative impact on the smooth flow of patients from clinic to hospital to home. Usually, however, with adequate fore-warning, these matters can be resolved and an operation can proceed in a timely fashion.

Developing New Teams

Economic pressures on surgical education have meant that in many institutions, including Mayo Clinic, fewer surgical residents are in the system but, at the same time, there are more consultant staff and more operations. As a result, nonresident team members, such as physicians' assistants and clinical nurse specialists, are assigned to many Mayo Clinic surgical services. They work not only in the out-patient setting but also in the operating rooms. Mayo Clinic faces the challenge of hiring and training individ-uals sufficiently expert and appropriately imbued with the Mayo Clinic way of caring to continue to provide the expected standard of patient care. In general, this approach has worked well, but it has meant an adaptation of the Mayo Clinic approach to practice in recent years.

Expanding Role of Philanthropy

While the practice at Mayo Clinic has continued to expand, compensation for the care of patients by outside providers,

particularly by Medicare, has grown little and thus has not kept up with inflation. Thus, fewer funds are left over from the clinical practice to support important programs in education and research. Therefore, Mayo Clinic has had to rely on the generous support of philanthropists, foundations, and granting agencies to maintain its com-mitment to education and research. These fiscal pressures on the support of education and research likely will continue into the future.

Continuing the Commitment to Ideals

In 1957, Mr. Harwick offered his observations on the future of Mayo Clinic after 44 years of service:

> The formation of cliques and special interest groups could harm the Mayo Clinic. The placing of individual ambition above the collective good could hurt the Clinic, seriously. A radical departure from the high ideals and standards that have pre-vailed in the past could destroy it.[23]

According to Dr. Will Mayo, these high ideals and standards are "an active ideal of service instead of per-sonal profit, a primary and serious concern for the care of the individual patient and an unselfish interest of every member of the group in the professional progress of every other member."[24] Continuity of experience, identified by Dr. Kirklin as the essence of his service to patients as a Mayo Clinic surgeon, represents the integration and perpetuation of the Mayos' ideals. As "an experiment in cooperative individualism," Mayo Clinic constantly tests this continuity with the forces of change. In responding to these forces, Mayo Clinic surgeons find inspiration in the words of Dr. Will Mayo:

> *Youth and age should travel together; each needs the other for orderly scientific advancement....*[25]

Each day as I go through the hospitals surrounded by younger men, they give me of their dreams and I give them of my experience, and I get the better of the exchange...As I see the younger men picking up the torch and carrying it on, I realize that scientific truth which I formerly thought of as fixed, as though it could be weighed and measured, is changeable. Add a fact, change the outlook, and you have a new truth. Truth is a constant variable. We seek it, we find it, our viewpoint changes, and the truth changes to meet it.[26]

This will be ever true.

REFERENCES

1. Clapesattle H: The Doctors Mayo. First edition. Minneapolis, University of Minnesota Press, 1941, p 709
2. Beck CS: Teamwork at Mayo: An Experiment in Cooperative Individualism. Rochester, Minnesota, Mayo Press, 1998
3. Clapesattle H: The Doctors Mayo. First edition. Minneapolis, University of Minnesota Press, 1941, p 148
4. Mayo WJ: If I had my teens to live over: a series of brief, practical messages to scholastic readers by distinguished American leaders. Scholastic 17:10, 1930
5. Mayo WJ: The necessity of cooperation in the practice of medicine. Coll Papers Staff St Mary's Hosp Mayo Clin 2:561; 565-566, 1910
6. Clagett OT: General Surgery at the Mayo Clinic 1900-1970. Rochester, Minnesota, 1980, pp 13-14
7. Clagett OT: General Surgery at the Mayo Clinic 1900-1970. Rochester, Minnesota, 1980, pp 27; 30; 44-45
8. Division of Publications Mayo Clinic: Sketch of the History of the Mayo Clinic and the Mayo Foundation. Philadelphia, WB Saunders Company, 1926, p viii
9. Harwick HJ: Forty-Four Years With the Mayo Clinic: 1908-1952. Rochester, Minnesota, 1957, p 44
10. Braasch WF: Early Days in the Mayo Clinic. Springfield, Illinois, Charles C Thomas, 1969, pp 34-35
11. Harwick HJ: Forty-Four Years With the Mayo Clinic: 1908-1952. Rochester, Minnesota, 1957, p 1
12. Braasch WF: Early Days in the Mayo Clinic. Springfield, Illinois, Charles C Thomas, 1969, pp 114-115
13. Clagett OT: General Surgery at the Mayo Clinic 1900-1970. Rochester, Minnesota, 1980, p 123
14. Kirklin JW: The sixth Reynolds historical lecture: lessons learned from the history of the Mayo Clinic, presented on February 22, 1985. In The Reynolds Historical Lectures 1980-1991. Birmingham, University of Alabama at Birmingham, 1993, pp 135-136
15. Harwick HJ: Forty-Four Years With the Mayo Clinic: 1908-1952. Rochester, Minnesota 1957, p 44
16. Harwick HJ: Forty-Four Years With the Mayo Clinic: 1908-1952. Rochester, Minnesota 1957, pp 21; 48
17. Clagett OT: General Surgery at the Mayo Clinic 1900-1970. Rochester, Minnesota, 1980, pp 119-120
18. Harwick HJ: Forty-Four Years With the Mayo Clinic: 1908-1952. Rochester, Minnesota 1957, pp 23-24
19. Harwick HJ: Forty-Four Years With the Mayo Clinic: 1908-1952. Rochester, Minnesota 1957, pp 57-58
20. Mayovox. January 1978, p 4
21. Division of Publications Mayo Clinic: Sketch of the History of the Mayo Clinic and the Mayo Foundation. Philadelphia, WB Saunders Company, 1926, p 19
22. Braasch WF: Early Days in the Mayo Clinic. Springfield, Illinois, Charles C Thomas, 1969, p 45
23. Harwick HJ: Forty-Four Years With the Mayo Clinic: 1908-1952. Rochester, Minnesota 1957, p 36
24. Clapesattle H: The Doctors Mayo. First edition. Minneapolis, University of Minnesota Press, 1941, pp 708-709
25. Mayo WJ: The beginning of education. Milwaukee Med Times 9:22-23, 1936
26. Mayo WJ: Seventieth birthday anniversary of William J Mayo. Ann Surg 94:799-800, 1931

COMMENTARY

As I reflect on gastrointestinal surgery at Mayo Clinic, I am aware of many important changes. In the earliest years of their practice, William W. Mayo, M.D., and his two sons, William (Will) J. Mayo, M.D., and Charles (Charlie) H. Mayo, M.D., were indeed "general surgeons." They performed whatever operation was necessary to treat a patient. Nonetheless, gastrointestinal surgery was a prominent part of the practice from the very beginning.

A patient once asked Dr. Will Mayo, "Who is the head doctor around here?" His response was "Charlie is; I'm the belly doctor." This was true. Dr. Will's area of interest was the stomach, and Dr. Charlie's was the eye, the thyroid, and all things about the head and elsewhere.

As surgical knowledge expanded, the Doctors Mayo recognized the need for surgeons to specialize and to be identified by a particular field of interest. Thus, the surgical staff of Mayo Clinic expanded with the addition of surgeons who developed specialties, including gastrointestinal surgery. Even subspecialties of fields of surgery were developed. For example, although most of the gastrointestinal surgery has remained within the field of general surgery, much of the esophageal surgery at Mayo Clinic was developed by thoracic surgeons.

For years, surgeons were appointed to Mayo Clinic staff as head of an independent section of general surgery. The surgeons were, however, frequently identified by an area of special interest, such as gastrointestinal surgery. Each surgeon practiced on the basis of his or her training and experience. Senior surgeons took on necessary related activities, such as education, research, and administration. When the Mayo brothers were practicing, Mayo Clinic surgeons were not formally organized into a department with a chair, as they were in many academic practices.

As the number of Mayo Clinic surgeons increased, the Board of Governors recognized the need for new organization. In 1964, the Board established a Department of Surgery, naming John W. Kirklin, M.D., as chair. The department was comprised of several divisions, including the Division of Gastroenterologic and General Surgery. Since that time, the rapidly developing recognition and certification of specialists have led to more specialization at earlier stages of surgical training. Today, Mayo Clinic surgeons begin their careers in a specialty within a division of the Department of Surgery and most often restrict their work to that specialty throughout their careers.

Increasing specialization and many other changes have necessitated innovation in practice, education, and research at Mayo Clinic. Helen Clapesattle's interpretation of Mayo Clinic as "an experiment in cooperative individualism," highlighted in the preceding chapter, points out the essential mechanism in Mayo Clinic's successful response to the growth of specialization.

I have experienced cooperative individualism as productive of both soundness and flexibility in times of change. On the basis of my experience, the Mayo Clinic approach requires that individualism and specialization always be balanced with cooperation and congeniality. Over the years, I have observed how this approach works. Because of the active intervention of the surgeon in the patient's illness, the surgeon is exposed to the "ups and downs" of treatment more acutely than are other physicians. The surgeon not only participates in establishing the clinical diagnosis but also has to make the decision, alone, whether to operate. Each surgeon decides how best to perform an operation on the basis of his or her training and experience and the disease process presented. Fundamentally, human anatomy does not change. Each surgeon approaches human anatomy as he or she thinks best to accomplish the operation being undertaken. For this reason, no single "Mayo way" has evolved as the only way to perform an operation at Mayo Clinic.

One of my teachers always did a gastric resection smoothly, accurately, and quickly, using an approach that was entirely different from that of other Mayo Clinic surgeons. His approach did not appeal to me, and so I asked him whether he always did the operation the same way. His response was, "Is there any other way to do it?" Even though this technique varied from that of other surgeons, the patients did not have different results. Another teacher taught me how to do an operation in which he did not expose and protect an important nerve. He seldom injured the nerve. This, too, was my early experience with the operation. Still, I altered the way I did the procedure by always identifying the nerve and protecting it so there was no risk of it being injured. The operation was modified in "my way."

Nonetheless, although the technical aspects of an operation varied among Mayo Clinic surgeons, and they still do, the surgical judgment that is used to decide whether to operate for a condition is almost uniform at Mayo Clinic. Congenial reasoning among Mayo Clinic surgeons results in universal judgment regarding surgical problems and their management. Individualism is balanced by cooperation and congeniality.

With independence of thought and action comes great responsibility and, with specialization, the need to develop medicine as a cooperative science. Teamwork is seen best in the union of physician and surgeon, and of surgeon and surgeon, and not as an occasional event but as part of the daily routine. In the surgical environment at Mayo Clinic, close cooperation exists among the physicians and surgeons and among surgeons, not only in the hallway and at the bedside but also in the operating room.

In 1910, Dr. Will Mayo said, "The best interest of the patient is the only interest to be considered, and in order that the sick may have the benefit of advancing knowledge, union of forces is necessary." He further said, "Jealousy in the medical profession is proverbial and it has done more to retard development than all other restricting influences combined." I have been privileged to participate in teamwork at its best—the union of physician and surgeon, and of surgeon and surgeon—not as an occasional event but as part of the daily routine.

Another major Mayo Clinic strength, "continuity of experience," was identified by Dr. Kirklin in an address at the University of Alabama. His interpretation of this characteristic is more fully developed in the preceding chapter. At Mayo Clinic, "continuity of experience" connects surgeons with their contemporaries and with their predecessors. It also renders individualism and cooperation as ultimately inseparable.

Oliver H. Beahrs, M.D.

COMMENTARY

Time, as defined in Webster's dictionary, is "a continuum which lacks spatial dimensions and in which events succeed one another from past through present to the future." Surgical past at Mayo Clinic began in 1883, when William W. Mayo, M.D., and his son, William J. Mayo, M.D., performed the first abdominal operation in Rochester, Minnesota, with the removal of a 24-pound multilocular ovarian cyst from a young woman.

The preceding chapter chronicles phases in the continuum of surgery at Mayo Clinic since that beginning event 120 years ago by reporting the historical and cultural perspectives of Mayo Clinic and the daily life of a Mayo Clinic surgeon from past to present. The authors also note the current forces of change and speculate that the high ideals, concern for the care of the individual patient, and unselfish interest in every member of the group will be paramount in maintaining outstanding surgical care at Mayo Clinic in the future.

As an emeritus surgeon of Mayo Clinic, who spent 36 years in practice there, I agree with the authors that the environment was and is unique. The atmosphere, particularly the collegiality of the institution, stimulates one's best possible efforts in all aspects of surgical practice, education, and research.

Changes in clinical practice during the past several years are staggering. There have been not only amazing technologic advancements but also a tremendous proliferation of new high-tech procedures. Pressure from managed care systems, federal intervention, integrated networks, insurance regulations, and many other escalating market forces are altering our daily professional lives. Such changes in practice are inevitable. We must keep abreast, adapt, and assert leadership to influence the process of change in the future while maintaining the strengths of our group practice.

I am optimistic that the men and women in training today and the future generations of surgeons will match or exceed the remarkable accomplishments of the past.

Donald C. McIlrath, M.D.

Chapter 2

Gastroesophageal Reflux and Esophageal Hiatal Hernia

Alexander Klaus, M.D.
Ronald A. Hinder, M.D.

Gastroesophageal reflux disease (GERD) is the most common pathologic condition of the esophagus, accounting for 75% of esophageal diseases.[1] It occurs mainly in the Western world; the incidence is low in Africa and Asia. Several studies have reported physiologic gastroesophageal reflux in normal individuals, especially postprandially[2-4] and at night.[5,6] However, when such reflux becomes excessive, gastrointestinal symptoms, such as heartburn, regurgitation, dysphagia, nausea, abdominal pain, vomiting, or respiratory symptoms may occur. These may result in the need for continuous medical therapy. When severe esophagitis is unresponsive to medication or when hemorrhage, chronic respiratory symptoms, ulceration, esophageal strictures, Barrett's esophagus, and adenocarcinoma of the esophagus occur, operation is usually required.[7]

The peak incidence of GERD occurs in patients between 30 and 40 years old, and there is equal distribution between the sexes. However, the mean age at which severe esophagitis is diagnosed is older than 60 years. More than half of all patients with Barrett's disease of the esophagus are older than 70 years.[8,9] This indicates that there is a relationship between the duration of disease and its complications.

In most patients, GERD can be sufficiently controlled by self-medication or intermittent antireflux medication. In a small number of patients, medication may not be adequate or may be required continuously to control symptoms. In these patients, an antireflux operation should be considered to avoid further esophageal damage and to control gastroesophageal reflux. In the United States, the introduction of laparoscopic cholecystectomy for diseases

of the gallbladder in 1989 heralded the use of the new techniques of minimally invasive surgery for esophageal diseases. The laparoscopic surgical management of GERD was reported in 1991.[10,11] The laparoscopic approach has proved its value in comparison with the open approach, in that efficacy is equivalent at 5 to 8 years. In addition, laparoscopic antireflux procedures are associated with less morbidity and mortality than open operations and, therefore, have a high patient acceptance.

PHYSIOLOGY AND PATHOLOGY

For a better understanding of esophageal and supraesophageal abnormalities due to gastroesophageal reflux and their treatment, it is important to understand the physiology of the antireflux mechanism at the cardia. Because the luminal environment of the stomach with a low pH content is totally different from the neutral pH of the esophagus, a functioning barrier between the stomach and the esophagus is required to separate these two locations in healthy individuals. This antireflux mechanism acts as a valve and protects the esophageal mucosa from gastric acid and other noxious secretions such as pepsin, trypsin, alkaline secretions from the duodenum, and bile acids. Dysfunction of the antireflux barrier is the most common cause of gastroesophageal reflux.

The physiologic barrier consists of the lower esophageal sphincter (LES), the esophageal hiatus of the diaphragm, the phrenicoesophageal ligaments, and the angle of His. The most important part is the LES, which is a thickening of the circular muscle layer, especially on the greater curvature side of the esophagus. The collar of

Helvetius is a band of oblique gastric smooth muscle fibers running from the angle of His toward the lesser curvature of the stomach. It also takes part in creating a high-pressure zone at the LES. The LES has a total length of more than 2 cm and lies partly within the chest and partly within the abdomen. In normal individuals, the abdominal portion measures more than 1 cm.

In addition to the length of the sphincter, the resting pressure of the sphincter plays a pivotal role in the pathophysiology of GERD. At the respiratory inversion point, the point where the positive-pressure deflection on inspiration becomes negative, the pressure should be more than 6 mm Hg to be effective in functioning as an antireflux barrier. Sufficient resting pressure is of particular importance during periods of increased intra-abdominal and intragastric pressure, delayed gastric emptying, and gastric distention, all of which make postprandial reflux more likely.

The diaphragmatic crura and the intra-abdominal pressure also aid in the prevention of gastroesophageal reflux. Dislocation of the LES into the chest shortens the intra-abdominal part of the sphincter and separates high-pressure zones of the LES and the diaphragmatic crura. This process occurs in patients with hiatal hernia. Failure of the LES mechanism can be due to several reasons, including primary weakness of the esophageal smooth muscles, short length of the sphincter, defective control mechanisms, an abnormally large number of transient relaxations of the LES, and dislocation of the LES into the chest. Weak esophageal body motility can lead to prolonged and more frequent episodes of esophageal acid exposure with poor clearance of acid from the esophagus, which predisposes its mucosa to injury.

Approximately 10% of the North American population has an esophageal hiatal hernia. There are different types of hiatal hernias: the sliding type in which the esophagogastric junction and the LES have slid superiorly into the thorax (type I), the type in which the gastric fundus herniates into the thorax so that it lies superior to the LES (paraesophageal hiatal hernia, type II), and the mixed type of paraesophageal hernia in which both the LES and the fundus of the stomach move into the chest (type III). The most common symptoms of paraesophageal hiatal hernias are regurgitation, heartburn, and dysphagia. Complications can have severe consequences. Volvulus of the stomach (either organoaxial or mesentericoaxial), venous obstruction caused by an incarcerated hernia, gastric ulceration, strangulation, and perforation can lead to emergency surgical procedures, which are associated with a higher mortality than elective procedures. Operation should therefore be recommended for symptomatic patients to prevent complications, whereas asymptomatic patients should be followed closely.

DIAGNOSIS AND IMAGING

Because the success of antireflux operation depends on identifying patients most likely to benefit from the procedure, every patient who is considered for operation must have a confirmed diagnosis of GERD. A properly taken history with detailed questions elicits the character and timing of esophageal and atypical symptoms. All patients who present with obvious symptoms of GERD and patients with an atypical presentation should undergo clinical testing to confirm the diagnosis and to exclude other causes of their symptoms.

Esophageal manometry is an essential preoperative test. The exact location of the LES in relation to the diaphragm, the overall length of the LES, its resting pressure, and its ability to relax can be evaluated with esophageal manometry. In patients with a large esophageal hiatal hernia, esophageal manometry may be difficult to perform because in some cases the manometric catheter cannot be passed into the stomach. A typical manometric finding in patients with hiatal hernia is the "double hump" configuration. Two peaks of increased pressure occur when a pressure-sensitive catheter is drawn from the stomach into the lower esophagus. This phenomenon is due to herniation of the stomach into the chest and thereby separation of the resting pressure of the LES from the high-pressure zone created by the diaphragmatic crura.

In addition to gathering information about the LES, esophageal manometry is able to assess esophageal body motility. Impaired esophageal body motility may lead to delayed esophageal clearance and prolonged acid exposure of the esophageal mucosa. Impaired esophageal body motility may lead to the need for a partial (270°) posterior fundoplication instead of a full (360°) fundoplication to avoid functional obstruction at the fundoplication. Poor esophageal body motility also has been shown to have an impact on the development and persistence of reflux-associated respiratory symptoms.

Esophagogastroduodenoscopy with biopsies should be performed to evaluate patients with GERD and to exclude or identify esophageal complications. These tests are useful to grade the severity of esophagitis, to identify esophageal diverticula and esophageal strictures, and to establish the size of a hiatal hernia. Biopsy specimens have to be obtained to exclude Barrett's esophagus and esophageal cancer. Additionally, esophagogastroduodenoscopy can be used to dilate strictures.

The most important diagnostic test to confirm the presence of acid reflux in patients with GERD is *24-hour esophageal pH monitoring*. Prolonged pH monitoring has shown a sensitivity of approximately 90% in diagnosing GERD. Proton pump inhibitor therapy has to be stopped at least 7 days before pH monitoring, and histamine$_2$

(H_2)-receptor blocker therapy has to be stopped for 48 hours before the test to ensure that drug effects do not influence the results. Under these circumstances, if the esophageal mucosa is exposed to a pH less than 4 for more than 5% of the duration of the test, pathologic acid reflux is present. A positive reflux score (determined by including the time that the distal esophagus is exposed to pH less than 4 during the total time, in the upright and supine positions, the number of reflux episodes with pH less than 4, the number of episodes lasting longer than 5 minutes, and the length of the longest episode) is also suggestive of pathologic acid reflux. However, one has to keep in mind that the refluxate from the stomach may be alkaline, resulting in a negative 24-hour acid pH score. In that case, an intraluminal probe for identifying bile salts in the esophageal lumen may be useful.

Barium esophagography is of importance for establishing the morphologic features of the esophagus, particularly the distal part. It can define the type of hiatal hernia, an intrathoracic stomach, and any concomitant esophagogastric abnormality such as esophageal strictures and malignancies. An upper gastroesophageal series also can help rule out esophageal motility disturbances. In some cases, gastric emptying is assessed, because some patients with GERD may present with delayed gastric emptying preoperatively. An antireflux operation speeds gastric emptying.

Upright *chest radiography* can establish whether there are GERD-related respiratory problems. It may reveal an air-fluid level behind the heart, indicating air in a hiatal hernia or in an intrathoracic stomach. For patients with supraesophageal complications, more precise investigation of the ear, nose, throat, and respiratory tract should be done with bronchoscopy, sinus radiography, allergy evaluation, spirometry before and after use of bronchodilators, sputum microbiologic or cytologic studies, and chest computed tomography.

INDICATIONS FOR OPERATION

In most patients, symptoms of GERD can easily be controlled with intermittent standard medication such as proton pump inhibitors, H_2-receptor antagonists, and promotility agents. These patients do not require surgical therapy. However, some patients do not respond to even high-dose medical therapy. Long-term therapy is ineffective in these patients. Therefore, they should be considered for surgical therapy early in the course of their disease to avoid esophageal complications such as motor disturbances or shortening of the esophagus due to chronic reflux-induced esophagitis and esophageal stricture. The need for aggressive long-term medical therapy, particularly in young patients, is another indication for operation. Inconvenience, ineffectiveness, and side effects of medication can result in poor patient compliance. Patients with GERD who present with severe esophagitis (grade III or IV) are most likely to require aggressive long-term therapy. However, medical therapy often fails in this patient population. Duodenogastroesophageal reflux, which is composed of acid and alkaline material, occurs frequently. Therefore, acid-suppressive therapy may be ineffective.

Patients with symptomatic GERD who present with a mechanically deficient LES and concomitant low-grade esophagitis (grade I or II) are suitable for operation, because in most cases their symptoms persist during medical therapy. Patients with a large hiatal hernia are also often refractory to medical therapy. In these patients, it seems to be important to restore the esophagogastric junction to its normal position to obtain persistent relief of symptoms.

Patients with GERD who have severe complications, such as esophageal stricture, ulceration, Barrett's esophagus, and severe pulmonary symptoms, obtain considerable benefit from surgical therapy. Most can stop medical therapy after operation and have substantial improvement of symptoms. Finally, patients with atypical symptoms, including aspiration, recurrent pneumonia, and chronic laryngitis, should be considered for antireflux operation. In these patients, dual esophageal pH probe measurements may reveal gastric acid in both the upper and the lower esophagus. However, it might be difficult to confirm a connection of these symptoms with GERD, especially in patients who present with only atypical symptoms.

Besides the appropriate indication for operation and choosing the appropriate surgical approach, another factor that determines the outcome of fundoplication is the quality of the operative procedure. In 1912, Giffin, a Mayo Clinic surgeon, described the first repair of a hiatal hernia.[12] After the poor results of surgical therapy for GERD with the Allison crural repair,[13] Nissen, in 1956, described the 360° fundoplication, a procedure that, after some modification, remains effective and popular.[14] Since then, a multitude of other operative procedures have been developed which can be performed laparoscopically or thoracoscopically. Performing an antireflux operation with minimally invasive techniques offers the advantage of rapid patient recovery, less mortality, low morbidity, better cosmetic results, low overall cost, and decreased pain. The operation often necessitates only an overnight stay in the hospital or can be performed as an outpatient procedure. Only symptomatic patients undergo operation.

Barrett's esophagus is defined as the presence of endoscopically visible columnar epithelium of any length with biopsy-proven intestinal metaplasia in the lower esophagus. Approximately 10% to 15% of patients with chronic

GERD have Barrett's metaplasia in the esophagus. It is known to be a premalignant condition with a strong association with esophageal adenocarcinoma.[7] Barrett's esophagus is the most severe form of chronic GERD; affected patients have more manometric and esophageal pH abnormalities and a longer duration of symptoms than other patients with GERD.

Barrett's esophagus is an uncommon finding after antireflux operation, and progression of Barrett's esophagus toward carcinoma is less common postoperatively. It can take several years for Barrett's esophagus with low-grade dysplasia to progress to adenocarcinoma. However, adenocarcinoma can proceed directly from low-grade dysplasia within 1 to 2 years after first diagnosis, skipping the intermediate stages of dysplasia. Therefore, young patients with Barrett's esophagus should be considered for surgical treatment, because the probability for development of Barrett's carcinoma increases proportionally with years. Indications for redo operations are breakdown of the fundoplication or the crural repair, a slipped Nissen fundoplication, a wrap that is too tight or too loose, misdiagnosis, or a displaced Angelchick prosthesis (Fig. 1).

Laparoscopic repair in patients with medically refractory esophageal strictures results in a good clinical outcome with minimal complications. In a Mayo Clinic study,[15] 15% of patients undergoing laparoscopic fundoplication had a stricture. The stricture could always be dilated preoperatively. The need for dilation decreased substantially after laparoscopic fundoplication. In a mean observation time of 26 months preoperatively, 252 dilations

were performed, whereas in a mean observation time of 25 months postoperatively, 29 dilations were performed.

THE PROCEDURES

Laparoscopic Nissen Fundoplication

The laparoscopic Nissen procedure is the standard procedure for GERD. The patient is placed in the lithotomy or inverted Y steep reverse Trendelenburg position. After establishment of a pneumoperitoneum with a needle inserted above the umbilicus, the first port is inserted at this site. If there has been a previous midline operation, the pneumoperitoneum may be established with the open technique or with a needle in the left hypochondrium. The surgeon, who stands between the legs of the patient, inspects the abdominal cavity with the laparoscope. This position offers the best comfort for the surgeon. Under visual control, four more ports are placed in a subcostal arc. The surgeon operates using the epigastric and left subcostal ports.

The liver can be retracted with a retractor placed through a right subcostal port. The extreme left port is used to manipulate the stomach with an atraumatic Babcock grasper. If necessary, another port can be inserted to the left of the lower midline port to enable better exposure. After retraction of the left lobe of the liver superiorly to prevent it from dropping into the operative field, the gastrohepatic omentum is incised. The hepatic branches of the vagi, which can be seen through the lesser omentum in thin patients, are preserved intact. Care must be taken to

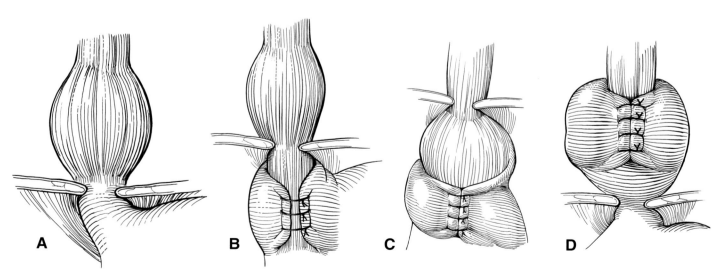

Fig. 1. Surgical failures after antireflux operation. (A), Type I, complete disruption of the wrap. (B), Type II, slippage of part of the stomach above the diaphragm. (C), Type III, "slipped Nissen"—part of the stomach lies above and part lies below the fundoplication. (D), Type IV, the intact wrap herniates through the esophageal hiatus into the chest. (Modified from Hinder.[9] By permission of Lippincott Williams & Wilkins.)

avoid damage to an aberrant left hepatic artery, which may pass through the lesser omentum in 8% to 23% of patients. In these patients, two windows should be created above and below the vessel. The surgeon then has access to the esophagogastric junction (Fig. 2).

The anterior edge of the right crus of the diaphragm should be identified and dissected free of the esophagus. Care must be taken not to damage large blood vessels or the anterior trunk of the vagal nerve, which is usually adjacent to the smooth muscle of the anterior wall of the esophagus. The posterior vagal trunk should be identified and preserved intact. It can be separated from the posterior esophageal wall. Usually the right crus and the anterior part of the left crus of the diaphragm can easily be dissected off the esophagus. The esophagus and the stomach have to be retracted to the right so that the posterior part of the left crus can be mobilized off the left side of the esophagus (Fig. 3). It is important to fully free the left crus posterior to the esophagus to allow for subsequent creation of a window behind the esophagus from the right-sided approach.

Next, the esophagus is elevated to allow dissection of the retroesophageal space from the right. The tissue behind the esophagus is loose and can be separated from the esophagus with blunt dissection. Through that window the left crus can be identified, and care is taken to identify the posterior vagus nerve, which may be allowed to remain fixed to the posterior wall of the esophagus or to fall posteriorly. Dissection too far superiorly into the mediastinum has the risk of damaging the left pleura, whereas dissection too far inferiorly may cause gastric or esophageal perforation. It is

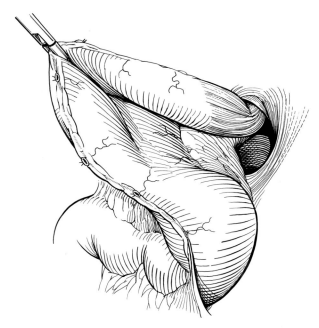

Fig. 3. The left crus of the diaphragmatic hiatus with the stomach and the esophagus retracted to the right.

important to continue dissection of the esophagus until the lower 2 to 3 cm is comfortably mobilized below the diaphragm. The dilated esophageal hiatus between the left and right crura should be cleared of overlying connective tissue until the muscle of both crura is exposed.

Several nonabsorbable sutures are used to loosely approximate the crura, beginning as far inferiorly as possible and then moving superiorly (Fig. 4). If the crural defect is very wide, pledgets may be used to buttress the sutures. Approximation of the crura is of great importance to add to the antireflux properties of the operation and to prevent slippage of the fundoplication into the chest. The approximation should allow for an adequate opening for the esophagus with only a small space around it. Some surgeons place a 56F to 60F Maloney bougie into the esophagus during crural approximation to size the space adequately. Because this step has a risk of esophageal perforation, we do not recommend its use.

The gastric fundus is next mobilized by dividing the short gastric vessels with a harmonic scalpel. This is begun 10 to 15 cm distal to the angle of His at the superior part of the greater curve of the stomach. The stomach is lifted and retracted to the right, and the vessels are held on tension with the Babcock dissector (Fig. 5). The fundus must be completely mobilized to avoid torsion of the esophagus, tension of the wrap, or inclusion of gastric corpus in the wrap. Failing to do so may result in delayed esophageal clearance and dysphagia in the postoperative period. During mobilization of the gastric fundus, the surgeon should

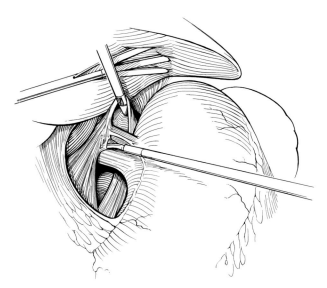

Fig. 2. Laparoscopic view of the esophagogastric junction with the liver retracted.

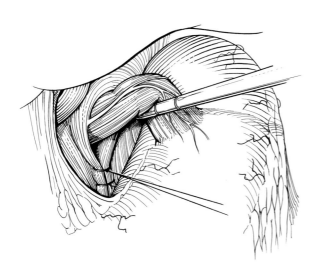

Fig. 4. Approximation of the crura during laparoscopic Nissen fundoplication.

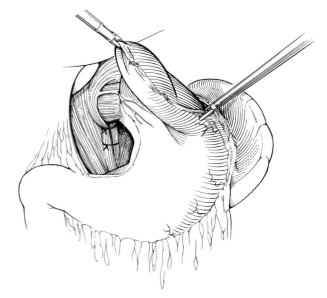

Fig. 5. The mobilized gastric fundus.

take care not to injure the stomach or spleen, particularly when dissecting around the upper pole of the spleen. Perforation or bleeding should be immediately repaired, a procedure that often requires advanced laparoscopic skills.

Finally, the fundoplication is performed. The posterior wall of the fundus is grasped about 8 cm distal to the angle of His at the level of the divided short gastric vessels with a Babcock grasper, which is passed from the right side posterior to the esophagus (Fig. 6). The posterior fundal wall is then brought behind the esophagus and finally to the right of the esophagus. Similarly, the anterior wall of the fundus is grasped on the left side of the esophagus at the level of the divided short gastric vessels and approximated to the posterior wall on the right of the esophagus. The fundus is rocked back and forth behind

the esophagus to assess its continuity and length (Fig. 7). In this way, a loose wrap is created. Some surgeons again pass a 56F to 60F Maloney bougie to assess the tightness of the wrap; we do not.

The fundoplication is secured with a U-shaped nonabsorbable suture with two polytef felt pledgets on either side (Fig. 8). The stitch includes a nearly full thickness of stomach and a partial thickness of esophageal wall. The latter is taken on the right side of the esophagus to avoid damage to the anterior vagus. This suture prevents telescoping of the stomach through the wrap into the chest. A second suture may be added either above or below to secure the wrap further. The wrap must not be too tight or longer than 2 cm; otherwise, dysphagia occurs. With experience, the appropriate tightness of

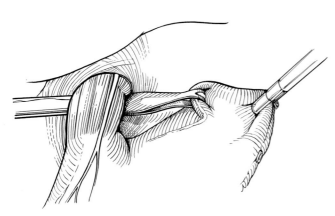

Fig. 6. Grasping the gastric fundus with a Babcock grasper passed from the right behind the esophagus.

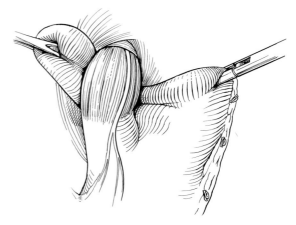

Fig. 7. The fundus of the stomach being brought behind the esophagus to form the wrap.

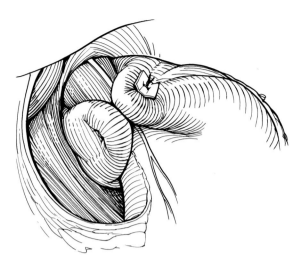

Fig. 8. The completed Nissen fundoplication.

the wrap can be assessed visually by the surgeon. The ports are then removed under vision to make sure that there is no substantial bleeding from the port sites. The fascia is sutured at all 10-mm port sites. The skin is closed with a subcuticular absorbable suture and adhesive strips are applied.

Laparoscopic Toupet Partial Posterior Fundoplication

The Toupet fundoplication is a wrap that encompasses only the posterior 180° to 270° of the esophagus. It is generally used in patients with poor esophageal body motility in whom a Nissen fundoplication might cause postoperative dysphagia. It is also used in patients after an esophageal myotomy to treat achalasia, diffuse esophageal spasm, or the nutcracker esophagus. The disadvantage of this procedure is that there is less increase in LES pressure than after the Nissen fundoplication and consequently reflux is more likely after operation.

The patient is placed in the same position used for the Nissen fundoplication. After establishment of a pneumoperitoneum, the ports are placed similarly. The gastrohepatic ligament is divided, and the esophagus and the crura are dissected as described for the Nissen fundoplication. The hiatal hernia is reduced, and the crura are approximated. After mobilization of the fundus by dividing the short gastric vessels, a Babcock grasper is passed behind the esophagus from the right to the left. The fundus is then passed posterior to the esophagus. The fundus is fixed to the left crus with one silk stitch and to the adjacent right crus with two more silk sutures. The fundus is sutured to the right side of the anterior esophagus and to the left side of the esophagus with three more sutures on each side. This creates a partial 270° fundoplication (Fig. 9).

Laparoscopic Paraesophageal Hernia Repair

Paraesophageal hernias generally occur in older patients. Fortunately, laparoscopic repair of these hernias can be done in elderly patients. This approach is safer, causes less surgical trauma with less blood loss and less loss of intravascular fluid into tissues, and results in a lower mortality and less morbidity than an open procedure. The laparoscopic approach also offers better visibility of the esophageal hiatus than the open approach. Moreover, it allows for better direct visualization of the hiatal hernia sac in the chest than with the open approach.

Patient and surgeon are positioned similar to the positions used for the Nissen procedure. The ports are inserted in the same fashion. The herniated stomach is gently pulled inferiorly from the chest into the abdomen (Fig. 10). After the gastrohepatic ligament is divided, the esophageal hiatus and the paraesophageal defect can be identified by dissecting the parietal peritoneum off the free edge of the right and left crura and adjacent diaphragm. Blunt and sharp dissection is used to gently tease the entire hernia sac out of the mediastinum. Both the surgeon and the anesthesiologist should be aware of the potential risk of a pneumothorax at this time. The hernia sac is left attached to the front of the stomach so as to avoid damage to the vagal nerves or blood vessels. A window is created behind the esophagus, as with a type I hernia, followed by crural repair and an antireflux procedure, as described for the Nissen procedure. The crural repair incorporates the paraesophageal hernia defect. Pledgets may be used to buttress these sutures. In most cases, a Nissen fundoplication is also done to prevent subsequent reflux. The extensive dissection around the cardia causes disruption of the phrenicoesophageal ligament and posterior esophageal attachments. The dissection

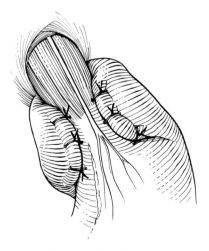

Fig. 9. The completed Toupet fundoplication.

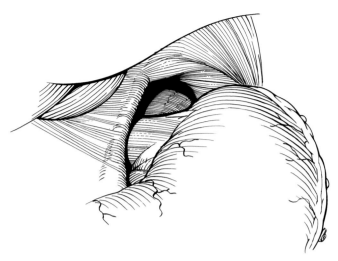

Fig. 10. Large paraesophageal hernial defect after reduction of the stomach into the abdomen.

may lead to subsequent reflux. Another issue is that the fundoplication helps to prevent hernia recurrence by fixing the stomach in the abdominal cavity. Adding an antireflux procedure does not increase the morbidity or mortality associated with the laparoscopic paraesophageal hernia repair.[16]

Other Procedures

Several other antireflux procedures with various success rates have been described. In patients with a long history of GERD, preoperative testing may show reflux-induced esophageal shortening. These patients may be treated with the *Collis esophageal lengthening procedure* (Fig. 11). This approach lengthens the intra-abdominal esophagus. The lengthening is combined with an appropriate antireflux procedure. The lengthening is created by firing a laparoscopic stapler along the cardia on the left side of the esophagus parallel to the lesser curve of the stomach. The stapler can be introduced either by way of the abdomen or blindly through a small incision in the axilla. The gastric fundus is then wrapped around the neoesophagus. The disadvantage of this procedure is that either a thoracotomy or simultaneous laparoscopy and thoracoscopy have to be performed.

Because perioperative and postoperative morbidity are higher and the time to return to work is longer than with the laparoscopic approach, antireflux procedures through the chest are reserved for special indications only. Besides esophageal shortening, a transthoracic antireflux procedure is indicated in patients who have had multiple failed transabdominal antireflux operations. Dissection of the hiatus and mobilizing a huge hiatal hernia sac might be easier through the chest, but performing the wrap,

dividing short gastric vessels, and controlling abdominal blood vessels are more challenging with this approach.

Another procedure is the *Hill repair*, which has been performed since 1959. This can be done laparoscopically. The procedure aims to fix the LES in the abdomen and to attach the lesser curvature of the stomach to the preaortic fascia. In this way it creates an angulation of the lower esophagus and so prevents reflux. However, it is not widely used because it is time-consuming and technically challenging.

With the *Dor partial anterior fundoplication*, the anterior portion of the fundus is fixed laparoscopically to the anterior wall of the distal esophagus and to the right crus of the diaphragm. This procedure is not commonly accepted, because it is not as successful for preventing reflux as a posterior or full fundoplication. Some surgeons use this type of fundoplication after esophageal myotomy for achalasia. However, we recommend the Toupet posterior fundoplication in this circumstance, because it has been shown to be superior for preventing reflux and dysphagia.

Redo Laparoscopic Antireflux Procedures

The ability to perform a redo antireflux procedure laparoscopically has encouraged many patients with a failed primary procedure to be re-treated surgically. Even though the need for reoperation is generally low, the increasing number of patients undergoing antireflux operations has led to a continuing need for redo operations. These can be done laparoscopically even after a previous open antireflux operation. The first step during laparoscopic redo fundoplication is to identify the esophageal hiatus and the crura. Once this is done, in most patients the previous wrap has to be taken down. This can be most challenging because sharp dissection may be required because of extensive adhesions. Care must be taken not to perforate the esophagus or the stomach during this phase of the procedure. If the LES does not lie below the diaphragm, esophageal lengthening may be necessary with the Collis procedure. A Toupet partial posterior fundoplication is often used because most patients who require redo antireflux procedures have poor esophageal body motility. The success rate after a redo laparoscopic antireflux operation is less than after a first operation. However, it may still be as high as 80%. In a third or even a fourth procedure, the success rate decreases to 50% to 66%. These technically difficult procedures should be attempted only by skilled and experienced laparoscopic esophageal surgeons.

SURGICAL OUTCOME

Laparoscopic antireflux operations can be performed in an average time of 1 to 2 hours. Difficult procedures may take longer. The mean blood loss is usually less than 50 mL.

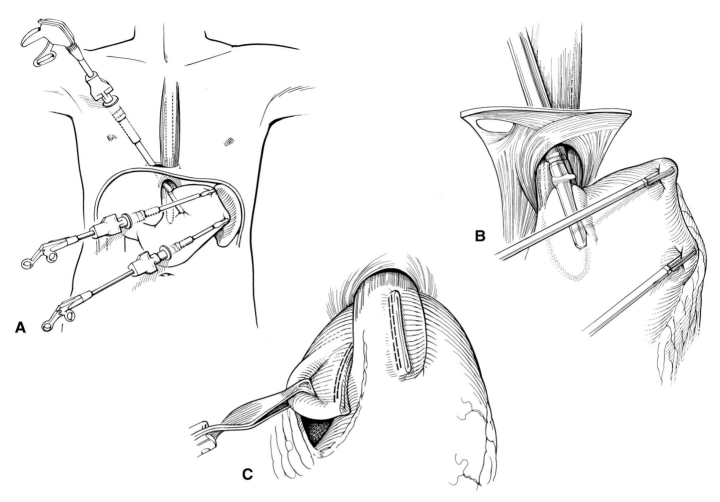

Fig. 11. Laparoscopic Collis gastroplasty for esophageal lengthening. Both the laparoscopic and the thoracoscopic approaches are used simultaneously.

Patients are encouraged to ambulate soon after the operation. They do not require nasogastric decompression. We allow our patients to take clear liquids immediately after the operation. The following morning they are advanced to a pureed diet. A radiographic meglumine diatrizoate (Gastrografin) swallow is useful in patients who have difficulty swallowing when their diet is advanced. It also may be indicated after a difficult procedure, when sharp dissection was used, or after repair of an intraoperative perforation. Most patients require only a few doses of parenteral analgesics and can soon start receiving oral analgesics. The median hospital stay is 1 day.

Perioperative Complications

Complications occur less frequently during laparoscopic antireflux procedures than during open procedures. Splenic injury rarely occurs during laparoscopic fundoplication. Another intraoperative complication is bleeding from the short gastric vessels or the liver. This can be controlled immediately, either by electrocoagulation or by clipping the offending blood vessel. The most important risk of the procedure is perforation of the esophagus or the stomach. To minimize this risk, we do not use a bougie for sizing the wrap. It is imperative to recognize immediately an esophageal or gastric perforation and to staple or oversew it immediately. Occasionally, a pneumothorax may occur, especially when extended dissection into the mediastinum is necessary. Only rarely is a pleural chest tube required. Most instances can be effectively controlled by lowering the pressure of the pneumoperitoneum and continuing with positive-pressure ventilation. Postoperative continuous positive airway pressure is recommended to support lung function.

Intra-abdominal or intrathoracic abscesses rarely occur. Computed tomography-guided or sonography-guided drainage may be needed. The surgeon should ascertain that there is no unsuspected esophageal or gastric leakage, which would require further operation. An infrequent, but serious, complication is acute gastric herniation through the hiatus. It occurs in less than 1% of patients,[17] but it requires operative correction. Further perioperative complications are pulmonary complications and deep vein thrombosis. Because of the advantage of rapid postoperative mobilization and early ambulation of patients after laparoscopic procedures, the incidence of these complications is close to zero.

The conversion rate from a laparoscopic to an open procedure has been reported to be about 4.2% during the learning curve of a surgeon,[11,18,19] but with increasing experience the conversion rate is as low as 1:600. The mortality rate after laparoscopic antireflux operations is about 0.2%.[20]

Postoperative Complications and Short-term Outcome
Early- and long-term follow-up studies after conventional open antireflux operations have shown excellent results related to quality of life and satisfaction rate.[21,22] The aim of laparoscopic antireflux procedures was to reach a similar outcome. Early results have demonstrated a success rate similar to that of the open procedure. A failure rate of only 3.4% was shown at 3 years after the laparoscopic approach.[23] The most common postoperative symptom is transient dysphagia. It occurs in 20% of cases.[20] Endoscopy or esophagography should be done in patients with dysphagia to identify the underlying problem. Postoperative edema due to manipulation at the gastroesophageal junction is the most frequent cause for this complaint. It usually resolves within 1 to 3 weeks or after esophageal dilation. Less than 5% of patients with dysphagia have persistent symptoms that last more than 6 months.[23-27] If the wrap is too tight and dilation does not improve the symptoms, revision operation may be needed.

Recurrent reflux after operation is usually less severe than it was preoperatively. In most patients it can be controlled with medications such as H_2-receptor blockers or proton pump inhibitors. Less than 1% of patients require further surgical intervention for recurrent reflux during the first 3 years after operation. Most of these patients had severe esophagitis, esophageal strictures, or esophageal ulceration before their first operation.[19]

Many patients with GERD are habitual air swallowers who clear their esophagus of refluxed acid or food. This habit may be responsible for postoperative gas bloat if patients continue to swallow gas and are unable to belch. Bloating is one of the most common symptoms after Nissen fundoplication.[11,24,27] It is rare after the Toupet fundoplication.[28] Medical therapy with gas-binding agents or prokinetics is often successful.

Other common symptoms after laparoscopic antireflux operation include early satiety, nausea, and diarrhea. Diarrhea is thought to be due to the speeding of gastric

emptying after fundoplication, change of diet, or the postvagotomy syndrome. Most of these symptoms disappear several weeks postoperatively. However, 17.8% of patients report new onset of diarrhea after fundoplication, but this is of minor consequence in most patients.

Some patients experience chronic, sometimes severe, upper abdominal epigastric pain postoperatively. Careful evaluation may identify gastritis with an excessive amount of bile in the stomach. Fundoplication has effectively controlled the gastroesophageal reflux, but duodenogastric reflux, likely present before operation, persists. In a small number of patients, a bile diversion operation may therefore be required at a later date to control the gastritis. Figure 12 shows the result of short-term follow-up after laparoscopic Nissen fundoplication. Typical symptoms of GERD, such as heartburn and regurgitation, are well controlled; however, atypical symptoms are not. Figure 13 shows the incidence of atypical symptoms before and 1 year after laparoscopic Nissen fundoplication.

Long-term Outcome
Three factors determine the outcome and success of laparoscopic antireflux operation: operation performed for a strict surgical indication, correct choice of the surgical procedure, and performance of a good-quality operation. If these factors are met, postoperative results will be good. It had to be proved that laparoscopic long-term results are as good as results after the open approach. After a 5- to 8-year follow-up, 96% of the patients who had the laparoscopic approach remained satisfied with the result.[29] Laparoscopic fundoplication appears to be as good as the open operation, which has a success of 91% after 10 years. GERD symptoms, such as regurgitation, heartburn, chest pain, and cough, persist in less than 6% of patients. Preoperative and postoperative symptoms of GERD after a follow-up of 5 to 8 years are shown in Figure 14.

One of the most common symptoms during follow-up is dysphagia. This occurred in 27% of our patients.[29] The rather high incidence was likely due to our strict definition of dysphagia. None of the patients required continued dilation and could manage with mild dietary modification. Abdominal bloating is another of the more common postoperative symptoms and occurs in about 20% of patients after 5 to 8 years. Up to 12% of patients have diarrhea. Most of them can control the diarrhea with medication. During long-term follow-up, a seventh of our patients were receiving continuous proton pump inhibitor therapy.[29] Careful analysis of the indications for proton pump inhibitors showed that they were being used for vague, nonspecific symptoms in the vast majority of patients. Only 6% had evidence of GERD necessitating therapy.

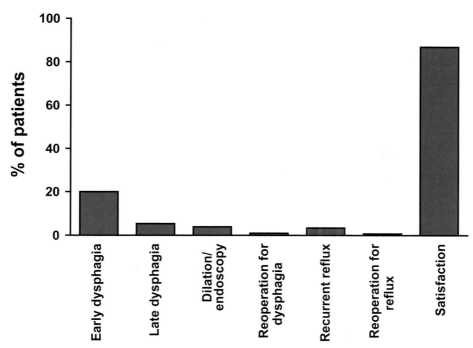

Fig. 12. Short-term cumulative experience after laparoscopic Nissen fundoplication in 2,453 patients. (Modified from Perdikis et al.[20] By permission of Lippincott Williams & Wilkins.)

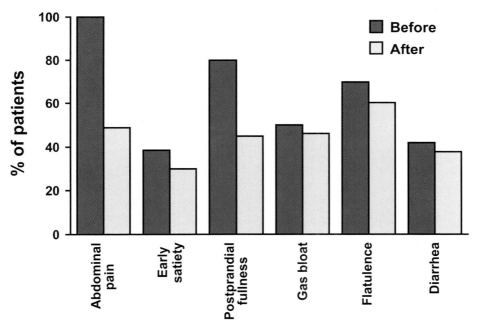

Fig. 13. Atypical symptoms before and 1 year after laparoscopic fundoplication.

The laparoscopic approach has emerged as being superior to open operation because of its safety, equal efficacy, minimal pain, early mobilization, and rapid postoperative recovery compared with the open procedure. Laparoscopic fundoplication is therefore an excellent long-term treatment for GERD and has good success in long-term follow-up. Choosing the right patient and having a surgeon with a solid understanding of the principles of antireflux surgery are the best predictors for good long-term success.

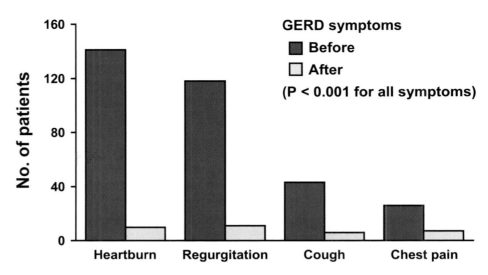

Fig. 14. Improvement of symptoms of gastroesophageal reflux disease (GERD) 5 to 8 years after laparoscopic Nissen fundoplication.[28] (From Bammer et al.[29] By permission of The Society for Surgery of the Alimentary Tract.)

CONCLUSION

Patients with GERD usually can be effectively treated with antacids, H_2-receptor blockers, or proton pump inhibitors. Symptoms often recur after cessation of medical therapy, and, therefore, many patients require lifelong medication. Some patients do not want to be dependent on medications for the rest of their lives, some fail to obtain permanent relief of symptoms, and some have complications of their disease. Antireflux operations restore a mechanically deficient LES to a competent LES, thus reestablishing a barrier to the reflux of gastric and duodenal contents across the sphincter into the esophagus. They are, therefore, effective treatments of GERD. The laparoscopic Nissen fundoplication has become the standard procedure. Laparoscopic antireflux operation is technically demanding, but it can be performed accurately and effectively. It has all the advantages of a minimally invasive operation, which include less pain, shorter hospitalization, and more rapid recovery. Short- and long-term results are excellent after laparoscopic procedures, and improvement of GERD symptoms usually frees patients from the need for long-term use of medications.

REFERENCES

1. Trus TL, Hunter JG: Minimally invasive surgery of the esophagus and stomach. Am J Surg 173:242-255, 1997
2. Mackie C, Hulks G, Cuschieri A: Enterogastric reflux and gastric clearance of refluxate in normal subjects and in patients with and without bile vomiting following peptic ulcer surgery. Ann Surg 204:537-542, 1986
3. Muller-Lissner SA, Fimmel CJ, Sonnenberg A, Will N, Muller-Duysing W, Heinzel F, Muller R, Blum AL: Novel approach to quantify duodenogastric reflux in healthy volunteers and in patients with type I gastric ulcer. Gut 24:510-518, 1983
4. Schindlbeck NE, Heinrich C, Stellaard F, Paumgartner G, Muller-Lissner SA: Healthy controls have as much bile reflux as gastric ulcer patients. Gut 28:1577-1583, 1987
5. Gotley DC, Morgan AP, Ball D, Owen RW, Cooper MJ: Composition of gastro-oesophageal refluxate. Gut 32:1093-1099, 1991
6. Gotley DC, Morgan AP, Cooper MJ: Bile acid concentrations in the refluxate of patients with reflux oesophagitis. Br J Surg 75:587-590, 1988
7. Brunnen PL, Karmody AM, Needham CD: Severe peptic oesophagitis. Gut 10:831-837, 1969
8. Khoury GA, Bolton J: Age: an important factor in Barrett's oesophagus. Ann R Coll Surg Engl 71:50-53, 1989
9. Hinder RA: Gastroesophageal reflux disease. In Digestive Tract Surgery: A Text and Atlas. Edited by RH Bell Jr, LF Rikkers, MM Mulholland. Philadelphia, Lippincott-Raven Publishers, 1996, pp 3-26
10. Dallemagne B, Weerts JM, Jehaes C, Markiewicz S, Lombard R: Laparoscopic Nissen fundoplication: preliminary report. Surg Laparosc Endosc 1:138-143, 1991
11. Hinder RA, Filipi CJ, Wetscher G, Neary P, DeMeester TR, Perdikis G: Laparoscopic Nissen fundoplication is an effective treatment for gastroesophageal reflux disease. Ann Surg 220:472-481, 1994
12. Giffin HZ: The diagnosis of diaphragmatic hernia. Ann Surg 55:388-399, 1912
13. Allison PR: Reflux esophagitis, sliding hiatal hernia, and anatomy of repair. Surg Gynecol Obstet 92:419-431, 1951
14. Nissen R: Eine einfache Operation zur Beeinflussung der Reflux-oesophagitis. Schweiz Med Wchnschr 86:590-592, 1956
15. Klingler PJ, Hinder RA, Cina RA, DeVault KR, Floch NR, Branton SA, Seelig MH: Laparoscopic antireflux surgery for the treatment of esophageal strictures refractory to medical therapy. Am J Gastroenterol 94:-632-636, 1999
16. Huntington TR: Laparoscopic mesh repair of the esophageal hiatus. J Am Coll Surg 184:399-400, 1997
17. Seelig MH, Hinder RA, Klingler PJ, Floch NR, Branton SA, Smith SL: Paraesophageal herniation as a complication following laparoscopic antireflux surgery. J Gastrointest Surg 3:95-99, 1999
18. Hunger JG, Trus TL, Branum GD, Waring JP, Wood WC: A physiologic approach to laparoscopic fundoplication for gastroesophageal reflux disease. Ann Surg 223:673-685, 1996
19. Jamieson GG, Watson DI, Britten-Jones R, Mitchell PC, Anvari M: Laparoscopic Nissen fundoplication. Ann Surg 220:137-145, 1994
20. Perdikis G, Hinder RA, Lund RJ, Raiser F, Katada N: Laparoscopic Nissen fundoplication: Where do we stand? Surg Laparosc Endosc 7:17-21, 1997
21. DeMeester TR, Bonavina L, Albertucci M: Nissen fundoplication for gastroesophageal reflux disease: evaluation of primary repair in 100 consecutive patients. Ann Surg 204:9-20, 1986
22. Grande L, Toledo-Pimentel V, Manterola C, Lacima G, Ros E, Garcia-Valdecasas JC, Fuster J, Visa J, Pera C: Value of Nissen fundoplication in patients with gastro-oesophageal reflux judged by long-term symptom control. Br J Surg 81:548-550, 1994
23. Hinder RA (editor): Gastroesophageal Reflux Disease. Austin, RG Landes, 1993
24. Leggett PL, Churchman-Winn R, Ahn C: Resolving gastroesophageal reflux with laparoscopic fundoplication: findings in 138 cases. Surg Endosc 12:142-147, 1998
25. Jamieson GG: The results of anti-reflux surgery and re-operative anti-reflux surgery. Gullett 3:41-45, 1993
26. Fuchs KH, Freys SM, Heimbucher J, Thiede A: Experiences with laparoscopic technique in anti-reflux surgery [German]. Chirurg 64:317-323, 1993
27. Klingler PJ, Hinder RA, DeVault KR: Laparoscopic antireflux surgery—experience and outcomes. Chirurgische Gastroenterologie 13:138-142, 1997
28. Lund RJ, Wetcher GJ, Raiser F, Glaser K, Perdikis G, Gadenstatter M, Katada N, Filipi CJ, Hinder RA: Laparoscopic Toupet fundoplication for gastroesophageal reflux disease with poor esophageal body motility. J Gastrointest Surg 1:301-308, 1997
29. Bammer T, Hinder RA, Klaus A, Klingler PJ: Five- to eight-year outcome of the first laparoscopic Nissen fundoplications. J Gastrointest Surg 5:42-48, 2001

Chapter 3

ACHALASIA AND OTHER ESOPHAGEAL MOTILITY DISORDERS

Jessica S. Donington, M.D.
Mark S. Allen, M.D.

ACHALASIA

Achalasia is a primary motility disorder of the esophagus. It is a well-recognized disorder and was originally described more than 300 years ago. The main pathologic feature is an abnormality of the lower esophageal sphincter (LES), which does not relax properly with swallowing. The abnormal relaxation of the LES is accompanied by abnormal peristalsis of the smooth muscle in the esophagus. If the condition is left untreated, the esophagus eventually dilates, leading to further food stasis. Therapy is directed at relieving the functional obstruction of the lower esophagus.

Epidemiology and Pathophysiology

Achalasia is a relatively uncommon disorder in North America and Europe; its incidence is approximately 1 per 200,000 persons. In North America, most patients are between 20 and 40 years old. Most series report that an equal number of males and females are affected. In South America, the incidence is higher. There, the parasitic protozoan *Trypanosoma cruzi* is endemic. This parasite causes Chagas' disease, an achalasia-like condition that is present in one of every eight Brazilian people, 5% of whom have serious esophageal symptoms.

The cause of achalasia in North America is not understood. The pathophysiology is related to loss of vagal innervation to the esophagus. Decreased vagal innervation can be attributed to abnormalities at three different levels of the esophageal innervation (Fig. 1). First, autopsy studies have demonstrated that the number of cells in the dorsal motor nucleus in the brain stem in patients with achalasia is 40% less than that in normal people. Cassella et al.[1] were able to reproduce achalasia in cats with bilateral destruction of the dorsal motor nerve of the vagus. Second, there is evidence of wallerian degeneration in the vagal nerve. Third, there is a degeneration or absence or both of the ganglion cells in the myenteric plexus of the esophagus. The changes in the myenteric plexus may be the result of neuronal degeneration, the primary pathologic disorder being in neural cell bodies at sites external to the esophagus. The result of this neuronal degeneration is a decrease of postganglionic cells, which are responsible for esophageal relaxation through release of vasoactive intestinal peptide, nitric oxide, and perhaps other neural inhibitory transmitters.[2] This results in an LES that is supersensitive to cholinergic agonists and that contracts paradoxically in response to cholecystokinin.[3] The cause of these neuronal changes is unknown. Different causes have been hypothesized, including genetic, autoimmune, viral infection, and primary degeneration.

Patient Evaluation

The primary symptom of achalasia is dysphagia. Most patients experience an indolent course, during which the diagnosis of achalasia may be missed, sometimes for many years. Initially, dysphagia is episodic and not related to the mechanical properties of the material ingested. Over time, symptoms worsen but may continue to be irregular and unpredictable. Another common symptom is effortless regurgitation of undigested food immediately or hours after eating. This may lead to frequent respiratory infections as a result of aspiration. If this condition persists, chronic lung disease can occur.

The diagnosis of achalasia cannot be established by clinical symptoms alone. Therefore, radiographic studies,

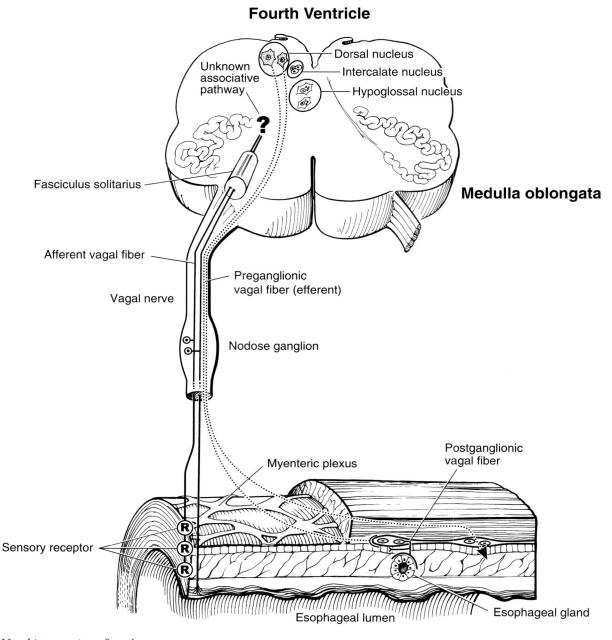

Fourth Ventricle

Dorsal nucleus

Intercalate nucleus

Hypoglossal nucleus

Unknown associative pathway

Medulla oblongata

Fasciculus solitarius

Afferent vagal fiber

Preganglionic vagal fiber (efferent)

Vagal nerve

Nodose ganglion

Postganglionic vagal fiber

Myenteric plexus

Sensory receptor

Esophageal lumen

Esophageal gland

Fig. 1. Vagal innervation of esophagus.

manometry, and endoscopy should be performed before any intervention. Abnormalities on plain chest radiography include a widened mediastinum, a posterior mediastinal air-fluid level, and the absence of a gastric air bubble. Barium contrast esophageal radiography often shows esophageal dilatation with a "bird's beak" deformity at the level of the gastroesophageal junction, retained food and secretions, and an absence of peristalsis (Fig. 2). Vigorous achalasia can result in diverticula or pseudodiverticula seen on contrast studies, and long-standing achalasia can result in a sigmoid-shaped esophagus with an enormous capacity to retain food

and secretions. Although there are scales that can be used to grade achalasia on the basis of the esophageal dilatation seen on radiography, there appears to be only a weak correlation between the degree of dilatation and tortuosity on radiography and the duration and severity of symptoms.

A manometric study, with either a perfusion catheter or a solid-state catheter system, is critical for the diagnosis of achalasia. Because the diagnosis affects esophageal smooth muscle, manometry will show a lack of peristaltic contractions in the lower two-thirds of the esophagus. Usually, wet-to-dry swallows are followed by simultaneous

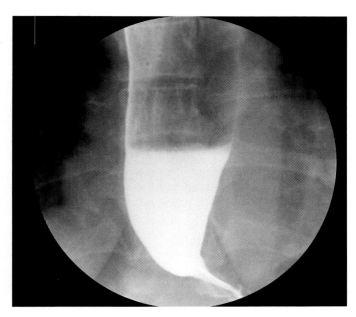

Fig. 2. Barium esophagogram of patient with achalasia.

esophageal contractions.[4] The contractions are of low amplitude (< 40 mm Hg), but occasionally are vigorous. The LES pressure is increased or normal but is never zero in an untreated patient with achalasia. The LES also does not relax properly. Usually, there is no or incomplete relaxation with swallowing; however, in 20% to 30% of patients, the LES pressure decreases to baseline, but only for a short time.

The term "pseudoachalasia" is applied to symptoms and radiographic findings similar to those of achalasia, but it is caused by a tumor at or near the gastroesophageal junction. Pseudoachalasia is suspected in patients with a short history, weight loss, and increased age. Endoscopy with biopsy always should be performed to rule out the presence of a malignancy. Typical endoscopic findings in true achalasia include a patulous and dilated esophageal body that ends in a smooth tapering funnel at the esophagogastric junction. There may be retained material adherent to the esophageal mucosa, mucosal thickening, yeast esophagitis, and cobblestoning of the mucosa due to contact esophagitis. Biopsy should be done on mucosal abnormalities in this area, and yeast esophagitis, if found, should be treated aggressively before intervention. The gastroesophageal junction fails to open in response to air insufflation, but it is usually easy to traverse the junction with the endoscope. As the endoscope traverses the gastroesophageal junction, a characteristic "pop" is felt. This is the relaxation of the LES, allowing passage of the endoscope. Carcinoma does not yield to the endoscope in this manner. If carcinoma is still suspected after endoscopy, esophageal ultrasonography or computed tomography should be performed.

Several additional studies are occasionally required before intervention. Ambulatory 24-hour esophageal pH monitoring may be necessary for patients with achalasia who have gastroesophageal reflux. Poor clearance of small amounts of acid is thought to lead to complaints of heartburn. Affected patients frequently have low pH in their esophagus, but the pattern is very different from that in reflux disease. In achalasia, there can be considerable fermentation of retained esophageal contents, which leads to lactic acid production and a decrease in pH. The pH is consistently low throughout the day and does not fluctuate, as it typically does in gastroesophageal reflux.

Esophageal transit studies with nuclear scintigraphy have been used to demonstrate impaired esophageal transit. They may be the best test to assess physiologically the results of treatments such as balloon dilation or cardiomyotomy, because radiographic improvement is not consistently seen. This study is generally not necessary to establish the diagnosis of achalasia.[4]

Treatment

There is currently no cure for achalasia, but there are many options available for palliation. The goal of treatment in patients with achalasia is relief of their obstructive symptoms by weakening the LES to improve esophageal emptying without causing gastroesophageal reflux. Currently used methods for the palliation of achalasia include pharmacologic therapy, botulinum toxin injection, pneumatic dilation, and surgical myotomy. Although each of these treatments has been studied in depth and the risks and success of each are fairly well understood, there is still considerable controversy about which treatment is best for patients with achalasia.

Pharmacologic

Many pharmacologic agents have been used for the treatment of achalasia, and they have had only moderate success. All share the goal of lowering LES pressure. The most widely used substances include anticholinergics, nitrates, calcium channel blockers, β-adrenergic agonists, and theophylline. Symptomatic relief can be obtained with nifedipine and isosorbide dinitrate in 50% to 80% of patients. These medicines have both been shown to cause a substantial decrease in LES resting pressure. Unfortunately, long-term results have been disappointing, and their profound side effects, including hypotension and headache, have limited their usefulness. Pharmacologic therapy is generally reserved for patients who are not candidates for other forms of treatment.[5,6]

Botulinum Toxin

Since the first reports of intersphincteric botulinum toxin

(Botox) injection for the treatment of achalasia, this treatment has generated excitement and controversy. Botulinum toxin is a potent inhibitor of neuromuscular transmission by inhibiting acetylcholine release from nerve endings. Injection of botulinum toxin seems to provide a safe treatment option for patients with achalasia. The main controversy with the use of botulinum toxin therapy revolves around its duration of action. Initial reports on its use were encouraging,[7] but, unfortunately, the improvement does not seem to last. The response lasts an average of 1.2 years, and most patients require repeated injections.[8,9] Currently, botulinum toxin is a reasonable treatment choice for high-risk, elderly patients to provide short-term relief.[10]

Pneumatic Dilation

Forceful dilation of the LES has been used for centuries for palliation in patients with achalasia. The devices used for dilation have included mercury-weighted bougies, hydrostatic dilators, and pneumatic dilators made of rubber or cloth. Today, pneumatic dilators with polyurethane balloons are most commonly used. Balloons with various compliances are available, but no difference in complications or outcomes has been found between the high- and low-compliance systems.[11] The technique of pneumatic dilation varies; however, typically the balloon of the pneumatic dilator is placed across the gastroesophageal junction under either fluoroscopic or endoscopic guidance. The balloon is then rapidly inflated and maintained in position for 2 to 3 minutes at a pressure of 300 mm Hg (10-12 psi) (Fig. 3). Efficacy is increased when the esophagus is dilated to a diameter of at least 3.0 cm.[12,13] Pneumatic dilation can be performed as an outpatient procedure if patients are observed briefly to assess response to therapy and to rule out perforation.[14]

The immediate success rate of a single dilation is 55% to 70%, but the rate has been reported to be up to 90% with multiple dilations. Subsequent dilation is required in almost half of patients, and about 8% of these patients experience no further benefit.[15]

Long-term results of pneumatic dilation are less encouraging. At 5 years after dilation, more than 50% of patients have recurrence of symptoms. In patients who had a good response to initial dilation, a second dilation is usually successful, but patients in whom initial treatment failed are unlikely to respond to a second dilation.

Minor complications of pneumatic dilation include aspiration pneumonia, prolonged pain, bleeding, and intramucosal hematoma; however, the most important and life-threatening complication is esophageal perforation. Perforations occur predominantly above the cardia on the left side of the esophagus. Perforation rates as high as 15% have been reported in the past, but with polyurethane pneumatic dilating catheters the rates range from 2.5% to 5.2%.[16] "Early" achalasia with less esophageal dilation and some retention of esophageal body motility is associated with a higher rate of perforation. In a retrospective review of 178 patients who underwent pneumatic dilation for achalasia, prior dilation and inflation pressure of more than 11 psi were independent risk factors for the development of a perforation.[17]

Esophagography with a water-soluble contrast agent should be performed in all patients when perforation is suspected. If a perforation is found, immediate surgical repair is the appropriate treatment. The esophagus should be repaired in layers with careful mucosal reapproximation. After repair, a myotomy is performed on the opposite side of the esophagus from the injury, and a partial wrap of gastric fundus around the esophagogastric junction may be added if reflux is a concern. If the perforation is found expediently and treated properly, patients do very well.

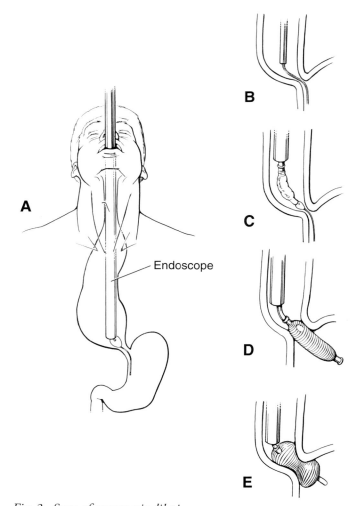

Endoscope

Fig. 3. Steps of pneumatic dilation.

Pneumatic dilation is a safe and effective treatment for achalasia which does not require a hospital stay, as surgical intervention does. The choice between the two treatment techniques is difficult. To date, only one prospective randomized trial has compared pneumatic dilation with esophagomyotomy for the treatment of achalasia. Csendes et al.[18] presented their late results in 81 patients: 39 had pneumatic dilation and 42 had myotomy by left thoracotomy. Results were considered good to excellent in 65% of patients after dilation and in 95% after myotomy; however, acid reflux was abnormal in 28% of patients after operation and only 8% of patients after dilation.

Surgical Myotomy

There still remains debate between surgeons and gastroenterologists about which patients should be offered surgical treatment. In general, surgical myotomy is considered appropriate in four groups of patients. The first group consists of younger patients, because the success of pneumatic dilation is somewhat age-dependent. In patients younger than 40 years, pneumatic dilation is only 40% to 70% effective and the concomitant risk of perforation is 2% to 7%.[19] Cardiomyotomy in this age group is approximately 90% effective and there is almost no mortality. The age-related failure of pneumatic dilation is difficult to explain but may be due to greater elasticity in the younger tissues which allows the tissues to stretch and return to their original shape after dilation rather than disrupt. The second and largest group of patients includes those with recurrent symptoms of achalasia after pneumatic dilation. Although repeat dilation may be attempted, 15% to 35% of these patients will require myotomy.[19,20] It still remains to be determined how many attempts are considered sensible before surgical intervention. The third group consists of patients for whom pneumatic dilation is considered too high a risk. This includes patients with a tortuous distal esophagus, esophageal diverticula, or previous operation at the gastroesophageal junction. Although these patients can be treated with botulinum toxin injections, endoscopic identification of the gastroesophageal junction is nearly impossible. Therefore, the odds of proper placement of the injection are poor. The fourth group is patients who choose cardiomyotomy over pneumatic dilation or botulinum toxin injection because of the better long-term results of cardiomyotomy or the fear of esophageal perforation.

Many questions have been raised about the feasibility of surgical myotomy after botulinum toxin injection. This therapy can cause considerable scarring between the mucosa and muscularis and obliteration of the dissection plane used at myotomy. Scarring is usually most severe at the level of the gastroesophageal junction after multiple injections. Although surgeons describe myotomy after botulinum toxin injection to be technically more difficult than myotomy without injection, the injection has not resulted in an increased complication rate in these patients.[21]

Heller's Contribution

Ernst Heller was a 36-year-old surgical assistant at the University Surgical Clinic in Leipzig, Germany, in 1914 when he made his contribution to the surgical treatment of achalasia.[22] The great German surgeons of the first half of the 20th century championed anastomotic cardioplasties. These cardioplasties resembled the pyloroplasties described by Heineke-Mikulicz, Jaboulay, and Finney. The late and devastating consequence of reflux caused by these operations was not recognized until the report from Barrett and Franklin in 1949.[23]

In 1913, Heller took a 51-year-old man with a 30-year history of dysphagia and radiographic evidence of achalasia to the operating room with the full intent of performing a side-to-side anastomotic esophagogastrostomy to bypass the spastic LES. As a result of his observations in the operating room, he abandoned his initial plan and instead performed a transabdominal double (anterior and posterior) vertical esophagomyotomy. Contrary to the apparent impulsive nature of this decision, Heller was quick to point out that the concept for such an operation had not been new to him. He had considered its possibility after his discussions with Gottsiem regarding his technique for pyloromyotomy. The patient did well postoperatively and took solids the day after the procedure. The patient had no subsequent treatment, and at last follow-up 8 years postoperatively he was in good health and subjectively had normal esophageal function.

Heller described his new procedure in a 1914 article titled "Extramukose Cardioplastik."[24] A Dutch surgeon later modified the procedure, eliminating the posterior myotomy. Although Heller continued to perform his operation, his work was essentially ignored in Europe until after World War I because of his young age and junior status. Heller's revolutionary technique was not widely accepted until Barrett and Franklin published their article in 1949.[23]

Subsequent work by Ripley et al.[25,26] in North America firmly established myotomy as the surgical treatment of choice for achalasia. Although Heller was denied immediate recognition for his important contribution to the treatment of achalasia, recognition eventually came during his long and successful career.

Esophagomyotomy

As described above, esophagomyotomy has been a successful treatment of achalasia for decades. In nearly 1,200 patients who had operation between 1980 and 1990, the overall success rate was 89%, the mortality rate was less than 1%, and the reoperation rate was less than 3%.[27] Once the decision is made to proceed with myotomy, many controversies surround the technical aspects of the procedure, the first of which is approach—abdominal versus thoracic, minimally invasive versus open, and thoracoscopic versus laparoscopic. There is also debate about the extent of myotomy in both the proximal and the distal direction and the need for the addition of an antireflux procedure to the operation.

Transabdominal Cardiomyotomy
Transabdominal cardiomyotomy is the most commonly performed procedure in the world for the treatment of achalasia. It is used frequently in Europe and in Brazil, where infectious achalasia is endemic. The world's largest series of myotomies comes from Pinotti et al.[28] in Sao Paulo. After transabdominal myotomy in 722 patients, they reported excellent long-term results in 95% and no mortality. They actually performed a cardiomyectomy, removing a 6.0- x 0.5-cm strip of esophageal muscle, followed by a 180° anterior hemifundoplication.

We do not perform a myectomy but rather merely divide the muscle along the anterior aspect of the esophagus. The myotomy is started 1.0 to 2.0 cm above the gastroesophageal junction, where the LES muscle is thickened and the risk of esophageal perforation is the least. The longitudinal muscles are divided first, exposing the circular fibers, which are bluntly dissected and divided. This step should expose a plane between mucosa and muscularis. This plane is usually easily identified, but botulinum toxin injection can severely obscure visualization of the plane. The circular fibers are elevated off the mucosa and divided with scissors. The myotomy is carried proximally approximately 6.0 cm superiorly, through the hiatus, and into the mediastinum. Ideally, the distal end of the myotomy extends just beyond the end of the LES, stopping just distal to the esophagogastric junction. Once the myotomy is complete, the mucosa is bluntly dissected free of the muscularis for at least 50% of the esophageal circumference.

Unfortunately, it can be very difficult to determine where the distal extent of the myotomy should extend to provide relief of dysphagia and not allow gastroesophageal reflux disease. Some surgeons extend the myotomy 1.0 to 2.0 cm down onto the stomach to ensure division of all the fibers of the LES, knowing that at the same time they are disrupting the normal antireflux mechanism of the hiatus. An antireflux procedure is then added to eliminate the reflux that otherwise would occur.

If an antireflux procedure is not added to an abdominal myotomy, 14% of patients will have symptomatic reflux and 28% of patients will have abnormal reflux by 24-hour pH study.[29] Peptic esophageal strictures can develop in patients with achalasia, even asymptomatic patients, because they have poor esophageal clearance. This complication occurs in approximately 3% of patients after myotomy and usually necessitates an esophagectomy to treat. Although fundoplication may not be complete protection against reflux and subsequent stricture formation, the frequency of reflux substantially decreases on 24-hour pH study when a fundoplication is performed at the time of myotomy.[29]

After completion of the myotomy, the diaphragmatic crura are reapproximated over a 60F bougie, and a partial fundoplication is performed. Floppy or loose Nissen fundoplications have been advocated by some, but a partial fundoplication is recommended as the best way to avoid reflux without causing dysphagia. A Toupet fundoplication, or posterior fundoplication, brings the fundus of the stomach behind the esophagus and secures it to the posterior edges of the esophageal muscularis which were divided (Fig. 4).[30] It has the advantage of holding those edges apart and creating a barrier to reflux at the gastroesophageal junction. The anterior hemifundoplication, or Dor fundoplication, places the fundus of the stomach anteriorly over the esophagus and secures it to the divided edges of muscularis of the myotomy.[29] We recommend the Toupet procedure for most patients.

Transthoracic Cardiomyotomy
The thoracic approach for surgical repair of achalasia permits a myotomy to be performed with minimal dissection

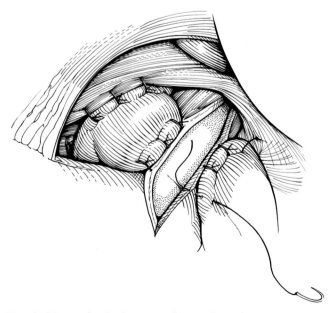

Fig. 4. Toupet fundoplication after esophageal myotomy.

of the esophageal hiatus, thereby preserving the native antireflux mechanism. A thoracic approach also permits easy visualization of the proximal portion of myotomy and treatment of associated abnormalities such as esophageal diverticula. An antireflux procedure also can be added to the thoracic approach if indicated. Ellis,[30] at Mayo Clinic, championed transthoracic esophagomyotomy without an antireflux procedure for many years. He believed an antireflux procedure was an unnecessary addition to the myotomy. He reported excellent results in 90% of patients and reflux in only 5%. A review of more than 5,000 patients in the worldwide literature demonstrated that reflux was twice as common when myotomy was performed transabdominally as opposed to transthoracically.[29]

Transthoracic myotomy is performed through a left posterolateral thoracotomy. After mobilization of the inferior pulmonary ligament and identification and protection of the vagal nerves, the longitudinal myotomy is performed. It begins at the gastroesophageal junction and extends 7.0 to 10.0 cm proximally up to the level of the left inferior pulmonary vein (Fig. 5). Care is taken to avoid undue traction on the esophagus and disruption of the esophageal hiatus. When the myotomy is complete, the mucosa is bluntly freed from the muscularis to approximately 50% of the esophageal circumference. If a hiatal hernia is present, it is repaired. The esophagus is returned to its mediastinal bed, and the mediastinal pleura is reapproximated. The lung is re-expanded, and

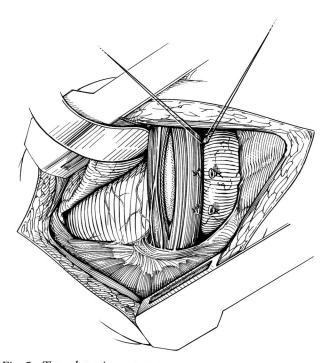

Fig. 5. Transthoracic myotomy.

chest tubes and a nasogastric tube are placed. The nasogastric tube can be removed the morning after operation and a soft diet begun. A meglumine diatrizoate (Gastrografin) swallow can be done in the postoperative period as a baseline for follow-up.

In a large series from the Mayo Clinic, 468 patients were evaluated after a transthoracic myotomy. Results were good to excellent in 85% of patients.[31] There was one death from malignant hyperthermia and five postoperative esophageal leaks, three of which necessitated reoperation. Unfortunately, the transthoracic approach causes considerable postoperative chest pain and a long hospital stay, so we do not use this approach often today.

Thoracoscopic Myotomy

The development of minimally invasive techniques has led surgeons to try to achieve outcomes equal to those of the transthoracic or transabdominal approach without pain and a prolonged hospitalization. Pellegrini et al.[32] first reported on thoracoscopic myotomy in 1992. The approach differs from the open thoracic procedure only by mode of access. A double-lumen endotracheal tube is used for selective ventilation of the right lung during the procedure. The patient is placed in the right lateral decubitus position. Five or six ports are placed for adequate retraction and exposure, and a 30° scope is used for better visualization. Identification of the esophagus is aided by the placement of an endoscope in the distal esophagus, which illuminates and displaces the esophagus to the left. The operation then proceeds in a fashion similar to its open equivalent. One key to the myotomy is that the surgeon needs to work with both hands, grasping the edge of muscularis with the left hand and retracting cephalad while dividing the muscle with a scissors or cautery hook in the right hand to extend the myotomy distally. This technique not only expedites the myotomy but also provides the best exposure of the gastroesophageal junction. A chest tube and nasogastric tube are placed at the completion of the procedure. Most surgeons routinely obtain a contrast esophagogram the morning after operation to rule out an unsuspected mucosal injury. Patients are then given a soft diet and released from the hospital after chest tube removal the day after operation.

Laparoscopic Myotomy

We now believe that laparoscopic myotomy is the operation of choice for achalasia. It has many of the same benefits as thoracoscopic myotomy with several additional advantages. The thoracoscopic approach has several limitations. It requires a double-lumen endotracheal tube, decubitus positioning, and intraoperative endoscopy. It also can be difficult to retract the lung and diaphragm properly to expose the esophagus. Finally, a chest tube is required, resulting in more pain than an abdominal approach.

Laparoscopic esophageal myotomy is performed with tools and skills similar to those used for laparoscopic fundoplication. Patients are placed supine in a modified lithotomy position. The operating surgeon stands between the legs and the assistant stands on the left. Port sites are chosen as shown in Figure 6. The right and left diaphragmatic crura are dissected free, and the lower esophagus is freed from the surrounding areolar tissue. It is necessary to identify and protect the anterior vagal nerve before myotomy. The fat pad at the gastroesophageal junction is removed to identify the gastroesophageal junction confidently. The myotomy is begun by gently pulling the longitudinal muscles apart and then carefully dividing the circular fibers. It is begun just above the gastroesophageal junction and continued cephalad and caudad (Fig. 7). Any bleeding usually stops spontaneously or with gentle cautery. "Peanuts" can be used to facilitate the dissection. The myotomy is extended 1.0 to 2.0 cm onto the stomach and 8.0 to 10.0 cm up on the esophagus. An antireflux procedure is performed after the myotomy, most frequently a partial Toupet fundoplication. Patients are given a soft diet and can be released from the hospital the day after operation.

Results

Laparoscopic myotomy, like thoracoscopic myotomy, is a new procedure, so no long-term results are yet available, in contradistinction to the results for open procedures. The Mayo Clinic reported results in 468 patients after open thoracic myotomy,[31] and Pinotti et al.[28] reported results in 722 patients after open abdominal myotomy. Both studies had more than 12 years of follow-up. These two studies and others reported excellent results in 85% to 95% of patients and reflux in only 5% to 10%. Unlike the results of pneumatic dilation, these results hold up over time with almost no late failures.

Historically, results were assessed according to symptomatic response with the Van Trappen scoring criteria. Today, elegant quantitative techniques are available to assess response to therapy. Manometry and 24-hour pH monitoring provide much more exact quantification of response to treatment. Even under this more scrutinous examination, thoracoscopic and laparoscopic myotomies improve esophageal outflow obstruction and relieve symptoms of dysphagia in 85% to 95% of patients, and they have minimal risk of perforation. Reflux occurs in less than 5% of patients when an antireflux procedure is performed. These results compare favorably with the results of pneumatic dilation, in that pain is increased minimally, hospital stay is short, and return to work is rapid.

The most frequent late complication of cardiomyotomy is gastroesophageal reflux. Some surgeons report a reflux rate of only 3% to 5% without an antireflux procedure.[30] Unfortunately, the incidence of reflux after myotomy seems to depend on the frequency of adequate testing for it. Although fewer patients actually complain of reflux symptoms, abnormal pH profiles can be detected in up to 48% of patients after myotomy without an antireflux procedure and in approximately 25% of patients after pneumatic dilation. The addition of a partial fundoplication reduces the rate of reflux on pH profiles after myotomy to 5% to 10%.

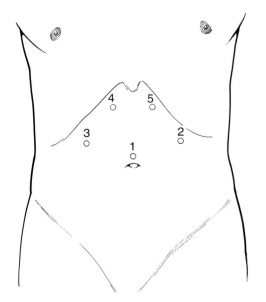

Fig. 6. Location of port sites for laparoscopic myotomy.

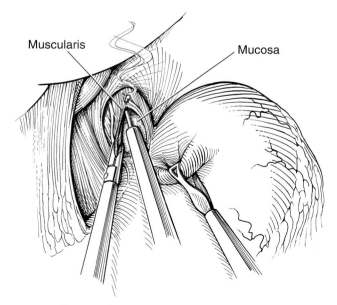

Fig. 7. Technique of myotomy.

Esophageal Resection

Symptoms recur or persist in 10% to 15% of patients after treatment. They are attributed to a wide variety of causes, including inadequate myotomy, healing of the myotomy, stricture due to gastroesophageal reflux, obstruction due to fundoplication, incorrect initial diagnosis, carcinoma, and paraesophageal hernia. Regardless of the reason for failure, it represents a therapeutic dilemma for the esophageal surgeon. Before reoperation is considered, it is useful to investigate thoroughly the suspected underlying pathophysiologic mechanism with barium swallow testing, manometry, 24-hour pH monitoring, and endoscopy with or without esophageal ultrasonography and biopsy. These studies can usually define the reason for the continued or persistent symptoms and more accurately guide therapy.

The approach for reoperation for achalasia has been variable and includes repeat myotomy with or without fundoplication, takedown, addition or revision of fundoplication, or esophageal resection. Ellis et al.[33] reported that only two-thirds of patients undergoing repeat esophagomyotomy had improvement of their symptoms, and the addition of a fundoplication did not further improve their outcome. However, all patients who had an esophageal resection reported symptomatic improvement. Although Ellis and others advocate proceeding immediately to resection after failed myotomy, each patient's problem should be thoroughly investigated and treatment individualized. In some patients, completion of a myotomy or the addition of a fundoplication may provide substantial relief from symptoms. In other patients with a markedly dilated esophagus, resection is often a better treatment option.

The method of esophageal resection is also a topic of debate. Orringer and Stirling[34] and Pinotti et al.[28] recommended transhiatal esophagectomy, but it is associated with a higher risk of mediastinal bleeding than a transthoracic esophagectomy. In a large series of more than 400 transhiatal esophagectomies reported by Orringer and Stirling,[34] the only two patients requiring reoperation for bleeding both had reoperation for achalasia. The esophageal arteries arising from the aorta, which supply the hypertrophied esophageal muscle, are larger in patients with achalasia than in normal patients and, therefore, are prone to increased bleeding in comparison with patients undergoing esophageal resection for other reasons. Pinotti et al.[28] reported similar problems with transhiatal esophagectomy, with a 2% mortality rate due to mediastinal hemorrhage. Our preference is to perform a transthoracic esophagectomy with high intrathoracic esophageal anastomosis. We have been able to accomplish this with low operative morbidity and mortality.[35] This procedure has excellent long-term functional results,

because almost all of the nonfunctional esophagus is removed. Although the method of resection seems to affect the outcome, the choice of conduit for reconstruction does not affect long-term function. The stomach is used most frequently because of its reliable blood supply, ease of use, and need for only one anastomosis. When stomach is not available, colon or small bowel can be used as conduits. Although they are technically more difficult to use, both yield good long-term results.

Conclusion

Achalasia is a rare neuromuscular disorder of unknown cause. It is characterized by a primary disorder of relaxation of the LES. Patients present with dysphagia and frequent regurgitation. Essential work-up before intervention includes radiographic contrast studies, manometry, and endoscopy. The approach for treatment must be individualized. For patients who do not want or will not tolerate operation, medical therapy including endoscopic botulinum toxin injection may provide some short-term palliation. Pneumatic dilation is more likely to result in long-term successful treatment, but it does have a higher risk of perforation than operation. Our preferred method of treatment is laparoscopic esophageal myotomy. This seems to be a safe and durable approach to the treatment of achalasia, providing successful relief of dysphagia in 85% to 90% of patients with low complication rates and minimal postoperative reflux when a partial fundoplication is added at the time of the procedure. In rare cases of persistent or recurrent symptoms after myotomy, a thorough investigation is warranted before intervention, when an esophageal resection may be a safe and reasonable treatment option.

OTHER ESOPHAGEAL MOTILITY DISORDERS

Functional disorders of the esophageal body may produce dysphagia and pain or interfere with normal swallowing without any organic obstruction of the esophagus. Although each disorder has characteristic clinical, radiographic, and manometric findings, there is considerable overlap between them. Every effort should be made to make a precise diagnosis before any intervention, because proper patient selection is necessary to ensure a good outcome.

Diffuse Esophageal Spasm

This is a rare disorder characterized by abnormal esophageal motility, chest pain, and dysphagia. It differs from achalasia in that it is a primary abnormality of the esophageal body, and the LES has normal resting pressure and normal relaxation with deglutition. Patients show a characteristic image on barium study with segmentation and pseudodiverticula or a "corkscrew" appearance. Manometric criteria for diagnosis require the presence of an increased frequency of simultaneous (nonperistaltic) contractions with abnormally high amplitude and long duration in the body of the esophagus with some preservation of normal peristaltic function.[36] Medical management involves the use of nitrates or calcium channel blockers. Patients who do not respond to medical therapy require dilation or long myotomy.

The goal of a surgical myotomy is to improve symptoms. A long myotomy reduces simultaneous contractions and improves the compliance of the esophagus but at the expense of decreasing peristalsis. On 24-hour ambulatory motility study, the presence of more than 75% simultaneous waveforms during meals is currently considered an accurate predictor of patients who will benefit from a myotomy.[37] The proximal extent of myotomy is determined with preoperative manometry, and distally the myotomy should extend across the sphincter and onto the stomach, necessitating the addition of an antireflux procedure.

Myotomy is performed through the left chest in a fashion similar to that for achalasia, but the myotomy is extended up proximal to the beginning of the manometric abnormality. Thoracoscopically, exposure can be difficult and requires placement of the patient almost into the prone position to allow the lung to fall forward out of the surgical field. Patti et al.[38] described 10 patients in whom thoracoscopic long surgical myotomies had good results and improvement of symptoms in 80%. The results of long surgical myotomy for diffuse esophageal spasm have improved in parallel with the improvements in preoperative diagnosis afforded by 24-hour manometry. Reports estimate 85% palliation of dysphagia at 5 years.[39]

Nutcracker Esophagus

This is a manometrically defined syndrome characterized by high-amplitude (> 180 mm Hg) peristaltic contractions in the body of the esophagus. Patients complain of dysphagia and chest pain, often indistinguishable from cardiac chest pain. Although barium studies and esophagoscopy should be performed to rule out other problems, manometry is required to confirm the diagnosis. Calcium channel blockers and anticholinergics are first-line therapy. In general, dilation and surgical myotomy are not reliably helpful in this disorder. They may increase or add dysphagia to the problem.

Nonspecific and Secondary Esophageal Motility Disorders

Nonspecific motility disorders are diagnoses of exclusion in patients who complain of dysphagia and chest pain. Results of manometry are abnormal, showing multipeaked, repetitive, spontaneous, and prolonged contractions, but the contractions do not meet the criteria for one of the other defined disorders. It is important to rule out secondary causes of esophageal dysfunction. A surgical myotomy is unlikely to be helpful in the treatment of this motility disorder unless there is an associated diverticulum.

Gastroesophageal reflux disease is the most common disorder leading to esophageal body dysfunction. It may be difficult to distinguish preoperatively from a primary motility disorder. The cause of gastroesophageal reflux disease is multifactorial, but the LES is incompetent in 60% to 70% of patients. Effective antireflux therapy can improve secondary esophageal motility disorders.

Associated systemic diseases that can produce motility disorders of the esophagus include scleroderma, diabetes mellitus, amyloidosis, dermatomyositis, and mixed connective tissue diseases. It is important to consider these diseases when evaluating patients with nonspecific esophageal motility disorders.

THE FUTURE

Achalasia and other motility disorders of the esophagus continue to be a challenging group of diseases to treat. With improved diagnostic accuracy, it is hoped that specific therapy can be aimed at correction. With careful surgical management, outcomes should be successful in most patients.

REFERENCES

1. Cassella RR, Brown AL Jr, Sayre GP, Ellis FH Jr: Achalasia of the esophagus: pathologic and etiologic considerations. Ann Surg 160:474-486, 1964
2. Aggestrup S, Uddman R, Sundler F, Fahrenkrug J, Hakanson R, Sorensen HR, Hambraeus G: Lack of vasoactive intestinal polypeptide nerves in esophageal achalasia. Gastroenterology 84:924-927, 1983
3. Dodds WJ, Dent J, Hogan WJ, Patel GK, Toouli J, Arndorfer RC: Paradoxical lower esophageal sphincter contraction induced by cholecystokinin-octapeptide in patients with achalasia. Gastroenterology 80:327-333, 1981
4. Stein HF, Korn O: Pathophysiology of esophageal motor disorders and gastroesophageal reflux disease. *In* Modern Approaches to Benign Esophageal Disease: Diagnosis and Surgical Therapy. Edited by CG Bremmer, TR DeMeester, A Peracchia. St Louis, Quality Medical Publishing, 1995, pp 1-16
5. Berger K, McCallum RW: Nifedipine in the treatment of achalasia. Ann Intern Med 96:61-62, 1982
6. Traube M, Dubovik S, Lange RC, McCallum RW: The role of nifedipine therapy in achalasia: results of a randomized, double-blind, placebo-controlled study. Am J Gastroenterol 84:1259-1262, 1989
7. Pasricha PJ, Ravich WJ, Hendrix TR, Sostre S, Jones B, Kalloo AN: Treatment of achalasia with intrasphincteric injection of botulinum toxin. A pilot trial. Ann Intern Med 121:590-591, 1994
8. Pasricha PJ, Rai R, Ravich WJ, Hendrix TR, Kalloo AN: Botulinum toxin for achalasia: long-term outcome and predictors of response. Gastroenterology 110:1410-1415, 1996
9. Fishman VM, Parkman HP, Schiano TD, Hills C, Dabezies MA, Cohen S, Fisher RS, Miller LS: Symptomatic improvement in achalasia after botulinum toxin injection of the lower esophageal sphincter. Am J Gastroenterol 91:1724-1730, 1996
10. Gordon JM, Eaker EY: Prospective study of esophageal botulinum toxin injection in high-risk achalasia patients. Am J Gastroenterol 92:1812-1817, 1997
11. Muehldorfer SM, Hahn EG, Ell C: High- and low-compliance balloon dilators in patients with achalasia: a randomized prospective comparative trial. Gastrointest Endosc 44:398-403, 1996
12. Gelfand MD, Kozarek RA: An experience with polyethylene balloons for pneumatic dilation in achalasia. Am J Gastroenterol 84:924-927, 1989
13. Eckardt VF, Aignherr C, Bernhard G: Predictors of outcome in patients with achalasia treated by pneumatic dilation. Gastroenterology 103:1732-1738, 1992
14. Barkin JS, Guelrud M, Reiner DK, Goldberg RI, Phillips RS: Forceful balloon dilation: an outpatient procedure for achalasia. Gastrointest Endosc 36:123-126, 1990
15. Wehrmann T, Jacobi V, Jung M, Lembcke B, Caspary WF: Pneumatic dilation in achalasia with a low-compliance balloon: results of a 5-year prospective evaluation. Gastrointest Endosc 42:31-36, 1995
16. Bell RC: Laparoscopic closure of esophageal perforation following pneumatic dilatation for achalasia: report of two cases. Surg Endosc 11:476-478, 1997
17. Nair LA, Reynolds JC, Parkman HP, Ouyang A, Strom BL, Rosato EF, Cohen S: Complications during pneumatic dilation for achalasia or diffuse esophageal spasm: analysis of risk factors, early clinical characteristics, and outcome. Dig Dis Sci 38:1893-1904, 1993
18. Csendes A, Braghetto I, Henriquez A, Cortes C: Late results of a prospective randomised study comparing forceful dilatation and oesophagomyotomy in patients with achalasia. Gut 30:299-304, 1989
19. Hunter JG, Richardson WS: Surgical management of achalasia. Surg Clin North Am 77:993-1015, 1997
20. Sauer L, Pellegrini CA, Way LW: The treatment of achalasia: a current perspective. Arch Surg 124:929-931, 1989
21. Horgan S, Hudda K, Eubanks T, McAllister J, Pellegrini CA: Does botulinum toxin injection make esophagomyotomy a more difficult operation? Surg Endosc 13:576-579, 1999
22. Payne WS: Heller's contribution to the surgical treatment of achalasia of the esophagus. 1914. Ann Thorac Surg 48:876-881, 1989
23. Barrett NR, Franklin RH: Concerning unfavorable late results of operations performed in treatment of cardiospasm. Br J Surg 37:194-202, 1949
24. Heller E: Extramuköse Cardioplastik beim chronischen Cardiospasmus mit Dilatation des Oesophagus. Mitt Grenzgeb Med Chir 27:141-149, 1913
25. Ripley HR, Olsen AM, Kirklin JW: Esophagitis after esophagogastric anastomosis. Surgery 32:1-9, 1952
26. Ripley HR, Leary WV, Grindlay JH, Seybold WD, Code CF: Experimental studies of peptic ulceration and stricture of the lower part of the esophagus. Surg Forum 1:60-64, 1950
27. Ferguson MK: Achalasia: current evaluation and therapy. Ann Thorac Surg 52:336-342, 1991
28. Pinotti HW, Felix VN, Zilberstein B, Cecconello I: Surgical complications of Chagas' disease: megaesophagus, achalasia of the pylorus, and cholelithiasis. World J Surg 15:198-204, 1991
29. Andreollo NA, Earlam RJ: Heller's myotomy for achalasia: Is an added anti-reflux procedure necessary? Br J Surg 74:765-769, 1987
30. Ellis FH Jr: Treatment of achalasia: a continuing controversy. Ann Thorac Surg 45:473, 1988
31. Okike N, Payne WS, Neufeld DM, Bernatz PE, Pairolero PC, Sanderson DR: Esophagomyotomy versus forceful dilation for achalasia of the esophagus: results in 899 patients. Ann Thorac Surg 28:119-125, 1979
32. Pellegrini C, Wetter LA, Patti M, Leichter R, Mussan G, Mori T, Bernstein G, Way L: Thoracoscopic esophagomyotomy: initial experience with a new approach for the treatment of achalasia. Ann Surg 216:291-296, 1992
33. Ellis FH Jr, Crozier RE, Gibb SP: Reoperative achalasia surgery. J Thorac Cardiovasc Surg 92:859-865, 1986
34. Orringer MB, Stirling MC: Esophageal resection for achalasia: indications and results. Ann Thorac Surg 47:340-345, 1989
35. Miller DL, Allen MS, Trastek VF, Deschamps C, Pairolero PC: Esophageal resection for recurrent achalasia. Ann Thorac Surg 60:922-925, 1995
36. Eypasch EP, DeMeester TR, Klingman RR, Stein HJ: Physiologic assessment and surgical management of diffuse esophageal spasm. J Thorac Cardiovasc Surg 104:859-868, 1992
37. Bremner RM, DeMeester TR: Current management of patients with esophageal motor abnormalities. Adv Surg 30:349-384, 1997
38. Patti MG, Pellegrini CA, Arcerito M, Tong J, Mulvihill SJ, Way LW: Comparison of medical and minimally invasive surgical therapy for primary esophageal motility disorders. Arch Surg 130:609-615, 1995
39. DeMeester TR: Surgery for esophageal motor disorders. Ann Thorac Surg 34:225-229, 1982

Chapter 4

EPIPHRENIC ESOPHAGEAL DIVERTICULA

Ronald A. Hinder, M.D.
Joaquin A. Rodriguez, M.D.

Epiphrenic esophageal diverticula occur in the lower one-third of the esophagus (Fig. 1 and 2). They are mucosal outpouchings that are muscle-covered when small and free of muscle when large.[1] One or more can be found in a single patient. They occur equally on the left or right side of the esophagus. These diverticula are uncommon, having an incidence of less than 1 per 100,000 persons.

ETIOLOGY AND PATHOPHYSIOLOGY

Theories about the cause of esophageal diverticula include traction by surrounding inflammation (as described for midesophageal diverticula caused by inflamed paratracheal lymph glands) or pulsion caused by an increase in intraluminal pressure. The latter is the most likely cause of lower esophageal diverticula. This theory is supported by the finding of a motility disorder, such as achalasia, diffuse esophageal spasm, hypertensive lower esophageal sphincter (LES), nonspecific motor abnormalities, or nutcracker esophagus, in most patients.[2] Multiple esophageal diverticula have been reported in patients with scleroderma.

SYMPTOMS AND DIAGNOSIS

Most diverticula are asymptomatic or cause minimal symptoms, such as mild dysphagia or occasional regurgitation of food. Accumulation of food and debris in a diverticulum can result in inflammation of its wall and in the adjacent mediastinum. The inflammation aggravates symptoms. Approximately 36% of patients with epiphrenic diverticula have severe dysphagia, regurgitation, or aspiration.[1] Other symptoms include chest pain and halitosis. Sometimes it

is difficult to distinguish the symptoms caused by a motor abnormality associated with a diverticulum from those caused by the diverticulum itself.

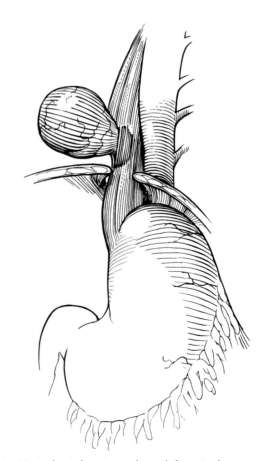

Fig. 1. Typical epiphrenic esophageal diverticulum.

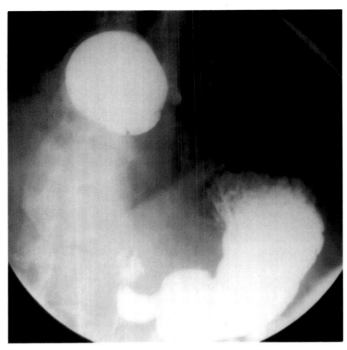

Fig. 2. Barium esophagogram, showing a large epiphrenic esophageal diverticulum.

Diagnosis is usually confirmed by contrast radiography with barium sulfate (Fig. 2) or by the discovery of a retrocardiac shadow containing gas and a fluid level on chest radiography. Diverticula may be evident at endoscopy. Care must be exercised during endoscopy to prevent inadvertent perforation of a thin-walled diverticulum by the endoscope. If a motor disorder of the esophagus is suspected, esophageal manometry should be done.

OPERATIVE TREATMENT

Small or asymptomatic diverticula do not require surgical treatment. Most will not cause problems. Operation is the only effective long-term treatment for symptomatic esophageal diverticula. Small diverticula can be inverted into the esophageal lumen, and the esophageal muscle at the site of the inversion closed with sutures. However, the type of operation advised for large diverticula remains controversial. Some surgeons, such as Streitz et al.,[3] propose diverticulectomy with selective use of myotomy to areas of demonstrated esophageal dysmotility, sparing the lower esophageal sphincter (when it is normal) to prevent subsequent reflux. We and others advocate diverticulectomy and routine "long" esophageal myotomy through the lower esophageal sphincter to decrease the risk of recurrence of the diverticulum and the risk of leakage from the site of diverticulectomy caused by high intraesophageal pressures associated with unsuspected spastic motor disorders.[4] We

also add a partial fundoplication to our procedure. Some argue that a fundoplication is not required;[3] however, our experience indicates that it is needed. This view is supported by the fact that after an esophageal myotomy for achalasia, the avoidance of a fundoplication results in symptomatic reflux in 15% of patients. This rate can be decreased to 5% by adding a partial fundoplication with little or no increase in the incidence of dysphagia.

The operation can be performed through an open thoracotomy or celiotomy or thoracoscopically or laparoscopically. In an effort to decrease postoperative pain and hospital stay after open thoracotomy, Peracchia et al.[5,6] suggested the thoracoscopic approach. However, a chest tube is then required, and the fundoplication is difficult to perform. We have found the laparoscopic approach to be best. It allows dissection and excision of the diverticulum, treatment of the motility disorder with a myotomy, and prevention of gastroesophageal reflux by creating a partial fundoplication. All of these can be safely accomplished laparoscopically with the benefits of decreased postoperative pain, a shorter hospital stay, and earlier return to normal activities compared with the other techniques.

Laparoscopic Esophageal Myotomy, Diverticulectomy, and Fundoplication

The procedure is performed with the patient under general anesthesia in the lithotomy position. The surgeon stands between the legs of the patient. A pneumoperitoneum is established with a Veress needle placed in the midline 2 cm above the umbilicus. A 10-mm port is then placed at this location, and the laparoscope is introduced. After laparoscopic exploration of the abdomen, the patient is placed in the steep, reverse Trendelenburg position. Four additional ports are placed. Two 5-mm ports are placed under direct vision in the midepigastrium and left upper quadrant. These are the main working ports of the surgeon. Additionally, two 10-mm ports are placed for the assistants. One is placed in the right midclavicular line below the costal margin and is used to retract the liver. The other is placed in the subcostal area in the left anterior axillary line and is used to provide countertraction of the esophagus. The lesser curvature of the stomach is grasped and retracted inferiorly, thus causing tenting of the gastrohepatic ligament, which is incised with electrocautery. Care is taken to look for an aberrant left hepatic artery running in this usually avascular ligament. If small, such an accessory hepatic artery can be clipped and divided.

Next, the right crus of the diaphragm is identified, and the avascular plane between it and the esophagus is developed (Fig. 3). The dissection is carried anteriorly over the esophagus onto the left crus. In a similar fashion, the left crus is dissected off the esophagus until it is found to curve under the esophagus. From the right side of the esophagus,

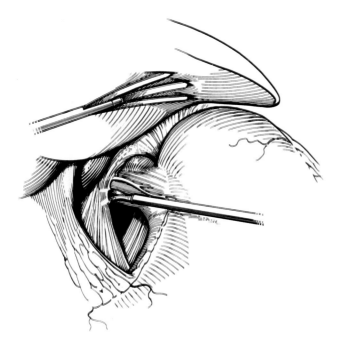

Fig. 3. Dissection of the esophageal hiatus.

the left crus is identified and a wide retroesophageal window is created. The posterior vagal nerve is identified and allowed to remain adherent to the posterior esophagus. A Penrose drain may be used to retract the esophagus inferiorly, so pulling the lower thoracic esophagus into the abdomen and putting tension on the left, or anterior, vagal nerve. Once the left nerve is identified, it is dissected off the anterior wall of the esophagus and cardia to prevent its injury during dissection of the diverticulum and performance of the myotomy. The nerve will be found to run from the left side of the esophagus in the mediastinum down toward the upper lesser curvature of the stomach. The lower 10 cm of esophagus is then mobilized within the mediastinum, and the diverticulum is identified.

Most diverticula have strong fibrous attachments to the mediastinum and may be difficult to identify. The diverticulum is freed of all of its mediastinal attachments by sharp dissection and firm inferior traction (Fig. 4). An endoscope placed in the esophageal lumen may be used to transilluminate the diverticulum, aiding its identification and dissection. The diverticulum is manipulated with care to avoid perforation, and its neck is clearly identified. While an assistant retracts the apex of the diverticulum laterally, the surgeon places a laparoscopic stapling device across the neck of the diverticulum parallel to the esophagus, being careful not to narrow the esophageal lumen or to damage the anterior vagal nerve (Fig. 5). A bougie may be placed in the esophagus to achieve this goal. Multiple firings of the stapler may be required to transect the neck. The resected diverticulum

is then placed in an endobag and removed from the abdomen (Fig. 5).

The myotomy is then accomplished with the electrocautery hook by dividing the outer longitudinal and inner circular esophageal muscle fibers from the level of the diverticulum to a point inferior to the LES. The esophageal mucosa should pout through the myotomy when the full thickness of esophageal muscle has been divided. The mucosa is gently dissected from the posterior aspect of the inner circular muscle layer with a blunt probe. The muscular layers are separated or cut with electrocautery proximally up to the distal edge of the staple line at the neck of the excised diverticulum and distally onto the cardia of the stomach for a length of about 2 cm (Fig. 6). The muscular fibers on the stomach are more difficult to dissect than those of the esophagus, and bleeding from the veins in the area may be encountered. It is important to cut through the entire muscular collar of Helvetius at the cardia to ensure a full myotomy. The consequence of not accomplishing this task, especially in patients with achalasia, is that continued resistance to the forward flow of esophageal content would be present at the LES, resulting in an increased risk of leakage at the site of the diverticulectomy.

At this point, the integrity of the closure is tested by insufflating air into the esophagus and stomach via the endoscope, while observing for escaping air into the abdomen. To assist with this, the lower esophagus may be bathed in saline while observing for bubbling from the esophageal incision. Because of the extensive dissection around the hiatus and the myotomy across the LES, an antireflux procedure is necessary.

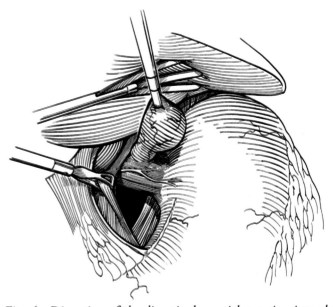

Fig. 4. Dissection of the diverticulum with traction into the abdomen.

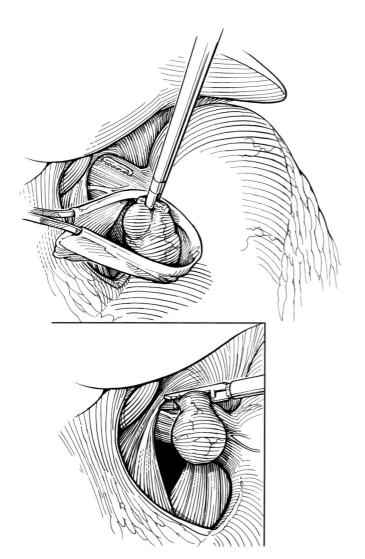

Fig. 5. Stapling of the neck of the diverticulum and placement of the resected diverticulum in an endobag.

Thoracoscopic Esophageal Myotomy, Diverticulectomy, and Fundoplication

The procedure is performed with the patient under general anesthesia with double-lumen endotracheal intubation. The patient is placed in either the right or the left lateral position, depending on which side promises to provide easiest access to the diverticulum. The lung on the affected side is deflated, and three 10-mm intercostal ports are placed: one each in the anterior axillary line of the 6th and 8th intercostal spaces, and one in the posterior axillary line of the 10th intercostal space. Two or three additional 6-mm intercostal ports may be placed as required. Endoscopic transillumination of the diverticulum aids in its identification and dissection. The dissection begins by dividing the inferior pulmonary ligament up to the pulmonary vein. The pleura over the esophagus is incised, and the esophagus is mobilized from the cardia to a point superior to the diverticulum, damage to the vagal nerves being avoided.

The diverticulum is grasped with a Babcock clamp and put under gentle tension. With use of an electrocautery hook, the diverticulum and its neck are dissected free from the adjacent mediastinal tissues. Once the neck is clearly defined, it is stapled with a laparoscopic stapling device introduced through the port that provides the nearest-to-parallel alignment with the esophagus (Fig. 8). This may take two or three firings, the first involving only a small section of the neck but the remainder allowing better subsequent alignment of the stapler. The excised diverticulum is placed

A partial fundoplication (Toupet operation) is performed by first dividing the upper short gastric vessels with the harmonic scalpel. The fundus is then brought through the retroesophageal window and fixed to the left crus of the diaphragm with one silk suture and to the right crus with two or three silk sutures (Fig. 6). Three silk sutures are used to fix the fundus to the right-cut margin of the myotomy. The fundus on the left side is similarly fixed to the left cut edge of the myotomy, creating a 270° posterior fundoplication (Fig. 7).

On the first postoperative day, meglumine diatrizoate (Gastrografin) esophagography is performed. If no leak is demonstrated, the patient is allowed to commence a clear liquid diet by mouth. Dismissal from the hospital usually takes place on day 2 after operation.

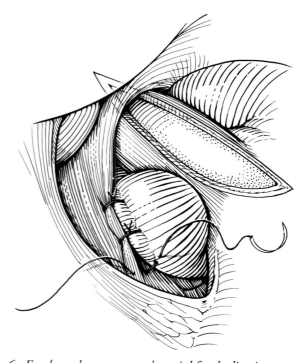

Fig. 6. Esophageal myotomy and partial fundoplication.

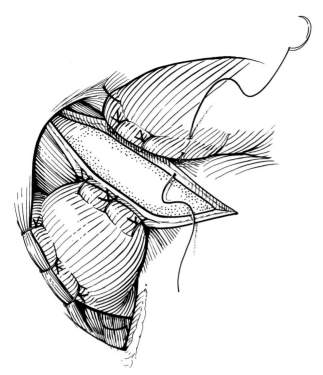

Fig. 7. Completed partial fundoplication.

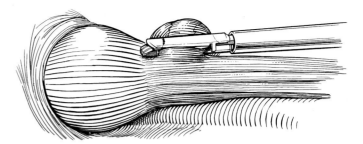

Fig. 8. Thoracoscopic stapling of epiphrenic diverticulum.

in an endobag and removed. Next, the esophageal hiatus is opened and the peritoneal cavity is entered. The cardia of the stomach is pulled into the chest.

A myotomy is performed beginning at the inferior margin of the staple line and is carried onto the stomach for 2 cm with a combination of blunt and sharp dissection (Fig. 9 A). The integrity of the mucosa is tested by insufflation of air through an esophageal endoscope. If no leakage is present, a modified Belsey fundoplication is performed (Fig. 9 B). With the use of two U-shaped nonabsorbable sutures, the gastric fundus below the cardia is sutured to the esophagus on either side of the myotomy. Third and fourth sutures can be used to tack the wrapped fundus to the diaphragm and to close the hiatus loosely (Fig. 9 B). A chest tube is placed through the lowest port. The ports are removed, and the lung is reexpanded. The chest tube is removed on the second postoperative day if no leakage is demonstrated on meglumine diatrizoate (Gastrografin) esophagogram. The patient is given a liquid diet.

RESULTS

Benacci et al.,[4] from our clinic, reported that good or excellent results can be achieved with surgical treatment in symptomatic patients. They studied 112 patients, 33 of whom had severe symptoms and underwent open surgical repair. These patients all had an open thoracic repair, because this series was conducted before the use of

laparoscopic or thoracoscopic procedures for esophageal disease. Most of the 33 patients were treated with a diverticulectomy and myotomy carried out through a left thoracotomy. The median hospital stay in these patients was 13 days. Leakage at the site of the diverticulectomy was the most serious early postoperative complication. In six patients, a leak developed from the site of resection, which closed spontaneously in four, and the patients remained asymptomatic during follow-up. Three patients had operative deaths: two had an esophageal leak, and one died of a cardiac arrhythmia. During a median follow-up of 6.9 years, 48.2% of patients had an excellent result, 27.6% had a good result, 17.2% had a fair result, and 6.9% were considered to have a poor result. Altorki et al.[7] reported their experience with the open transthoracic approach for epiphrenic diverticula in 17 patients. There was one postoperative death after a rupture of the mucosa at the myotomy site. The long-term results in that series seem to be good. All but one of their patients was symptom-free 2 years postoperatively.

Results after thoracoscopic and laparoscopic approaches seem to be as good as those after open operations, but patients have not as yet been followed as long.[5,6] Certainly, their hospitalization time is shorter, and their early recovery is associated with decreased postoperative pain. Return to their usual activities is faster. Our experience at Mayo Clinic in Jacksonville, Florida, during the 4-year period from 1996 to 2000 includes 17 patients. Six of these patients were asymptomatic or had a small diverticulum (less than 2 cm). In five patients the diverticula were incidentally found during antireflux operation or during esophageal myotomy for achalasia. These were all small and were inverted, and the overlying muscle was plicated. Six patients had significant symptoms, including regurgitation, reflux, heartburn, and dysphagia. All six underwent operation, and the diverticulum was excised. Two of the patients had concomitant achalasia defined by manometry preoperatively. One of the patients had an attempted thoracoscopic resection; this operation was

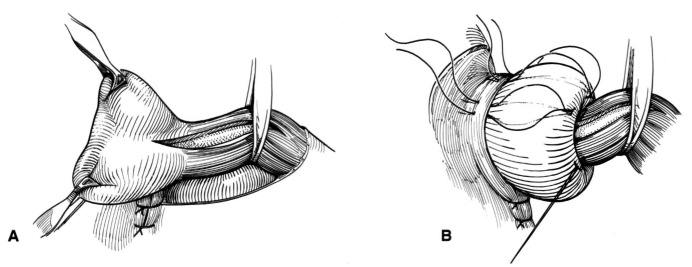

Fig. 9. (A), *Thoracoscopic myotomy.* (B), *Modified Belsey fundoplication.*

converted to a thoracotomy because of difficulty with dissection of the diverticulum.

In our experience, these operations can be achieved easily by the laparoscopic route, and good visualization and the performance of both diverticulectomy and esophageal myotomy are possible at laparoscopy. One patient had an esophageal leak from the staple line on the fourth day after a laparoscopic diverticulectomy. This required a thoracotomy to oversew the leak and to add a myotomy. This patient had normal results on esophageal manometry preoperatively and had not had an earlier myotomy. Subsequently, we decided to do a myotomy routinely, because we believe that manometry may not always exclude a motility disorder. In another patient, pneumonia developed 4 weeks postoperatively with empyema that required surgical drainage. A meglumine diatrizoate (Gastrografin) esophagogram indicated no leakage from the esophagus.

Long-term follow-up (mean, 26 months) of the 11 surgical patients indicates that only 1 patient has had to modify his diet postoperatively. Two patients are receiving proton pump inhibitors for reflux symptoms. One of these patients did not have an antireflux procedure. When we compared the long-term outcome of the surgical patients with that of patients not treated surgically, clearly the patients who had operation had a significantly better symptom outcome. The surgical patients had less dysphagia for liquids and solids, less regurgitation, and less chest pain than the patients who were not treated surgically.

CONCLUSION

Laparoscopic diverticulectomy, esophageal myotomy, and Toupet fundoplication compose our current operative approach to patients with symptomatic epiphrenic esophageal diverticula. Generally, asymptomatic diverticula and small diverticula that are minimally symptomatic can be treated nonsurgically. For symptomatic patients, surgical treatment seems to be the option of choice. Large diverticula are excised, and smaller diverticula may be inverted and the overlying muscle oversewn. The laparoscopic approach is our procedure of choice, because thoracoscopy seems to be associated with greater difficulty in achieving an adequate myotomy and diverticulectomy. The gastroesophageal junction is better visualized by laparoscopy than thoracoscopy and allows for a more accurate antireflux procedure. We have had no need for conversion to the open procedure during our laparoscopic experience.

Our one patient with an esophageal leak from the staple line had not had a myotomy performed during the initial operation. We believe that high intraluminal pressures may have been caused by a motility disorder that failed to reveal itself during preoperative manometry. For this reason, we now routinely perform a myotomy to reduce the intraluminal pressure at the staple line. If a myotomy is added, a fundoplication should be done to prevent gastroesophageal reflux. We prefer a partial Toupet fundoplication for this purpose because of the potentially altered esophageal motility after the myotomy. However, if esophageal motility is normal, a Nissen fundoplication may be done.

Esophageal diverticula are uncommon, and symptoms seem to be related to their size. Operation should be considered for all diverticula that are symptomatic or larger than 5 cm. We prefer the laparoscopic approach with diverticulectomy accompanied by a long myotomy and an antireflux procedure. This offers patients all the advantages of the minimally invasive approach with good long-term control of symptoms.

REFERENCES

1. Achkar E: Esophageal diverticula. *In* The Esophagus. Edited by DO Castell, JE Richter. Philadelphia, Lippincott Williams & Wilkins, 1999, pp 301-314
2. Anselmino M, Hinder RA, Filipi CJ, Wilson P: Laparoscopic Heller cardiomyotomy and thoracoscopic esophageal long myotomy for the treatment of primary esophageal motor disorders. Surg Laparosc Endosc 3:437-441, 1993
3. Streitz JM Jr, Glick ME, Ellis FH Jr: Selective use of myotomy for treatment of epiphrenic diverticula: manometric and clinical analysis. Arch Surg 127:585-587, 1992
4. Benacci JC, Deschamps C, Trastek VF, Allen MS, Daly RC, Pairolero PC: Epiphrenic diverticulum: results of surgical treatment. Ann Thorac Surg 55:1109-1113, 1993
5. Peracchia A, Bonavina L, Rosati R, Bona S: Thoracoscopic resection of epiphrenic esophageal diverticula. *In* Minimally Invasive Surgery of the Foregut. Edited by JH Peters, TR DeMeester. St Louis, Quality Medical Publishing, 1995, pp 110-116
6. Rosati R, Fumagalli U, Bona S, Bonavina L, Peracchia A: Diverticulectomy, myotomy, and fundoplication through laparoscopy: a new option to treat epiphrenic esophageal diverticula? Ann Surg 227:174-178, 1998
7. Altorki NK, Sunagawa M, Skinner DB: Thoracic esophageal diverticula: Why is operation necessary? J Thorac Cardiovasc Surg 105:260-264, 1993

Cancer of the Esophagus

Dawn E. Jaroszewski, M.D.
Claude Deschamps, M.D.
Leonard L. Gunderson, M.D.
Louis A. Lanza, M.D.
Victor F. Trastek, M.D.
Peter C. Pairolero, M.D.

The prognosis for patients with esophageal carcinoma is usually grim. Survival is directly related to the stage of the disease at the time of treatment. Unfortunately, fewer than 5% of patients present with localized disease, and fewer than 10% survive beyond 5 years despite having what appears to be a resectable lesion.[1,2] Early detection and surgical resection provide the best chance for cure. Even though cancer screening techniques have steadily improved during the past 2 decades, additional progress in this area will be needed to improve outcomes. Also, new approaches combining surgical resection with chemotherapy and radiation therapy need to be developed to assess their potential for improving survival. This chapter describes Mayo Clinic's management of esophageal cancer and emphasizes our current multidisciplinary approach.

ETIOLOGY AND EPIDEMIOLOGY

Carcinoma of the esophagus accounts for approximately 5% of all gastrointestinal malignancies and is predominantly a disease of men older than 60 years. The incidence in men is 3 times greater than that in women. The white person:black person ratio is 3.5:1 for adenocarcinoma of the esophagus, whereas the reverse is true for squamous cell carcinoma of the esophagus.[3] Most cancers occur in the mid or distal third of the esophagus. Only 15% occur in the proximal third.

Direct causative factors for esophageal carcinoma have not been identified. Several studies have implicated Barrett's disease of the esophagus, esophageal achalasia, and caustic strictures as lesions predisposing to the development of esophageal cancer.[4-7] Alcohol and smoking are major risk factors for squamous cell carcinoma of the esophagus, but their role in the development of adenocarcinoma of the esophagus and at the gastric cardia is less certain. For adenocarcinoma, an increased risk among current cigarette smokers is reported, but not among past smokers or alcoholics. Patients with Plummer-Vinson syndrome, first described at Mayo Clinic, have a predilection for development of squamous cell esophageal cancer. Patients with tylosis, an autosomal dominant disorder, inherit a propensity for esophageal cancer. Among such patients, about a third will have squamous cell carcinoma of the esophagus.[8]

In the United States, the incidence of cancer of the distal esophagus and gastric cardia has increased during the past 2 decades.[9] Interestingly, the incidence of adenocarcinoma in the noncardiac portions of the stomach has remained unchanged or decreased.[3,4,6,10] Today, adenocarcinoma is the most common esophageal cancer, especially in white men, accounting for more than 70% of esophageal carcinomas.[4] Currently, the majority of the esophageal cancers treated at Mayo Clinic are adenocarcinomas. Other institutions have reported similar trends, with half to three-fourths of recent patients with esophageal cancer presenting with adenocarcinoma. Adenocarcinomas arising in Barrett's esophagus are reported frequently and perhaps account for the increasing incidence of distal esophageal cancers.[9]

PATHOLOGY AND PATHOGENESIS

Adenocarcinoma, squamous cell carcinoma, adenosquamous variants, small cell carcinoma, sarcoma, and lymphoma are the major types of esophageal cancer. Adenocarcinomas are the most prevalent in the distal esophagus and cardia, and squamous cell carcinomas are the most prevalent in the proximal and mid esophagus. This chapter mainly addresses adenocarcinomas and squamous cell carcinomas.

Most adenocarcinomas appear in columnar mucosa (Barrett's mucosa) that arises at the cardia and in the distal esophagus in patients with gastroesophageal reflux disease. It is theorized that the reflux of gastric juice, bile, and pancreatic juice from the stomach into the distal esophagus causes a metaplasia of the distal esophageal mucosa from a squamous mucosa to a columnar mucosa. The metaplastic, columnar mucosa can become dysplastic (Fig. 1), after which an invasive adenocarcinoma can appear.[11] The bacterium *Helicobacter pylori* does not seem to facilitate, and may even combat, this malignant transformation.[12] In contrast, the bacterium causes inflammation, ulceration, and the appearance of mucosa-associated lymphoid tumors in the stomach. Pathologically, adenocarcinomas of the distal esophagus and those arising in the gastric cardia are remarkably similar. Whether distal esophageal cancers are true esophageal cancers or gastric cancers that have invaded the esophagus has been questioned. The presence of Barrett's epithelium at the cardia or in the distal esophagus is the most convincing evidence that these tumors arise at the cardia or in the distal esophagus and are not gastric cancers invading the cardia and esophagus. The association of Barrett's epithelium with distal esophageal adenocarcinoma is reported to be as high as 100% of cases.[5,6,9,10]

Adenocarcinomas and squamous cell carcinomas invade extensively in mucosal and submucosal planes.

This growth pattern contributes to treatment failure and necessitates resection of a minimum of 6 cm of grossly disease-free margin during a surgical resection.

SYMPTOMS AND SIGNS

The most common early symptoms of esophageal carcinoma are dysphagia, odynophagia, and weight loss. When the disease invades adjacent structures, pain, hoarseness (with recurrent laryngeal nerve involvement), superior vena caval syndrome, malignant pleural effusions, hematemesis, and cough related to tracheal-esophageal or bronchial-esophageal fistulas appear.

DIAGNOSIS

In addition to history, physical examination, and blood tests, including complete blood count, serum electrolyte determinations, and liver function tests, preoperative evaluation focuses on determining the size and depth of invasion of the tumor, the presence or absence of local, regional, or distant metastases, and the patient's mental and physical ability to tolerate a major surgical procedure. Preoperative evaluation includes esophagogastric endoscopy with biopsy or brushings (Fig. 2), endoscopic esophageal ultrasonography for evaluation of the extent of invasion of the lesion and to look for metastases in the regional lymph nodes, and computed tomography of the chest and abdomen (Fig. 3, Table 1). Endoscopic ultrasonography with fine-needle aspiration of regional nodes suspected of harboring malignancy can increase the sensitivity and specificity of diagnosis to 93% and 100%,

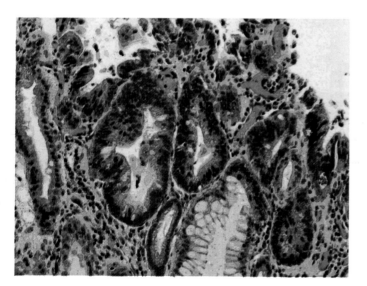

Fig. 1. Distal esophageal mucosal biopsy specimen, showing low-grade mucosal dysplasia in a patient with Barrett's esophagus. (Optical magnification, hematoxylin-eosin; x400.)

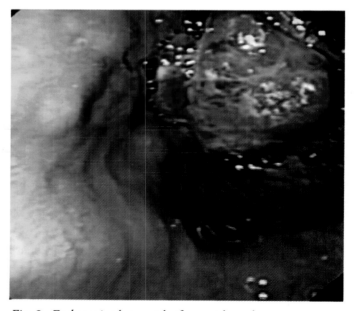

Fig. 2. Endoscopic photograph of an esophageal cancer.

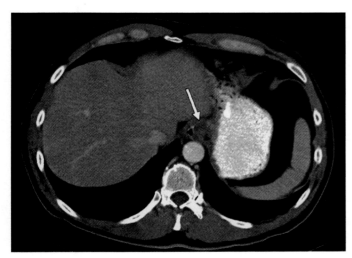

Fig. 3. Computed tomogram of an esophageal cancer causing thickening of distal esophageal wall just above esophagogastric junction (arrow).

respectively.[13] Radiologic examination of the esophagus with barium sulfate is sometimes used (Fig. 4). In addition to these tests, we have used positron emission tomography for further evaluation of patients in whom metastatic disease is suspected but not revealed in the standard work-up (Fig. 5). Staging laparoscopy and thoracoscopy are rarely used at our institution, because their role is still undetermined and their cost substantial. Moreover, unless tracheal or bronchial invasion is suspected in proximal or mid esophageal lesions, bronchoscopy usually is not performed.

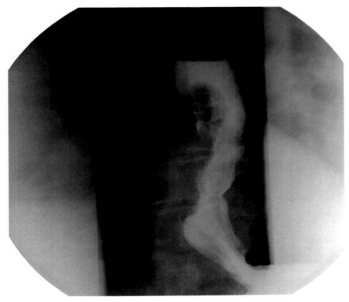

Fig. 4. Esophageal radiograph, intraluminal barium sulfate used for contrast. A mid esophageal cancer is present that distorts the wall of the esophagus and projects into its lumen.

Table 1.—Tests Used for Diagnosis of Esophageal Cancer

Test	Capabilities
Endoscopy with biopsy	Most useful to detect and confirm the diagnosis by biopsy
Barium swallow radiography	Provides information about level, length of tumor and degree of obstruction. Less useful for detecting small tumors. No biopsy can be done
Endoscopic ultrasonography with or without FNA biopsy	Most accurate preoperative assessment for depth of tumor invasion and involvement of local lymph nodes, which can be biopsied by FNA. Inability to pass probe beyond malignant strictures with more advanced tumors
Computed tomography	Evaluate local invasion (i.e., loss of fat plane relative to adjacent structures), regional node status, and metastasis
Magnetic resonance imaging	Evaluate local invasion, regional node status, and metastasis
Bronchoscopy	Rule out invasion of left main-stem bronchus for mid esophageal lesions
Positron emission tomography	Identify focal areas of increased metabolism for detection of distant metastases and metastases in local and regional nodes
Diagnostic laparoscopy	Biopsy of suspicious celiac nodes or sites of possible distant spread

FNA, fine-needle aspiration.

Once patients are deemed to have a potentially resectable esophageal lesion, they undergo a medical work-up to determine their suitability for operation. Evaluating pulmonary and cardiac function and nutrition is paramount. Feeding with a percutaneous endoscopic gastrostomy tube for 3 to 4 weeks preoperatively may be necessary for patients with weight loss of more than 25% of body weight or serum albumin levels less than 2.0 g/dL.

STAGING

Clinical staging with the tumor (T), lymph node (N), distant metastases (M) classification (cTNM) is based on the growth and spread of the primary tumor, as determined by pretreatment studies.[14]

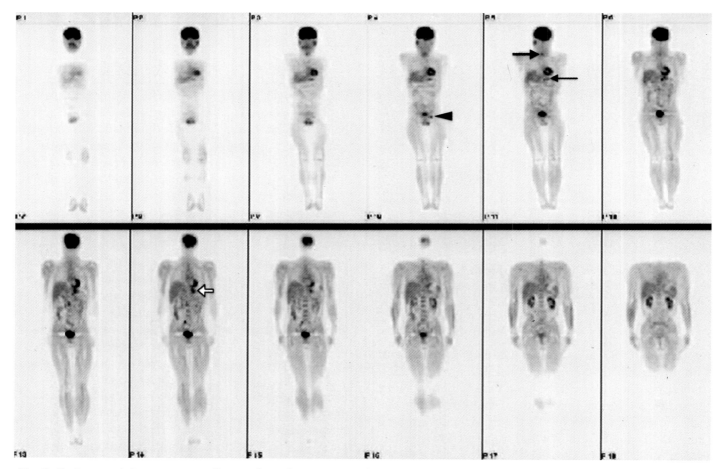

Fig. 5. Positron emission tomogram of an esophageal cancer at esophagogastric junction (lower panel, open arrow) *with metastases to regional lymph nodes* (upper panel, thin arrow) *and a left inguinal lymph node* (arrowhead). *A thyroid nodule is also present* (thick arrow).

Pathologic staging is based on data acquired clinically, during surgical exploration, and during histologic examination of the removed pathologic specimen, including the regional lymph nodes. A single staging classification serves both clinical and pathologic staging for all regions of the esophagus. Although celiac lymph node involvement constitutes metastatic disease (M1a) in the American Joint Committee on Cancer (AJCC) staging system, for distal-third esophageal lesions it amounts to regional node disease. In the AJCC system, supraclavicular lymph node involvement is considered regional nodal disease for patients with cervical and upper thoracic esophageal lesions but distant metastasis in patients with mid and distal esophageal cancers (Table 2).

CHOICE OF TREATMENT

Esophageal cancer is rarely localized at diagnosis and is characterized by a high incidence of local, regional, and distant spread at death. Any successful treatment strategy must address these issues. Even among patients who present with apparent localized disease, a multidisciplinary approach is often necessary to achieve desirable outcomes.

The goals of treatment are to restore and preserve the ability to take oral nourishment and to provide an opportunity to achieve long-term survival. If the patient is not deemed a surgical candidate, then palliation is necessary. Several successful palliative options are available and are discussed later in this chapter.

The preoperative work-up is designed to determine which patients are candidates for surgical resection. The TNM classification is most important for determining the choice of treatment and the prognosis.[14]

T1-2 N0 M0
Surgical resection with reconstruction is the primary treatment of patients with T1-2 N0 M0 disease (Table 3). Chemoradiation alone is the best option for patients who are not candidates for operation because of severe medical comorbidities.

Table 2.—TNM Staging for Esophageal Cancer

Primary tumor (T)
- TX   Primary tumor cannot be assessed
- T0   No evidence of primary tumor
- Tis   Carcinoma in situ (into mucosa only)*
- T1   Tumor invades lamina propria or submucosa
- T2   Tumor invades muscularis propria
- T3   Tumor invades adventitia
- T4   Tumor invades adjacent structures (or adherent to)*

Regional lymph nodes (N)
- NX   Regional lymph nodes cannot be assessed
- N0   No regional lymph node metastases
- N1   Regional lymph node metastasis

Distant metastases (M)
- MX   Distant metastasis cannot be assessed
- M0   No distant metastasis
- M1   Distant metastasis†

Stage grouping

Stage	T	N	M
0	Tis	N0	M0
I	T1	N0	M0
IIA	T2-T3	N0	M0
IIB	T1-T2	N1	M0
III	T3	N1	M0
	T4	Any N	M0
IV	Any T	Any N	M1

*Items in parentheses were added by authors.
†Lower thoracic tumors: M1a, celiac nodes; M1b, other distant metastases. Upper thoracic tumors: M1a, cervical nodes; M1b, other distant metastases. Mid thoracic, only M1b applicable.
From Fleming et al.[14] By permission of the American Joint Committee on Cancer.

T1-2 N1 M0; T3 N0 M0

Preoperative chemoradiation followed by esophageal resection is our preferred approach to treatment of patients with T1-2 N1 M0 disease with biopsy-positive nodes. This approach may decrease the local relapse rate after resection. In some, but not all, randomized studies, the decreased relapse rate has been shown to improve overall survival. For patients with T3 N0 M0 lesions, we prefer the same approach of preoperative chemotherapy and external beam radiation followed by resection in view of the technical challenges of delivering both preoperative and postoperative chemotherapy and external beam radiation in such patients. Responders to preoperative therapy and radiation plus operation may have a survival advantage after resection compared with nonresponders. Postoperative adjuvant chemoradiation is used for patients who have T1-2 N1 M0 or T3 N0 M0 lesions at the time of resection but did not have preoperative chemoradiation. A phase II study at Mayo Clinic showed satisfactory tolerance to postoperative external beam radiation plus concurrent 5-fluorouracil and cisplatin after resection.

T3 N1 M0

Preoperative chemotherapy and external beam radiation is also our preferred approach for T3 N1 M0 disease with biopsy-positive nodes. This therapy is followed by resection.

T4 N0-1 M0

We also usually recommend preoperative chemoradiation for patients with T4 N0-1 M0 lesions. Although chemoradiation alone can achieve significant palliation, we usually proceed to restaging after the chemoradiation, followed by resection and intraoperative electron irradiation. This approach applies to patients who have no evidence of hematogenous or peritoneal metastases after restaging and have adequate performance status.

Any T Any N M1

Chemotherapy in the setting of protocol treatment is our treatment of choice. Palliative chemoradiation may be indicated for local symptoms. Radical operation is contraindicated for patients with disseminated disease, but a bypass procedure may be appropriate for severe obstruction. Stents placed at endoscopy also can be used to allow food and drink to pass through obstructing lesions and may be preferable to surgical bypass. Laser therapy is being selectively evaluated for palliation of these patients.

SURGICAL THERAPY

Surgical resection continues to play a key role in the treatment of esophageal cancer. In centers where many operations are performed for esophageal carcinoma, the mortality rate associated with the procedures is 3% or less. Esophagogastric resection can be performed in several ways. The two main surgical techniques we use are the transthoracic (Ivor Lewis) approach and the transhiatal approach. Each of these two approaches has its advocates, but no statistical evidence, either in retrospective comparative series or in prospective randomized trials, shows a difference in survival between the two approaches. Ideally, surgeons dealing with esophageal carcinoma should be expert in both approaches and should select the best approach for an individual patient.

For a large majority of distal esophageal carcinomas, the procedure of choice at Mayo Clinic remains the one-stage Ivor Lewis operation. However, patients who have

Table 3.—Treatment Plan for Esophageal Cancer*

TNM class	Operation	Radiotherapy	Chemotherapy
T1-2 N0 M0	Esophagectomy and anastomosis	None[†]	None[†]
T1-2 N1 M0 T3 N0 M0	Esophagectomy and anastomosis	Preop or postop, 45-50 Gy	5-Fluorouracil, cisplatin concurrent with radiation and maintenance or alternative chemotherapy
T3 N1 M0	Esophagectomy and anastomosis	Preop, 45-50 Gy, attempt resection	As above or alternative chemotherapy
T4 N0-1 M0	Esophagectomy and anastomosis	Preop, 45-50 Gy, attempt resection and intraoperative electron radiation	As above or alternative chemotherapy
Any T Any N M1	Bypass if obstruction is severe; esophageal stent or PEG tube may be preferable	Palliative, 50 Gy, as indicated	As above or investigational phase I or II chemotherapy

PEG, percutaneous endoscopic gastrostomy; TNM, tumor, node, metastases.
*Protocol treatment is preferable, if available. Consider esophageal stent, feeding jejunostomy, or percutaneous endoscopic gastrostomy tube before radiation and chemotherapy for patients with dysphagia and evidence of, or risk for, malnutrition.
†Except for squamous cell cancer adjacent to aorta when radiation (50-60 Gy) and chemotherapy (5-fluorouracil, cisplatin) are given preoperatively or postoperatively.

had this operation for esophageal carcinoma and who have survived 5 or more years not uncommonly have symptoms of reflux, dumping, and dysphagia.[15,16] Fewer symptoms of gastroesophageal reflux are present postoperatively among patients who have had a transhiatal esophagectomy, although they often have more dumping than patients who have the Ivor Lewis procedure. Thus, we use the transhiatal approach in patients who are younger, have dysplasia as their primary diagnosis, and have a long life expectancy. We believe that the transhiatal approach reduces the risk of postoperative symptomatic reflux esophagitis and may improve the quality of life compared with the Ivor Lewis operation.

Ivor Lewis Esophagogastrectomy
In 1946, Ivor Lewis, while presenting the Hunterian Lecture at the Royal College of Surgeons in London, described a new operative approach for neoplasms in the distal esophagus. He proposed an abdominal procedure to assess for metastases and free the stomach, followed by a right thoracotomy to resect the involved esophagus and stomach and reestablish enteric continuity with an esophagogastric anastomosis. Although he initially proposed this as a two-stage procedure, it is currently done in one stage. We often use an Ivor Lewis approach for patients with distal esophageal and esophagogastric junction carcinomas for several reasons.[17,18] This approach allows complete visualization and removal of all perigastric and periesophageal lymph tissue, including that in the chest. It also allows direct visualization and dissection of the thoracic esophagus, thus virtually eliminating the uncommon but potentially disastrous damage to adjacent structures that can occur with transhiatal esophagectomy. We favor the Ivor Lewis approach over the left thoracoabdominal approach because construction of the anastomosis high in the right chest is technically easier than performing an anastomosis high in the left chest.

Setup and Incision
To improve ventilation during the thoracic portion of the procedure, a double-lumen endotracheal tube is placed. The patient is positioned supine on the operating table, and the skin is prepared from the chin to the pubis in case a transition to a transhiatal approach is indicated after the exploration. An upper midline incision is begun just to the left of the xiphoid process and extended to just cephalad of the umbilicus. A retractor is positioned to elevate the costal arch, and a second retractor spreads the caudal end of the incision (Fig. 6). The patient is placed in the reverse Trendelenburg position to enhance exposure to the upper abdomen. Abdominal exploration is performed, and the liver, peritoneum, and periaortic areas are carefully assessed for metastases.

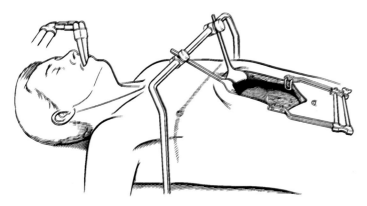

Fig. 6. Upper abdominal incision and inserted retractors.

Assessing Local Resectability

Once metastatic disease is ruled out, local resectability is assessed. The gastroesophageal junction is mobilized to determine whether the tumor is adherent to or invading the vertebral column, aorta, or pericardium (Fig. 7). The left lobe of the liver is mobilized and retracted laterally, and the left triangular ligament is divided. With blunt dissection, and care taken not to transgress the tumor, the esophagus is circled with a Penrose drain. A portion of the crura of the diaphragm can be resected with the tumor, if necessary. With manual palpation, adherence to mediastinal structures is assessed. If the tumor is mobile, the resection is begun.

Mobilization of Stomach

The portion of the esophagus that is removed will be replaced with a gastric tube made from the greater curvature of the stomach. The goal of the abdominal portion of the operation is to mobilize the stomach. With the stomach retracted cephalad and the colon caudad, the lesser sac is entered caudad to the right gastroepiploic arcade. The omentum is divided, with careful preservation of the right gastroepiploic vessels. The colonic attachments to the stomach and duodenum are divided so that the greater curvature of the stomach has no connection to the colon. The stomach is then mobilized from the spleen, all short gastric vessels being taken until the esophageal hiatus is reached. No attempt is made to leave extra tissue with the short gastric vessels. With the greater curvature of the stomach lifted cephalad and the pancreas and celiac axis retracted caudad, the left gastric artery and vein are exposed, ligated, and divided (Fig. 8). All nodal tissue along the cephalad border of the pancreas is swept toward the stomach and removed. The remaining tissue along the aorta cephalad to the hiatus is also taken with the specimen. The stomach is then retracted laterally to the left, allowing division of the hepatic branches of the vagal nerves and any associated vessels. The stomach is confirmed to be free from the hiatus to the pylorus by passing the Penrose drain in ring fashion over it. The hiatus is enlarged to four

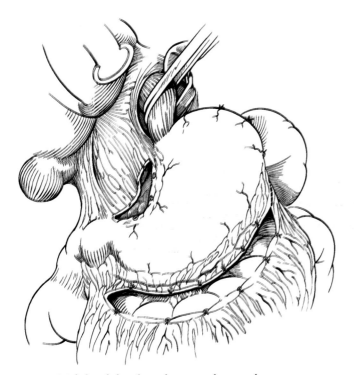

Fig. 7. Mobilized distal esophagus and stomach.

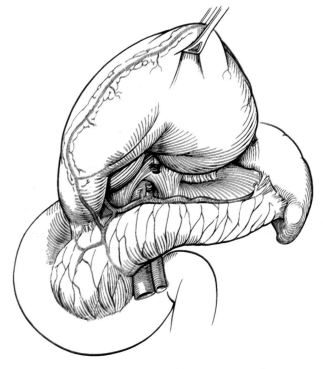

Fig. 8. Ligated left gastric artery, lesser sac approach.

fingerbreadths by dividing a portion of the right crus so that there is no ledge effect that may cause future gastric outlet obstruction. The lesser curve area is prepared by dividing all of the blood vessels to a level between the third and fourth branches of the left gastric artery. The resulting bare area ends up in the chest when the stomach is later pulled into the chest for anastomosis to the proximal esophagus. A pyloromyotomy or a pyloroplasty is then performed (Fig. 9), after which the abdominal wall is closed.

When the stomach is not available, the colon or the small bowel can act as an appropriate replacement for the esophagus.[19] A left colon or small bowel interposition is favored for a short conduit. A long left colon interposition is recommended for a subtotal or total esophagectomy. A long-limb Roux-en-Y jejunum interposition is favored after a total gastrectomy. The ultimate goal should be to restore swallowing with minimal morbidity and mortality. Most surgeons no longer place a jejunostomy tube because of the

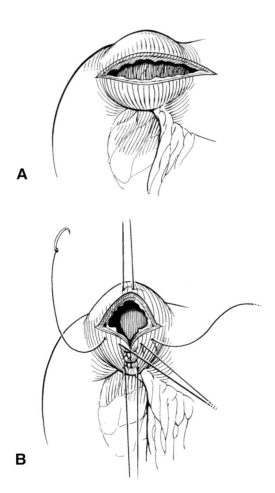

Fig. 9. Heinecke-Mikulicz pyloroplasty, accomplished by making a longitudinal incision centered at the pylorus (A), which is closed transversely with interrupted sutures (B).

potential morbidity from it. The abdomen is irrigated and hemostasis is ensured, after which the abdomen is closed.

Right Thoracotomy
The patient is placed in the left lateral decubitus position and the right lung is collapsed. The fourth intercostal space is entered through an incision over the right fifth rib (Fig. 10). This approach allows excellent access to the apex of the chest so that a proximal esophagogastric anastomosis can be performed. The chest is explored for metastatic disease.

Mobilization of Esophagus
The mediastinal pleura overlying the esophagus is divided laterally along the hemiazygos vein, across the hiatus, then back cephalad along the pericardium to the azygos vein. The entire envelope of tissue around the esophagus, including lymph nodes, fatty tissue, and the thoracic duct, is freed by developing a plane between the esophagus and the aorta. The thoracic duct is doubly clipped and divided. A Penrose drain is placed around the esophagus for traction. Lymph nodes are removed from the distal paraesophageal, inferior pulmonary ligamental, subcarinal, and proximal paraesophageal and paratracheal areas. The azygos vein is ligated and divided at its junction with the superior vena cava. A suture ligature of 3-0 polypropylene is used on the end of the vein that joins the superior vena cava. A pleural flap is incised up to the apex of the chest in an inverted J fashion. The proximal esophagus is then freed to the apex of the chest, with care taken to stay close to the wall of the esophagus to avoid injury to both the right and the left recurrent laryngeal nerves. When the esophagus has been freed to the apex of the thoracic cavity, a Satinski clamp is placed across it at this level,

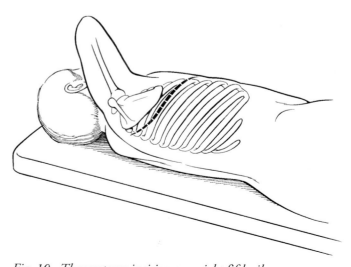

Fig. 10. Thoracotomy incision over right fifth rib.

and the esophagus is divided 1.5 cm caudad to the clamp. The excised specimen is removed and sent for frozen section microscopy to determine the completeness of resection of the tumor.

Preparation of Gastric Tube and Esophagogastric Anastomosis

The stomach is transposed through the hiatus into the chest. Hemostasis is carefully achieved along the posterior mediastinum where the esophagus was removed. Once the proximal esophageal margin is shown to be free of tumor by the pathologist, a gastric tube is made based on the greater curvature of the stomach. The fundus of the stomach is stretched out, and the distance from the distal cut end of the proximal esophagus to the esophageal hiatus is measured along the greater curvature. At this point, a linear stapler is placed transversely across the stomach to make a 5-cm cut. A gastric tube is then fashioned by additional stapler applications parallel to the greater curvature to the site at the "bare" area that had been previously prepared on the lesser curvature (Fig. 11). The fundus of

the stomach is removed along with a good portion of the lesser curve and the lymph nodes in this area. The staple lines of the gastric tube are oversewn with running 4-0 polypropylene. An end-to-side esophagogastric anastomosis is performed, the gastric tube being placed posterior to the esophagus. The anastomosis is done in two layers with interrupted 3-0 polyglycolic acid or 3-0 silk sutures (Fig. 12). The anastomosis is covered with a mediastinal pleural flap and the gastric tube is secured to the mediastinum with interrupted 3-0 silk. A nasogastric tube is placed through the anastomosis and advanced to the level of the esophageal hiatus. A chest tube is placed, and the incision is closed.

Postoperative Care

The patient recovers in a step-down intensive care unit for one night. The nasogastric tube and chest tubes are removed on the third or fourth postoperative day. A water-soluble radiographic contrast swallow test is performed on the sixth postoperative day; if no leakage or obstruction is noted, the patient begins oral feedings, which are advanced to soft solids over the next 3 to 4 days.

Outcome

An Ivor Lewis esophagogastrectomy is a safe surgical approach for esophageal cancer. It can be performed with low mortality, provides adequate palliation, and results in satisfactory long-term survival for patients with more favorable stages of cancer. Our experience with the operation

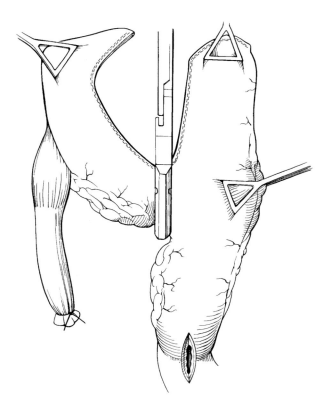

Fig. 11. Removal of mid and distal esophagus, containing the cancer, and gastric fundus and proximal lesser curve of the gastric corpus. Gastric wall along lesser curve is divided with a stapler. Greater curve of proximal stomach is preserved. The Heinecke-Mikulicz incision at the pylorus is also shown.

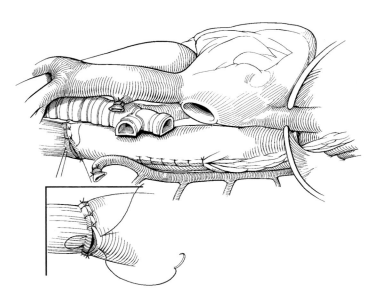

Fig. 12. Stomach is pulled into chest, and anastomosis is made between distal end of remaining esophagus and proximal end of remaining stomach. Inset shows interrupted horizontal mattress sutures used to complete seromuscular layer of anastomosis.

at Mayo Clinic showed that 5-year survival was 86% in patients with stage I disease, 34% to 50% with stage II, and 15% with stage III.[1,18] Patients with unresectable stage IV disease usually survived less than 6 months after operation. Functional outcome after the Ivor Lewis operation at Mayo Clinic was worse in older patients and men than in younger patients and women. Even though long-term survival after esophagectomy for stage I and stage II carcinoma was less than that expected in a normal population, quality of life after resection as assessed by the patients themselves was similar to that of healthy persons.

Transhiatal Esophagogastrectomy

The technique of transhiatal esophagogastrectomy is applicable to patients with carcinoma limited to the cardia and proximal stomach. It is generally possible to resect the distal esophagus, cardia, and proximal stomach in such a way that 4 to 6 cm of proximal gastric corpus still exists. For this operation, the upper esophagus should not be divided until the surgeon is certain that it is possible to preserve almost all of the entire greater curvature of the stomach while performing the proximal gastrectomy. Otherwise, the remaining stomach may not reach to the neck. As long as the entire greater curvature of the stomach can be preserved, the stomach should reach the neck for construction of the cervical anastomosis.[20]

Setup and Incision

The transhiatal esophagectomy is performed through a celiotomy and a cervical incision. The anesthetic management and placement of the patient are unchanged from that described for the Ivor Lewis operation, with the exception of the head being turned to the patient's right to maximize exposure through a left lateral cervical incision. Also, a double-lumen endotracheal tube is not used.

Abdominal Phase

As described above, assessment for resectability should be performed before initiation of any resection. After the stomach is completely mobilized, as described for the Ivor Lewis operation, the abdominal esophagus is dissected and encircled with tape or a rubber drain for use in retracting. This phase is identical to that described for the Ivor Lewis procedure.

Mediastinal Phase

The xiphisternum is elevated, and the mediastinal dissection of the esophagus is begun under direct vision by sharply or bluntly dividing esophageal attachments to the prevertebral fascia posteriorly and the pericardium anteriorly. As the esophagus is mobilized away from the pericardium and the tracheal carina, care must be taken to avoid injury to the posterior membranous trachea. The dissection is extended manually to the level of the carina or the aortic arch. Subcarinal lymph nodes may be included with the specimen as the dissection proceeds. Surgical experience in intrathoracic operations is of benefit when performing the mediastinal dissection without direct visualization.

Cervical Phase

A cervical incision 6 cm in length is made along the anterior border of the left sternocleidomastoid muscle beginning at the level of the cricoid cartilage and extending caudally toward the clavicle. The platysma and omohyoid are divided, and the sternocleidomastoid and carotid sheath are retracted laterally. Care is taken to avoid injury to the recurrent laryngeal nerve either during direct dissection of tissues or with retractor pressure. The dissection is carried down to the prevertebral space behind the cervical esophagus with blunt dissection. The tracheoesophageal groove is developed, and the cervical esophagus is encircled with a rubber drain and retracted superiorly. Blunt dissection is used to mobilize the esophagus down to the level of the carina. The use of a "sponge stick" can greatly facilitate dissection along the prevertebral fascia.

When the surgeon's hands meet through the two incisions near the level of the aortic arch, two fingers of the lower hand are used to strip lateral attachments from the esophagus along its anterolateral surfaces. Hypotension can be induced when the hand inserted through the diaphragmatic hiatus displaces the heart. A flattened hand posteriorly is best tolerated. A similar blunt dissection of the lateral attachments is performed from posterior with two fingers of the surgeon's lower hand to complete the mobilization of the esophagus. The vagal fibers passing from the hilum of the lungs onto the esophagus may be hooked by the index finger, divided, and ligated.

The esophagus is divided obliquely in the neck with a surgical stapler, and then the more distal esophagus is withdrawn through the abdominal incision. The mobilized stomach and attached esophagus are evaluated. For tumors of the distal esophagus and cardia, an area along the lesser curvature of the stomach at the level of the second vascular arcade from the cardia is cleared of fat and blood vessels between clamps and ties. The stomach is progressively divided near the lesser curvature with sequential applications of the 5-cm gastrointestinal anastomosis stapler beginning approximately 4 to 6 cm distal to palpable tumor. For tumors of the upper and middle esophagus and in cases of benign disease requiring esophagectomy, as little stomach as possible is sacrificed to preserve gastric submucosal collateral circulation to the fundus. The esophagus, esophagogastric junction, and lesser curvature of the stomach are then removed en bloc and sent for pathologic confirmation that disease-free margins have been obtained.

The newly constructed gastric tube is then carefully guided through the posterior mediastinum to the cervical incision with the help of a Penrose drain. A Babcock clamp, inserted into the superior mediastinum through the cervical wound, is used to grasp the proximal end of the stomach and guide it gently upward into the neck. Careful attention should be made to ensure that the stomach and its blood supply are not twisted. Towels are placed to protect the wound from contamination.

The cervical esophagogastric anastomosis is now performed through the cervical incision by an end-to-end anastomosis with sutures (Fig. 13) or a side-to-side anastomosis with a 3-cm stapler and 3.5-mm staples. A nasogastric tube is then inserted across the anastomosis and into the intrathoracic stomach for postoperative gastric decompression. The cervical wound is closed loosely with absorbable suture over a small rubber drain.

Outcome

We have found that transhiatal esophagectomy is an excellent, safe procedure for patients with dysplasia or early lesions when long-term survival is expected. The main advantage is an anastomosis located in the neck, which avoids a thoracotomy. Limitations are the length of the stomach required to reach the neck and the inability to perform mediastinal lymph node dissection. Quality of life may be improved with less gastroesophageal reflux. However, symptoms of dumping are reportedly higher after transhiatal esophagectomy than after the Ivor Lewis operation.[15,16]

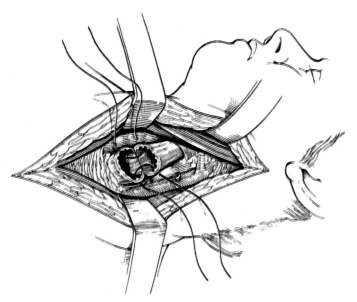

Fig. 13. Cervical esophagogastric anastomosis done with an incision in left neck after transhiatal esophagectomy has been accomplished.

Analysis of outcomes among patients treated at Mayo Clinic with transhiatal esophagectomy[20] showed operative morbidity and mortality rates and long-term survival rates similar, by cancer stage, to those among patients who had the Ivor Lewis operation. Long-term quality of life in patients who survived more than 5 years after resection of esophageal carcinoma was good.

Overall Surgical Outcomes

Functional outcome after esophagectomy is affected by age, sex, and type of resection. In our study of 107 patients surviving 5 or more years after esophagectomy (Ivor Lewis done in 72% of patients, transhiatal esophagectomy in 13%, extended esophagectomy in 4%, transthoracoabdominal esophagectomy and other in 11%), gastroesophageal reflux was the predominant complaint in 60%.[15] Fifty percent of patients had symptoms of dumping and 25% had dysphagia to solid food. Patients who had a cervical anastomosis had considerably fewer reflux symptoms. Dumping syndrome occurred more frequently in younger patients and women. Despite these symptoms, quality of life after resection, as assessed by the patients themselves, was similar to the national norm, including the ability to work, social interaction, daily activities, emotional function scores, and perception of health. Results from other centers also suggest that when surgeons have extensive experience in the treatment of esophageal cancer, mortality can be kept to a minimum, and long-term survivors do well.

COMBINED TREATMENT

For patients with resectable early cancers who are suitable surgical candidates (Tis through T2 N0 M0), operation alone remains the standard of treatment in the United States. However, in an effort to improve the results obtained by operation alone, various combinations of radiation, operation, and chemotherapy have been applied at Mayo Clinic. For patients with a high probability that the tumor has extended beyond the muscularis propria (T3 or T4) or into the regional lymph nodes (N1 or M1a), trimodality therapy, although controversial, may be preferable to operation alone. This hypothesis is based on results of the study by Walsh et al.[21] for adenocarcinoma of the esophagus and gastric cardia and on the results of the University of Michigan studies for squamous cell and adenocarcinomas of the esophagus[22-24] (Table 4). However, combined therapy in any form subjects patients to the toxicity of more than one type of treatment. Thus, the benefits of trimodality therapy have remained controversial. The results of several randomized and nonrandomized trials are discussed here.

Preoperative Chemotherapy

Preoperative chemotherapy as a single adjuvant has been tested in single institutions[27-29] and randomized trials.[25,30,31] Neither the three small randomized trials nor a larger intergroup phase III trial[32] demonstrated a survival benefit for preoperative chemotherapy. The Radiation Therapy Oncology Group trial[33] established that external beam radiation plus 5-fluorouracil and cisplatin is the current standard of care for the nonsurgical management of esophageal cancer, as discussed in a subsequent section.

Given reports of activity both as a single agent and in combination with cisplatin and 5-fluorouracil, paclitaxel is being evaluated in several pilot regimens for locally advanced and potentially resectable disease (concurrent with electron beam radiation and as maintenance chemotherapy). Ongoing trials are evaluating new agents such as irinotecan, vinorelbine, and gemcitabine in combination with cisplatin for patients with metastatic disease.

Thus, systemic chemotherapy is applicable in three areas of our practice: metastatic disease, preoperatively with irradiation, and in combination with irradiation as primary treatment for patients with localized disease who are poor candidates for, or refuse, surgical resection.

Preoperative External Beam Radiation

Preoperative external beam radiation therapy (EBRT) alone has been used in an attempt to improve the results of conventional therapy. Some retrospective comparisons of

Table 4.—Results of Trimodality Phase III Trials for Esophageal Cancer

Randomized trials	No. of patients	Preoperative treatment	Path. CR rate	Survival Median, mo	Survival 3-y overall	P value
Dublin						
Walsh et al.[21]	55	Operation alone	...	11	6%	
		vs.				0.01
	58	EBRT, 40 Gy in 15 Fx; 5-FU, CDDP	13 of 52, 25%	16	32%	
University of Michigan						
Urba et al.[22]	50	Operation alone	...	18	16	
Forastiere et al.[23]		vs.				0.15*
Urba et al.[24]						
	50	EBRT 45 Gy in 30 Fx; 5-FU, CDDP, VBL	14 of 50, 28%	17	30	(Cox regression)
Scandinavia						
Nygaard et al.[25]	91	Operation ± CDDP, bleo	...	7.2†	6	
		vs.				0.009
	95	EBRT 35 Gy in 20 Fx ± CDDP, bleo	...	9.2†	19	
France & EORTC						
Bosset et al.[26]	139	Operation alone	...	19	28 (DFS)	
		vs.				0.003
	143	EBRT 37 Gy in 10 Fx; CDDP 0-2 d before EBRT	29 of 112, 26%	19	40 (DFS)	

bleo, bleomycin; CDDP, cisplatin; DFS, disease-free survival; EBRT, external beam radiation therapy; EORTC, European Organization for Research and Treatment of Cancer Data Center, Belgium; 5-FU, 5-fluorouracil; Fx, fractions; Path. CR, pathologically complete resection; VBL, vinblastine.

*In multivariate analysis, trimodality treatment results in 31% lower risk of death ($P = 0.09$).

†Data taken from published figure.

EBRT plus operation versus operation alone do suggest improvement in survival with this combination therapy.

In the report by Akakura et al.,[34] 5-year survival was 25% among patients receiving EBRT plus operation and 14% among patients treated with operation alone. Fatal complications were higher among patients receiving combination therapy, however (21% of patients vs. 13%). Other retrospective studies suggest worse survival with EBRT plus operation in comparison with operation alone.[35,36]

Four prospective randomized studies of operation versus preoperative EBRT plus operation have been performed in patients with esophageal cancer. Three of these studies have not shown any difference in survival.[37-40] A study from Scandinavia comparing results in patients randomized to 35 Gy preoperative EBRT (with or without chemotherapy) followed by operation versus operation (with or without preoperative chemotherapy) without preoperative EBRT suggested a survival benefit for patients who received preoperative EBRT.[25] An imbalance in prognostic factors favored the preoperatively irradiated patients. Nearly twice as many patients with T1 disease received EBRT.

Preoperative EBRT Plus Chemotherapy

An important study of preoperative chemotherapy and radiation therapy was recently published by Walsh et al.[21] (Table 4). Patients with adenocarcinoma of the esophagus were randomized to receive preoperative EBRT (40 Gy in 15 fractions), 5-fluorouracil (15 mg/kg per day continuous infusion, equivalent to about 600 mg/m^2 per day for 5 days, weeks 1 and 6), and cisplatin (75 mg/m^2 on the first day of each infusion of 5-fluorouracil). This was followed by surgical resection 8 weeks after completion of radiation therapy or immediate operation. A highly significant difference in survival was observed with combination therapy (intent to treat principle: median survival 16 months vs. 11 months, 3-year survival 32% vs. 6%, $P = 0.01$; actual treatment: median survival 32 months vs. 11 months, $P = 0.001$; 3-year survival 37% vs. 7%, $P = 0.006$). However, the study has been criticized because of the unusually high operative mortality rate (9%) and poor survival rate (6%) in the surgical control arm and the short follow-up (3 years). These factors likely contributed to the observed results.

Urba et al.[22] found a trend toward a survival advantage for patients treated with preoperative chemoradiation compared with operation alone. Preoperative treatment involved 5-fluorouracil, cisplatin, and vinblastine given concurrently with radiation. Patients with either squamous or adenocarcinomas were eligible, but a majority of the 100 randomized patients had adenocarcinoma. Survival differences favoring trimodality treatment did not appear until after several years of follow-up; the 3-year survival was 16% for operation alone and 30% for multimodality treatment ($P = 0.15$, Cox regression; $P = 0.09$, log rank in multivariate analysis). Longer follow-up, however, failed to show a survival advantage in the combination treatment group compared with the operation-alone group. A confirmatory intergroup trial was performed in North America in an attempt to validate the positive results found in the small trials by Walsh et al.[21] and Urba et al.[22] The intergroup trial was closed prematurely because of poor accrual.

In a trial conducted by the French Foundation of Digestive Cancer and the European Organization for Research and Treatment of Cancer, 297 patients were randomized to operation alone or preoperative chemoradiation.[26] Of the 282 eligible patients, 139 were assigned to operation alone and 143 to preoperative adjuvant treatment. Those randomized to receive preoperative treatment had longer disease-free survival at 3 years ($P = 0.003$), improved local control ($P = 0.01$), a lower rate of cancer-related deaths ($P = 0.002$), and a higher rate of curative resection ($P = 0.017$). The rate of postoperative death was also higher in the preoperative chemoradiation group ($P = 0.012$), which, along with the lack of maintenance chemotherapy, likely contributed to a lack of difference in both median and long-term survival.

Given currently available data, preoperative chemoradiation is warranted only within the confines of investigational trials. Until further trials show a survival advantage compared with operation alone, the substantial costs and morbidity of preoperative chemoradiation make this approach problematic for widespread application.

Postoperative EBRT With or Without Chemotherapy

Postoperative EBRT has been advocated as yet another method of improving the dismal results of single-method therapy. Such treatment has been advocated for patients with adverse prognostic factors such as positive mediastinal lymph nodes, invasion of tumor through the entire esophageal wall, or close surgical margins. Published data on this topic, however, show lack of benefit for postoperative EBRT as a single adjuvant for patients with surgical-pathologic stage III esophageal cancer. Kasai et al.,[41] for example, found the 5-year survival rate was 18% in patients with node-positive disease who had operation alone and only 11% in patients who had postoperative EBRT. Although the results in node-negative disease were more optimistic (survival rate of 27% with operation alone and 85% with operation plus postoperative EBRT), such results have not been evaluated in detail in another series. Other randomized trials have either shown no benefit for postoperative EBRT or have indicated that postoperative EBRT may result in decreased survival.[42,43] On the basis of available evidence, postoperative EBRT as a single adjuvant fails to provide any additional benefits and subjects patients to additional toxic effects and expense.

In summary, we believe that neither postoperative adjuvant EBRT nor adjuvant chemotherapy should be used as a single adjuvant. At Mayo Clinic, we are evaluating the use of postoperative EBRT in conjunction with interrupted infusion of 5-fluorouracil plus cisplatin in a controlled phase I/II clinical trial.

Chemoradiation Without Operation

For unresected and unresectable lesions, the chemoradiotherapy approach seems to improve both local control and survival in nonrandomized trials.[44-54] Such benefits have also been shown in randomized trials.[25,55-58]

The landmark studies in esophageal cancer were the phase III trials by the Radiation Therapy Oncology Group, in which EBRT alone (64 Gy) was compared with EBRT (50 Gy) plus concomitant and maintenance 5-fluorouracil and cisplatin.[25,59] A marked survival and disease-control benefit was noted among the patients who had combination therapy.[59] Actuarial 2-year survival was 42% vs. 10% ($P = 0.0009$), and actuarial local control at 2 years was 53% vs. 30%, favoring chemoradiation ($P = 0.01$). The final results of this study have been reported.[25] With a minimum follow-up of 5 years, the 5-year survival rate was 27% in the patients who had combination therapy and 0% in the patients who had EBRT alone ($P < 0.0001$). Results in the combination therapy arm of the study are comparable to some of the best single-institution results in the surgical literature.

PALLIATIVE THERAPY

In most patients who present with esophageal cancer, surgical cure is not possible, and the focus of treatment is palliation. Operation, chemoradiation, and various endoscopic methods are used to relieve dysphagia. In any patient with malignant dysphagia, the specific treatment must be selected according to the severity of the problem and the site of the tumor. In esophageal cancer, the cell type does not directly influence therapy.[44]

Chemoradiation

Radiation alone or in conjunction with chemotherapy also has been successful for palliating pain and improving dysphagia in 65% to 80% of cases. In 1.8- to 2.0-Gy fractions, the palliation dose is close to the definitive dose of 50 to 60 Gy. Combination chemoradiation has improved disease control and survival over that with radiation alone. However, radiation alone can provide excellent relief of dysphagia for patients who are too ill to undergo combination chemoradiation.

Esophagectomy and Bypass

Esophagectomy for palliation in patients with poor functional status has a mortality rate of more than 20%.[60] Numerous esophageal and gastric bypass procedures are described in the literature but rarely are used at our institution because so many low-risk minimally invasive procedures are available. Because of the high operative mortality and complication rates associated with these surgical procedures, most institutions have abandoned their use, except for a few rare patients in whom radiation therapy is contraindicated or palliative therapies are unsuccessful. Percutaneous endoscopic gastrostomy tubes or jejunal feeding tubes are preferable, however, and are associated with considerably fewer complications than surgical bypass procedures.

Dilation and Stents

Esophageal dilation alone provides only temporary relief, and stent placement is usually required. Repeat dilation can improve dysphagia for a few days to weeks at the most. Because expandable metal stents have a small diameter before deployment, aggressive dilation of the esophagus is rarely necessary. In the United States, expandable metal stents have replaced plastic stents for use in the esophagus.[61] Dysphagia is safely and immediately relieved in most patients who receive expandable metal stents. In the distal esophagus, newer stents with a one-way flap valve on the gastric side of the stent can prevent gastroesophageal reflux and aspiration. For patients with persistent weight loss and dysphagia, percutaneous endoscopic gastrostomy tube placement through a preexisting esophageal stent is still possible, although stent migration may occur.

NEWER THERAPEUTIC APPROACHES

Photodynamic Therapy

Photodynamic therapy is a novel endoscopic technique that combines a photosensitizing agent and laser light to destroy target cells.[62] There is no thermal injury to other cells and tissues. The agent accumulates in malignant tissue but is inactive until exposure to specific wavelengths of light, when it becomes activated and generates cytotoxic singlet oxygen. Compared with laser therapy, photodynamic therapy seems to produce longer lasting relief from dysphagia, and patient survival is similar. It is also useful for tumor ingrowth and overgrowth into expandable metal stents.[44] Photodynamic therapy is being evaluated at Mayo Clinic as a therapeutic technique for patients with Barrett's esophagus, providing the lesion has not invaded deeper than the mucosa.

Endoscopic Laser Therapy

Laser therapy uses the direct application of laser light to burn and vaporize tissue under endoscopic visualization. The neodymium:yttrium-aluminum-garnet laser has been used for almost 20 years for palliation of malignant dysphagia. Complications of laser therapy include tracheoesophageal fistulas, bleeding, and perforation. It is most effective for exophytic, short-segment, discrete malignant strictures.

Intraoperative Electron Irradiation

Intraoperative electron irradiation has been evaluated as a component of treatment for patients with T4 esophageal cancer or bulky nodal disease in whom resection alone with negative margins is unlikely. Patients usually receive preoperative EBRT (45-50.4 Gy in 1.8-Gy fractions) plus concurrent 5-fluorouracil and cisplatin followed in 5 to 6 weeks by resection and intraoperative electron irradiation if restaging shows no evidence of metastatic cancer. Most patients recover so slowly that additional cycles of chemotherapy have not been feasible postoperatively. The addition of electron beam radiation to preoperative EBRT plus concurrent chemotherapy and resection appears to improve the local control of esophageal cancer that is locally "unresectable for cure." However, this has not translated into long-term survival benefits because of high rates of systemic relapse (about 75% at 1 year) in initial analyses (Miller RC, Gunderson LL, Haddock MG, Trastek VF, Donohue JH, read at the Third International Meeting of the International Society of Intraoperative Radiation Therapy, Aachen, Germany, 2002). Additional cycles of maintenance chemotherapy probably are needed to decrease systemic risks. It may be necessary to give the additional chemotherapy before, rather than with, preoperative radiation.

Thoracoscopic Operations

The use of thoracoscopic operations for treatment of esophageal cancer is being explored at Mayo Clinic. To date, these operations have not had a major role in our surgical armamentarium.

PREVENTION

Increasing efforts toward endoscopic surveillance for Barrett's disease are hoped to lead to earlier detection and possibly improved long-term survival for patients with premalignant, dysplastic lesions or early malignancies. Aggressive medical and surgical management of Barrett's esophagus may decrease the frequency of cancers arising from the lesion.

CONCLUSION

Surgical resection remains the standard of care for patients with resectable esophageal cancer. Despite noted advances in treatment, long-term results remain less than optimal regardless of the method. Clinical trials are essential to define the role of chemotherapy, radiation, and operation in the treatment of esophageal cancer. Refinements in trimodality therapy will necessitate continued enrollment of patients in clinical trials to allow development of the most effective and best-tolerated treatment strategies for the future. Continued enthusiasm within the surgical community is necessary for accrual and completion of trials within a reasonable time. Future efforts will continue toward improvement of multimodality therapies, earlier detection methods, and identification of biochemical tumor markers that may be predictive of chemotherapy response or tumor resistance.

REFERENCES

1. King RM, Pairolero PC, Trastek VF, Payne WS, Bernatz PE: Ivor Lewis esophagogastrectomy for carcinoma of the esophagus: early and late functional results. Ann Thorac Surg 44:119-122, 1987

2. Lund O, Hasenkam JM, Aagaard MT, Kimose HH: Time-related changes in characteristics of prognostic significance in carcinomas of the oesophagus and cardia. Br J Surg 76:1301-1307, 1989

3. Parkin DM, Pisani P, Ferlay J: Global cancer statistics. CA Cancer J Clin 49:33-64, 1999

4. Blot WJ, McLaughlin JK: The changing epidemiology of esophageal cancer. Semin Oncol 26 Suppl 15:2-8, 1999

5. Cameron AJ, Ott BJ, Payne WS: The incidence of adenocarcinoma in columnar-lined (Barrett's) esophagus. N Engl J Med 313:857-859, 1985

6. Pera M, Cameron AJ, Trastek VF, Carpenter HA, Zinsmeister AR: Increasing incidence of adenocarcinoma of the esophagus and esophagogastric junction. Gastroenterology 104:510-513, 1993

7. Schottenfeld D: Epidemiology of cancer of the esophagus. Semin Oncol 11:92-100, 1984

8. DeMeester TR, Barlow AP: Surgery and current management for cancer of the esophagus and cardia. Curr Probl Cancer 12:243-328, 1988

9. Hesketh PJ, Clapp RW, Doos WG, Spechler SJ: The increasing frequency of adenocarcinoma of the esophagus. Cancer 64:526-530, 1989

10. Blot WJ, Devesa SS, Kneller RW, Fraumeni JF Jr: Rising incidence of adenocarcinoma of the esophagus and gastric cardia. JAMA 265:1287-1289, 1991

11. Pera M, Trastek VF, Carpenter HA, Allen MS, Deschamps C, Pairolero PC: Barrett's esophagus with high-grade dysplasia: an indication for esophagectomy? Ann Thorac Surg 54:199-204, 1992

12. Jones AD, Bacon KD, Jobe BA, Sheppard BC, Deveney CW, Rutten MJ: *Helicobacter pylori* induces apoptosis in Barrett's-derived esophageal adenocarcinoma cells. J Gastrointest Surg 7:68-76, 2003

13. Vazquez-Sequeiros E, Norton ID, Clain JE, Wang KK, Affi A, Allen M, Deschamps C, Miller D, Salomao D, Wiersema MJ: Impact of EUS-guided fine-needle aspiration on lymph node staging in patients with esophageal carcinoma. Gastrointest Endosc 53:751-757, 2001

14. Fleming ID, Cooper JS, Henson DE, Hutter RVP, Kennedy BJ, Murphy GP, O'Sullivan B, Sobin LH, Yarbro JW: AJCC Cancer Staging Manual. Fifth edition. Philadelphia, Lippincott-Raven Publishers, 1997

15. McLarty AJ, Deschamps C, Trastek VF, Allen MS, Pairolero PC, Harmsen WS: Esophageal resection for cancer of the esophagus: long-term function and quality of life. Ann Thorac Surg 63:1568-1572, 1997

16. Headrick JR, Nichols FC III, Miller DL, Allen MS, Trastek VF, Deschamps C, Schleck CD, Thompson AM, Pairolero PC: High-grade esophageal dysplasia: long-term survival and quality of life after esophagectomy. Ann Thorac Surg 73:1697-1702, 2002

17. Trastek VF: Esophagectomy: Ivor Lewis. *In* Atlas of Surgical Oncology. Edited by JH Donohue, JA van Heerden, JRT Monson. Cambridge, Blackwell Science, 1995, pp 126-130

18. Visbal AL, Allen MS, Miller DL, Deschamps C, Trastek VF, Pairolero PC: Ivor Lewis esophagogastrectomy for esophageal cancer. Ann Thorac Surg 71:1803-1808, 2001

19. Deschamps C: Use of colon and jejunum as possible esophageal replacements. Chest Surg Clin N Am 5:555-569, 1995

20. Vigneswaran WT, Trastek VF, Pairolero PC, Deschamps C, Daly RC, Allen MS: Transhiatal esophagectomy for carcinoma of the esophagus. Ann Thorac Surg 56:838-844, 1993

21. Walsh TN, Noonan N, Hollywood D, Kelly A, Keeling N, Hennessy TP: A comparison of multimodal therapy and surgery for esophageal adenocarcinoma. N Engl J Med 335:462-467, 1996

22. Urba S, Orringer M, Turrisi A, Whyte R, Iannettoni M, Forastiere A: A randomized trial comparing surgery (S) to preoperative concomitant chemoirradiation plus surgery in patients (pts) with resectable esophageal cancer (CA): updated analysis (abstract). Program/Proc Am Soc Clin Oncol 16:277a, 1997

23. Forastiere AA, Orringer MB, Perez-Tamayo C, Urba SG, Husted S, Takasugi BJ, Zahurak M: Concurrent chemotherapy and radiation therapy followed by transhiatal esophagectomy for local-regional cancer of the esophagus. J Clin Oncol 8:119-127, 1990

24. Urba SG, Orringer MB, Turrisi A, Iannettoni M, Forastiere A, Strawderman M: Randomized trial of preoperative chemoradiation versus surgery alone in patients with locoregional esophageal carcinoma. J Clin Oncol 19:305-313, 2001

25. Nygaard K, Hagen S, Hansen HS, Hatlevoll R, Hultborn R, Jakobsen A, Mantyla M, Modig H, Munck-Wikland E, Rosengren B: Pre-operative radiotherapy prolongs survival in operable esophageal carcinoma: a randomized, multicenter study of pre-operative radiotherapy and chemotherapy. The second Scandinavian trial in esophageal cancer. World J Surg 16:1104-1109, 1992

26. Bosset JF, Gignoux M, Triboulet JP, Tiret E, Mantion G, Elias D, Lozach P, Ollier JC, Pavy JJ, Mercier M, Sahmoud T: Chemoradiotherapy followed by surgery compared with surgery alone in squamous-cell cancer of the esophagus. N Engl J Med 337:161-167, 1997

27. Kelsen D: Neoadjuvant therapy of esophageal cancer. Can J Surg 32:410-414, 1989

28. Kelsen DP, Ahuja R, Hopfan S, Bains MS, Kosloff C, Martini N, McCormack P, Golbey RB: Combined modality therapy of esophageal carcinoma. Cancer 48:31-37, 1981

29. Kelsen DP, Bains M, Burt M: Neoadjuvant chemotherapy and surgery of cancer of the esophagus. Semin Surg Oncol 6:268-273, 1990

30. Roth JA, Pass HI, Flanagan MM, Graeber GM, Rosenberg JC, Steinberg S: Randomized clinical trial of preoperative and post-operative adjuvant chemotherapy with cisplatin, vindesine, and bleomycin for carcinoma of the esophagus. J Thorac Cardiovasc Surg 96:242-248, 1988

31. Schlag PM: Randomized trial of preoperative chemotherapy for squamous cell cancer of the esophagus. The Chirurgische Arbeitsgemeinschaft Fuer Onkologie der Deutschen Gesellschaft Fuer Chirurgie Study Group. Arch Surg 127:1446-1450, 1992

32. Kelsen DP, Ginsberg R, Pajak TF, Sheahan DG, Gunderson L, Mortimer J, Estes N, Haller DG, Ajani J, Kocha W, Minsky BD, Roth JA: Chemotherapy followed by surgery compared with surgery alone for localized esophageal cancer. N Engl J Med 339:1979-1984, 1998

33. al-Sarraf M, Martz K, Herskovic A, Leichman L, Brindle JS, Vaitkevicius VK, Cooper J, Byhardt R, Davis L, Emami B: Progress report of combined chemoradiotherapy versus radiotherapy alone in patients with esophageal cancer: an intergroup study. J Clin Oncol 15:277-284, 1997

34. Akakura I, Nakamura Y, Kakegawa T, Nakayama R, Watanabe H, Yamashita H: Surgery of carcinoma of the esophagus with preoperative radiation. Chest 57:47-57, 1970

35. Sugimachi K, Matsufuji H, Kai H, Masuda H, Ueo H, Inokuchi K, Jingu K: Preoperative irradiation for carcinoma of the esophagus. Surg Gynecol Obstet 162:174-176, 1986

36. Sugimachi K, Matsuoka H, Matsufuji H, Maekawa S, Kai H, Okudaira Y: Survival rates of women with carcinoma of the esophagus exceed those of men. Surg Gynecol Obstet 164:541-544, 1987

37. Gignoux M, Roussel A, Paillot B, Gillet M, Schlag P, Dalesio O, Buyse M, Duez N: The value of preoperative radiotherapy in esophageal cancer: results of a study by the EORTC. Recent Results Cancer Res 110:1-13, 1988

38. Gignoux M, Roussel A, Paillot B, Gillet M, Schlag P, Favre JP, Dalesio O, Buyse M, Duez N: The value of preoperative radiotherapy in esophageal cancer: results of a study of the E.O.R.T.C. World J Surg 11:426-432, 1987

39. Launois B, Delarue D, Campion JP, Kerbaol M: Preoperative radiotherapy for carcinoma of the esophagus. Surg Gynecol Obstet 153:690-692, 1981

40. Mei W, Xian-Zhi G, Weibo Y, Guojun H, Liang-Jun W, Da-Weiz: Randomized clinical trial on the combination of preoperative irradiation and surgery in the treatment of esophageal carcinoma: report on 206 patients. Int J Radiat Oncol Biol Phys 16;325-327, 1989

41. Kasai M, Mori S, Watanabe T: Follow-up results after resection of thoracic esophageal carcinoma. World J Surg 2:543-551, 1978

42. Vokes EE, Mauer AM: Multimodality therapy for esophageal cancer: an emerging role. Cancer J Sci Am 4:226-229, 1998

43. Kok TC: Chemotherapy in oesophageal cancer. Cancer Treat Rev 23:65-85, 1997

44. Adler DG, Baron TH: Endoscopic palliation of malignant dysphagia. Mayo Clin Proc 76:731-738, 2001

45. Pringle R, Winsey HS: The palliation of oesophageal carcinoma. J R Coll Surg Edinb 18:188-190, 1973

46. Keane TJ, Harwood AR, Rider WD, Cummings BJ, Thomas GM: Concomitant radiation and chemotherapy for squamous cell carcinoma (SCC) esophagus (abstract). Int J Radiat Oncol Biol Phys 10 Suppl 2:89, 1984

47. Herskovic A, Leichman L, Lattin P, Han I, Ahmad K, Leichman G, Rosenberg J, Steiger Z, Bendal C, White B, Seydel G, Seyedsadr M, Vaitkevicius V: Chemo/radiation with and without surgery in the thoracic esophagus: the Wayne State experience. Int J Radiat Oncol Biol Phys 15:655-662, 1988

48. Seydel HG, Leichman L, Byhardt R, Cooper J, Herskovic A, Libnock J, Pazdur R, Speyer J, Tschan J: Preoperative radiation and chemotherapy for localized squamous cell carcinoma of the esophagus: a RTOG Study. Int J Radiat Oncol Biol Phys 14:33-35, 1988

49. Byfield JE, Barone R, Mendelsohn J, Frankel S, Quinol L, Sharp T, Seagren S: Infusional 5-fluorouracil and X-ray therapy for non-resectable esophageal cancer. Cancer 45:703-708, 1980

50. Coia LR, Engstrom PF, Paul A: Nonsurgical management of esophageal cancer: report of a study of combined radiotherapy and chemotherapy. J Clin Oncol 5:1783-1790, 1987

51. Coia LR, Engstrom PF, Paul AR, Stafford PM, Hanks GE: Long-term results of infusional 5-FU, mitomycin-C and radiation as primary management of esophageal carcinoma. Int J Radiat Oncol Biol Phys 20:29-36, 1991

52. Coia LR, Paul AR, Engstrom PF: Combined radiation and chemotherapy as primary management of adenocarcinoma of the esophagus and gastroesophageal junction. Cancer 61:643-649, 1988

53. Lokich JJ, Shea M, Chaffey J: Sequential infusional 5-fluorouracil followed by concomitant radiation for tumors of the esophagus and gastroesophageal junction. Cancer 60:275-279, 1987

54. Richmond J, Seydel HG, Bae Y, Lewis J, Burdakin J, Jacobsen G: Comparison of three treatment strategies for esophageal cancer within a single institution. Int J Radiat Oncol Biol Phys 13:1617-1620, 1987

55. Hishikawa Y, Kurisu K, Taniguchi M, Kamikonya N, Miura T: High-dose-rate intraluminal brachytherapy (HDRIBT) for esophageal cancer. Int J Radiat Oncol Biol Phys 21:1133-1135, 1991

56. Sischy B, Ryan L, Haller D, Smith T, Dayal Y, Schutt A, Hinson J: Interim report of EST 1282 phase III protocol for the evaluation of combined modalities in the treatment of patients with carcinoma of the esophagus, stage I and II (abstract). Program/Proc Am Soc Clin Oncol 9:105, 1990

57. Smith TJ, Ryan LM, Douglass HOJ, Haller DG, Dayal Y, Kirkwood J, Tormey DC, Schutt AJ, Hinson J, Sischy B: Combined chemoradiotherapy vs. radiotherapy alone for early stage squamous cell carcinoma of the esophagus: a study of the Eastern Cooperative Oncology Group. Int J Radiat Oncol Biol Phys 42:269-276, 1998

58. Araujo CM, Souhami L, Gil RA, Carvalho R, Garcia JA, Froimtchuk MJ, Pinto LH, Canary PC: A randomized trial comparing radiation therapy versus concomitant radiation therapy and chemotherapy in carcinoma of the thoracic esophagus. Cancer 67:2258-2261, 1991

59. Herskovic A, Martz K, al-Sarraf M, Leichman L, Brindle J, Vaitkevicius V, Cooper J, Byhardt R, Davis L, Emami B: Combined chemotherapy and radiotherapy compared with radiotherapy alone in patients with cancer of the esophagus. N Engl J Med 326:1593-1598, 1992

60. Conlan AA, Nicolaou N, Hammond CA, Pool R, de Nobrega C, Mistry BD: Retrosternal gastric bypass for inoperable esophageal cancer: a report of 71 patients. Ann Thorac Surg 36:396-401, 1983

61. Baron TH: Expandable metal stents for the treatment of cancerous obstruction of the gastrointestinal tract. N Engl J Med 344:1681-1687, 2001

62. Saidi RF, Marcon NE: Nonthermal ablation of malignant esophageal strictures: photodynamic therapy, endoscopic intratumoral injections, and novel modalities. Gastrointest Endosc Clin N Am 8:465-491, 1998

Chapter 6

GASTRIC ADENOCARCINOMA

Barbara A. Pockaj, M.D.

The treatment of gastric cancer has a long history at Mayo Clinic. William J. Mayo, M.D., one of the well-known and respected medical pioneers of the early 20th century, advocated new and aggressive surgical treatments for gastric cancer. He was only too well acquainted with this disease, diagnosing it in himself and dying of it soon thereafter.

Carcinoma of the stomach remains a leading cause of death from cancer worldwide. The incidence of gastric cancer is highest in Japan, South America, and Eastern Europe. In Japan, gastric cancer, remarkably, is the most frequently diagnosed cancer in both men and women.[1] In the United States in 2002, gastric cancer developed in an estimated 21,600 persons, and 12,400 died of the disease.[2] For still unknown reasons, gastric cancer has dramatically declined in the United States. In 1950, gastric cancer was the leading cause of death from cancer among men in the United States; in contrast, in 2000, it was the seventh cause of cancer-related death in men.[2] Approximately two-thirds of patients are older than 65 years at diagnosis, and the diagnosis is infrequent before the age of 40 years. The disease occurs more commonly in men than in women and is also more common in African Americans, Hispanic Americans, and American Indians than in Anglo-Americans.[1-3]

Even though the incidence of gastric cancer has declined, several controversies and challenges confront the surgeon. Because the symptoms of gastric carcinoma are usually insidious, diagnosis is often made only at a late stage. A 1995 study by the American College of Surgeons found that 66% of patients with gastric cancer had locally advanced or metastatic disease at diagnosis. This phenomenon led to resection rates of only 30% to 50% and, not unexpectedly, poor 5- and 10-year survival rates.[3] The 5-year survival rate is highly stage-dependent and ranges from 7% to 78%. The overall 10-year survival rate is a dismal 20%.[4] The role of the surgeon is crucial to the care of patients with gastric cancer. Controversy remains as to the proper preoperative work-up and appropriate procedure. Considerable data, largely from Japan, suggest that the extent of operation has an important impact on survival, but several larger, multicenter trials in the Western world fail to confirm the Japanese data. The use of adjuvant and neoadjuvant therapy has only recently shown promising results, but further investigation is needed.

EPIDEMIOLOGY AND RISK FACTORS

One of the most dramatic changes in the epidemiology of gastric cancer is related to the distribution of the primary lesion within the stomach. There has been a shifting proportion to more proximal cancers during the past 3 decades.[5,6] According to a study by the American College of Surgeons, the distribution of the lesions was as follows: upper third, 30%; middle third, 14%; distal third, 26%; entire stomach, 10%; and unknown, 19%.[5] Interestingly, there has been a concurrent increase in distal esophageal carcinoma.[7]

The cause of gastric cancer is still unknown. Environmental factors have been strongly implicated in its development. People who have a high risk, such as the Japanese or Eastern Europeans, and migrate to a low-risk area such as the United States continue to have a high risk even after they have adopted a Western diet, but the risk for the second- and third-generation populations decreases markedly to that of the native population.[8,9]

Dietary habits and preservatives have been implicated as risk factors for the development of cancer. Reasons postulated for the decline in the incidence of gastric cancer in the United States have been related to changes in diet and food preservation practices.[10] Diets rich in salt, smoked or poorly preserved foods, nitrates, and nitrites are associated with an increased risk of gastric cancer.[10,11] Large consumption of highly salty foods may lead to atrophic gastritis, which is a risk factor for gastric carcinoma.[1,11] Nitrates and nitrites increase the risk of gastric cancer in animals as a result of the formation of N-nitroso compounds.[11] Other investigators believe that nitrites decrease the ascorbate:nitrite ratio, which may lead to an increase of gastric cancer.[12] However, newer epidemiologic studies have failed to confirm an association between nitrates or salts and an increased risk of gastric cancer.[13,14] Several studies have found that a diet high in fruits, vegetables, and fiber may have a protective effect against gastric cancer, an effect postulated to be due to vitamin C or carotenes.[15,16] In contrast, other studies have not shown any change in the risk of gastric cancer with such a diet.[17,18] Future epidemiologic and chemoprevention studies may give us a better insight into the role of nutrition in the pathogenesis of gastric cancer.

Tobacco and alcohol have been implicated in the development of gastric cancer. A recent meta-analysis reviewed 40 studies. Smokers had a relative risk of 1.5 to 1.6 compared with nonsmokers.[19] Studies of the use of alcohol and the risk of gastric cancer have been inconclusive; some demonstrate an increased risk, whereas others find no increase in risk. There is some suggestion that alcohol intake may increase the risk of cancer in smokers.[20,21]

Several precursor conditions definitely increase the risk of gastric cancer. These include chronic atrophic and hypersecretory gastritis, pernicious anemia, Ménétrier's disease, partial gastrectomy for benign causes, and gastric polyps.[5] Chronic gastric mucosal injury is theorized to be the initiating event leading to the progression of intestinal metaplasia to dysplasia and then to possible invasive carcinoma. Atrophic gastritis and invasive carcinoma share similar risk factors. Atrophic gastritis is prevalent in areas with a high incidence of gastric cancer. Chronic atrophic gastritis has two forms: type A and type B. Gastric cancer will develop in approximately 10% of patients with chronic atrophic gastritis type B within 10 to 20 years.[22] Patients with pernicious anemia have a twofold to threefold higher risk for development of gastric cancer. The mechanism is thought to be due to achlorhydria, which leads to intestinal metaplasia.[23,24] Ménétrier's disease is a rare disorder characterized by rugal-fold hypertrophy,

hypochlorhydria, and protein-losing enteropathy. Several case reports demonstrate a link between gastric cancer and Ménétrier's disease.[25,26] Patients who have undergone partial gastrectomies are at increased risk for the development of cancer in the gastric remnant. The risk increases with time and becomes statistically significant 15 to 20 years after the operation. Previous diagnoses of gastric versus duodenal ulcer, male sex, and a Billroth II type reconstruction increase the risk of carcinoma development. The pathophysiologic mechanism is believed to be related to achlorhydria, enterogastric reflux, and bacterial overgrowth.[27]

Gastric polyps can be precancerous lesions or a marker of a precancerous condition elsewhere in the gastric mucosa, depending on the type of polyp. Adenomatous polyps are classified as tubular, villous, and tubulovillous. Their biologic significance is similar to that of adenomas found in the colon. The risk of carcinoma increases with the size of the polyp. Polyps more than 2 cm in size harbor a focus of carcinoma in 40% of specimens. Malignant degeneration occurs at a rate of 11% at 4 years.[28,29] New polyps will develop in 25% to 33% of patients who have had endoscopic removal of an adenoma; thus, lifelong endoscopic surveillance is indicated.[29] Hyperplastic polyps are not believed to degenerate into malignancy, but for patients who harbor multiple hyperplastic polyps, there is an 8% incidence of development of a gastric cancer in the normal mucosa. Thus, these patients also need endoscopic surveillance.[30] Several genetic polyposis syndromes manifest polyps in the stomach. Patients with the Gardner variant of familial polyposis coli have a 35% to 100% chance for development of polyps (often multiple) in the distal stomach and duodenum. The duodenal polyps are more likely to undergo malignant degeneration.[31,32] Patients with hereditary, nonpolyposis colorectal cancer (Lynch syndrome) also manifest an increased risk of gastric cancer.[33]

Other hereditary conditions associated with gastric cancer include an increased risk for the development of carcinoma in people with blood type A.[34] Patients with a positive family history of a first-degree relative with gastric cancer have a twofold to threefold increase in the risk of gastric cancer.[35,36] Recently, families have been described with an autosomal dominant inherited predisposition to gastric cancer. Although rare, mutations in E-cadherin have been identified in most of these pedigrees; diffuse gastric cancers usually develop, often before the age of 50 years, and thus prophylactic gastrectomy is warranted in selected patients.[37]

The importance of *Helicobacter pylori* in the pathogenesis of peptic ulcer disease has been recognized. There is also compelling evidence that links chronic *H. pylori* infection to gastric cancer. *H. pylori* is a gram-negative, microaerophilic bacterial rod that induces a chronic active gastritis in most infected individuals. The magnitude of the infection varies between strains of *H. pylori* and hosts. Most *H. pylori* infections are of no clinical consequence.[38] Initial studies demonstrated an increased risk of gastric cancer in patients with *H. pylori* infection in the United States and Britain.[39-41] Another study found that the greater the prevalence of *H. pylori* infection, the higher the incidence of gastric cancer.[42] A recent meta-analysis confirmed a twofold increased risk of gastric cancer for patients with *H. pylori* infections, and the risk was greatest in young patients and decreased with age.[43] Interestingly, people with *H. pylori*-induced duodenal ulcer disease are less likely to have gastric carcinoma than the average population, a finding implying that several interacting factors probably have a role in the pathogenesis of the cancer.[44] Chronic recurrent epithelial injury can induce tumorigenesis in many tissues. The atrophic gastritis that develops due to *H. pylori* infection is believed to be a precursor to the development of cancer. The mechanism by which *H. pylori* induces tumorigenesis and the cofactors that are necessary have not been elicited yet. *H. pylori* strains that are cag (cytotoxic-associated gene)–positive are more virulent. Cag-positive strains induce visible gastric damage, whereas cag-negative strains fail to incite such changes.[45] There is a strong correlation with cag-positive *H. pylori* strains and the development of peptic ulcer disease and cancer.[46]

PATHOLOGY

In 1997, the American Joint Committee on Cancer (AJCC) and the Union Internationale Contre le Cancer (UICC) redefined the staging of nodal (N) disease in gastric cancer. The new TNM staging system relies on the number of lymph nodes involved and not on the location of the lymph nodes, as had been done historically. The removal of a minimum of 15 lymph nodes was recommended for adequate staging. The staging system defined by the AJCC is summarized in Table 1.[47,48]

The new staging system has been validated by several investigators.[49,50] Because it focuses on the number of lymph nodes involved by metastatic cancer, it is a better reflection of prognosis and more reproducible than using the location of the metastatic lymph nodes. Removal of more than 15 lymph nodes often led to stage migration and, thus, more accurate staging. Both the extent of tumor invasion (T stage) and lymph node involvement (N stage) have been shown to have prognostic significance. The depth of the tumor correlates closely with lymph node involvement.[50]

Controversy currently persists regarding how to report the histologic type and grade. The World Health

Table 1.—American Joint Committee on Cancer Staging System for Gastric Carcinoma

Primary tumor (T)
  Tis Tumor in situ
  T1   Tumor invades lamina propria or submucosa
  T2   Tumor invades muscularis propria or subserosa
  T3   Tumor penetrates serosa
  T4   Tumor invades adjacent structures
Regional lymph nodes (N)
  N0   No metastasis to regional lymph nodes
  N1   Metastasis in 1-6 regional lymph nodes
  N2   Metastasis in 7-15 regional lymph nodes
  N3   Metastasis in >15 regional lymph nodes
Distant metastases (M)
  M0   No distant metastasis
  M1   Distant metastasis

Stage grouping

Stage	T	N	M
IA	T1	N0	M0
IB	T1	N1	M0
	T2	N0	M0
II	T1	N2	M0
	T2	N1	M0
	T3	N0	M0
IIIA	T2	N2	M0
	T3	N1	M0
	T4	N0	M0
IIIB	T3	N2	M0
IV	T4	N1	M0
	T1	N3	M0
	T3	N3	M0
	T4	N2	M0
	T4	N3	M0
	Any T	Any N	M1

R category
  R0   No residual tumor
  R1   Microscopic residual tumor
  R2   Macroscopic residual tumor

From Fleming et al.[47] By permission of the American Joint Committee on Cancer.

Organization (WHO) International Histologic Classification on gastric cancer reviewed the various types of classifications. Traditional tumor typing (tubular or mucinous adenocarcinoma, signet cell, small cell, or undifferentiated carcinoma), the Lauren classification (intestinal versus nonintestinal type), and the Ming classification (expanding versus infiltrative type) had no impact on prognosis. Many of the previous differences suggested by some investigators generally can be explained by different tumor stages.[51] Recently, the new Goseki histologic classification was introduced. The Goseki classification described a histologic grading system based on tubular differentiation and mucous quality. Subsequently, one group of investigators compared the new Goseki system with the WHO, Lauren, and tumor differentiation classifications.[52] They also evaluated the prognostic implication of a lymphocytic and eosinophilic infiltrate. The most important factor for survival was still the TNM stage. Although the Goseki classification appeared to add further prognostic information to the TNM stage, further studies are needed to verify this finding.

DIAGNOSIS AND PREOPERATIVE EVALUATION

The initial symptoms of gastric cancer are usually insidious. The American College of Surgeons reviewed the symptoms in more than 18,000 patients with gastric cancer. The symptoms included weight loss in 62%, abdominal pain in 52%, nausea in 34%, anorexia in 32%, dysphagia in 26%, melena in 20%, early satiety in 18%, ulcer-type pain in 17%, and lower extremity swelling in 6%.[5]

Endoscopy is the diagnostic method of choice, because it allows direct visualization of the tumor, assessment of its extent, and biopsy for histologic diagnosis. In Japan, screening leads to earlier diagnosis of gastric cancer and an overall better prognosis because of earlier detection at a less advanced stage.[53] Indeed, with the very high incidence in Japan, such screening has led to the current situation, in which about 40% of patients with a diagnosis of gastric cancer have "early gastric cancer" (i.e., disease confined to the mucosa). In contrast, less than 5% of patients in Western countries have early gastric cancer. An evaluation of the use of endoscopy as a screening tool in patients with a history of dyspepsia was performed in England. Patients older than 40 years were referred for endoscopy if they had a 2-week history of dyspepsia. An esophageal, gastric, or duodenal malignancy was found in 115 (4%) of 2,700 patients. Gastric cancer was found in 2% of this population, all but one of whom were older than 55 years; interestingly, 26% of these "screened" patients had early gastric cancer. The investigators believed that the study supported the recommendation that patients older than 55 with a history of dyspepsia should undergo upper gastrointestinal endoscopy.[54]

Laboratory evaluation is usually neither helpful nor pathognomonic. Anemia is a common finding (42%)

and may be the initiating event for endoscopy. Liver function tests are usually unrevealing unless significant metastatic disease (26%) is present, as manifested by an increased alkaline phosphatase level. The tumor may cause malnutrition due to early satiety and pain, resulting in hypoalbuminemia.[55] There are no useful tumor markers. Carcinoembryonic antigen, α-fetoprotein, and carbohydrate antigen (CA 19-9) values are increased in about 30% of patients. These tumor markers are more commonly increased in patients with metastatic or unresectable disease.[56]

Abdominal and pelvic computed tomography (CT) is the most common initial staging tool. The use of helical CT with intravenous contrast provides more information than traditional CT. Helical CT scanning can accurately suggest serosal involvement in 70% to 80% of patients and lymph node metastases in 25% to 70% of patients.[57] Another study correlated the size of lymph nodes and metastatic disease and found that lymph nodes 15 mm or more in size had an 80% risk of containing cancer, although metastatic disease can be found in lymph nodes smaller than 5 mm.[58] The limitations of CT are its failure to visualize small liver metastases and small peritoneal implants.

Endoscopic ultrasonography (EUS) may increase sensitivity for evaluation of the depth of gastric wall penetration (80%-90%) and lymph node metastases (70%-90%). The use of EUS can aid in determining the extent of the tumor and contiguous organ invasion.[57] EUS is most helpful for evaluating patients who have T3 or T4 lesions and are candidates for neoadjuvant protocols.

The use of staging laparoscopy before formal celiotomy has improved patient management tremendously. Three large studies found that metastatic disease was present at laparoscopy in 23% to 37% of patients who had negative results on preoperative staging work-up. Patients who were found to harbor metastatic disease did not undergo an operation. Only 0% to 20% of these patients required a subsequent operation for obstruction or bleeding. Patients found to have metastatic disease at laparoscopy versus laparotomy have a shorter hospital stay and fewer complications. Because no survival advantage is associated with palliative resection, pain, complications, and the convalescence of celiotomy are prevented. The authors advocated preoperative laparoscopic evaluation in all patients with a negative staging work-up who are not bleeding and have no obstructive symptoms preventing oral intake.[59-61]

The use of peritoneal lavage at preoperative laparoscopy or at operation is still controversial. Several studies have demonstrated a worse survival in patients with positive results on peritoneal lavage. They found that a positive peritoneal lavage correlated with serosal invasion and lymph node involvement metastases.[62,63] The use of immunohistochemical staining further improved the ability to detect positive peritoneal washings, which also proved to be a negative prognostic variable.[62] The standard use of peritoneal cytologic evaluation in the work-up of gastric carcinoma, however, remains under investigation. Positive cytologic results should not prohibit surgical resection.

SURGICAL MANAGEMENT

The surgical therapy of gastric cancer continues to be controversial. The primary aim of operation is to perform a complete resection of all tumor, leaving no residual tumor behind. This is defined as an R0 resection. An R1 resection leaves microscopic disease, and an R2 resection leaves macroscopic disease. Continued debate and surgical trials are focused on the extent of gastrectomy and lymph node dissection.

There are two surgical options for cancers of the middle or distal stomach: total gastrectomy or subtotal (near-total) gastrectomy. Two randomized trials evaluated total versus subtotal gastrectomy as the surgical treatment in this patient population. The first study randomized 169 patients with antral carcinoma to either total or subtotal

gastrectomy. Postoperative mortality, morbidity, and 5-year survival were identical in both groups.[64] A larger trial randomized 624 patients with cancers in the distal half of the stomach to total or subtotal gastrectomy. Both groups underwent a D2 lymph node dissection (see next page for a discussion of the extent of lymph node dissection of the D component of the operation). No statistical difference in postoperative morbidity or mortality was found between the two surgical options. Therefore, we most commonly use a subtotal gastrectomy at Mayo Clinic (Fig. 1). Both groups had an increase in morbidity if a splenectomy or resection of adjacent organs (e.g., distal pancreatectomy to accomplish a D2 lymphadenectomy) was performed. Again, there was no difference in survival.[65,66]

The surgical options for proximal gastric cancers include transabdominal total gastrectomy, proximal gastrectomy, esophagogastrectomy (Ivor-Lewis procedure), and transhiatal esophagectomy with a cervical esophageal-gastric anastomosis. No randomized trials have evaluated these different surgical options. The largest prospective study compared total with proximal gastrectomy in 98 patients. Postoperative mortality and overall 5-year survival were not statistically different. The study did not address postoperative morbidity or long-term functioning after the two operations.[67]

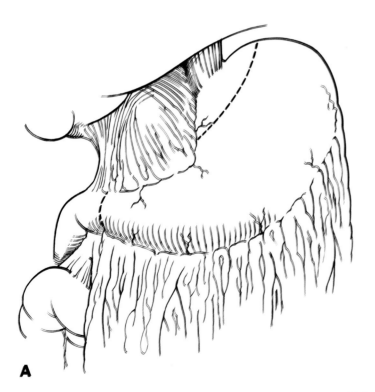

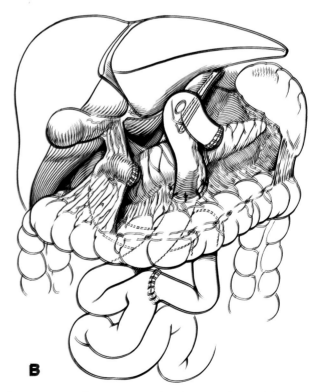

Fig. 1. **(A)**, *Margins of resection of subtotal gastrectomy.* **(B)**, *Establishment of gastrointestinal continuity with a Roux-en-Y gastrojejunostomy.*

In addition to the importance of the type of resection, the ability to obtain negative surgical margins is crucial. Traditionally, a 6-cm margin away from the grossly visible tumor was the standard surgical dogma. Investigators noted that if 6-cm margins were obtained, there was little or no risk of microscopic involvement at the margin of resection.[68] A more recent evaluation from the American College of Surgeons found that the 5-year survival rate was 35% for patients with negative margins, 13% for patients with microscopically positive margins, and 3% for those with grossly involved margins.[5] New studies reveal that margin status plays a more significant role in patients with limited lymph node involvement. In a study from the Memorial Sloan-Kettering Cancer Center, there was a significant overall survival difference favoring patients with negative margins. In subset analysis, this difference was not found in patients with more than five metastatically involved lymph nodes.[69] The attainment of negative margins probably plays a larger role in early-stage disease. The extent of negative margins is less important than obtaining negative margins. Frozen section can be useful to guide the extent of resection. The use of frozen section to determine margin status is recommended for patients undergoing gastric resection. It is used routinely at Mayo Clinic.

The extent of the lymph node dissection (D extent) has been controversial. The Japanese Research Society for Gastric Cancer classified lymph nodes into anatomical stations (Fig. 2, Table 2).[70,71] The N1 lymph nodes are located in the perigastric areas and include stations 1-6. The N1 lymph nodes are removed with D1 lymph node

Table 2.—Japanese Classification of Regional Gastric Lymph Nodes*

Perigastric lymph nodes
1. Right pericardial
2. Left pericardial
3. Lesser curvature
4. Greater curvature
5. Suprapyloric
6. Infrapyloric

Extraperigastric lymph nodes
7. Left gastric arterial
8. Common hepatic arterial
9. Celiac arterial
10. Splenic hilar
11. Splenic arterial
12. Hepatic arterial
13. Retropancreatic
14. Mesenteric root
15. Middle colic arterial
16. Para-aortic

*See Figure 2 for anatomical depiction of lymph nodes.
Modified from Kajitani.[70] By permission of the Japan Surgical Society.

dissections. The N2 lymph nodes include stations 7-11 and involve the nodes that accompany the named arteries to the stomach (common hepatic, left gastric, celiac, and splenic arteries) and splenic hilum; these are removed with D2

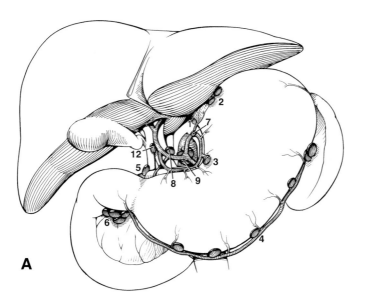

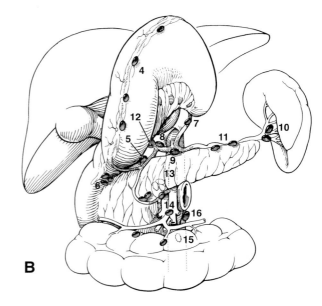

Fig. 2. Anatomical location of N1, N2, and N3 lymph nodes. (A), Anterior view. (B), Posterior view.

lymph node dissections. The N3 nodes include stations 12-16 and generally include more distant lymph nodes located in the base of the small bowel mesentery, middle colic artery, aorta, and retroperitoneum. The removal of N3 nodes is performed in Japan, but it is not routinely included in D2 dissections. Which specific lymph node stations are removed depends on the location of the primary tumor (Fig. 3 and Table 3).[71]

The rationale for an extended lymph node dissection is that it achieves an R0 resection because of clearance of the metastatic extraperigastric lymph nodes, which would not be removed with a typical perigastric resection (D1 lymph node dissection). The removal of all disease would then lead to better survival rates. An evaluation of the pattern of lymph node metastases in more than 1,900 patients demonstrated that most metastases occurred in N1 (perigastric) lymph nodes, but additional spread to the N2 lymph nodes, especially those surrounding the celiac vessels, was also common. A total of 11% of patients with positive nodes had metastases that "skipped" the level 1 (D1) perigastric nodes. On the basis of this analysis, it was proposed that a D2 resection should be performed in all patients; otherwise, metastatic disease would be missed.[72] Initial retrospective studies from Japan repeatedly revealed that patients who underwent an extended lymph node dissection had a better overall survival than those who did not.[73] Extended lymphadenectomy has become and remains the surgical standard of care for patients with gastric cancer in Japan.

Results from Japan demonstrating improved survival with a D2 lymph node dissection led to four randomized trials. A small trial from South Africa evaluated 43 patients randomized to a D1 or D2 lymph node dissection. There was no difference in overall survival, but the patients who underwent a D2 lymph node dissection had a longer

Table 3.—Lymph Node Removal According to Location of Gastric Tumor*

Lymph node group	Anatomical station of lymph nodes, by location of gastric tumor			
	Entire stomach	Lower third	Middle third	Upper third
N1[†]	1-6	3-6	1, 3-6	1-4
N2[‡]	7-11	1, 7-9	2, 7-11	5-11
N3[§]	12-14	2, 10-14	12-14	12-14

*See Figure 2 for anatomical depiction of lymph nodes.
[†]D1 dissection, removal of N1 lymph nodes.
[‡]D2 dissection, removal of N1 + N2 lymph nodes.
[§]D3 dissection, removal of N1 + N2 + N3 lymph nodes.

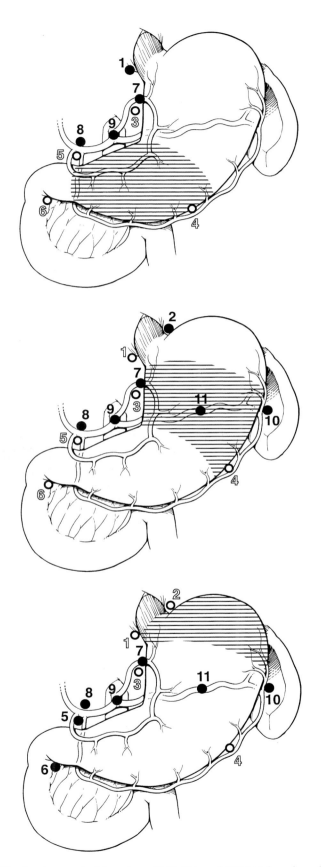

Fig. 3. Anatomical location of N1 (O) and N2 (●) lymph nodes in relation to location of primary tumor (shaded area).

operating time, more blood transfusions, longer hospital stay, and more reoperations. The authors recommended that larger trials be performed to validate their findings.[74] Another small trial performed in Hong Kong randomized 55 patients to undergo either an R1 subtotal resection with omentectomy or an R3 total gastrectomy (omentectomy, splenectomy, distal pancreatectomy, lymphatic clearance of the celiac axis, and skeletonization of the porta hepatis). The R3 group had significantly longer operating times, more transfusion requirements, longer hospital stay, and development of subphrenic abscesses. Overall survival was significantly better for patients with an R1 resection (1,511 days) than for those with an R3 resection (922 days) ($P = 0.05$).[75]

Two large European randomized trials were then performed.[76-80] The Dutch trial randomized 991 patients, 711 of whom underwent the allocated treatment, and the other patients received palliative therapy. Patients who had a D2 resection had a higher operative mortality (D2 10% vs. D1 4%, $P = 0.004$) and a higher operative morbidity (D2 43% vs. D1 25%, $P < 0.001$). Hemorrhage, anastomotic leak, and intra-abdominal infections occurred more frequently after D2 resection. Most importantly, however, was that overall survival was not different between the two groups (D2 47% and D1 45%). The increased operative mortality and morbidity were in large part related to the splenectomy and distal pancreatectomy included as part of the D2 dissection.[76,77] These investigators subsequently published a report identifying several protocol violations, which included contamination (removing selected D2 lymph nodes in patients randomized to D1 lymph node dissection) and noncompliance (not removing enough of the N2 lymph nodes during the D2 dissection). The problem with noncompliance was more common.[78] These protocol violations are not uncommon in a randomized surgical protocol but may influence the results and need to be kept in mind. This study also exemplifies the difficulty in standardizing complex surgical procedures among surgeons with varied experience.

A similar trial was performed in the United Kingdom.[79,80] Four hundred patients were randomized to a D1 or D2 lymph node dissection. Patients who underwent a D2 dissection had a higher operative mortality (D2 13% vs. D1 6.5%, $P = 0.04$) and higher operative morbidity (D2 46% vs. D1 28%, $P < 0.001$), related to a higher incidence of anastomotic leak, cardiac complications, and respiratory complications. Again, patients undergoing D2 dissections had an increased incidence of splenectomy and distal pancreatectomy, which have been implicated in the increased morbidity and mortality. Overall 5-year survival, however, was not different between the two groups (D2 33% vs. D1 35%).

In contrast, several prospective nonrandomized series have demonstrated that a D2 dissection can be performed with minimal morbidity and apparently improved overall survival. The German Gastric Carcinoma Study Group prospectively followed 2,394 patients with gastric carcinoma. Of the 1,654 patients who underwent surgical resection, 558 had a standard lymph node dissection (< 26 lymph nodes removed) and 1,096 underwent an extended lymph node dissection. Postoperative mortality was the same for both groups (5%), and postoperative morbidity did not differ either (standard 27% vs. extended 31%). The study, however, suggested an improved survival in certain subgroups, including stage II (standard 27% vs. extended 55%, $P < 0.01$) and stage IIIA (standard 25% vs. extended 38%, $P = 0.03$). There was no survival advantage for patients with stage I, stage IIIB, or stage IV disease.[81] Siewert et al.[82] reanalyzed the German data at 10 years and found that lymph node ratio and lymph node status were the most important prognostic factors in patients with resected gastric cancer. The improved survival was most pronounced in the pT2 N1 and pT3 N0 patient subgroups, in whom a more extended lymph node dissection was performed. Subsequent cytokeratin immunohistologic evaluation of the lymph node dissection of 100 patients revealed that up to 45% of the patients harbored micrometastatic disease that correlated with tumor stage. The micrometastatic disease had a negative impact on prognosis.[83]

In a study from Memorial Sloan-Kettering Cancer Center, patients with pN0 gastric carcinoma, identified from a prospective gastric database, were reevaluated. The survivals of patients who underwent a D2 or D1 resection were compared. Overall, there was no difference in survival between the two groups; however, when the patients were stratified by tumor stage, patients with a T3 tumor had improved survival if they underwent a D2 dissection (D1 39% vs. D2 54%, $P = 0.05$). The authors concluded that excision of N2 lymph nodes may remove microscopic disease and thus contribute to an improvement in survival.[84] Similar findings were demonstrated by investigators in Italy[50] who evaluated patients with gastric cancer who had potentially curative resections. Patients who were lymph node-negative and had more than 15 lymph nodes removed had a better 5-year survival than those who had a less complete lymph node dissection, 82% and 59%, respectively. This finding also supports the theory that removal of micrometastatic disease may have an important role in overall prognosis.[85]

The effect of extended lymphadenectomy was analyzed by the American Commission on Cancer. In a comparison of patients who had 15 or more lymph nodes removed with patients who had a less extensive lymphadenectomy, survival increased for those with a more extended lymph-adenectomy. The largest increase in survival (10%) occurred in patients with stage IB and II disease. If more than 25 lymph nodes were evaluated, patients with IIIB disease had a survival advantage. The difference in survival appears to be due to stage migration; the more lymph nodes evaluated, the higher the chance of finding metastatic disease and increasing the stage.[4] Most surgeons agree that an extended lymph node dissection results in more accurate staging. The extended lymph node dissection probably increases the rate of an R0 dissection. Both of these factors have a role in accurately reflecting the prognosis and removing all locoregional disease at operation.

For patients with early gastric cancer, lymph node metastases are uncommon. In patients with intramucosal tumors and submucosal tumors, lymph node metastases develop in less than 5% and 25% of cases, respectively. In both clinical situations, the incidence of N2 lymph node involvement is rare (< 5%).[86,87] Most patients with early gastric cancer are adequately treated with just a D1 resection. The patients at risk for N2 disease are those with a submucosal lesion that is larger than 2 cm; in these patients, a D2 dissection can be considered.[88]

Issues about quality of life should be addressed when discussing surgical options with patients who have gastric cancer. Overall function relating to disease-related symptoms and physical functioning seem to be better with subtotal gastrectomy than with total gastrectomy. Most patients experience better food tolerance, fewer gastrointestinal complaints, and less weight loss with a subtotal gastrectomy.[89-91] The additional D2 lymph node resection does not seem to change any quality-of-life factors.[90,92] Most authors believe, as do we at Mayo Clinic,[93,94] that a subtotal gastrectomy should be performed if the oncologic results would not be compromised. An extended lymphadenectomy has no bearing on quality of life. As demonstrated in reported randomized trials, the addition of splenectomy or distal pancreatectomy has a negative impact on postoperative morbidity and mortality, and more recent techniques allow for a splenic artery lymphadenectomy without the need for distal pancreatectomy or splenectomy.

OPERATIVE APPROACH AT MAYO CLINIC

Our current operative approach at Mayo Clinic is a subtotal gastrectomy, which removes more than half of the stomach (Fig. 1). Resection usually extends to within 2 cm of the esophagogastric junction along the lesser curvature to remove the perigastric lesser curvature nodes but to a variable location along the greater curvature, depending on the site of origin of the primary tumor (commonly just below the short gastric arteries). This extent of gastrectomy allows for preservation of the blood supply to the gastric remnant via the short gastric arteries and removal of all the D1 lymph nodes. Because the left gastric artery is divided, care needs to be taken to preserve the most proximal short gastric arteries, if possible. The number of short gastric arteries varies between 2 and 10 and, therefore, the number needs to be determined before ligation. The distal margin of resection extends just beyond the pylorus, the extent of which also varies with the location of the primary tumor, and a negative duodenal margin is confirmed by frozen-section analysis. If an extended lymph node dissection is performed (surgeon- and disease-specific), then the dissection usually begins at the gastroduodenal artery.

The dissection continues along the common and proper hepatic artery. The right gastric artery is ligated. The dissection includes all the tissue around the hepatic artery and porta hepatis and should include the area up to the bifurcation of the hepatic artery. The dissection extends to the celiac plexus and includes celiac plexus nodes. The multiple small lymphatic vessels in this area should be ligated with suture or microclips. Medially, the left gastric artery and adjacent vein are ligated at the site of origin of the artery from the celiac artery. The lymph nodes surrounding the celiac axis are removed (Fig. 4). Again, care should be taken to ligate small lymphatics in this area. The lesser and greater omenta are removed with the gastrectomy specimen. The superior leaf of the transverse mesocolon may be resected with the greater omentum. At this point, care is taken to dissect the lymph nodes along the superior border of the pancreas along the splenic artery and up to and including the splenic hilum.

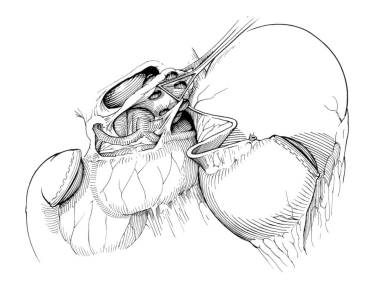

Fig. 4. Dissection of N2 lymph nodes around the hepatic artery and celiac axis.

Gastrointestinal continuity is restored with a Billroth II-like gastrojejunostomy if there is a sufficient volume remaining in the gastric remnant (usually for less than 80% gastrectomies) or with a Roux-en-Y gastrojejunostomy for more extensive subtotal gastrectomies (Fig. 1). In the latter situation, at least a 40-cm Roux limb (and probably preferably a 60-cm limb) should be used to prevent bile reflux, gastritis, and esophagitis in the postoperative period.

Most surgeons prefer the dissection to begin with mobilization of the omentum off the transverse colon. The lesser omentum is then divided at the liver. The right gastric artery is identified and divided. The duodenum is divided, and the dissection proceeds as described above. Another alternative is to mobilize the omentum and then dissect the splenic hilum and pancreatic lymph nodes (Fig. 5). The surgeon carries the dissection superiorly to the celiac axis lymph nodes, working medially around the hepatic artery toward the porta hepatis. The method of dissection should be individualized to the location of the tumor and patient's anatomy.

A total gastrectomy extends the resection to above the gastroesophageal junction for tumors located in the proximal stomach. The short gastric arteries are ligated individually, progressing upward from below. The phreno-esophageal membrane is divided on the right and left of the esophagus. Mobilization of the left lobe of the liver by division of the left triangular ligament may facilitate exposure to this area. There are many options to restore

gastrointestinal continuity. The most common is a Roux-en-Y esophagojejunostomy. Again, at least a 40- to 60-cm Roux limb is recommended. Handsewn or stapled (with a circular stapler) anastomoses appear to work equally well. Some believe that the incidence of anastomotic stricture is greater with a stapled anastomosis. Some surgeons advocate construction of a jejunal pouch after total gastrectomy; we have not been convinced that such pouches add to quality of life, and we usually do not use them.

Several studies have demonstrated that routine resection of adjacent organs does not lead to increased survival. If tumor invasion is found into adjacent organs at operation, we do consider en bloc resection, especially if it involves the spleen or transverse colon or both. Many midbody tumors necessitate a splenectomy because of technical considerations. Distal pancreatectomy is considered only if the tumor invades the distal pancreas. If there is more extensive invasion, a curative resection is not performed. Invasion into the retroperitoneum also precludes a curative resection.

ADJUVANT AND NEOADJUVANT THERAPY

One of the problems in Western countries is that most patients present with locally advanced disease. Even with an R0 resection, the rate of local and systemic recurrence is high. Because of the poor prognosis in most patients with gastric cancer, various forms of adjuvant therapy have been studied in attempts to improve prognosis.

In patients with curatively resected gastric cancers but who are at a high risk for recurrence, the use of post-operative radiation therapy alone has no impact on overall survival.[95,96] The use of intraoperative radiation also has failed to demonstrate a survival advantage.[97] Although local control rates are high for both external beam or intraoperative radiation, overall survival is not affected.

The use of adjuvant chemotherapy after R0 resection of gastric cancer has been controversial. The many phase II studies performed have had varying results. A meta-analysis of 11 studies involving more than 2,000 patients did not demonstrate a statistically significant survival benefit to adjuvant therapy, despite a slight "trend" to improved survival with adjuvant therapy.[98] A more recent meta-analysis that included 13 randomized trials in non-Asian countries did demonstrate a small but relatively unimpressive survival advantage.[99] In Japan, several studies have shown a survival advantage with adjuvant chemotherapy, and it has become standard in the East.[100] Various chemotherapy regimens have been used and include FAM (5-fluorouracil, Adriamycin [doxorubicin], mitomycin C), FAMTX (5-fluorouracil, Adriamycin, methotrexate), FEP (5-fluorouracil, etoposide, cisplatin), and FAP (5-fluorouracil, epirubicin,

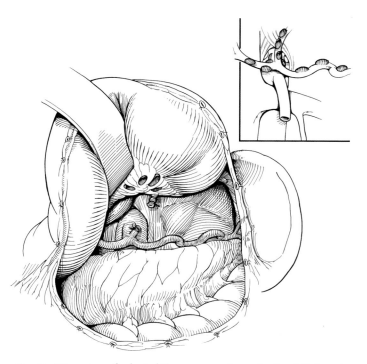

Fig. 5. Dissection of splenic hilar, pancreatic, and celiac N2 lymph nodes.

cisplatin). Newer agents, such as paclitaxel, have demonstrated a response rate in gastric cancer but have yet to be tested in an adjuvant setting.[101]

Some small phase II and phase III trials comparing adjuvant chemoradiation therapy have suggested a benefit to this approach. Recently, a large Intergroup trial randomized 603 patients with stage IB to IV, M0 gastric cancer to operation alone or to operation with postoperative chemoradiation therapy. The adjuvant regimen included 5-fluorouracil and leucovorin in combination with 4,500 cGy of radiation. After 3 years of follow-up, the study demonstrated an improvement in disease-free survival in the treatment group (49% vs. 32%, P = 0.001) and improvement in overall survival (52% vs. 41%, P = 0.03). Median survival was also significantly better in the chemoradiation group (42 months vs. 27 months).[102]

Because the majority of patients with gastric cancer in the United States and other Western countries have locally advanced disease at diagnosis, only about 50% have resectable disease at diagnosis, and those who have resection for cure have a high recurrence rate. Because of the locally advanced nature of most cases of gastric cancer, neoadjuvant (before operation) chemotherapy has been increasingly used and studied. Theoretic benefits include downstaging of the tumor to enhance resectability and possibly an increase in overall survival. Some phase II studies suggest an increased resectability rate in patients with locally advanced gastric cancer after neoadjuvant chemotherapy with various regimens.[103,104] Certain centers have found that response to chemotherapy is related to better overall survival.[104] A Dutch randomized neoadjuvant therapy trial was closed early because of poor accrual, and an interim analysis failed to suggest a difference in curative resectability rates.[105] Many centers are evaluating various neoadjuvant therapies for patients with locally advanced gastric cancer to determine whether resectability and overall survival are indeed affected. Because of the recent positive finding with use of adjuvant chemoradiation therapy, this combination treatment is also being studied at various centers in a neoadjuvant setting.

Recurrence locally and to the peritoneum are common after curative resection for gastric cancer.[106] Because of this pattern of recurrence, intraperitoneal chemotherapy as an adjuvant to surgical resection has been studied in patients at high risk. A prospective, randomized trial evaluating operation alone compared with operation and intraoperative chemotherapy did not demonstrate a difference in 5-year survival, except in a post-hoc subset analysis in which patients with stage III gastric cancer had a statistically improved overall survival when the chemotherapy was added.[107] Other groups have found more disappointing results with no improvement in survival and an increase in postoperative morbidity after intraperitoneal adjuvant chemotherapy.[108]

CURRENT APPROACH TO NEOADJUVANT AND ADJUVANT THERAPY AT MAYO CLINIC

Because of the recent studies, we refer patients for adjuvant chemoradiation if they have cancer that is T1 or higher or lymph node-positive or both. The use of neoadjuvant chemotherapy, however, is still considered investigational. Neoadjuvant chemotherapy is best used in a protocol setting. A patient who has locally advanced disease is evaluated for neoadjuvant chemotherapy. Patients placed in a protocol are those who are thought to have unresectable disease for cure at the time of initial evaluation.

LONG-TERM FOLLOW-UP

Overall survival is based on stage of disease at diagnosis. Our most recent study[93] found an overall 5-year survival rate of 48%. In a large study of patients who underwent resection for cure and had 15 lymph nodes evaluated, the 5-year survival rate based on stage was IA 95%, IB 85%, II 54%, IIIA 37%, IIIB 11%, and IV 7%.[50] Recently, the use of adjuvant chemoradiation therapy was shown to be effective, and we may begin to see overall improved survival rates in the future.[102]

Locoregional recurrence is common after the treatment of advanced gastric cancer. A study evaluating second-look laparotomy after surgical resection for advanced gastric cancer demonstrated a local and regional (lymph node) recurrence rate of 54%, and 88% of patients manifested localized peritoneal metastases.[109] A recent Japanese study of more than 2,000 patients who underwent curative operations for gastric cancer found that 508 patients had recurrence. The most common site of recurrence was the peritoneal surface (46%). Peritoneal recurrence was related to serosal invasion and lymph node metastasis at the time of initial surgical resection. Local recurrence was found in 33% of the patients. Hematogenous metastases occurred in 34% of patients; liver was the most common (19%), followed by lung (7%) and bone (7%). Extra-abdominal lymph node metastases (supraclavicular, axillary, and inguinal) were found in 5% of patients.[106]

Follow-up for patients with gastric cancer should address nutritional issues and adjustments caused by gastric resection. Most patients lose weight immediately (approximately 10% of total body weight) after operation, and the weight loss is often permanent. Diarrhea, dumping syndrome, and bile reflux are common. These symptoms are usually mild and tend to resolve with time, but occasionally these symptoms are permanent.[92,110] Certain dietary recommendations may help in the postoperative period. The patient should start a diet of pureed food and then advance slowly to a mechanically soft diet and then to a normal diet. Usually the patient starts with 6 small meals a day, and, as the body adjusts, the amount of food at each meal can be increased as the number of meals per day is decreased. Patients should concentrate on consuming protein-rich food during meals. To avoid dumping, the patient should restrict the intake of foods high in sugar content and fluid intake during meals. Rather, they should drink fluids between meals. Oral multivitamin, iron, and calcium supplements are recommended, along with lifelong vitamin B_{12} supplements. Calcium supplements are especially important in women, because a Billroth II or Roux gastrectomy bypasses the duodenum, which is the major site of calcium absorption.

There are currently no accepted standards for the follow-up of gastric cancer. Most patients are at high risk of recurrence. Operation alone usually has only a palliative role in most patients with recurrence. Recurrence is best treated with supportive care, chemotherapy, radiation, or a combination of these. Placement of intraluminal stents in patients with obstructing lesions from locally recurrent or nonoperable locally advanced disease has had good symptomatic results and minimal complications.[111]

The National Comprehensive Cancer Network published its guidelines for clinical follow-up in 1998. The recommendations are a history and physical examination every 3 months for 2 years, then every 6 months for 3 to 5 years. A complete blood count and blood chemistry studies, including liver function tests, are advised every 6 months for 3 years, and abdominal CT or endoscopy is performed as clinically indicated.[112] Whether this close follow-up will improve outcome is uncertain.

CONCLUSION

Mayo Clinic has a long history in the treatment of gastric cancer. Gastric carcinoma is still challenging for the surgeon. The cause worldwide may be related to *H. pylori* infection. Early detection is difficult because of the ambiguous nature of the symptoms. Liberal use of endoscopy in patients with dyspepsia may increase the number of patients in whom gastric cancer is diagnosed early. The disease should be diagnosed with endoscopy and biopsy, and additional staging information is gained by endoscopic ultrasonography and abdominal CT. Preoperative staging laparoscopy decreases the number of patients undergoing nontherapeutic celiotomies for unresectable disease. The combined use of all these methods helps guide clinical management.

Even though the extent of operation is still controversial, a curative (R0) resection is essential for long-term survival. The gastric resection needs to include the tumor and a negative margin of tumor-free tissue. Randomized studies have not demonstrated a survival advantage with routine D2 resection, but several prospective studies have found that removal of at least 15 lymph nodes is important in surgical therapy. Removal of 15 or more lymph nodes ensures that staging is adequate. Moreover, the data suggest that removal of lymph nodes containing microscopic disease may improve prognosis. Removal of the spleen or pancreas adds significantly to postoperative morbidity and mortality but not to survival. Patients with locally advanced disease may be considered for preoperative neoadjuvant chemoradiation. This approach may increase the resectability rate. Even when it does not, it spares patients with rapidly progressing disease from operation. The use of adjuvant chemoradiation therapy after operation is effective in selected patients. Postoperatively, all patients should be referred to an oncologist for consideration of adjuvant therapy.

REFERENCES

1. Fuchs CS, Mayer RJ: Gastric carcinoma. N Engl J Med 333:32-41, 1995
2. Jemal A, Thomas A, Murray T, Thun M: Cancer statistics, 2002. CA Cancer J Clin 52:23-47, 2002
3. Lawrence W Jr, Menck HR, Steele GD Jr, Winchester DP: The National Cancer Data Base report on gastric cancer. Cancer 75:1734-1744, 1995
4. Hundahl SA, Phillips JL, Menck HR: The National Cancer Data Base report on poor survival of U.S. gastric carcinoma patients treated with gastrectomy: Fifth Edition American Joint Committee on Cancer Staging, proximal disease, and the "different disease" hypothesis. Cancer 88:921-932, 2000
5. Wanebo HJ, Kennedy BJ, Chmiel J, Steele G Jr, Winchester D, Osteen R: Cancer of the stomach: a patient care study by the American College of Surgeons. Ann Surg 218:583-592, 1993
6. Salvon-Harman JC, Cady B, Nikulasson S, Khettry U, Stone MD, Lavin P: Shifting proportions of gastric adenocarcinomas. Arch Surg 129:381-388, 1994
7. Blot WJ, Devesa SS, Kneller RW, Fraumeni JF Jr: Rising incidence of adenocarcinoma of the esophagus and gastric cardia. JAMA 265:1287-1289, 1991
8. Staszewski J: Migrant studies in alimentary tract cancer. Rec Results Cancer Res 39:85-97, 1972
9. Kamineni A, Williams MA, Schwartz SM, Cook LS, Weiss NS: The incidence of gastric carcinoma in Asian migrants to the United States and their descendants. Cancer Causes Control 10:77-83, 1999
10. Ramon JM, Serra L, Cerdo C, Oromi J: Dietary factors and gastric cancer risk: a case-control study in Spain. Cancer 71:1731-1735, 1993
11. Ames BN: Dietary carcinogens and anticarcinogens: oxygen radicals and degenerative diseases. Science 221:1256-1264, 1983
12. Mowat C, Carswell A, Wirz A, McColl KE: Omeprazole and dietary nitrate independently affect levels of vitamin C and nitrite in gastric juice. Gastroenterology 116:813-822, 1999
13. Knekt P, Jarvinen R, Dich J, Hakulinen T: Risk of colorectal and other gastro-intestinal cancers after exposure to nitrate, nitrite and N-nitroso compounds: a follow-up study. Int J Cancer 80:852-856, 1999
14. Eichholzer M, Gutzwiller F: Dietary nitrates, nitrites, and N-nitroso compounds and cancer risk: a review of the epidemiologic evidence. Nutr Rev 56:95-105, 1998
15. Gonzalez CA, Riboli E, Badosa J, Batiste E, Cardona T, Pita S, Sanz JM, Torrent M, Agudo A: Nutritional factors and gastric cancer in Spain. Am J Epidemiol 139:466-473, 1994
16. Chyou PH, Nomura AM, Hankin JH, Stemmermann GN: A case-cohort study of diet and stomach cancer. Cancer Res 50:7501-7504, 1990
17. Botterweck AA, van den Brandt PA, Goldbohm RA: Vitamins, carotenoids, dietary fiber, and the risk of gastric carcinoma: results from a prospective study after 6.3 years of follow-up. Cancer 88:737-748, 2000
18. Zheng W, Sellers TA, Doyle TJ, Kushi LH, Potter JD, Folsom AR: Retinol, antioxidant vitamins, and cancers of the upper digestive tract in a prospective cohort study of postmenopausal women. Am J Epidemiol 142:955-960, 1995
19. Tredaniel J, Boffetta P, Buiatti E, Saracci R, Hirsch A: Tobacco smoking and gastric cancer: review and meta-analysis. Int J Cancer 72:565-573, 1997
20. Nomura A, Grove JS, Stemmermann GN, Severson RK: A prospective study of stomach cancer and its relation to diet, cigarettes, and alcohol consumption. Cancer Res 50:627-631, 1990
21. Hansson LE, Baron J, Nyren O, Bergstrom R, Wolk A, Adami HO: Tobacco, alcohol and the risk of gastric cancer: a population-based case-control study in Sweden. Int J Cancer 57:26-31, 1994
22. Antonioli DA: Gastric carcinoma and its precursors. Monogr Pathol 31:144-180, 1990
23. Brinton LA, Gridley G, Hrubec Z, Hoover R, Fraumeni JF Jr: Cancer risk following pernicious anaemia. Br J Cancer 59:810-813, 1989
24. Hsing AW, Hansson LE, McLaughlin JK, Nyren O, Blot WJ, Ekbom A, Fraumeni JF Jr: Pernicious anemia and subsequent cancer: a population-based cohort study. Cancer 71:745-750, 1993
25. Hsu CT, Ito M, Kawase Y, Sekine I, Ohmagari T, Hashimoto S: Early gastric cancer arising from localized Ménétrier's disease. Gastroenterol Jpn 26:213-217, 1991
26. Simson JN, Jass JR, McColl I: Ménétrier's disease and gastric carcinoma. J R Coll Surg Edinb 32:134-136, 1987
27. Safatle-Ribeiro AV, Ribeiro U Jr, Reynolds JC: Gastric stump cancer: What is the risk? Dig Dis 16:159-168, 1998
28. Kamiya T, Morishita T, Asakura H, Miura S, Munakata Y, Tsuchiya M: Long-term follow-up study on gastric adenoma and its relation to gastric protruded carcinoma. Cancer 50:2496-2503, 1982
29. Ginsberg GG, Al-Kawas FH, Fleischer DE, Reilly HF, Benjamin SB: Gastric polyps: relationship of size and histology to cancer risk. Am J Gastroenterol 91:714-717, 1996
30. Seifert E, Gail K, Weismuller J: Gastric polypectomy: long-term results (survey of 23 centres in Germany). Endoscopy 15:8-11, 1983
31. Iida M, Yao T, Itoh H, Watanabe H, Kohrogi N, Shigematsu A, Iwashita A, Fujishima M: Natural history of fundic gland polyposis in patients with familial adenomatosis coli/Gardner's syndrome. Gastroenterology 89:1021-1025, 1985
32. Wallace MH, Phillips RK: Upper gastrointestinal disease in patients with familial adenomatous polyposis. Br J Surg 85:742-750, 1998
33. Lynch HT, Smyrk TC, Watson P, Lanspa SJ, Lynch JF, Lynch PM, Cavalieri RJ, Boland CR: Genetics, natural history, tumor spectrum, and pathology of hereditary nonpolyposis colorectal cancer: an updated review. Gastroenterology 104:1535-1549, 1993
34. Haenszel W, Kurihara M, Locke FB, Shimuzu K, Segi M: Stomach cancer in Japan. J Natl Cancer Inst 56:265-274, 1976
35. Zanghieri G, Di Gregorio C, Sacchetti C, Fante R, Sassatelli R, Cannizzo G, Carriero A, Ponz de Leon M: Familial occurrence of gastric cancer in the 2-year experience of a population-based registry. Cancer 66:2047-2051, 1990
36. La Vecchia C, Negri E, Franceschi S, Gentile A: Family history and the risk of stomach and colorectal cancer. Cancer 70:50-55, 1992
37. Caldas C, Carneiro F, Lynch HT, Yokota J, Wiesner GL, Powell SM, Lewis FR, Huntsman DG, Pharoah PD, Jankowski JA, MacLeod P, Vogelsang H, Keller G, Park KG, Richards FM, Maher ER, Gayther SA, Oliveira C, Grehan N, Wight D, Seruca R, Roviello F, Ponder BA, Jackson CE: Familial gastric cancer: overview and guidelines for management. J Med Genet 36:873-880, 1999

38. Parsonnet J: *Helicobacter pylori*: the size of the problem. Gut 43 Suppl 1:S6-S9, 1998

39. Nomura A, Stemmermann GN, Chyou PH, Kato I, Perez-Perez GI, Blaser MJ: *Helicobacter pylori* infection and gastric carcinoma among Japanese Americans in Hawaii. N Engl J Med 325:1132-1136, 1991

40. Forman D, Newell DG, Fullerton F, Yarnell JW, Stacey AR, Wald N, Sitas F: Association between infection with *Helicobacter pylori* and risk of gastric cancer: evidence from a prospective investigation. BMJ 302:1302-1305, 1991

41. Parsonnet J, Friedman GD, Vandersteen DP, Chang Y, Vogelman JH, Orentreich N, Sibley RK: *Helicobacter pylori* infection and the risk of gastric carcinoma. N Engl J Med 325:1127-1131, 1991

42. The EUROGAST Study Group: an international association between *Helicobacter pylori* infection and gastric cancer. Lancet 341:1359-1362, 1993

43. Huang JQ, Sridhar S, Chen Y, Hunt RH: Meta-analysis of the relationship between *Helicobacter pylori* seropositivity and gastric cancer. Gastroenterology 114:1169-1179, 1998

44. Hansson LE, Nyren O, Hsing AW, Bergstrom R, Josefsson S, Chow WH, Fraumeni JF Jr, Adami HO: The risk of stomach cancer in patients with gastric or duodenal ulcer disease. N Engl J Med 335:242-249, 1996

45. Marchetti M, Arico B, Burroni D, Figura N, Rappuoli R, Ghiara P: Development of a mouse model of *Helicobacter pylori* infection that mimics human disease. Science 267:1655-1658, 1995

46. Maeda S, Ogura K, Yoshida H, Kanai F, Ikenoue T, Kato N, Shiratori Y, Omata M: Major virulence factors, VacA and CagA, are commonly positive in *Helicobacter pylori* isolates in Japan. Gut 42:338-343, 1998

47. Fleming ID, Cooper JS, Henson DE, Hutter RVP, Kennedy BJ, Murphy GP, O'Sullivan B, Sobin LH, Yarbro JW (editors): AJCC Cancer Staging Manual. Fifth edition. Philadelphia, Lippincott-Raven Publishers, 1997

48. Sobin LH, Wittekind CH (editors): TNM Classification of Malignant Tumours. Fifth edition. New York, J Wiley, 1997

49. Roder JD, Bottcher K, Busch R, Wittekind C, Hermanek P, Siewert JR: Classification of regional lymph node metastasis from gastric carcinoma. German Gastric Cancer Study Group. Cancer 82:621-631, 1998

50. Karpeh MS, Leon L, Klimstra D, Brennan MF: Lymph node staging in gastric cancer: Is location more important than number? An analysis of 1,038 patients. Ann Surg 232:362-371, 2000

51. Watanabe H, Jass JR, Sobin LH: Histological Typing of Oesophageal and Gastric Tumours. Second edition. Berlin, Springer-Verlag, 1990

52. Songun I, van de Velde CJ, Arends JW, Blok P, Grond AJ, Offerhaus GJ, Hermans J, van Krieken JH: Classification of gastric carcinoma using the Goseki system provides prognostic information additional to TNM staging. Cancer 85:2114-2118, 1999

53. Kampschoer GH, Fujii A, Masuda Y: Gastric cancer detected by mass survey: comparison between mass survey and outpatient detection. Scand J Gastroenterol 24:813-817, 1989

54. Hallissey MT, Allum WH, Jewkes AJ, Ellis DJ, Fielding JW: Early detection of gastric cancer. BMJ 301:513-515, 1990

55. Weed TE, Nuessle W, Ochsner A: Carcinoma of the stomach: Why are we failing to improve survival? Ann Surg 193:407-413, 1981

56. Posner MR, Mayer RJ: The use of serologic tumor markers in gastrointestinal malignancies. Hematol Oncol Clin North Am 8:533-553, 1994

57. Miller FH, Kochman ML, Talamonti MS, Ghahremani GG, Gore RM: Gastric cancer: radiologic staging. Radiol Clin North Am 35:331-349, 1997

58. Fukuya T, Honda H, Hayashi T, Kaneko K, Tateshi Y, Ro T, Maehara Y, Tanaka M, Tsuneyoshi M, Masuda K: Lymph-node metastases: efficacy for detection with helical CT in patients with gastric cancer. Radiology 197:705-711, 1995

59. O'Brien MG, Fitzgerald EF, Lee G, Crowley M, Shanahan F, O'Sullivan GC: A prospective comparison of laparoscopy and imaging in the staging of esophagogastric cancer before surgery. Am J Gastroenterol 90:2191-2194, 1995

60. Lowy AM, Mansfield PF, Leach SD, Ajani J: Laparoscopic staging for gastric cancer. Surgery 119:611-614, 1996

61. Burke EC, Karpeh MS, Conlon KC, Brennan MF: Laparoscopy in the management of gastric adenocarcinoma. Ann Surg 225:262-267, 1997

62. Benevolo M, Mottolese M, Cosimelli M, Tedesco M, Giannarelli D, Vasselli S, Carlini M, Garofalo A, Natali PG: Diagnostic and prognostic value of peritoneal immunocytology in gastric cancer. J Clin Oncol 16:3406-3411, 1998

63. Kodera Y, Yamamura Y, Shimizu Y, Torii A, Hirai T, Yasui K, Morimoto T, Kato T: Peritoneal washing cytology: prognostic value of positive findings in patients with gastric carcinoma undergoing a potentially curative resection. J Surg Oncol 72:60-64, 1999

64. Gouzi JL, Hufuier M, Fagniez PL, Launois B, Flamant Y, Lacaine F, Paquet JC, Hay JM: Total versus subtotal gastrectomy for adenocarcinoma of the gastric antrum: a French prospective controlled study. Ann Surg 209:162-166, 1989

65. Bozzetti F, Marubini E, Bonfanti G, Miceli R, Piano C, Crose N, Gennari L: Total versus subtotal gastrectomy: surgical morbidity and mortality rates in a multicenter Italian randomized trial. The Italian Gastrointestinal Tumor Study Group. Ann Surg 226:613-620, 1997

66. Bozzetti F, Marubini E, Bonfanti G, Miceli R, Piano C, Gennari L: Subtotal versus total gastrectomy for gastric cancer: five-year survival rates in multicenter randomized Italian trial. Italian Gastrointestinal Tumor Study Group. Ann Surg 230:170-178, 1999

67. Harrison LE, Karpeh MS, Brennan MF: Total gastrectomy is not necessary for proximal gastric cancer. Surgery 123:127-130, 1998

68. Bozzetti F, Bonfanti G, Bufalino R, Menotti V, Persano S, Andreola S, Doci R, Gennari L: Adequacy of margins of resection in gastrectomy for cancer. Ann Surg 196:685-690, 1982

69. Kim SH, Karpeh MS, Klimstra DS, Leung D, Brennan MF: Effect of microscopic resection line disease on gastric cancer survival. J Gastrointest Surg 3:24-33, 1999

70. Kajitani T: The general rules for the gastric cancer study in surgery and pathology. Part I. Clinical classification. Jpn J Surg 11:127-139, 1981

71. Behrns KE, Dalton RR, van Heerden JA, Sarr MG: Extended lymph node dissection for gastric cancer: Is it of value? Surg Clin North Am 72:433-443, 1992

72. Maruyama K, Gunven P, Okabayashi K, Sasako M, Kinoshita T: Lymph node metastases of gastric cancer: general pattern in 1931 patients. Ann Surg 210:596-602, 1989

73. Maruyama K, Okabayashi K, Kinoshita T: Progress in gastric cancer surgery in Japan and its limits of radicality. World J Surg 11:418-425, 1987

74. Dent DM, Madden MV, Price SK: Randomized comparison of R1 and R2 gastrectomy for gastric carcinoma. Br J Surg 75:110-112, 1988

75. Robertson CS, Chung SC, Woods SD, Griffin SM, Raimes SA, Lau JT, Li AK: A prospective randomized trial comparing R1 subtotal gastrectomy with R3 total gastrectomy for antral cancer. Ann Surg 220:176-182, 1994

76. Bonenkamp JJ, Songun I, Hermans J, Sasako M, Welvaart K, Plukker JT, van Elk P, Obertop H, Gouma DJ, Taac CW: Randomised comparison of morbidity after D1 and D2 dissection for gastric cancer in 996 Dutch patients. Lancet 345:745-748, 1995

77. Bonenkamp JJ, Hermans J, Sasako M, van de Velde CJ: Extended lymph-node dissection for gastric cancer. Dutch Gastric Cancer Group. N Engl J Med 340:908-914, 1999

78. Bunt AM, Hermans J, Smit VT, van de Velde CJ, Fleuren GJ, Bruijn JA: Surgical/pathologic-stage migration confounds comparisons of gastric cancer survival rates between Japan and Western countries. J Clin Oncol 13:19-25, 1995

79. Cuschieri A, Fayers P, Fielding J, Craven J, Bancewicz J, Joypaul V, Cook P: Postoperative morbidity and mortality after D1 and D2 resections for gastric cancer: preliminary results of the MRC randomised controlled surgical trial. The Surgical Cooperative Group. Lancet 347:995-999, 1996

80. Cuschieri A, Weeden S, Fielding J, Bancewicz J, Craven J, Joypaul V, Sydes M, Fayers P: Patient survival after D1 and D2 resections for gastric cancer: long-term results of the MRC randomized surgical trial. Surgical Co-operative Group. Br J Cancer 79:1522-1530, 1999

81. Siewert JR, Bottcher K, Roder JD, Busch R, Hermanek P, Meyer HJ: Prognostic relevance of systematic lymph node dissection in gastric carcinoma. German Gastric Carcinoma Study Group. Br J Surg 80:1015-1018, 1993

82. Siewert JR, Bottcher K, Stein HJ, Roder JD: Relevant prognostic factors in gastric cancer: ten-year results of the German Gastric Cancer Study. Ann Surg 228:449-461, 1998

83. Siewert JR, Kestlmeier R, Busch R, Bottcher K, Roder JD, Muller J, Fellbaum C, Hofler H: Benefits of D2 lymph node dissection for patients with gastric cancer and pN0 and pN1 lymph node metastases. Br J Surg 83:1144-1147, 1996

84. Harrison LE, Karpeh MS, Brennan MF: Extended lymph-adenectomy is associated with a survival benefit for node-negative gastric cancer. J Gastrointest Surg 2:126-131, 1998

85. Bruno L, Nesi G, Montinaro F, Carassale G, Boddi V, Bechi P, Cortesini C: Clinicopathologic characteristics and outcome indicators in node-negative gastric cancer. J Surg Oncol 74:30-32, 2000

86. Sasako M, McCulloch P, Kinoshita T, Maruyama K: New method to evaluate the therapeutic value of lymph node dissection for gastric cancer. Br J Surg 82:346-351, 1995

87. Kitamura K, Yamaguchi T, Taniguchi H, Hagiwara A, Sawai K, Takahashi T: Analysis of lymph node metastasis in early gastric cancer: rationale of limited surgery. J Surg Oncol 64:42-47, 1997

88. Tsujitani S, Oka S, Saito H, Kondo A, Ikeguchi M, Maeta M, Kaibara N: Less invasive surgery for early gastric cancer based on the low probability of lymph node metastasis. Surgery 125:148-154, 1999

89. Thybusch-Bernhardt A, Schmidt C, Kuchler T, Schmid A, Henne-Bruns D, Kremer B: Quality of life following radical surgical treatment of gastric carcinoma. World J Surg 23:503-508, 1999

90. Wu CW, Hsieh MC, Lo SS, Lui WY, P'Eng FK: Quality of life of patients with gastric adenocarcinoma after curative gastrectomy. World J Surg 21:777-782, 1997

91. Jentschura D, Winkler M, Strohmeier N, Rumstadt B, Hagmuller E: Quality-of-life after curative surgery for gastric cancer: a comparison between total gastrectomy and subtotal gastric resection. Hepatogastroenterology 44:1137-1142, 1997

92. Svedlund J, Sullivan M, Liedman B, Lundell L, Sjodin I: Quality of life after gastrectomy for gastric carcinoma: controlled study of reconstructive procedures. World J Surg 21:422-433, 1997

93. Soreide JA, van Heerden JA, Burgart LJ, Donohue JH, Sarr MG, Ilstrup DM: Surgical aspects of patients with adenocarcinoma of the stomach operated on for cure. Arch Surg 131:481-486, 1996

94. Thompson GB, van Heerden JA, Sarr MG: Adenocarcinoma of the stomach: Are we making progress? Lancet 342:713-718, 1993

95. Yu CC, Levison DA, Dunn JA, Ward LC, Demonakou M, Allum WH, Hallisey MT: Pathological prognostic factors in the second British Stomach Cancer Group trial of adjuvant therapy in resectable gastric cancer. Br J Cancer 71:1106-1110, 1995

96. Gunderson LL, Burch PA, Donohue JH: The role of irradiation as a component of combined modality treatment for gastric cancer. J Infus Chemother 5:117-124, 1995

97. Sindelar WF: Intraoperative radiotherapy in carcinoma of the stomach and pancreas. Recent Results Cancer Res 110:226-243, 1988

98. Hermans J, Bonenkamp JJ, Boon MC, Bunt AM, Ohyama S, Sasako M, Van de Velde CJ: Adjuvant therapy after curative resection for gastric cancer: meta-analysis of randomized trials. J Clin Oncol 11:1441-1447, 1993

99. Earle CC, Maroun JA: Adjuvant chemotherapy after curative resection for gastric cancer in non-Asian patients: revisiting a meta-analysis of randomised trials. Eur J Cancer 35:1059-1064, 1999

100. Nakajima T: Review of adjuvant chemotherapy for gastric cancer. World J Surg 19:570-574, 1995

101. Ajani JA, Fairweather J, Dumas P, Patt YZ, Pazdur R, Mansfield PF: Phase II study of Taxol in patients with advanced gastric carcinoma. Cancer J Sci Am 4:269-274, 1998

102. Macdonald JS, Smalley S, Benedetti J, Estes N, Haller DG, Ajani JA, Gunderson LL, Jessup M, Martenson JA Jr: Postoperative combined radiation and chemotherapy improves disease-free survival (DFS) and overall survival (OS) in resected adenocarcinoma of the stomach and GE junction. Results of Intergroup study INT-0116 (abstract). Prog/Proc Am Soc Clin Oncol 19:1A, 2000

103. Fink U, Schuhmacher C, Stein HJ, Busch R, Feussner H, Dittler HJ, Helmberger A, Bottcher K, Siewert JR: Preoperative chemotherapy for stage III-IV gastric carcinoma: feasibility, response and outcome after complete resection. Br J Surg 82:1248-1252, 1995

104. Lowy AM, Mansfield PF, Leach SD, Pazdur R, Dumas P, Ajani JA: Response to neoadjuvant chemotherapy best predicts survival after curative resection of gastric cancer. Ann Surg 229:303-308, 1999

105. Songun I, Keizer HJ, Hermans J, Klemetschitsch P, van de Velde CJH: Preoperative chemotherapy (CT) for operable gastric cancer (POCOM): results of the Dutch randomized trial (abstract). Proc Am Soc Clin Oncol 16:277A, 1997

106. Yoo CH, Noh SH, Shin DW, Choi SH, Min JS: Recurrence following curative resection for gastric carcinoma. Br J Surg 87:236-242, 2000

107. Yu W, Whang I, Suh I, Averbach A, Chang D, Sugarbaker PH: Prospective randomized trial of early postoperative intraperitoneal chemotherapy as an adjuvant to resectable gastric cancer. Ann Surg 228:347-354, 1998

108. Samel S, Singal A, Becker H, Post S: Problems with intraoperative hyperthermic peritoneal chemotherapy for advanced gastric cancer. Eur J Surg Oncol 26:222-226, 2000

109. Gunderson LL, Sosin H: Adenocarcinoma of the stomach: areas of failure in a re-operation series (second or symptomatic look). Clinicopathologic correlation and implications for adjuvant therapy. Int J Radiat Oncol Biol Phys 8:1-11, 1982

110. Liedman B: Symptoms after total gastrectomy on food intake, body composition, bone metabolism, and quality of life in gastric cancer patients—is reconstruction with a reservoir worthwhile? Nutrition 15:677-682, 1999

111. Park HS, Do YS, Suh SW, Choo SW, Lim HK, Kim SH, Shim YM, Park KC, Choo IW: Upper gastrointestinal tract malignant obstruction: initial results of palliation with a flexible covered stent. Radiology 210:865-870, 1999

112. NCCN practice guidelines for upper gastrointestinal carcinomas. National Comprehensive Cancer Network. Oncology (Huntingt) 12:179-223, 1998

Chapter 7

Primary Gastric Lymphoma

Clive S. Grant, M.D.
Thomas M. Habermann, M.D.

Primary gastric lymphoma (PGL) serves as a model to demonstrate the rather dramatic changes and advances that have occurred in non-Hodgkin's lymphoma. New entities have been defined. New classification schemes have evolved. New treatment strategies have been validated.

There is no lymphoid tissue in the normal stomach. The majority of cases of PGL continue to be classified as diffuse large-cell non-Hodgkin's lymphoma. However, with the advent of immunophenotyping, previously considered benign lymphoid infiltrates (gastric "pseudolymphoma") have been reclassified as low-grade B-cell non-Hodgkin's lymphoma. The clinicopathologic features of PGL are more closely associated in structure and function to the so-called mucosa-associated lymphoid tissue (MALT) lymphoma than to lymphomas derived from peripheral lymph nodes. The association of *Helicobacter pylori* with MALT and the use of antibiotics to treat this entity have led to a change in the paradigm of certain lymphomas. Clarifying the mechanism for development of these low-grade lymphomas has contributed to the understanding of the biology and natural history of the disease. It seems clear now that a bacterial infection is the primary cause of this malignancy, and in certain circumstances treatment with antibiotics can be successful. The diagnosis is now regularly established with upper gastrointestinal endoscopy. Systemic chemotherapy has been used in the management of PGL.

The management of PGL has been evolving. Optimal treatment of PGL has become more complex and controversial. The role of surgical resection alone, classically the keystone of treatment, has been supplanted at Mayo Clinic and elsewhere by other approaches. During the 1950s

and 1960s, the 5-year survival rate at our institution was only 50% for patients with PGL overall and 64% for those who underwent resection.[1] Subsequently, Rosen et al.[2] from Mayo Clinic found that complete excision of gastric lymphoma increased the 5-year survival rate to 75%. Still, relapse occurred too frequently, and new methods of treatment were sought.

Few prospective studies have been published, and the conclusions are sometimes conflicting.[3-6] No prospective randomized trials have been published. Many retrospective experiences have been reported, but the inclusion of widely different stages, heterogeneous histologic types, various treatment combinations, and many other factors confound resolution of treatment recommendations. Despite these limitations, considerable data exist that, when considered together, support a rational approach to diagnosis and treatment.

DEFINITION

Lymphomatous involvement of the stomach can occur in two distinctly different settings with markedly different treatments and prognoses. As part of a systemic process, involvement of the stomach by lymphoma may occur in up to 60% of cases,[7] often as a late or preterminal event. The *primary* form, first defined by Dawson et al.,[8] relates to 1) a gastric lesion without palpable superficial lymphadenopathy on initial presentation, 2) no mediastinal nodal involvement, 3) normal leukocyte and differential counts, 4) disease, if present, limited to adjacent lymph nodes, and 5) no tumor in the spleen or liver. Only this primary form is addressed in this review.

EPIDEMIOLOGY

Even though PGL accounts for less than 5% of gastric malignancies,[7,9] the incidence of PGL, the most common type of extranodal lymphoma, has been increasing in the past decade. Data from the Surveillance, Epidemiology and End Results study confirm a true increase in the incidence rates in both men and women.[10-12] The median age in most series is the sixth or seventh decade of life. The occurrence of gastric lymphoma is greater in men than in women, with a predominance in men of up to 2.1:1; women outnumbered men in only one report.[1,13]

CLINICAL FEATURES

Presenting complaints of patients with PGL are often vague and nonspecific and lack distinguishing features from gastric adenocarcinoma or even from benign peptic ulcer disease. The median duration of symptoms ranges from 4 to 15 months. The most common symptom is epigastric pain that can be associated with other symptoms, including nausea, vomiting, anorexia, early satiety, fatigue, and weight loss. Weight loss is the most common constitutional symptom.[1,14-16] In contrast to nodal lymphoma, fever and night sweats are uncommon. Epigastric pain associated with PGL can sometimes be relieved temporarily with histamine$_2$-receptor antagonists, a characteristic that further mimics benign ulcer disease. An abdominal mass has been reported to be present in approximately 25%.[17] Obstruction, perforation, and massive bleeding are uncommon presenting symptoms. Anemia from occult bleeding may be present in at least 25% of patients.

DIAGNOSIS

Because gastric lymphomas originate in the submucosal layer, they may escape detection because they do not result in a mucosal defect that can always be detected with radiographic studies or endoscopic inspection. Esophagogastroduodenoscopy is the procedure of choice for establishing the diagnosis. This procedure offers direct visualization and the possibility of a tissue diagnosis. The accuracy of diagnosis with endoscopic biopsy can surpass 90%,[18] although the rate of a positive biopsy result usually ranges from only 60% to 80%. However, even in a recent series, the initial endoscopy was nondiagnostic in 53% of patients,[19] emphasizing the need for repeated endoscopy or, less likely, laparotomy to establish the diagnosis. Multiple biopsy specimens in the range of 8 to 12 or more and deep bites are important.[20]

Upper gastrointestinal radiographs may show various abnormalities, ranging from a normal-appearing mucosa to a diffusely infiltrating lesion to a large mass with one or multiple ulcers. The appearance is not sufficiently characteristic to differentiate PGL from adenocarcinoma. Computed tomography may be normal or abnormal, demonstrating gastric wall thickening, a gastric mass, or perigastric lymphadenopathy. It often can delineate the extent of the primary tumor and regional nodal and extranodal involvement.

CLINICAL STAGING

Positive lymph nodes on both sides of the diaphragm (stage III) and any evidence of dissemination of lymphoma to non-gastrointestinal tract organs or tissues (stage IV) are findings consistent with systemic disease, not PGL. After the history, physical examination, and establishment of the diagnosis, clinical staging should encompass a complete blood count, chemistry analysis (liver and renal function, albumin, and lactate dehydrogenase), and chest radiography. Extranodal lymphomas, including those involving the gastrointestinal tract, are common in patients infected with the human immunodeficiency virus (HIV), but most of these patients have advanced-stage disease at the time of the diagnosis.[21] A bone marrow biopsy is indicated in many patients to further stage the extent of the disease. An evaluation of the head and neck to delineate concurrent involvement of Waldeyer's ring is essential to complete the evaluation of patients before therapeutic interventions.

Computed tomography is routinely used to assess the extent of the primary lesion and the presence of other nodal disease. If the results are abnormal before treatment, then computed tomography may be used to monitor treatment response. Endoscopic ultrasonography has received recent support for initial staging of PGL and is generally considered to be the most sensitive and accurate method to determine the local extent of the nodal and gastric wall disease.[22-24] After upper gastrointestinal endoscopy, the combination of computed tomography and endoscopic ultrasonography usually provides accurate enough staging information to preclude laparotomy.[25,26] However, other reports note that although the depth of tumor invasion can be accurately defined, distinguishing lymph nodes involved with lymphoma from enlarged but hyperplastic perigastric lymph nodes remains problematic. In the absence of disseminated lesions, however, the standard for differentiating stages IE and IIE of PGL remains laparotomy,[3] but surgical staging is no longer routinely used in the management of PGL. Except for isolated indications, magnetic resonance imaging, radionuclide scanning, and lymphangiography are not routinely used in the staging of PGL.

Complete clinical staging is recommended at the time of diagnosis. In one study, 54 of 158 patients with MALT lymphoma, not merely PGL, presented with disseminated disease at the time of diagnosis.[27]

PATHOLOGY

General

The pathologic classification of non-Hodgkin's lymphoma is complex. Previous classifications, including the TNM classification,[28] the Kiel classification,[29] the Working Formulation for Clinical Usage,[30] the Revised European-American Lymphoma (REAL) Classification,[31] and others, have been replaced by the World Health Organization (WHO) Classification of Neoplastic Diseases of the Hematopoietic and Lymphoid Tissues.[32] The Working Formulation had three major subdivisions: low grade (small lymphocytic), intermediate grade (diffuse large cell), and high grade. The Working Formulation did not have MALT lymphoma in the classification. Most cases were likely defined as small lymphocytic lymphoma. The Working Formulation included diffuse mixed histologic types in the intermediate-grade category, an entity not classified as such in the REAL and WHO classifications.

With these classification systems, not all categories could be directly translated from one classification system to another. Thus, interpretation of previous reports was difficult. The REAL and WHO classifications are based not only on morphologic features but also on immunohistochemical, cytogenetic, and molecular genetic data. From a practical standpoint, the WHO classification recognizes the two most common histologic types in gastric lymphoma, categorized under mature (peripheral) B-cell neoplasms: extranodal marginal zone B-cell lymphoma of MALT type and diffuse large B-cell lymphoma (Table 1).

Marginal Zone B-Cell Lymphoma of MALT Type

MALT, which closely resembles normal Peyer patches, is absent in the normal gastric mucosa. Acquired MALT may develop within the gastric mucosa in response to *H. pylori* infection.[33] MALT lymphoma has been associated with *H. pylori* infection in up to 92% of cases.[34] In lymphomas limited to mucosa and submucosa, 76% were positive for *H. pylori*, as opposed to only 48% of lymphomas invading deeper into the muscularis or beyond.[35] Cases of MALT lymphoma have shown complete regression in response to antibiotic eradication of *H. pylori*, first in five of six patients so treated in 1993[36] and then in 16 of 26 patients in subsequent series.[37,38] Eradication of *H. pylori* is first-line therapy in patients affected by low-grade B-cell MALT lymphoma.[38] However, relapse of MALT lymphoma has been reported after treatment with antibiotics.[39] Re-treatment with antibiotic regimens has been

Table 1.—Proposed WHO Classification of Lymphoid Neoplasms*

B-cell neoplasms
  Precursor B-cell neoplasm
    Precursor B-lymphoblastic leukemia/lymphoma (precursor B-cell acute lymphoblastic leukemia)
  Mature (peripheral) B-cell neoplasms
    B-cell chronic lymphocytic leukemia/small lymphocytic lymphoma
    B-cell prolymphocytic lymphoma
    Lymphoblastic lymphoma
    Splenic marginal zone B-cell lymphoma (± villous lymphocytes)
    Hairy cell leukemia
    Plasma cell myeloma/plasmacytoma
    Extranodal marginal zone B-cell lymphoma of MALT type
    Nodal marginal zone B-cell lymphoma (± monocytoid B cells)
    Follicular lymphoma
    Mantle cell lymphoma
    Diffuse large B-cell lymphoma
      Mediastinal large B-cell lymphoma
      Primary effusion lymphoma
    Burkitt's lymphoma/Burkitt's cell leukemia

MALT, mucosa-associated lymphoid tissue; WHO, World Health Organization.
B- and T-NK-cell neoplasms are grouped according to major clinical presentations (predominantly disseminated/leukemic, primary extranodal, predominantly nodal).
*T-cell and NK-cell neoplasms and Hodgkin's lymphoma are omitted from this table but are a part of the WHO classification. The most common types are in boldface.

successful. Any enthusiasm directed to prevent PGL by clearing the population of *H. pylori* is tempered by the fact that 50% of the world population is reportedly infected with the bacteria.[40] Moreover, the frequency of encountering mucosa-limited MALT lymphoma with *H. pylori* infection in the usual practice is uncommon—in one prospective study,[41] only 1 of 12 patients with PGL was so affected.

From a pathophysiologic perspective, *H. pylori* infection, which induces chronic gastritis within the gastric mucosa normally devoid of lymphoid follicles, activates an immune T-cell–mediated response from which results a gastric epithelial clonal outgrowth of low-grade B-cell MALT lymphoma. The key pathologic characteristic of these lymphomas is a lymphoepithelial lesion with unequivocal invasion and partial destruction of gastric glands or crypts by aggregates of tumor cells. These lesions are composed of plasma cells, reactive follicles, and centrocyte-like cells (Fig. 1).

The key characteristics of this disease entity are as follows.[40,42-44] Gastric MALT lymphomas are often indolent and remain localized, with a very favorable prognosis. They seldom disseminate. Monoclonality of the lymphoma cells is usually demonstrable by gene rearrangement studies.[36] Relapse of disease may occur exclusively in other sites along the gastrointestinal tract, and up to one-third of patients have multicentric areas within the stomach. Low-grade MALT lymphomas, even those traversing the gastric wall, may regress after antibiotic-based eradication of H. pylori.[45] Molecular genetic studies of MALT lymphomas show that they do not share common features of nodal lymphomas. Polymerase chain reaction (PCR) molecular analysis for mutations may enable strong suspicion of the diagnosis even before histologic changes are apparent.[46] Moreover, PCR posttreatment screening may be possible as a means of follow-up. However, ongoing mutations

have persisted in 70% to 75% of patients with MALT lymphoma in whom H. pylori was eradicated.[47,48] This finding has raised questions about the long-term efficacy of antibiotic treatment alone for low-grade B-cell MALT lymphoma. Histologic transformation may occur with progression into a high-grade lymphoma.[49]

H. pylori may be detected with serum antibodies or histologic examination. In most patients with gastric MALT lymphoma, serum antibodies are detectable. However, H. pylori may be found in only 78% of patients on histologic examination.[50]

Diffuse Large B-Cell Lymphoma

Diffuse large B-cell lymphoma is the most common histologic type of PGL. It also represents about a third of all non-Hodgkin's lymphoma histologic types. It is immunohistochemically characterized by staining positive for anti-CD20 antibody and typically demonstrates light-chain restriction. MALT lymphoma may convert to diffuse large B-cell lymphoma.[51]

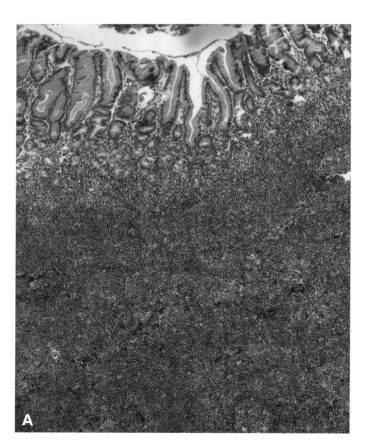
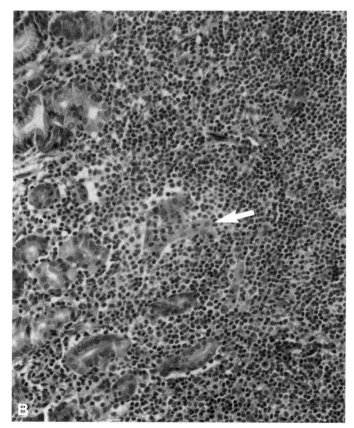

Fig. 1. Extranodal marginal zone B-cell gastric lymphoma of mucosa-associated lymphoid tissue (MALT) type. (A), Lower-power photomicrograph demonstrates typical architecture of low-grade MALT lymphoma, including presence of nonneoplastic germinal centers deep in the lesion and an infiltrate that fills the submucosa and focally impinges on mucosa. (B), Higher-power view shows cytologic characteristics of neoplastic lymphocytes. In the center of the field is a lymphoepithelial lesion (arrow), a histologic hallmark with this type of lymphoma. (This lymphoma was associated with Helicobacter pylori.)

STAGING

Staging is defined according to the Ann Arbor staging system,[52] which was subsequently modified by Musshoff (Table 2).[53] Most reports use a variant of the Ann Arbor staging system, adapted for gastric lymphomas with the letter "E" indicating extranodal origin of the tumor. Of

Table 2.—Staging System

IE	Localized involvement of one or more gastrointestinal sites on one side of the diaphragm without lymph node infiltration
	IE1 Lymphoma confined to mucosa and submucosa
	IE2 Lymphoma extending beyond submucosa
IIE	Localized involvement of one or more gastrointestinal sites on one side of the diaphragm with lymph node infiltration; any depth of lymphoma infiltration into the gut wall
	IIE1 Infiltration of regional lymph nodes
	IIE2 Infiltration of lymph nodes beyond regional area

Modified from Musshoff.[53] By permission of Urban & Vogel Medien und Medizin Verlagsgesellschaft mbH & Company.

particular importance is the depth of penetration into the gastric wall (Fig. 2) and whether involved nodes reside in proximity to the stomach or are distant. Thus, stage IIE is subdivided into those involving proximal (IIE1) and distant (IIE2) abdominal lymph nodes according to Musshoff's modification of the Ann Arbor system. This staging system has shown a good correlation with patient survival, but an adverse prognosis based on tumor involvement of the serosa or adjacent organs has caused some groups to adapt the modified TNM staging system proposed by Lim and colleagues.[54]

TREATMENT

General

The mainstay of treatment for all histologic types of PGL 25 years ago was surgical resection, and controversy revolved around the need for and advisability of adding radiation therapy. Today, the treatment of PGL has undergone a major shift. Recognizing the cause and mechanism of gastric lymphomagenesis has dramatically altered treatment algorithms. This change includes introducing

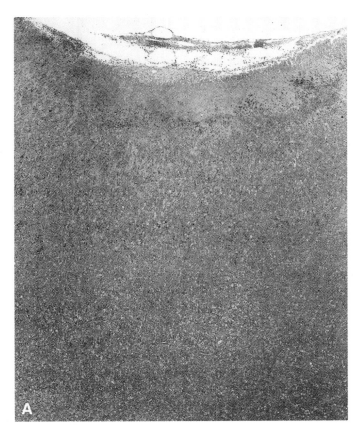 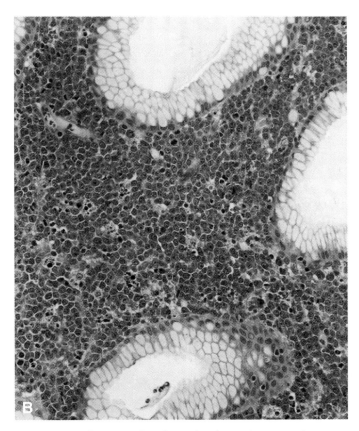

Fig. 2. Diffuse large B-cell lymphoma. (A), Transmural infiltration of gastric wall, and associated with an ulcer base. (Hematoxylin-eosin; x40.) (B), Large neoplastic lymphoid cells infiltrating between the glands of the gastric lamina propria. (Hematoxylin-eosin; x250.)

the revolutionary concept of treating a malignancy with antibiotics and using external beam radiation or chemotherapy as front-line therapy. Certainly, surgical resection retains an important role in emergency situations such as perforation and severe bleeding, but increasing emphasis on gastric-preserving treatment has gained considerable favor. The initial approach to PGL is primarily dependent on the histologic findings of the lesion.

Surgical

In addition to providing potentially curative treatment of the lymphoma, operative management provides 1) the most accurate form of staging; 2) debulking of gross disease that may be resistant to other treatments; 3) palliation of the tumor-related signs and symptoms of hemorrhage, obstruction, and perforation; and 4) a means of avoiding the bleeding or gastric rupture that can accompany tumor necrosis after radiation therapy or chemotherapy.[55-58]

In the elective setting, when the diagnosis has been firmly established, certain surgical considerations should be weighed to judge the extent of gastrectomy, the advisability of proceeding surgically at all, comorbid medical conditions, disease status, and other conditions. Paramount in these considerations, which are associated with significant morbidity, should be whether an extensive subtotal or a total gastrectomy would be required to extirpate the PGL completely. A second concern is the intraoperative decision regarding a microscopically involved surgical margin. To take full advantage of staging afforded by laparotomy, perigastric and distant nodes should usually be removed in the course of gastric resection. However, full abdominal nodal sampling, splenectomy, and liver biopsy in the absence of gross involvement are not necessary. Surgical debulking of gastric lymphomas, when gross tumor is left unresected, is not valuable.

In PGL, subtotal or total gastrectomy is frequently necessary to excise the entire tumor. Transmural invasion and adherence to adjacent organs, such as the pancreas, liver, spleen, and transverse colon, can, in selected patients, be treated with en bloc resection, but frequently these lesions are not resectable. Distal extension into the duodenum or proximally into the esophagus also may limit complete resection of the lymphoma. ReMine[59] summarized the results in nearly 700 Mayo Clinic patients with gastric lymphoma treated predominantly with extirpation, but many patients were treated with adjuvant radiation in the later postoperative years. In most series the 4-year survival in patients with PGL treated with operation alone was 50% (range, 35%-75%). Over time, it became clear that treatment other than operation, even when a curative resection had been performed, was indicated for most patients.

Stage IE1, Low-Grade MALT Lymphoma, *H. pylori*-Positive

Wotherspoon et al.[36] first reported in 1993 that eradication of *H. pylori* led to regression of low-grade gastric MALT lymphoma in five of six patients. Most importantly, these lesions had a positive gene rearrangement that converted to a negative gene rearrangement. Since that report, several other groups have confirmed this finding. In another study, acquired MALT disappeared in 21 of 25 cases, prompting the authors to conclude that "anti-*H. pylori* treatment is first-line therapy in patients affected by low-grade B-cell MALT lymphoma."[38] Other groups have reported lymphoma regression in only 60%[37] and 50%.[45] A late relapse was observed in 6 of 76 patients in one series.[60] These and other data suggest that eradication of *H. pylori* may take 12 months. Even though regression is not always complete and a response may not be documented for months, antibiotic treatment is the initial choice in gastric MALT that has not transformed into large-cell lymphoma. In most patients, disease remains in complete remission over a median follow-up of 24 months.[61]

In one study, 97 patients were treated and PCR was performed.[62] Seventy-seven patients obtained a complete endoscopic and histologic remission. Forty-four patients had PCR monoclonality at diagnosis. Twenty patients continued to have PCR monoclonality for a median of 20.5 months (range, 0-50.4 months) after a complete remission. Local relapse occurred in four patients. All four patients had monoclonal PCR before relapse, and three of the four had ongoing monoclonality throughout follow-up. These data suggest that PCR negativity may indicate cure of the disease, but half of patients continue to have long-term monoclonality. Therefore, these patients should be observed and followed closely with upper gastrointestinal endoscopy. In the study described, patients were followed every 6 months with endoscopy, which is a reasonable plan of follow-up.

The associated cytogenetic abnormalities are t(11;18)(q21;q21) and t(1;14)(p22q32).[63,64] The t(11;18) may be demonstrated by fluorescent in situ hybridization.[65] Patients with t(11;18) do not respond to *H. pylori* therapy.[66] Analysis for t(11;18) should be performed before therapeutic intervention. Patients with the translocation should be managed with other therapeutic approaches.

PGL MALT may occur in posttransplantation-related lymphomas.[67] The management of these disorders is complex.[68] At this time, *H. pylori* eradication should be the initial treatment of choice.

Stage IE1, Low-Grade MALT Lymphoma, *H. pylori* Eradication Fails or Cytogenetic Abnormalities

Gastric MALT lymphomas refractory to antibiotic therapy may be treated with radiation alone. Yahalom et al.[69] achieved a 100% complete response in 30 patients with gastric MALT lymphoma treated with a median dose of only 30 Gy. One treatment failure occurred with follow-up of 30 months. Similarly, with local therapy consisting of operation or radiation but without additional chemotherapy, 12 of 13 patients remained disease-free at 10 years, and 1 patient had a salvage treatment and a disease-free survival of 100% at 10 years.[70] Of these patients, only four received radiation alone, but the authors supported the concept of radiation in preference to operation.

Oral chemotherapy also has been shown to be efficacious in this setting.[71] Seventeen patients with stage I disease and seven with stage IV disease were treated with daily oral cyclophosphamide or chlorambucil for 12 to 24 months. The complete remission rate was 75%.

Diffuse Large B-Cell Lymphoma, Stage IE, Intermediate- and High-Grade MALT Lymphoma, *H. pylori*-Positive

From a clinical perspective, *H. pylori* eradication may result in a complete remission in approximately 75% of patients with *low-grade* MALT lymphoma with no evidence of transformation. The remission rates in primary *intermediate-* and *high-grade* B-cell gastric lymphoma after cure of *H. pylori* infection remain a question. Eight patients with high-grade lymphoma received *H. pylori* eradication therapy.[72] The effect was assessed surgically in two patients and with endoscopic biopsy in six patients. A complete remission was achieved in seven patients. In four patients, no further therapy was administered. In six patients, complete remission continued at 6 to 66 months. Further prospective trials are required. However, *H. pylori* eradication should be considered as the initial treatment.

The role of anthracycline-based doxorubicin chemotherapy was reported in diffuse large B-cell PGL in 45 patients.[73] Eleven patients received chemotherapy alone, and 34 patients received chemotherapy plus involved-field radiation therapy. In 43 patients, a complete remission was achieved. The 5-year overall disease-specific survival was 90% and the failure-free survival was 87%. Chemotherapy, with or without radiation therapy, is associated with high response rates and an excellent survival.

Currently, no randomized trials support a single specific approach in diffuse large B-cell PGL. The response rates and survival rates in selected patients are high with different therapeutic approaches. The trend is now toward systemic combination chemotherapy with cyclophosphamide (Cytoxan), doxorubicin (hydroxydaunomycin, Adriamycin), vincristine (Oncovin), and prednisone (CHOP) or with rituximab (Rituxan)-CHOP.[74,75]

Stage IE1, Resectable With Subtotal Gastrectomy, Resection Margin Negative

Data to support curative operation are abundant. In selected series of patients with stage IE disease, 5-year survival rates in excess of 80% have been reported.[54,76,77] Of 34 patients treated at Memorial Sloan-Kettering Cancer Center, 15 underwent surgical resection only, and survival was 100%.[19] In another series of 25 patients with stage IE disease treated with only resection, 3 (12%) had relapse and a complete response was achieved with salvage chemotherapy.[78] The authors suggested that for early-stage disease, operation alone will cure the majority of patients and avoid the toxic effects of systemic chemotherapy, except for patients who have relapse. Current regimens of chemotherapy are reasonably safe, but induction chemotherapy for aggressive gastrointestinal disease incurred a 6% mortality rate in one series[79] and 10% in another series.[80] However, a mortality of only 1% has been reported with CHOP.[74]

Depth of gastric wall penetration has been identified as a high-risk prognostic factor,[76,81] significantly correlating with lymph node infiltration.[82] Radaszkiewicz et al.[42] provided convincing evidence that stage IE1, with a 90% 5-year survival, has a better prognosis than stage IE2, which had only a 54% 5-year survival. This observation was further supported by Cogliatti et al.,[17] who noted that penetration beyond the serosa decreased the 5-year survival from 80% to 54%.

Surgical mortality and morbidity must be addressed. Perioperative mortality rates in recent series, however, have been highly acceptable, from 0% to 7%.[17,19,83-85] Resection of the entire stomach adversely affects nutritional status,[86] risks significant postgastrectomy sequelae with consequent deterioration in quality of life compared with subtotal gastrectomy, and may interfere with compliance with subsequent chemotherapy.[59]

Stage IE1, Resected With Subtotal Gastrectomy, Resection Margin Microscopically Positive

Involved resection margins certainly do not preclude cure in PGL, as they almost certainly would in adenocarcinoma. Whether to add radiation therapy, which, in combination with surgical resection, has been associated with an exceptional 9-year disease-free survival of 93%,[85] or chemotherapy remains debatable. Clearly, the surgical margins must not be so heavily infiltrated with tumor as to risk a safe anastomosis.

Stage IE2, IIE1, Resectable With Subtotal Gastrectomy

Patients with full-thickness gastric wall involvement or local node disease can still benefit from combination treatment with surgical resection and chemotherapy. Bartlett et al.[19] achieved a 5-year survival of 82% for stage IIE1 disease with combination treatment. However, they did note a distinct and sharp decline in survival between stage IIE1 and IIE2 disease, the latter faring more like stage III. In concurrence, 10-year survival was 47% in stage IIE1 and 0% in IIE2 in another series.[42] An improvement of 50% was estimated if operation was followed by chemotherapy in stage IIE in one report,[18] and 10-year survival was improved from 60% to 92% when chemotherapy was added to operation in another series combining stages IE and IIE disease.[18]

Two prospective nonrandomized German multicenter trials of stages IE and IIE PGL initially reported the outcome of 190 patients.[87] The data were subsequently updated.[88] The goal of these studies was to address the question of combined surgical and conservative management or conservative treatment alone. For low-grade lymphoma, IE and IIE disease were treated with either resection or total abdominal radiation (30 Gy) with a 10-Gy boost if residual disease was present or extended-field radiation (30 Gy plus 10-Gy boost). The patients with IIE disease also received six cycles of COP chemotherapy (cyclophosphamide, vincristine [Oncovin], and prednisone) before the radiation. In intermediate- and high-grade lymphoma, patients with stage IE were managed with four cycles of CHOP followed by extended-field radiation (30 Gy plus 10-Gy boost), and patients with stage IIE were treated with six cycles of CHOP and 40 Gy of radiation. At last report, 184 and 185 patients were evaluable. Histologic status did not significantly influence survival. There was no significant difference in survival between the surgically and nonsurgically managed patients. The conclusion from these two studies was that "the operative approach seems not to be advantageous compared to conservative treatment and should be critically reconsidered."

In contrast, a somewhat similar prospective multicenter study from the German-Austrian Gastrointestinal Lymphoma Study Group, studying 266 patients with PGL, concluded that "with the exception of eradication therapy in *H. pylori*-positive low-grade lymphoma of stage EI and the subgroup of locally advanced high-grade lymphoma, resection remains the treatment of choice."[89]

Stage IIE2, III, IV or Appearance That Disease of Any Stage Would Require a Total Gastrectomy

Stage IIE2 disease tends to follow a clinical course and outcome more like those of stage III disease than the more typical, localized PGL. Defining IIE2 nodes as histologically positive in the absence of more extensive distant adenopathy or stage IV involvement has usually required surgical exploration. The combination of computed tomography and endoscopic ultrasonography may provide accurate enough clinical staging to avoid laparotomy.

Also, the avoidance of a total gastrectomy in favor of gastric preservation and primary chemotherapy is an important issue.

CONCLUSION

The intriguing evidence that a malignancy has the potential to be cured by antibiotic therapy is remarkable. Radiation therapy, chemotherapy, and surgical resection all have a role in the management of the individual patient. The role of surgical resection has been reduced in the past decade. Our current treatment recommendations are summarized in Table 3.

Table 3.—Current Treatment Recommendations

Extranodal marginal zone B-cell lymphoma of MALT type
  Stage IE1, low-grade MALT lymphoma, *H. pylori*-positive
  Treatment: Antibiotic double- or triple-drug therapy to eradicate *H. pylori*
    Amoxicillin (750 mg 3 times daily), omeprazole (40 mg 3 times daily) for 2 weeks
    Metronidazole (400 mg 2 times daily), clarithromycin (250 mg 2 times daily), omeprazole (20 mg 2 times daily) for 7 days
  Stage IE1, low-grade MALT lymphoma, *H. pylori* eradication fails
  Treatment alternatives:
    Radiation
    Oral chlorambucil
    Surgical resection, including regional lymph nodes
    Anti-CD20 antibody therapy (rituximab, Rituxan)
    Cyclophosphamide and prednisone chemotherapy
Diffuse large B-cell lymphoma, mature (peripheral) B-cell neoplasm
  Stage IE1, IIE1
  Treatment considerations:
    Systemic chemotherapy as primary treatment—CHOP (cyclophosphamide, doxorubicin [hydroxydaunomycin, Adriamycin], vincristine [Oncovin], and prednisone) with or without anti-CD20 monoclonal antibody (rituximab, Rituxan)
    Surgical resection with radiation
    Surgical resection followed by chemotherapy
  Stage IIE2, III, IV or appearance that disease of any stage would require a total gastrectomy
  Treatment: Primary chemotherapy (CHOP)—with or without anti-CD20 antibody therapy

MALT, mucosa-associated lymphoid tissue.

REFERENCES

1. Burgess JN, Dockerty MB, ReMine WH: Sarcomatous lesions of the stomach. Ann Surg 173:758-766, 1971
2. Rosen CB, van Heerden JA, Martin JK Jr, Wold LE, Ilstrup DM: Is an aggressive surgical approach to the patient with gastric lymphoma warranted? Ann Surg 205:634-640, 1987
3. Ruskone-Fourmestraux A, Aegerter P, Delmer A, Brousse N, Galian A, Rambaud JC: Primary digestive tract lymphoma: a prospective multicentric study of 91 patients. Groupe d'Etude des Lymphomes Digestifs. Gastroenterology 105:1662-1671, 1993
4. Avilés A, Díaz-Maqueo JC, de la Torre A, Rodriguez L, Guzmán R, Talavera A, García EL: Is surgery necessary in the treatment of primary gastric non-Hodgkin lymphoma? Leuk Lymphoma 5:365-369, 1991
5. Steward WP, Harris M, Wagstaff J, Scarffe JH, Deakin DP, Todd ID, Crowther D: A prospective study of the treatment of high-grade histology non-Hodgkin's lymphoma involving the gastrointestinal tract. Eur J Cancer Clin Oncol 21:1195-1200, 1985
6. Sheridan WP, Medley G, Brodie GN: Non-Hodgkin's lymphoma of the stomach: a prospective pilot study of surgery plus chemotherapy in early and advanced disease. J Clin Oncol 3:495-500, 1985
7. Haber DA, Mayer RJ: Primary gastrointestinal lymphoma. Semin Oncol 15:154-169, 1988
8. Dawson IM, Cornes JS, Morson BC: Primary malignant lymphoid tumours of the intestinal tract: report of 37 cases with a study of factors influencing prognosis. Br J Surg 49:80-89, 1961
9. Frazee RC, Roberts J: Gastric lymphoma treatment: medical versus surgical. Surg Clin North Am 72:423-431, 1992
10. Severson RK, Davis S: Increasing incidence of primary gastric lymphoma. Cancer 66:1283-1287, 1990
11. Hayes J, Dunn E: Has the incidence of primary gastric lymphoma increased? Cancer 63:2073-2076, 1989
12. Schechter NR, Yahalom J: Low-grade MALT lymphoma of the stomach: a review of treatment options. Int J Radiat Oncol Biol Phys 46:1093-1103, 2000
13. Solidoro A, Payet C, Sanchez-Lihon J, Montalbetti JA: Gastric lymphomas: chemotherapy as a primary treatment. Semin Surg Oncol 6:218-225, 1990
14. Jung SS, Wieman TJ, Lindberg RD: Primary gastric lymphoma and pseudolymphoma. Am Surg 54:594-597, 1988
15. Loehr WJ, Mujahed Z, Zahn FD, Gray GF, Thorbjarnarson B: Primary lymphoma of the gastrointestinal tract: a review of 100 cases. Ann Surg 170:232-238, 1969
16. Moore I, Wright DH: Primary gastric lymphoma—a tumour of mucosa-associated lymphoid tissue: a histological and immuno-histochemical study of 36 cases. Histopathology 8:1025-1039, 1984
17. Cogliatti SB, Schmid U, Schumacher U, Eckert F, Hansmann ML, Hedderich J, Takahashi H, Lennert K: Primary B-cell gastric lymphoma: a clinicopathological study of 145 patients. Gastroenterology 101:1159-1170, 1991
18. Bozzetti F, Audisio RA, Giardini R, Gennari L: Role of surgery in patients with primary non-Hodgkin's lymphoma of the stomach: an old problem revisited. Br J Surg 80:1101-1106, 1993
19. Bartlett DL, Karpeh MS Jr, Filippa DA, Brennan MF: Long-term follow-up after curative surgery for early gastric lymphoma. Ann Surg 223:53-62, 1996
20. Lin HJ, Lee FY, Tsai YT, Lee SD, Lin CY, Tsay SH, Chiang H: A prospective evaluation of biopsy site in the diagnosis of gastric malignancy: The margin or the base? J Gastroenterol Hepatol 4:137-141, 1989
21. Safai B, Diaz B, Schwartz J: Malignant neoplasms associated with human immunodeficiency virus infection. CA Cancer J Clin 42:74-95, 1992
22. de Jong D, Aleman BM, Taal BG, Boot H: Controversies and consensus in the diagnosis, work-up and treatment of gastric lymphoma: an international survey. Ann Oncol 10:275-280, 1999
23. Caletti GC, Lorena Z, Bolondi L, Guizzardi G, Brocchi E, Barbara L: Impact of endoscopic ultrasonography on diagnosis and treatment of primary gastric lymphoma. Surgery 103:315-320, 1988
24. Taal BG, den Hartog Jager FC, Tytgat GN: The endoscopic spectrum of primary non-Hodgkin's lymphoma of the stomach. Endoscopy 19:190-192, 1987
25. Taal BG, den Hartog Jager FC, Burgers JM, van Heerde P, Tio TL: Primary non-Hodgkin's lymphoma of the stomach: changing aspects and therapeutic choices. Eur J Cancer Clin Oncol 25:439-450, 1989
26. Caletti G, Barbara L: Gastric lymphoma: Difficult to diagnose, difficult to stage? Endoscopy 25:528-530, 1993
27. Thieblemont C, Berger F, Dumontet C, Moullet I, Bouafia F, Felman P, Salles G, Coiffier B: Mucosa-associated lymphoid tissue lymphoma is a disseminated disease in one third of 158 patients analyzed. Blood 95:802-806, 2000
28. Hermanek P, Sobin LH (editors): TNM Classification of Malignant Tumours/UICC, International Union Against Cancer. Fourth edition. Berlin, Springer-Verlag, 1987
29. Stansfeld AG, Diebold J, Noel H, Kapanci Y, Rilke F, Kelenyi G, Sundstrom C, Lennert K, van Unnik JA, Mioduszewska O, Wright DH: Updated Kiel classification for lymphomas (letter to the editor). Lancet 1:292-293, 1988
30. The Non-Hodgkin's Lymphoma Pathologic Classification Project: National Cancer Institute sponsored study of classifications of non-Hodgkin's lymphomas: summary and description of a working formulation for clinical usage. Cancer 49:2112-2135, 1982
31. Harris NL, Jaffe ES, Stein H, Banks PM, Chan JK, Cleary ML, Delsol G, De Wolf-Peeters C, Falini B, Gatter KC: A revised European-American classification of lymphoid neoplasms: a proposal from the International Lymphoma Study Group. Blood 84:1361-1392, 1994
32. Harris NL, Jaffe ES, Diebold J, Flandrin G, Muller-Hermelink HK, Vardiman J, Lister TA, Bloomfield CD: World Health Organization classification of neoplastic diseases of the hematopoietic and lymphoid tissues: report of the Clinical Advisory Committee meeting—Airlie House, Virginia, November 1997. J Clin Oncol 17:3835-3849, 1999
33. Stolte M, Eidt S: Lymphoid follicles in antral mucosa: immune response to Campylobacter pylori? J Clin Pathol 42:1269-1271, 1989
34. Wotherspoon AC, Ortiz-Hidalgo C, Falzon MR, Isaacson PG: Helicobacter pylori-associated gastritis and primary B-cell gastric lymphoma. Lancet 338:1175-1176, 1991
35. Nakamura S, Yao T, Aoyagi K, Iida M, Fujishima M, Tsuneyoshi M: Helicobacter pylori and primary gastric lymphoma: a histopathologic and immunohistochemical analysis of 237 patients. Cancer 79:3-11, 1997
36. Wotherspoon AC, Doglioni C, Diss TC, Pan L, Moschini A, de Boni M, Isaacson PG: Regression of primary low-grade B-cell gastric lymphoma of mucosa-associated lymphoid tissue type after eradication of Helicobacter pylori. Lancet 342:575-577, 1993

37. Roggero E, Zucca E, Pinotti G, Pascarella A, Capella C, Savio A, Pedrinis E, Paterlini A, Venco A, Cavalli F: Eradication of *Helicobacter pylori* infection in primary low-grade gastric lymphoma of mucosa-associated lymphoid tissue. Ann Intern Med 122:767-769, 1995

38. Cammarota G, Tursi A, Montalto M, Papa A, Branca G, Vecchio FM, Renzi C, Verzi A, Armuzzi A, Pretolani S, Fedeli G, Gasbarrini G: Prevention and treatment of low-grade B-cell primary gastric lymphoma by anti-*H. pylori* therapy. J Clin Gastroenterol 21:118-122, 1995

39. Horstmann M, Erttmann R, Winkler K: Relapse of MALT lymphoma associated with *Helicobacter pylori* after antibiotic treatment. Lancet 343:1098-1099, 1994

40. Parsonnet J, Hansen S, Rodriguez L, Gelb AB, Warnke RA, Jellum E, Orentreich N, Vogelman JH, Friedman GD: *Helicobacter pylori* infection and gastric lymphoma. N Engl J Med 330:1267-1271, 1994

41. Karat D, O'Hanlon DM, Hayes N, Scott D, Raimes SA, Griffin SM: Prospective study of *Helicobacter pylori* infection in primary gastric lymphoma. Br J Surg 82:1369-1370, 1995

42. Radaszkiewicz T, Dragosics B, Bauer P: Gastrointestinal malignant lymphomas of the mucosa-associated lymphoid tissue: factors relevant to prognosis. Gastroenterology 102:1628-1638, 1992

43. Isaacson PG: Recent developments in our understanding of gastric lymphomas. Am J Surg Pathol 20 Suppl 1:S1-S7, 1996

44. Nizze H, Cogliatti SB, von Schilling C, Feller AC, Lennert K: Monocytoid B-cell lymphoma: morphological variants and relationship to low-grade B-cell lymphoma of the mucosa-associated lymphoid tissue. Histopathology 18:403-414, 1991

45. Steinbach G, Ford R, Glober G, Sample D, Hagemeister FB, Lynch PM, McLaughlin PW, Rodriguez MA, Romaguera JE, Sarris AH, Younes A, Luthra R, Manning JT, Johnson CM, Lahoti S, Shen Y, Lee JE, Winn RJ, Genta RM, Graham DY, Cabanillas FF: Antibiotic treatment of gastric lymphoma of mucosa-associated lymphoid tissue: an uncontrolled trial. Ann Intern Med 131:88-95, 1999

46. Savio A, Franzin G, Wotherspoon AC, Zamboni G, Negrini R, Buffoli F, Diss TC, Pan L, Isaacson PG: Diagnosis and posttreatment follow-up of *Helicobacter pylori*-positive gastric lymphoma of mucosa-associated lymphoid tissue: Histology, polymerase chain reaction, or both? Blood 87:1255-1260, 1996

47. Thiede C, Alpen B, Morgner A, Schmidt M, Ritter M, Ehninger G, Stolte M, Bayerdorffer E, Neubauer A: Ongoing somatic mutations and clonal expansions after cure of *Helicobacter pylori* infection in gastric mucosa-associated lymphoid tissue B-cell lymphoma. J Clin Oncol 16:3822-3831, 1998

48. Neubauer A, Thiede C, Morgner A, Alpen B, Ritter M, Neubauer B, Wundisch T, Ehninger G, Stolte M, Bayerdorffer E: Cure of *Helicobacter pylori* infection and duration of remission of low-grade gastric mucosa-associated lymphoid tissue lymphoma. J Natl Cancer Inst 89:1350-1355, 1997

49. Montalban C, Manzanal A, Castrillo JM, Escribano L, Bellas C: Low grade gastric B-cell MALT lymphoma progressing into high grade lymphoma: clonal identity of the two stages of the tumour, unusual bone involvement and leukemic dissemination. Histopathology 27:89-91, 1995

50. Eck M, Schmausser B, Greiner A, Muller-Hermelink HK: *Helicobacter pylori* in gastric mucosa-associated lymphoid tissue type lymphoma. Recent Results Cancer Res 156:9-18, 2000

51. Hsi ED, Eisbruch A, Greenson JK, Singleton TP, Ross CW, Schnitzer B: Classification of primary gastric lymphomas according to histologic features. Am J Surg Pathol 22:17-27, 1998

52. Carbone PP, Kaplan HS, Musshoff K, Smithers DW, Tubiana M: Report of the Committee on Hodgkin's Disease Staging Classification. Cancer Res 31:1860-1861, 1971

53. Musshoff K: [Clinical staging classification of non-Hodgkin's lymphomas (author's translation).] Strahlentherapie 153:218-221, 1977

54. Lim FE, Hartman AS, Tan EG, Cady B, Meissner WA: Factors in the prognosis of gastric lymphoma. Cancer 39:1715-1720, 1977

55. Bonadonna G, Valagussa P: Should lymphomas of gastrointestinal tract be treated differently from other disease presentations? Eur J Cancer Clin Oncol 22:1295-1299, 1986

56. Hande KR, Fisher RI, DeVita VT, Chabner BA, Young RC: Diffuse histiocytic lymphoma involving the gastrointestinal tract. Cancer 41:1984-1989, 1978

57. List AF, Greer JP, Cousar JC, Stein RS, Johnson DH, Reynolds VH, Greco FA, Flexner JM, Hande KR: Non-Hodgkin's lymphoma of the gastrointestinal tract: an analysis of clinical and pathologic features affecting outcome. J Clin Oncol 6:1125-1133, 1988

58. Talamonti MS, Dawes LG, Joehl RJ, Nahrwold DL: Gastrointestinal lymphoma: a case for primary surgical resection. Arch Surg 125:972-976, 1990

59. ReMine SG: Abdominal lymphoma: role of surgery. Surg Clin North Am 65:301-313, 1985

60. Savio A, Zamboni G, Capelli P, Negrini R, Santandrea G, Scarpa A, Fuini A, Pasini F, Ambrosetti A, Paterlini A, Buffoli F, Angelini GP, Cesari P, Rolfi F, Graffeo M, Pascarella A, Valli M, Mombello A, Ederle A, Franzin G: Relapse of low-grade gastric MALT lymphoma after *Helicobacter pylori* eradication: True relapse or persistence? Long-term post-treatment follow-up of a multicenter trial in the north-east of Italy and evaluation of the diagnostic protocol's adequacy. Recent Results Cancer Res 156:116-124, 2000

61. Kuipers EJ: *Helicobacter pylori* and the risk and management of associated diseases: gastritis, ulcer disease, atrophic gastritis and gastric cancer. Aliment Pharmacol Ther 11 Suppl 1:71-88, 1997

62. Thiede C, Wundisch T, Alpen B, Neubauer B, Morgner A, Schmitz M, Ehninger G, Stolte M, Bayerdorffer E, Neubauer A: Long-term persistence of monoclonal B cells after cure of *Helicobacter pylori* infection and complete histologic remission in gastric mucosa-associated lymphoid tissue B-cell lymphoma. J Clin Oncol 19:1600-1609, 2001

63. Levine EG, Arthur DC, Machnicki J, Frizzera G, Hurd D, Peterson B, Gajl-Peczalska KJ, Bloomfield CD: Four new recurring translocations in non-Hodgkin lymphoma. Blood 74:1796-1800, 1989

64. Wotherspoon AC, Pan LX, Diss TC, Isaacson PG: Cytogenetic study of B-cell lymphoma of mucosa-associated lymphoid tissue. Cancer Genet Cytogenet 58:35-38, 1992

65. Remstein ED, Kurtin PJ, James CD, Wang X, Meyer RG, Dewald GW: Detection of t(11;18)(q21;q21) in extranodal marginal zone B-cell lymphomas of malt type by two-color fluorescence in situ hybridization (abstract). Mod Pathol 81:177A, 2001

66. Liu H, Ruskon-Fourmestraux A, Lavergne-Slove A, Ye H, Molina T, Bouhnik Y, Hamoudi RA, Diss TC, Dogan A, Megraud F, Rambaud JC, Du MQ, Isaacson PG: Resistance of t(11;18) positive gastric mucosa-associated lymphoid tissue lymphoma to

Helicobacter pylori eradication therapy. Lancet 357:39-40, 2001

67. Le Meur Y, Pontoizeau-Potelune N, Jaccard A, Paraf F, Leroux-Robert C: Regression of a gastric lymphoma of mucosa-associated lymphoid tissue after eradication of *Helicobacter pylori* in a kidney graft recipient. Am J Med 107:530, 1999

68. Paya CV, Fung JJ, Nalesnik MA, Kieff E, Green M, Gores G, Habermann TM, Wiesner PH, Swinnen JL, Woodle ES, Bromberg JS: Epstein-Barr virus-induced posttransplant lymphoproliferative disorders. ASTS/ASTP EBV-PTLD Task Force and The Mayo Clinic Organized International Consensus Development Meeting. Transplantation 68:1517-1525, 1999

69. Yahalom J, Schechter NR, Portlock CS: Effective treatment of MALT lymphoma of the stomach with radiation alone (abstract). Int J Radiat Oncol Biol Phys 42 Suppl:129, 1998

70. Fung CY, Grossbard ML, Linggood RM, Younger J, Flieder A, Harris NL, Graeme-Cook F: Mucosa-associated lymphoid tissue lymphoma of the stomach: long term outcome after local treatment. Cancer 85:9-17, 1999

71. Hammel P, Haioun C, Chaumette MT, Gaulard P, Divine M, Reyes F, Delchier JC: Efficacy of single-agent chemotherapy in low-grade B-cell mucosa-associated lymphoid tissue lymphoma with prominent gastric expression. J Clin Oncol 13:2524-2529, 1995

72. Morgner A, Miehlke S, Fischbach W, Schmitt W, Muller-Hermelink H, Greiner A, Thiede C, Schetelig J, Neubauer A, Stolte M, Ehninger G, Bayerdorffer E: Complete remission of primary high-grade B-cell gastric lymphoma after cure of *Helicobacter pylori* infection. J Clin Oncol 19:2041-2048, 2001

73. Pro B, Hagemeister FB, Rodriguez MA, Hess M, Romaguera J, McLaughlin P, Younes A, Sarris AH, Ha C, Cox J, Cabanillas F: Early stage primary gastric lymphoma: excellent cure rates without surgery (abstract). Prog/Proc Am Soc Clin Oncol 20:297a, 2001

74. Fisher RI, Gaynor ER, Dahlberg S, Oken MM, Grogan TM, Mize EM, Glick JH, Coltman CA Jr, Miller TP: Comparison of a standard regimen (CHOP) with three intensive chemotherapy regimens for advanced non-Hodgkin's lymphoma. N Engl J Med 328:1002-1006, 1993

75. Miller TP, Dahlberg S, Cassady JR, Adelstein DJ, Spier CM, Grogan TM, LeBlanc M, Carlin S, Chase E, Fisher RI: Chemotherapy alone compared with chemotherapy plus radiotherapy for localized intermediate- and high-grade non-Hodgkin's lymphoma. N Engl J Med 339:21-26, 1998

76. Weingrad DN, Decosse JJ, Sherlock P, Straus D, Lieberman PH, Filippa DA. Primary gastrointestinal lymphoma: a 30-year review. Cancer 49:1258-1265, 1982

77. Paulson S, Sheehan RG, Stone MJ, Frenkel EP: Large cell lymphomas of the stomach: improved prognosis with complete resection of all intrinsic gastrointestinal disease. J Clin Oncol 1:263-269, 1983

78. Jelic S, Kovcin V, Jovanovic V, Opric M, Milanovic N: Primary gastric non-Hodgkin's lymphoma localized to the gastric wall: no adjuvant treatment following radical surgery. Oncology 51:270-272, 1994

79. Maor MH, Maddux B, Osborne BM, Fuller LM, Sullivan JA, Nelson RS, Martin RG, Libshitz HI, Velasquez WS, Bennett RW: Stages IE and IIE non-Hodgkin's lymphomas of the stomach. Comparison of treatment modalities. Cancer 54:2330-2337, 1984

80. Salles G, Herbrecht R, Tilly H, Berger F, Brousse N, Gisselbrecht C, Coiffier B: Aggressive primary gastrointestinal lymphomas: review of 91 patients treated with the LNH-84 regimen. A study of the Groupe d'Etude des Lymphomes Agressifs. Am J Med 90:77-84, 1991

81. Pasini F, Ambrosetti A, Sabbioni R, Todeschini G, Santo A, Meneghini V, Perona G, Cetto GL: Postoperative chemotherapy increases the disease-free survival rate in primary gastric lymphomas stage IE and IIE. Eur J Cancer 1:33-36, 1994

82. Eidt S, Stolte M, Fischer R: Factors influencing lymph node infiltration in primary gastric malignant lymphoma of the mucosa-associated lymphoid tissue. Pathol Res Pract 190:1077-1081, 1994

83. Durr ED, Bonner JA, Strickler JG, Martenson JA, Chen MG, Habermann TM, Donohue JH, Earle JD, Grill JP: Management of stage IE primary gastric lymphoma. Acta Haematol 94:59-68, 1995

84. Roukos DH, Hottenrott C, Encke A, Baltogiannis G, Casioumis D: Primary gastric lymphomas: a clinicopathologic study with literature review. Surg Oncol 3:115-125, 1994

85. Zinzani PL, Frezza G, Bendandi M, Barbieri E, Gherlinzoni F, Neri S, Baldissera A, Salvucci M, Babini L, Tura S: Primary gastric lymphoma: a clinical and therapeutic evaluation of 82 patients. Leuk Lymphoma 19:461-466, 1995

86. Bozzetti F, Ravera E, Cozzaglio L, Dossena G, Agradi E, Bonfanti G, Koukouras D, Gennari L: Comparison of nutritional status after total or subtotal gastrectomy. Nutrition 6:371-375, 1990

87. Willich NA, Reinartz G, Horst EJ, Delker G, Reers B, Hiddemann W, Tiemann M, Parwaresch R, Grothaus-Pinke B, Kocik J, Koch P: Operative and conservative management of primary gastric lymphoma: interim results of a German multicenter study. Int J Radiat Oncol Biol Phys 46:895-901, 2000

88. Koch P, Willich N, Jen B, Tiemann M, Berdel WE: Localized primary gastric lymphoma (PGL): treatment results in 369 patients from two consecutive multicentre studies (abstract). Prog/Proc Am Soc Clin Oncol 20:297a, 2001

89. Fischbach W, Dragosics B, Kolve-Goebeler ME, Ohmann C, Greiner A, Yang Q, Bohm S, Verreet P, Horstmann O, Busch M, Duhmke E, Muller-Hermelink HK, Wilms K: Primary gastric B-cell lymphoma: results of a prospective multicenter study. The German-Austrian Gastrointestinal Lymphoma Study Group. Gastroenterology 119:1191-1202, 2000

Chapter 8

PEPTIC ULCER

Richard J. Gray, M.D.
Keith A. Kelly, M.D.

Peptic ulcers are lesions of the digestive tract caused by an imbalance between the caustic effects of acid and pepsin and the healing effects of the mucosal defense mechanisms. The disease can affect the mucosa only (gastritis, duodenitis, esophagitis), or it can extend into the submucosa and beyond (true ulceration). Approximately 300,000 to 500,000 persons are newly affected by peptic ulcer each year in the United States. Another 4 million experience persistent or recurrent peptic ulcer annually. As many as 14% of men and 11% of women in the U.S. population will be affected during their lifetimes.

The role of the surgeon in the management of peptic ulcer has been lessened dramatically by new, effective medical and endoscopic therapies for the disease. Despite this, surgeons continue to have an important role in the care of affected patients. Surgeons treating peptic ulcer must possess a thorough understanding of the pathogenesis, diagnostic methods, and therapeutic options for peptic ulcer in order to provide the most effective surgical therapy with the least morbidity.

BACKGROUND

Peptic ulcer has long been the subject of scientific investigation. Through these investigations, our understanding of this disease's pathophysiology has progressed greatly. Certain milestones are of special note. The initial report of peptic ulcer appeared in 1688.[1] In 1824, Prout was the first to identify hydrochloric acid in gastric juice,[2] and Beaumont in 1833 further detailed the presence of hydrochloric acid and defined its role in gastric digestion in his pioneering studies on his patient Alexis St. Martin.[3] Around that same time, Brodie[4]

became the first to recognize the importance of the vagal nerve in gastric secretion, and nearly 100 years later Pavlov established the pivotal role of the vagi in the cephalic phase of gastric secretion.

In 1921, Latarjet described the anatomy of the lesser curve gastric vagal branches[3] and subsequently used vagotomy in the surgical therapy of peptic ulceration. He later recognized the deleterious effects of vagotomy on gastric emptying and added gastrojejunostomy for drainage in subsequent patients. His work did not, however, gain widespread acceptance for more than 2 decades.

Many individuals theorized on the relationship between gastric acid and the genesis of peptic ulcer. Schwartz stated in the early 1900s, "No acid, no ulcer." Dragstedt and colleagues,[5] in 1951, delineated the relationship between vagal secretory function and increased acid secretion in patients with duodenal ulcers. They went on to perform truncal vagotomy for duodenal ulcer and later combined vagotomy with gastrojejunostomy, as had Latarjet before them.[6]

The history of gastrin begins with its discovery by Edkins,[7] who named it and showed its effect on acid secretion. Other investigators at the time, however, questioned Edkins' claim. They showed evidence that the stimulation of acid secretion which Edkins attributed to gastrin might have been caused by histamine, which also was present within his extracts. It was not until 1938 that Komarov[8] showed gastrin's effect to be separate from that of histamine. Zollinger and Ellison identified that the hypersecretion of acid caused by pancreatic gastrinomas resulted in severe peptic ulceration. The syndrome they described in 1955 now bears their name. Finally, in 1962, Gregory and Tracy were able to isolate gastrin and identify its chemical composition.[9]

The development of more effective medical treatment has greatly affected the management of peptic ulcer. Antacids have been used for centuries in the treatment of acid-peptic disease. A breakthrough was made in 1972 when Black and colleagues[10] identified the histamine$_2$ (H$_2$) receptor on the gastric oxyntic cell and discovered a receptor blocker that inhibited histamine-induced acid secretion. The early H$_2$-receptor antagonists had substantial side effects, but, by 1975, cimetidine, a drug with few side effects, was developed. It greatly improved the management of peptic ulcer by markedly decreasing acid secretion. Four years later, it became possible to inhibit the final common pathway of acid secretion, the "proton pump" of the oxyntic cell, with the development of another new drug, omeprazole.

Finally, true revolution in the medical therapy of peptic ulcer was brought about by the recognition in 1975 that a bacterium, *Helicobacter pylori*, has a causal role in the development of the disease. This gram-negative bacterium was found on the gastric mucosa of 80% of patients with gastric ulcer and nearly all patients with duodenal ulcer. In 1983, Warren and Marshall[11] published their landmark study characterizing the organism and its relationship to gastritis. Although there is still debate about the exact role of *H. pylori*, these discoveries and subsequent studies have led us to view much of peptic ulceration as an infectious disease.

EPIDEMIOLOGY

Before the 20th century, duodenal ulcer was unusual. Gastric ulcer was the predominant form of peptic ulcer, particularly in women. In the early 20th century, however, the incidence of duodenal ulcer increased steadily, especially in men. By the mid-1940s, it was estimated that 10% of the U.S. male population would be affected before the age of 65 years.[12] This frequency held until the mid 1960s, when decreases in the incidence and mortality were noted.[13] Subsequent studies confirmed a decrease in the incidence of peptic ulcers of nearly 50% from 1960 to 1972.[14] In Sweden, elective operations for peptic ulcer decreased from 72.1 per 100,000 persons in 1956 to 10.7 per 100,000 persons in 1986. Emergency operations declined from 12.8 per 100,000 persons to 6.4 per 100,000 persons during the same period.[15] Elective operations decreased at Mayo Clinic from 49.1 per 100,000 persons in 1956-1960 to 6.3 per 100,000 persons in 1981-1985.[16] Because peptic ulcer is a complex disease, involving multiple genetic and environmental factors, the reason for the increase and subsequent decrease in incidence is unclear.

Changes in diet, smoking habits, societal roles, and socioeconomic status and the use of ulcerogenic drugs, such as nonsteroidal anti-inflammatory drugs (NSAIDs), have all been proposed as possible factors.[17]

Some investigators have postulated that the introduction of cimetidine is responsible for the decreasing incidence of peptic ulcer in recent years. There are few data, however, to support this view. The decline in incidence antedated the use of H$_2$-receptor antagonists by at least 2 decades.[12] The decrease in operations began before the introduction of cimetidine or the fiberoptic endoscope. The majority of the decrease has been in men. Current incidence figures are approximately 400,000 new cases of duodenal ulcer per year and 90,000 new cases of gastric ulcer. The current 1-year prevalence of duodenal and gastric ulcer is 1.8%. The lifetime prevalence is 11% to 14% for men and 8% to 11% for women in the United States. The peak incidence of duodenal ulcer is in the fourth decade of life, whereas that of gastric ulcer is most commonly between the ages of 50 and 65 years.

PATHOGENESIS

Understanding the pathophysiology of peptic ulcer allows the surgeon to select appropriate therapy. Historically, the role of acid has been the focus of the pathogenesis and therapy of this disease. Indeed, central to the initiation of peptic ulceration is an imbalance between the caustic activity of acid and pepsin and the mucosal defense mechanisms. Recent discoveries have made it clear, though, that three etiologic factors cause this imbalance in the vast majority of patients with peptic ulcer: infection with *H. pylori*, the use of NSAIDs, and smoking. Zollinger-Ellison syndrome is another, less common factor.

Acid Secretion and Mucosal Defense

Knowledge of the physiology of acid secretion is essential for surgeons managing peptic ulcer. A comprehensive review of gastric secretory physiology is beyond the scope of this chapter, but certain factors are worth emphasizing. Three known substances act on specific receptors of gastric oxyntic cells to stimulate acid secretion: acetylcholine, histamine, and gastrin. Gastrin receptors also exist on the enterochromaffin-like cells within the mucosa of the stomach which, when stimulated, cause the release of histamine. Histamine acts on neighboring oxyntic cells, causing them to secrete acid. Histamine and the other two agents are synergistic rather than additive, so that stimulation by one increases the effect of stimulation by the others by more than just an additive factor. The gastric acid proton pump, H$^+$-K$^+$ adenosine triphosphatase (ATPase), is present in its active form in the canalicular membrane of the oxyntic cell. H$^+$-K$^+$ ATPase is responsible for hydrogen ion secretion and potassium ion reabsorption. This proton pump is the final common pathway for acid secretion.

A complex system of mucosal defense resists the caustic action of acid and pepsin. Surface epithelial cells secrete mucus. The unstirred layer of mucus adjacent to the epithelial surface acts as a barrier to luminal pepsin and, to a lesser extent, acid. Acid is secreted in a pulsatile fashion through channels in this mucous layer. The channels then close quickly to prevent back-diffusion. The secretion of mucus is stimulated by prostaglandins. Gastric epithelial cells also secrete bicarbonate to keep the mucous layer at a pH of approximately 7.[18] Bicarbonate secretion is stimulated by both prostaglandins and luminal acid. Markedly diminished bicarbonate secretion within the duodenal bulb is a prevalent abnormality in patients with duodenal ulcer. No alterations in bicarbonate production have been demonstrated in patients with gastric ulcer.[18] Bicarbonate secretion is dependent on the presence of bicarbonate anion at the basolateral membrane of the epithelial cell. In states of mucosal acidosis, bicarbonate secretion is impaired. This likely plays an important role in stress ulceration. Prostaglandins play a central role in mucosal defense not only through stimulation of mucus and bicarbonate secretion but also through stimulation of mucosal blood flow.[19] Gastric surfactant provides an additional layer of defense for the gastric mucosa.

In addition to these systems to prevent injury, the gastroduodenal mucosa readily repairs itself. Damage to the mucosa results in formation of a cap of gelatinous mucus, fibrin, and cellular debris, referred to as the mucoid cap. This provides an environment conducive to restitution and regeneration. Restitution is a process whereby epithelial cells migrate along the basal membrane to an area of injury. This allows healing of small defects before they become ulcerations. This process is blocked in the presence of mucosal ischemia or acidosis. Regeneration, which requires cellular proliferation, is the process by which larger mucosal defects, like ulcers, heal. This process is at least partially dependent on prostaglandins and growth factors.

Helicobacter pylori

An important causative factor in peptic ulcer disease is *H. pylori*. This organism is found in the stomachs of 90% to 95% of patients with duodenal ulcer and 70% to 90% of patients with gastric ulcer.[20-24] It is the principal cause of chronic antral gastritis.[22] This bacterium does not invade the mucosa, but it does incite an inflammatory response, chronic gastritis, which is found in virtually all patients with peptic ulcer.[25] It is associated with a decrease in the resistance of the mucous layer to acid permeation and an increase in acid and gastrin secretion.

Eradication of *H. pylori* has been shown to decrease acid secretion[26] and increase duodenal bicarbonate secretion[27] in some patients with duodenal ulcers. *H. pylori*-associated gastritis occurs in a large segment of the general population; the rate approaches 50% in persons older than 60 years. However, a clinical peptic ulcer develops in only 10% to 20% of those colonized with *H. pylori*.[28] Although other factors clearly are acting in patients with ulcers, the impact of treatment for *H. pylori* is remarkable. Eradication of the organism is associated with healing of peptic ulcers and with a rate of ulcer recurrence of less than 10%. In contrast, treatment with only acid-reducing medications results in recurrence rates of 60% to 100% once use of these medications is discontinued. *H. pylori* also appears to have a role in the development of gastric lymphoma[29] and adenocarcinoma.[30,31]

Nonsteroidal Anti-inflammatory Drugs

Chronic use of NSAIDs is associated with an 8-fold increase in the risk of duodenal ulceration and a 40-fold increase in the risk of gastric ulceration.[32,33] Thus, most NSAID-associated ulcers occur in the stomach. Approximately 20% to 25% of chronic users of NSAIDs will have mucosal ulceration at a rate of 2% to 4% per year of exposure. The risk of hemorrhage or perforation from an ulcer is increased by 300% to 700%.[34,35] NSAID-associated peptic ulcers account for 48% of all cases of nonvariceal upper gastrointestinal hemorrhage.[36] The primary mechanism of injury in NSAID-associated ulceration is inhibition of cyclooxygenase-1 (COX-1). COX-1 is the rate-limiting enzyme in the production of gastrointestinal prostaglandins, whose central role in mucosal defense was reviewed above. These prostaglandins inhibit acid secretion, increase mucosal blood flow, and promote production of mucus and bicarbonate. NSAIDs have been found to induce mucosal microvascular ischemia.

Smoking

Smoking is a risk factor for peptic ulcer disease. Smoking does not substantially alter gastric acid secretion, but it is associated with an increased risk of *H. pylori* infection in patients with and without peptic ulceration.[37] It has been found to increase the incidence and complication rates of peptic ulcers and also to retard ulcer healing and promote recurrence. The mechanism is unknown.

Zollinger-Ellison Syndrome

The constellation of a non-β islet cell tumor of the pancreas, a gastrinoma producing gastric hypersecretion, and a peptic ulceration is termed the Zollinger-Ellison syndrome, after the two men who first reported it. It can occur sporadically (80%) or as a part of the multiple endocrine neoplasia (MEN) syndrome type I (20%). Among patients with peptic ulcer, 0.1% to 1% have Zollinger-Ellison syndrome. In these patients, gastrinomas secrete gastrin in an unregulated fashion, which, in turn, stimulates the stomach to secrete acid, which causes the ulcers. This syndrome is more fully discussed in Chapter 19.

Other Etiologic Factors

Up to 20% of peptic ulcers occur in patients who are *H. pylori*-negative, have no history of NSAID use, do not smoke, and have normal serum gastrin. Some of these patients have been found to be taking NSAIDs surreptitiously, but certainly not all. Patients with duodenal and pyloric channel ulcers generally secrete more acid, both at rest and when stimulated, than healthy controls. There is, however, considerable overlap between patients and healthy subjects who do not have peptic ulceration. Moreover, no direct relationship exists between the degree of acid hypersecretion and the severity of ulcer disease. Although the role of acid in duodenal ulceration is undeniable, only about one-third of patients are true acid hypersecretors.[38] Some of these patients have hyperhistaminemia caused by systemic mastocytosis or chronic basophilic leukemia, but the majority have no known reason for their acid hypersecretion. As stated earlier, *H. pylori* may play a role in acid hypersecretion in many of these patients, and elimination of *H. pylori* causes a reduction of acid secretion to normal levels in some. Patients with gastric ulcers tend to have normal or decreased acid secretion, but the presence of acid and pepsin is still necessary to cause gastric ulceration.

Studies before the recognition of *H. pylori* suggested that genetic factors have a role in peptic ulcer disease. Much of the increased incidence of peptic ulcers within families likely is due to clustering of *H. pylori* infection. This notwithstanding, various physiologic abnormalities are found in some patients with ulcer which may be genetically determined. These include enlarged parietal cell mass, hyperpepsinogenemia, postprandial hypergastrinemia, and rapid gastric emptying. Uncommonly, several genetic diseases are associated with peptic ulceration, including systemic mastocytosis, gastrin cell hyperplasia, and MEN type I. As with other disease entities, genetic factors likely have some role in the pathogenesis of peptic ulcer, but these factors are much less important than the acquired factors discussed above.

Alterations in motility may predispose some patients to peptic ulcer. Duodenal ulceration is associated with rapid gastric emptying and slowed duodenal transit, resulting in longer exposure of the duodenal mucosa to acid and pepsin. In contrast, patients with gastric ulcer often have slow gastric emptying and longer exposure of the gastric mucosa to acid and pepsin. Duodenogastric reflux may have a role in gastric ulcer. Resting and stimulated pyloric sphincter pressure is decreased in some patients with gastric ulcer. It is theorized that this allows reflux of duodenal contents into the stomach, which produces gastritis and eventual ulceration. This remains an unproved theory, one that is disputed by the uncommon development of gastric ulcer in patients with loop gastrojejunostomy. The gastrojejunostomy often leads to copious reflux of bile and pancreatic and duodenal secretions into the stomach, and yet gastric ulcer is seldom found in this setting.

Still other factors may have lesser roles in the pathogenesis of peptic ulcer. Although there is mixed evidence, emotional stress may be related to peptic ulcers.[39,40] Corticosteroids, although not ulcerogenic themselves, increase the risk of NSAID-induced ulceration, impair ulcer healing, and mask the symptoms of perforation and penetration by peptic ulcers. Several dietary products have been shown to be mild stimulants of acid secretion, including beer, coffee, tea, colas, and milk. None of these, however, have been demonstrated to be associated with peptic ulcer. Bland diets are of no benefit in preventing or treating ulcer disease.

PRESENTATION AND DIAGNOSIS

Uncomplicated Ulcers

Peptic ulcers cause a burning or gnawing pain in the epigastrium. In gastric ulcer, the pain is often brought on by or closely follows eating. In duodenal ulcer, pain often develops several hours after a meal, when the duodenum has emptied and the ulcer crater is exposed to unbuffered gastric secretions. Food or alkali commonly relieves the pain. Whether a patient's pain is from a duodenal ulcer or a gastric ulcer cannot be reliably distinguished.

The mechanism of ulcer pain is unknown but may be due to acidic luminal contents stimulating afferent nerves within the ulcer crater or to muscular contractions passing through the ulcer producing irritation. The pain is generally chronic and recurrent. The pain in peptic ulcer is nonspecific, and the severity of pain does not correlate with the degree or even the presence of ulceration. Other common signs and symptoms include nausea, weight loss, and mild epigastric tenderness.

The diagnosis of uncomplicated peptic ulcer disease is usually straightforward. A thorough history and physical examination must be performed. The history should include questioning for NSAID use, use of tobacco, personal and family history of peptic ulceration, and factors suggesting Zollinger-Ellison syndrome. In young patients with symptoms suspicious for peptic ulcer, in whom the risk of malignancy is low, some investigators advocate a trial of therapy without further testing. In most cases, however, diagnostic testing should be undertaken.

The best initial examination in patients suspected of having peptic ulcer disease is either contrast radiography or upper gastrointestinal endoscopy. Double-contrast radiographs of the upper gastrointestinal tract detect more than 90% of gastric or duodenal ulcers. This is comparable to the sensitivity achieved with endoscopic examination. However, endoscopy has several advantages over radiography. The specificity of radiographs is approximately 92%, whereas that of upper endoscopy approaches 100%. Of gastric malignancies, 3% to 7% will appear benign on radiographs; therefore, endoscopy and biopsy are recommended for all gastric lesions. In these cases, radiography becomes superfluous. Also, at endoscopy, biopsy specimens can be obtained and examined for the presence of H. pylori and malignant cells.

After a peptic ulcer is found, further diagnostic efforts should be directed at identifying the underlying cause of the ulceration. Because H. pylori plays a central role in peptic ulcer disease, detection of this organism is important. H. pylori can be detected by breath testing, serologic antibody testing, or subjecting endoscopically obtained biopsy specimens to histologic examination or urease testing. Histologic examination can show the organisms directly or can demonstrate gastritis. Active chronic gastritis is virtually diagnostic of infection, whereas its absence excludes H. pylori. Each of the available tests has equivalent sensitivities and specificities of more than 90% in most circumstances. If a patient has been previously treated for H. pylori, serologic testing is less reliable. The breath test is less reliable if patients have been taking proton pump inhibitors within 2 weeks of the test. The rapid urease test and histologic results are less reliable if there is blood in the stomach.[41] Therefore, serologic testing should be used if hemorrhage is present and the patient has not been previously treated for H. pylori.

Many practitioners advocate empiric treatment for H. pylori in certain circumstances. With the presence of a duodenal ulcer, the chances of infection are 90% to 95%. In patients with nonvariceal upper gastrointestinal bleeding who have not been taking NSAIDs, the rate of H. pylori positivity is 96%.[42] Although empirically treating these patients saves the expense and risk of testing, this approach must be balanced against the expense and complications of the treatment. In addition, with the increased frequency of H. pylori treatment, it is likely that the epidemiologic features of H. pylori will change. Therefore, the most reasonable course is to test nearly all patients. If endoscopy is being performed, biopsy specimens should be taken for histologic or urease testing. Otherwise, breath testing or serologic testing should be done.

Patients who have no history of NSAID use, who are negative for H. pylori infection, and who have symptoms and signs suggestive of Zollinger-Ellison syndrome should have serum gastrin measurements. If the serum gastrin value is more than 1,000 pg/mL with a duodenal ulcer present, gastrinoma can be diagnosed. In those with a serum gastrin value less than 150 pg/mL, gastrinoma is rare and can be cautiously excluded in the appropriate clinical circumstances. Patients with the signs and symptoms or with a serum gastrin value of 150 to 1,000 pg/mL should undergo provocative testing with secretin. An increase in the serum gastrin value of more than 200 pg/mL after secretin is administered intravenously is 90% to 95% sensitive and more than 95% specific for gastrinoma. In patients with hypergastrinemia and no duodenal ulcer, basal acid output or pH should be measured, because achlorhydria or hypochlorhydria can increase the serum gastrin level as a result of loss of feedback inhibition of gastrin secretion by acid. For more details on the diagnosis of Zollinger-Ellison syndrome, see the later section of this chapter and Chapter 19.

Tests for levels of acid secretion are rarely indicated in patients without hypergastrinemia because of the overlap in secretory rates between patients with ulcer and controls and because secretory studies are not usually helpful for directing therapy. Similarly, tests of vagal integrity, such as the Hollander test and the sham feeding test, are indicated in only select patients, such as those who have previously undergone vagotomy but who have recurrent ulcer disease.[43]

Ulcers With Complications

Despite increasingly effective medical therapy, the incidence of ulcer complications has not been significantly reduced during the past 20 years.[44,45] In many patients, bleeding, perforation, or even obstruction occurs as the initial presentation.

Hemorrhage

Hemorrhage is the most common complication of peptic ulcer, occurring in 15% of patients. In 10% to 20% of patients, hemorrhage is the presenting symptom. It is also the most common indication for operation today and the principal cause of death from peptic ulcer. Bleeding from an ulcer spontaneously stops in 80% of patients,[12] but approximately 5% of patients with transfusion-requiring bleeding will need an operation.[46] Patients with bleeding ulcers require aggressive resuscitation, blood transfusions as necessary, and early upper gastrointestinal endoscopy. Combining these measures with an aggressive operative approach can decrease the overall mortality to less than 6%.[46,47]

Endoscopy is the most important first intervention to determine the site of hemorrhage and rule out other sources necessitating specific medical therapy, such as esophageal varices. Endoscopic localization of bleeding ulcers is helpful to distinguish gastric from duodenal sources, but we have found that the endoscopist's description of the exact location of ulcers within these organs differs from the location found by the surgeon 53% of the time.[48] Therapeutic measures for bleeding peptic ulcers are often feasible with use of the flexible endoscope. Endoscopic hemostatic procedures are indicated for active bleeding or a visible vessel at the ulcer base. The availability of therapeutic endoscopy reduces the need for transfusion[49] and the likelihood that emergency operation will be required to control the hemorrhage.[49-53] Although approximately 20% of patients with endoscopic control of hemorrhage have bleeding again, in half of these the bleeding can be controlled with another endoscopic treatment. Therapeutic endoscopy has not been shown to decrease mortality.[48,49]

Despite the ability of acid neutralization to prevent clot lysis in vitro, antacids and H_2-receptor antagonists do not decrease the risk of rebleeding in peptic ulcer.[54] Alternatively, omeprazole, a proton pump inhibitor, decreases the risk of rebleeding and the need for operation in patients with a clot or visible vessel at the ulcer base.[54] In a meta-analysis, octreotide was shown to lower slightly the risk of rebleeding from peptic ulcer in comparison with H_2-receptor antagonists or placebo.[55]

Perforation

Perforation occurs in up to 10% of patients with peptic ulcer and can be the initial presentation.[12] Peptic ulcers that penetrate the full thickness of the gastric or duodenal wall generally cause a free perforation into the peritoneal cavity. Uncommonly, an ulcer perforates into an adjacent organ and creates a fistula or sinus. Free perforation of a peptic ulcer usually causes acute abdominal pain as a result of a chemical peritonitis created by gastric or duodenal content escaping through the perforation. The pain is sudden, severe, and located in the epigastrium. It remains constant and commonly radiates to the right scapula because of a right subphrenic collection of gastric or duodenal contents. Patients who are elderly and debilitated or those taking corticosteroids may have more minor symptoms from the chemical peritonitis and present late with septic shock.

Physical examination reveals a low-grade fever and peritoneal signs. Perforated peptic ulcer must be considered in any patient with unexplained peritonitis. Free air

in the abdominal cavity is detected on plain radiographs in 67% to 80% of patients with a perforated ulcer. Uncommonly, adjacent omentum or liver seals the perforation before extensive peritoneal soiling. Patients may have atypical symptoms and an absence of free air on plain radiographs. Water-soluble upper gastrointestinal contrast radiographs can help in demonstrating a sealed perforation in these circumstances.

Obstruction

Gastric outlet obstruction occurs in 2% of patients with peptic ulcer and historically has been the indication for operation in up to 10% to 15% of patients with duodenal ulcer treated surgically.[12] Most of these patients will have intermittent symptoms of pain, bloating, early satiety, nausea, and vomiting. Others have unrelenting emesis of gastric contents and present with dehydration and hypochloremic, metabolic alkalosis. Of those with acute, unrelenting emesis who are admitted to the hospital, the majority have obstruction caused by ulcer-induced edema or impaired antral motility rather than a fixed outlet obstruction. These patients are treated with nasogastric suction, intravenous hydration, and an intravenous H_2-receptor antagonist or a proton pump inhibitor. Parenteral nutrition is instituted early because they are usually malnourished.

Endoscopy is essential to confirm the nature of the obstruction and to rule out malignancy. In addition, endoscopic dilation can relieve the obstruction in 85% of patients, and the relief is long-lasting in about half of these. Approximately 72 hours after treatment, patients are reevaluated with a saline load test. In this test, 750 mL of saline is instilled into the patient's stomach through a nasogastric tube, and 30 minutes later the nasogastric tube is returned to suction. Return of 400 mL or more of residual gastric contents suggests a fixed obstruction requiring operation. If the obstruction resolves with endoscopic dilation, a proton pump inhibitor should be prescribed, but recurrence of obstruction occurs in up to 50% of patients. Operation is advised if, after 7 to 10 days, antisecretory treatment and nasogastric suction have been unsuccessful.

MEDICAL THERAPY

The medical treatment of peptic ulcer is designed to decrease secretion or enhance mucosal defense or both. Each patient's therapy should be targeted at the underlying cause. Often, simply eliminating the pathogenic factor, e.g., *H. pylori* or NSAID use, will result in ulcer healing. However, medications can hasten the healing process.

Lifestyle Modifications

Lifestyle modifications are seemingly the simplest mode of therapy, but compliance rates are low. Cessation of smoking is clearly of great benefit for healing duodenal ulcers and probably is beneficial for gastric ulcer also.[18] Elimination of smoking also decreases the risk of ulcer recurrence. Alcohol, coffee, tea, colas, and milk all stimulate acid secretion somewhat, but there is no evidence that elimination of these or any other products from one's diet is helpful in ulcer treatment or prevention.[18]

Drug Therapy

Drug therapy for peptic ulcer disease is remarkably effective and has greatly diminished the need for surgical therapy. Chronic ulcer pain, once common, has been virtually eliminated with medical intervention. The vast array of medications available are reviewed in Table 1 and in the following text.

Antacids, the oldest drugs used, are effective. Their use is limited by the necessity of dosing four times per day and potential side effects. Low-dose antacids do not appear to have any advantage over other available medications.

Sucralfate and *bismuth* are also effective in the treatment of ulcers. Their use is limited by dosing four times per day. Neither produces any identifiable systemic side effects with short courses of treatment.

Prostaglandin analogues have a limited role because of their overall decreased effectiveness and increased side effects in comparison with other commonly used medications. The only agent in this class currently approved for use by the Food and Drug Administration is misoprostol. This agent is useful for the prevention of gastric ulceration in patients taking NSAIDs on a chronic basis.

Although the effectiveness of *anticholinergic agents* is similar or superior to that of the H_2-receptor antagonists at equivalent doses, they have many more side effects,

Table 1.—Medications for Peptic Ulcer

Class	Mechanism	Effectiveness
Antacids	Neutralize luminal acid. Stimulate mucus and HCO_3^- secretion, mucosal blood flow, prostaglandin release, and mucosal regeneration	4 weeks: DU healing 75% / GU healing 60% / 8 weeks: DU healing 85% / GU healing 85%
Sucralfate	Protective barrier, trophic effect on mucosa, binds EGF, and stimulates mucus, HCO_3^-, and PGE_2 secretion	4 weeks: DU healing 75% / GU healing 60% / 8 weeks: DU healing 85% / GU healing 85%
Colloidal bismuth	Similar to sucralfate, anti-*Helicobacter pylori* action	4 weeks: DU healing 75% / GU healing 60% / 8 weeks: DU healing 90% / GU healing 85%
Prostaglandin analogues	Stimulate mucosal blood flow and secretion of mucus and HCO_3^-. Inhibit acid secretion	Limited, except misoprostol, for prevention of ulceration in patients with chronic use of NSAIDs
Anticholinergic agents	Decrease acid secretion by inhibiting acetylcholine action at oxyntic cell muscarinic receptors	Good at high doses, but dosing is limited by side effects
H_2-Receptor antagonists	Decrease acid secretion by competitive inhibition of oxyntic cell H_2-receptor	4 weeks: DU healing 75% / GU healing 60% / 8 weeks: DU healing 90% / GU healing 85%
Proton pump inhibitors	Decrease acid secretion by binding covalently to H^+-K^+ ATPase pump, inhibiting the enzyme	4 weeks: DU healing 93% / GU healing 70% / 8 weeks: DU healing 98% / GU healing 92%

ATPase, adenosine triphosphatase; DU, duodenal ulcer; EGF, epidermal growth factor; GU, gastric ulcer; HCO_3^-, bicarbonate; NSAIDs, nonsteroidal anti-inflammatory drugs; PGE_2, prostaglandin E_2.

including urinary retention, blurred vision, dry mouth, delayed gastric emptying, and mental disturbances. These effects obviously limit the use of these agents.

The *H₂-receptor antagonists* are remarkably effective and have few side effects. The newer agents require less frequent dosing and have side effect rates of less than 3%.

The *proton pump inhibitors* are the most potent class of secretory inhibitors. These agents decrease acid secretion by 90% at standard doses (versus 37% to 68% with H₂-receptor antagonists) and by nearly 100% at higher doses.[18] The rate of minor side effects such as headache, nausea, or diarrhea is similar to that of the H₂-receptor antagonists or placebo. The risk of gastric carcinoid from use of these drugs, as described in animals, does not appear to be clinically relevant, except in patients with Zollinger-Ellison syndrome and those with chronic atrophic gastritis.

Treatment of *Helicobacter pylori*
Medical therapy of peptic ulcer should include eradicating *H. pylori* when it is present. As mentioned, this organism is found in 90% to 95% of patients with duodenal ulcer and 70% to 90% of patients with gastric ulcer.[21-24] Antibiotics generally are used in combination with bismuth or a proton pump inhibitor. Both of these medications suppress *H. pylori* without eliminating it. The effectiveness of these treatments for eradicating *H. pylori* varies from 65% to 80%. More effective are the "triple" therapies, in which bismuth and a proton pump inhibitor are used in combination with an antibiotic. These regimens clear *H. pylori* in 85% to 90% of patients.

After treatment, a urea breath test to confirm eradication of the organism is indicated in all patients with complicated peptic ulcer. Routine posttreatment testing for *H. pylori* is controversial but seems prudent given the substantial rate of treatment failures and the high risk of recurrence when the organism is not eradicated. Reinfection with *H. pylori* after eradication is uncommon, occurring at a rate of 1% per year.

Treatment of Duodenal Ulcer
The medical management of an uncomplicated duodenal ulcer entails general lifestyle modifications, as noted above, and then treatment directed at the underlying cause of the ulcer. *H. pylori*-associated ulcers are treated with one of the anti-*H. pylori* regimens outlined above. After this regimen is completed, therapy with an antisecretory drug is continued to facilitate ulcer healing.

Before recognition of the causal role of *H. pylori*, the rate of recurrent duodenal ulcer was 80% at 6 months after discontinuation of therapy. Because of this, maintenance therapy with anti-ulcer drugs was once standard. With eradication of *H. pylori*, however, recurrence rates

are less than 10% and maintenance therapy is not recommended. For NSAID-associated duodenal ulcers in patients who are *H. pylori*-negative, use of the offending medication should be discontinued, or perhaps it can be replaced with a selective COX-2 inhibitor. Antisecretory therapy is then given to facilitate ulcer healing. If use of the NSAID must be continued, a proton pump inhibitor is the most effective agent. In the unusual patient with no identifiable cause for duodenal ulcer, antisecretory therapy is given, followed by a maintenance regimen such as an H₂-receptor antagonist at bedtime.

If the patient's symptoms abate, endoscopy to ensure healing is not necessary for uncomplicated duodenal ulcer disease. If a duodenal ulcer does not heal with these regimens, *H. pylori* negativity must be ensured, and the patient should be questioned carefully for compliance. Healing then can be accomplished by prolonging treatment, converting to or increasing the dose of a proton pump inhibitor, or combining these approaches. If recurrent duodenal ulcer develops, the clinician must ensure eradication of *H. pylori* and institute maintenance H₂-receptor antagonist therapy at bedtime. If recurrent ulcer develops despite maintenance therapy (whether or not due to noncompliance) or the patient does not want chronic therapy with medications, operative therapy is indicated.

Treatment of Gastric Ulcers
Medical therapy for gastric ulcers is also remarkably effective (Table 1). An analysis of the factors influencing gastric ulcer healing reveals some differences from duodenal ulcers. With active treatment or placebo therapy, there is a strong correlation between ulcer healing and the length of observation.[56] Healing rates with placebo approach 60% by 8 weeks. Like duodenal ulcers, healing rates in gastric ulcers increase with the duration of treatment, but gastric ulcers require, on average, 2 to 4 weeks longer to heal.[56-58] This difference may be related to gastric ulcers being larger.

As in the treatment of duodenal ulcer, antisecretory medications are given to aid gastric ulcer healing, specific therapy is directed at *H. pylori,* and the use of NSAIDs is discontinued, as outlined above. If there is no identifiable cause for a gastric ulcer and the patient has a type II or a type III gastric ulcer (see Fig. 4), a maintenance antisecretory regimen should be instituted.

Follow-up endoscopy to ensure healing is essential for gastric ulcers, because up to 3% harbor malignancy,[58] which can be misdiagnosed as a benign ulcer on the basis of endoscopic appearance and even biopsy.[22] If the ulcer is not healed at 8 weeks with treatment, possible causes of resistance to treatment should be reviewed, especially noncompliance, undetected *H. pylori*, or the use of

NSAIDs. Repeat endoscopy should be done with repeat biopsies and brushings. A proton pump inhibitor should then be given at twice the standard dose for 6 to 8 weeks. If the ulcer still does not heal and the patient is a reasonable operative risk, operation is then indicated to rule out malignancy.

The patient with a recurrent gastric ulcer should have repeat endoscopy, biopsies, and brushings and a clinical review seeking reasons for the recurrence. The recurrent ulcer is treated as appropriate for a first ulcer, unless this treatment failed previously. Operative intervention is indicated when recurrence is frequent (more than 3 per year) or healing is prolonged (requiring longer than 12 weeks of treatment).

Prophylaxis for NSAID-Associated Ulcers

As noted previously, patients taking NSAIDs are at increased risk for peptic ulceration. Prevention of ulcers in these patients is important, but the risk and cost of giving prophylactic medications to the millions of people taking NSAIDs are substantial.

Misoprostol is the only agent approved by the Food and Drug Administration for the prevention of NSAID-associated peptic ulcer disease. It is the most effective medication available, being slightly superior to proton pump inhibitors. Interestingly, H_2-receptor antagonists may be the most common class of medication given to prevent NSAID-associated ulceration, but they are ineffective. The cost-effectiveness of prophylaxis with misoprostol or proton pump inhibitors is poor overall. Studies to identify which patients will benefit most are needed.

Current recommendations for patients with chronic NSAID use are to test for *H. pylori* and to treat if the organism is present. If the patient has a history of ulcer disease, prophylaxis with misoprostol is reasonable. If the patient has a history of complicated peptic ulcer disease, misoprostol is strongly indicated. If misoprostol is not tolerated, a proton pump inhibitor can be substituted. For patients with no history of ulcer disease, it is probably not cost-effective to give prophylaxis.

SURGICAL THERAPY: GENERAL APPROACH

Many patients with peptic ulcer disease treat themselves with over-the-counter medications. Of those seeking professional treatment, approximately 95% are effectively treated with pharmacologic intervention. The remaining 5% require operative intervention. Indications for elective operation for peptic ulcers include intractability, inability to exclude malignancy, and obstruction. Indications for emergency operation include severe hemorrhage and perforation.

Operative Trends

An important evolution in the operative management of peptic ulcer has occurred at Mayo Clinic and elsewhere. These changes have paralleled both the increasing knowledge of gastric physiology and the changing epidemiology of the disease. In the late 1800s and early 1900s, gastrojejunostomy was the procedure of choice for peptic ulcer in the United States and at Mayo Clinic. In fact, the success of gastroenterostomy for peptic ulcer at Mayo Clinic did much to establish the institution as a leading gastrointestinal surgical center in the early 1900s. The benefit of gastrojejunostomy likely was due to partial diversion of acidic chyme away from the ulcer and neutralization of gastric juice by refluxing jejunal contents. Likely beneficial also was the net slowing of gastric emptying that we have shown occurs with this operation.[59] However, the cumulative frequency of stomal ulcer after gastrojejunostomy reached 34% by 20 years after operation.[60]

Because of the high rate of recurrent ulcer after gastrojejunostomy, interest in gastric resection for peptic ulcer increased in the 1920s and 1930s. By the late 1930s, Walters reported that subtotal gastrectomy including the ulcer was the procedure of choice at Mayo Clinic.[61] In the 1950s, truncal vagotomy was introduced as a surgical treatment of duodenal ulcer at Mayo Clinic, based on the pioneering work of Dragstedt. In the 1950s and 1960s, vagotomy and antrectomy were used increasingly by Mayo Clinic surgeons as the role of gastrin became better understood. The concept of proximal gastric vagotomy, developed by Griffith and Harkins in dogs in 1957,[62] was applied to humans by Holle,[63] who performed the procedure with pyloromyotomy. Use of proximal gastric vagotomy without a drainage procedure was reported by Amdrup and Jensen[64] and by Johnston and Wilkinson in 1970.[65] It was first performed at Mayo Clinic in 1973. Proximal gastric vagotomy slowly increased in popularity until, by the 1980s, it had become the most common elective procedure for duodenal ulcer at Mayo Clinic. With the decrease in the frequency of peptic ulcer, the increased effectiveness of medical therapy, and the increased recognition of postvagotomy syndromes, we and others have gradually moved away from emergency anti-ulcer operations and toward treating only the complications of ulcer at operation. Operation is then followed by medical therapy.[66]

Operative Techniques

Several operations have been used in the treatment of peptic ulcer (Table 2). *Truncal vagotomy* entails mobilization of the gastroesophageal junction and identification of the anterior and posterior vagal trunks. These are then divided at the esophageal hiatus. If identification of the nerves is uncertain, a portion of each should be sent for frozen-section

Table 2.—Operations for Peptic Ulcer

Pyloroplasty*
Gastrojejunostomy*
Gastric resection
    Total
    Wedge*
    Subtotal
    Proximal
    Sleeve
    Distal*
    Gastroduodenostomy (Billroth I)
    Gastrojejunostomy (Billroth II)*
Vagotomy + antrectomy*
    Truncal* or selective vagotomy
    Billroth I or II*
Vagotomy + "drainage"*
    Truncal* or selective vagotomy
    Pyloromyotomy*
    Pyloroplasty*
    Gastrojejunostomy*
Proximal gastric vagotomy*
    With "drainage"
    Without "drainage"
    With antrectomy

*Techniques that have been performed laparoscopically.

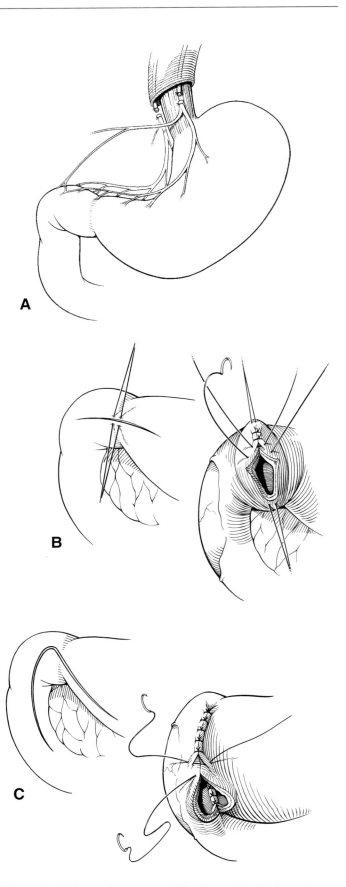

Fig. 1. (A), *Truncal vagotomy.* (B), *Heineke-Mikulicz pyloroplasty.* (C), *Finney pyloroplasty.*

analysis. If, on inspection, small accessory vagal trunks are found, they are also divided. A "drainage" procedure is then done (Fig. 1). The one we use most often is the Heineke-Mikulicz pyloroplasty. In this operation, the pylorus is divided longitudinally with the incision extending 3.5 cm onto the antrum and 3.5 cm onto the duodenum. The incision is then closed transversely with one layer of sutures to enlarge the diameter of the pylorus. In the Finney pyloroplasty, the medial proximal duodenum and the greater curve of the distal antrum are sutured together and then a curved incision is made across the pylorus to create a gastroduodenostomy with destruction of the pyloric mechanism. The Jaboulay gastroduodenostomy is similar, but, instead of a curved incision, two separate incisions are made to create a side-to-side gastroduodenostomy. The essential difference between the Jaboulay and Finney procedures is that the incision is not carried through the pylorus in the Jaboulay gastroduodenostomy. These pyloroplasties are usually used only when the pylorus is so scarred and inflamed as to prevent use of the Heineke-Mikulicz pyloroplasty. Finally, a gastrojejunostomy can be created if a pyloroplasty is not feasible.

In a *proximal gastric vagotomy* (also referred to as highly selective vagotomy, superselective vagotomy, or parietal cell vagotomy), division of vagal branches is begun 7 cm proximal to the pylorus along the lesser curve of the stomach. From this point, the blood vessels and nerves at the junction of the lesser omentum and the anterior gastric wall are divided and ligated proceeding proximally to the esophagogastric junction, and the vagal nerves to the antrum and pylorus (the nerves of Latarjet) are preserved (Fig. 2). After this step, a similar dissection is done on middle and posterior layers of vessels and nerves along the lesser curve. Then, any remaining branches at the esophagogastric junction or along the

proximal greater curve (the nerves of Grassi) are divided. Finally, the right gastroepiploic vessels are divided and ligated at the antral-corporeal junction, because recurrent vagal fibers can course along these vessels from the antrum to the corpus. Proximal gastric vagotomy is technically challenging, but it is safe and effective, including when used in surgical training programs.[67]

Selective vagotomy is rarely used at Mayo Clinic. In this operation, the vagal nerves to the stomach, including the nerves of Latarjet, are divided, but the hepatic and celiac vagal branches are preserved. This technique denervates the gastric antrum and pylorus and so results in postoperative side effects similar to those after truncal vagotomy.[68]

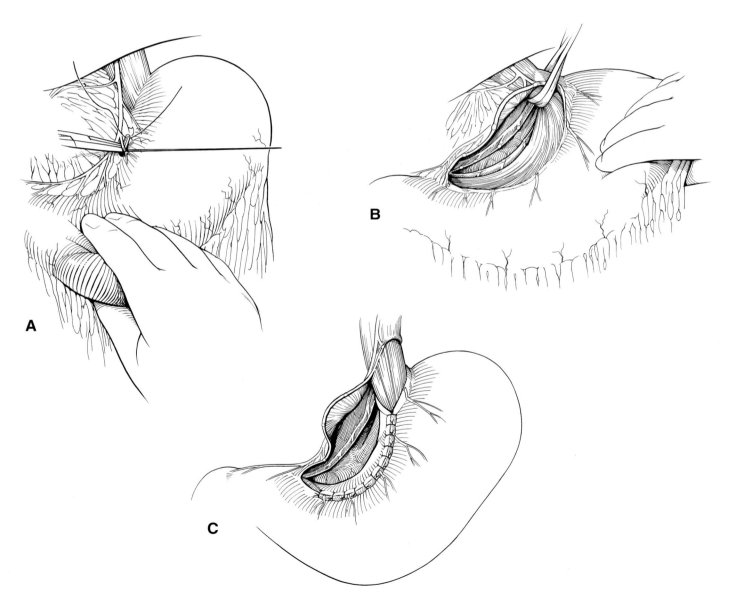

Fig. 2. Proximal gastric vagotomy. (A), *Division of neurovascular bundles to the gastric corpus along the lesser curve.* (B), *Division of all lesser curve neurovascular bundles to the gastric fundus and corpus.* (C), *Closure of gastric serosa over area of lesser curve dissection.*

Distal gastric resection, or antrectomy, can be performed alone for the treatment of gastric ulcer or added to truncal vagotomy in the treatment of duodenal ulcer. The operation is begun by mobilizing the proximal duodenum and the distal stomach. The right gastric and right gastroepiploic vessels are divided. The stomach is transected from a line just proximal to the incisura angularis to a point on the greater curve about two-thirds of the way from the esophagogastric junction to the pylorus. A 5-mm cuff of proximal duodenum is resected with the specimen. If inflammation and fibrosis make identification of the pylorus difficult, frozen-section examination of the distal margin of resection is essential. Verification of duodenal Brunner glands at the distal margin ensures that the entire distal antrum has been resected and avoids leaving antral mucosa attached to the duodenal stump. The opening at the divided end of the remaining proximal stomach is narrowed along the lesser curve with staples or sutures, after which gastrointestinal continuity is restored by anastomosing the remaining opening on the greater curve to the small intestine. If a gastroduodenostomy (Billroth I) is not feasible, the anastomosis is made to a loop of proximal jejunum (Billroth II) and the duodenal stump is closed (Fig. 3). We prefer gastroduodenostomy because it is more "physiologic" and avoids the risk of possible duodenal stump leak, afferent loop syndrome, and the retained antrum syndrome.

All of these procedures have been effectively performed laparoscopically.[69-74] Long-term results of gastric laparoscopic procedures are not known, but the current results are similar to those of open procedures. As these laparoscopic techniques are perfected and morbidity is reduced, there could be a resurgence in elective operations for peptic ulcer.

Physiologic Effects of Operation

The various forms of vagotomy are intended to eliminate acetylcholine-induced stimulation of gastric acid secretion. This effect also reduces the sensitivity of the oxyntic cells to histamine and gastrin.[75,76] The result is a reduction of 75% in basal acid output and of 50% in stimulated acid output.[77] Distal gastrectomy, or antrectomy, can be added to truncal vagotomy to decrease gastrin release and, hence, gastrin-stimulated acid production.[78] The addition of antrectomy to truncal vagotomy reduces stimulated acid secretion by 85%. Truncal vagotomy interrupts the parasympathetic innervation of the stomach, small intestine, proximal colon, and hepatobiliary tract and, therefore, causes decreases in pancreatic exocrine secretion, biliary secretion, and the release of several gastrointestinal hormones. Proximal gastric vagotomy reduces acid output to approximately the same degree as truncal vagotomy, but patients may be somewhat more susceptible to recovery of acid secretion over time.[79]

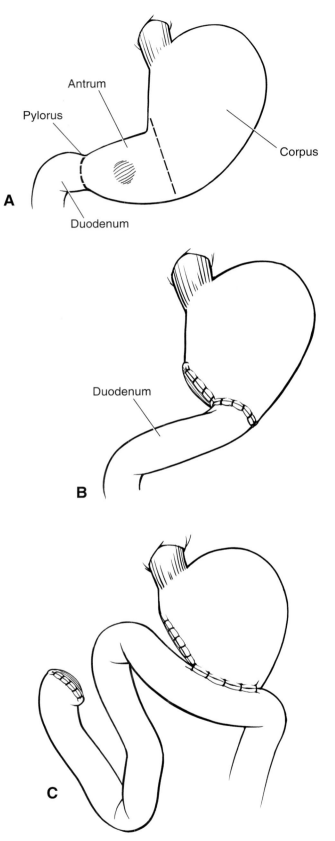

Fig. 3. Antrectomy. (A), Dotted lines outline area of resection, including the ulcer (shaded area). (B), Gastroduodenal reconstruction. (C), Gastrojejunal reconstruction.

Truncal vagotomy and proximal gastric vagotomy produce postoperative hypergastrinemia. Fasting serum gastrin levels are twice normal after operation, and the release of gastrin in response to a meal is exaggerated. The early increase is due to increased gastric luminal pH causing a loss of feedback inhibition of gastrin release. Loss of direct vagal inhibition of gastrin release also may play a role. Chronically, G-cell hyperplasia occurs and sustains the hypergastrinemia. With the addition of antrectomy, basal gastrin levels are reduced by 50% compared with preoperative levels. After antrectomy, some gastrin is still secreted by the duodenum.

Truncal vagotomy abolishes receptive relaxation and impairs accommodation and storage in the proximal stomach.[80] This produces increased intragastric pressure for a given volume of ingesta and, therefore, more rapid emptying of liquids. Further, truncal vagotomy weakens distal gastric peristalsis and impairs trituration, thus delaying the gastric emptying of solids.[81-83] These effects necessitate a "drainage" procedure. The net effect of truncal vagotomy plus any "drainage" procedure is more rapid emptying of both solids and liquids, unless a Roux-en-Y gastrojejunostomy is constructed, in which case gastric emptying is slowed.[78,84] Truncal vagotomy with antrectomy also produces more rapid emptying of liquids but variable emptying of solids. Unregulated, rapid gastric emptying predisposes patients to the dumping syndrome and diarrhea.[85] In addition, patients who have had vagotomy and antrectomy have an increased risk of duodenogastric or jejunogastric reflux. This can lead to bilious vomiting, gastritis, and possibly an increased risk of gastric cancer. Alkaline reflux gastritis occurs in 5% to 15% of patients after antrectomy or "drainage" procedures.[86] The following procedures are listed in order of highest to lowest incidence of reflux gastritis: Billroth II gastrojejunostomy, loop gastrojejunostomy, Billroth I gastroduodenostomy, and pyloroplasty. The denervation of the hepatobiliary tract, the pancreas, and the small and proximal large intestine increases the risk of gallstones, pancreatic insufficiency, and rapid intestinal transit,[85] respectively.

We have shown that proximal gastric vagotomy decreases receptive relaxation, accommodation, and storage in the proximal stomach, just as truncal vagotomy does.[87] Thus, proximal gastric vagotomy also leads to more rapid emptying of liquids.[88] These changes are less profound than with truncal vagotomy.[89] The major advantage of proximal gastric vagotomy is that the strength of antral peristaltic contractions and gastric trituration are not altered.[90] This means that gastric emptying of solids is not changed. The risk of dumping syndrome, diarrhea, gastric atony, and reflux gastritis is, therefore, less after

proximal gastric vagotomy than after truncal vagotomy. The motor effects of gastric operations are discussed in more detail in Chapter 9.

OPERATION FOR DUODENAL ULCER

Elective Operations

Indications for Operation
Patients with chronic duodenal ulcers that do not heal after approximately 3 months of therapy (a result nearly always due to noncompliance), patients who have more than three recurrences per year despite maintenance therapy with H_2-receptor antagonists and eradication of *H. pylori*, and patients who need maintenance therapy to prevent recurrences but who do not want to take medications for life should be considered for operation.

Choice of Operation
Emphasis should be given to avoiding operative morbidity and mortality and to maintaining normal or near-normal gastrointestinal function in patients undergoing elective operation for duodenal ulcer. Because these patients are treated electively, the duration of the operation is not among the most important considerations.

The operation best suited to meeting these goals is proximal gastric vagotomy. This procedure provides good relief of symptoms, relatively low recurrence rates, negligible mortality, and low rates of postoperative complications. Truncal vagotomy with drainage has a higher complication rate and a similar rate of recurrent ulcer, and so it cannot be advocated in this setting. Truncal vagotomy with antrectomy has considerably lower recurrence rates than proximal gastric vagotomy, but at the cost of a fourfold increase in postoperative gastric atony, dumping, and diarrhea. Because duodenal ulcers are treated so effectively with medications, the use of an elective procedure with complication rates higher than those associated with proximal gastric vagotomy is difficult to justify.

Results
When the results of these procedures are compared, lowering the risk of postoperative ulcer recurrence increases, to an extent, the risk of postoperative morbidity (Table 3). Although the data represented in Table 3 were collected before the era of *H. pylori* treatment, they still provide a relevant comparison. The addition of antrectomy to truncal vagotomy decreases recurrence rates from 5%-15% to 1%-2%, and there is no substantial change in mortality or long-term side effects in the elective setting.[1] In several randomized prospective trials, recurrence rates with

Table 3.—Results of Operation for Chronic Duodenal Ulcer Without Postoperative Therapy for *Helicobacter pylori*

Category	Operation		
	TV + antrectomy	TV + pyloroplasty	PGV
Ulcer recurrence, % of patients	1-2	5-15	5-16
Mortality, % of patients	0.6-1.8	0.5-1.4	0-0.3
Postoperative motor disorder, % of patients	13-29	11-26	3-8
Gastric emptying			
Liquids	Accelerated	Accelerated	Accelerated
Solids	Variable	Variable	Unchanged
Acid reduction, %			
Basal	85	75	75
Stimulated	85	50	50

PGV, proximal gastric vagotomy; TV, truncal vagotomy.

proximal gastric vagotomy are comparable to those with truncal vagotomy plus drainage but inferior to those with truncal vagotomy plus antrectomy.[91-93] At Mayo Clinic, proximal gastric vagotomy had a 5-year recurrence rate of 6% and a 10-year recurrence rate of 12% in the period before *H. pylori* therapy.[94] However, proximal gastric vagotomy was associated with no operative mortality and markedly decreased side effects. Substantial diarrhea or dumping occurred in only 1% of patients, bile reflux gastritis in 0.5%, and gastroesophageal reflux in 0.8%.[94]

Operations for Complications of Duodenal Ulcer

For emergency operations in duodenal ulcer, the patient's history of ulcer disease and treatment are extremely important in directing therapy, as are the patient's stability and overall health status. For patients with a definable cause for their ulcer, such as *H. pylori* or a history of NSAID use and no history of treatment for peptic ulcer, emergency operations should be directed at controlling the complication only. The operation is then followed by medical therapy for the underlying disease. In stable patients who do not have a known treatable cause for their ulcer or who have a history of chronic ulcer, the operation should not only correct the complication but also be therapeutic for the underlying peptic ulcer. Interestingly, one study from Taiwan found a lower rate of *H. pylori* in patients requiring emergency operations (56%) than in those treated medically (87% for duodenal ulcers and 76% for gastric ulcers) or those with elective operations (89%).[95] Unstable patients need only the most rapid and reliable procedure to control the ulcer complication regardless of their ulcer history.

After medical, endoscopic, or operative control of the complication, medical treatment should be directed at the underlying cause, as outlined in "Medical Therapy" (page

108). Follow-up endoscopy and, if applicable, *H. pylori* testing are indicated in all patients with peptic ulcer complications to ensure healing and organism eradication.

Hemorrhage

The indications for operation in a patient with a bleeding duodenal ulcer are 1) severe hemorrhage unresponsive to resuscitation, 2) prolonged bleeding with loss of approximately half of estimated blood volume, 3) recurrent hemorrhage after initial control with medical or endoscopic interventions, 4) a second hospitalization for ulcer hemorrhage, or 5) a coexisting indication for operation. Several factors predict a need for operative intervention. Endoscopic identification of a visible vessel, pulsatile bleeding, an oozing red clot, or a duodenal ulcer crater larger than 1 cm correlate highly with the eventual need for operation.[46,96] Clinical risk factors for rebleeding include age older than 60 years, shock at presentation, and chronic renal failure.[46]

Several operations are acceptable in a patient with hemorrhage due to duodenal ulcer, and these must be judiciously applied to the individual patient. All patients should undergo immediate longitudinal duodenotomy and ligation of the bleeding vessel to control the hemorrhage. Bleeding duodenal ulcers that require operation are usually situated on the posterior wall of the duodenal bulb, where they penetrate into the gastroduodenal artery or one of its branches. If the patient is unstable, ligation of this artery is all that should be done at this operation. However, if the patient is stable and has no known treatable cause for the ulcer, an acid-reducing procedure should be considered.

The acid-reducing procedure of choice is proximal gastric vagotomy. At Mayo Clinic, even before *H. pylori* treatment, proximal gastric vagotomy for hemorrhage from a duodenal ulcer had a 2% rebleeding rate (none requiring reoperation), an 11% ulcer recurrence rate, no operative mortality, and no occurrence of postvagotomy syndromes.[97] Others have reported similarly good results.[1] In elderly patients with significant comorbid conditions who are otherwise stable, truncal vagotomy with pyloroplasty can be considered. This operation is quick and easy in these high-risk patients and can lower rebleeding rates to 8%, but it is followed by postvagotomy sequelae in about 25% of patients.[98]

Perforation
Initial management of patients with perforated duodenal ulcer entails fluid resuscitation and broad-spectrum antibiotics. Ulcer perforation is an indication for emergency operation in almost all cases. Some have advocated nonoperative management for patients without generalized peritonitis or ongoing leak through the perforation and for patients with irreversible shock or other contraindications to laparotomy.[99] These patients are treated with nasogastric suction, antisecretory medications, and broad-spectrum antibiotics. Nonoperative treatment should be used only in extraordinary circumstances, however, because urgent laparotomy usually provides the greatest hope of survival. Especially high mortality rates in patients older than 70 years when operative treatment is delayed by unsuccessful nonoperative management suggest that this group is particularly unsuited for this treatment plan.[100]

Operations for perforated duodenal ulcer can be performed either at celiotomy or by laparoscopy. Laparoscopy is best limited to simple procedures such as omental patch closure in this emergency setting. Peritoneal toilet and operative results with laparoscopy are equivalent to those obtained with open procedures.[101-104]

Surgical judgment is required to decide whether treatment for the underlying ulcer disease is indicated. All patients treated operatively should undergo prompt closure of the perforation with sutures reinforced by an omental (Graham) patch. In patients who are unstable, have significant comorbidity, or have a medically treatable cause for their ulcer, this is all that should be done. Closure of perforation without an acid-reducing procedure previously was associated with an ulcer recurrence rate of nearly 80%, but this is now much lower.[16] Closure only, however, does have a higher rate of recurrence than when a proximal gastric vagotomy is added. Performing a proximal gastric vagotomy lowers recurrence rates to 3%[16] and should be considered in stable patients.

Proximal gastric vagotomy is preferred over truncal vagotomy with drainage because the rate of ulcer recurrence after operation is as good as that with truncal vagotomy and its operative and long-term morbidity rates are considerably lower. The avoidance of an incision or anastomosis that is at risk for suture line breakdown in the presence of peritonitis is a great advantage of proximal gastric vagotomy.[105,106] The primary advantage of truncal vagotomy is that it can be performed quickly. This factor could be important in the rare setting of a patient who is known to be *H. pylori*-negative and free from NSAID use and is too unstable to undergo proximal gastric vagotomy. This type of patient has a higher risk of failure with medical therapy alone. Truncal vagotomy with pyloroplasty may provide a reduction in recurrence risk while still allowing a relatively rapid completion of the operation. Truncal vagotomy with antrectomy is rarely indicated in the setting of a perforation because of the additional time required for the operation and the increased morbidity and mortality.

Our preferred management of a peptic ulcer with perforation resulting in a fistula is endoscopic biopsy to rule out malignancy followed by standard medical therapy, as outlined above. Usually, healing of the ulcer is associated with closure of the fistula. If the fistula persists despite ulcer healing, operative intervention is indicated only for complications of the fistula (e.g., recurrent cholangitis from duodenal-choledochal fistula or diarrhea from a gastrocolonic fistula).

Obstruction
For patients with chronic duodenal ulcer and gastric outlet obstruction, the goals of operation are similar to those in intractable ulcers with the added importance of restoring proper gastric emptying. There are several reasonable alternatives for this circumstance depending on the patient's history. In patients who are *H. pylori*-positive or have been using NSAIDs but are unable to have their obstruction dilated endoscopically, an acceptable alternative is pyloroplasty or gastrojejunostomy alone followed by medical ulcer therapy. This provides relief of the obstruction with the lowest risk of postoperative morbidity. In this setting, the likelihood of being able to control the ulcer disease with a proper medical regimen is high. This is obviously a less attractive option for patients who are anticipated to have poor compliance or in whom a readily treatable cause for their ulcer cannot be identified. The treatment of choice in these patients is proximal gastric vagotomy with intraoperative mechanical dilation, pyloroplasty, or gastrojejunostomy.[107-111] This relieves the obstruction and treats the underlying ulcer disease while maintaining low rates of postoperative sequelae. In nearly half of patients, mechanical dilation intraoperatively is successful, and thus the intestinal tract need not be entered.[107,108,112] Mechanical dilation and even pyloroplasty may not be feasible if the pylorus is severely scarred. If this is the case,

gastrojejunostomy is an appropriate alternative. Although bypass or destruction of the pylorus would be suspected to negate many of the advantages of proximal gastric vagotomy, dumping syndromes still occur much less frequently than with truncal vagotomy.[111,113] Again, truncal vagotomy with drainage has higher complication rates and similar recurrence rates. Truncal vagotomy with antrectomy has lower recurrence rates but a much higher risk of dumping and diarrhea. In addition, the distortion of the pyloroduodenal anatomy increases the risk of pancreatic and bile duct injuries and makes duodenal stump closure more difficult and hazardous.

OPERATION FOR GASTRIC ULCER

Types of Ulcer

There are four types of gastric ulcer, based on location (Fig. 4). Type I gastric ulcers occur in the antrum, most often along the lesser curve. They almost always occur in non–acid-secreting antral mucosa at or just distal to the border with the more proximal acid-secreting corporeal mucosa. They are invariably associated with chronic gastritis. Type II gastric ulcers also occur in the antrum but are associated with either active ulcers or scars indicative of previous ulceration within the duodenum. The duodenal ulcer generally precedes the gastric ulcer, and the disease features increased acid secretion similar to that found in simple duodenal ulcer. Type III gastric ulcers are located in the antrum, are often multiple, and are usually associated with use of NSAIDs. Type IV gastric ulcers are located on the lesser curve near the esophagogastric junction. These proximal ulcers, which would be expected to reside in oxyntic gland mucosa, actually occur in metaplastic antral mucosa in this area. Types I and IV ulcers are associated with normal or low gastric acid secretion and have higher rates of recurrence.

A giant gastric ulcer is defined as having a diameter

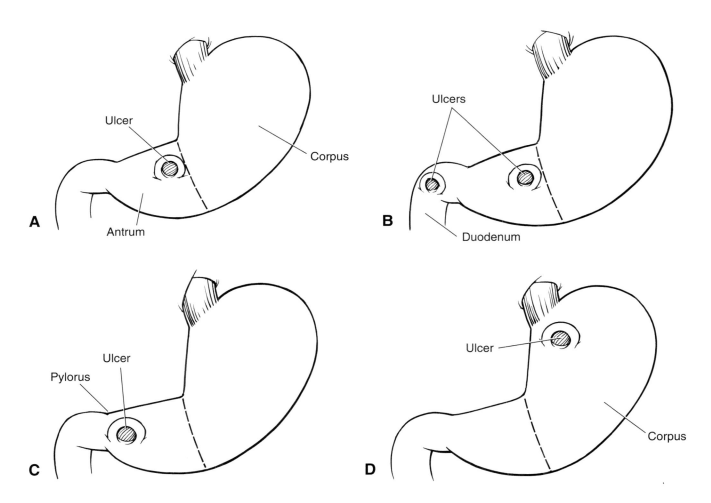

Fig. 4. Types of gastric ulcer. (A), Type I. (B), Type II. (C), Type III. (D), Type IV. Dashed line is the gastric, antral-corporeal, mucosal junction.

more than 3 cm. More than 95% of giant gastric ulcers occur along the lesser curve. These ulcers often penetrate into adjacent organs and can be mistakenly diagnosed as unresectable malignancies. We have shown that they have a higher rate of bleeding and malignancy than non-giant gastric ulcers.[114] Operative therapy is more often necessary. They are approached in the same manner as type I or III ulcer.

Patients with gastric ulcers tend to be older and have more comorbid conditions than those with duodenal ulcers. They are more often hospitalized for their disease, and complications of their gastric ulcers more often require operative intervention. These factors may reflect a difference in the virulence of the two diseases or may be due to differences in the demographics of the two groups.

Indications for Operation

As recently as 1985, 17% of patients with gastric ulcers required operation.[115] The rate is certainly lower now, but patients with gastric ulcers continue to come to operation earlier and more often than those with duodenal ulcers. This difference is partially related to the increased risk of malignancy but also to the fact that complications of gastric ulcers require operation more often than do those of duodenal ulcers.[1] Operative indications for patients with gastric ulcers are the same as for those with duodenal ulcers: intractability, inability to exclude malignancy, obstruction, severe hemorrhage, and perforation. Intractability is uncommon with modern medical therapy, but inability to rule out malignancy is a major indication for operation in gastric ulcer because of the 3% rate of underlying malignancy. A gastric ulcer can be considered intractable if it does not heal after 12 to 16 weeks of therapy, as discussed in "Medical Therapy" (page 108).

Choice of Elective Operation

The operations available for the treatment of gastric ulcer must be tailored to the individual patient. The operative treatment of gastric ulcer is largely directed at removing the ulcerated tissue. The surgeon must know and consider the physiologic effects of the contemplated procedures, the risk of recurrent ulcer, and the potential postoperative sequelae. Patients undergoing gastric operations should discontinue use of antisecretory medications for approximately 72 hours before the procedure to restore gastric acidity and minimize bacterial overgrowth in the gastric lumen.

For patients undergoing an elective operation for gastric ulcer, the choice of operation depends on the ulcer location and whether there is an associated duodenal ulcer. For patients with ulcers in the gastric body, antrum, or pylorus (types I, II, and III), distal gastric resection inclusive of the ulcer is our procedure of choice. Reconstruction with gastroduodenostomy (Billroth I) is preferred because it is more "physiologic" than gastrojejunostomy (Billroth II), it avoids the need to suture the duodenum closed, and it does not create an afferent jejunal limb. Proximal gastric vagotomy with excision of the ulcer also may be an option.[116] This procedure is associated with recurrent ulcer rates comparable to those of distal gastric resection, but the number of patients so treated has been small to date. Unless there is an associated duodenal ulcer (type II), truncal vagotomy provides no additional benefit for these types of ulcers. For type II ulcers, recurrence rates are lower with truncal vagotomy and antrectomy but at a cost of a fourfold increase in long-term sequelae. This rate of morbidity is unacceptable in the modern therapy of peptic ulcers. Local excision with or without truncal vagotomy and drainage has higher recurrence rates than distal gastrectomy or proximal gastric vagotomy with excision.[117,118]

For type IV ulcers, we perform a distal gastrectomy including a tongue of the lesser curve to include the ulcer (Pauchet procedure) with Billroth I gastroduodenostomy. Antrectomy with the ulcer left in situ has recurrence rates as high as 30% and does not allow for complete histologic examination of the ulcer. Similar to types I and III ulcers, truncal vagotomy provides no additional benefit. A more aggressive alternative for type IV ulcers is the Csendes procedure.[119] This operation entails subtotal gastrectomy with the proximal margin reaching the esophagogastric junction at the lesser curve. Reconstruction is carried out with a Roux-en-Y esophagogastrojejunostomy. This is occasionally the only viable option when the ulcer is located at the esophagogastric junction.

Operation for Complications of Gastric Ulcers

Hemorrhage

Patients with hemorrhage from a gastric ulcer more often require operative intervention than do patients with bleeding duodenal ulcers. Gastric ulcers are 3 times as likely as duodenal ulcers to rebleed after initial control.[120] The surgeon must again decide whether the goal of operation is to control bleeding only or to treat the underlying disease, as outlined in "Operations for Complications of Duodenal Ulcer" (page 108).

In all patients, initial identification and control of the bleeding site are done through a longitudinal gastrotomy that is placed with endoscopic localization. The recommended operation directed at controlling the hemorrhage only is wedge excision of the bleeding ulcer. Simple oversewing of the ulcer may be considered in an unstable patient but results in higher rates of rebleeding and limits histologic examination for malignancy. If a stable patient is deemed to need a procedure for long-term therapy of the underlying ulcer disease, we use distal gastrectomy inclusive of the ulcer with Billroth I gastroduodenostomy. Addition of a vagotomy does not provide significant benefit but does increase long-term complication rates. If a stable patient has substantial comorbid conditions that preclude a distal gastrectomy but definitive ulcer procedure is strongly thought to be needed, a reasonable alternative is truncal vagotomy, pyloroplasty, and excision of the ulcer.[116]

Perforation

Perforated gastric ulcers are associated with a mortality of 5% to 10%. Simple control of the perforation is best achieved with wedge excision of the ulcer. Closure of the perforation with an omental patch is an alternative in this situation but has the disadvantage of leaving behind a perforating gastric ulcer that might harbor carcinoma. If operative treatment of the underlying ulcer disease is deemed necessary, distal gastrectomy with Billroth I gastroduodenostomy should be performed.

Obstruction

Gastric outlet obstruction due to gastric ulcer usually occurs with a type II ulcer but occasionally can occur with a type III ulcer. The recommended operative management is distal gastric resection with Billroth I gastroduodenostomy. Although pyloroduodenal inflammation and fibrosis make this procedure more difficult, distal gastrectomy provides the most reliable long-term therapy for the ulcer while relieving the obstruction. A vagotomy should be added for pyloric or pre-pyloric ulcers.

ADVERSE OUTCOMES OF ULCER OPERATIONS

Anastomotic Ulcer

Anastomotic or stomal ulcer was first described by Braun in 1891 and refers to mucosal ulceration at the site of an anastomosis, usually in the jejunal mucosa after gastrojejunostomy. This complication occurs at its highest rate after operations for duodenal ulcer. Associated risk factors include smoking, failure to eradicate *H. pylori* after operations, and the use of NSAIDs. Other contributing factors are retained antrum attached to the duodenal stump after Billroth II gastrojejunostomy, incomplete vagotomy, inadequate gastric resection, and the Zollinger-Ellison syndrome.

The most common symptom of a stomal ulcer is pain, present in 74% of patients. Hemorrhage is also frequent, occurring in 40% to 56%. Other signs and symptoms

include perforation (5%-8%) and stenosis (0.4%-5%). Stomal ulcer is diagnosed with contrast radiography or endoscopy. Because these ulcers are closely associated with gastric mucosa, which can harbor malignancy, endoscopic inspection, biopsy, and brushings are indicated in all cases. In addition, affected patients usually have had some form of acid-reducing procedure in the past and, therefore, by definition, now have complicated ulcer disease. Because of this, serum gastrin testing must be performed to rule out Zollinger-Ellison syndrome. Interpretation of the baseline serum gastrin test result can be misleading if the patient has had a Billroth II gastrectomy. Retained gastric antrum in the duodenal stump causes hypergastrinemia. Thus, provocative testing with secretin must be performed to diagnose or rule out gastrinoma. Also, if the patient has had a previous vagotomy, testing is indicated to determine whether the vagotomy has been complete.

Medical Management

The medical management of stomal ulcer is the same as that described for duodenal ulcer with the exception that healing must be endoscopically confirmed, as in gastric ulcer. As in other forms of peptic ulcer, medical regimens are extremely effective, with healing rates of 70% to 90%. These rates were achieved with H_2-receptor antagonists only. Current therapy with proton pump inhibitors and anti-*H. pylori* regimens may provide even better rates of healing. If no underlying cause, such as *H. pylori* or NSAID use, is identified and eliminated, maintenance therapy should be instituted after healing.

Surgical Management

The operative management of anastomotic ulcers is more difficult than that of other forms of peptic ulcer disease. In these patients, not only have upper abdominal procedures been done previously but also the physiology has already been altered. Because complications such as hemorrhage and perforation are so common in these ulcers, preoperative physiologic testing is often not feasible. For chronic intractable anastomotic ulcers in which vagotomy is incomplete, repeat vagotomy is an appropriate option. This can be accomplished either transabdominally or transthoracically. Transthoracic vagotomy offers the advantage of avoidance of a previously operated field and often can be accomplished thoracoscopically. If the serum gastrin level is increased and secretin testing is negative for a gastrinoma, an exploratory procedure should be done to look for a retained gastric antrum attached to the duodenal stump. Preoperative technetium 99m scanning may confirm the diagnosis. For refractory anastomotic ulcers in patients who have not had an acid-reducing procedure, antrectomy and Billroth II gastrojejunostomy with truncal vagotomy is the procedure of choice.

Metabolic Disorders

Several metabolic disorders can occur after gastric operations, particularly after gastrectomy. Chronic diarrhea after truncal vagotomy can result in derangements of fluid volume and sodium and chloride homeostasis. Patients who have had subtotal gastrectomy may have disorders of calcium homeostasis or anemia due to iron or vitamin B_{12} deficiency. Rarely, celiac disease can be unmasked by ulcer operations.

Gastric Cancer

Adenocarcinoma of the proximal gastric stump is a time-dependent complication after distal gastrectomy. The pathogenesis of the late development of gastric cancer is not well understood. Hypochlorhydria, alkaline reflux, decreased gastrin production, gastric stress, and bacterial proliferation have all been proposed as possible contributing factors. The frequency has been reported to be 1% to 4% of patients at risk, and the risk increases with years after operation. Endoscopic screening is recommended given this considerable risk. If adenocarcinoma is discovered, the treatment is completion gastrectomy or esophagogastrectomy.

Postoperative Gastric Motor Disorders

Changes in gastric motility and emptying produced by operations for chronic gastric and duodenal ulcer result in postoperative gastric motor disorders in about 25% of patients. The cause, diagnosis, and treatment of these disorders are discussed in Chapter 9.

Zollinger-Ellison Syndrome

The Zollinger-Ellison syndrome is discussed in Chapter 19.

ACUTE STRESS ULCERS

General Considerations and Pathogenesis

Acute stress erosions and ulcers are relatively common in patients with serious illnesses. They almost always manifest in the stomach. Patients at risk include those experiencing head injuries (Cushing ulcers), severe burns (Curling ulcers), major operation with substantial blood loss, shock, respiratory failure, sepsis, or jaundice.

The pathogenesis of acute stress ulcers has not been fully elucidated. The major factors seem to be local tissue hypoxia and acidosis. Contributing factors include systemic hypoxia and acidosis, anemia, hypotension, and decreased cardiac output. The resultant gastrointestinal mucosal hypoxia and acidosis cause decreased bicarbonate availability, impaired cellular metabolism, and decreased secretion of mucosal protective factors. The resultant acute mucosal erosions are generally asymptomatic, but about 10% to 25% cause hemorrhage.

The current estimate of the rate of clinically important gastrointestinal bleeding in critically ill patients is about 2%.[121] The two strongest independent risk factors that have been identified for gastrointestinal bleeding from stress ulcers are respiratory failure requiring mechanical ventilation for longer than 48 hours and coagulopathy.[122] These risk factors remain predictive whether or not the patient receives prophylaxis for stress ulcer.

Prophylaxis for Stress Ulcers

Prophylaxis for stress ulcers became routine for critically ill patients in the 1980s. More recent studies have suggested that stress ulcer prophylaxis is not necessary in all of these patients.[121-124] Current evidence supports the use of stress ulcer prophylaxis for patients with the following conditions or situations: mechanical ventilation, coagulopathy, shock, severe sepsis, jaundice, head trauma, neurosurgical procedures, tetraplegia, multiple organ failure, and burns affecting more than 30% of body surface area.[124]

Antacids, sucralfate, and H_2-receptor antagonists have all been shown to decrease the rate of gastrointestinal hemorrhage from stress ulceration when compared with placebo.[125] Proton pump inhibitors have been shown to be effective in small trials.[126] Antacids are effective prophylactic agents only if given at a frequency of every 1 to 2 hours. Also, they have substantial side effects, including constipation, diarrhea, rebound hyperacidity, and electrolyte imbalances. One advantage of sucralfate is that it does not alter intragastric pH and, thus, does not potentiate gastric bacterial overgrowth. This appears to decrease the risk of hospital-acquired pneumonia.

In a multicenter, randomized, placebo-controlled study, clinically important stress ulcer hemorrhage developed in 1.7% of patients receiving H_2-receptor antagonist prophylaxis and in 3.8% of patients receiving sucralfate. The sucralfate group had a trend toward a lower rate of pneumonia, but it did not reach statistical significance.[127] A meta-analysis of 63 trials showed no statistically significant difference in stress ulcer bleeding among patients receiving antacids, sucralfate, or H_2-receptor antagonists but did show a lower incidence of pneumonia in those treated with sucralfate.[125]

The frequent dosing and potential side effects of antacids make their use impractical in the intensive care unit. The imminent availability of intravenous proton pump inhibitors in the United States should lead to trials comparing these agents with sucralfate and H_2-receptor antagonists, but currently their relative effectiveness remains unproved. The choice between sucralfate and H_2-receptor antagonists is not clear. Both provide effective prophylaxis with few side effects. The H_2-receptor antagonists have the advantage of ease of administration, and sucralfate has the advantages of lower cost and a potential reduction in the risk for pneumonia.

Management of Stress Ulcer Hemorrhage

The initial management of hemorrhage from stress ulcers is vigorous resuscitation and early upper endoscopy, as outlined for peptic ulcer hemorrhage. Medical treatment should be begun if not already in place prophylactically. Increased doses of these medications are of unproven benefit unless the gastric pH is less than 5. On endoscopic examination, multiple discrete areas of erythema with hemorrhage are seen throughout the gastric mucosa. Endoscopic therapy can be used, but the diffuse nature and large number of lesions make this difficult. The stomach is lavaged with saline to remove the blood and excess clot so that fibrinolysis is minimized at the bleeding sites. More than 80% of patients will have their hemorrhage controlled with these measures.

For patients with ongoing bleeding, the therapeutic options are limited. Selective arterial catheterization has been used to administer vasopressin through the left gastric artery. This can be given for 48 to 72 hours. Vasopressin is contraindicated in patients with considerable coronary vascular disease. Angioembolization also has been attempted. Success rates with both of these interventions are variable.

For patients in whom operative therapy is required, the preferred approach is not well established, in large part because no operation provides effective treatment with low mortality. Mortality, regardless of operative approach, is 30% to 60%. Acid-reducing procedures, gastric devascularization, and gastric resection have all been used.

It seems imprudent to approach patients with an acid-reducing procedure because this does not address the pathophysiologic aspect of the disease. Gastric devascularization, in which all arterial blood supply to the stomach is divided except the short gastric arteries, has a low rebleeding rate but a mortality rate comparable to that with gastrectomy. Gastric resection is the only procedure that addresses the diseased mucosa. It is, therefore, the preferred treatment. Unfortunately, the hemorrhage nearly always arises from lesions throughout the stomach, so that near-total or total gastrectomy is required to control the bleeding.

THE DIEULAFOY LESION

Dieulafoy lesions are vascular abnormalities most commonly found in the proximal stomach. The condition has also been called Dieulafoy ulcer, Dieulafoy disease, gastric aneurysm, caliber-persistent artery, and solitary exulceration simplex. This lesion presents acutely with massive upper gastrointestinal hemorrhage resulting from a small submucosal artery rupturing into the gastric lumen. It occurs twice as frequently in men as in women, and its peak incidence is in the sixth decade of life. It is the cause of up to 1% to 2% of upper gastrointestinal hemorrhage.[128] The mortality rate with Dieulafoy ulcer hemorrhage only recently has decreased to less than 25%.[129] Rebleeding in the postoperative setting is associated with an even worse prognosis.

Etiology

The underlying cause of Dieulafoy lesion is unknown, but the principal cause is thought to be an abnormally large artery traversing the gastric submucosa.[130] The vessel is usually 1 to 3 mm in size without aneurysmal dilatation. It runs with its wall in intimate contact with the gastric mucosa, so that any overlying mucosal defect can cause erosion into the artery. Whether this is a true acid-peptic disorder is debated. There is a lack of inflammation at the site of rupture, suggesting that mucosal ulceration may not be the cause of arterial rupture. In addition, no vasculitis is present, as is the usual case in peptic ulceration. There is, however, no other evident process that would explain the defect necessary for hemorrhage to ensue. Some investigators have theorized that thrombosis within the artery leads to necrosis of the wall and subsequent bleeding.[130] There is no convincing evidence that this is the underlying process. The true cause of hemorrhage remains unknown.

Presentation and Diagnosis

Massive hemorrhage is the usual presentation, and recurrent episodes of hemorrhage over several days are not uncommon. Typically, patients with Dieulafoy lesions do not have symptoms of peptic ulcer. Similar bleeding lesions have been reported in other areas of the gastrointestinal tract, but the stomach is clearly the most common site.

Diagnostic work-up is the same as that for all upper gastrointestinal hemorrhage, and the diagnosis is usually made by endoscopic examination. Because these lesions are small, repeated endoscopic procedures are often needed to localize the site of bleeding. In more than 80% of cases, the lesion is located along the proximal 6 cm of the stomach near the lesser curve.[129] Rarely, multiple sites of bleeding have been described.[131]

Management

These lesions should be managed with aggressive resuscitation, transfusion as needed, and early endoscopy. Spontaneous cessation of hemorrhage is less common with these lesions than with bleeding peptic ulcers, and about 80% of patients are effectively treated with endoscopic coagulation methods.[128,129,132,133] This is the preferred initial treatment. As with bleeding peptic ulcers, bleeding unable to be controlled endoscopically necessitates operative exploration.

At operation, the entire gastric mucosal surface must be carefully examined for the site of bleeding, particularly along the proximal lesser curve. Once the site of bleeding is identified, a wedge resection of this area provides the most secure treatment. Reports of rebleeding after simple ligation make this option less attractive than wedge resection. Bleeding in sites other than the stomach is controlled with suture ligation and wedge or segmental resection.

REFERENCES

1. Stabile BE: Current surgical management of duodenal ulcers. Surg Clin North Am 72:335-356, 1992
2. Baron JH: One-hundred-and-fifty years of measurements of hydrochloric acid in gastric juice. Br Med J 4:600-601, 1973
3. Modlin IM: From Prout to the proton pump—a history of the science of gastric acid secretion and the surgery of peptic ulcer. Surg Gynecol Obstet 170:81-96, 1990
4. Brodie B: Experiments and observations on the influence of the nerves of the eighth pair on the secretions of the stomach. Philos Trans R Soc Lond 104:102, 1814
5. Dragstedt LR, Oberhelman HA Jr, Woodward ER: Physiology of gastric secretion and its relation to the ulcer problem. JAMA 147:1615-1620, 1951
6. Dragstedt LR, Fournier HJ, Woodward ER, Tovee EB, Harper PV Jr: Transabdominal gastric vagotomy: a study of the anatomy and surgery of the vagus nerves at the lower portion of the esophagus. Surg Gynecol Obstet 85:461-466, 1947
7. Edkins JS: The chemical mechanism of gastric secretion. J Physiol (Lond) 34:133-144, 1906
8. Komarov SA: Gastrin. Proc Soc Exp Biol Med 38:514-516, 1938
9. Gregory RA: Memorial lecture: the isolation and chemistry of gastrin. Gastroenterology 54 Suppl:723-726, 1968
10. Black JW, Duncan WA, Durant CJ, Ganellin CR, Parsons EM: Definition and antagonism of histamine H₂-receptors. Nature 236:385-390, 1972
11. Warren JR, Marshall B: Unidentified curved bacilli on gastric epithelium in active chronic gastritis. Lancet 1:1273-1275, 1983
12. Stabile BE, Passaro E Jr: Duodenal ulcer: a disease in evolution. Curr Probl Surg 21:1-79, 1984
13. Kurata JH: Ulcer epidemiology: an overview and proposed research framework. Gastroenterology 96:569-580, 1989
14. Mendeloff AI: What has been happening to duodenal ulcer? Gastroenterology 67:1020-1022, 1974
15. Gustavsson S, Nyren O: Time trends in peptic ulcer surgery, 1956 to 1986: a nation-wide survey in Sweden. Ann Surg 210:704-709, 1989
16. Gustavsson S, Kelly KA, Melton LJ III, Zinsmeister AR: Trends in peptic ulcer surgery: a population-based study in Rochester, Minnesota, 1956-1985. Gastroenterology 94:688-694, 1988
17. Weinberg JA, Stempien SJ, Movius HJ, Dagradi AE: Vagotomy and pyloroplasty in the treatment of duodenal ulcer. Am J Surg 92:202-206, 1956
18. McQuaid KR, Isenberg JI: Medical therapy of peptic ulcer disease. Surg Clin North Am 72:285-316, 1992
19. Rask-Madsen J: The role of eicosanoids in the gastrointestinal tract. Scand J Gastroenterol Suppl 127:7-19, 1987
20. Silen W: Experimental models of gastric ulceration and injury. Am J Physiol 255:G395-G402, 1988
21. Dooley CP, Cohen H: The clinical significance of *Campylobacter pylori*. Ann Intern Med 108:70-79, 1988
22. Isenberg JI, McQuaid KR, Laine L, Rubin W: Acid-peptic disorders. *In* Textbook of Gastroenterology. Vol 1. Edited by T Yamada. Philadelphia, JB Lippincott Company, 1991, pp 1241-1339
23. Peterson WL: *Helicobacter pylori* and peptic ulcer disease. N Engl J Med 324:1043-1048, 1991
24. Graham DY, Klein PD, Opekun AR, Boutton TW: Effect of age on the frequency of active *Campylobacter pylori* infection diagnosed by the [13C]urea breath test in normal subjects and patients with peptic ulcer disease. J Infect Dis 157:777-780, 1988
25. Steer HW: The gastro-duodenal epithelium in peptic ulceration. J Pathol 146:355-362, 1985
26. el-Omar EM, Penman ID, Ardill JE, Chittajallu RS, Howie C, McColl KE: *Helicobacter pylori* infection and abnormalities of acid secretion in patients with duodenal ulcer disease. Gastroenterology 109:681-691, 1995
27. Hogan DL, Rapier RC, Dreilinger A, Koss MA, Basuk PM, Weinstein WM, Nyberg LM, Isenberg JI: Duodenal bicarbonate secretion: eradication of *Helicobacter pylori* and duodenal structure and function in humans. Gastroenterology 110:705-716, 1996
28. Walsh JH, Peterson WL: The treatment of *Helicobacter pylori* infection in the management of peptic ulcer disease. N Engl J Med 333:984-991, 1995

29. Ohashi S, Segawa K, Okamura S, Urano H, Kanamori S, Ishikawa H, Hara K, Hukutomi A, Shirai K, Maeda M: A clinicopathologic study of gastric mucosa-associated lymphoid tissue lymphoma. Cancer 88:2210-2219, 2000

30. Saito K, Arai K, Mori M, Kobayashi R, Ohki I: Effect of *Helicobacter pylori* eradication on malignant transformation of gastric adenoma. Gastrointest Endosc 52:27-32, 2000

31. El-Omar EM, Oien K, Murray LS, El-Nujumi A, Wirz A, Gillen D, Williams C, Fullarton G, McColl KE: Increased prevalence of precancerous changes in relatives of gastric cancer patients: critical role of *H. pylori*. Gastroenterology 118:22-30, 2000

32. Soll AH, Kurata J, McGuigan JE: Ulcers, nonsteroidal antiinflammatory drugs, and related matters. Gastroenterology 96:561-568, 1989

33. Soll AH, Weinstein WM, Kurata J, McCarthy D: Nonsteroidal anti-inflammatory drugs and peptic ulcer disease. Ann Intern Med 114:307-319, 1991

34. Fries JF, Miller SR, Spitz PW, Williams CA, Hubert HB, Bloch DA: Toward an epidemiology of gastropathy associated with nonsteroidal antiinflammatory drug use. Gastroenterology 96:647-655, 1989

35. Griffin MR, Piper JM, Daugherty JR, Snowden M, Ray WA: Nonsteroidal anti-inflammatory drug use and increased risk for peptic ulcer disease in elderly persons. Ann Intern Med 114:257-263, 1991

36. Peura DA, Lanza FL, Gostout CJ, Foutch PG: The American College of Gastroenterology Bleeding Registry: preliminary findings. Am J Gastroenterol 92:924-928, 1997

37. Kurata JH, Nogawa AN: Meta-analysis of risk factors for peptic ulcer: nonsteroidal antiinflammatory drugs, *Helicobacter pylori*, and smoking. J Clin Gastroenterol 24:2-17, 1997

38. Soll AH: Pathogenesis of peptic ulcer and implications for therapy. N Engl J Med 322:909-916, 1990

39. Feldman M: Mental stress and peptic ulcers: an earthshaking association. Am J Gastroenterol 93:291-292, 1998

40. Jess P: The personality pattern in peptic ulcer disease. Dan Med Bull 43:330-335, 1996

41. Hirschl AM, Glupczynski Y: Diagnosis. Curr Opin Gastroenterol 15 Suppl:S5-S9, 1999

42. Tu TC, Lee CL, Wu CH, Chen TK, Chan CC, Huang SH, Lee MS: Comparison of invasive and noninvasive tests for detecting *Helicobacter pylori* infection in bleeding peptic ulcers. Gastrointest Endosc 49:302-306, 1999

43. Feldman M, Richardson CT, Fordtran JS: Experience with sham feeding as a test for vagotomy. Gastroenterology 79:792-795, 1980

44. Christensen A, Bousfield R, Christiansen J: Incidence of perforated and bleeding peptic ulcers before and after the introduction of H₂-receptor antagonists. Ann Surg 207:4-6, 1988

45. McConnell DB, Baba GC, Deveney CW: Changes in surgical treatment of peptic ulcer disease within a veterans hospital in the 1970s and the 1980s. Arch Surg 124:1164-1167, 1989

46. Branicki FJ, Boey J, Fok PJ, Pritchett CJ, Fan ST, Lai EC, Mok FP, Wong WS, Lam SK, Hui WM: Bleeding duodenal ulcer: a prospective evaluation of risk factors for rebleeding and death. Ann Surg 211:411-418, 1990

47. Hunt PS: Bleeding gastroduodenal ulcers: selection of patients for surgery. World J Surg 11:289-294, 1987

48. Miller AR, Farnell MB, Kelly KA, Gostout CJ, Benson JT: Impact of therapeutic endoscopy on the treatment of bleeding duodenal ulcers: 1980-1990. World J Surg 19:89-94, 1995

49. Laine L, Peterson WL: Bleeding peptic ulcer. N Engl J Med 331:717-727, 1994

50. Laine L: Multipolar electrocoagulation in the treatment of peptic ulcers with nonbleeding visible vessels: a prospective, controlled trial. Ann Intern Med 110:510-514, 1989

51. Lin HJ, Lee FY, Chan CY, Huang ZC, Kang WM, Lee CH, Lee SD, Tsai YT: Heat probe thermocoagulation as a substitute for surgical intervention to arrest massive peptic ulcer hemorrhage: an experience in 153 cases. Surgery 108:18-21, 1990

52. Lin HJ, Lee FY, Kang WM, Tsai YT, Lee SD, Lee CH: A controlled study of therapeutic endoscopy for peptic ulcer with nonbleeding visible vessel. Gastrointest Endosc 36:241-246, 1990

53. Cook DJ, Guyatt GH, Salena BJ, Laine LA: Endoscopic therapy for acute nonvariceal upper gastrointestinal hemorrhage: a meta-analysis. Gastroenterology 102:139-148, 1992

54. Khuroo MS, Yattoo GN, Javid G, Khan BA, Shah AA, Gulzar GM, Sodi JS: A comparison of omeprazole and placebo for bleeding peptic ulcer. N Engl J Med 336:1054-1058, 1997

55. Imperiale TF, Birgisson S: Somatostatin or octreotide compared with H₂ antagonists and placebo in the management of acute nonvariceal upper gastrointestinal hemorrhage: a meta-analysis. Ann Intern Med 127:1062-1071, 1997

56. Howden CW, Hunt RH: The relationship between suppression of acidity and gastric ulcer healing rates. Aliment Pharmacol Ther 4:25-33, 1990

57. Chiverton SG, Hunt RH: Relationship between inhibition of acid secretion and healing of peptic ulcers. Scand J Gastroenterol Suppl 166:43-47, 1989

58. Bauerfeind P, Koelz HR, Blum AL: Ulcer treatment: regimens and duration of inhibition of acid secretion: how long to dose. Scand J Gastroenterol 23 Suppl 153:23-24, 1988

59. Kelly KA, Morley KD, Wilbur BG: Effect of corporal and antral gastrojejunostomy on canine gastric emptying of solid spheres and liquids. Br J Surg 60:880-884, 1973

60. Lewisohn R: The frequency of gastrojejunal ulcers. Surg Gynecol Obstet 40:70-76, 1925

61. Herrington JL Jr: Gastroduodenal ulcer: overview of 150 papers presented before the Southern Surgical Association 1888-1986. Ann Surg 207:754-769, 1988

62. Griffith CA, Harkins HN: Partial gastric vagotomy: an experimental study. Gastroenterology 32:96-102, 1957

63. Holle F: New method for surgical treatment of gastroduodenal ulceration. *In* Surgery of the Stomach and Duodenum. Third edition. Edited by LM Nyhus, C Wastell. Boston, Little Brown, 1977, pp 329-338

64. Amdrup E, Jensen HE: Selective vagotomy of the parietal cell mass preserving innervation of the undrained antrum: a preliminary report of results in patients with duodenal ulcer. Gastroenterology 59:522-527, 1970

65. Johnston D, Wilkinson AR: Highly selective vagotomy without a drainage procedure in the treatment of duodenal ulcer. Br J Surg 57:289-296, 1970

66. Feliciano DV: Do perforated duodenal ulcers need an acid-decreasing surgical procedure now that omeprazole is available? Surg Clin North Am 72:369-380, 1992

67. Weger RV, Meier DE, Richardson CT, Feldman M, McClelland RN: Parietal cell vagotomy in a surgical training program. Am J Surg 144:689-693, 1982

68. Sawyers JL, Scott HW Jr, Edwards WH, Shull HJ, Law DH IV: Comparative studies of the clinical effects of truncal and selective gastric vagotomy. Am J Surg 115:165-172, 1968

69. Werscher GJ, Hinder RA, Redmond EJ, et al: Laparoscopic highly selective vagotomy. Contemp Surg 44:153, 1994

70. Casas AT, Gadacz TR: Laparoscopic management of peptic ulcer disease. Surg Clin North Am 76:515-522, 1996

71. Pietrafitta JJ, Schultz LS, Graber JN, Hickok DF: Laser laparoscopic vagotomy and pyloromyotomy. Gastrointest Endosc 37:338-343, 1991

72. Anvari M, Park A: Laparoscopic-assisted vagotomy and distal gastrectomy. Surg Endosc 8:1312-1315, 1994

73. Goh P, Tekant Y, Isaac J, Kum CK, Ngoi SS: The technique of laparoscopic Billroth II gastrectomy. Surg Laparosc Endosc 2:258-260, 1992

74. Goh PM, Alponat A, Mak K, Kum CK: Early international results of laparoscopic gastrectomies. Surg Endosc 11:650-652, 1997

75. Gillespie IE, McCusker VI, Gillespie G: The effect of vagotomy on gastric secretion elicited by pentagastrin in man: a multicenter study. Lancet 2:534-536, 1967

76. Konturek SJ, Wysocki A, Oleksy J: Effect of medical and surgical vagotomy on gastric response to graded doses of pentagastrin and histamine. Gastroenterology 54:392-400, 1968

77. Debas HT: Peripheral regulation of gastric acid secretion. In Physiology of the Gastrointestinal Tract. Vol 2. Second edition. Edited by LR Johnson. New York, Raven Press, 1987, pp 931-945

78. Cranley B, Kelly KA, Go VL, McNichols LA: Enhancing the anti-dumping effect of Roux gastrojejunostomy with intestinal pacing. Ann Surg 198:516-524, 1983

79. Byrne DJ, Brock BM, Morgan AG, McAdam WA: Highly selective vagotomy: a 14-year experience. Br J Surg 75:869-872, 1988

80. Wilbur BG, Kelly KA: Effect of proximal gastric, complete gastric, and truncal vagotomy on canine gastric electric activity, motility, and emptying. Ann Surg 178:295-303, 1973

81. Dozois RR, Kelly KA: Gastric secretion and motility in duodenal ulcer: effect of current vagotomies. Surg Clin North Am 56:1267-1276, 1976

82. Kelly KA, Code CF: Effect of transthoracic vagotomy on canine gastric electrical activity. Gastroenterology 57:51-58, 1969

83. Mroz CT, Kelly KA: The role of the extrinsic antral nerves in the regulation of gastric emptying. Surg Gynecol Obstet 145:369-377, 1977

84. Cullen JJ, Kelly KA: Functional characteristics of canine pylorus in health, with pyloroplasty, and after pyloric reconstruction. Dig Dis Sci 41:711-719, 1996

85. Passaro E Jr, Stabile BE: Late complications of vagotomy in relation to alterations in physiology. Postgrad Med 63:135-137, 1978

86. Delcore R, Cheung LY: Surgical options in postgastrectomy syndromes. Surg Clin North Am 71:57-75, 1991

87. Kelly KA: Neural control of gastric electric and motor activity. In Nerves and the Gut. Edited by FP Brooks, PW Evers. Thorofare, New Jersey, Charles B Slack, 1977, pp 223-232

88. Kelly KA: Motility of the stomach and gastroduodenal junction. In Physiology of the Gastrointestinal Tract. Vol 1. Edited by LR Johnson. New York, Raven Press, 1981, pp 393-410

89. Morimoto H, Kelly KA: Mechanisms of insulin-induced relaxation of the canine proximal stomach after proximal gastric vagotomy. J Gastrointest Surg 1:386-394, 1997

90. Hould FS, Cullen JJ, Kelly KA: Influence of proximal gastric vagotomy on canine gastric motility and emptying. Surgery 116:83-89, 1994

91. Johnston D, Blackett RL: Recurrent peptic ulcers. World J Surg 11:274-282, 1987

92. Johnston D, Blackett RL: A new look at selective vagotomies. Am J Surg 156:416-427, 1988

93. Jordan PH Jr: Surgery for peptic ulcer disease. Curr Probl Surg 28:265-330, 1991

94. Soper NJ, Kelly KA, van Heerden JA, Ilstrup DM: Long term clinical results after proximal gastric vagotomy. Surg Gynecol Obstet 169:488-494, 1989

95. Lee WJ, Wu MS, Chen CN, Yuan RH, Lin JT, Chang KJ: Seroprevalence of Helicobacter pylori in patients with surgical peptic ulcer. Arch Surg 132:430-433, 1997

96. Laurence BH, Cotton PB: Bleeding gastroduodenal ulcers: nonoperative treatment. World J Surg 11:295-303, 1987

97. Miedema BW, Torres PR, Farnell MB, van Heerden JA, Kelly KA: Proximal gastric vagotomy in the emergency treatment of bleeding duodenal ulcer. Am J Surg 161:64-66, 1991

98. Farris JM, Smith GK: Appraisal of the long-term results of vagotomy and pyloroplasty in 100 patients with bleeding duodenal ulcer. Ann Surg 166:630-639, 1967

99. Donovan AJ, Vinson TL, Maulsby GO, Gewin JR: Selective treatment of duodenal ulcer with perforation. Ann Surg 189:627-636, 1979

100. Crofts TJ, Park KG, Steele RJ, Chung SS, Li AK: A randomized trial of nonoperative treatment for perforated peptic ulcer. N Engl J Med 320:970-973, 1989

101. Takeuchi H, Kawano T, Toda T, Minamisono Y, Nagasaki S, Sugimachi K: Laparoscopic repair for perforation of duodenal ulcer with omental patch: report of initial six cases. Surg Laparosc Endosc 8:153-156, 1998

102. Nathanson LK, Easter DW, Cuschieri A: Laparoscopic repair/peritoneal toilet of perforated duodenal ulcer. Surg Endosc 4:232-233, 1990

103. Urbano D, Rossi M, De Simone P, Berloco P, Alfani D, Cortesini R: Alternative laparoscopic management of perforated peptic ulcers. Surg Endosc 8:1208-1211, 1994

104. Thompson AR, Hall TJ, Anglin BA, Scott-Conner CE: Laparoscopic plication of perforated ulcer: results of a selective approach. South Med J 88:185-189, 1995

105. Jordan PH Jr, Morrow C: Perforated peptic ulcer. Surg Clin North Am 68:315-329, 1988

106. Boey J, Branicki FJ, Alagaratnam TT, Fok PJ, Choi S, Poon A, Wong J: Proximal gastric vagotomy: the preferred operation for perforations in acute duodenal ulcer. Ann Surg 208:169-174, 1988

107. Pollard SG, Friend PJ, Dunn DC, Hunter JO: Highly selective vagotomy with duodenal dilatation in patients with duodenal ulceration and gastric outlet obstruction. Br J Surg 77:1365-1366, 1990

108. Mentes AS: Parietal cell vagotomy and dilatation for peptic duodenal stricture. Ann Surg 212:597-601, 1990

109. Hooks VH III, Bowden TA Jr, Sisley JF III, Mansberger AR Jr: Highly selective vagotomy with dilatation or duodenoplasty: a surgical alternative for obstructing duodenal ulcer. Ann Surg 203:545-550, 1986

110. Lunde OC, Liavag I, Roland M: Proximal gastric vagotomy and pyloroplasty for duodenal ulcer with pyloric stenosis: a thirteen-year experience. World J Surg 9:165-170, 1985

111. Donahue PE, Yoshida J, Richter HM, Liu K, Bombeck CT, Nyhus LM: Proximal gastric vagotomy with drainage for obstructing duodenal ulcer. Surgery 104:757-764, 1988

112. Hom S, Sarr MG, Kelly KA, Hench V: Postoperative gastric atony after vagotomy for obstructing peptic ulcer. Am J Surg 157:282-286, 1989

113. Csendes A, Maluenda F, Braghetto I, Schutte H, Burdiles P, Diaz JC: Prospective randomized study comparing three surgical techniques for the treatment of gastric outlet obstruction secondary to duodenal ulcer. Am J Surg 166:45-49, 1993

114. Gustavsson S, Kelly KA, Hench VS, Melton LJ III: Giant gastric and duodenal ulcers: a population-based study with a comparison to nongiant ulcers. World J Surg 11:333-338, 1987

115. Adkins RB Jr, DeLozier JB III, Scott HW Jr, Sawyers JL: The management of gastric ulcers: a current review. Ann Surg 201:741-751, 1985

116. Kelly KA, Malagelada JR: Medical and surgical treatment of chronic gastric ulcer. Clin Gastroenterol 13:621-634, 1984

117. Greenall MJ, Lehnert T: Vagotomy or gastrectomy for elective treatment of benign gastric ulceration? Dig Dis Sci 30:353-361, 1985

118. de Miguel J: Recurrence of gastric ulcer after selective vagotomy and pyloroplasty for chronic uncomplicated gastric ulcer: a 5-10 year follow-up. Br J Surg 62:875-878, 1975

119. Csendes A, Braghetto I, Calvo F, De la Cuadra R, Velasco N, Schutte H, Sepulveda A, Lazo M: Surgical treatment of high gastric ulcer. Am J Surg 149:765-770, 1985

120. Sugawa C, Joseph AL: Endoscopic interventional management of bleeding duodenal and gastric ulcers. Surg Clin North Am 72:317-334, 1992

121. Cook DJ, Fuller HD, Guyatt GH, Marshall JC, Leasa D, Hall R, Winton TL, Rutledge F, Todd TJ, Roy P, Lacroix J, Griffith L, Willan A: Risk factors for gastrointestinal bleeding in critically ill patients: Canadian Critical Care Trials Group. N Engl J Med 330:377-381, 1994

122. Tryba M, Cook D: Current guidelines on stress ulcer prophylaxis. Drugs 54:581-596, 1997

123. Marrone GC, Silen W: Pathogenesis, diagnosis and treatment of acute gastric mucosal lesions. Clin Gastroenterol 13:635-650, 1984

124. Navab F, Steingrub J: Stress ulcer: Is routine prophylaxis necessary? Am J Gastroenterol 90:708-712, 1995

125. Cook DJ, Reeve BK, Guyatt GH, Heyland DK, Griffith LE, Buckingham L, Tryba M: Stress ulcer prophylaxis in critically ill patients: resolving discordant meta-analyses. JAMA 275:308-314, 1996

126. Phillips JO, Metzler MH, Palmieri MT, Huckfeldt RE, Dahl NG: A prospective study of simplified omeprazole suspension for the prophylaxis of stress-related mucosal damage. Crit Care Med 24:1793-1800, 1996

127. Cook D, Guyatt G, Marshall J, Leasa D, Fuller H, Hall R, Peters S, Rutledge F, Griffith L, McLellan A, Wood G, Kirby A: A comparison of sucralfate and ranitidine for the prevention of upper gastrointestinal bleeding in patients requiring mechanical ventilation: Canadian Critical Care Trials Group. N Engl J Med 338:791-797, 1998

128. Lin HJ, Lee FY, Tsai YT, Lee SD, Lee CH, Kang WM: Therapeutic endoscopy for Dieulafoy's disease. J Clin Gastroenterol 11:507-510, 1989

129. Stark ME, Gostout CJ, Balm RK: Clinical features and endoscopic management of Dieulafoy's disease. Gastrointest Endosc 38:545-550, 1992

130. Veldhuyzen van Zanten SJ, Bartelsman JF, Schipper ME, Tytgat GN: Recurrent massive haematemesis from Dieulafoy vascular malformations—a review of 101 cases. Gut 27:213-222, 1986

131. Juler GL, Labitzke HG, Lamb R, Allen R: The pathogenesis of Dieulafoy's gastric erosion. Am J Gastroenterol 79:195-200, 1984

132. Sherman L, Shenoy SS, Satchidanand SK, Neumann PR, Barrios GG, Peer RM: Arteriovenous malformation of the stomach. Am J Gastroenterol 72:160-164, 1979

133. Pointner R, Schwab G, Konigsrainer A, Dietze O: Endoscopic treatment of Dieulafoy's disease. Gastroenterology 94:563-566, 1988

Chapter 9

DISORDERS OF GASTROINTESTINAL MOTILITY AND EMPTYING AFTER GASTRIC OPERATIONS

Keith A. Kelly, M.D.
Michael G. Sarr, M.D.
Ronald A. Hinder, M.D.

The need for operative treatment of peptic ulcer has decreased markedly in the past 40 years.[1] The recent introduction of more effective and potent medical therapy and a better understanding of the role of *Helicobacter pylori* in the pathogenesis of this disease have contributed to this decrease. Moreover, when operation is necessary, proximal gastric vagotomy, an operation with minimal postoperative morbidity, has gained acceptance as a suitable procedure, especially for duodenal ulcer.[2] Thus, with fewer gastric operations being done and with fewer morbid procedures being used when operative treatment is necessary, fewer patients with postoperative gastric syndromes are requiring treatment.

Nonetheless, operations more radical than proximal gastric vagotomy, such as truncal vagotomy and drainage or gastric resection, are still sometimes being used to treat peptic ulcer, especially to manage the acute complications of the disease. Also, subtotal or total gastrectomy continues to be required for patients who have resectable gastric cancer. These more radical gastric operations are associated with considerable long-term morbidity in up to 25% of patients. Much of this morbidity relates to postoperative derangements in the pattern of gastrointestinal motility and emptying. Symptoms such as abdominal pain, bloating, nausea, vomiting, and diarrhea can be understood best in terms of the abnormal gastrointestinal motility and emptying resulting from the operations. Also, postoperative reflux of bile from the small intestine into the stomach may cause alkaline reflux gastritis, and chronic postoperative gastric stasis and bile reflux may predispose to gastric cancer.

The pathophysiologic mechanisms underlying the various syndromes after gastric operations can be better understood by knowing the physiology of gastric motility and emptying in health. The information in this chapter is based largely on work done at Mayo Clinic, but the work of others is also used.

PHYSIOLOGY OF GASTRIC MOTILITY AND EMPTYING

The development and application of radiologic and radionuclide studies of gastric emptying during the past 20 years have provided an elegant, noninvasive means of defining the emptying of solid and liquid ingesta by the healthy stomach. Modern radiopharmaceutical methods allow different isotopes with distinct emission spectra to be attached separately to the liquid and solid components of a meal.[3] A gamma camera then can be used to record simultaneously the separate patterns of emptying of the liquid component and the solid component over time.

Ingesta generally are categorized as liquids, digestible solids, and indigestible solids. Nonnutrient liquids empty most rapidly initially, and as the volume remaining in the stomach decreases the rate slows (Fig. 1). Nonnutrient liquids follow a pattern of exponential emptying. In contrast, the emptying of nutrient-rich liquids is characterized by a relatively constant rate of delivery to the duodenum.[4] Hence, the emptying of nutrient-rich liquids follows a linear pattern. Digestible solids are retained in the stomach and mechanically triturated by the antrum into particles less than 1 mm in diameter before they are emptied. The emptying of digestible solids thus has an initial lag phase, during which little or no emptying takes place, because few or no particles less than 1 mm in size are present. Once the small particles

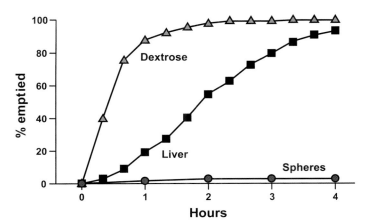

Fig. 1. Gastric emptying of a meal consisting of a liquid (400 mL 1% dextrose), a digestible solid (50 g cubed liver), and indigestible solids (40 plastic spheres) in a healthy dog. The liver was diced into 1-cm cubes. The plastic spheres were 7 mm in diameter.[4]

begin to appear, a pattern of slow, linear emptying occurs. In contrast, indigestible solids are retained within the stomach until the nutrients have emptied and the fasting state returns. They are then emptied rapidly and in boluses by cyclically recurring, large-amplitude, proximal and distal gastric contractions characteristic of the motility of the fasting stomach.

Although gastric emptying has been well described in health, the sensory and effector mechanisms responsible for the close regulation of the emptying need to be understood. To do so, it is helpful to remember that the stomach is divided functionally into two parts, a proximal part, consisting of the gastric fundus and the proximal corpus, and a distal part, consisting of the distal corpus, the antrum, and the pylorus. The proximal stomach serves as a reservoir, and the distal stomach serves as a grinder and a pump. Each part may be disturbed by gastric operations.[5]

Variations in the tone of the proximal stomach are important in receiving and storing food and in regulating the rate of gastric emptying of liquids. Proximal gastric tone decreases with swallowing (receptive relaxation) or with gastric distention (accommodation), both of which are vagally mediated reflexes. This decrease in tone permits the fundus and upper body of the stomach to function as a reservoir, which relaxes as the stomach fills. The relaxation keeps intragastric pressure low and prevents excessively rapid gastric emptying, especially of liquids. Proximal gastric tone, however, does create a small but important gradient in pressure between the gastric lumen and the duodenal lumen. This gradient drives gastric content steadily from the stomach toward the duodenum. The pylorus, which remains open much of the time, offers little resistance to the flow of liquids into the duodenum. In contrast, the small opening usually present at the

pylorus does block the passage of solids that are more than 1 mm in diameter out of the stomach.

The peristaltic contractions of the distal stomach have a pivotal role in the grinding and emptying of solid food. Their frequency and direction of propagation are controlled by the gastric pacemaker located in the proximal gastric corpus near the greater curve. The pacemaker generates electrical signals, the electrical slow waves or pacesetter potentials, at a frequency of 3 per minute. The signals are propagated distally from the pacemaker to the pylorus, phasing the onset of peristaltic contractions as they go. These peristaltic contractions propel liquid, and the suspension of tiny solid particles within it, from the stomach into the duodenum. When particles larger than 1 mm appear at the pylorus, however, the pylorus closes to prevent their passage. The distal antrum then squeezes down on them, grinding them together and repelling them back toward the more proximal stomach. The sequence of propulsion, grinding, and retropulsion gradually breaks down the larger solids into tiny particles that are finally allowed to pass into the duodenum.

This same antropyloric mechanism also helps to prevent the reflux of potentially injurious duodenal content, such as bile and pancreatic juice, into the stomach. The pylorus closes as the duodenum contracts, preventing the reflux. Finally, the small bowel offers a mechanical resistance to the inflow of ingesta. This resistance may contribute to the slowing of gastric emptying, particularly if gastric operations have destroyed one or more of the usual mechanisms controlling the emptying. Also, the small bowel releases hormones, for example, cholecystokinin and gastric inhibitory peptide, in response to the presence of hydrochloric acid, fats, osmolytes, and amino acids in its lumen. The hormones decrease the strength of gastric contractions and relax the proximal stomach, thereby slowing gastric emptying.

GASTRIC EMPTYING AFTER GASTRIC OPERATIONS

After Proximal Gastric Vagotomy

Proximal gastric vagotomy (PGV) is the ulcer operation that causes the least disturbance in the normal pattern of gastric motility and emptying. The most characteristic alteration it does cause is an increase in the rate of initial emptying of liquids.[6] This acceleration of early liquid emptying has been attributed to loss of vagally mediated receptive relaxation of the proximal stomach and to impairment of gastric accommodation after PGV, even though vagally enhanced hormonal accommodation still occurs.[6-8] The loss of gastric accommodation also may explain the mild satiety and sensation of gastric distention with eating experienced by approximately 25% of patients early after PGV (Table 1). The acceleration of the early phase of liquid emptying after PGV rarely results in symptoms of dumping, presumably because pyloric compensatory mechanisms prevent excessively rapid emptying of liquids. When pyloroplasty or gastroenterostomy is added to any form of PGV or truncal vagotomy, the compensatory mechanism is lost, and dumping is more likely to occur. Interestingly, dumping is extremely uncommon when pyloroplasty or gastroenterostomy is performed in the absence of a previous vagotomy, probably because gastric accommodation and receptive relaxation remain intact, slowing emptying of liquids.

Because the antropyloric mechanism and its innervation remain intact, gastric emptying of solids is largely unchanged after PGV.[6] Furthermore, the maintenance of an intact, innervated distal antrum and pylorus virtually eliminates reflux of duodenal content into the stomach.

After Truncal Vagotomy and Pyloroplasty

The pyloroplasty used with truncal vagotomy destroys the pyloric sphincter, creating a wide opening between the stomach and the duodenum.[9] The reduction in resistance across the pylorus caused by the pyloroplasty, in addition to the loss of proximal gastric receptive relaxation and accommodation due to the truncal vagotomy, produces rapid and unregulated emptying of liquids from the stomach (Table 1).

Gastric emptying of solids after truncal vagotomy and pyloroplasty is varied; patients cannot be categorized into a single group. The vagotomy usually results in weak,

Table 1.—Types of Gastric Motor Disorders Found After Gastric Operation

Operation	Gastric motor disorder	Resulting syndrome
Proximal gastric vagotomy	Rapid emptying of liquids	Early satiety
Truncal vagotomy	Rapid emptying of liquids, slow emptying of solids	Dumping, diarrhea, or gastroparesis
Pyloroplasty, gastrojejunostomy	Enterogastric reflux	Alkaline reflux gastritis
Roux-en-Y gastro-jejunostomy	Slow emptying of liquids and solids	Roux stasis syndrome
Gastrectomy	Rapid emptying of liquids and solids, enterogastric reflux	Dumping, diarrhea, alkaline reflux gastritis

infrequent, distal gastric contractions after a meal. The diminished grinding function results in a prolonged lag phase and a slow, linear emptying of solids, especially in patients with antecedent gastric dilatation from an obstructing duodenal ulcer.[10] Other patients are more influenced by destruction of the pyloric mechanism and have rapid gastric emptying of solids, which are no longer held back by the pylorus. Solids are emptied prematurely as large chunks (more than 1 mm in diameter) that have not been triturated into smaller particles, as occurs in the healthy stomach. Destruction of the pylorus also allows the free reflux of duodenal content into the stomach, which can incite alkaline reflux gastritis.

After Distal Gastrectomy

Distal gastrectomy removes the pylorus, the antrum, and a variable portion of the body of the stomach. A gastroduodenostomy or gastrojejunostomy is then created that decreases the resistance to gastric outflow compared with the resistance offered by the antropyloric mechanism in health. The increased release of antral gastrin, which normally enhances gastric accommodation after a meal, is abolished after antrectomy. These factors speed gastric emptying of liquids slightly.[11] When distal gastrectomy is combined with a Billroth II reconstruction (gastrojejunostomy), gastric chyme bypasses receptors in the duodenal mucosa. Thus, the negative feedback that slows gastric emptying when acidic, hyperosmolar, fatty, or nutrient-rich fluid reaches the duodenum is impaired. All of these changes produce an increase in the rate of gastric emptying of liquids. The addition of vagotomy to distal gastrectomy results in the loss of receptive relaxation and accommodation, which further increases the speed of gastric emptying of liquids.

With loss of the normal antropyloric grinding mechanism after distal gastrectomy, a rapid emptying of large solids often occurs.[11] Abnormal retention of solids after distal gastrectomy is unusual, although the addition of vagotomy increases the risk for this problem.[10] Reconstruction with either a gastroduodenostomy or a gastrojejunostomy results in the free reflux of enteric content into the stomach. Alkaline reflux gastritis can occur after the operation (Table 1).

After Roux-en-Y Gastrojejunostomy

The Roux operation diverts duodenal content and bile away from the gastric remnant. The Roux-en-Y gastrojejunostomy is performed by transecting the proximal jejunum about 25 cm distal to the ligament of Treitz. The distal cut end of the jejunum is then anastomosed to the gastric remnant, and the proximal cut end is anastomosed to the mid jejunum approximately 45 cm distal to the gastroenterostomy (Fig. 2). Truncal vagotomy is usually added, if this has not already been done, to reduce the risk of postoperative jejunal ulcer at the gastrojejunal anastomosis. Unlike with a Billroth II anastomosis, the jejunal mucosa at the site of a Roux-en-Y gastrojejunostomy is "unprotected," because it is not bathed in alkaline pancreatic and biliary secretions present in the upper small intestinal lumen; hence, it is more susceptible to acid-peptic corrosion.

Disordered motility of the Roux limb is in part due to the jejunal transection required for the Roux-en-Y construction. The transection separates the Roux limb from the duodenal pacemaker. In health, the duodenal pacemaker drives the contractions of the jejunum to a more rapid frequency than the jejunum can achieve on its own. After the transection, the frequency distal to the cut decreases. Ectopic pacemakers then appear in the Roux limb, but they beat at a frequency about 25% slower than before the transection. Also, they often appear downstream from the site of the transection, so they produce orally propagating electrical waves and, hence, orally propagating contractions in the proximal part of the limb, at least in dogs (Fig. 3).[12,13]

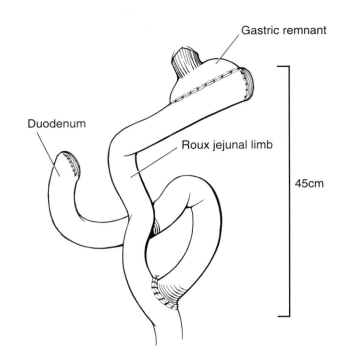

Fig. 2. Near-total distal gastrectomy with standard Roux-en-Y gastrojejunostomy.

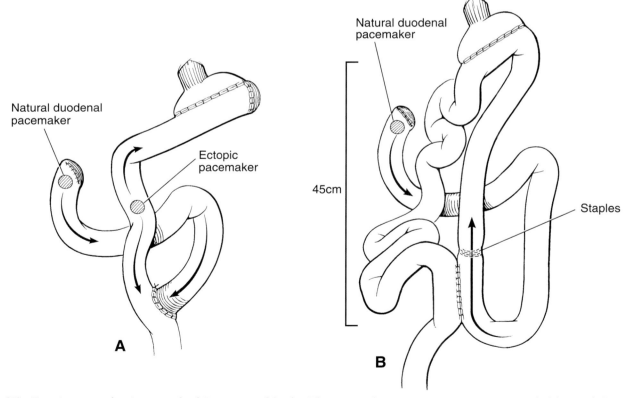

Fig. 3. (A), *Ectopic pacemaker in a standard Roux jejunal limb. This pacemaker generates pacesetter potentials (electrical slow waves) at a slower frequency than the natural duodenal pacemaker and drives those of the proximal part of the limb (hence, the contractions in this area) in an oral direction toward the stomach* (upper arrow). (B), *In contrast, the natural duodenal pacemaker maintains the frequency and aboral propagation of pacesetter potentials* (arrows) *in an uncut Roux limb, just as it does in the healthy, intact bowel. No ectopic pacemakers appear.*

This is in contrast to the consistent distally progressing electrical and contractile sequences present in the healthy, intact bowel. Small intestinal content driven in a proximal direction by the ectopic pacemakers in the Roux limb increases the resistance to outflow from the gastric remnant. The result is that both gastric emptying and transit through the jejunal limb are slowed after Roux gastrojejunostomy (Table 1).[13-16] Many patients who have the procedure are abusers of nonsteroidal anti-inflammatory drugs. Stasis of these pills in the stomach or Roux limb can cause inflammation, ulcers, and strictures in the stomach or Roux limb.

After Proximal Gastrectomy

Resection of the proximal stomach decreases the reservoir function of the stomach. Greater increases in intragastric pressure then occur after a meal, leading to an increased rate of gastric emptying of liquids.[17] Gastric emptying of solids has not received careful study after proximal gastrectomy. The grinding function of the antrum is maintained, but antral contractions are slower because the gastric pacemaker usually has been resected. The ectopic pacemakers that then appear beat more slowly. Also, the peristaltic waves in the distal gastric remnant are smaller in amplitude, weakened by the vagotomy that usually accompanies these resections.

Summary

Gastric operations can cause rapid or slow emptying from the stomach and can result in enterogastric reflux. Each of these three main pathophysiologic disturbances may cause symptoms, although, remarkably, they fail to do so in a majority of patients.

MAJOR POSTOPERATIVE SYNDROMES AFTER GASTRIC OPERATIONS

Slow Gastric Emptying

Slow gastric emptying, or gastroparesis, is one of the most serious complications of gastric operations. Fortunately, it is uncommon. For example, gastroparesis occurs in less than 1% of patients after PGV. Truncal vagotomy increases the risk of slow gastric emptying at least twofold. Procedures that combine truncal vagotomy and Roux-en-Y gastrojejunostomy result in the greatest incidence of slow gastric emptying. Symptoms of upper-gut stasis appear in 30% of patients after this combination of operations.[18,19] Some patients with diseases affecting the gastrointestinal tract are at increased risk for development of postoperative gastric stasis. Patients with diabetes mellitus, hypothyroidism, autonomic neurologic disorders, or pancreatic cancer are particularly susceptible. Preoperative

gastric outlet obstruction also increases the risk of slow emptying, especially in the early postoperative period.

Patients with gastroparesis have upper abdominal pain, postprandial epigastric fullness, nausea, and vomiting of food ingested hours or even days beforehand.[20] Gastric bezoars can form and aggravate symptoms. Most patients with the condition tolerate liquids better than solids. Many can ingest adequate calories and fluid from a liquid diet, but the addition of solids leads to symptoms. Patients with more severe symptoms cannot ingest adequate nourishment in either liquid or solid form, and so they lose weight. Severe postvagotomy, postgastrectomy gastroparesis can lead to life-threatening malnutrition requiring aggressive intervention with enteral or parenteral feedings.

Rapid Gastric Emptying, Dumping, and Diarrhea

The rapid gastric emptying of liquids that may occur after gastric operations is well tolerated by most patients. However, the rapid emptying of nutrient-rich liquids, especially hyperosmolar carbohydrates, can produce the dumping syndrome.[21] There are two types of dumping: early dumping and the more uncommon late dumping. Both occur as a result of hyperosmolar, carbohydrate-rich meals passing too quickly into the small intestine. In early dumping, symptoms occur 10 to 30 minutes after a meal, whereas in late dumping, symptoms appear 2 to 3 hours after a meal. Both conditions produce vasomotor symptoms, including diaphoresis, weakness, dizziness, flushing, and palpitations.

In addition, early dumping produces the gastrointestinal symptoms of nausea, abdominal cramps, and diarrhea. In early dumping, the changes begin with the rapid shifts of fluid from the blood into the small bowel lumen to dilute the hyperosmolar chyme emptied into the small bowel from the stomach. The resultant loss of intravascular volume and the hyperosmolar intestinal content cause the release of serotonin, gastric inhibitory peptide, vasoactive inhibitory peptide, neurotensin, and other vasoregulatory substances, all of which contribute to vasomotor symptoms.

In late dumping, release of enteroglucagon and probably other "incretins" in response to the high carbohydrate concentrations in the small bowel is believed to sensitize the pancreatic B cell to stimuli, causing a relative hypersecretion of insulin. This hyperinsulinemia produces a subsequent "reactive" hypoglycemia, which is the primary causal factor of the late dumping symptoms. Increased release of epinephrine in response to hypovolemia in early dumping and in response to hypoglycemia in late dumping also contributes to symptoms.

Up to 50% of patients experience some degree of dumping after truncal vagotomy and a drainage operation, but in most patients the dumping is mild and responds to dietary manipulation. Women appear to be more susceptible to dumping and to another condition, postvagotomy diarrhea.

The frequency of postvagotomy diarrhea is 10% to 20% in patients after truncal vagotomy and 2% to 4% after PGV. Usually the postvagotomy diarrhea is mild, but rarely (about 1% of cases) it can be severe and debilitating. The mechanism is unknown, but the decrease in frequency with the more selective vagotomy, which preserves the vagal innervation to the small bowel, suggests that the vagal denervation of the small bowel, biliary tree, and pancreas after truncal vagotomy has a role. Rapid gastric emptying of liquids also has been correlated with postvagotomy diarrhea. Other factors that may contribute to the diarrhea include decreased intestinal transit time, decreased absorption, decrease in biliary and pancreatic secretion, and release of humoral factors capable of inducing diarrhea.

Alkaline Reflux Gastritis

Alkaline reflux gastritis is an uncommon syndrome of upper abdominal pain, nausea, and bilious vomiting occurring in patients after gastrectomy, pyloroplasty, gastroenterostomy, or, rarely, cholecystectomy. The syndrome develops when bile refluxes into the stomach from the small intestine, usually through a surgically created gastroenterostomy or pyloroplasty.[22] The bile acids in bile damage the gastric mucosa and disrupt the barrier to back diffusion of acid from the gastric lumen into the gastric wall. Gastritis results, and symptoms appear. The triad of constant (not postprandial) epigastric pain, nausea, and bilious vomiting develops and is associated with endoscopic evidence of bile reflux into the stomach and sometimes macroscopic and histologic evidence of gastritis. This triad can occur after gastric resection or a gastric "drainage" procedure for peptic ulcer. Although the precise component of the refluxate that causes mucosal injury is unknown, bile salts are most commonly implicated. It is unclear why this syndrome is not more common, given that all patients who have had a gastrectomy or a gastric drainage operation have reflux of duodenal content to some degree.

The quantity of bile entering the stomach does not seem to be important for determining symptoms, but slow gastric emptying of the refluxed bile does correlate with symptoms.[11] Slow gastric emptying results in delayed clearing of bile from the stomach, prolonging contact of the refluxed bile with the gastric mucosa.

Cancer of the Gastric Remnant

Adenocarcinoma can appear in the gastric remnant after gastrectomy and vagotomy (see Chapter 8). The interval between the initial operation and the appearance of the

cancer is usually long, a mean of 10 years or more. The cause is thought to be related to a combination of stasis, hypoacidity, bile acid-induced mucosal injury, and bacterial overgrowth in the gastric lumen of the gastric remnant. The stasis also prolongs the exposure of the gastric mucosa to nitrosamines, nitrosamides, and other carcinogenic agents, and the bacterial overgrowth enhances the conversion of nitrates to N-nitroso compounds. Cancers of the gastric remnant are often asymptomatic at first, but as they grow larger and spread, symptoms of abdominal pain, early satiety, nausea, anorexia, and weight loss ensue. With further growth, ulceration, bleeding, obstruction, and perforation can occur.

DIAGNOSIS OF POSTOPERATIVE GASTRIC MOTOR DISORDERS

The patient with substantial symptoms after gastric operation poses a challenging clinical problem in diagnosis and clinical management. The history should focus particularly on the indication for the original gastric operation, the symptoms preceding that operation, the details of the preceding operation(s), and the presenting symptoms, their relationship to eating or drinking, and their progression or improvement with time. The patient's previous illness-related behavior and the presence of behaviors that may exacerbate the symptoms, such as alcohol, tobacco, or analgesic abuse, also need to be addressed.

On the basis of the history, it is usually possible to identify a likely postoperative gastric syndrome and to postulate a possible pathophysiologic mechanism. In addition to a disorder of gastric emptying, the diagnosis of recurrent ulcer, stomal stenosis, partial afferent limb obstruction, or partial small bowel obstruction should always be considered, because effective treatment for each is available. A combination of endoscopy and radiologic imaging with barium sulfate as the contrast agent can help identify these complications and can detect cancer in the gastric remnant. However, more commonly, the symptoms fit into one of the postoperative syndromes described above. In this case, decisions regarding operative intervention should be made judiciously, because symptoms usually improve with time or with medical and dietary manipulations, especially symptoms that develop in the early postoperative period. Moreover, operative revision does not always lead to improvement.

Rapid and slow gastric emptying and transit through the upper gut can be readily diagnosed with radioisotope tests of gastric emptying (scintiscanning). Severe, incapacitating diarrhea after vagotomy is unusual, occurring in only about 1% of patients at risk. The diagnosis is one of exclusion. All other causes of diarrhea should be ruled out before this diagnosis is made. Radionuclide or contrast imaging tests often show rapid gastrointestinal transit.

For evaluation of the patient with presumed alkaline reflux gastritis, the anatomy should be defined with endoscopy and radiologically with a barium meal and a small bowel follow-through. A solid-liquid radionuclide meal should be given to determine the current pattern of gastric emptying of both solids and liquids. This test is an essential diagnostic examination, because symptoms are poor predictors of gastric emptying unless the patient vomits food eaten the day before; this is virtually pathognomonic of delayed gastric emptying, of either a functional or a mechanical cause. The diagnosis of alkaline reflux gastritis is often problematic, however, and can be made only when recurrent ulcer, biliary, and pancreatic disease and afferent loop syndrome have been ruled out. The diagnosis can be aided by observation of reflux of an intravenously administered biliary tracer into the stomach on hepato-iminodiacetic acid scintiscanning and with the alkaline Bernstein test. In a positive Bernstein test, intragastric infusion of NaOH reproduces the patient's pain, but acid infusion does not. On endoscopy, a pool of bile is found in the stomach, and bile is seen refluxing through a surgically created stoma between the duodenum or jejunum and the stomach. The gastric mucosa often is reddish and friable and may contain small pinpoint ulcers.

Gastric cancers appearing after operation are best diagnosed with endoscopy and biopsy.

MEDICAL AND DIETARY INTERVENTIONS

Slow Gastric Emptying
Medical and dietary interventions for slow gastric emptying include metoclopramide (effective only when the antrum is intact) and erythromycin in combination with the choice of more frequent liquid, well-chewed, smaller meals. Some patients must avoid solid food entirely and subsist on a high-calorie liquid diet.

After a standard Roux gastrojejunostomy in experimental animals (dogs), we have successfully treated the slow gastric emptying and slow jejunal transit with small intestinal electrical pacing.[23] The pacing suppresses the abnormal ectopic pacers in the Roux limb and drives or paces the electrical waves of the limb in their usual aboral or distal direction at their usual frequency. In dogs, pacing restores gastric emptying and transit through the Roux limb to a healthy pattern. Unfortunately, the technique of small intestinal pacing is not yet ready for application to humans.

Dumping and Diarrhea
Dumping usually can be effectively treated with dietary and medical means.[21] Dietary manipulations involve the use of small, frequent, dry, high-fiber meals, the avoidance of hyperosmolar, carbohydrate-rich liquids, and a reduction in fluid intake with meals. Increased dietary fiber or ingestion of a nonabsorbable bulking agent such as kaolin-pectin has been proposed as a means of slowing emptying and ameliorating dumping symptoms. Similarly, the use of the amylase inhibitor acarbose to slow the chemical breakdown of starch into simple sugars has had variable success in some patients. Posture during the meal also may be important. An upright posture may hasten gastric emptying and symptoms. In contrast, recumbency after a meal may reduce dumping symptoms. Octreotide also has been used. Subcutaneous injections of 75 μg or 100 μg of this drug, given 20 minutes before eating, have been effective in slowing gastric emptying and ameliorating the dumping syndrome in some of our patients. The long-acting forms of octreotide are most beneficial.

Postvagotomy diarrhea is unusual, but when present it is difficult or impossible to treat effectively. Affected patients are miserable because of rapid gastrointestinal transit, often with an element of functional malabsorption. Dietary manipulations are of little benefit, and pharmacologic agents have proved to be of essentially no use. Attempts to slow transit with bulking agents or various narcotics (such as codeine, tincture of opium, loperamide) are generally ineffective. Similarly, octreotide has proved ineffective. In summary, no good or effective dietary or pharmacologic agents are available to treat this type of diarrhea.

Alkaline Reflux Gastritis
Alkaline reflux gastritis may respond to frequent meals, including a bedtime snack, magnesium and aluminum hydroxides, and cholestyramine, all of which bind bile salts and neutralize hydrogen ions in the gastric lumen, thus aiding healing of the gastritis. Coating the gastric mucosa with sucralfate may minimize damage by bile salts. However, these pharmacologic approaches often have little success.

PREOPERATIVE CONSIDERATIONS

If the patient's postoperative symptoms persist despite medical and dietary interventions, and operative intervention is contemplated, the clinician should evaluate gastric emptying carefully before operation to decide which type of revisional procedure is needed. This evaluation is extremely important, because our experience has shown that many patients in whom alkaline reflux gastritis is diagnosed actually have gastroparesis. This differential diagnosis is crucial, because operative conversion to a Roux-en-Y gastrojejunostomy will worsen symptoms in patients with gastroparesis.

Also, clinicians should remember that spontaneous improvement often occurs with time. For example, after operations that cause dumping and diarrhea, conservative management for at least 1 year is prudent before offering any revisionary operation. During that year, dumping or diarrhea may resolve spontaneously or improve to the point that operative management is not needed.

OPERATIVE TREATMENT OF POSTOPERATIVE DISORDERS

Delayed Gastric Emptying

Patients with delayed gastric emptying of solids after gastric operations generally do not respond well to chronic prokinetic medication. Some success has been reported with gastric pacing or electrical stimulation. A pacemaker is implanted in the subcutaneous tissues. Electrical impulses from the pacemaker are delivered to the tunica muscularis of the stomach by wire leads attached to the gastric wall, a process similar in principle to cardiac pacing. The results have been inconsistent. We are not convinced of the efficacy and have not adopted this technique in our practice.

Accordingly, many of our patients come to revisional operation. After truncal vagotomy and pyloroplasty, partial gastrectomy and gastroenterostomy may alleviate the stasis if the primary problem is loss of effective antropyloric contractions. However, the failure rate is also high, because the cause of the stasis may also in large part be related to vagal denervation of the proximal stomach, which will not be helped by antrectomy or gastroenterostomy. In patients with gastric atony after vagotomy and partial gastrectomy, and in selected patients after truncal vagotomy and pyloroplasty, the best current surgical option is near-total gastrectomy (Table 2). Roux-en-Y reconstruction is then necessary to divert bile from the gastric remnant and esophagus to prevent the development of alkaline reflux esophagitis (Fig. 2). However, both surgeon and patient must understand that this operation is not always successful. Extensive gastric resection for delayed gastric emptying offers some improvement in about 50% of patients, but only 25% are returned to excellent health.

We recently reviewed 62 patients (51 females, 11 males) who underwent near-total gastrectomy with Roux-en-Y gastrojejunostomy for postvagotomy, postgastrectomy gastroparesis.[24] All patients were moderately or severely symptomatic, and all had nutritional failure requiring some form of intervention. They complained of nausea, vomiting, and pain, and many had become chemically dependent

Table 2.—Corrective Operations for Gastric Motor Disorders After Gastric Operation

Disorder	Corrective operation
Gastroparesis	Near-total gastrectomy, standard or uncut Roux-en-Y gastrojejunostomy
Dumping, diarrhea	
Antropyloric nerves intact	Pyloric reconstruction
Antropyloric nerves severed	Antrectomy, standard Roux-en-Y gastrojejunostomy
Alkaline reflux gastritis	Antrectomy, standard or uncut Roux-en-Y gastrojejunostomy
Gastric cancer	Total gastrectomy with standard or uncut Roux-en-Y gastrojejunostomy

because of chronic narcotic use. All had undergone a previous vagotomy, and many had had four or more previous gastric operations, often progressing from vagotomy and pyloroplasty to Billroth I gastrectomy to Billroth II gastrectomy and finally to Roux-en-Y gastrojejunostomy, all without improvement.

No early postoperative deaths occurred after the near-total gastrectomy, but 40% of patients had early postoperative complications, the most common of which were due to postoperative ileus and to narcotic withdrawal in patients who were dependent on narcotics preoperatively. On long-term follow-up a mean of 5.4 years later, only 43% of patients had relief of all or most of their preoperative symptoms, and 57% continued to have abdominal pain, nausea, and vomiting and had little objective relief. About 50% maintained their nutrition with oral feedings, and 50% required supplemental enteral or parenteral nutrition or both. Patients with the combination of nausea and vomiting, retained food in the stomach, and the need for total parenteral nutrition preoperatively usually had a poor long-term outcome. Because of these unsatisfactory results, we strongly recommend placing a feeding jejunostomy at the time of the near-total gastrectomy.

We wondered whether the poor long-term outcome after near-total gastrectomy and Roux-en-Y gastrojejunostomy in these patients might be due, in part, to the retrograde or orally moving contractions in the Roux limb used to reconstruct enteric continuity after the near-total gastrectomy (i.e., the Roux stasis syndrome).[18] Ectopic pacemakers and orally moving contractions in the Roux limb after operation slow emptying from the small remaining gastric remnant and retard transit through the Roux limb itself. To prevent the Roux stasis, we evaluated a new type of Roux limb, a so-called uncut Roux limb.[23,25,26]

In this procedure the gastric remnant is joined end-to-side to an uncut loop of jejunum, as in a conventional end-to-side gastrojejunostomy (Fig. 3). A side-to-side jejunojejunostomy is then made between the afferent and efferent jejunal limbs at a site 45 cm distal to the gastroenterostomy. The lumen of the afferent jejunal limb leading to the stomach is then occluded with rows of stainless steel staples placed by a noncutting linear stapler just distal to the jejunojejunostomy. This procedure totally diverts bile and jejunal chyme through the jejunojejunostomy and into the efferent limb, where it passes downstream away from the stomach. The occluding staple lines are designed both to prevent reflux of bile into the gastric remnant and esophagus and to preserve normal propagation of electrical signals from the duodenum across the staple line into the afferent jejunal limb and, thence, aborally down the efferent jejunal limb.

In an early series of these operations done at Mayo Clinic, no sign of gastric stasis occurred in any of the 14 patients who underwent the procedure.[27] However, in 5 of the 14 patients, bile reflux esophagitis developed from breakdown of the staple lines that had been used to occlude the afferent jejunal limb. The breakdown allowed bile and enteric content to pass into the afferent jejunal limb and up into the gastric remnant, where it refluxed into the esophagus. Because of these results, we now occlude the afferent jejunal limb with two cartridges of staples (four rows of staples) instead of one cartridge of staples (two rows of staples). This occlusion provides a more secure, long-term closure and yet preserves the propagation of electrical signals across the staple lines. Other investigators also have reported excellent results with a similar modification of an uncut Roux limb for the relief of gastroparesis.[28] Still others have used a purse-string suture to occlude the lumen of the afferent limb;[29] no bile reflux appeared after operation in a series of 11 patients who had the procedure for gastroparesis.

What about the patients who already have the Roux stasis syndrome after a standard Roux-en-Y reconstruction operation? As stated, electrical pacing of the Roux limb in dogs abolished ectopic pacemakers and improved gastric emptying,[23] but pacing has not yet achieved clinical reality.[13,20] We have wondered whether a new type of reconstructive operation might work. We have shown in experimental animals that after a conventional jejunal transection, as is done in making a Roux limb, a careful end-to-end, layer-by-layer anastomosis of the two cut ends with microsurgical techniques can at least partially restore propagation of pacesetter potentials across the anastomosis, thus preventing ectopic pacemakers from appearing in the bowel distal to the transection and maintaining pacing of the jejunum by the duodenal pacemaker.[30] Thus, a possible operative approach to patients

with the Roux stasis syndrome would be to take down the Roux gastrojejunostomy, to use operative microscopy to reanastomose the jejunum with an end-to-end jejunojejunostomy, and then to reconstruct with an uncut Roux gastrojejunostomy at a site distal to the end-to-end jejunojejunostomy (Fig. 4). An operation similar to this has been done in dogs,[31] but it awaits trial in humans.

Rapid Gastric Emptying, Dumping, and Diarrhea

Various surgical reconstructions have been recommended in patients with dumping and diarrhea refractory to medical and dietary therapy. Interposition of a jejunal segment between the stomach and the duodenum, conversion of the gastrojejunostomy to a gastroduodenostomy, and reversal of a 10-cm to 15-cm segment of proximal jejunum have all been done at Mayo Clinic with rather mixed, inconsistent results.

Some groups have reported excellent results with pyloric reconstruction for dumping after vagotomy and pyloroplasty, but the results of this operation in our hands have sometimes been disappointing.[22] The successes we have had with it have been in patients who have retained some vagal innervation of the distal stomach and pylorus. In these patients, gastric emptying has been restored by pyloric reconstruction to a pattern found in health (Table 2). In contrast, those who have gastric vagal denervation of the distal stomach will have gastric stasis after pyloric reconstruction and continue to have symptoms from it. Among eight such patients who had operation at Mayo Clinic, six had a poor postoperative result.

Because of the less than optimal results with other procedures, we prefer that most patients who need operation for dumping and diarrhea have conversion to a distal gastrectomy and a standard Roux-en-Y gastrojejunostomy.[22] In contrast to the deleterious effects produced by the Roux limb in patients with gastroparesis, the slow gastric emptying produced by the Roux limb in patients with rapid gastric emptying, dumping, and diarrhea may have a beneficial effect. In one report, the Roux-en-Y reconstruction diminished symptoms in 86% of patients with dumping, albeit the delay in emptying was sufficient to cause new symptoms of gastric stasis in 23% of patients.[32] The rare patients with severe, incapacitating diarrhea present an especially difficult problem. These patients have extremely rapid gastrointestinal transit, often measured in minutes rather than hours. No one and no institution has more than very limited experience with this condition, because it is so rare. Anecdotal reports of using a 10-cm reversed jejunal limb 100 cm from the ligament of Treitz or even two separate, reversed segments at 100-cm intervals should be viewed with caution. Many gastrointestinal surgeons, including ourselves, have not had encouraging, long-lasting success with this procedure.

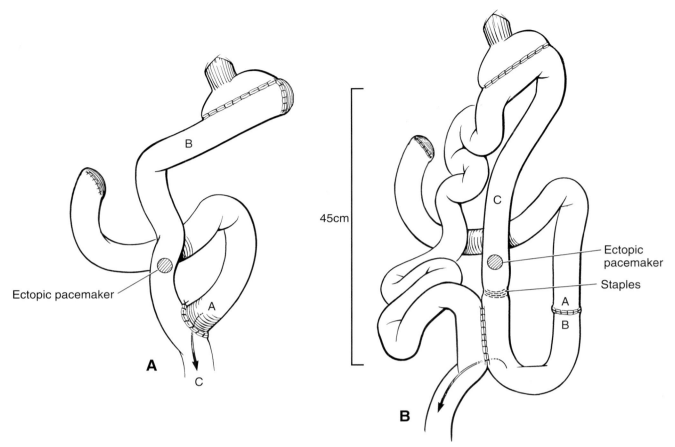

Fig. 4. Treatment of the Roux stasis syndrome with takedown of the gastrojejunostomy and the end-to-side jejunojejunostomy (A), *followed by end-to-end jejunojejunostomy and construction of an uncut Roux gastrojejunostomy at a site distal to the jejunojejunostomy* (B).

Alkaline Reflux Gastritis

The medical treatment of this syndrome is generally ineffective. If symptoms are severe enough to justify revisionary operation, a Roux-en-Y, end-to-side gastrojejunostomy appears to be the best procedure to divert bile and other small bowel content away from the gastric remnant (Table 2). The Roux procedure in our hands has helped about 75% of patients.[18] However, bilious vomiting is the only symptom consistently abolished. The abdominal pain and nausea experienced by many patients after Roux gastrectomy is probably related to continued or worsened upper gut stasis of solids after the Roux operation. The preoperative slow gastric emptying often present with this syndrome may contribute to the symptoms postoperatively, as may the retardant effect of the Roux limb. As stated, the surgeon must carefully exclude the presence of considerable gastroparesis preoperatively, because the Roux operation will predictably fail and worsen this condition.

Because of the slowing of gastrointestinal transit produced by a conventional Roux-en-Y gastrojejunostomy, we are now exploring use of the uncut Roux-en-Y technique for

this condition. Also, some surgeons recommend a near-total gastrectomy as part of the Roux procedure for patients with alkaline reflux gastritis who also have delayed gastric emptying. However, which patients will have gastric stasis after Roux gastrectomy cannot be fully predicted by the preoperative gastric emptying rate, unless markedly slow gastric emptying is present. Thus, prophylactic near-total gastrectomy at the time of Roux-en-Y gastrojejunostomy is probably not justified in most patients.

Gastric Remnant Cancer

Cancer of the gastric remnant almost always necessitates a total gastrectomy to remove all the gastric mucosa at risk. Excision of the regional lymph nodes should be accomplished with the gastrectomy. Reconstruction is then accomplished with an esophagojejunostomy with a Roux-en-Y jejunal limb (Table 2). Again, we are exploring the uncut Roux limb in this situation. The use of an uncut Roux limb in patients with cancer, however, may not be as important as in patients with functional disorders, such as peptic ulcer. Patients with cancer have fewer postgastrectomy disorders than patients with peptic ulcer.

Prognosis after operation depends mainly on whether the tumor and the lymph nodes to which it may have metastasized can be completely resected. With spread of the tumor to distant lymph nodes or distant sites or with transmural growth and direct invasion of the tumor into other organs, the prognosis is grim (see Chapter 6).

PREVENTION OF DISORDERS

The morbidity of gastric operation can be decreased in several ways. Elective operation for uncomplicated peptic ulcer should be considered only after aggressive medical therapy fails. This situation is extremely rare today. Operations with minimal long-term sequelae, such as PGV, should be used whenever possible. A decision to perform a specific operation based solely on the reported incidence of ulcer recurrence postoperatively is inappropriate, because the somewhat greater incidence of recurrent ulcer after less extensive operations, such as PGV (about 10%), as opposed to antrectomy and truncal vagotomy (about 2%), must be weighed against the much lower incidence of serious postoperative morbidity with the more selective vagotomy and by avoiding gastrectomy. Furthermore, recurrent ulcer can be readily managed with medical therapy. The healing effects of PGV and medical therapy are synergistic. In addition, attention should always be paid to factors exacerbating ulcer disease, such as smoking, nonsteroidal anti-inflammatory drugs, and infection with *Helicobacter pylori*. Supplements of oral iron, oral calcium, and parenteral vitamin B_{12} should be taken after gastric operations to prevent the later appearance of anemias and osteoporosis. Finally, when significant postoperative morbidity does occur and fails to resolve with medical and dietary therapy, further intervention should be based on a clear understanding of the pathophysiologic mechanisms underlying the disordered gastric emptying.

CONCLUSION

Gastric operations predispose the patient to three main adverse patterns of postoperative gastric emptying: delayed emptying, rapid emptying, and reflux of small bowel content into the stomach. These abnormal emptying patterns can be explained by postoperative disturbances in gastric motility and emptying.

Delayed gastric emptying is often due in large part to weakened motor activity of the stomach after vagotomy. When gastrectomy accompanies the vagotomy, the use of a Roux limb in the reconstruction can worsen the slow emptying caused by the vagotomy. The surgical treatment of gastroparesis is a near-total gastrectomy to remove the atonic gastric remnant. Unfortunately, reconstruction with a Roux-en-Y gastrojejunostomy often has been deemed necessary to avoid subsequent postoperative reflux esophagitis. We are exploring the use of an uncut Roux-en-Y gastrojejunostomy, rather than a standard Roux operation, because we believe the uncut procedure causes less slowing of gastric emptying than the standard operation. *Rapid gastric emptying* can result in the dumping syndrome and diarrhea. This syndrome usually can be controlled with dietary and medical measures but may require treatment with octreotide. In the unusual patient who requires operative intervention, conversion to conventional Roux-en-Y gastrojejunostomy is our procedure of choice.

Enterogastric reflux is best treated with a Roux-en-Y gastrojejunostomy. Again, we are exploring use of the uncut Roux limb for this condition. Approximately 70% of patients can be improved with revisional gastric operation. Preventing postoperative gastric emptying disorders is enhanced by adhering to stringent indications for ulcer or cancer operation and by using more physiologic operations, such as PGV, when operation is necessary.

REFERENCES

1. Gustavsson S, Kelly KA, Melton LJ III, Zinsmeister AR: Trends in peptic ulcer surgery: a population-based study in Rochester, Minnesota, 1956-1985. Gastroenterology 94:688-694, 1988

2. Soper NJ, Kelly KA, van Heerden JA, Ilstrup DM: Long term clinical results after proximal gastric vagotomy. Surg Gynecol Obstet 169:488-494, 1989

3. Miedema BW, Heddle R, Kelly KA: Postoperative gastric emptying disorders. Resident Staff Phys 38:111-122, 1992

4. Hinder RA, Kelly KA: Canine gastric emptying of solids and liquids. Am J Physiol 233:E335-E340, 1977

5. Cullen JJ, Kelly KA: Gastric motor physiology and pathophysiology. Surg Clin North Am 73:1145-1160, 1993

6. Wilbur BG, Kelly KA: Effect of proximal gastric, complete gastric, and truncal vagotomy on canine gastric electric activity, motility, and emptying. Ann Surg 178:295-303, 1973

7. Hould FS, Cullen JJ, Kelly KA: Influence of proximal gastric vagotomy on canine gastric motility and emptying. Surgery 116:83-89, 1994

8. Morimoto H, Kelly KA: Mechanisms of insulin-induced relaxation of the canine proximal stomach after proximal gastric vagotomy. J Gastrointest Surg 1:386-394, 1997

9. Cullen JJ, Kelly KA: Functional characteristics of canine pylorus in health, with pyloroplasty, and after pyloric reconstruction. Dig Dis Sci 41:711-719, 1996

10. Hom S, Sarr MG, Kelly KA, Hench V: Postoperative gastric atony after vagotomy for obstructing peptic ulcer. Am J Surg 157:282-286, 1989

11. Dozois RR, Kelly KA, Code CF: Effect of distal antrectomy on gastric emptying of liquids and solids. Gastroenterology 61:675-681, 1971

12. Karlstrom LH, Soper NJ, Kelly KA, Phillips SF: Ectopic jejunal pacemakers and enterogastric reflux after Roux gastrectomy: effect of intestinal pacing. Surgery 106:486-495, 1989

13. Karlstrom L, Kelly KA: Ectopic jejunal pacemakers and gastric emptying after Roux gastrectomy: effect of intestinal pacing. Surgery 106:867-871, 1989

14. Morrison P, Miedema BW, Kohler L, Kelly KA: Electrical dysrhythmias in the Roux jejunal limb: cause and treatment. Am J Surg 160:252-256, 1990

15. Cullen JJ, Eagon JC, Hould FS, Hanson RB, Kelly KA: Ectopic jejunal pacemakers after jejunal transection and their relationship to transit. Am J Physiol 268:G959-G967, 1995

16. Miedema BW, Kelly KA, Camilleri M, Hanson RB, Zinsmeister AR, O'Connor MK, Brown ML: Human gastric and jejunal transit and motility after Roux gastrojejunostomy. Gastroenterology 103:1133-1143, 1992

17. Wilbur BG, Kelly KA, Code CF: Effect of gastric fundectomy on canine gastric electrical and motor activity. Am J Physiol 226:1445-1449, 1974

18. Gustafsson S, Ilstrup DM, Morrison P, Kelly KA: Roux-Y stasis syndrome after gastrectomy. Am J Surg 155:490-494, 1988

19. Eagon JC, Miedema BW, Kelly KA: Postgastrectomy syndromes. Surg Clin North Am 72:445-465, 1992

20. Fich A, Neri M, Camilleri M, Kelly KA, Phillips SF: Stasis syndromes following gastric surgery: clinical and motility features of 60 symptomatic patients. J Clin Gastroenterol 12:505-512, 1990

21. Eagon JC, Cullen JJ, Hould F-S, Kelly KA: Dumping syndrome in a 54-year-old woman. Postgrad Gen Surg 4:210-213, 1992

22. Kelly KA, Becker JM, van Heerde JA: Reconstructive gastric surgery. Br J Surg 68:687-691, 1981

23. Miedema BW, Kelly KA: The Roux stasis syndrome: treatment by pacing and prevention by use of an 'uncut' Roux limb. Arch Surg 127:295-300, 1992

24. Forstner-Barthell AW, Murr MM, Nitecki S, Camilleri M, Prather CM, Kelly KA, Sarr MG: Near-total completion gastrectomy for severe postvagotomy gastric stasis: analysis of early and long-term results in 62 patients. J Gastrointest Surg 3:15-21, 1999

25. Miedema BW, Kelly KA: The Roux operation for postgastrectomy syndromes. Am J Surg 161:256-261, 1991

26. Tu BN, Kelly KA: Elimination of the Roux stasis syndrome using a new type of "uncut Roux" limb. Am J Surg 170:381-386, 1995

27. Tu BN, Sarr MG, Kelly KA: Early clinical results with the uncut Roux reconstruction after gastrectomy: limitations of the stapling technique. Am J Surg 170:262-264, 1995

28. Mon RA, Cullen JJ: Standard Roux-en-Y gastrojejunostomy vs. "uncut" Roux-en-Y gastrojejunostomy: a matched cohort study. J Gastrointest Surg 4:298-303, 2000

29. Noh SM: Improvement of the Roux limb function using a new type of "uncut Roux" limb. Am J Surg 180:37-40, 2000

30. Hart SC, Nguyen-Tu BL, Hould FS, Hanson RB, Kelly KA: Restoration of myoelectric propagation across a jejunal transection using microsurgical anastomosis. J Gastrointest Surg 3:524-532, 1999

31. Tu BL, Kelly KA: Surgical treatment of Roux stasis syndrome. J Gastrointest Surg 3:613-617, 1999

32. Vogel SB, Hocking MP, Woodward ER: Clinical and radionuclide evaluation of Roux-Y diversion for postgastrectomy dumping. Am J Surg 155:57-62, 1988

Chapter 10

MORBID OBESITY

Michael G. Sarr, M.D.
Keith A. Kelly, M.D.
Geoffrey B. Thompson, M.D.
Florencia G. Que, M.D.

In the United States, obesity has become a health crisis of epidemic proportions. Obesity is defined as a body mass index (BMI, weight in kg ÷ height in meters²) of 27 or more; a normal BMI is 25 or less. According to this definition, nearly 90 million Americans are affected by obesity to some extent. Within this context is the subset of Americans with morbid obesity (BMI > 35), which includes about 7% of all women and 3% of all men. One need only imagine the implications of obesity to the health care dollar to understand the enormity of this health care crisis. In 1990, more than a decade ago, weight-related morbidity accounted for an estimated increase of $69 billion in the health care budget alone.[1]

This chapter addresses obesity from the aspect of the surgical health care provider. Although only a minority of general or gastrointestinal surgeons perform bariatric surgery, most physicians and surgeons will encounter patients who are or should be considered candidates for operative treatment or who have problems or complications directly related to a previous bariatric procedure. Moreover, although bariatric surgery suffers from a somewhat jaded history, interest in this topic has been renewed by surgical investigators. Indeed, a National Institutes of Health consensus conference in 1991[2] concluded that bariatric intervention is an acceptable, established, and effective treatment option in selected patients. Thus, bariatric surgery, at least into the near future, is here to stay. This chapter discusses the problem, the medical complications of obesity, the history of bariatric surgery and the lessons learned, the current surgical approach at Mayo Clinic, and the future.

THE PROBLEM

Although mild to moderate obesity (BMI 28-35) is inconsistently associated with medical morbidity, a BMI more than 35 and especially more than 40 (usually a weight of more than 250 lb in women and more than 280 lb in men) renders the vast majority of affected subjects at risk for considerable morbidity directly related to their weight (morbid obesity). This chapter considers specifically morbid obesity and its management. A few cautions are needed in regard to use of the term "morbid obesity." First, the term should not be used indiscriminately. The insightful health care provider understands that this term means weight-related morbidity due to excess weight. However, the naive subject or patient may think you are calling them "morbid," to some a perjurious term, to many an embarrassment, and to others a call to fight. A better term is "medically complicated obesity." Second, not all persons with a BMI more than 35 have morbid obesity. For instance, a health care provider would not refer to the defensive end of a professional football team as having morbid obesity. In contrast, morbid obesity should not require a minimal weight or a minimal BMI. For instance, a 40-year-old man with coronary artery disease caused by hyperlipidemia, insulin-resistant diabetes mellitus, hypertension, incapacitating degenerative joint disease, and severe sleep apnea but who weighs "only" 230 lb and has a BMI of 33 does have morbid obesity, (i.e., direct weight-related morbidity), much of which is reversible with substantial weight loss.

MEDICAL COMPLICATIONS OF OBESITY (TABLE 1)

Numerous studies have clearly documented an increased mortality rate in patients with morbid obesity. Men between the ages of 25 and 34 years with a BMI more than 40 have a documented 12-fold higher risk of early death than men of normal weight.[3] The similar relative risk for women with morbid obesity is not well known but is obviously greater than that for women of normal weight. Weight loss with weight management reduces the prevalence of overall cardiovascular risk factors and thereby reduces the overall mortality rate. Probably the most common and most directly debilitating complication of morbid obesity is *premature degenerative joint disease*. The degenerative joint disease is not really an arthritis as such but rather a mechanical arthropathy. It develops with age—in some people at a younger age—but with morbid obesity the wear and tear on articulating cartilaginous, weight-bearing surfaces can be unrelenting. The most commonly involved joints are the knees and hips, but the lower back and the ankles are involved also. Low back pain or frank lumbar disk disease has a markedly increased prevalence in the patient with morbid obesity and, even with considerable weight reduction, can be difficult to treat effectively. Unfortunately, most people with morbid obesity never consider themselves (or are never considered by their physicians) as realistic candidates for bariatric surgery until symptoms develop—usually pain on walking—and by that time the degenerative joint disease is advanced. Many symptomatic patients first consult an orthopedic surgeon only to be told they are too heavy to undergo arthroplasty—thus, the referral for weight loss. The key is to intervene before irreversible damage has occurred.

Adult-onset *diabetes mellitus* of the insulin-resistant type is a common complication of morbid obesity and is

Table 1.—Medical Complications of Obesity

Degenerative joint disease (mechanical arthropathy)
Insulin-resistant diabetes mellitus
Hypertension
Coronary artery disease
Hyperlipidemia
Sleep apnea
Malignancy (endometrial, breast, colon)
Gallstones
Varicose veins
Lower extremity lymphedema
Accidents (at home and at work)
Psychosocial ostracism
Discrimination in the workplace

24 times more frequent in obese patients than in the general population. The presence of diabetes then introduces its own related morbidity. This form of diabetes is commonly genetic. Most patients will relate a history of diabetes in overweight first- and second-degree relatives, and this can be predictive of whether diabetes will develop later in life in younger, markedly overweight, presymptomatic subjects. "Chemical" diabetes (fasting blood glucose value of 120-140 mg/dL) is relatively common in patients in their 30s who have morbid obesity, but hyperglycemia severe enough to require insulin administration usually begins in the 40s. Daily insulin requirements are often more than 50 U per day (normal daily endogenous insulin secretion is 10-12 U per day) and not infrequently 100 to 200 U per day. Extreme obesity establishes a poorly understood insulin resistance at the end organs. Affected patients have higher than normal circulating insulin levels yet maintain a persistent hyperglycemia.

Although insulin resistance is a factor in the diabetes of obesity, the oral intake of carbohydrates and other caloric substances also is an important factor. Even early after a bariatric operation the need for insulin promptly and markedly decreases when food intake is acutely restricted. Often within a few days or weeks after operation, insulin requirements are reduced to one-half or less of the preoperative values. Normalization of serum glucose concentrations preoperatively, believed important for preventing or ameliorating the renal, cardiac, vascular, neurologic, and ophthalmologic consequences of diabetes, thus requires pharmacologic levels of insulin. However, the insulin-resistant diabetes of morbid obesity is imminently treatable and usually curable with substantial weight loss. Elegant studies by Pories et al.[4] showed that this form of diabetes responds to successful bariatric operation rapidly and virtually completely in more than 95% of patients. Thus, the patient with morbid obesity and insulin-resistant diabetes has a surgically treatable form of diabetes and should be strongly considered for a bariatric operation.

Hypertension affects 30% to 40% of patients with morbid obesity. The cause is probably multifactorial, including hyperlipidemia (see page 141) and diabetes mellitus, and may even be "iatrogenic" (falsely increased because of use of a normal-sized blood pressure cuff instead of the more appropriate large cuff). Hypertension predisposes to the risk of stroke and cardiac disease. Most studies have shown that satisfactory weight loss will reverse hypertension in about 50% of patients with morbid obesity; the remaining patients probably have a form of essential hypertension.

Coronary artery disease affects virtually all patients with morbid obesity to some extent, in part related to the coexistent hyperlipidemia of obesity. Angina is 37

times more frequent in this population; sudden unexplained cardiac arrest also has a high prevalence (see sleep apnea, below). The extent of obesity undoubtedly is not the only relevant factor, but cardiovascular morbidity and mortality decrease markedly with successful maintenance of weight loss.

Hyperlipidemia can be a real problem in the patient with morbid obesity because it also predisposes to cardiac and vascular complications. Most prevalent is hypertriglyceridemia, especially in persons with diabetes. The cause of this dyslipidemia is multifactorial, but weight loss and maintenance of weight loss in conjunction with a decrease in both calorie intake and the relative percentage of fat result in a marked decrease in serum lipid levels and an increase in the "good" HDL cholesterol.

Sleep apnea is a major problem in the population of patients with morbid obesity, especially in men. Sleep apnea in the patient with morbid obesity represents a central deregulation of the respiratory center. No longer is breathing regulated by the PaO_2 but rather by blood pH caused by CO_2 buildup. Instead of nighttime breathing being closely controlled by minor decreases in PaO_2, in the obese patient with sleep apnea the PaO_2 can decrease to low levels before the blood pH decreases sufficiently to trigger onset of inspiration. With persistent sleep apnea, the sleep center becomes deconditioned, leading to potentially serious hypoxia during sleep. Before public and physician awareness of sleep apnea in the past decade, nighttime sudden death during sleep was a common cause of death in patients with morbid obesity.

Similarly, it was not uncommon for the 40- to 50-year-old man with the classic "beer belly" to die during sleep. On first glance, this occurrence seems strange, because at night during sleep, heart rate and oxygen consumption decrease, and thus the reason for an increased incidence of myocardial infarction is unclear. Several factors are important. First, the classic "beer belly," or truncal form of obesity, is associated with a more virulent cardiovascular disease, much more so than the female, or gynecoid, fat distribution (i.e., big thighs and a more normal-sized torso). Truncal obesity involves a different type of fat metabolism with a greater prevalence of dyslipidemia and a higher prevalence of sleep apnea. Second, many patients with morbid obesity have extensive underlying, but asymptomatic, coronary artery disease and a relatively sedentary lifestyle. At night, the coexistent sleep apnea and central respiratory deconditioning lead to severe hypoxia that, in combination with a critical coronary artery stenosis, eventuates in insufficient oxygen delivery to the myocardium with subsequent myocardial infarction or severe arrhythmia leading to death.

Because of the increased postoperative morbidity in patients with untreated sleep apnea, all patients with morbid

obesity should be screened preoperatively for sleep apnea. Symptoms include restless sleep, a feeling of still being tired in the morning, severe snoring, and apneic spells during sleep (witnessed by another observer—the patient may be unaware of the problem). Many times the bed sheets are scattered all over because of the restless sleep pattern. Other telltale signs are severe drowsiness in the late afternoon, falling asleep during daytime driving, or excessive snoozing in the evening before retiring to bed. Some patients may appear "slow-on-the-draw" when interviewed. This process may come on gradually such that the patient or the family does not fully appreciate the changes. Recognition of sleep apnea preoperatively is important, because in the postoperative period affected patients may "desaturate" when they sleep or doze; the increased cardiac irritability induced by an anesthetic thus puts the patient at much higher risk for a cardiac arrhythmia during these periods of relative hypoxia. Preoperative treatment with continuous positive airway pressure at night for at least 1 to 2 months tends to decrease the extent of these hypoxic periods and "reconditions" the central respiratory mechanism such that without the continuous positive airway pressure the hypoxic episodes are markedly diminished.

Some *malignancies* occur at an increased frequency in patients with morbid obesity. Endometrial carcinoma is the most notable. If endometrial carcinoma occurs in a woman younger than 35 years, she is almost certainly markedly overweight. Some investigators also believe that breast cancer in women and colon cancer are also somewhat more common in the patient with morbid obesity.

Many other medical and social problems are also related to obesity. *Venous stasis disease* and *lymphedema* are common complaints that improve markedly with weight loss. The incidence of *gallstones* also is increased. *Social and work-related ostracism and discrimination* are less well appreciated but are common complaints of the patients. *Accidents* at work and home also occur at a higher rate as a result of restrictions in mobility of the patient with morbid obesity.

Several other unique situations in patients with morbid obesity should be mentioned, all of which are indications for bariatric surgery (Table 2). Patients with multiply recurrent incisional hernias often have associated morbid obesity; in this clinical situation, the obesity predisposes to recurrence of the ventral hernia. Similarly, elderly patients

Table 2.—Unique Indications for Bariatric Surgery

Huge abdominal wall hernias
Incapacitating degenerative joint disease in elderly patients
Hypothalamic disorders of hyperphagia in adolescents

with severe degenerative joint disease who are obese are often denied arthroplasty because of their weight; in this clinical situation, bariatric surgery should be considered, not necessarily to increase longevity but rather to improve quality of life by allowing eventual joint replacement. Finally, the rare genetic disorder leading to hypothalamic hyperphagia in children, such as the Prader-Willi syndrome, or the development of centrally mediated hyperphagia after neurosurgical procedures (e.g., excision of a craniopharyngioma), may warrant a bariatric surgical approach.

HISTORY OF BARIATRIC SURGERY

The history of bariatric surgery is checkered. Although the concept of surgical treatment of obesity started in the mid-1950s with good intention, the operation originally designed (the small bowel bypass) was taken up by many surgeons with no focused interest in obesity and especially without a well-designed program for postoperative evaluation of long-term results. Too many of these operations were performed without adequate provisions for metabolic surveillance; results were (predictably, in retrospect) bad, and the subsequent problems related to global malabsorption often went unheeded, ignored, unexplained, or unappreciated. Similarly, conversion from small intestinal bypass to the technically simple gastroplasties was embraced with equally poorly prepared enthusiasm. Just as for the small bowel bypass, which was technically more difficult, far too many "unbanded" gastroplasties (see page 145) were performed by physicians, often by non–board-certified or even non–board-eligible "surgeons" without any formal program for, or appreciation of a need for, medical follow-up. It took many years and many operative failures for the unsatisfactory results of these preliminary operations to be fully appreciated. Much of the blame should be placed on academic centers for not accepting the concept of bariatric surgery and closely evaluating the results. Bariatric surgery was considered distasteful, without academic merit, and not "macho" enough for serious interest. Also, the challenge of performing a complex gastrointestinal operation on a patient with such severe obesity did not appeal to many academic surgeons.

Fortunately, these black marks in the history of bariatric surgery seem to have been overcome. Increasing public and physician awareness and appreciation of the health crisis of obesity have altered the field of bariatric surgery. Many academic centers (including Mayo Clinic) have developed formal multidisciplinary programs in obesity and are closely evaluating outcomes, complications, and the ever-new procedures being developed (e.g., minimal-access gastric bypass, gastric banding). It is hoped that the future will be more complimentary than the past.

Although a discussion of the history of bariatric surgery may not seem relevant to the practicing surgeon who does not perform bariatric operations, many patients in the United States (and the world) have undergone these operations during the past 40 years and problems have developed related to their postoperative anatomy. Many of these problems are both predictable and preventable. Thus, all general surgeons should have at least a rudimentary knowledge of the anatomy and function of the procedures such that he or she can provide appropriate intervention or referral to a bariatric center for patients who have previously undergone a bariatric procedure and who present electively or under emergency conditions.

Small Intestinal Bypass

The first bariatric procedure was the small bowel bypass with a jejunocolic anastomosis. This operation transected the jejunum about 250 cm from the ligament of Treitz with closure of the distal jejunal stump and an end-to-side jejunotransverse colostomy (Fig. 1 *A*). This operation effectively bypassed all the ileum and ascending colon. It induced a severe fat malabsorption, because the bypass of the ileum prevented reabsorption of bile salts with depletion of the bile salt pool. In addition, the bile salts entering the colon caused a severe, bile salt-induced diarrhea. Problems with dehydration, severe steatorrhea, and malabsorption of all the fat-soluble vitamins rapidly led surgeons to abandon this operation in favor of the jejunoileal bypass (Fig. 1 *B* and 1 *C*). Most of these jejunocolic operations were done in the late 1950s and the 1960s; thus, many patients with this anatomy are not alive today. However, one of the authors (M.G.S.) recently (1998) took down one of these operations and restored intestinal continuity in a patient who had severe metabolic problems 39 years after the operation.

Jejunoileal Bypass

Two versions of jejunoileal bypass were the most common, often referred to as the 14/4 procedures (i.e., 14 inches of proximal jejunum and 4 inches of ileum left in continuity with complete enteric isolation of the remainder of the jejunoileum). With the end-to-end version (Fig. 1 *B*), the proximal end of the bypassed segment (proximal jejunum) was sewn closed, and the distal end (distal ileum) was reanastomosed to the ascending, transverse, or sigmoid colon. The end-to-side version (Fig. 1 *C*) involved transecting only the proximal jejunum, closing the distal end, and performing an end-to-side jejunoileostomy 14 inches proximal to the ileocecal junction. Some surgeons believed (on the basis of little objective data) that weight loss was less after the end-to-side version because of absorption of "refluxed" proximal enteric content up into the

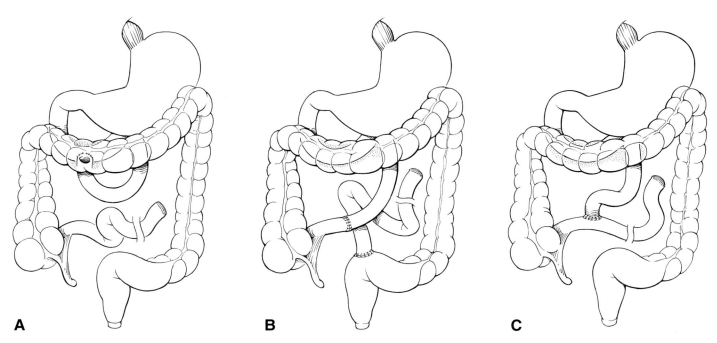

Fig. 1. Small bowel bypasses. (A), *Jejunocolic bypass.* (B), *End-to-end jejunoileal bypass.* (C), *End-to-side jejunoileal bypass.*

"bypassed" distal ileum and that this refluxate also might be involved in many of the metabolic and immunologic complications of the jejunoileal bypass. One group even advocated creating an antireflux valve just proximal to the end-to-side jejunoileal anastomosis to prevent this reflux.

The jejunoileal bypass worked well in terms of weight loss. Its anatomy set up both a functional malabsorption by limiting the available mucosal surface area for absorption (all duodenum, 14 inches of jejunum, 4 inches of ileum). Moreover, the jejunoileal bypass also induced a relative maldigestion. With only 4 inches of ileum, bile salts were malabsorbed and lost in the stool; the body's bile salt pool became depleted, and emulsification, digestion, and absorption of fats were markedly disrupted. However, the jejunoileal bypass had advantages. One psychologic benefit was that the patient would not have to change eating habits markedly—except that the more one ate (especially fats), the more diarrhea or steatorrhea occurred. Overall, the jejunoileal bypass was a theoretically attractive operation— global malabsorption led to decreased use of ingested calories and severe diarrhea, presumably leading to a type of behavior modification to decrease oral intake, especially of high-calorie fats.

Unfortunately, the jejunoileal bypass anatomy often both worked too well in establishing a global malabsorption and introduced new, unforeseen problems in the bypassed segment (Table 3). Metabolic problems were and continue to be problematic. Protein and calorie malnutrition occurred occasionally from inability to absorb the requisite minimal calorie and protein requirements.

Electrolyte abnormalities were common as a result of severe diarrhea. Most common were potassium deficiency and chronic metabolic acidosis caused by overwhelming loss of potassium and bicarbonate in the stool. A baseline contraction dehydration was not uncommon.

As should have been expected, vitamin and mineral deficiencies were rampant. The steatorrhea predisposed to deficiencies of the fat-soluble vitamins A, D, E, and K. Night blindness occurred, but most prominent was the long-term development of metabolic bone disease caused by abnormally low vitamin D levels and subsequent decreased absorption of calcium. Often this complication became evident only years later. Vitamin deficiencies were not limited to the fat-soluble vitamins. Folate deficiency was reported in association with symptoms of the Wernicke-Korsakoff syndrome. In addition, many other bizarre and not fully understood neurologic disorders ensued—believed related to some combination of vitamin and mineral deficiency.

The short-gut anatomy had other side effects. Oxalate absorption was markedly enhanced, leading to a marked hyperoxaluria. Recurrent oxalate kidney stones developed in more than 30% of patients. More worrisome, however, was the development of oxalate nephropathy, possibly related to oxalate deposition in the renal interstitium; if left untreated, a progressive, irreversible renal failure occurs.[5]

Several unpredictable abnormalities in hepatic function were noted. All groups noted a 10% to 15% frequency of acute hepatic dysfunction—sometimes severe enough to classify as acute hepatic failure and mandate reversal of

Table 3.—Complications of Small Bowel Bypass

Metabolic
    Protein and calorie malnutrition
    Potassium deficiency
    Chronic metabolic acidosis
    Contraction dehydration
    Lactic acid encephalopathy
    Oxalate kidney stone
    Oxalate nephropathy
    Acute hepatic failure
    Chronic hepatic cirrhosis
    Gallstones
Vitamin deficiencies
    Fat-soluble vitamins A, D, E, K
    Metabolic bone disease
    Folate deficiency
    Bizarre neurologic disorders
Bypass enteropathy
    Bypass enteritis
    Intestinal pseudo-obstruction
    Intussusception
Immunologic disorders
    Immune complex migratory arthritis

the jejunoileal bypass. Attempts to reverse this acute hepatic failure with total parenteral nutrition were often misguided and ineffective. This serious complication was and still remains poorly understood; the hepatic dysfunction is presumed to be due to some combination of protein deficiency, bacterial overgrowth in the bypassed segment with release of hepatotoxins, and the decreased release of hepatotrophic factors from the gut.

A potentially related problem recognized only recently is the occult development of hepatic cirrhosis, probably multifactorial in origin from the chronic nutritional deficiencies in combination with the bypassed segment. Although the incidence of chronic cirrhosis is unknown, the authors have seen this complication of occult unsuspected cirrhosis several times in the past 15 years.

Jejunoileal bypass also is associated with a spectrum of disorders believed related to the bypassed jejunoileum. One group of disorders is classified as bypass enteropathy (i.e., disorders localized to the bypassed segment). An unusual but well-described complication was intussusception, with the closed end of the proximal jejunum serving as the lead point. The most prominent disorder, however, was bypass enteritis (i.e., a chronic low-grade bacterial overgrowth in the bypassed, defunctionalized gut). This problem presented with fever, abdominal cramps, distention, and worsening diarrhea. Rarely, this bypass enteritis manifested as a motility disorder mimicking intestinal pseudo-obstruction with marked abdominal distention due to dilatation of the bypassed segment. Because patients were also subject to mechanical small bowel obstruction from development of often intense adhesions, exploration for presumed mechanical obstruction was done in many patients with this pseudo-obstruction, but only dilated bowel without any evident cause was found.

Related in part to bypass enteritis is the development of a poorly understood migratory polyarthritis. This inflammatory arthritis is believed to be due to the deposition of immune complexes in the joint from cross-reaction to bacterial antigens in the defunctionalized lumen. Most worrisome is that this arthritis is not always reversible with takedown of the jejunoileal bypass.

Currently, most general surgeons will be asked to evaluate patients because of chronic metabolic disorders, such as recurrent oxalate nephrolithiasis, development of oxalate nephropathy, polyarthritis, intractable metabolic bone disease, and nutritional deficiencies. Depending on the severity of the disease, takedown of the jejunoileal bypass and the simultaneous conversion to another, more current type of bariatric anatomy should be considered (preferably a Roux-en-Y gastric bypass), because about 90% of patients will regain their pre-procedure weight if intestinal continuity alone is restored. In contrast, if the metabolic deficiency is severe and the overall health is seriously compromised, only takedown of the jejunoileal bypass should be done.

Restoration of intestinal continuity is complicated. The bypassed jejunoileum is often very atrophic, with a thin wall and a diameter of 1 cm or less, and the jejunoileum in continuity is hypertrophic with a thick wall (1/4 to 3/8 cm) and a large diameter of 8 to 12 cm. Restoration of normal jejunal continuity usually requires a very careful end-to-side jejunojejunostomy. The ileal end of the bypassed segment is usually somewhat dilated, and thus the ileoileostomy is relatively straightforward.

Gastroplasty

With all the problems of the jejunoileal bypass, the approach toward bariatric procedures changed from a global malabsorptive procedure to a "restrictive" approach—commonly called a "gastric stapling" or "stomach stapling." This procedure was markedly facilitated by the introduction of surgical stapling devices. The concept of this spectrum of operations was to separate or "partition" the stomach into a small proximal pouch (≤ 50 mL) that communicated with the remainder of the stomach through a narrow channel, or "stoma," about 1 cm in diameter. The proximal pouch had a volume small enough to cause an early satiety. In addition, the narrow stoma retarded emptying of the proximal pouch, especially of solid food. The need for marked chewing of solid food to the consistency of pulp, in theory, slowed ingestion of meals and served as a form of forced behavior modification. If the patient failed to chew well enough, ate too much, or ate too quickly, the proximal gastric pouch distended and did not empty quickly, and the patient either needed to vomit or experienced rather severe epigastric discomfort. In concept, restrictive gastroplasty was theoretically very attractive.[6] There were no gastrointestinal anastomoses and no gastrointestinal bypasses, and everything that made its way through the stoma into the distal stomach was absorbed normally.

Many different versions of restrictive gastroplasties were introduced without quality control or detailed objective follow-up. Most gastroplasties involved a horizontal stapling with removal of several staples along the lesser or greater curvature of the stomach or somewhere in the middle of the staple line (Fig. 2). These operations were technically easy and often were performed by poorly trained surgeons and even by some general practitioners who practiced some basic surgical techniques. These procedures were performed in the late 1960s through the mid 1980s. Unfortunately, follow-up to determine long-term outcome was unsatisfactory, and many surgical groups did not adequately assess their results.

Long-term results, when carefully evaluated, proved unsatisfactory for several reasons. The stoma between the upper and lower gastric pouches tended to enlarge; once it reached a diameter of more than 1.5 cm, the restrictive nature of the anatomy disappeared, and weight again increased. In addition, patients rapidly realized that if they ate semisolid foods (such as ice cream and milkshakes) rather than "meat and potatoes," they would not have early satiety, epigastric pain, or vomiting. Because most of these semisolid foods were high-calorie, their body weight increased. This "maladaptive" eating behavior persisted despite attempts at postoperative counseling. The concept of preoperative education in eating habits and behavior modification was not well developed in the 1970s or was not available in many small centers. For these reasons, the results measured in terms of weight loss and reversal of weight-related comorbidity were unsatisfactory in most centers with these forms of gastroplasty. In general, more than 50% of patients had poor outcomes.

In an attempt to prevent stomal dilatation, the concept of a "banded gastroplasty" was developed by Mason at the University of Iowa.[7] He introduced the vertical banded

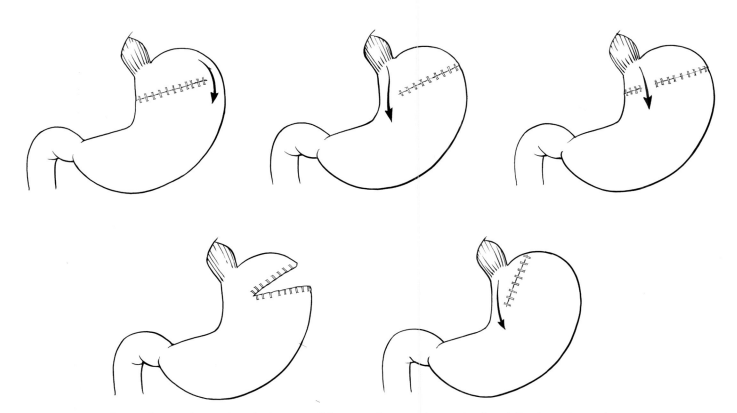

Fig. 2. Various forms of gastroplasty. Note the location of the stoma between the proximal and distal gastric pouches.

gastroplasty (Fig. 3). This operation, still popular today, involves use of an intraluminal circular stapler to create a doughnut hole near the lesser curvature of the stomach, a *vertical* application of a noncutting linear stapler inserted through the doughnut hole up to the angle of His to create the gastric partition, and then "banding" of the stoma between the upper gastric pouch and the remainder of the stomach with a nonabsorbable prosthetic material, usually polypropylene, polytetrafluoroethylene, or, more recently, a silicone ring, leaving an outside diameter of about 1.6 cm and an inside diameter of about 1.1 cm. The vertically oriented staple line was easier to construct, because it did not require ligating or dividing any short gastric vessels, and the banded stoma prevented stomal enlargement. Early results with weight loss were very encouraging,[6] and many groups rapidly embraced this operation. Indeed, a National Institutes of Health consensus conference[2] sanctioned this operation as effective. However, in our evaluation, long-term results have proved very disappointing and unsatisfactory because of failure to maintain long-term weight loss.[8,9] Indeed, a satisfactory weight loss has been maintained by only 39% of patients at 3 years postoperatively and by only 22% at 10 years postoperatively.

All the gastroplasties, however, are associated with potential problems (Table 4). Most of the severe nutritional sequelae of the jejunoileal bypass have been notably absent. However, many complications have led to unsatisfactory results with weight loss and inadequate reversal of weight-related comorbid conditions and quality of life. With the unbanded gastroplasties, stomal dilatation was very

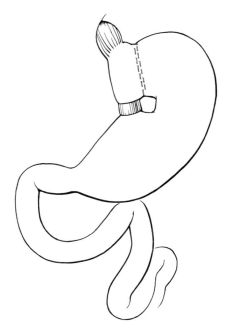

Fig. 3. Vertical banded gastroplasty.

Table 4.—Complications of Restrictive Gastroplasties

Stomal dilatation (nonbanded gastroplasties)*
Stomal stenosis†
Prosthetic erosion of stoma (only "banded" gastroplasties)
Staple line dehiscence*
Dilatation of proximal pouch*‡
Maladaptive eating behavior*
Persistent vomiting‡
Gastroesophageal reflux‡

---

*Unsatisfactory weight loss.
†Too much weight loss.
‡With and without stomal stenosis.

frequent; stomal stenosis also occurred, but less commonly. In contrast, with the banded gastroplasties, either a mechanical or a functional stomal stenosis has been common, leading to severe acute weight loss (protein and calorie malnutrition), recurrent intractable vomiting, or maladaptive eating with change to a liquid-type diet. In many patients, palliation could be achieved with endoscopic dilatation of the stoma. However, in some patients, the stenosis recurred (or persisted), was related to erosion of the band into the lumen, or was due to "angling" of the band such that the effective diameter of the channel between the proximal pouch and the distal stomach was much less than with the band at its usual axis of 90° to the channel. These stomal problems often required reoperation.[10]

Another problem proved to be dehiscence of the staple line that "partitioned" the stomach into the two compartments. This staple line breakdown abolished the restrictive nature of the procedure. Although not well investigated, some degree of staple line dehiscence probably occurs in as many as 40% to 50% of patients after a banded gastroplasty.

Several other problems unique to the gastroplasty concept also occur. Dilatation of the proximal pouch can occur, even in the absence of mechanical stenosis of the stoma. This enlargement of the gastric reservoir allows patients to ingest larger and larger quantities of food at any one sitting. Also, symptoms of severe gastroesophageal reflux may develop. Although one group has claimed that a vertical banded gastroplasty is an antireflux procedure because it "effectively" lengthens the functional intra-abdominal "esophagus" and establishes a new high-pressure zone (the stoma),[11] this has not been our experience.[12,13] Indeed, 3 years after vertical banded gastroplasty, we noted that 20% of patients had symptoms of gastroesophageal reflux that were not present preoperatively.[8] With the horizontal gastroplasties, dilatation of the proximal pouch would provide a larger acid-secreting surface, allowing symptomatic acid reflux. Whether the gastroplasty alters function of the lower esophageal sphincter is unknown.

Currently, vertical banded gastroplasty remains one of the accepted and National Institutes of Health-sanctioned bariatric procedures and is still used as the primary bariatric procedure in many surgical practices. Although our initial enthusiasm for this procedure arose from a very unsatisfactory experience with a nonbanded gastroplasty[14] and the theoretically attractive concept of a banded, restrictive, nonmalabsorptive procedure,[6] our experience with it has proved unsatisfactory. Early experience at 3 years postoperatively showed that about 60% of patients failed to lose and maintain a weight loss of at least 50% of their excess body weight.[8] Many patients (> 50%) had multiple difficulties eating meats and breads, and an additional 30% to 50% had vomiting once or more per week. We abandoned vertical banded gastroplasty in 1989 for another procedure (Roux-en-Y gastric bypass). A long-term follow-up (> 10 years) after vertical banded gastroplasty showed a progressive decline in satisfactory results: only about 20% of patients had maintained a weight loss of more than 50% of excess body weight, and 20% had had reoperation for inadequate weight loss or gastroesophageal reflux and vomiting.[9] In addition, vomiting and symptoms of gastroesophageal reflux continue to be a problem.[12,13] Clearly, results with vertical banded gastroplasty in our practice have been unsatisfactory, and we no longer perform the procedure.

Gastric Bypass

In 1969, Mason and Ito[15] described the gastric bypass operation. This procedure, a modification of which is still popular today (see "Current Bariatric Approach at Mayo Clinic," page 150), incorporated a combination of a gastric restrictive anatomy, a selective malabsorptive anatomy, and a dumping-type physiology (Fig. 4). These operations were originally designed with a horizontal partition (staple line), thereby completely separating the upper gastric pouch from enteric continuity with the distal, "bypassed" stomach (and duodenum). The proximal gastric pouch was then drained into a loop of proximal jejunum (Fig. 4 A), and later into a Roux-en-Y limb (Fig. 4 B); the Roux anatomy was adopted because of frequent problems with bile reflux esophagitis after the loop anatomy. This operation works by preventing the ingestion of large quantities of food at one sitting (restrictive component) and by causing dumping symptoms if high-calorie sweets are ingested, because these high osmolar meals rapidly enter the jejunum without being hindered from emptying by the pylorus, as with the gastroplasties. This dumping physiology functions as a form of behavior modification and prevents the maladaptive eating behavior

that is so common after vertical banded gastroplasty. Unfortunately, the dumping often resolves more than 1 year postoperatively. This procedure also may induce or function to maintain a weight loss by disrupting the normal postprandial hormonal milieu established by release of gastrointestinal hormones from the pancreatoduodenal axis, because ingested foods "bypass" the distal stomach and duodenum.

Roux-en-Y gastric bypass also has been sanctioned by the National Institutes of Health as one of the two acceptable and effective bariatric procedures.[2] Results

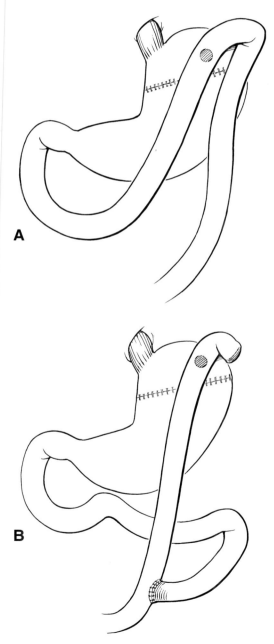

Fig. 4. Gastric bypass. (A), *Loop.* (B), *Roux-en-Y.*

with gastric bypass generally have been much better than with gastroplasties such as the vertical banded gastroplasty. At least one randomized, prospective study showed superior results in terms of weight loss with gastric bypass compared with vertical banded gastroplasty.[16] In addition, gastric bypass has been well documented to reverse weight-related insulin-resistant diabetes mellitus.[4] This therapeutic effect is probably related primarily to decreased calorie ingestion and weight loss, but the bypass of the gastroduodenal axis also may play a role in this effect by altering the postprandial hormonal milieu.

Gastric bypass also is associated with mechanical complications relevant to the practicing general surgeon (Table 5). With the original loop gastric bypass, pancreatobiliary secretions from the afferent limb would enter (and leave) the small proximal gastric pouch. About 20% to 30% of patients had considerable bile reflux esophagitis, often necessitating conversion to a Roux-en-Y anatomy—an easily solvable problem but one necessitating reoperation. Other stomal problems also occurred. Stomal stenosis developed in 5% to 10% of patients but was usually related to a stomal ulcer. With the original horizontally oriented staple line, stomal ulcers were a complication in 3% to 5% of patients. Acid-producing mucosa (gastric fundus) was present in the proximal gastric pouch, and the Roux anatomy brought an "unprotected" jejunal mucosa in contact with the stomach. In addition, if the staple line dehisced, acid from the distal stomach could reflux into the proximal pouch and lead to stomal ulcer. Finally, an adhesive bowel obstruction in the proximal jejunum, proximal to the jejunojejunostomy, occasionally led to an afferent limb obstruction of the "bypassed" gastroduodenum. The diagnosis was difficult, often necessitating computed tomography to visualize the duodenum, because bilious vomiting of the obstructed duodenum cannot occur in that the distal stomach does not communicate with the esophagus. Symptoms of postprandial pain, bloating, and upper abdominal distention (dilated stomach) or episodes of acute pancreatitis should suggest the diagnosis.

Metabolic problems can occur after a gastric bypass, but fortunately they are not very common. Absorption of divalent cations is abnormal. Because iron absorption takes place predominantly in the duodenum, and a gastric bypass effectively bypasses the duodenum, an element of iron malabsorption occurs. Usually this is of relevance only in menstruating women, and usually only in women with heavy menses. Oral iron replacement often suffices, but on occasion intravenous iron dextran is necessary to replenish the iron stores. Calcium absorption also is decreased. Vitamin B_{12} deficiency, although also uncommon, may occur. The cause of vitamin B_{12} deficiency is multifactorial. Absorption of cyanocobalamin requires acid (from stomach) to dissociate the pteryl groups from the cyanocobalamin in foods, then the cyanocobalamin binds to intraluminal R factor (secreted from gastric mucosa). R factor is dissociated by enzymes in the duodenal lumen so that cyanocobalamin can bind to intrinsic factor (also secreted from gastric mucosa). The intrinsic factor-cyanocobalamin complex then is absorbed specifically and *only* in the distal ileum. Gastric bypass anatomy interferes with the normal upper gut processes involved in breakdown and absorption of vitamin B_{12} in the diet.[17] Although unusual, vitamin B_{12} deficiency may occur years after the gastric bypass (the liver can store vitamin B_{12} for 2 to 3 years), and many physicians will not consider this diagnosis as a possibility years after the operation.

Selective Malabsorptive Procedures

These operations were designed to increase effective weight loss without establishing a global malabsorption. The original procedure, called the partial biliopancreatic bypass, as popularized initially in Italy by Scopinaro et al.,[18] was designed to establish a partially restrictive gastric anatomy (80% gastrectomy), divert the pancreatobiliary (digestive) secretions to the distal ileum 50 cm proximal to the ileocecal junction, and drain the proximal gastric pouch into the proximal ileum (Fig. 5 *A*). This anatomy functionally bypassed all the duodenum, jejunum, and some of the proximal ileum; but, unlike the jejunoileal bypass, this bypassed segment still had all the pancreatobiliary secretions passing through it, and the problems of a blind bypassed segment (such as bypass enteropathies, acute hepatic failure) did not occur. All digestion of complex carbohydrates, proteins, and lipids occurred in the distal 50 cm of ileum—the so-called common channel. As might be expected, this form of selective malabsorption was directed primarily at fats, in that this 50 cm did not allow satisfactory length and surface area for lipid digestion or for complete bile salt reabsorption. Results in terms of weight

Table 5.—Complications of Gastric Bypass

Mechanical
　Bile reflux esophagitis (only with loop gastric bypass)
　Stomal stenosis of gastrojejunostomy
　Stomal ulcer at gastrojejunostomy*
　Staple line dehiscence
　Afferent limb obstruction
Metabolic
　Iron deficiency anemia (usually premenopausal women)
　Vitamin B_{12} deficiency

*Beware of staple line dehiscence.

loss were good. Patients lost a mean of 80% of their excess body weight, and this operation was embraced strongly on the west coast of the United States in the mid to late 1980s.

Unfortunately, this rather severe form of selective fat malabsorption introduced a new set of metabolic complications, related primarily to the fat-soluble vitamins. Most patients who underwent this operation had impressive steatorrhea, and many complained bitterly of greasy and extremely foul-smelling stools, usually 4 to 6 per day. Subsequent protein and calorie malnutrition occurred in a substantial percentage of patients. Others had metabolic bone disease presumably related to a protein deficiency in combination with vitamin D deficiency. Other complex vitamin and mineral deficiencies also occurred. For these reasons, most surgeons in the United States no longer perform this operation.[19]

Two other forms of selective malabsorptive procedures are currently done. The first is called the duodenal-switch with distal bypass (Fig. 5 B). This procedure preserves the lesser curvature and pylorus of the stomach by excising the greater curvature of the stomach, thereby inducing a different form of gastric restriction. The duodenum proximal to the entry of pancreatobiliary secretions is transected, the distal end is oversewn, and the proximal duodenum is sewn to a Roux-en-Y limb, similar in principle to a biliopancreatic bypass. The distal "bypassed" biliopancreatic limb is sewn into the distal ileum about 100 cm proximal to the ileocecal junction. The 100-cm "common channel" appears to minimize the metabolic problems noted with the original biliopancreatic bypass, and maintaining the pylorus is presumed to prevent dumping symptoms. This operation is popular in Canada and in some areas along the west coast of the United States.

A modification of the concept of a biliopancreatic bypass and the Roux-en-Y gastric bypass is the so-called distal gastric bypass (Fig. 5 C). This procedure involves creation of a very small proximal gastric pouch (the gastric restrictive aspect); gastrointestinal continuity is restored by a gastrojejunostomy to the proximal jejunum (as with a typical gastric bypass). However, instead of a Roux limb of 60 to 150 cm, the proximal jejunum is anastomosed to the distal ileum 100 cm proximal to the ileocecal junction, thereby diverting all the pancreatobiliary digestive secretions to the distal ileum. This procedure leaves a very long Roux-en-Y limb (300-400 cm) and a 100-cm common channel in which digestion and absorption of complex nutrients can occur. Results with this procedure are good in selected patients (i.e., those with extreme obesity—weights > 225% above ideal body weight or BMI > 50).[19]

BARIATRIC SURGERY AT MAYO CLINIC

Interest in bariatric surgery at Mayo Clinic began in about 1981 and stemmed from a concern about our potential

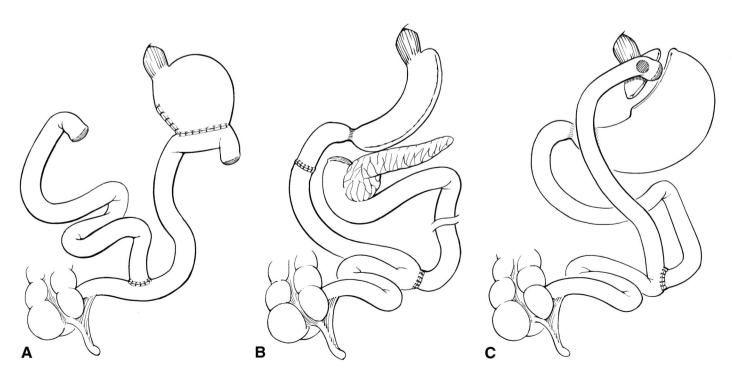

Fig. 5. Selective malabsorptive procedures. (A), *Biliopancreatic bypass.* (B), *Duodenal switch with gastric restriction and partial biliopancreatic distal bypass.* (C), *Very, very long-limb Roux-en-Y gastric bypass.*

role as surgical physicians in addressing the metabolic problem of obesity. We first adopted a modification of gastric stapling (a primary gastric restrictive procedure without any anatomical bypass). This gastric partitioning was created with a vertical staple line with three individual staples near the lesser curvature removed from the stapler, thereby leaving a "stoma" or communication between the proximal and distal stomach with a diameter about 1 cm. An attempt at externally buttressing this stoma with a heavy suture and pledgets was used to prevent stomal enlargement (Fig. 6 A). Results with our first patients were unsatisfactory.[14]

In 1985, we switched to the vertical banded gastroplasty (Fig. 3), again to ensure a nondilating stoma and to minimize metabolic complications by avoiding any gastrointestinal bypass. Although results appeared encouraging initially,[6] the 3-year results in our first 70 patients were unsatisfactory;[8] only 40% of patients had lost and maintained a weight loss of 50% or more of their excess body weight. Moreover, vomiting once or more per week, inability to eat meats and bread, and an increase in symptoms of gastroesophageal reflux convinced us to adopt and prospectively evaluate another bariatric procedure—vertical banded Roux-en-Y gastric bypass.

Our initial approach to Roux-en-Y gastric bypass began in 1989. We used two rows of linear staples to partition the stomach completely. We used a TA9OB stapler (US Surgical, Inc., Norwalk, CT), which automatically places two rows of staples rather than the conventional single row (Fig. 6 B). However, in our first 70 patients, we noted a dehiscence of this staple line in 2; thus, after 1992 we started to routinely divide the stomach between two separate staple lines placed with two different staplers (Fig. 6 C). Since then, the only substantial modification is that three of the four authors routinely use a 150-cm Roux-en-Y limb, a so-called very long-limb Roux-en-Y gastric bypass rather than a 50- to 100-cm Roux limb. Our results have been much better than after vertical banded gastroplasty; 75% of patients lose and maintain a weight loss of 50% or more of excess body weight at 4 years and have minimal vomiting, little food intolerance, and no symptoms of gastroesophageal reflux.[20]

In about 1987, we began to evaluate use of selective malabsorptive procedures in very selected, very obese patients. We initially tried the partial biliopancreatic bypass in 11 such patients (BMI > 50) who had failed a previous anatomically intact vertical banded gastroplasty, or who had such a "malignant" form of obesity that maximal weight loss and a decrease in hyperlipidemia were imperative (Fig. 5 A). Although the weight loss was impressive, during the ensuing 10 years one patient who failed to maintain the requisite medical follow-up died 1.5 years

later of multiple nutritional and vitamin deficiencies complicated by liver failure, two had symptomatic metabolic bone disease, and the rest all described very foul-smelling stool that interfered with their social life.[19] For these reasons, we no longer support this operative procedure.

Currently, we perform what we call a very, very long-limb, vertical, disconnected Roux-en-Y gastric bypass in selected patients (Fig. 5 C). Weight loss after this operation is superior to that with our standard gastric bypass, and metabolic complications have been few.[19] We remain pleased with these results in selected patients, but we are careful to reinforce the need for lifelong medical follow-up with monthly parenteral vitamin B_{12} (1,000 µg), oral multivitamins, oral calcium supplements, and yearly evaluation of serum vitamin D levels. Not only the patients but also the patients' primary health care providers are so instructed.

Current Bariatric Approach at Mayo Clinic

Our current primary bariatric procedure is the vertical disconnected very long-limb Roux-en-Y gastric bypass[20] (Fig. 6 C). We use this for most patients as the first-line bariatric procedure, except in selected patients (BMI > 50, "malignant" obesity with imminently life-threatening weight-related comorbidity) in whom we strongly consider a very, very long-limb, vertical, disconnected Roux-en-Y gastric bypass provided they appear to be reliable and compliant (Fig. 5 C). Occasionally, we have made poor choices (in retrospect) by performing a selective malabsorptive procedure in a nonreliable patient and have (again, in retrospect) regretted our decision. Therefore, we try hard, through our multidisciplinary approach, to make judicious decisions about patient selection.[21]

In brief, all prospective patients first see an endocrinologist with a dedicated interest in obesity. If they meet appropriate criteria (Table 6), they are then screened by a psychologist or psychiatrist interested in obesity (not just eating disorders such as bulimia), a dietitian familiar with bariatric surgical considerations, and a bariatric surgeon. If the consensus is that a patient is an appropriate candidate, the endocrinologist (not the surgeon) writes a letter of support to the insurance provider. Once the approval is obtained, the patient is scheduled for the operation, and the surgeon usually sees the patient again, just before the proposed date of operation.

Several other considerations apply. First, if there are any signs of sleep apnea, a detailed sleep evaluation is done. If sleep apnea is present, some form of continuous positive airway pressure is begun, preferably for at least 2 months preoperatively to "recondition" the respiratory center. Second, if the psychologic evaluator believes that a course of preoperative behavior modification or behavior insight is

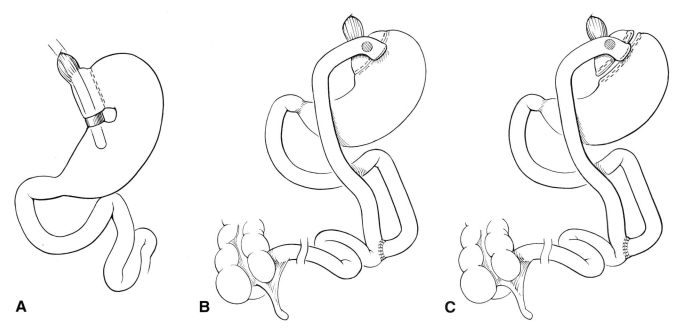

Fig. 6. Bariatric operations performed at Mayo Clinic. (A), Vertical banded gastroplasty (1985-1989). (B), Vertical Roux-en-Y gastric bypass (1989-1992). (C), Vertical disconnected Roux-en-Y gastric bypass (1992-current); note the physical separation of the proximal gastric pouch of cardia from remainder of stomach.

appropriate, we arrange this with a psychologist near the patient's home. Third, we do not undertake any formal gastrointestinal evaluation unless there is some clinical indicator suggesting a pertinent problem. For instance, three of the four authors routinely perform a cholecystectomy even if we can feel no gallstones in the gallbladder. We do this because about 30% of patients with morbid obesity have concomitant gallstones; in addition, gallstones will develop in 30% of patients during their rapid weight loss, and the primary risk of performing a cholecystectomy is "getting there," and we are already "there" at the time of operation. Also, if the patient has

Table 6.—Criteria for Bariatric Operation

BMI > 40, or BMI > 35 with weight-related morbidity[*]
BMI < 35 but with severe weight-related morbidity
Failure of previous controlled dietary programs
No active, uncontrolled psychiatric problems[†]
No active substance abuse or chemical dependency (other than tobacco)
Weight-related morbidity
Insight into cause of obesity
Some type of social support system

BMI, body mass index.
[*]Insurance providers prefer a BMI ≥ 35 for 5 years.
[†]Beware of the patient with a borderline personality disorder.

considerable gastroesophageal reflux preoperatively, an extensive work-up is not needed, provided there is no evidence of an esophageal stricture. Roux-en-Y gastric bypass may very well be the most effective antireflux procedure available, because it completely prevents acid-peptic reflux into the esophagus from the stomach (the proximal gastric pouch of cardia has essentially no acid or peptic production)[22] and the 150-cm Roux-en-Y limb also prevents any biliopancreatic esophageal reflux.[13]

Technique of Gastric Bypass

We believe strongly that epidural analgesia postoperatively not only maximizes pain control but also promotes deep breathing and ambulation. Also, in patients with sleep apnea, the need for systemic narcotics that might further depress the respiratory drive is minimized. We administer perioperative antibiotic coverage for *Staphylococcus aureus* and mini-dose heparin in combination with sequential lower-extremity compression devices activated in the operating room. We proceed with a midline incision from just below the xiphoid to the umbilicus. Cutting into the xiphoid provides no better exposure, makes the rostral end of the fascial incision difficult to close securely, and increases the chance of potentially painful ectopic calcification in the rostral end of the fascial closure. We always check for an umbilical hernia, because about 20% of patients have one. In women, we carefully evaluate the pelvic organs, and in both men and women we examine the colon. Three of the four authors perform a cholecystectomy whether or not stones are palpable; the other author removes the gallbladder only if stones are present.

Our technique has been described in depth.[23] In brief, we enter the lesser sac through the lesser omentum (gastrohepatic ligament) in the avascular plane caudal to the left gastric artery. After elevating the fat pad draping over the cardia of the stomach, we bluntly develop a retrogastric tunnel from the lesser omentum to the angle of His. This area of the greater curvature is relatively avascular, because the first short gastric vessels from the splenic artery arise 3 cm or more from the angle of His. After two 18F catheters are passed through this tunnel, the catheters are then repositioned at the edge of the lesser curvature after a 1-cm window is sharply developed between the lesser curvature of the stomach and the neurovascular arcade (vagal nerves of Latarjet, ascending arterial branches from right gastric artery and descending branches from left gastric artery) (Fig. 7 A).

With the catheters used as guides, two separate 90-mm linear staplers are passed across the proximal stomach, both are fired, and the gastric wall between the staplers is transected. This maneuver physically separates a very small proximal pouch of cardia (< 15 mL) from the remainder of the stomach. The staple lines are oversewn in a further attempt to prevent fistulization between the proximal gastric pouch and the more distal stomach. One trick in placement of the proximal stapler is not to apply it exactly at 90° but rather to apply it at an angle, thereby

leaving more anterior wall of the cardia than posterior wall. This keeps the pouch of small volume but maximizes the area of the anterior wall of the cardia for the jejunal anastomosis. An alternative technique used by one author (K.A.K.) involves two applications of the linear stapler, one over the other, thereby applying four rows of staples; the gastric wall is not divided.

Next, a Roux limb is constructed. We prefer to go about 50 to 70 cm distal to the ligament of Treitz because the mesenteric arteries become less close to one another, and more length of the Roux limb can be gained to minimize any tension at the gastric anastomosis. The limb is then brought retrocolic (to avoid having to drape the Roux limb over an often very fat omentum), but antegastric, through the gastrocolic ligament. Some groups prefer to bring the Roux limb retrogastric, but we see no advantage to this technique. The minimal shorter overall length (1-2 cm) seems outweighed by the increased technical difficulties in performing the cardiojejunostomy

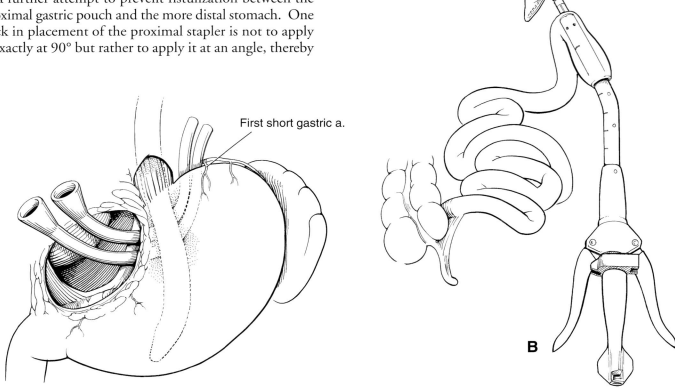

First short gastric a.

A

B

Fig. 7. Mayo Clinic technique of Roux-en-Y gastric bypass. (A), Retrogastric tunnel created through lesser sac to angle of His via gastrohepatic ligament; 18F catheters facilitate passing the linear stapler. Orogastric tube in place. (B), Circular stapler of 21 mm in circumference is inserted through end of Roux limb to accomplish cardiojejunostomy. (From Sarr.[23] By permission of S Karger.)

with a relatively immobile Roux limb; moreover, any need to reoperate will make mobilization of this Roux limb unnecessarily difficult.

We then perform the cardiojejunostomy. Three of the authors prefer to use a 21-mm circular stapler passed through the end of the Roux limb (Fig. 7 *B*). Use of a circular stapler is fast and easy and creates an anastomosis that should not dilate over time. If the tissue donuts are not complete, we carefully search for the area of disruption and reapproximate the mucosal areas with interrupted transmural sutures. In addition, the entire circular staple line is oversewn with Lembert-type seromuscular sutures. One author continues to hand sew this anastomosis with a formal two-layer side-to-side technique. In more than 500 of these anastomoses, we have had only two anastomotic leaks, only one of which required reoperation.

After the redundant proximal end of the Roux limb is excised and stapled closed, an end-to-side jejunojejunostomy is performed 100 to 150 cm distally in the Roux limb (or 100 cm proximal to the ileocecal junction if a very, very long-limb gastric bypass is being performed) (Fig. 5 *C*). The defects in the mesocolon, the jejunal mesentery, and the infracolic space posterior to the mesentery of the Roux limb (the site of a Petersen hernia) are closed with sutures. Any redundant Roux limb rostral to the mesenteric defect in the mesocolon is brought below the mesocolon, and this mesenteric defect is obliterated with sutures. A closed-suction drain is variably left at the cardiojejunostomy. In addition, a temporary gastrostomy may be left in the defunctionalized distal stomach for several reasons. No longer can the distal stomach be intubated with a nasogastric tube should gastric stasis and stomach distention develop. Also, the gastrostomy can be used to give medications, additional fluids, or even nutrition if a problem arises at the cardiojejunostomy which prevents oral intake. We used to also place a needle catheter jejunostomy,[24] but we have found this to be of little benefit in most patients.

Results of Bariatric Surgery at Mayo Clinic

Hospital Mortality and Morbidity

Because of our unsatisfactory results with unbanded gastroplasty[14] and the short-term and long-term results with vertical banded gastroplasty,[8,9] we have maintained a primary approach of Roux-en-Y gastric bypass.[20] The hospital mortality rate has remained low for primary procedures of all types (2/400, <1%). Hospital morbidity included wound infections (about 8%), intra-abdominal abscess (<1%), anastomotic leak (<1%), abdominal dehiscence (about 1%), and other comorbid conditions, such as pulmonary embolus, deep vein thrombosis, and cardiorespiratory problems (<5%). Despite the severe extent of obesity in patients, operative risks and complications remained low and acceptable.

Weight Loss

With the primary operation of very long vertical Roux-en-Y gastric bypass, mean weight loss at 3-year follow-up was 51 kg; BMI decreased from a mean (± SEM) of 49 ± 5 preoperatively to 34 ± 1 postoperatively; 66% of patients lost, and maintained a loss of, 50% or more of excess body weight at 3 years.[20] Of the patients evaluable at 7 years postoperatively, mean BMI was 33, and 60% maintained a weight loss of more than 50% excess body weight. Weight loss after use of the very, very long-limb Roux-en-Y gastric bypass for the severely obese[19] has been, of course, more extensive. Mean weight loss (*n* = 26) has been 71% ± 5% of excess body weight, and mean BMI decreased from 67 ± 3 to 42 ± 2 at a mean follow-up of 2 years.

Long-term Sequelae

As with any operative procedure, several potential problems can arise. Most common has been incisional hernia; 17% of patients return with an incisional hernia.[20] This frequency has been virtually everyone's experience with a fully open method. Many of these hernias have been large, involving the entire incision, or ostensibly localized, only to turn out to be of a Swiss-cheese–like pattern with other smaller fascial defects along the extent of the incision. For this reason, we prefer a Stoppa-type mesh repair of these hernias.[25] We believe that the origin of these hernias and their increased frequency over that normally expected after primary celiotomy (2%-3%) is multifactorial. The patient's obesity has a definite role, but equally important is the relative protein and calorie malnutrition to which these patients are obligated in the first 3 or 4 postoperative months because of their bariatric anatomy; most patients lose 15 to 30 kg during this early interval.

Other postoperative sequelae include symptoms of dumping, early satiety, epigastric pain, and vomiting. Dumping is usually not bothersome unless very high-calorie sweets are ingested. Even this dumping tends to abate (unfortunately) after the first year postoperatively. Dumping with regular diets is distinctly uncommon; it was symptomatic enough to warrant repeated patient complaints in only 2 of more than 500 patients. Early satiety is frequently expected and reassuring. Many patients, however, do not experience the typical premonitory symptoms of "getting full" and, after ingesting an additional (often small) amount of food, notice an intense substernal or epigastric pain or pressure that usually takes 20 to 30 minutes to abate or is relieved by vomiting. They usually learn quickly how to avoid this unpleasant feeling. Repeated vomiting (at least once per week) is unusual (<10%), in contrast to late results with vertical banded gastroplasty, in which up to 50% of patients continued to vomit.[8]

Small bowel obstruction can and does occur after bariatric operation. Several caveats exist. The obstruction may occur in the afferent "bypassed" segment. Patients present with postprandial abdominal pain that may not be cramping, upper abdominal distention, and nonproductive vomiting. Pancreatitis may occur. Often an abdominal radiograph may be unrevealing unless one can appreciate a dilated (bypassed) stomach or duodenum. An upper gastrointestinal contrast study may help if a contrast agent will reflux into a markedly dilated duodenum, but often such reflux does not occur. The best means of diagnosis is computed tomography, which shows a markedly dilated stomach and duodenum. Temporary treatment involves percutaneous drainage of the stomach and, if resolution fails to occur, reoperation either for adhesiolysis or for a simple bypass with duodenojejunostomy. Obstruction of the Roux limb can occur either above or below the mesocolon or at the site of the mesocolic defect; usually these obstructions present as nonbilious vomiting of recently ingested food. Radiographs will not show a dilated Roux limb because it easily decompresses proximally. Internal hernias can occur either at the site of the retrocolic Roux limb or at the jejunojejunostomy. A more typical distal adhesive small bowel obstruction will present routinely with cramping pain, bilious vomiting, and abdominal distention; abdominal radiographs are pathognomonic.

Comorbidity

Virtually all patients have reversal of their insulin resistance and no longer require oral hyperglycemic agents or exogenous insulin. Hypertension is either abolished (about 50%) or the number of medications or the dosage required is decreased.[20] Sleep apnea is much harder to evaluate, because we have not been able to initiate a formal program of reevaluation; anecdotally, many patients have stopped using their continuous positive airway pressure machines, because they no longer feel they need this nighttime treatment.

Degenerative joint disease is a special category. The degenerative joint disease of morbid obesity is primarily a mechanical arthropathy related to extreme weight. Chronic weight-related articular damage is largely irreversible, but the discomfort unquestionably decreases. Best results have been obtained in patients whose mobility was severely hampered by irreversible painful arthropathy but who were too heavy to be considered candidates for total arthroplasty (hip, knee). Substantial loss of weight has allowed safe, effective, and long-lasting total hip and knee arthroplasties, but at a

body weight ensuring both safe anesthesia and a longer-lasting artificial joint.[26] Severe low back pain generally improves, but often not to the extent of joint complaints related to the hips, knees, or ankles.

Special Situations

Children

Although serious obesity often begins in childhood, we have generally been reluctant to offer surgical treatment before the age of 21 years. Because many psychologic changes and adjustments are needed to prepare for the operation and for the postoperative state, we believe that the patient's decision to proceed needs to be made with considerable insight. We have performed bariatric procedures in only a handful of patients younger than 25 years, all of whom had both active weight-related comorbidity and a strong family history of obesity and serious morbidity directly related to weight. Some form of objective and interested social support system also is required. Special situations involve children with a hyperphagia condition, such as the Prader-Willi syndrome. Our experience is limited to two patients. We strongly suggest a selective malabsorptive procedure, but we require a guarantee of closely supervised medical follow-up.

Elderly

Should a bariatric operation be offered to patients older than 50 years or even older than 60 years? In general, the aim of bariatric operations is to increase survival and maximize health by inducing weight loss and to abolish, stabilize, or partially reverse the weight-related morbidity. In patients older than 50 years and especially older than 65 years, the indications for weight loss are directed more at quality of life. If they have already reached age 65 at a weight considered to be morbid obesity, effective weight loss may not be expected to affect future survival to the extent that it might in a 30-year-old person. However, quality of life, if limited by severe degenerative joint disease, now becomes the prime indication. Some people are homebound or wheelchair-bound because orthopedic surgeons have understandably turned them down for joint arthroplasty. Under these conditions, age itself is not an absolute contraindication for a bariatric operation. Indeed, our results have been very rewarding,[27] albeit at a somewhat increased risk of perioperative morbidity. Total joint arthroplasty has restored nonpainful and unaided mobility in many such patients.[26]

Extremely Heavy Patients (Body Weight > 600 lb)

Somewhat surprisingly, operative exposure in these patients is not proportionally more difficult, although a specially modified retractor is needed. Some form of selective malabsorptive procedure, obviously, is indicated. Again, we prefer a very, very long-limb Roux-en-Y gastric bypass leaving a "common channel" of only 100 cm of the distal ileum for both digestion and absorption of complex ingested proteins, fats, and carbohydrates.[19] However, other potentially unforeseen problems may arise when operating on the severely obese, and the wary surgeon and nursing staff will need to be prepared.[28] For instance, simple transport of the patient to and from the operating room requires a special heavy-duty wheelchair and stretchers. Likewise, transferring the still partially anesthetized patient postoperatively from the operating room table to the stretcher requires multiple personnel unless the hospital has an airbag slide transport system (Air-Pal Patient Lift, Patient Transfer Systems, Allentown, PA). Other mundane considerations involve special operating tables, modified retractor systems, chairs to sit in postoperatively, and even concern about the toilets to be used. Toilet stools suspended from the wall will not support such weight, and heavy-duty combination chair-commodes are the best solution.

Huge Ventral Hernias

Umbilical or recurrent incisional hernias in patients with morbid obesity can reach enormous size. The reasons are multifactorial. Primary operative repairs of abdominal wall hernias in morbidly obese patients are associated with a high recurrence rate. Once the hernias recur, many surgeons are reluctant (rightfully so) to attempt repair until the patient loses weight. Although this concept is medically correct, the chance of considerable spontaneous weight loss is very unlikely. Often the hernia then further increases in size, and the surgeon is even less likely to offer repair. The situation becomes a vicious circle and, up to this point, the patient, the primary care physician, and the general surgeon have not aggressively addressed the real problem, that is, the patient's weight. Under this condition, our approach has been to "ignore" the huge hernia, perform a bariatric procedure preferably through a celiotomy within good, intact fascia, and let the patient's weight decrease and stabilize. We then repair the still-huge hernia defect with prosthetic material (usually polypropylene mesh) in a Stoppa-like fashion 12 to 16 months later. Results have been rewarding in the few patients we have so managed.[25]

Plastic Surgical Reconstruction

As the patients lose weight, they lose subcutaneous and visceral fat and muscle mass but not skin. Thus, very large patients have much redundant skin—most prominent as an abdominal panniculus (or abdominal "apron") but also evident around the high thigh region, the upper arms, and under the chin. The breasts in women may become very ptotic. Although socially embarrassing and, by common standards, unsightly, these areas of redundant skin are not medical problems, as such, and thus insurance providers do not provide health care reimbursement for what they term "aesthetic" surgery. Several exceptions, however, do exist. First, if the abdominal panniculus overhangs the groin area and causes stasis dermatitis, insurance coverage is usually provided. We encourage patients with this secondary inguinal dermatitis to consult a physician immediately to document its presence and to have pictures taken of the inguinal areas as further objective documentation to support their insurance application. Second, very large pendulous breasts also can cause a stasis dermatitis in the inframammary folds; arguments for insurance coverage are similar to those described above. In addition, such large pendulous breasts can cause considerable shoulder and upper back discomfort that is best managed with a reduction mammoplasty.

Bariatric Reoperation

The topic of reoperation for obesity has become a bit of a "hot potato," for several reasons. First, there is a much quoted misconception that operative mortality and morbidity rates are exorbitant. Second, many investigators believe that reoperation will not work because the patient "out-ate" or "ate-through" the previous operation. Third, insurance providers are reluctant to approve financial coverage for correction of previous unsuccessful procedures. All of these reasons are unfortunate, because we have had good results with very low mortality and morbidity rates (albeit somewhat greater than with primary operations).[10]

One might consider bariatric reoperation similar to vascular reoperation and cardiac reoperation. The concept of bariatric reoperation may be even more prominent, because so many ineffective operations were done without sufficient long-term data to objectively support their use (e.g., jejunoileal bypass, nonbanded gastroplasty, loop gastric bypass, biliopancreatic bypass, and, even currently, vertical banded gastroplasty).[9] As discussed on page 156 ("The Future"), some of the newer hot topics, such as laparoscopic gastric banding (a minimal-access operation) are attractive, at least theoretically, to the consumer. However, to some inexperienced bariatric surgeons, these newer operations, if unproved in efficacy, may result in many patients with unsatisfactory results requesting reoperation. All patients in whom previous bariatric operations were ineffective but in whom active, directly weight-related comorbid conditions exist remain potential candidates for bariatric reoperation.

Another situation involves correction of complications or side effects of previous bariatric procedures. Such complications include anastomotic breakdown with entero-cutaneous fistulas, staple line dehiscence abolishing the gastric partition, stomal problems (stenosis, dilatation, ulceration, band erosion), gastroesophageal reflux, or severe protein and calorie deficiency caused by an anatomical bypass that was too severe (jejunoileal bypass, biliopan-creatic bypass, or duodenal switch with a common channel that is too short). Another type of problem includes an intact bariatric anatomy but a completely inadequate weight loss due to modifications of diet with maladaptive eating habits with any of the gastroplasties. Although the examining physician and surgeon must maintain a high standard of care and require that patients meet appropri-ate criteria, reoperation should not be denied solely on the basis of a previous failed operation.

Bariatric reoperation involves insight and experience in understanding why the previous operation failed and an armamentarium of many surgical options to deal with the diverse types of problems and complications that arise. Most reoperations should be done in a center of excel-lence with considerable experience with reoperation.

THE FUTURE

Undoubtedly, new procedures and minimally invasive techniques will be introduced. Currently, many talent-ed surgeons have advocated a laparoscopic approach of Roux-en-Y gastric bypass.[29,30] Our group is interested and has followed the literature closely. Current tech-niques require advanced laparoscopic skills, the learning curve is steep, and the operations, at least as currently described, do not fully reproduce our open technique. The true frequency of anastomotic leak has been hard to glean from reports; anything more than 1% would be unacceptable, because this is a life-threatening compli-cation. The low rate of ventral hernia is, however, a very attractive aspect of the laparoscopic approach. As expe-rience grows, laparoscopic Roux-en-Y gastric bypass is becoming state of the art for many patients and will undoubtedly grow in prominence in the next decade.

Of more worry, however, is the attraction of laparo-scopic adjustable gastric banding.[31] This operation is currently popular in Europe. It is theoretically attractive, because it does not involve a gastrointestinal bypass, is technically easy to insert, and is very marketable to the public (i.e., small incision, short hospital stay, "adjustable" technology, and effective weight loss procedure). How-ever, surgical history has repeatedly shown *all* primary restrictive procedures to be largely unsuccessful. Sequelae include maladaptive eating, later weight gain, gastro-esophageal reflux, and the worry of a foreign body eroding or migrating. Until reliable long-term results are available, we continue to watch the experience of others before we become enthusiastic for this type of approach.[32]

REFERENCES

1. Rippe JM: The obesity epidemic: challenges and opportunities. J Am Diet Assoc 98 Suppl 2:S5, 1998

2. Consensus Development Conference Panel: NIH conference: gastrointestinal surgery for severe obesity. Ann Intern Med 115:956-961, 1991

3. Drenick EJ, Bale GS, Seltzer F, Johnson DG: Excessive mortality and causes of death in morbidly obese men. JAMA 243:443-445, 1980

4. Pories WJ, Caro JF, Flickinger EG, Meelheim HD, Swanson MS: The control of diabetes mellitus (NIDDM) in the morbidly obese with the Greenville Gastric Bypass. Ann Surg 206:316-323, 1987

5. Hassan I, Juncos LA, Milliner DS, Sarmiento JM, Sarr MG: Chronic renal failure secondary to oxalate nephropathy: a preventable complication after jejunoileal bypass. Mayo Clin Proc 76:758-760, 2001

6. Sarr MG: Surgical treatment for obesity (bariatric surgery). Viewpoints Dig Dis 20:5-8, 1988

7. Mason EE: Vertical banded gastroplasty for obesity. Arch Surg 117:701-706, 1982

8. Nightengale ML, Sarr MG, Kelly KA, Jensen MD, Zinsmeister AR, Palumbo PJ: Prospective evaluation of vertical banded gastroplasty as the primary operation for morbid obesity. Mayo Clin Proc 66:773-782, 1991

9. Balsiger BM, Poggio JL, Mai J, Kelly KA, Sarr MG: Ten and more years after vertical banded gastroplasty as primary operation for morbid obesity. J Gastrointest Surg 4:598-605, 2000

10. Behrns KE, Smith CD, Kelly KA, Sarr MG: Reoperative bariatric surgery: lessons learned to improve patient selection and results. Ann Surg 218:646-653, 1993

11. Deitel M, Khanna RK, Hagen J, Ilves R: Vertical banded gastroplasty as an antireflux procedure. Am J Surg 155:512-516, 1988

12. Kim CH, Sarr MG: Severe reflux esophagitis after vertical banded gastroplasty for treatment of morbid obesity. Mayo Clin Proc 67:33-35, 1992

13. Balsiger BM, Murr MM, Mai J, Sarr MG: Gastroesophageal reflux after intact vertical banded gastroplasty: correction by conversion to Roux-en-Y gastric bypass. J Gastrointest Surg 4:276-281, 2000

14. Hocking MP, Kelly KA, Callaway CW: Vertical gastroplasty for morbid obesity: clinical experience. Mayo Clin Proc 61:287-291, 1986

15. Mason EE, Ito C: Gastric bypass. Ann Surg 170:329-339, 1969

16. Sugerman HJ, Starkey JV, Birkenhauer R: A randomized prospective trial of gastric bypass versus vertical banded gastroplasty for morbid obesity and their effects on sweets versus non-sweets eaters. Ann Surg 205:613-624, 1987

17. Smith CD, Herkes SB, Behrns KE, Fairbanks VF, Kelly KA, Sarr MG: Gastric acid secretion and vitamin B_{12} absorption after vertical Roux-en-Y gastric bypass for morbid obesity. Ann Surg 218:91-96, 1993

18. Scopinaro N, Gianetta E, Civalleri D, Bonalumi U, Bachi V: Bilio-pancreatic bypass for obesity. II. Initial experience in man. Br J Surg 66:618-620, 1979

19. Murr MM, Balsiger BM, Kennedy FP, Mai JL, Sarr MG: Malabsorptive procedures for severe obesity: comparison of pancreaticobiliary bypass and very very long limb Roux-en-Y gastric bypass. J Gastrointest Surg 3:607-612, 1999

20. Balsiger BM, Kennedy FP, Abu-Lebdeh HS, Collazo-Clavell M, Jensen MD, O'Brien T, Hensrud DD, Dinneen SF, Thompson GB, Que FG, Williams DE, Clark MM, Grant JE, Frick MS, Mueller RA, Mai JL, Sarr MG: Prospective evaluation of Roux-en-Y gastric bypass as primary operation for medically complicated obesity. Mayo Clin Proc 75:673-680, 2000

21. Balsiger BM, Luque de Leon E, Sarr MG: Surgical treatment of obesity: Who is an appropriate candidate? Mayo Clin Proc 72:551-558, 1997

22. Behrns KE, Smith CD, Sarr MG: Prospective evaluation of gastric acid secretion and cobalamin absorption following gastric bypass for clinically severe obesity. Dig Dis Sci 39:315-320, 1994

23. Sarr MG: Vertical disconnected Roux-en-Y gastric bypass. Dig Surg 13:45-49, 1996

24. Sarr MG: Needle catheter jejunostomy: an aid to postoperative care of the morbidly obese patient. Am Surg 54:510-512, 1988

25. Temudom T, Siadati M, Sarr MG: Repair of complex giant or recurrent ventral hernias by using tension-free intraparietal prosthetic mesh (Stoppa technique): lessons learned from our initial experience (fifty patients). Surgery 120:738-743, 1996

26. Parvizi J, Trousdale RT, Sarr MG: Total joint arthroplasty in patients surgically treated for morbid obesity. J Arthroplasty 15:1003-1008, 2000

27. Murr MM, Siadati MR, Sarr MG: Results of bariatric surgery for morbid obesity in patients older than 50 years. Obes Surg 5:399-402, 1995

28. Sarr MG, Felty CL, Hilmer DM, Urban DL, O'Connor G, Hall BA, Rooke TW, Jensen MD: Technical and practical considerations involved in operations on patients weighing more than 270 kg. Arch Surg 130:102-105, 1995

29. Wittgrove AC, Clark GW: Laparoscopic gastric bypass, Roux-en-Y: experience of 27 cases, with 3-18 months follow-up. Obes Surg 6:54-57, 1996

30. Schauer PR, Ikramuddin S, Gourash WF: Laparoscopic Roux-en-Y gastric bypass: a case report at one-year follow-up. J Laparoendosc Adv Surg Tech A 9:101-106, 1999

31. O'Brien PE, Brown WA, Smith A, McMurrick PJ, Stephens M: Prospective study of a laparoscopically placed, adjustable gastric band in the treatment of morbid obesity. Br J Surg 86:113-118, 1999

32. Balsiger BM, Murr MM, Poggio JL, Sarr MG: Bariatric surgery: surgery for weight control in patients with morbid obesity. Med Clin North Am 84:477-489, 2000

Chapter 11

HEPATOCELLULAR CARCINOMA AND INTRAHEPATIC CHOLANGIOCARCINOMA

Juan M. Sarmiento, M.D.
David M. Nagorney, M.D.

Hepatocellular carcinoma (HCC) is one of the most common cancers and a leading cause of death worldwide. Although recent surveillance programs in patients at risk for HCC have allowed early diagnosis, overall survival remains poor. Advanced stage of disease and concomitant chronic liver disease continue to confound the management of patients with HCC. Partial hepatic resection remains the predominant treatment used for curative intent. However, the role of total hepatectomy and hepatic transplantation has been revisited, and this approach has emerged as an attractive and effective therapy for both HCC and its failing organ of origin—the liver. The last quarter of the 20th century witnessed significant advances in hepatic imaging and operative techniques on the liver and the evolution of chemoembolization and hepatic tumor ablation, which have expanded treatment options for patients with HCC.

Mayo Clinic in Rochester, Minnesota, has been on the forefront of hepatic surgery through the pioneering work of John Waugh, M.D., and Martin A. Adson, M.D. Even though they lacked the sophisticated imaging, perioperative hardware, and anesthetic support that are common today, their approach and outcomes are as laudable today as they were during their years of practice. Their influence has been integral to the evolution of our current management approach to HCC.

This chapter reviews the basic epidemiology, clinicopathology, and management of HCC and describes our current multidisciplinary algorithm for management.[1]

EPIDEMIOLOGY

There are marked geographic differences in the incidence of HCC. HCC is estimated to affect nearly 1,000,000 patients a year worldwide.[2] It is the most common solid tumor in Southeast Asia and sub-Saharan Africa. The annual age-adjusted incidence per 100,000 people is 100-160 in Korea, 80 in Taiwan, 28.4 in Hong Kong, 25.8 in Japan, and 28.4 in South Africa. In contrast, the incidence in the Western world is far less, ranging from 1.8 in the United States, 2 in Canada, 2.6 in Norway, to 3.4 in Germany.[3] However, a report[4] from the Surveillance, Epidemiology, and End Results database showed an increase in HCC in the United States from 1.4 to 2.4 per 100,000 population between 1976-1980 and 1991-1995. This increase has been attributed to hepatitis viral infections, predominantly with hepatitis C virus. Interestingly, HCC typically occurs a decade earlier in patients from the West than in those from the East. Differences in regional incidence imply various causes and, consequently, may affect the management and overall outcome of patients with HCC.

ETIOLOGY

Hepatitis B Virus
The association of HCC and hepatitis B virus (HBV) infection is one of the most well-recognized etiologic relationships in cancer biology.[5] Epidemiologically, geographic areas with the highest prevalence of HBV coincide with the highest incidence of HCC.[6] For example, the prevalence of HBV carriers (positive for hepatitis B surface antigen) in the United States and Europe is less than 1%, and the autopsy prevalence of HCC is 0.25%.[7] In contrast, the HBV carrier prevalence in Asia is 10% and the frequency of HCC ranges from 2% to 8%. In a

prospective study of HBV carriers, a 200-fold increased risk for HCC was found.[8] As expected, HBV carriers, even in low-prevalence areas, also have a significantly greater incidence of HCC. Exclusive of HBV carriers, patients with past HBV infection (positive for hepatitis B surface antibody) also have a greater frequency of HCC.[9,10]

HBV DNA and RNA have been identified in HCC from patients with prior HBV infection. The presumed key oncogenic event is the integration of HBV DNA into the host with activation or suppression of cellular genes involved in cell growth and proliferation or apoptosis.[11] This integration generates alteration of functional proteins and genetic expression leading to cancer. If HBV integration could be prevented, hepatocarcinogenesis would be thwarted; thus, prophylaxis for HCC would be through HBV immunization. This clinical hypothesis was tested in Taiwan, a hyperendemic area of HBV and HCC.[12] Through an HBV immunization program in children, the HBV carrier rate was reduced 10-fold. Preliminary findings also suggest reduction in the incidence of HCC. This landmark epidemiologic study strengthens the cause-effect relationship between HBV and HCC and attests to the rationale for HBV immunization programs for prevention of HCC.

Hepatitis C Virus

Hepatitis C virus (HCV) infection may portend a greater risk for HCC than does HBV. HCV is the other major candidate for viral hepatocarcinogenesis,[13] particularly in areas where HBV infection is low.[14] HCV infection is increasing in the United States. In most patients with HCV, cirrhosis will eventually develop, and each year HCC will develop in 2% to 5% of patients with cirrhosis. The relative risk of HCC in patients with chronic HCV infection is at least 100 times the risk in noninfected persons. The increased incidence of HCV has coincided with an increase in the incidence of HCC in the United States after an interim of 2 to 3 decades.[15] In Japan, where HBV infection has been more controlled, HCV is associated with nearly 70% of patients with HCC.[16] In the United States, HCV is associated with 30% to 50% of patients with HCC.

The molecular mechanisms for hepatocarcinogenesis by HCV are unknown. HCV is a single-stranded RNA virus that does not integrate with host DNA. However, repeated HCV hepatocyte injury and inflammation with regeneration and cirrhosis are the presumed venues for HCC. Other cocarcinogenic factors, such as alcohol, hasten hepatocellular injury leading to HCC. Immunization against HCV is an attractive prophylaxis against HCC, but immunization against this virus is not yet available.

Aflatoxins

Some toxins in food also can produce HCC. Aflatoxins (produced by *Aspergillus flavus*), which are found in corn, peanuts, and rice, are metabolized in the liver to intermediates that bind selectively to guanine residues in the DNA of the hepatocytes, with resultant mutations in the p53 tumor-suppressor gene.[17] After inactivation of this gene, there is unregulated cell proliferation potentially leading to HCC. This carcinogen is active in Africa and Thailand. Although aflatoxins do not cause chronic hepatitis, they are proven experimental carcinogens for HCC. Clinically, aflatoxins probably act as major cocarcinogens in the pathogenesis of HCC in patients with underlying cirrhosis or hepatitis.

Cirrhosis

Cirrhosis is a major factor in the development of HCC. More than 75% of patients with HCC have underlying cirrhosis regardless of cause. Macronodular patterns of cirrhosis are associated with a greater frequency of HCC than micronodular patterns. Alcoholism is the predominant cause of cirrhosis in the West. Repetitive or chronic exposure to the hepatocyte offender leads to cellular injury and abnormal regeneration, which best account for HCC development.[18] The degree of association between cirrhosis and HCC depends on the primary condition. HCC is uncommon in patients with autoimmune hepatitis, primary biliary cirrhosis, cirrhosis associated with inflammatory bowel disease, α_1-antitrypsin deficiency, and Wilson's disease, although the relative risk of HCC is increased. Other causes of cirrhosis, particularly cirrhosis from hemochromatosis, alcohol abuse, HCV, and HBV, are associated with a marked increase in HCC.[19]

PATHOLOGY

HCC usually arises within cirrhotic liver. The tumors can be solitary (Fig. 1), but they are usually multifocal. The gross tumor characteristics of HCC can be broadly divided into a nodular, expansile type or a spreading, infiltrating type. The former may be pseudoencapsulated. Overlapping gross patterns may occur. Either type may be associated with areas of necrosis, hemorrhage, and vascular or biliary invasion. Bile pigmentation is common. HCC in cirrhotic liver is often softer than the surrounding parenchyma, and the converse is true in noncirrhotic liver.

Microscopically, HCC usually demonstrates some hepatocellular differentiation. HCC cells usually present in a trabecular pattern without portal tracts. Bile is often evident in HCC cells. Vascular invasion into some divisions of the hepatic or portal veins is frequent. Multiple HCCs may represent either intrahepatic metastases

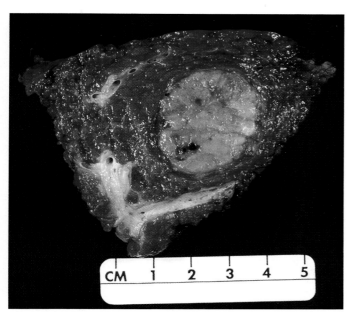

Fig. 1. Hepatocellular carcinoma in a patient with cirrhosis.

(usually via portal venous invasion) or actual multicentric primary HCC. Although numerous histologic subtypes have been recognized, the fibrolamellar variant and the epithelioid hemangioendothelioma are noteworthy. Both of these tumors almost always occur in noncirrhotic livers and may be associated with a prolonged overall survival compared with conventional HCC because of their early stage at presentation.

CLINICAL FEATURES

Patients with HCC generally present with either constitutional symptoms or abdominal complaints from advanced disease. Pain is characteristic in nearly half of patients, located either in the right upper quadrant or radiating to the back. Anorexia, nausea or vomiting, weight loss, and fatigue occur frequently. Many patients with cirrhosis present with hepatic decompensation manifested by abdominal distention from ascites, gastrointestinal hemorrhage, or increasing encephalopathy. Rarely, patients present acutely with hypotension and abdominal pain from HCC rupture and bleeding.

On physical examination, hepatomegaly is common, although in patients with cirrhosis the liver is often nodular and contracted. A discrete hepatic mass is often palpable in patients with large tumors. Ascites and other clinical stigmata of chronic hepatic disease occur in patients with cirrhosis. Jaundice may result from bile duct compression, intrabiliary tumor thrombi, or hepatic decompensation. Splenomegaly and fever may be present. Rarely, a bruit can be heard over the tumor, reflecting the hypervascular nature of HCC.

LABORATORY FINDINGS

Most routine hematologic, electrolyte, and clinical serum or blood values are normal in patients with HCC. Predominant abnormalities include abnormal increases in liver enzyme levels and prolonged coagulation levels due to chronic liver disease, decreased platelets from hypersplenism, and decreased serum albumin level from chronic liver disease.

Serum α-fetoprotein levels are increased in 60% to 80% of patients with HCC. Although α-fetoprotein is the most accurate tumor marker for HCC, its overall sensitivity approaches only 85%, although its specificity is 90%. The presence of a liver mass with an α-fetoprotein value of 500 ng/mL or more is virtually diagnostic of HCC. α-Fetoprotein values less than 500 ng/mL may be associated with various benign hepatic diseases, including acute or chronic hepatitis with or without cirrhosis or undifferentiated germ cell tumors. Serum des-γ-carboxyprothrombin, a prothrombin precursor, has had a frequency of increase similar to that of α-fetoprotein in patients with HCC. Its sensitivity, specificity, and accuracy are also similar to those of α-fetoprotein. Numerous other substances have been proposed as serum markers for HCC, but, in our opinion, none have the accuracy to warrant routine clinical use.

About 5% to 10% of patients present with unusual laboratory manifestations that should raise clinical suspicion for HCC, especially in patients with cirrhosis. Paraneoplastic syndromes include hypoglycemia, erythrocytosis, and hypercalcemia.[20]

Hypoglycemia occurs infrequently but usually indicates advanced disease. Two causes have been proposed. First, hypoglycemia can occur with advanced-stage HCC, leading to marked anorexia and depletion of glycogen reserves, which prevents hepatic glycogenesis. Second, and less common, glucose metabolism can be directly affected by HCC cells, which prevent glucose release from glycogen. This latter paraneoplastic syndrome is profoundly difficult to treat.

Erythrocytosis is due to increased production of erythropoietin or its precursor by HCC. Erythrocytosis in patients with cirrhosis, who usually have cytopenia from secondary hypersplenism, should prompt evaluation for HCC.

Hypercalcemia is related to production of parathormone-like hormones by HCC. Other, much less common manifestations include Cushing syndrome, porphyria, polycythemia, and dysfibrinogenemia.

NATURAL HISTORY

The natural history of HCC is the outcome to which the efficacy of resection must be compared. The survival of patients with untreated HCC, as expected, is strongly related to disease stage at diagnosis. Median survival for symptomatic patients with advanced-stage HCC (American Joint Committee on Cancer stage III or IV disease) and cirrhosis ranges from 1 to 4 months. Patients with HCC of similar stage without cirrhosis fare slightly better and have a survival of 6 to 9 months. Symptoms, poor clinical performance status, cirrhosis, and synthetic liver dysfunction adversely affect survival. In contrast, the natural history of small HCC (≤ 3 cm) is clearly prolonged compared with that of large, advanced-stage tumors. Median survival for patients with untreated small HCC ranges from 2 to 3 years. Finally, survival of patients with untreated HCC is affected by tumor doubling times. Doubling times for HCC are disparate, ranging from 1 to 14 months, and have a considerable potential to affect outcome. The longer the doubling time, the longer the survival.

SELECTION OF PATIENTS

Although partial hepatic resection is the preferred treatment for HCC worldwide, treatment choice has been confounded by the ever changing role of hepatic transplantation for patients with HCC. Patient selection for resection is limited to patients with HCC grossly limited to the liver and is primarily dependent on the intrahepatic extent of the HCC and the hepatic functional status. In general, multicentric, bilobar HCC, extrahepatic metastases, and clinically impaired hepatic function (cirrhosis) are the major factors precluding resection. Initial evaluation for resection should aim at technical assessment of resectability. Issues regarding functional assessment of resectability should be addressed subsequently. Technical resectability broadly implies the potential for gross total excision of tumor with preservation of the afferent and efferent vasculature to the remnant liver with or without bile duct resection, but with adequate bile ducts remaining to restore bilioenteric continuity.

Accurate assessment of the number, size, and location of HCCs is best obtained by using multiple complementary imaging studies. Abdominal ultrasonography is used initially. It is noninvasive and cost-effective. The number, size, and location of HCCs should be defined. The relationship of the HCCs to the major hepatic and portal veins and the major bile ducts also should be assessed. Major vascular or bile duct invasion may preclude resection or warrant additional imaging for definition. Recognition of cirrhosis, splenomegaly, ascites, and regional adenopathy is important because these conditions affect resectability and

warrant further imaging or functional assessment. Finally, preoperative ultrasonography provides a useful comparison for intraoperative ultrasonography.

After the basic characteristics of HCC are defined with ultrasonography, more extensive imaging with rapid contrast-enhanced computed tomography is recommended. This will corroborate ultrasonographic findings and provide a better dimensional depiction of HCC for planning resection. The chest and abdomen should be imaged with and without an intravenous contrast agent. In addition to confirming ultrasonographic findings, computed tomography can further define evidence of local invasion, vascular invasion, regional and distant metastases, and portal hypertension (Fig. 2 and 3). Importantly, computed tomography has the advantage of calculating accurately the resection volume inclusive of the HCC and the expected remnant volume of the nonmalignant liver. These calculations are essential for determining the functional resectability of HCC in patients with cirrhosis.

Magnetic resonance imaging of the liver has emerged as another accurate imaging method for HCC. Magnetic resonance imaging with or without contrast agents is particularly useful for defining tumor and vessel relationships, tumor vascularity, and bile duct anatomy. It has supplanted the need for hepatic angiography in our practice. Moreover, it is preferred over computed tomography in patients with impaired renal function. It is the best single imaging method of the liver and bile ducts, but it lacks the clarity of computed tomography for assessment of extrahepatic disease.

Hepatic angiography has an ever decreasing role in assessing the resectability of HCC. Currently, it is primarily

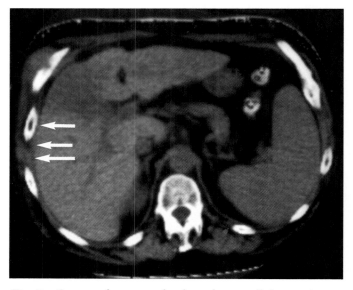

Fig. 2. Computed tomography shows hepatocellular carcinoma invading the chest wall (arrows).

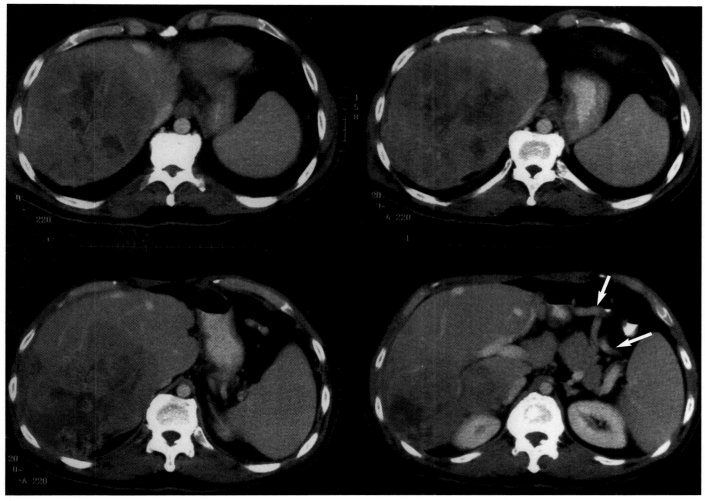

Fig. 3. Computed tomography shows large hepatocellular carcinoma creating hepatic venous outflow obstruction. Note large collateral veins (arrows).

directed at therapy rather than diagnosis. Hepatic angiography with the contrast agent iodized oil (Lipiodol) is particularly accurate for the diagnosis of small HCC when computed tomography and magnetic resonance imaging are indeterminate. Hepatic angiography with chemoembolization is used to reduce the size of HCC and thus increase resectability for patients with noncirrhotic liver or as neoadjuvant therapy in patients before transplantation. Portal vein embolization can be used to increase resectability. In general, it is used electively to induce hypertrophy of the lobe contralateral to the HCC when the predicted postresection remnant is small and the risk of hepatic failure is increased.

Assessment of functional hepatic capacity or reserve has been the focus of intense study. In patients without cirrhosis, anatomical assessment of resection is of primary importance because functional reserve of the hepatic remnant is generally limited by resection of only 75% to 80% of the functioning (nonmalignant) hepatic mass.

Currently, computed tomographic volumetry of the estimated postresection hepatic remnant can be evaluated and expressed as a ratio to total liver volume based on body surface area. If adequate remnant volumes are predicted in a patient with cirrhosis, resection is performed. Chronic biliary obstruction, parenchymal inflammation, and hepatic steatosis may reduce resection volumes in patients without cirrhosis and warrant more conservative resections.

In addition to determination of anatomical resectability in patients with cirrhosis, estimates of hepatic function and the probability of adequate functional reserve of the liver remnant are critical factors in determining resectability. Numerous tests of synthetic capacity or clearance capacity have been evaluated. No method of assessing liver function in patients with cirrhosis has been accepted as the standard. If anatomical resectability of HCC has been confirmed by imaging, functional assessment is best based on the modified Pugh-Child classification. This functional categorization of patients with chronic liver disease may be supplanted by more accurate models of survival in the near future. The Mayo end-stage liver disease model has been recently validated and stratifies patients by survival expectancy.[21] Computed tomographic volumetric calculation of the functional hepatic resection rate preoperatively and intraoperative ultrasonography are critical to the conduct of accurate resections in patients with cirrhosis.

Currently, hepatic resections for HCC in patients with cirrhosis in our practice are limited to patients with Pugh-Child A cirrhosis who are not candidates for liver transplantation. Importantly, the operative decision between partial hepatectomy and total hepatectomy with hepatic transplantation is critical for optimal outcome in patients with cirrhosis and must be assessed carefully. In general, all other patients with cirrhosis and HCC are considered for ablative therapies (thermal or chemical) or chemoembolization. Despite such efforts, hepatic decompensation remains the primary cause of mortality and morbidity postoperatively. Patients with Pugh-Child A liver disease with a normal bilirubin value and minimal portal hypertension ($\leq$ 10 mm Hg) are candidates for resection of up to 40% of the functional liver (i.e., expected postresection remnant > 60%). Partial hepatectomy is tolerated by some patients with Pugh-Child B disease. Resection should be limited to less than 20% to 25% of functional liver volume and undertaken only in patients who are not having transplantation. Currently, partial hepatectomy is not used in patients with Pugh-Child C disease because expected survival related to the liver disease is exceeded by the natural history (survival) of the untreated HCC.

LIVER BIOPSY

We do not advocate routine liver biopsy for suspected HCC. Liver biopsy has direct risks, is expensive, and has the oncologic risk of tumor seeding. In most patients, the combination of clinical, laboratory, and imaging features provides reliable diagnostic accuracy for HCC. Clearly, the presence of a new vascular hepatic mass on ultrasonography or computed tomography in a patient with cirrhosis or chronic liver disease and a serum α-fetoprotein value of 200 ng/mL or more is considered clinically diagnostic of HCC. In patients without cirrhosis, biopsy of a hepatic mass is performed only if a specific histopathologic finding would preclude resection or is necessary for institution of nonoperative therapy.

If liver biopsy is indicated, the biopsy should be performed with ultrasonographic or computed tomographic guidance and with fine-needle technology. The current state of practice prohibits blind large-core biopsy techniques.

Imaging-directed biopsy ensures appropriate tissue sampling and reduces the risk of visceral and vascular perforation. Moreover, a directed paracentesis can be performed concurrently to reduce the risk of bleeding or for symptoms. A review of more than 9,200 liver biopsies at Mayo Clinic in Rochester, Minnesota, showed an overall hemorrhage rate of 0.4%: 0.16% for fatal hemorrhage and 0.24% for nonfatal hemorrhage.[22] Malignancy, female sex, and number of biopsy passes (> 1) were associated with increased risk. Other complications such as bile leakage (0.1%) and septicemia (< 0.1%) are rare.[23] Alternatively, laparoscopic-guided biopsy is useful selectively for preoperative staging of suspected HCC.

A flowchart for managing patients with a suspected diagnosis of HCC is shown in Figure 4.

STAGING

HCC is staged according to either the American Joint Committee on Cancer or the International Union Against Cancer (UICC) scheme.[24] The current staging systems are cumbersome because of the various components of the T stage. The current staging system is defined in Table 1.

SURVEILLANCE

Because of the risk of HCC in patients with cirrhosis and the poor overall survival associated with HCC due to the common advanced stages at diagnosis, programs have been developed to focus on early diagnosis to reduce disease-specific mortality. Surveillance refers to the repeated use of screening tests for detection of subclinical disease over time. The major principles of screening and surveillance for cancer should be that they are inexpensive, easily applicable, safe, and acceptable to a well-defined target population and, finally, that they should be linked to an effective therapy. To date, surveillance for HCC has not been proven efficacious.[25] There have been no randomized, controlled trials of surveillance for HCC showing improved survival, cost-benefit, or cost-effectiveness. Nevertheless, surveillance has become accepted clinical practice for most patients with cirrhosis, regardless of cause, because any therapy for symptomatic patients has limited effectiveness. Surveillance usually involves hepatic ultrasonography and determining serum α-fetoprotein levels at 6-month intervals. The sensitivity and specificity of these tests for screening vary considerably, and thus the accuracy of each surveillance program is affected. Abnormal screening tests are corroborated by additional imaging with or without liver biopsy. Although HCC clearly can be detected earlier with surveillance, current data fail to demonstrate that disease-specific mortality is reduced. Many patients with

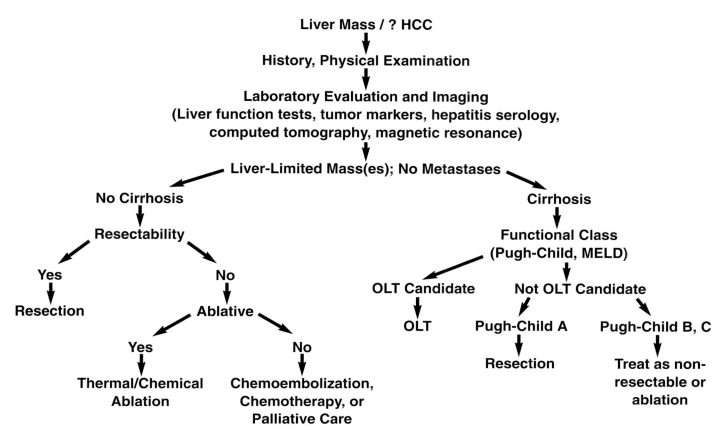

Fig. 4. Management of patients with hepatocellular carcinoma (HCC). MELD, Mayo end-stage liver disease model; OLT, orthotopic liver transplantation.

HCC found on surveillance have tumors that are unresectable because of disease stage or degree of hepatic failure. Moreover, lead-time bias (i.e., early detection of HCC) may account for changes in overall survival. Despite obvious limitations of surveillance, current practice dictates surveillance of high-risk patients who have cirrhosis with preserved hepatic function (Pugh-Child A or B disease) who would be candidates for resection or ablation of HCC if detected. Surveillance of patients with Pugh-Child C disease is not indicated because of the associated limited life expectancy.

TREATMENT

Surgical Treatment

Liver resection aimed at complete extirpation of the tumor offers the best hope for prolonged survival and potential cure for patients with HCC.[25] The criteria for resectability are exclusion of extrahepatic metastases, anatomical intrahepatic accessibility of the tumor, and adequate hepatic functional reserve. Importantly, underlying liver disease, despite resection of HCC, inevitably progresses and also

affects outcome. Quality-of-life assessment after resection of HCC in patients with chronic liver disease remains undetermined and will likely be a major issue in patient management in the future, especially with the evolution of ablative methods.

The overall frequency of survival of patients with HCC after partial hepatic resection has ranged from 25% to 50% at 5 years. Overall 5-year survival was 27% in our initial data from Mayo Clinic, Rochester, Minnesota,[26] and 31% in a recent update.[27] Overall perioperative mortality has ranged from 2% to 15%, which is consistent with our experience of 8%. Operative mortality is clearly less in large-volume specialty centers than in institutions with less experience. Perioperative mortality is adversely affected by the presence of cirrhosis, which is present in nearly 75% of patients in most reports. Overall operative morbidity has ranged from 10% to 20%. The most troublesome complications remain perioperative bleeding and liver failure, especially in patients with underlying liver disease.

Several caveats about interpreting reports on partial hepatic resection in patients with HCC warrant comment. First, each series of patients is highly selected. The

Table 1.—Staging of Primary Hepatocellular Carcinoma

	Primary tumor			
T class	No. of lesions	Size, cm	Site	Vascular invasion*
T1	Solitary	≤2	Unilobar	0
T2	Solitary	≤2		+
	Multiple	≤2	Unilobar	0
	Solitary	>2		0
T3	Solitary	>2		+
	Multiple	≤2	Unilobar	+
	Multiple	>2		0, +
T4	Multiple	Any	Bilobar or unilobar†	+pv, hv‡

	Stage grouping		
Stage	T class	Nodal status§	Distant metastases§
I	T1	N0	M0
II	T2	N0	M0
IIIA	T3	N0	M0
IIIB	T1	N1	M0
	T2	N1	M0
	T3	N1	M0
IVA	T4	Any N	M0
IVB	Any T	Any N	M1

*0, absent; +, present.
†With direct invasion of adjacent organs except gallbladder or perforating visceral peritoneum.
‡With major portal or hepatic vein invasion.
§Metastases present (1) or absent (0).
Modified from American Joint Committee on Cancer.[24] By permission of the American Joint Committee on Cancer.

overall resectability rate approaches only 10% of all patients with HCC. Second, the definition of resectability varies widely. Some groups categorically exclude patients from resection on the basis of, for example, size (more than 5 cm), vascular invasion, microscopic lymph node metastases, and degree of portal hypertension. Third, most patients with HCC who undergo resection have underlying cirrhosis; in fact, nearly 75% to 85% of the patients have cirrhosis. The degree of hepatic dysfunction, although inevitably progressive, may fluctuate and influence perioperative mortality and postoperative hepatic decompensation, which affects overall outcome. Moreover, as emphasized earlier, the cause of cirrhosis varies, and the natural history of the underlying liver disease varies widely. Clearly, there is substantial heterogeneity among patients with resected HCC, and overall comparison of patients undergoing resection generally neglects these differences.

The relationship of survival to various patient and tumor characteristics has been examined repeatedly. Factors associated with a more favorable prognosis include solitary HCC, small size (less than 3 cm), pseudocapsule, absence of vascular invasion, absence of lymph node metastases, early tumor stage, negative margins of resection, and absence of symptoms. Whether cirrhosis adversely affects disease-specific survival remains controversial. However, our data suggest that the degree of hepatic fibrosis does adversely affect overall survival.

Orthotopic Liver Transplantation
Oncologically, orthotopic liver transplantation (OLT) offers the patient the best chance for cure because both the HCC and the preneoplastic liver are removed. Despite early enthusiasm for OLT in patients with HCC, the lack of well-defined criteria resulted in 5-year survival rates of only 15%. The initial dismal results clearly highlighted the need for accurate selection. Moreover, although OLT remains an attractive treatment option, several practical problems exist, including the need for long-term immunosuppression; the interval between diagnosis and donor organ availability, during which intrahepatic metastases may occur; the risk of OLT itself; and the expense. Nevertheless, a patient population has been identified that might benefit from OLT. Clinical evidence shows that patients with preoperative stage I and II HCC or those with incidental tumors have better survival rates than patients with stage III or IV HCC, and this has led most transplant centers to revise their indications for OLT in HCC.

Several recent series on OLT for small HCC have shown better survival rates than previously.[28-30] Mazzaferro et al.[31] reported an overall survival rate at 4 years of 85% and a recurrence-free survival rate at 4 years of 92% in patients with a single tumor less than 5 cm in diameter or two or three tumors less than 3 cm each. Similar results with small HCC have been reported at other centers. Indeed, at Mayo Clinic, Rochester, Minnesota, 22 of 27 candidates have undergone OLT for HCC after preoperative chemoembolization.[32] With a median follow-up of 30 months, no patient has had an overt recurrence. Three patients have died of unrelated causes. Whether preoperative chemoembolization or any tumor-specific therapy is effective for ablating HCC and preventing intrahepatic progression of HCC during the interim to donor availability remains unproved.

Recurrence is a crucial event after OLT. Male sex, multicentricity, bilobar involvement, and vascular invasion are the major predictors of HCC recurrence. In a retrospective study of 178 patients, those with tumor less than 4 cm and no vascular invasion in the explanted liver showed no evidence of recurrence on follow-up.[33] In contrast, all patients with macrovascular invasion except one have had tumor recurrence. Additionally, male sex and multiple lesions were associated with a poor prognosis. Unfortunately, current imaging is not able to detect microvascular invasion, and preoperative staging is based solely on size.

Recent data from an international cooperative study (including both Western and Eastern institutions) addressed specific tumor features to predict microvascular invasion and, hence, select candidates for OLT. From a cohort of 245 patients with HCC, a multivariate analysis showed that tumors more than 4 cm (odds ratio 2.3) and high-tumor grade (odds ratio 6.1) were independent predictive factors for microvascular invasion. Thus, a pretransplantation liver biopsy could improve the selection of candidates for OLT by excluding patients with vascular invasion.[34]

Repeat Hepatic Resection for Recurrent HCC

The major drawback of partial hepatic resection as primary therapy for HCC has been the incidence of recurrence. Indeed, recurrence rates at 5 years have ranged from 50% to 70%.[34,35] Intrahepatic recurrence may result from metastases or multicentric tumors. Temporally, metastases present sooner than new or second primary HCCs. Intrahepatic metastases imply a poor prognosis because they represent an advanced stage of the primary tumor. Partial hepatic resection of either recurrent HCC or intrahepatic or new primary HCC still may offer chance for cure. Perioperative evaluation for repeat resection is similar to that for resection of the primary HCC. Resection is indicated for only focal recurrence. The caveats (described above) regarding resection of functional hepatic mass and the patient's current Pugh-Child class also must be considered. Interval deterioration in Pugh-Child class from the initial hepatectomy or an estimate of resection of total functional hepatic volume exceeding 50% (inclusive of both the initial and the planned repeat resections) is a contraindication to repeat resection and dictates alternative therapy. The frequency distribution of patterns of recurrent HCC—focal, multiple, or diffuse—suggests that 10% of patients with prior partial hepatic resection may be candidates for repeat resection. Clearly, early recognition of "recurrent" HCC (12-24 months) after initial resection portends reduced survival salvage. Although recurrent HCC is often distinguished from a new or neo-primary HCC, arbitrarily by temporal recognition, only DNA clonal analysis can determine whether an intrahepatic *recurrence* is a new primary tumor or a metastasis.

Intrahepatic metastases and portal invasion (at second hepatectomy) recently were described as prognostic factors for decreased survival after resection for recurrent HCC in a study of 48 patients. Number of tumors, bilaterality, size, degree of differentiation, and type of hepatitis did not affect survival significantly. Overall survival was not different from that in patients with resection of primary HCC.[36]

The overall 5-year survival from resection of the recurrence approaches 20% to 30%. Repeat resection rate is less than 10% in most series. The best candidates for repeat resection are patients with solitary recurrences at the resection margins or peripherally in the remnant liver. Repeat resections have proved safe in major hepatobiliary centers, and the perioperative mortality was approximately 1% in a collective literature review.[1] There are also reports of second and third repeat resections in selected patients, even those with cirrhosis. Ablation likely will supplant repeat resection as its efficacy is subsequently established.

Ablation

In situ ablation of HCC evolved as an alternative to partial hepatic resection for patients with hepatic dysfunction. Rationale for ablation was selective destruction of tumor with minimal destruction of adjacent functional liver. The two basic types of ablative approaches are chemical and thermal. Chemical ablation is based on direct intratumoral injection of either absolute ethanol or acetic acid. Thermal ablation uses either focal freezing (cryoablation) or heating (radiofrequency, microwave, or laser) through probes specifically designed for tumor destruction. Each ablative method is guided by imaging (primarily ultrasonography because it displays the tumor in real time). Diffusion of chemicals and thermal destruction should be monitored to ensure thorough ablation.

In general, chemical ablation is limited to smaller HCCs (< 3-4 cm), although repeated injections can be used for larger tumor (large volume). Large HCCs have been more frequently treated by thermal techniques. Each method can be performed percutaneously, laparoscopically, or during laparotomy. Procedure-related morbidity and mortality for each vary, but, in general, complications of any ablative technique are far less frequent than those after partial resection.

Chemical Ablation

Percutaneous Ethanol Injection

Percutaneous ethanol injection therapy was developed during the 1980s. Ethanol ablation results from diffusion into cells, producing immediate coagulation necrosis from cellular dehydration and protein denaturation, followed by fibrosis and small vessel thromboses. Tumors are localized with ultrasonography. Fine-needle (22-gauge) aspiration biopsy is performed, then absolute ethanol is injected slowly. Ethanol diffusion is easily observed with ultrasonography through the marked echogenicity of the microbubbles in ethanol. Surrounding cirrhotic liver usually contains the ethanol diffusion within the softer HCC. Overall survival after the procedure has ranged from 30% to 40% at 5 years for small HCCs (< 3-4 cm). This approaches the rates reported for partial resection of HCCs of similar size. However, recurrence of HCC after ethanol injection is approximately 65% at 2 years and is often in disparate sites throughout the liver. Recently, percutaneous acetic acid injection (15%-50% solution) has proved similarly effective.[37]

Thermal Ablation

Cryoablation
Freezing was the initial thermal technology used for HCC ablation. Cryoablation results from intracellular and extracellular ice formation, which causes denaturation of the cellular membrane, cellular dehydration, ionic shifts, and, finally, cell death. The cryoprobe is inserted into the tumor under ultrasonographic guidance. Double freeze-thaw cycles, which are more efficiently destructive, are monitored ultrasonographically to ensure that the freeze ball encompasses the HCC. The zone of frozen liver is very distinct on ultrasonography. Cryoprobe size is dictated directly by HCC size. Core body temperature is monitored and maintained. Limited data suggest that cryoablation as part of a multimethod approach (with chemoembolization and systemic chemotherapy) may achieve a 5-year survival of 10% to 20% depending on HCC size.[38] The reported operative mortality of 1% may be less with laparoscopic or percutaneous approaches. Recurrence of HCC within the liver has been similar to that with ethanol injection; however, local recurrence adjacent to major vessels may be greater because of incomplete freezing caused by warming by blood flow (i.e., heat-sink effect).

Heat Ablation
Recently, heat destruction of tumors has become applicable through technologic developments of microwave coagulation therapy,[39] laser-induced ablation,[40] and, the most currently practiced, radiofrequency ablation.[41] The source of heat production varies with each of these methods, but the tumor destruction is caused directly by heat denaturation of cellular components. Currently, achievable zones of tumor necrosis vary and range from a diameter of 1 to 2 cm for microwave and laser ablation to 3 to 5 cm for radiofrequency ablation, although repeated probe positioning can increase necrotic volume for each method.

Similar to cryoablation, probes are placed into the HCC with ultrasonographic guidance. Radiofrequency tines are used. Time of ablation is based on HCC size, and ablation is performed after the monitored temperature of destruction is achieved. Repeat ablation cycles are used for large tumors. Radiofrequency ablation can be performed percutaneously, laparoscopically, or at open laparotomy.[42] Early data suggest that it may be effective in selected patients with HCC.[41] Median survival was 15 months. Local recurrence at the ablation site was only 2%, but new HCC developed in 45% of patients. Overall morbidity was 12%, and mortality was nil. Although these data are encouraging and warrant further study, especially in patients with HCC and cirrhosis, long-term efficacy is currently unproved.

Adjuvant Therapy
Because the rate of recurrence of HCC after partial hepatic resection approaches 50% to 70% at 5 years, effective adjuvant therapy has been a major goal of overall management. Similar to the limitations imposed on resection, cirrhosis and frequently associated secondary hypersplenism limit patients' candidacy for chemotherapy trials. Despite such limitations, there is basically no evidence that any systemic chemotherapy, with either single or multiple agents, produces durable objective tumor responses, prolongs survival, or improves quality of life in patients with unresectable HCC. Combination chemotherapy with 5-fluorouracil, semustine, doxorubicin (Adriamycin), and streptozocin resulted in an overall response rate of only 13% and a 1-year survival of less than 25%.[43] Toxicity was considerable. Single-agent trials of mitomycin C and doxorubicin have been similarly disappointing, although doxorubicin is currently viewed as the most effective single agent for HCC. Regional infusional (hepatic arterial) chemotherapy, despite the potential for reduced systemic side effects, has not warranted routine clinical use. Indeed, because there is no standard chemotherapy for unresectable HCC, nearly all patients seeking treatment for unresectable HCC should be directed toward centers conducting investigational chemotherapeutic studies.

Despite lack of established efficacy, postoperative chemotherapy has been used adjuvantly (i.e., after total gross resection of HCC). In a prospective case-controlled study, postoperative systemic therapy with epirubicin and mitomycin was compared with no treatment as control.[44] The overall 5-year survival rate was 72% with therapy and 51% in controls, and the 5-year disease-specific survival rate was 63% with treatment and 32% in controls. Although these results are encouraging, confirmatory data are needed. In another prospective randomized trial, adjuvant therapy with systemic epirubicin and intra-arterial cisplatin and iodized oil (Lipiodol) was compared with no further treatment in patients who had partial resection of HCC with cirrhosis.[45] In contrast with the results of the study just described, the disease-specific 3-year survival was significantly less for the treated patients (18%) than for the controls (48%). Moreover, the recurrence rate was also greater for the treated patients (75% vs. 50%).

Two novel adjuvant approaches recently were reported from outside the United States: postoperative oral polyprenoic acid[46] and postoperative iodine [131]I Lipiodol arterial embolization.[47] Retinoids,[48] such as polyprenoic acid, inhibit carcinogenesis and induce apoptosis. Daily oral therapy with polyprenoic acid (600 mg) was compared with placebo in patients after resection or ethanol ablation of HCC. Polyprenoic acid reduced the rate of recurrence or new HCC at a median follow-up of 38 months (27% vs. 49%). Moreover, this therapy reduced the rate of subsequent primary HCC over controls (16% vs. 44%). Importantly, that study highlights the role of retinoids as *chemopreventive* therapy, which is particularly relevant in patients with cirrhosis or other chronic liver diseases. Intra-arterial [131]I Lipiodol may prove beneficial as a focal radiotherapeutic agent. Lipiodol is a fatty acid ester containing a large component of iodine. This compound is retained by the neovascularity of HCC for prolonged periods after intra-arterial injection. Thus, [131]I Lipiodol permits focal deposition of a radioactive emitter within the HCC. After safety of the agent was demonstrated and a 52% objective response rate was found in 26 patients with unresectable HCC, a prospective randomized trial was conducted in which intra-arterial [131]I Lipiodol (1,850 MBq dose) as adjuvant therapy was compared with no treatment after resection of HCC.[49] Median duration of survival was significantly increased after [131]I Lipiodol therapy (57 months) versus controls (14 months),[50] and the recurrence rate was reduced by half (29% vs. 59%). These strikingly positive findings prompted premature closure of this trial, and [131]I Lipiodol injection became the new standard adjuvant therapy after resection of HCC. These findings have been confirmed in a phase II study of [131]I Lipiodol (1,110 MBq dose).[51] In the near future, it is hoped that one or both of these novel approaches will be approved for clinical study or use in the United States.

PREVENTION

Prevention of progressive chronic liver disease would be the most significant prophylaxis for HCC. To date, only vaccination against HBV and the subsequent decrease in the rate of chronic infection (from 10% to < 1%) has substantially decreased the incidence of HCC. Importantly, a population-based study[12] confirmed the nature of HCC as a preventable condition when population strategies are considered. Similarly, strategies addressing environmental factors, such as reduction of aflatoxins in the food supply, where appropriate, may also reduce the incidence of HCC.

Treatment with interferon has had some efficacy in patients with chronic HCV. This finding may translate into a reduction of HCC. Recently, an analysis of 923 patients with chronic HCV, 224 of whom had undergone interferon treatment and 699 of whom did not, showed a 5-year cumulative incidence of HCC of 2.2% among treated patients and of 9.5% in untreated patients ($P = 0.01$).[52] Moreover, recurrence of HCC was reduced in patients with HCV after treatment with ethanol injection when patients received interferon beta compared with no interferon therapy.[53] These data support the possibility that interferon reduces the incidence of HCC by decreasing the activity of chronic hepatic disease.

FIBROLAMELLAR HCC

Fibrolamellar HCC (FL-HCC) is a distinct histopathologic subtype that repeatedly has been associated with a favorable prognosis. FL-HCC is characterized histologically by large eosinophilic polygonal cells with prominent macronuclei[54] dispersed throughout a fibrolamellar stroma (Fig. 5). Grossly, the presence of a central stellate scar in FL-HCC mimics focal nodular hyperplasia, although the latter is rarely as large as FL-HCC. Typically, FL-HCC tumors occur in young adults (approximate mean age, 26 years), are frequently resectable, and have a better prognosis based on T stage than non–FL-HCC. Most tumors (55%-65%) are large and solitary (Fig. 6).[55] Cirrhosis is conspicuous by its absence. Patients usually present with an

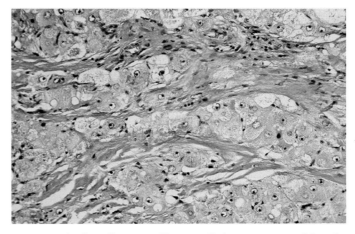

Fig. 5. Fibrolamellar type of hepatocellular carcinoma. Note the large polygonal cells with giant macronuclei dispersed throughout a dense fibrolamellar stroma.

abdominal mass and fullness. Constitutional symptoms of malignancy are uncommon.

Laboratory findings typical of most HCCs are absent. The α-fetoprotein level is increased in only 7% of patients. Other markers, however, are found with this tumor: serum neurotensin and vitamin B$_{12}$ binding capacity are increased. In one study, the serum descarboxyprothrombin level was abnormal in nearly 41% of patients with FL-HCC.[56] Positive HBV and HCV serologic results are infrequent (< 6%).

The overall resectability rate for FL-HCC is higher (75%) than for non–FL-HCC.[57] Overall survival has ranged from 40% to 65% at 5 years, and the median survival is between 33 and 50 months. Patients with focally unresectable FL-HCC are often candidates for OLT. Data have shown an estimated 38% survival at 5 years and a median survival of about 3 years after OLT.[30]

Differences in overall survival between FL-HCC and HCC are probably related to clinicopathologic heterogeneity of patients with HCC in regard to tumor stage and grade and the ages of the patient with FL-HCC.[57] Most FL-HCCs are stage II (T2 N0 M0), although tumor size is often large (> 2 cm). FL-HCCs typically do not present with vascular invasion, are not multicentric, are resectable, and lack lymphatic spread. However, stage-per-stage outcome is similar to that of typical HCC.

INTRAHEPATIC CHOLANGIOCARCINOMA

Among the primary liver carcinomas, intrahepatic cholangiocarcinoma (ICC) is second in frequency to HCC and has an estimated prevalence of 10% to 30%.[58,59] ICC is part of the spectrum of cholangiocarcinomas (intrahepatic,

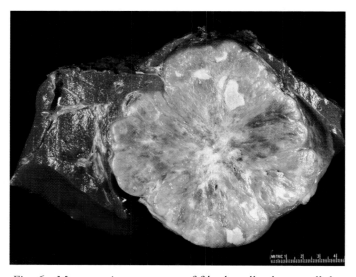

Fig. 6. Macroscopic appearance of fibrolamellar hepatocellular carcinoma. These tumors are typically large and solitary, arising in a noncirrhotic liver.

hilar [Klatskin's tumor], and distal) and is the least common of them; its estimated incidence is 6%.[60] The incidence of cholangiocarcinoma in the United States ranges from 0.01% to 0.46% in autopsy series.[61] The geographic prevalence of ICC is 10 times more frequent in the East than the West.

Etiology

The etiopathogenesis of ICC is distinct from that of HCC. Conditions associated with ICC predominantly relate to chronic biliary inflammation or anatomical abnormalities and include hepaticolithiasis, Caroli's disease, biliary dysplasia, primary sclerosing cholangitis, bile duct cysts, and infestation by *Clonorchis sinensis*. Additionally, ICC has been associated with intravenous administration of contrast medium (Thorotrast).

Patients with bile duct cysts have an increased incidence of cholangiocarcinoma (25%), although these tumors can occur intrahepatically and not within the usual extrahepatic cyst. Caroli's disease, a type of bile duct cystic disease, also is associated with ICC. Thorotrast also predisposes to ICC after a latent period of approximately 3 to 5 years. Lithiasis acts as a ductal irritant that creates chronic inflammation. Hepatolithiasis is found in 20% of patients with ICC.[62] Each etiologic factor associated with ICC occurs more frequently in the East than the West.

Clinical Features

In a review of 61 patients with ICC seen at Mayo Clinic in a 31-year period, the most common symptom was abdominal pain, followed by weight loss and anorexia; jaundice occurred in 15% of cases.[63] Abdominal mass was the most frequent sign (33%), and other signs included ascites, cachexia, and splenomegaly.[63] Usually, when patients with ICC are symptomatic, advanced disease is present, and the chance for curative resection is decreased.

Diagnostic Evaluation

Laboratory

Laboratory findings are usually normal in patients with ICC, except for minor increases in results of liver tests. Alkaline phosphatase and aspartate aminotransferase are often increased.[63] The tumor marker carcinoembryonic antigen is infrequently increased; α-fetoprotein was increased in 8% of the patients in our most recent series.[63] Most frequently, the carbohydrate antigen 19-9 has correlated most strongly with ICC.

Imaging

The imaging of ICC is similar to that of HCC. The only major imaging difference between ICC and HCC is the decreased vascularity of ICC resulting from its intense fibrosis.[64,65]

Pathology

There are three basic morphologic types of ICC: mass-forming, periductal infiltrating, and intraductal.[66] The mass-forming type is most common and in combination with periductal infiltration is associated with the worst prognosis of the various types.[66] The intraductal growth type has the most favorable prognosis.[67] All ICCs are adenocarcinomas.[68] Peripheral ICCs can be markedly anaplastic and behave very aggressively.[69] ICC produces mucin and rarely bile, in clear contrast to HCC. ICC spreads along ducts, by infiltration of Glisson's capsule and by microvascular invasion.[70] When tumor infiltrates Glisson's capsule, it accesses the lymphatics and the perineural spaces, which accounts for the frequent regional nodal involvement. The presence of microvascular (portal venous) invasion leads to intrahepatic metastases.[70]

Treatment

Resection is the only curative treatment in the management of ICC. Patients with resected ICC are the only long-term survivors in our experience.[63] Survival at 3 years was 60% after resection and 7% without resection. In most patients, however, ICC is not resectable at diagnosis or exploration because the disease is advanced. Of 61 patients seen at Mayo Clinic in a 31-year period, 12 were deemed to have unresectable disease preoperatively and 21 had unresectable disease at laparotomy.[63]

The aim of resection in patients with ICC is complete excision with negative margins. All types of resection, regardless of extent, have been used. Operative mortality has been low (< 2%), and morbidity is nearly 15%.[63] Factors associated with decreased survival are positive lymph nodes, intrahepatic metastases, vascular invasion, and stage.[63,71] Obviously, patients who have incomplete resection of tumors have a decreased survival compared with those who have complete resections.

OLT has been associated with a very low long-term survival (14% at 1 year),[58] although few patients with ICC have had OLT. Currently, overt ICC is considered a contraindication for OLT. Perhaps OLT can be considered for patients with small (≤ 1 cm) tumors who have primary sclerosing cholangitis.[72]

OPERATIVE TECHNIQUE

Partial hepatectomy is essential to the treatment of HCC. Because OLT is discussed in Chapter 14, only the most important steps in the performance of the most common types of hepatectomy are shown here. Nonanatomical resections, commonly used in our practice to treat HCC, are not described in this chapter because they do not require special techniques.

The operative steps in partial hepatectomy are illustrated in Figures 7 through 14.

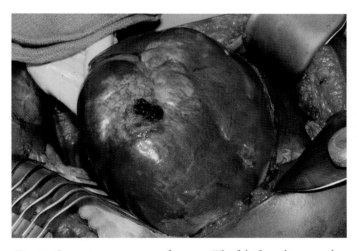

Fig. 7. Operative assessment of tumor. The falciform ligament has been sectioned, as have the right triangular and coronary ligaments. This approach allows for complete rotation of the liver, exposing the tumor (in this case located in segments 7-8). This mobilization is key for the performance of intraoperative ultrasonography and subsequent resection of the lesion.

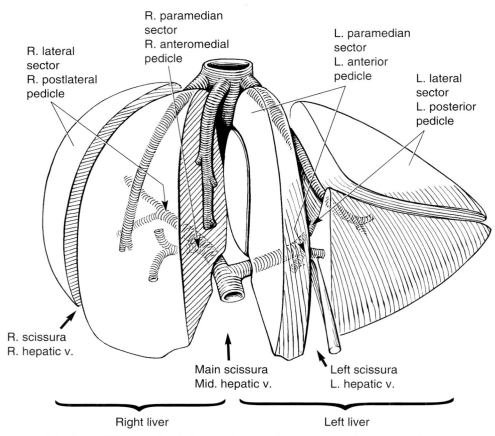

Fig. 8. Sectorial anatomy of the liver. The portal pedicles supplying each segment are shown. The hepatic veins (intersegmental) are seen emptying into the inferior vena cava. The main scissura divides the right and left lobes in the anatomical classification. L, left; R, right; v, vein. (From Nagorney DM: Hepatic resections. In Atlas of Surgical Oncology. Edited by JH Donohue, JA van Heerden, JRT Monson. Cambridge, Blackwell Science, 1995, p 190. By permission of Mayo Foundation.)

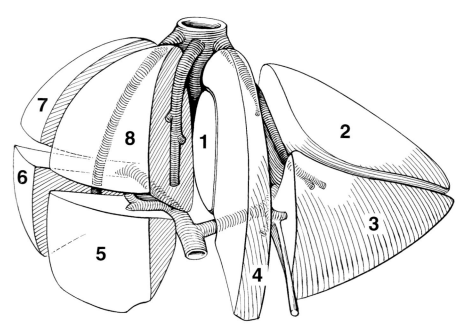

Fig. 9. Segmental anatomy of liver. All eight segments of the liver are shown. A specific portal branch supplies (and defines) each segment. (From Nagorney DM: Hepatic resections. In Atlas of Surgical Oncology. Edited by JH Donohue, JA van Heerden, JRT Monson. Cambridge, Blackwell Science, 1995, p 190. By permission of Mayo Foundation.)

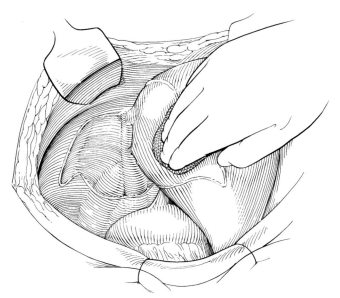

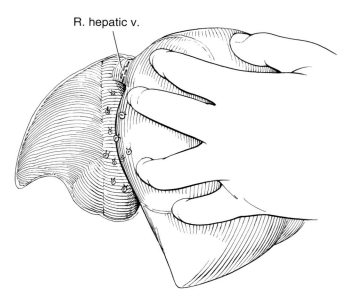

Fig. 10. *After a bilateral subcostal incision is made and metastatic disease has been ruled out, the falciform ligament is taken with electrocautery. When the posterior area is approached, care must be taken to avoid injury of the hepatic veins. These can be initially dissected and ligated from this position and the liver freed laterally and posteriorly from the inferior vena cava. (From Nagorney DM: Hepatic resections.* In *Atlas of Surgical Oncology. Edited by JH Donohue, JA van Heerden, JRT Monson. Cambridge, Blackwell Science, 1995, p 197. By permission of Mayo Foundation.)*

Fig. 11. *Immediately after the step shown in Figure 10, the triangular and coronary ligaments are taken on the right side. The same dissection is done on the contralateral side. Small draining veins can be seen at the most posterior aspect of the right lobe. Excessive traction can tear these fragile veins. We usually take these with single ties. Staples have been placed across the right hepatic vein (R. hepatic v.) before its division. (This step is done after ligation of the right hepatic artery, right portal vein, and right hepatic duct [Fig. 12].) (From Nagorney DM: Hepatic resections.* In *Atlas of Surgical Oncology. Edited by JH Donohue, JA van Heerden, JRT Monson. Cambridge, Blackwell Science, 1995, p 198. By permission of Mayo Foundation.)*

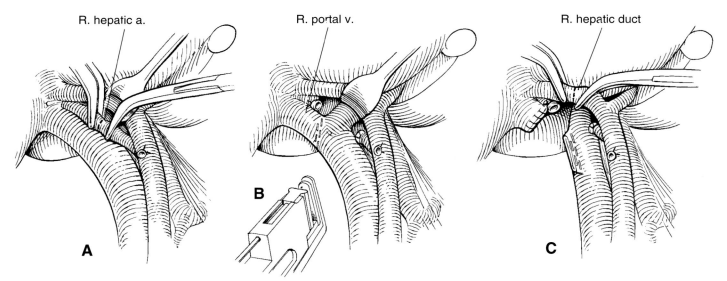

Fig. 12. *Dissection of portal triad. The structures in the triad follow a fairly constant arrangement. Artery, anterior on the left; bile duct, anterior to the right; portal vein, posterior. The steps for performing a right hepatectomy are shown. (A), The right hepatic artery (R. hepatic a.) is exposed anteriorly, clamped, and transected at dotted line. (B), Proximal double-ligation of the right hepatic artery with 2-0 silk sutures has been done. This maneuver exposes the right portal vein; some dissection of fibrous tissue posterior to the vein completes the isolation of the vein. The right portal vein (R. portal v.) is usually transected between lines of vascular staples. (C), Finally, the right (R.) hepatic duct is transected at the dotted line or, preferably, inside the liver. (From Nagorney DM: Hepatic resections.* In *Atlas of Surgical Oncology. Edited by JH Donohue, JA van Heerden, JRT Monson. Cambridge, Blackwell Science, 1995, p 196. By permission of Mayo Foundation.)*

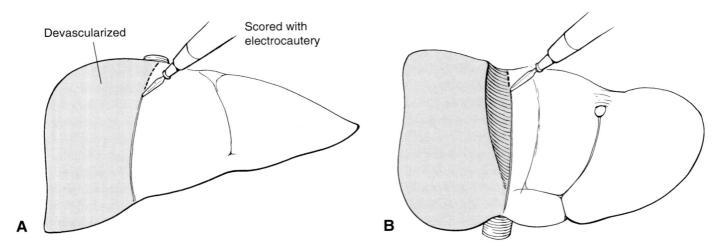

Fig. 13. *After the right hepatic pedicle is ligated, the interface between the right and left lobes is evident; the right lobe becomes ischemic and turns purple (shaded areas). We ligate the right hepatic vein (already isolated) with vascular staples (Fig. 11) to achieve a bloodless field and decrease operative bleeding. After Glisson's capsule is scored with electrocautery (A), the ultrasonic aspirator is used to transect the hepatic parenchyma (B). Fibrous structures (i.e., vessels and bile ducts) are ligated before transection. (From Nagorney DM: Hepatic resections. In Atlas of Surgical Oncology. Edited by JH Donohue, JA van Heerden, JRT Monson. Cambridge, Blackwell Science, 1995, p 197. By permission of Mayo Foundation.)*

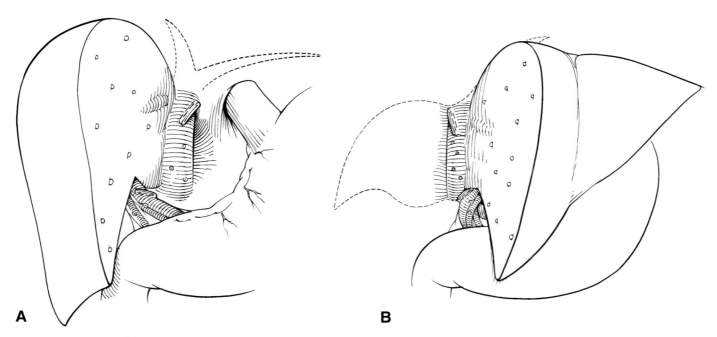

Fig. 14. *Appearance of the transected liver after a left lobar hepatectomy (A) and after a right lobar hepatectomy (B). Usually the middle hepatic vein is within the liver substance of the remaining liver, independent of the side of the hepatectomy. The corresponding stapled hepatic vein stump is seen joining the inferior vena cava. (From Nagorney DM: Hepatic resections. In Atlas of Surgical Oncology. Edited by JH Donohue, JA van Heerden, JRT Monson. Cambridge, Blackwell Science, 1995, p 200. By permission of Mayo Foundation.)*

REFERENCES

1. Nagorney DM, Gigot JF: Primary epithelial hepatic malignancies: etiology, epidemiology, and outcome after subtotal and total hepatic resection. Surg Oncol Clin N Am 5:283-300, 1996
2. Rustgi VK: Epidemiology of hepatocellular carcinoma. Gastroenterol Clin North Am 16:545-551, 1987
3. Simonetti RG, Camma C, Fiorello F, Politi F, D'Amico G, Pagliaro L: Hepatocellular carcinoma: a worldwide problem and the major risk factors. Dig Dis Sci 36:962-972, 1991
4. El-Serag HB, Mason AC: Rising incidence of hepatocellular carcinoma in the United States. N Engl J Med 340:745-750, 1999
5. Alberti A, Pontisso P: Hepatitis viruses as aetiological agents of hepatocellular carcinoma. Ital J Gastroenterol 23:452-456, 1991
6. Di Bisceglie AM, Rustgi VK, Hoofnagle JH, Dusheiko GM, Lotze MT: NIH conference: hepatocellular carcinoma. Ann Intern Med 108:390-401, 1988
7. Lefkowitch JH: The epidemiology and morphology of primary malignant liver tumors. Surg Clin North Am 61:169-180, 1981
8. Beasley RP: Hepatitis B virus. The major etiology of hepatocellular carcinoma. Cancer 61:1942-1956, 1988
9. Lee CS, Sung JL, Hwang LY, Sheu JC, Chen DS, Lin TY, Beasley RP: Surgical treatment of 109 patients with symptomatic and asymptomatic hepatocellular carcinoma. Surgery 99:481-490, 1986
10. Suenaga M, Nakao A, Harada A, Nonami T, Okada Y, Sugiura H, Uehara S, Takagi H: Hepatic resection for hepatocellular carcinoma. World J Surg 16:97-104, 1992
11. Zuckerman AJ: Prevention of primary liver cancer by immunization. N Engl J Med 336:1906-1907, 1997
12. Chang MH, Chen CJ, Lai MS, Hsu HM, Wu TC, Kong MS, Liang DC, Shau WY, Chen DS: Universal hepatitis B vaccination in Taiwan and the incidence of hepatocellular carcinoma in children: Taiwan Childhood Hepatoma Study Group. N Engl J Med 336:1855-1859, 1997
13. Tsukuma H, Hiyama T, Tanaka S, Nakao M, Yabuuchi T, Kitamura T, Nakanishi K, Fujimoto I, Inoue A, Yamazaki H, Kawashima T: Risk factors for hepatocellular carcinoma among patients with chronic liver disease. N Engl J Med 328:1797-1801, 1993
14. Tanaka K, Hirohata T, Koga S, Sugimachi K, Kanematsu T, Ohryohji F, Nawata H, Ishibashi H, Maeda Y, Kiyokawa H: Hepatitis C and hepatitis B in the etiology of hepatocellular carcinoma in the Japanese population. Cancer Res 51:2842-2847, 1991
15. Ince N, Wands JR: The increasing incidence of hepatocellular carcinoma. N Engl J Med 340:798-799, 1999
16. Heintges T, Wands JR: Hepatitis C virus: epidemiology and transmission. Hepatology 26:521-526, 1997
17. Ozturk M: p53 mutation in hepatocellular carcinoma after aflatoxin exposure. Lancet 338:1356-1359, 1991
18. Umeno M, McBride OW, Yang CS, Gelboin HV, Gonzalez FJ: Human ethanol-inducible P450IIE1: complete gene sequence, promoter characterization, chromosome mapping, and cDNA-directed expression. Biochemistry 27:9006-9013, 1988
19. Niederau C, Fischer R, Sonnenberg A, Stremmel W, Trampisch HJ, Strohmeyer G: Survival and causes of death in cirrhotic and in noncirrhotic patients with primary hemochromatosis. N Engl J Med 313:1256-1262, 1985
20. Cochrane M, Williams R: Humoral effects of hepatocellular carcinoma. *In* Hepatocellular Carcinoma. Edited by K Okuda, RL Peters. New York, Wiley, 1976, pp 333-352
21. Kamath PS, Wiesner RH, Malinchoc M, Kremers W, Therneau TM, Kosberg CL, D'Amico G, Dickson ER, Kim WR: A model to predict survival in patients with end-stage liver disease. Hepatology 33:464-470, 2001
22. McGill DB, Rakela J, Zinsmeister AR, Ott BJ: A 21-year experience with major hemorrhage after percutaneous liver biopsy. Gastroenterology 99:1396-1400, 1990
23. van Leeuwen DJ, Wilson L, Crowe DR: Liver biopsy in the mid-1990s: questions and answers. Semin Liver Dis 15:340-359, 1995
24. American Joint Committee on Cancer: AJCC Cancer Staging Manual. Fifth edition. Edited by ID Fleming, JS Cooper, DE Henson, RVP Hutter, BJ Kennedy, GP Murphy, B O'Sullivan, LH Sobin, JW Yarbro. Philadelphia, Lippincott-Raven Publishers, 1997, pp 97-101
25. Collier J, Sherman M: Screening for hepatocellular carcinoma. Hepatology 27:273-278, 1998
26. Nagorney DM, van Heerden JA, Ilstrup DM, Adson MA: Primary hepatic malignancy: surgical management and determinants of survival. Surgery 106:740-748, 1989
27. Que FG, Gigot JF, Harmsen WS, Nagorney DM: Hepatic resection of hepatocellular carcinoma (abstract). Hepatology 26:245A, 1997
28. Penn I: Hepatic transplantation for primary and metastatic cancers of the liver. Surgery 110:726-734, 1991
29. Gores GJ: Liver transplantation for malignant disease. Gastroenterol Clin North Am 22:285-299, 1993
30. Iwatsuki S, Starzl TE, Sheahan DG, Yokoyama I, Demetris AJ, Todo S, Tzakis AG, Van Thiel DH, Carr B, Selby R: Hepatic resection versus transplantation for hepatocellular carcinoma. Ann Surg 214:221-228, 1991
31. Mazzaferro V, Regalia E, Doci R, Andreola S, Pulvirenti A, Bozzetti F, Montalto F, Ammatuna M, Morabito A, Gennari L: Liver transplantation for the treatment of small hepatocellular carcinomas in patients with cirrhosis. N Engl J Med 334:693-699, 1996
32. Harnois DM, Steers J, Andrews JC, Rubin JC, Pitot HC, Burgart L, Wiesner RH, Gores GJ: Preoperative hepatic artery chemoembolization followed by orthotopic liver transplantation for hepatocellular carcinoma. Liver Transpl Surg 5:192-199, 1999
33. Marsh JW, Dvorchik I, Subotin M, Balan V, Rakela J, Popechitelev EP, Subbotin V, Casavilla A, Carr BI, Fung JJ, Iwatsuki S: The prediction of risk of recurrence and time to recurrence of hepatocellular carcinoma after orthotopic liver transplantation: a pilot study. Hepatology 26:444-450, 1997
34. Esnaola NF, Lauwers GY, Mirza NQ, Nagorney DM, Doherty DA, Ikai I, Belghiti J, Yamaoka Y, Curley SA, Ellis LM, Vauthey JN: Predictors of microvascular invasion in patients with hepatocellular carcinoma who are candidates for orthotopic liver transplantation (abstract). Gastroenterology 120 Suppl 1:A90, 2001
35. Nagasue N, Uchida M, Makino Y, Takemoto Y, Yamanoi A, Hayashi T, Chang YC, Kohno H, Nakamura T, Yukaya H: Incidence and factors associated with intrahepatic recurrence following resection of hepatocellular carcinoma. Gastroenterology 105:488-494, 1993
36. Minagawa M, Makuuchi M, Takayama T: Prognostic factors after repeat hepatectomy for recurrent hepatocellular carcinoma (abstract). Gastroenterology 120 Suppl 1:A560, 2001
37. Ohnishi K, Nomura F, Ito S, Fujiwara K: Prognosis of small hepatocellular carcinoma (less than 3 cm) after percutaneous acetic acid injection: study of 91 cases. Hepatology 23:994-1002, 1996
38. Zhou XD, Tang ZY, Yu YQ, Weng JM, Ma ZC, Zhang BH, Zheng YX: The role of cryosurgery in the treatment of hepatic cancer: a report of 113 cases. J Cancer Res Clin Oncol 120:100-102, 1993
39. Seki T, Wakabayashi M, Nakagawa T, Imamura M, Tamai T, Nishimura A, Yamashiki N, Inoue K: Percutaneous microwave coagulation therapy for solitary metastatic liver tumors from colorectal cancer: a pilot clinical study. Am J Gastroenterol 94:322-327, 1999

40. Vogl TJ, Mack MG, Roggan A, Straub R, Eichler KC, Muller PK, Knappe V, Felix R: Internally cooled power laser for MR-guided interstitial laser-induced thermotherapy of liver lesions: initial clinical results. Radiology 209:381-385, 1998

41. Curley SA, Izzo F, Ellis LM, Vauthey JN, Vallone P: Radiofrequency ablation of hepatocellular cancer in 110 patients with cirrhosis. Ann Surg 232:381-391, 2000

42. McGahan JP, Browning PD, Brock JM, Tesluk H: Hepatic ablation using radiofrequency electrocautery. Invest Radiol 25:267-270, 1990

43. Falkson G, MacIntyre JM, Moertel CG, Johnson LA, Scherman RC: Primary liver cancer: an Eastern Cooperative Oncology Group Trial. Cancer 54:970-977, 1984

44. Huang YH, Wu JC, Lui WY, Chau GY, Tsay SH, Chiang JH, King KL, Huo TI, Chang FY, Lee SD: Prospective case-controlled trial of adjuvant chemotherapy after resection of hepatocellular carcinoma. World J Surg 24:551-555, 2000

45. Lai EC, Lo CM, Fan ST, Liu CL, Wong J: Postoperative adjuvant chemotherapy after curative resection of hepatocellular carcinoma: a randomized controlled trial. Arch Surg 133:183-188, 1998

46. Yamada R, Kishi K, Terada M: Transcatheter arterial chemoembolization for unresectable hepatocellular carcinoma. In Primary Liver Cancer in Japan. Edited by T Tobe, H Kameda. Tokyo, Springer-Verlag, 1992, pp 259-271

47. Groupe d'Etude et de Traitement du Carcinome Hepatocellulaire: A comparison of Lipiodol chemoembolization and conservative treatment for unresectable hepatocellular carcinoma. N Engl J Med 332:1256-1261, 1995

48. Muto Y, Moriwaki H, Ninomiya M, Adachi S, Saito A, Takasaki KT, Tanaka T, Tsurumi K, Okuno M, Tomita E, Nakamura T, Kojima T: Prevention of second primary tumors by an acyclic retinoid, polyprenoic acid, in patients with hepatocellular carcinoma: Hepatoma Prevention Study Group. N Engl J Med 334:1561-1567, 1996

49. Leung WT, Lau WY, Ho S, Chan M, Leung N, Lin J, Ho KC, Metreweli C, Johnson PJ, Li AK: Selective internal radiation therapy with intra-arterial iodine-131-Lipiodol in inoperable hepatocellular carcinoma. J Nucl Med 35:1313-1318, 1994

50. Lau WY, Leung TW, Ho SK, Chan M, Machin D, Lau J, Chan AT, Yeo W, Mok TS, Yu SC, Leung NW, Johnson PJ: Adjuvant intra-arterial iodine-131-labelled lipiodol for resectable hepatocellular carcinoma: a prospective randomised trial. Lancet 353:797-801, 1999

51. Partensky C, Sassolas G, Henry L, Paliard P, Maddern GJ: Intra-arterial iodine 131-labeled lipiodol as adjuvant therapy after curative liver resection for hepatocellular carcinoma: a phase 2 clinical study. Arch Surg 135:1298-1300, 2000

52. Inoue A, Tsukuma H, Oshima A, Yabuuchi T, Nakao M, Matsunaga T, Kojima J, Tanaka S: Effectiveness of interferon therapy for reducing the incidence of hepatocellular carcinoma among patients with type C chronic hepatitis. J Epidemiol 10:234-240, 2000

53. Ikeda K, Arase Y, Saitoh S, Kobayashi M, Suzuki Y, Suzuki F, Tsubota A, Chayama K, Murashima N, Kumada H: Interferon beta prevents recurrence of hepatocellular carcinoma after complete resection or ablation of the primary tumor: a prospective randomized study of hepatitis C virus-related liver cancer. Hepatology 32:228-232, 2000

54. Burgart LJ, Martinez CJM, Batts KP: Fibrolamellar hepatoma: importance of using a strict definition (abstract). Mod Pathol 7:129A, 1994

55. Stevens WR, Johnson CD, Stephens DH, Nagorney DM: Fibrolamellar hepatocellular carcinoma: stage at presentation and results of aggressive surgical management. AJR Am J Roentgenol 164:1153-1158, 1995

56. Pinna AD, Iwatsuki S, Lee RG, Todo S, Madariaga JR, Marsh JW, Casavilla A, Dvorchik I, Fung JJ, Starzl TE: Treatment of fibrolamellar hepatoma with subtotal hepatectomy or transplantation. Hepatology 26:877-883, 1997

57. Nagorney DM, Adson MA, Weiland LH, Knight CD Jr, Smalley SR, Zinsmeister AR: Fibrolamellar hepatoma. Am J Surg 149:113-119, 1985

58. Pichlmayr R, Lamesch P, Weimann A, Tusch G, Ringe B: Surgical treatment of cholangiocellular carcinoma. World J Surg 19:83-88, 1995

59. Colombari R, Tsui WM: Biliary tumors of the liver. Semin Liver Dis 15:402-413, 1995

60. Nakeeb A, Pitt HA, Sohn TA, Coleman J, Abrams RA, Piantadosi S, Hruban RH, Lillemoe KD, Yeo CJ, Cameron JL: Cholangiocarcinoma: a spectrum of intrahepatic, perihilar, and distal tumors. Ann Surg 224:463-473, 1996

61. Yeo CJ, Pitt HA, Cameron JL: Cholangiocarcinoma. Surg Clin North Am 70:1429-1447, 1990

62. Yamanaka N, Okamoto E, Ando T, Oriyama T, Fujimoto J, Furukawa K, Tanaka T, Tanaka W, Nishigami T: Clinicopathologic spectrum of resected extraductal mass-forming intrahepatic cholangiocarcinoma. Cancer 76:2449-2456, 1995

63. Lieser MJ, Barry MK, Rowland C, Ilstrup DM, Nagorney DM: Surgical management of intrahepatic cholangiocarcinoma: a 31-year experience. J Hepatobiliary Pancreat Surg 5:41-47, 1998

64. Freeny PC: Computed tomography in the diagnosis and staging of cholangiocarcinoma and pancreatic carcinoma. Ann Oncol 10 Suppl 4:12-17, 1999

65. Lee MG, Jeong YK, Sung KB: Breath-hold contrast-enhanced 3D MR angiography in 19 seconds: value in the assessment of vascular invasion and pancreaticobiliary disease. In Proceedings of the 5th Annual Meeting of the International Society for Magnetic Resonance in Medicine. Vancouver, International Society for Magnetic Resonance in Medicine, 1997, pp 1-92

66. Nozaki Y, Yamamoto M, Ikai I, Yamamoto Y, Ozaki N, Fujii H, Nagahori K, Matsumoto Y, Yamaoka Y: Reconsideration of the lymph node metastasis pattern (N factor) from intrahepatic cholangiocarcinoma using the International Union Against Cancer TNM staging system for primary liver carcinoma. Cancer 83:1923-1929, 1998

67. Suh KS, Roh HR, Koh YT, Lee KU, Park YH, Kim SW: Clinicopathologic features of the intraductal growth type of peripheral cholangiocarcinoma. Hepatology 31:12-17, 2000

68. Marcos-Alvarez A, Jenkins RL: Cholangiocarcinoma. Surg Oncol Clin N Am 5:301-316, 1996

69. Nakajima T, Kondo Y, Miyazaki M, Okui K: A histopathologic study of 102 cases of intrahepatic cholangiocarcinoma: histologic classification and modes of spreading. Hum Pathol 19:1228-1234, 1988

70. Namieno T, Koito K, Takahashi M, Une Y, Yamashita K, Shimamura T: Survival-associated histologic spreading modes of operable intrahepatic, peripheral-type cholangiocarcinomas. World J Surg 25:572-577, 2001

71. Harrison LE, Fong Y, Klimstra DS, Zee SY, Blumgart LH: Surgical treatment of 32 patients with peripheral intrahepatic cholangiocarcinoma. Br J Surg 85:1068-1070, 1998

72. Goss JA, Shackleton CR, Farmer DG, Arnaout WS, Seu P, Markowitz JS, Martin P, Stribling RJ, Goldstein LI, Busuttil RW: Orthotopic liver transplantation for primary sclerosing cholangitis: a 12-year single center experience. Ann Surg 225:472-481, 1997

HEPATIC METASTASES FROM EXTRAHEPATIC CANCERS

Florencia G. Que, M.D.
John H. Donohue, M.D.
David M. Nagorney, M.D.

Because the liver is the natural "filter" of blood from the colon and rectum, the pancreas, and the upper gastrointestinal tract, it is a common organ to which metastases from cancers in these areas spread. Hepatic metastases from these and other sites cause major morbidity that usually results in death. In the past, patients with such metastases seldom survived for more than 3 years.[1] However, recent improvements in detection of these metastatic tumors, advances in surgical techniques for resection, and new chemotherapeutic agents and regional therapies have made it possible to achieve longer survival. The longer survival has occurred most often in the subset of patients with isolated hepatic metastases from colorectal cancers. Results in these patients have formed the basis for the current approach taken at Mayo Clinic in all patients with isolated liver metastases, namely, early detection of lesions and appropriately timed hepatic resection and adjuvant therapy. Today, hepatic resection is our treatment of choice for hepatic metastases from colorectal carcinoma and neuroendocrine cancers. However, the role of hepatic resection in the treatment of noncolorectal, nonneuroendocrine metastases is less well established.

SELECTING PATIENTS FOR OPERATION

The selection of patients for hepatic resection is influenced by several factors, including the time of discovery of the hepatic metastases, the status of the primary tumor, the extent of the hepatic metastases, the intent of resection (curative or palliative), and the overall health of the patient. Patients in good general health who have minimal organ comorbidities should be able to undergo hepatic resection with an expected operative mortality rate of less than 5%.

Metastases present temporally in three ways: synchronously with the primary cancer, metachronously after resection of the primary cancer, and metachronously after previous resection of metastases. Most operations are done for metachronous metastases. Undertaking synchronous bowel and hepatic resection requires thorough preoperative staging, inclusive of hepatic imaging, which often has not been done. If resections are undertaken synchronously, initial gross, thorough resection of the primary tumor and all gross regional disease is a prerequisite. Moreover, intraoperative ultrasonography should be done to check for nonpalpable, nonvisible hepatic metastases. When the extent of the hepatic metastases is in doubt, synchronous resection should not be done.

The status of the primary tumor clearly affects the decision to resect the hepatic metastases. Candidates for hepatic resection must have had complete excision of their primary cancer without gross residual extrahepatic disease. Standard resection of the primary tumor should have included tumor-free margins of resection and appropriate regional lymphadenectomy. Confirmation of an adequate locoregional resection allows the surgeon who is considering reoperation to focus on the metastases.

When patients are referred for resection of hepatic metastases, surgeons must be cognizant of the possibility that resection of the primary tumor may have been inadequate. This situation is particularly relevant for patients in whom hepatic metastases were recognized unexpectedly during a prior colorectal resection. The oncologic standards during the resection may have been unwisely compromised because of the stage of the disease. If objective documentation of an inadequate resection of the primary tumor is present, the original site of the primary tumor should be evaluated further. Although an inadequate resection of the primary tumor does not exclude reoperation for metastatic disease, the patient must be informed of the adverse effect residual primary disease has on survival. In fact, the surgeon who is undertaking hepatic resection must stress that reexcision of residual primary tumor may be required or, more ominously, that resection of the hepatic metastases may have to be aborted. Residual primary tumor may be unresectable at exploration, even if the hepatic metastases themselves are resectable.

Additional factors that may affect the selection of patients for resection of hepatic metastases are the gross pathologic features of the primary tumor and the operative technique used during resection of the primary tumor. For example, patients with large colorectal tumors that have been "peeled off" adjacent pelvic structures or major vascular structures with tumor extending microscopically to the margins may benefit from an initial period of postoperative adjuvant chemoradiation for optimal local control. Adjuvant treatment and subsequent restaging should precede operation for hepatic metastases. Other factors that influence the selection for reoperation are fracture of the primary tumor during resection and a prior incisional biopsy of hepatic metastases. Gross spillage of tumor cells during resection of the primary tumor or during hepatic biopsy dictates a longer observation before reoperation for hepatic metastases to allow detection of residual intraperitoneal disease. Positron emission tomography to assess for peritoneal disease and staging laparoscopy before open laparotomy for resection of metastases may be particularly useful in patients who may have had gross spillage of tumor cells.

Another important point is that hepatic resection for metastases should rarely be undertaken if any extrahepatic metastases exist, exclusive of residual regional lymph node metastases from the primary tumor. The exception to this caveat is that of hepatic metastases from hormonally functional neuroendocrine tumors, in which case debulking of the metastases may allow a substantial improvement in the patient's quality of life.

Operative intent also affects selection of patients. Resection of hepatic metastases from colorectal cancer is undertaken primarily for cure, which implies removal or ablation of all metastases. Rarely, resection may be offered as palliative treatment for refractory pain, infection, or bleeding caused by necrotic metastases.

The presence and extent of underlying hepatic disease influence the patient's ability to withstand hepatic resection. In brief, adequate postoperative hepatic function can be predicted in patients without chronic liver disease if two or more anatomically adjacent segments are preserved during the resection. If cirrhosis is present, the extent of resection must be reduced; ablation of metastases, rather than resection, may be a better choice. Extensive hepatic steatosis without cirrhosis, frequent in obese patients, also limits the extent of hepatic resection.

PREOPERATIVE CARE

Preoperative preparation of the patient for hepatic resection is similar to that undertaken for any major hepatopancreatobiliary procedure. A bowel preparation is given, abnormal coagulation profiles are corrected, and prophylactic antibiotics directed at upper gastrointestinal tract flora are administered. Importantly, if jaundice, cholangitis, and bile duct obstruction are present, biliary decompression by endoscopic or percutaneous intubation is preferred to improve hepatic function and control infection. In general, major hepatic resection is not undertaken unless the total serum bilirubin value is less than 5 mg/dL and clinical infection is controlled. If it is necessary to reduce the bilirubin level, biliary drainage is established in the planned hepatic remnant.

OPERATIVE TECHNIQUE

Safe hepatic resection is predicated on a clear understanding of hepatic anatomy. Although the regenerative capacities and metabolic reserve of the liver are great, anatomical hepatic resections reduce operative risk and optimize postoperative liver function. The major anatomical features of the liver relevant to resection have been detailed elsewhere.[2] Resection or ablation of metastases should never risk irreversible hepatic damage. The extent of resection depends on the tumor size and location and, importantly, on the relation of the tumor to the major afferent and efferent hepatic vasculature and to the bile ducts. Anatomical resections of segments or lobes are preferred in most patients. A 1- to 2-cm disease-free margin is considered optimal to reduce the risk of intrahepatic recurrence of the metastases, with the exception of tumors that originate from neuroendocrine malignancies. However, margins of resection should never risk damage to major hepatic vasculature. The afferent and efferent vasculature of the liver remnant must be scrupulously protected.

A major complement to the safety of hepatic resection is anesthetic management. The maintenance of low central venous pressure (5-7 mm Hg) reduces blood loss from the hepatic veins during resection. Large-bore intravenous access for rapid transfusion is essential.

The major pitfalls or danger points with hepatic resection include hemorrhage from hepatic or portal veins or hepatic arteries, air embolism from hepatic venous injury, injury to the biliary duct system with postoperative obstruction or fistula formation, portal or hepatic vein compromise with subsequent ischemia or portal hypertension, prolonged vascular inflow occlusion leading to refractory hepatic ischemia, and injury to the diaphragm, inferior vena cava, or intestine.

Incision and Exposure

A bilateral subcostal incision affords wide exposure for any hepatic resection. A long midline incision provides a satisfactory alternative, particularly for limited resections of segments 2 through 6 or if the patient has a narrow or acute costal angle (< 90°). However, tumors that involve segments 7 or 8 or extended lobar resections are approached more safely through a bilateral subcostal incision, which permits better exposure and control of the hepatic vein–inferior vena cava junction. Rarely, a right thoracic extension (thoracoabdominal incision) is necessary to excise bulky tumors that involve segments 7 and 8. Perihepatic adhesions are divided and the liver is mobilized by complete division of its ligamentous attachments (i.e., coronary, falciform, and triangular ligaments). The thin gastrohepatic omentum is incised adjacent to the hepatoduodenal ligament to provide access to the foramen of Winslow for subsequent inflow vascular occlusion. A self-supporting retractor should be used to elevate the rib cage anteriorly and cephalad, and additional retractors are used to retract the viscera caudally.

Division of Major Vessels and Hepatic Parenchyma

The hepatic artery, portal vein, and hepatic veins of the segment or lobe of the liver to be removed are ligated as the initial step. Major hepatic or portal veins are best occluded with vascular staples. The hepatic parenchyma is transected by the preferred method of the surgeon. At Mayo Clinic, various methods have been used, including compression (finger fracture [digitoclysis], clamp fracture [Kelly-clysis], or mechanical staples), contact techniques (Cavitron Ultrasonic Surgical Aspirator, Valleylab, Boulder, Colorado), or thermal techniques (electrocautery, laser, harmonic scalpel) (Fig. 1). Each approach has advantages and disadvantages. Each disrupts parenchyma to expose vessels and bile ducts for ligation. Although the extent of parenchymal necrosis adjacent to the transection plane varies among techniques, such devitalized parenchyma is insignificant clinically. Vessels or ducts more than 2 mm in diameter generally require ligation with sutures or clips.

Control of Bleeding and Bile Ducts

Intraoperative hemorrhage is reduced by digital compression of the liver bilateral to the transection plane. The

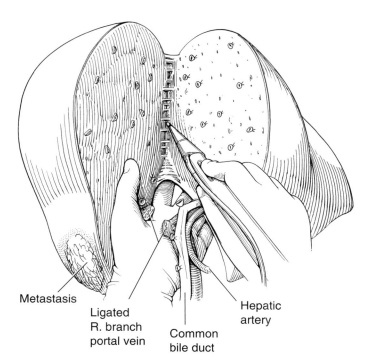

Fig. 1. Division of liver with an ultrasonic dissector during a right hepatic lobectomy for hepatic metastasis from a right colon cancer.

surgeon and the assistant compress the parenchyma on opposite sides of the transection plane. Typically, the assistant surgeon maintains hemostasis by electrocautery, and an additional assistant maintains field exposure by suctioning bile or blood from the transection interface. Bile ducts or vessels more than 2 mm in diameter are clamped with metal clips, ligated with sutures, or stapled. The surgeon should remember that suture ligation of vessels or ducts limits imaging artifacts postoperatively. The specific types of resection have been detailed elsewhere.[2] After local hemostasis and bile stasis are obtained, the abdomen is closed. Drainage is optional unless concurrent biliary tract reconstruction is performed. Closed, low-pressure suction drainage is preferred when drainage is used.

POSTOPERATIVE CARE

Postoperative care generally involves appropriate fluid administration. The addition of albumin to standard crystalloid solutions reduces postoperative weight gain and maintains adequate urine output. Most hepatic resections are associated with a mild acidosis and coagulation abnormalities in the immediate postoperative period. Neither acid-base abnormalities nor coagulation deficits are corrected postoperatively, unless they are clinically significant. Nasogastric intubation is continued overnight to reduce the risk of aspiration and then is discontinued the morning after operation. Postoperative epidural analgesia markedly improves pulmonary function and pain control. Urinary output is monitored until hemodynamic stability has been maintained for 24 hours.

COMPLICATIONS OF HEPATIC RESECTION AND THEIR MANAGEMENT

Intraoperative Complications

Hemorrhage is the most common intraoperative complication and usually results from major vessel trauma along the transection interface or from coagulopathy. Intermittent inflow occlusion or total hepatic vascular isolation has dramatically reduced the risk of life-threatening hemorrhage intraoperatively. A simple Pringle maneuver with an appropriate-sized vascular clamp easily controls hemorrhage from either the portal vein or the hepatic arteries. Traumatic injury to the extrahepatic bile duct from a vascular clamp is rare. The noncirrhotic, nonsteatotic liver tolerates warm ischemia periods for more than 1 hour without any measurable long-term consequences. Ischemia-reperfusion injury may be reduced by intermittent occlusion or ischemic preconditioning. Although ischemic hepatic injury causes increases of serum aspartate transaminase and bilirubin levels and prolongation of the prothrombin time, these changes reverse rapidly (< 7-10 days).

Diffuse hemorrhage from the transection interface usually results from increase of the central venous pressure to pressures more than 12 to 15 mm Hg. Continuous intraoperative monitoring of the central venous pressure and volume replacement to maintain central venous pressures less than 5 mm Hg reduce this risk but allow maintenance of adequate systemic hemodynamics. Persistent interface hemorrhage is best treated by coagulation with electrocautery or argon beam coagulator or by compression with laparotomy pads and topical hemostatic agents. Should interface bleeding persist after the use of these techniques, intraoperative evaluation for a coagulopathy must be undertaken.

Another important intraoperative complication is air embolus from hepatic vein damage. Although a potentially life-threatening source of cardiac arrhythmias and ventilation-perfusion defects, early recognition is possible through careful anesthetic monitoring. Air embolism can be detected with precordial Doppler sonography, right heart catheterization, capnography from mass spectroscopy, transcutaneous oxygen probes, and transesophageal echocardiography. Capnographic mass spectrometry provides the most practical recognition of venous air embolism. With an increasing volume of air embolism, initial gas exchange abnormalities are supplanted by deteriorating systemic hemodynamics. Venous air embolism should be suspected initially from decreases in arterial oxygen tension, transcutaneous oxygen pressure, and fractional end-tidal concentrations of carbon dioxide and from an increase in fractional end-tidal concentration of nitrogen. If an embolus is present, the arterial carbon dioxide tension and transcutaneous carbon dioxide pressures will increase rapidly. Advanced signs include a precordial machinery murmur, visible air in the hepatic vein or inferior vena cava, and decreases in cardiac output and blood pressure. Treatment consists of placing the patient in a Trendelenburg position, putting the head of the patient's bed down, suture closure of the hepatic vein, and aspiration of the intracardiac air through a central venous catheter with positive-pressure ventilation.

Postoperative Complications

Postoperative hemorrhage usually arises from loosened vascular clips or ligatures. Recognition should be obvious from depressed hemodynamic or bloody abdominal drainage. Any concurrent coagulopathy should be at least partially corrected before reoperation to control hemorrhage.

Serosanguineous drainage through intra-abdominal drains is expected postoperatively. The volume of drainage may vary widely. Large volumes may necessitate isotonic fluid replacement to maintain fluid and electrolyte balance postoperatively. In general, abdominal drains can be removed safely regardless of the volume unless the drainage is bilious. Usually, even high-output drainage volumes are resorbed rapidly through the peritoneum and diaphragm without the formation of focal fluid collections or ascites. In patients with cirrhosis, drains should be avoided after hepatic resection because of the probability of protracted ascitic fluid drainage and secondary infection of the ascites.

Bilious drainage through abdominal drains or after puncture of loculated perihepatic fluid collections is indicative of a biliary fistula. Fistulas are best managed conservatively with continuous closed suction drainage until resolution. Persistent fistulas usually resolve with continuous suction drainage and endoscopic biliary stenting. Reoperation for repair of biliary fistula is rarely indicated unless there is complete disruption of the major bile duct from the hepatic remnant and bilioenteric bile flow is completely absent.

Perihepatic intra-abdominal abscess may occur after any hepatic resection. Percutaneous drainage is the treatment of choice.

Hepatic insufficiency or failure can occur after hepatic resection. The most common cause of hepatic insufficiency after hepatic resection is inadequate residual functional hepatic reserve. Hepatic failure usually occurs in patients with chronic hepatitis or cirrhosis, especially after extended polysegmental resection. The treatment of hepatic failure is simply supportive. Orthotopic liver transplantation, which provides the only curative solution for refractory postoperative hepatic failure, is not applicable in the clinical setting of metastatic cancer in the liver.

Correctable causes of hepatic insufficiency should be sought postoperatively. These causes include major bile duct obstruction, infection, and efferent or afferent vascular compromise as a result of thrombosis. Color-flow Doppler ultrasonography and magnetic resonance imaging are the best screening techniques if thrombosis is suspected. Angiography further defines the extent of and vascular damage caused by thrombus. Once thromboses are recognized, thrombectomy and repair of the venous damage that precipitated the thrombus are indicated. Bile duct obstruction should be suspected from steadily increasing total and direct serum bilirubin levels. Endoscopic retrograde cholangiography best defines the location and extent of the injury. Percutaneous transhepatic cholangiography is less useful postoperatively because of delayed proximal bile duct dilatation and altered hepatic position after resection.

RESULTS OF HEPATIC RESECTION FOR COLORECTAL METASTASES

The reported 5-year survival rate after hepatic resection for colorectal metastases done at major centers has ranged from 26% to 39% (Table 1).[3-7] Most such centers have reported a perioperative mortality rate of less than 4%. Our most recent Mayo Clinic study of 662 patients showed

an overall 5-year survival rate of 37% and a disease-related 5-year survival rate of 42% (Table 1). Importantly, survival was actual; that is, there was a minimal follow-up of 5 years for each of the survivors. Our 30-day mortality rate was 2%, and the 60-day mortality rate was 3%. The probability of any recurrence was 65% at 5 years. Recurrence developed within 3 years of hepatic resection in 80% of patients who had recurrence. The liver was the site of recurrence in 50% of patients, and 12% of the patients underwent repeat hepatic resection with survival outcomes similar to those after the initial resections.

Numerous studies of outcomes have correlated clinical, pathologic, and interventional factors with survival to define more clearly the criteria for selection of patients for hepatic resection of colorectal metastases. Not unexpectedly, given the diversity of patient populations and various selection criteria used for resection, prognostic relationships have been inconsistent. Broadly, patients with a normal clinical performance, preserved hepatic function, and limited hepatic metastases fare best. Several large studies[6-8] have developed scoring systems based on clinicopathologic factors that correlate with survival to stratify patients by expected outcome for subsequent adjuvant therapy. These studies and our own identified similar but inconsistent risk factors. Although these scoring systems have applicabilities within their respective institutions, identification of the optimal model for widespread application is as yet unestablished. Figure 2 shows a colon cancer metastasis in a resected right hepatic lobe with a surgical margin more than 1 cm. A disease-free surgical margin more than 1 cm is associated with a better prognosis in some reports. Figure 3 shows a portion of liver removed for metastasis from a colon cancer; a portal

Table 1.—Results of Resection of Hepatic Metastases From Colorectal Cancers

Reference	Patients, no.	Operative mortality, % of patients	5-Year overall survival, % of patients
Hughes et al., 1986[3]	859	NS	33
Nordlinger et al., 1992[4]	1,818	2.4	26
Scheele et al., 1997[5]	471	4.5	39
Fong et al., 1999[6]	1,001	2.8	37
Iwatsuki et al., 1999[7]	305	1	32
Mayo Clinic, 2002	662	3	37

NS, not stated.

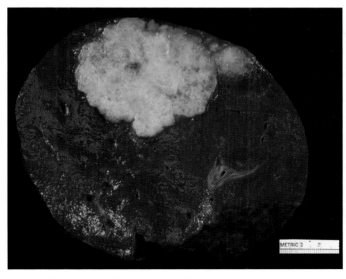

Fig. 2. Specimen of liver removed for metastatic colon cancer. An adequate disease-free surgical margin (> 1 cm) is present.

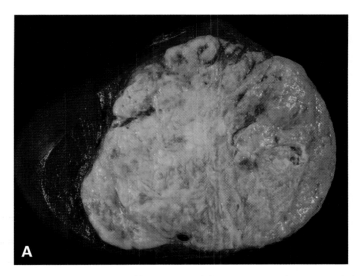
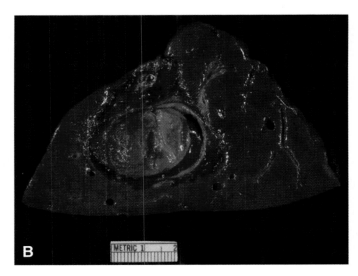

Fig. 3. (A), *Specimen of liver removed for metastatic colon cancer.* (B), *Tumor thrombus is present in an intrahepatic branch of the portal vein.*

vein tumor thrombus was found in the specimen. This is a negative prognostic factor. We imported our current database into each model and were unable to show similar stratification of outcomes for each model. Thus, the criteria for selection of patients for resection remain unchanged: complete surgical excision of the primary colorectal cancer, the absence of concurrent, extrahepatic colorectal metastases, and the expectation for complete resection of the hepatic metastases. The concurrent presence of any extrahepatic metastases, with the rare exception of a solitary pulmonary metastasis, essentially excludes curative resection.

NONRESECTIONAL SURGERY FOR HEPATIC COLORECTAL METASTASES

Hepatic Cryoablation and Radiofrequency Ablation
Ablative techniques for metastatic cancer to the liver have evolved as an alternative treatment for patients who cannot tolerate resection or as an adjunct to resection. Each ablative method attempts to destroy fully intrahepatic cancer in situ. Cryoablation involves the freezing and thawing of metastases with a cryoprobe. Freeze-thaw cycles cause intracellular and extracellular ice formation, which leads to tumor cell death. Radiofrequency ablation involves heating of the metastases with a radiofrequency electrode and cytotoxicity through coagulative necrosis. Both techniques are guided ultrasonographically for accurate positioning of the probe and assessment of the extent of tissue destruction. The techniques for each method have been detailed by others.

No comparative studies assess the efficacy of ablative techniques or compare ablative techniques with resection

for colorectal metastases. The long-term survival after either ablative method for colorectal metastases to the liver is unclear. Survival rates after cryoablation for unresectable metastases have approached 60% at 2 years (median survival, 25-32 months).[9-11] Estimated 5-year survival rates have ranged from 15% to 35%. Estimated survival rates after radiofrequency ablation of colorectal metastases have been similar, although the duration of follow-up is even more limited for this method.[12]

Hepatic Arterial Infusional Chemotherapy
Hepatic arterial infusional chemotherapy has been used primarily for unresectable hepatic metastases from colorectal carcinoma and adjuvantly after hepatic resection. Although combination systemic chemotherapy has produced objective responses in a minority of patients and has resulted in a slight but substantial improvement in patient survival compared with no therapy or single-agent chemotherapy, systemic chemotherapy remains primarily palliative. In contrast, regional chemotherapy for unresectable metastases has proved more effective. The theoretic rationale for regional or hepatic artery infusional chemotherapy is based on the nearly exclusive arterial blood supply of the metastases from the hepatic artery and first-past drug clearance kinetics, which support high local hepatic concentrations of the drug with reduced systemic toxicity.

Multiple studies have compared the use of regional hepatic arterial infusion of 5-fluorodeoxyuridine with systemic 5-fluorouracil. Meta-analyses of these trials have shown that objective tumor response rates are considerably greater with regional 5-fluorodeoxyuridine than with systemic 5-fluorouracil treatment but that there is minimal or no improvement in overall survival.[13,14] The use of regional infusional chemotherapy improved median survival times by only 3.2 months compared with systemic chemotherapy. The data from individual trials may have biased outcomes, because many patients randomized to regional therapy did not undergo or complete therapy because of technical problems with the infusion pump or toxicity. Subset analyses of patients who actually received regional therapy have shown improved survival compared with those treated systemically.

Hepatic arterial infusional chemotherapy has been used after hepatic resection to reduce hepatic recurrence and improve survival. Recent studies[15] have confirmed a 50% decrease in hepatic recurrences and a trend toward improved survival for combined regional and systemic chemotherapy compared with systemic chemotherapy alone. A more recent study[16] confirmed benefit for prolonging time to recurrence, especially in the liver, but not improved survival. Currently, investigations of combined systemic and regional adjuvant chemotherapy after hepatic resection are focusing on more effective systemic chemotherapeutic agents. Importantly, regional chemotherapy is used only in the absence of extrahepatic metastases.

Complications of hepatic arterial chemotherapy can be divided into two broad groups: pump-related (technical) complications and chemotherapy-related complications. Pump-related complications include pump malfunctions and pump site infections, whereas chemotherapy-related complications include hematologic and gastrointestinal toxicities. Gastrointestinal toxicity includes nausea, vomiting, and diarrhea, which occur infrequently with hepatic artery infusion of 5-fluorodeoxyuridine. When diarrhea does occur, misperfusion of chemotherapy to the gastrointestinal tract through an improperly placed catheter or hepatic arterial collateral vessels should be suspected. The most common problems of hepatic artery infusion therapy are gastroduodenal ulceration and hepatotoxicity. The ulcers usually result from misperfusion of the stomach and duodenum by way of small collateral branches of the hepatic artery or the right gastric artery. They are preventable with careful division of these collateral vessels during pump placement. Hepatobiliary toxicity is the most problematic toxicity. The bile ducts are particularly sensitive to regional chemoperfusion, because, like hepatic metastases, bile ducts derive their blood supply almost exclusively from the hepatic artery. Clinically, biliary toxicities manifest as an increase in the aspartate aminotransferase, alkaline phosphatase, and bilirubin levels. Biliary sclerosis mimicking sclerosing cholangitis is found on cholangiography. Hepatotoxicity is manifested by hepatitis. Dose reduction of 5-fluorodeoxyuridine and concurrent corticosteroid perfusion through the pump reduce hepatobiliary toxicity.

HEPATIC RESECTION FOR METASTASES FROM NEUROENDOCRINE TUMORS

Neuroendocrine tumors of the gastrointestinal tract are typically slow-growing and often metastasize to the liver.[17] Despite new chemotherapeutic and immunologic agents, surgical therapy remains the most effective approach to this type of metastatic disease and offers the longest-lasting benefits. Cytoreduction of the hepatic disease has been shown to improve survival.[18] When complete resection is not feasible, current recommendations dictate removal of at least 90% of the disease to achieve adequate palliation.[19]

Rationale for Cytoreductive Hepatic Surgery

Cytoreductive hepatic surgery refers to incomplete resection of tumor to reduce symptoms and facilitate the effect of nonoperative strategies.[20] Traditionally, this has been the mainstay of treatment for neuroendocrine metastases to the liver, because alternative therapies have failed to extend survival. Although the aim of any surgical intervention is to remove malignancy in its entirety, our group has defined a successful debulking as resection of at least 90% of the tumor. This approach allows us to achieve control of the endocrine symptoms in the majority of patients (90%).[21] For therapy in which control of symptoms, not extension of survival, is the primary goal, the risk-benefit ratio needs to be clearly defined in favor of surgical outcomes in order to be justified. If a cytoreductive operation can increase survival, then the application of operative interventions is doubly justified in a patient population that can survive many years with symptomatic disease.

Results

Data from Mayo Clinic and elsewhere have evaluated cytoreductive hepatic resection as a therapeutic and palliative treatment in patients with metastatic neuroendocrine disease. Two studies from Mayo Clinic[18,22] assessed alleviation of symptoms and survival in patients with metastases from islet cell tumors and carcinoid tumors. In addition to our own experience, a review of the scant cases reported in the literature supports cytoreductive hepatic operation as a valid method of treatment.

In our most recent experience,[22] 96% of patients had a partial or complete response with a decrease in their hormonal symptoms after cytoreductive operation. Symptoms had recurred in 59% of patients at 5 years (median interval between operation and recurrence, 45.5 months).

Tumor recurrence rates after partial hepatectomy with or without ablative techniques for metastatic neuroendocrine tumors were 84% at 5 years and 94% at 10 years. The median time to recurrence was 21 months after operation. Patients with complete resection of tumor had lower recurrence rates (complete vs. incomplete, 76% vs. 91%) at 5 years and a longer median time between operation and recurrence (complete vs. incomplete, 30 months vs. 6 months; $P < 0.0004$ by log-rank evaluation).

Overall survival of patients after partial hepatectomy for metastatic neuroendocrine tumors was 61% at 5 years and 36% at 10 years. Median survival was 6.4 years. Among patients with hepatic metastases from carcinoid tumors and those with metastases from islet cell tumors, there were no differences in survival, duration of symptomatic response, or recurrence of tumor. Also, survival was not different between asymptomatic and symptomatic patients with neuroendocrine metastases. In our series, the operative morbidity rate was 14% and the mortality rate was 1.2%. These data are similar to those reported by others.

Nonsurgical therapy is an inadequate means of treating metastatic neuroendocrine tumors.[23] The latest pharmacologic approach introduced the somatostatin analogues, which have been used for control of symptoms and also to slow the growth of the metastatic disease.[24] However, this medication, although useful as an adjuvant measure, has not had the expected success as a treatment of metastatic neuroendocrine tumors. Other agents have been equally ineffective.[25]

Surgical resection, thus, remains the most successful strategy for the treatment of these metastatic tumors.[22,26-29] In the most recent series on this topic (Table 2), 5-year survival rates generally exceed 50% and correspond with the findings reported here. Historical data on the survival of patients with untreated hepatic metastases from neuroendocrine tumors reveal a 5-year survival rate of 30% to 40% and a median survival of 2 to 4 years.[30,31] Our data provide evidence that survival rates can be increased to more than 60% at 5 years with a median survival of 6.5 years. We believe operation is justified because of the improved survival rates after operation.

Another issue in validating surgical therapy concerns treatment of the manifestations of the disease. Given the unpredictable response of hormonal symptoms to medical therapy, operation offers an additional benefit in the management of these symptoms. Naturally, reducing the tumor load lessens the need for medication compared with the preoperative period. Although symptoms eventually do recur, the majority of patients (59%) did not have a recurrence of symptoms until 5 years after operation (median time from operation to recurrent symptoms, almost 4 years).[22] We have not compared these results with those achieved with chemotherapeutic agents (including somatostatin analogues), but surgical treatment does offer an extended period of symptom control with minimal or no need for medical therapy. Because most patients become partially resistant to somatostatin analogues (after a median interval of 12 months for those with carcinoid and 3 months for those with islet cell tumors), we recommend a surgical approach.

Another argument in favor of cytoreductive therapy is our findings in asymptomatic patients, in whom, interestingly, the survival rate was similar to that in patients with symptoms.[22] Traditionally, we have not aggressively treated asymptomatic patients, but our findings that operative therapy improves survival strengthen our position that favors surgical management of metastatic neuroendocrine tumors in this subset of patients.

Surgical resection of neuroendocrine tumors is especially challenging in patients who present with carcinoid heart disease. This condition is characterized by stenosis of the tricuspid and pulmonary valves with a subsequent increase in central venous pressure. This increased pressure is difficult to overcome intraoperatively and can result in massive operative bleeding from the hepatic veins. Evidence attests to the benefit of maintaining low central venous pressure during the performance of major liver resections.[32] Another problem is the hypervascular nature of the neuroendocrine tumors, for which liberal use of extrahepatic vascular control during the hepatic resection is helpful.[18]

Table 2.—Results of Resection of Hepatic Metastases From Neuroendocrine Cancers

Reference	Patients, no.	Operative mortality, % of patients	Symptom control, % of patients	Survival, % of patients
Chamberlain et al., 2000[26]	34	6	90	76% at 5 y
Grazi et al., 2000[27]	19	0	NS	92% at 4 y
Jaeck et al., 2001[28]	13	0	NS	91% at 3 y
Nave et al., 2001[29]	31	0	NS	47% at 5 y
Mayo Clinic, 2003[22]	170	1.2	96	61% at 5 y

NS, not stated.

Ultimately, all patients with hepatic metastases from neuroendocrine tumors have recurrence of their disease.[22] This finding is in concordance with the natural history of these tumors. We cannot state that surgical therapy is curative in these patients (although there are anecdotal reports of long-term cures). Attempts at "cure" (complete resections) are simply means of achieving better disease control, and eventual recurrences are almost always responsible for the demise of these patients. However, this outcome does not diminish the benefit of surgical therapy. Doubling of the expected survival, better symptom control, and minimal surgical complications justify the operative approach.

Although experience with radiofrequency ablation has been limited in our patients,[22] we recognize that this could be a therapeutic option, especially to complete the treatment of metastases deep in the liver parenchyma or otherwise not amenable to surgical removal. Because the disease process in neuroendocrine tumors is widespread in most cases, we recently have been resecting most of the superficial disease and augmenting resection with radiofrequency ablation in deep tissues. This new strategy could increase the number of patients selected as suitable candidates for operation by permitting control of the metastatic lesions not amenable to surgical resection during the operation. Few series have reported this approach, and more time will be needed to generalize its application.[33] Hepatic arterial embolization also has been used by others for unresectable metastases from carcinoid tumors.[34,35] Prolonged survival times have been reported after this procedure. However, we seldom use it at Mayo Clinic.

In summary, we consider hepatic resection for neuroendocrine metastases to the liver to be a safe procedure that provides control of symptoms, reduces the need for pharmacologic therapy, and improves survival. Recurrence is high, and cure is usually not possible. Asymptomatic patients who are amenable to resection are also good candidates for operation. There is a definite role for palliation as long as the surgeon has the prospect of resecting at least 90% of the gross disease. New technologies, such as radiofrequency ablation, are being explored as an adjuvant treatment for these tumors.

HEPATIC RESECTION OF METASTASES FROM NONCOLORECTAL, NONNEUROENDOCRINE TUMORS

Since Foster's[36] 1978 review of published cases of hepatic resection of metastatic tumor, the curative potential of hepatectomy for metastasis from colorectal cancer and the palliative benefit of debulking for functional neuroendocrine metastasis have become well accepted.

For hepatic tumors metastatic from other primary cancers, the benefits are less certain. The criteria for such resections are poorly defined, largely because isolated hepatic metastases from these tumors are relatively rare.

General Principles

Several authors[37-39] have offered guidelines for resection of noncolorectal, nonneuroendocrine metastases. The Memorial Sloan-Kettering group[38] proposed selection criteria similar to those used for colorectal metastases, namely, no extrahepatic tumor and limited hepatic disease that is amenable to complete resection. Elias et al.[39] modify their recommendations for hepatectomy depending on the type of primary malignancy and the availability of effective adjuvant therapies. Many authors[38,40,41] have noted that longer disease-free intervals result in better survival, but strict guidelines have not been proposed regarding waiting a specific duration before proceeding with resection. Careful preoperative evaluation and diagnostic laparoscopy[42] are critical to the appropriate selection of patients who do not have disseminated cancers or extrahepatic spread.

Despite individual institutional experiences having small numbers of patients for analysis and collected series containing heterogeneous patient populations, most authors agree that some tumors are more treatable with hepatic resection than others. Wilms' tumor metastatic to the liver is thought to be ideal for resection,[36,37,43] with a 5-year survival rate of 39%.[37] Most series[38,39,41,43] have found good or intermediate survival rates with genitourinary cancer, with testicular cancer (5-year survival rates of up to 46%[39]) being especially responsive to operation plus chemotherapy. Soft tissue tumors including sarcomas, melanomas, and breast cancer have a lengthened survival time after hepatectomy in some reports.[37-40,44] However, Schwartz[43] did not conclude that liver metastasis from these cancers warranted resection. Resections of metastases from pancreatic and gastric carcinomas have been regarded as the least likely to benefit patients.[37-45]

Genitourinary Tumors

Among genitourinary malignancies, testicular cancer metastatic to the liver has the best results with treatment. Testicular cancer has become a highly curable disease, largely because of effective chemotherapy. Limited residual tumor masses are resected because necrotic tumor (52%) and benign teratoma (21%) cannot be distinguished from residual viable carcinoma (27%).[46] After chemotherapy for testicular cancers, resection is rarely performed for liver masses; Hahn et al.[46] reported that 57 hepatectomies were done in a total of 2,219 treated men (2.6%). More than 97% of patients were alive at 2 years; survival was shortest in the cohort with residual viable tumor and longest when only necrotic tissue was present. In another report on hepatic resection for testicular cancer,[47] 62% of patients (23 of 37) were alive and free of disease at a median follow-up of more than 5 years.

Chi et al.[48] reported their experience with hepatic resections in 12 women with various gynecologic cancers, more than half of which were papillary or serous ovarian carcinomas. Even though most women received additional chemotherapy, the median survival was only 27 months, and only 3 patients remained free of recurrent tumor at last follow-up. The authors recommended that hepatic resection be limited to selected patients without extrahepatic disease and no more than four hepatic metastases that were amenable to complete excision.

Solitary metastases from renal carcinoma occur in 2% to 7% of patients, and surgical resection results in 5-year survival rates of 25% to 35%.[49] Most experiences with hepatic resection for metastatic kidney cancer are limited to fewer than 10 patients. Stief et al.[50] described 17 patients with metachronous hepatic metastases from renal cancer (mean, 3.6 years after primary tumor resection), 11 (65%) of whom had resection with curative intent. The results were poor: the operative mortality rate was 31% and mean duration of survival was 4 months.[50] In general, the prognosis for metastasis from renal cell cancer is poor, but we would pursue resection of an isolated metachronous metastasis because some patients can enjoy a long disease-free interval.

Sarcomas

Hepatic metastases were diagnosed in only 7% of patients with sarcoma at Memorial Sloan-Kettering Cancer Center.[51] Almost all (94%) of the primary tumors were intra-abdominal, and 85% were high-grade leiomyosarcomas. (The majority of these would now be classified as gastrointestinal stomal tumors.) Only 22% of patients had hepatic resection, all of whom had tumor recurrence (79% in the liver remnant) with a median survival duration of 30 months.[51] In an update from the same institution, DeMatteo et al.[52] found no improvement in the hepatic resection rate (17%). Sixty-one percent of the patients with resection had primary gastrointestinal stomal tumors. Actuarial 5-year survival was 30% after hepatectomy (4% without resection). Ten patients (18%) were alive at least 5 years after liver operation and had an overall median survival duration of 39 months. A disease-free interval of more than 2 years was the only significant prognostic indication on multivariate analysis. Lang et al.,[53] from Hanover, Germany, reported results for hepatic resection in 26 patients with metastatic sarcomas. Their patient population and survival results (median survival of 32

months and 20% 5-year survival after complete resection) were comparable to those in the Sloan-Kettering group. More than a third of the patients had more than one operation for hepatic metastases. In the analysis by Lang et al., neither recurrent hepatic metastasis nor extra-hepatic tumor was a contraindication for hepatic resection.

Melanoma

Malignant melanoma is a capricious disease that can spread to nearly any site and appear even decades after treatment of the primary lesion. Uveal melanomas have a specific tendency to spread to the liver, usually with a diffuse, bilobar pattern of metastasis. In a combined experience with 75 patients from Europe, Salmon et al.[54] reported on an aggressive combination treatment (resection of all possible disease and intra-arterial chemotherapy) for metastatic uveal melanomas. Overall, the median duration of survival was only 9 months with this treatment and 5 months without operation. For the 61 patients who completed therapy, the median duration of survival was still only 10 months. However, for the 19 patients (28%) in whom all macroscopic tumor was resectable, the median duration of survival was 22 months. There were no 5-year survivors.[54] In an evaluation of 1,750 patients with melanoma metastatic to the liver, Rose et al.[55] found only 34 (2%) who had an exploration for liver resection, of whom only 52% (*n* = 18) had a potentially curative operation. Patients with complete resection had substantially better disease-free survival but not substantially improved overall survival. The median duration of survival for all patients with resection was 28 months, with an actuarial 5-year survival of 29%.[55] The median disease-free interval in the combined Sydney-Los Angeles experience was 58 months.[55] We have pursued hepatic resection for metastatic cutaneous melanoma, usually in patients with limited, liver-only metastases and a long disease-free interval.

Breast Cancer

Carcinoma of the breast metastasizes to the liver in more than 50% of women, but in only 5% to 6% of them is the liver the only site of distant disease.[56] Indicative of the natural biology of breast cancer are the findings from Maksan et al.[57] Of 90 patients with breast cancer referred for possible surgical management of liver metastases during 15 years, only 9 (10%) had hepatic resection with curative intent. The rest had extrahepatic spread or extensive bilobar metastases. The actuarial 5-year survival was 51% for women undergoing resection, and five patients were still alive at a median follow-up of 29 months. Patients with a long disease-free interval and node-negative primary breast cancer had the best prognosis. These same prognostic factors were noted in another experience with 52 hepatic resections for breast cancer from Paris, France.[58] The 3-year survival rate was 49%. Another report from France by Elias et al.[59] included 21 women undergoing liver resection. The liver was the most common site of recurrence (75% of patients) at a mean time of 15 months. Median duration of survival was 38.2 months, and the actuarial 5-year survival rate was 24%. No patients were disease-free at 5 years.

Chemotherapy was given to many patients in all these experiences,[56-59] and various treatment regimens were used. Both neoadjuvant and postoperative therapies were given, and there was no evidence of improved outcome. Selzner et al.[60] from Duke University, in a study of 17 women with hepatic metastases who had had resection, used neoadjuvant high-dose chemotherapy in most. There were two long-term survivors (actuarial 5-year survival of 22%). Although a disease-free interval of more than 1 year after treatment of the primary cancer predicted a better outcome, no improvement in survival was apparent after aggressive chemotherapy. In our practice, patients with breast cancer are treated when they have limited hepatic disease. Most have been younger women with long disease-free intervals. Despite complete resection and adjuvant systemic therapy, the tumor recurs in the liver and other sites in most women.

Pancreatic and Gastric Cancer

Hepatic metastases from pancreatic cancers are generally thought to have the worst prognosis among the group of tumors that metastasize to the liver. Resection usually is not done because of poor prognosis. Takada et al.[61] compared the results in 11 patients who had adenocarcinoma of the pancreas and synchronous hepatic metastases and underwent combined pancreaticoduodenectomy and hepatectomy with the results in 22 patients who had only palliative bypass. There was no difference in survival (median 6 months and 4 months, respectively), and all patients who had resection died with multiple recurrent liver metastases within 1 year. In another Japanese experience,[62] the results were slightly better for hepatic resection for metachronous liver metastases after Whipple procedure for periampullary malignancies, but the only 2-year survivors had atypical histologic findings (neuroendocrine cancer and leiomyosarcoma). We do not perform both a Whipple procedure and hepatic resection for synchronous metastases of periampullary cancers. Moreover, we have only a limited surgical experience with isolated small synchronous and metachronous hepatic metastases, most commonly of pancreatic histologic type other than ductal adenocarcinoma.

Gastric adenocarcinoma commonly metastasizes to the liver, but extensive nodal and peritoneal metastases are also usually present. Not surprisingly, because of the high rate of gastric cancer in Japan, the majority of reports on hepatectomy for metastases from gastric cancer originate from Japan. Okano et al.[63] performed hepatic resection in 21% of patients (19 of 90) with synchronous or metachronous liver metastases from gastric cancer. The actuarial 5-year survival rate was 34%, and there were 3 actual 5-year survivors. The most favorable outcomes occurred in patients with solitary, metachronous metastases that had a fibrous pseudocapsule. Ambiru et al.[64] found that metachronous presentation was the only significant prognostic factor in a multivariate analysis of 40 patients who had hepatectomy for metastatic gastric cancer (18% 5-year actuarial survival rate, and 6 patients were alive at more than 5 years). Similar results were noted by Ochiai et al.[65] who reported 4 long-term survivors among 21 patients who had hepatectomy. If serosal involvement by the primary cancer was present, the authors did not recommend hepatectomy for synchronous metastases. Bines et al.[66] reported one long-term survivor (74 months) after metachronous hepatectomy for metastatic gastric cancer ($n = 3$) but none after synchronous hepatic resection ($n = 4$). We agree that patients with limited metachronous hepatic metastases from gastric cancers without evidence of extrahepatic disease should be offered resection, but the expected 5-year survival rate likely will be only 10% to 20%.

CONCLUSION

In conclusion, resection of hepatic metastases from extrahepatic malignancies is a safe procedure that provides a potential for cure. Our data suggest that hepatic resection of colorectal metastases has a low operative mortality rate and can prolong life. In patients with neurohormonal symptoms related to neuroendocrine tumors metastatic to the liver, control of symptoms and increased longevity are achievable with hepatic resection. Although recurrence is high and cure may not be possible for these patients, hepatic resection improves their quality of life. The role of hepatic resection for noncolorectal, nonneuroendocrine tumors is less well established. New technologies, such as radiofrequency ablation and advances in adjuvant chemotherapy, may have a future role in the treatment of these tumors.

REFERENCES

1. Hughes K, Scheele J, Sugarbaker PH: Surgery for colorectal cancer metastatic to the liver: optimizing the results of treatment. Surg Clin North Am 69:339-359, 1989

2. Nagorney DM: Hepatic resections. *In* Atlas of Surgical Oncology. Edited by JH Donohue, JA van Heerden, JRT Monson. Cambridge, Blackwell Science, 1995, pp 189-200

3. Hughes KS, Simon R, Songhorabodi S, Adson MA, Ilstrup DM, Fortner JG, Maclean BJ, Foster JH, Daly JM, Fitzherbert D, et al: Resection of the liver for colorectal carcinoma metastases: a multi-institutional study of patterns of recurrence. Surgery 100:278-284, 1986

4. Nordlinger B, Jaeck D, Guiguet M, Vaillant JC, Balladur P, Schaal JC: Multicentric retrospective study by the French Surgical Association. *In* Treatment of Hepatic Metastases of Colorectal Cancer. Edited by B Nordlinger, D Jaeck. Paris, Springer-Verlag, 1992, pp 129-146

5. Scheele J, Rudroff C, Altendorf-Hofmann A: Resection of colorectal liver metastases revisited. J Gastrointest Surg 1:408-422, 1997

6. Fong Y, Fortner J, Sun RL, Brennan MF, Blumgart LH: Clinical score for predicting recurrence after hepatic resection for metastatic colorectal cancer: analysis of 1,001 consecutive cases. Ann Surg 230:309-318, 1999

7. Iwatsuki S, Dvorchik I, Madariaga JR, Marsh JW, Dodson F, Bonham AC, Geller DA, Gayowski TJ, Fung JJ, Starzl TE: Hepatic resection for metastatic colorectal adenocarcinoma: a proposal of a prognostic scoring system. J Am Coll Surg 189:291-299, 1999

8. Nordlinger B, Guiguet M, Vaillant JC, Balladur P, Boudjema K, Bachellier P, Jaeck D: Surgical resection of colorectal carcinoma metastases to the liver: a prognostic scoring system to improve case selection, based on 1,568 patients. Association Française de Chirurgie. Cancer 77:1254-1262, 1996

9. Ravikumar TS: The role of cryotherapy in the management of patients with liver tumors. Adv Surg 30:281-291, 1996

10. Ross WB, Horton M, Bertolino P, Morris DL: Cryotherapy of liver tumours—a practical guide. HPB Surg 8:167-173, 1995

11. Korpan NN: Hepatic cryosurgery for liver metastases: long-term follow-up. Ann Surg 225:193-201, 1997

12. Solbiati L, Livraghi T, Goldberg SN, Ierace T, Meloni F, Dellanoce M, Cova L, Halpern EF, Gazelle GS: Percutaneous radiofrequency ablation of hepatic metastases from colorectal cancer: long-term results in 117 patients. Radiology 221:159-166, 2001

13. Vauthey JN, de W Marsh R, Cendan JC, Chu NM, Copeland EM: Arterial therapy for hepatic colorectal metastases. Br J Surg 83:447-455, 1996

14. Meta-Analysis Group in Cancer: Reappraisal of hepatic arterial infusion in the treatment of nonresectable liver metastases from colorectal cancer. J Natl Cancer Inst 88:252-258, 1996

15. Kemeny N, Huang Y, Cohen AM, Shi W, Conti JA, Brennan MF, Bertino JR, Turnbull AD, Sullivan D, Stockman J, Blumgart LH, Fong Y: Hepatic arterial infusion of chemotherapy after resection of hepatic metastases from colorectal cancer. N Engl J Med 341:2039-2048, 1999

16. Kemeny MM, Adak S, Gray B, Macdonald JS, Smith T, Lipsitz S, Sigurdson ER, O'Dwyer PJ, Benson AB III: Combined-modality treatment for resectable metastatic colorectal carcinoma to the liver: surgical resection of hepatic metastases in combination with continuous infusion of chemotherapy—an intergroup study. J Clin Oncol 20:1499-1505, 2002

17. Moertel CG: Karnofsky memorial lecture: an odyssey in the land of small tumors. J Clin Oncol 5:1502-1522, 1987

18. Que FG, Nagorney DM, Batts KP, Linz LJ, Kvols LK: Hepatic resection for metastatic neuroendocrine carcinomas. Am J Surg 169:36-42, 1995

19. McEntee GP, Nagorney DM, Kvols LK, Moertel CG, Grant CS: Cytoreductive hepatic surgery for neuroendocrine tumors. Surgery 108:1091-1096, 1990

20. Wong RJ, DeCosse JJ: Cytoreductive surgery. Surg Gynecol Obstet 170:276-281, 1990

21. Que FG, Sarmiento JM, Nagorney DM: Hepatic surgery for metastatic gastrointestinal neuroendocrine tumors. Cancer Control 9:67-79, 2002

22. Sarmiento JM, Que FG: Hepatic surgery for metastases from neuroendocrine tumors. Surg Oncol Clin N Am 12:231-242, 2003

23. Moertel CG, Johnson CM, McKusick MA, Martin JK Jr, Nagorney DM, Kvols LK, Rubin J, Kunselman S: The management of patients with advanced carcinoid tumors and islet cell carcinomas. Ann Intern Med 120:302-309, 1994

24. Maton PN, Gardner JD, Jensen RT: Use of long-acting somatostatin analog SMS 201-995 in patients with pancreatic islet cell tumors. Dig Dis Sci 34 Suppl:28S-39S, 1989

25. Dousset B, Saint-Marc O, Pitre J, Soubrane O, Houssin D, Chapuis Y: Metastatic endocrine tumors: medical treatment, surgical resection, or liver transplantation. World J Surg 20:908-914, 1996

26. Chamberlain RS, Canes D, Brown KT, Saltz L, Jarnagin W, Fong Y, Blumgart LH: Hepatic neuroendocrine metastases: Does intervention alter outcomes? J Am Coll Surg 190:432-445, 2000

27. Grazi GL, Cescon M, Pierangeli F, Ercolani G, Gardini A, Cavallari A, Mazziotti A: Highly aggressive policy of hepatic resections for neuroendocrine liver metastases. Hepatogastroenterology 47:481-486, 2000

28. Jaeck D, Oussoultzoglou E, Bachellier P, Lemarque P, Weber JC, Nakano H, Wolf P: Hepatic metastases of gastroenteropancreatic neuroendocrine tumors: safe hepatic surgery. World J Surg 25:689-692, 2001

29. Nave H, Mossinger E, Feist H, Lang H, Raab H: Surgery as primary treatment in patients with liver metastases from carcinoid tumors: a retrospective, unicentric study over 13 years. Surgery 129:170-175, 2001

30. Chen H, Hardacre JM, Uzar A, Cameron JL, Choti MA: Isolated liver metastases from neuroendocrine tumors: Does resection prolong survival? J Am Coll Surg 187:88-92, 1998

31. Thompson GB, van Heerden JA, Grant CS, Carney JA, Ilstrup DM: Islet cell carcinomas of the pancreas: a twenty-year experience. Surgery 104:1011-1017, 1988

32. Melendez JA, Arslan V, Fischer ME, Wuest D, Jarnagin WR, Fong Y, Blumgart LH: Perioperative outcomes of major hepatic resections under low central venous pressure anesthesia: blood loss, blood transfusion, and the risk of postoperative renal dysfunction. J Am Coll Surg 187:620-625, 1998

33. Siperstein AE, Berber E: Cryoablation, percutaneous alcohol injection, and radiofrequency ablation for treatment of neuroendocrine liver metastases. World J Surg 25:693-696, 2001

34. Eriksson BK, Larsson EG, Skogseid BM, Lofberg AM, Lorelius LE, Oberg KE: Liver embolizations of patients with malignant neuroendocrine gastrointestinal tumors. Cancer 83:2293-2301, 1998

35. Azimuddin K, Chamberlain RS: The surgical management of pancreatic neuroendocrine tumors. Surg Clin North Am 81:511-525, 2001

36. Foster JH: Survival after liver resection for secondary tumors. Am J Surg 135:389-394, 1978

37. Wolf RF, Goodnight JE, Krag DE, Schneider PD: Results of resection and proposed guidelines for patient selection in instances of non-colorectal hepatic metastases. Surg Gynecol Obstet 173:454-460, 1991

38. Harrison LE, Brennan MF, Newman E, Fortner JG, Picardo A, Blumgart LH, Fong Y: Hepatic resection for noncolorectal, nonneuroendocrine metastases: a fifteen-year experience with ninety-six patients. Surgery 121:625-632, 1997

39. Elias D, Cavalcanti de Albuquerque A, Eggenspieler P, Plaud B, Ducreux M, Spielmann M, Theodore C, Bonvalot S, Lasser P: Resection of liver metastases from a noncolorectal primary: indications and results based on 147 monocentric patients. J Am Coll Surg 187:487-493, 1998

40. Berney T, Mentha G, Roth AD, Morel P: Results of surgical resection of liver metastases from non-colorectal primaries. Br J Surg 85:1423-1427, 1998

41. Laurent C, Rullier E, Feyler A, Masson B, Saric J: Resection of noncolorectal and nonneuroendocrine liver metastases: late metastases are the only chance of cure. World J Surg 25:1532-1536, 2001

42. D'Angelica M, Jarnagin W, Dematteo R, Conlon K, Blumgart LH, Fong Y: Staging laparoscopy for potentially resectable noncolorectal, nonneuroendocrine liver metastases. Ann Surg Oncol 9:204-209, 2002

43. Schwartz SI: Hepatic resection for noncolorectal nonneuroendocrine metastases. World J Surg 19:72-75, 1995

44. Hamy AP, Paineau JR, Mirallie EC, Bizouarn P, Visset JP: Hepatic resections for non-colorectal metastases: forty resections in 35 patients. Hepatogastroenterology 47:1090-1094, 2000

45. Hemming AW, Sielaff TD, Gallinger S, Cattral MS, Taylor BR, Greig PD, Langer B: Hepatic resection of noncolorectal nonneuroendocrine metastases. Liver Transpl 6:97-101, 2000

46. Hahn TL, Jacobson L, Einhorn LH, Foster R, Goulet RJ Jr: Hepatic resection of metastatic testicular carcinoma: a further update. Ann Surg Oncol 6:640-644, 1999

47. Rivoire M, Elias D, De Cian F, Kaemmerlen P, Theodore C, Droz JP: Multimodality treatment of patients with liver metastases from germ cell tumors: the role of surgery. Cancer 92:578-587, 2001

48. Chi DS, Fong Y, Venkatraman ES, Barakat RR: Hepatic resection for metastatic gynecologic carcinomas. Gynecol Oncol 66:45-51, 1997

49. Tongaonkar HB, Kulkarni JN, Kamat MR: Solitary metastases from renal cell carcinoma: a review. J Surg Oncol 49:45-48, 1992

50. Stief CG, Jahne J, Hagemann JH, Kuczyk M, Jonas U: Surgery for metachronous solitary liver metastases of renal cell carcinoma. J Urol 158:375-377, 1997

51. Jaques DP, Coit DG, Casper ES, Brennan MF: Hepatic metastases from soft-tissue sarcoma. Ann Surg 221:392-397, 1995

52. DeMatteo RP, Shah A, Fong Y, Jarnagin WR, Blumgart LH, Brennan MF: Results of hepatic resection for sarcoma metastatic to liver. Ann Surg 234:540-547, 2001

53. Lang H, Nussbaum KT, Kaudel P, Fruhauf N, Flemming P, Raab R: Hepatic metastases from leiomyosarcoma: a single-center experience with 34 liver resections during a 15-year period. Ann Surg 231:500-505, 2000

54. Salmon RJ, Levy C, Plancher C, Dorval T, Desjardins L, Leyvraz S, Pouillart P, Schlienger P, Servois V, Asselain B: Treatment of liver metastases from uveal melanoma by combined surgery-chemotherapy. Eur J Surg Oncol 24:127-130, 1998

55. Rose DM, Essner R, Hughes TM, Tang PC, Bilchik A, Wanek LA, Thompson JF, Morton DL: Surgical resection for metastatic melanoma to the liver: the John Wayne Cancer Institute and Sydney Melanoma Unit experience. Arch Surg 136:950-955, 2001

56. Raab R, Nussbaum KT, Behrend M, Weimann A: Liver metastases of breast cancer: results of liver resection. Anticancer Res 18:2231-2233, 1998

57. Maksan SM, Lehnert T, Bastert G, Herfarth C: Curative liver resection for metastatic breast cancer. Eur J Surg Oncol 26:209-212, 2000

58. Pocard M, Pouillart P, Asselain B, Salmon R: Hepatic resection in metastatic breast cancer: results and prognostic factors. Eur J Surg Oncol 26:155-159, 2000

59. Elias D, Lasser PH, Montrucolli D, Bonvallot S, Spielmann M: Hepatectomy for liver metastases from breast cancer. Eur J Surg Oncol 21:510-513, 1995

60. Selzner M, Morse MA, Vredenburgh JJ, Meyers WC, Clavien PA: Liver metastases from breast cancer: long-term survival after curative resection. Surgery 127:383-389, 2000

61. Takada T, Yasuda H, Amano H, Yoshida M, Uchida T: Simultaneous hepatic resection with pancreato-duodenectomy for metastatic pancreatic head carcinoma: Does it improve survival? Hepatogastroenterology 44:567-573, 1997

62. Fujii K, Yamamoto J, Shimada K, Kosuge T, Yamasaki S, Kanai Y: Resection of liver metastases after pancreatoduodenectomy: report of seven cases. Hepatogastroenterology 46:2429-2433, 1999

63. Okano K, Maeba T, Ishimura K, Karasawa Y, Goda F, Wakabayashi H, Usuki H, Maeta H: Hepatic resection for metastatic tumors from gastric cancer. Ann Surg 235:86-91, 2002

64. Ambiru S, Miyazaki M, Ito H, Nakagawa K, Shimizu H, Yoshidome H, Shimizu Y, Nakajima N: Benefits and limits of hepatic resection for gastric metastases. Am J Surg 181:279-283, 2001

65. Ochiai T, Sasako M, Mizuno S, Kinoshita T, Takayama T, Kosuge T, Yamazaki S, Maruyama K: Hepatic resection for metastatic tumours from gastric cancer: analysis of prognostic factors. Br J Surg 81:1175-1178, 1994

66. Bines SD, England G, Deziel DJ, Witt TR, Doolas A, Roseman DL: Synchronous, metachronous, and multiple hepatic resections of liver tumors originating from primary gastric tumors. Surgery 114:799-805, 1993

BENIGN TUMORS AND CYSTS OF THE LIVER

Glenroy Heywood, M.D.
Florencia G. Que, M.D.

Benign neoplasms and cysts of the liver are encountered commonly in clinical practice. Improvement in and availability of newer techniques of liver imaging, such as computed tomography (CT), ultrasonography, and magnetic resonance imaging (MRI), have increased our recognition of these often-asymptomatic hepatic lesions. The discovery of benign hepatic neoplasms often poses diagnostic and therapeutic challenges, although most cysts can be diagnosed reliably on the basis of radiographic imaging features and do not require therapeutic intervention. In general, management of these lesions depends on the histologic findings, the natural history, and the associated symptoms.

When symptoms occur, they develop insidiously as a consequence of expansion leading to compression of adjacent organs. Vague upper abdominal pain or a sensation of fullness occurs in one-third of patients. Jaundice is rare but may develop from bile duct compression. Appropriate management of these lesions requires the surgeon to be thoroughly familiar with their gross appearances, radiologic characteristics, clinical significance, and natural history. Resection is usually indicated for relief of symptoms, when the risk of spontaneous hemorrhage or malignant transformation is present, and when the diagnosis is unclear.

This chapter describes the cause, pathology, diagnosis, and management of benign neoplasms and nonparasitic cystic lesions of the liver.

CLASSIFICATION

Benign primary neoplasms of the liver have been recognized for more than a century but were only formally classified by Ishak and Rabin[1] in 1975. The most common benign, solid primary hepatic tumors are focal nodular hyperplasia (FNH), hepatocellular adenomas (HAs), hemangiomas, and bile duct adenomas, but there are many others (Table 1).

Cystic lesions of the liver also can be broadly divided into four groups: congenital, inflammatory, neoplastic, and traumatic (Table 2). Congenital cysts are the most common form and include simple cysts and polycystic liver disease. Inflammatory cysts of the liver generally are related to infectious etiologies and will not be discussed here. Primary cystic neoplasms are the rare cystadenomas. Traumatic cysts arise from an injury to the liver which causes either a subcapsular hematoma or a transected biliary duct.

DIAGNOSIS AND IMAGING

With the exception of those instances when discovery of benign neoplasms and cysts of the liver is incidental to the surgical procedure, most patients who are referred to the surgeon have undergone a vast array of diagnostic investigations. Unfortunately, these investigations often lack specificity and leave the diagnosis uncertain despite considerable cost to the patient. To make an intelligent decision about which diagnostic method to use for a particular patient, the surgeon must understand the limitations of each.

Imaging Tests

Spiral CT is the imaging technique of choice for evaluating the liver and detecting hepatic masses. Unlike conventional dynamic CT, it uses rapid subsecond radiologic scanning of the different phases (arterial, portal, delayed) of hepatic enhancement.[2] Particular lesions may have characteristic dynamic enhancement patterns. MRI provides superior

Table 1.—Classification of Benign Solid Lesions of the Liver

Hepatocellular tumors
    Nodular regeneration or transformation
    Focal nodular hyperplasia
    Hepatocellular adenoma
Cholangiocellular tumors
    Bile duct adenoma
    Biliary hamartoma
    Biliary cystadenoma
Vascular tumors
    Hemangioma
    Lymphangioma
Mesenchymal tumors
    Lipoma
    Myelolipoma
    Angiomyolipoma
    Pseudolipoma
    Leiomyoma
    Chondroma
    Benign mesothelioma
Mixed mesenchymal tumors
    Mesenchymal hamartoma
    Benign teratoma
Neural tumors
    Schwannoma
Miscellaneous tumors
    Adrenal rest tumor
    Pancreatic heterotopia
    Inflammatory pseudotumor
    Hepatic splenosis
    Peliosis hepatis
    Focal fatty change

Table 2.—Classification of Benign Cystic Lesions of the Liver

Congenital cysts
    Simple
    Polycystic liver disease
Inflammatory cysts
    Parasitic
    Bacterial
Neoplastic cysts
    Cystadenoma
Traumatic cysts
    Subcapsular hematoma
    Transected biliary duct

contrast resolution without ionizing radiation and is also an important diagnostic tool in detecting and characterizing focal hepatic lesions. Imaging characteristics of lesions such as hemangioma, FNH, HA, and hepatic cyst are well known. Familiarity with these imaging features can help the surgeon to characterize particular lesions. Hepatic scintigraphy also may be helpful.

Laboratory Evaluation
We obtain selective laboratory tests to screen for evidence of organ system dysfunction, coagulation abnormalities, and gastrointestinal blood loss. Liver function test results are usually normal; however, increases in the concentrations of serum transaminases may occur with secondary hemorrhage and necrosis of a lesion. Serologic testing may help exclude the diagnosis of parasitic disease.

Biomolecular Markers
Serum tumor markers (e.g., α-fetoprotein, carcinoembryonic antigen, carbohydrate antigen) are usually normal. However, there are reports of increased concentrations of carbohydrate antigen in patients with benign hepatic neoplasms[3] and cysts[4] that falsely suggest malignancy.

Preoperative Biopsy
We base our decision about whether to perform a resection primarily on the patient's clinical presentation and radiographic findings. Percutaneous needle biopsy of a hepatic lesion has an inherent risk of hemorrhage, sampling error, misdiagnosis, and needle tract seeding, should the lesion prove to be malignant. The risk of intraperitoneal, intrahepatic, and needle track seeding can significantly worsen the prognosis of a patient who has a malignant lesion.[5,6] Therefore, we do not require preoperative histologic confirmation before resection in a good-risk patient with a presumed benign hepatic mass. Instead, we reserve percutaneous biopsy for patients who are not candidates for surgical exploration and whose biopsy results may influence patient management.

BENIGN TUMORS

Hepatocellular Tumors

Focal Nodular Hyperplasia
FNH is the most common benign hepatocellular lesion encountered in clinical practice. It can occur at any age. However, it is often observed between the third and fifth decades of life, with a male-to-female ratio of about 1:2.[7] FNH is typically an incidental diagnosis, because 50% to 90% of patients lack symptoms.[8-12] FNH has been

associated with the long-term use of exogenous contraceptive steroids.[12-14] However, the incidence of FNH has not increased despite the increased and widespread use of oral contraceptives.[13] Interestingly, symptoms occur more frequently in women using contraceptive steroids.[12] Symptomatic patients usually present with nonspecific upper abdominal discomfort or pain of 1 to 9 months' duration.[8] Patients rarely present with sudden severe pain,[1,15] portal hypertension,[1] hemorrhage, or necrosis.[16]

FNH is usually a peripheral, superficial, solitary, well-circumscribed lesion without a capsule, measuring 1 cm to 15 cm in diameter (mean diameter, 5.6 cm) (Fig. 1).[8] FNH is multifocal in 10% to 20% of patients.[9,11] The cut surface typically has a whitish depressed area of central fibrosis, with broad stellate strands radiating to the periphery (Fig. 1). The central scar probably results from associated vascular malformation and thrombosis.[17] Microscopically, FNH has no true lobular structure. The lesions are composed of normal hepatocytes, supplied by large arteries and fibrous septa. Bile duct proliferation and abnormal interlobular bile ducts are also present. Focal hemorrhage or necrosis is rare.

On CT scan, FNH exhibits a characteristic pattern of enhancement.[18] The lesions usually are enhanced on early-phase images and subsequently wash out on delayed images, with the lesion appearing imperceptible except for any mass effect.[2] A central scar, if present, may demonstrate delayed enhancement (Fig. 2 A). On MRI, FNH appears isointense in relation to a normal liver. However, the central scar may appear of variable hypointensity on T1-weighted images and hyperintense on T2-weighted images (Fig. 2 B, 3 A and B).[2]

Technetium ^{99m}Tc-disofenin scintigraphy has proved useful in the diagnosis of FNH, with an accuracy of about 90% in one report.[19] It also can help differentiate FNH from HA. Unlike HA, FNH contains Kupffer cells that can accumulate disofenin, which CT scans can detect as a normal or an increased uptake.[19-21] However, 30% of FNH lesions do show focal defects, unlike HA, which sometimes has normal uptake of colloid.[22,23]

Conservative management of FNH is recommended, because malignant transformation is unlikely. Moreover, only a few patients have symptoms, and these are rarely severe. Lesions that are diagnosed incidentally during laparotomy for other indications usually are excised. In most cases of FNH, the small size and peripheral location allow simple wedge excision or enucleation with minimal operative risk.[8,10,11] Large or central lesions should be examined by biopsy. Further therapy should be based on the development and severity of symptoms or complications. Asymptomatic or minimally symptomatic patients with incidental FNH detected by abdominal imaging can be managed either by observation or by resection. However, resection may be preferable in young women of childbearing age, given the unpredictable changes in the liver during pregnancy.[12]

Hepatocellular Adenoma

HA is the second most common hepatocellular lesion encountered in clinical practice, and, like FNH, it is more prevalent in women.[8,10,12] It does occur in men, however, especially those who use anabolic steroids, or in patients with glycogen storage disease.

Like FNH, HA is usually a solitary subcapsular lesion. The lesions vary in size from 5 cm to 15 cm in diameter (mean, 9 cm). The cut surface has a yellowish or hemorrhagic color (Fig. 4 and 5). Microscopically, HA is a proliferation of normal-appearing hepatocytes without the normal hepatic lobular structure. When more than four nodules are present, the condition is referred to as hepatic adenomatosis (Fig. 6). HA may undergo malignant transformation.[24-26]

In contrast to FNH, the incidence of HA has definitely increased since the widespread use of oral contraceptive steroids.[8,27-31] The causal relationship between contraceptive steroids and HA has been strongly supported clinically by the prevalence of HA in women who have engaged in long-standing contraceptive steroid use,[27,29,30] regression of HA after discontinuation of contraceptive steroids,[8,11,13,32] recurrence of HA after resumption of

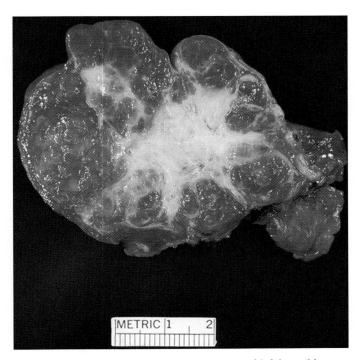

Fig. 1. Focal nodular hyperplasia of the resected left lateral hepatic lobe. The lesion has a prominent central scar. The lesion also is sharply demarcated from the normal liver yet has no true capsule.

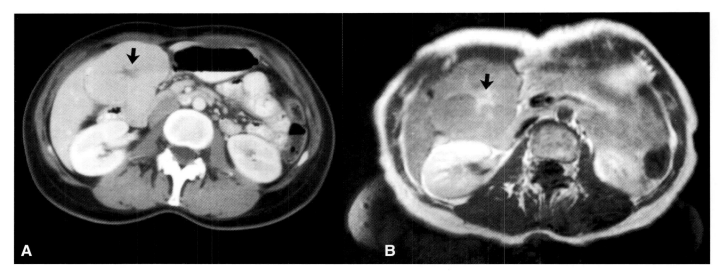

Fig. 2. (A), *Computed tomography of the abdomen depicting a large 7- x 7-cm area of focal nodular hyperplasia arising from the medial segment of the left hepatic lobe. Lesion has a hypovascular central scar* (arrow). (B), *Same mass on T1-weighted magnetic resonance imaging showing the hyperintense central scar.*

contraceptive steroid use,[33] and growth of HA during pregnancy.[34]

Unlike patients with FNH, most patients with HA are symptomatic at presentation, with abdominal pain the predominant symptom.[8] Nearly 30% of patients present with acute symptoms from hemorrhage or rupture of the HA.[8,10-12,27,33,35,36] HA size, location, or number has not been correlated significantly with complications.

On CT, HA appears as a well-defined, hypoattenuating mass, because the surrounding capsule defines the borders (Fig. 7 *A*).[2] The presence of hemorrhage and heterogeneous attenuation is usually the key to correct diagnosis (Fig. 7 *A* and *B*).[18] The appearance of HA on MRI also is influenced by the presence of hemorrhage.[2] HAs are supplied by the hepatic artery and, thus, exhibit early enhancement on CT scan.[2,18]

Resection rather than observation or selective intervention is recommended for patients with HA, because the clinical course of these lesions is unpredictable. Malignant transformation, rupture, hemoperitoneum, shock,

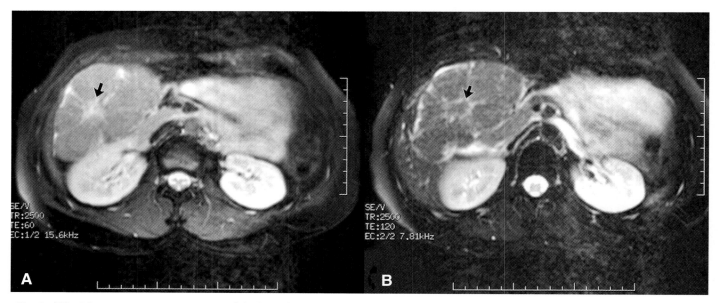

Fig. 3. (A), *Magnetic resonance imaging of the liver demonstrating a large, 10-cm area of focal nodular hyperplasia occupying most of the right hepatic lobe. The lesion has a central scar* (arrow) *that has a high-signal intensity on the T2-weighted image.* (B), *The scar becomes isointense* (arrow) *compared with the normal liver on the more heavily T2-weighted image.*

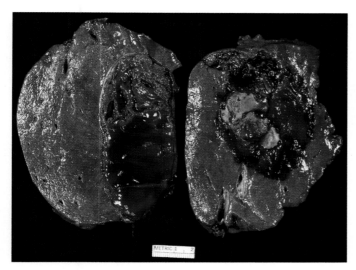

Fig. 4. Hepatocellular adenoma with associated hemorrhagic necrosis.

and death can occur. Permanent discontinuation of oral contraceptive steroid use is mandatory.

Of 45 consecutive patients treated with surgical resection of benign hepatic tumors at Mayo Clinic, 21 had FNH and 24 had HA.[8] In the FNH group, 10 patients were symptomatic. Resection was performed and resulted in no mortality and minimal morbidity. Fifteen of 21 patients had a central scar. Fourteen of these patients had excision. In the HA group, 19 of 24 patients were symptomatic, with abdominal pain the predominant symptom. Oral contraceptives were used by 9 of the 22 female patients. Nineteen patients were managed with resection, and five were treated conservatively with observation. Of the patients treated conservatively, none have had subsequent HA growth or rupture. One female patient had CT-documented regression that occurred after discontinuation of oral contraceptive use.

Nodular Regenerative Hyperplasia

Nodular regenerative hyperplasia is a diffuse nodular lesion of the entire liver parenchyma. It is a rare liver lesion whose etiology may be similar to that of FNH. It usually is associated with portal hypertension or with collagen diseases such as polyarteritis nodosa, rheumatoid vasculitis, and Felty's syndrome.

These lesions appear as multiple small whitish nodules on the cut surface of the liver. They may be mistaken for metastatic carcinoma. Microscopically, the nodules are composed of hyperplastic hepatocytes arranged in rows. These abnormal hepatocytes compress the surrounding atrophic parenchyma.[37-39] These lesions may have premalignant potential, because they sometimes show atypia. There have been documented cases of hepatocellular carcinoma arising in livers with nodular regenerative hyperplasia.[37-41] Surgical resection may be indicated because of the risk of malignant transformation.

Cholangiocellular Tumors

Bile Duct Adenoma

Intrahepatic bile duct adenomas are rare benign tumors that generally present as well-circumscribed, solitary, whitish subcapsular nodules, less than 2 cm in diameter, and characterized by small tubules in a variable amount of stroma. These small lesions usually are located in the periphery of the liver, are hypervascular on angiography, and show prolonged enhancement on CT. They can

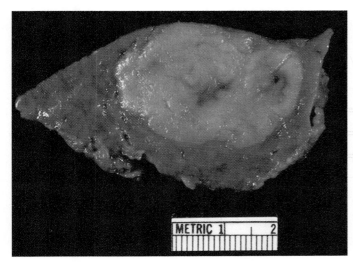

Fig. 5. Cross-section of hepatocellular adenoma shows it as a soft tan lesion with a central area of hemorrhagic necrosis.

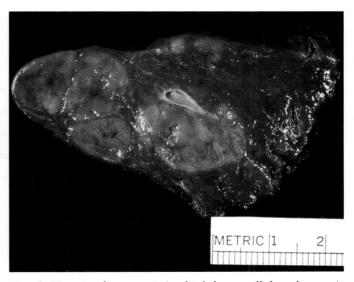

Fig. 6. Hepatic adenomatosis (multiple hepatocellular adenomas).

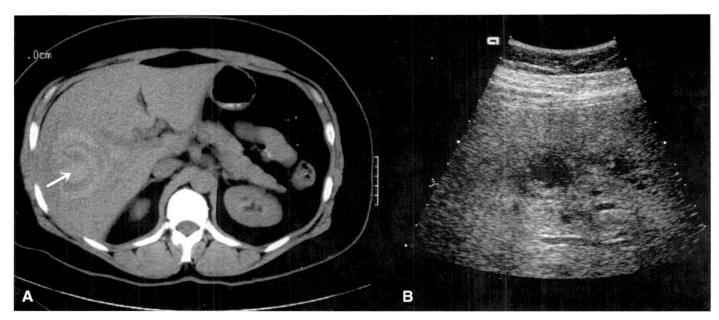

Fig. 7. (A), *Precontrast computed tomography of the abdomen showing an 8-cm hepatic adenoma in the right lobe of the liver that contains high attenuation material representing hemorrhage* (arrow). (B), *Transabdominal ultrasonography of the same mass.*

be mistaken for hepatic metastases. There are no reports of malignant transformation, so surgical resection is indicated only when diagnosis is uncertain or symptoms are present.

Biliary Hamartoma

Biliary hamartoma, also known as von Meyenburg's or Moschcowitz's complex, is a rare benign malformation of the biliary tract that presents as a fibrolipocystic disease of the liver. These lesions are considered a precursor to autosomal-dominant polycystic liver disease (see page 201). The lesions usually are discovered at autopsy or confused with metastases or other cystic hepatic lesions. They generally present as multiple small, whitish, subcapsular nodules, scattered throughout the liver.[42] The lesions usually are hypodense on contrast-enhanced CT scans and hypoechoic on sonograms. When single or multiple small hepatic lesions are present, regardless of uniformity of size or distribution, the diagnosis of biliary hamartoma should be considered in patients suspected of a primary malignant tumor. Malignant transformation of these lesions is so rare[43,44] that routine surgical resection of them is not warranted.

Vascular Tumors

Hemangioma

Cavernous hemangiomas are the most common benign tumors of the liver found at autopsy, occurring in 2% to 7% of livers examined.[1] In most cases, they are found incidentally. The lesions are usually solitary and less than 4 cm in diameter. They consist of dilated vascular spaces lined by flat endothelial cells in a fibrous stroma. Small hemangiomas, which do not require therapy, are almost always asymptomatic and relatively free from complications. Giant hemangiomas (diameter, ≥ 4 cm) (Fig. 8) can cause symptoms such as abdominal pain, nausea, and increased girth. Rare cases of rupture,[45,46] jaundice, or consumptive coagulopathy (Kasabach-Merritt syndrome) have resulted from sequestration and destruction of platelets within these tumors.[47-49]

Hemangiomas are hypodense on unenhanced CT and have characteristic peripheral puddling of contrast early after its injection. They then subsequently fill in from the periphery. Therefore, on delayed images, there is central filling of the previous hypodense lesion, which may become isoattenuated or slightly hyperattenuated (Fig. 9).[2] On CT, hemangiomas demonstrate a similar postcontrast pattern of enhancement (Fig. 10 *A*). On ultrasonography, they appear as hyperechoic masses clearly demarcated from the surrounding liver (Fig. 10 *B*).

Because most patients with hepatic hemangiomas are asymptomatic, nonoperative management is usually pursued. However, current indications for surgical resection of giant cavernous hemangiomas include severe abdominal pain, rapid enlargement of the tumor, rupture or potential for rupture, or indeterminate diagnosis. These hepatic lesions can be removed safely by either resection or enucleation.[50] There is usually a "delightfully friendly" plane between the cavernous hemangioma

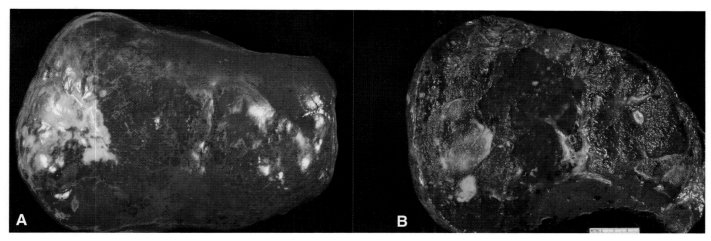

Fig. 8. (A), *Gross appearance of a large cavernous hemangioma viewed from the surface. Note the typical red or purple blotches with central whitish scarring.* (B), *On the cut section, the lesion has a characteristic spongelike histologic appearance due to venous lakes.*

and the normal hepatic parenchyma. This plane of somewhat fibrotic, compressed liver tissue is typically avascular, allowing safe enucleation and thus decreasing the risk of severe hemorrhage. Although no margin of normal tissue is required, it may be safer and wiser to perform a standard segmental or lobar hepatic resection in certain instances.[10]

In a retrospective review of 122 patients who presented to Mayo Clinic over a 20-year period with the diagnosis of cavernous hemangioma,[45] we found that these tumors were more than 4 cm in diameter in 49 patients, of whom 36 were female. Of the 49 patients, 41% were symptomatic at presentation. The diagnosis of cavernous hemangioma was suspected in 32 patients. In the other 17, the lesions were found incidentally during surgical evaluation or with imaging techniques. Resection was performed in 13

patients, and 36 were observed. Two patients were lost to follow-up. Four patients had postoperative complications, but no deaths occurred. The benign course of most of these lesions favors watchful waiting rather than operation, especially for lesions that are asymptomatic or that are large enough to pose a major operative risk.

Lymphangioma

In 1892, Ziegler (Enzinger) first described hepatic lymphangioma. These lesions are extremely rare; only a few cases have been described.[51-53] They may present either as a solitary hepatic tumor or as diffuse lymphangiomatosis. The lesions are usually spongy, soft, well circumscribed, and composed of endothelial-lined lymphatic channels filled with lymphocytes. Because malignant transformation has not been reported, no treatment is necessary

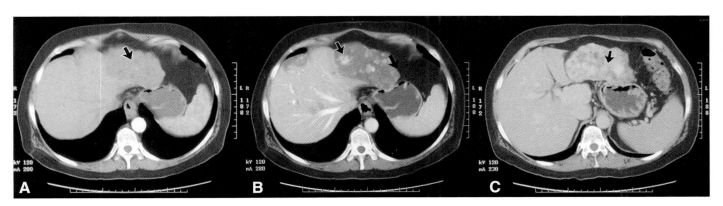

Fig. 9. Computed tomography of the abdomen shows four hemangiomas in the liver, the largest occupying most of the lateral segment of the left hepatic lobe. (A), *On the precontrast image, the lesion* (arrow) *has the same attenuation as blood and, therefore, appears isodense.* (B), *Soon after administration of contrast, the mass demonstrates globular or nodular peripheral enhancement* (arrow). (C), *The delayed image demonstrates progressive enhancement* (arrow), *similar to the spread of drops of ink in water due to an accumulation of contrast within the dilated vascular spaces.*

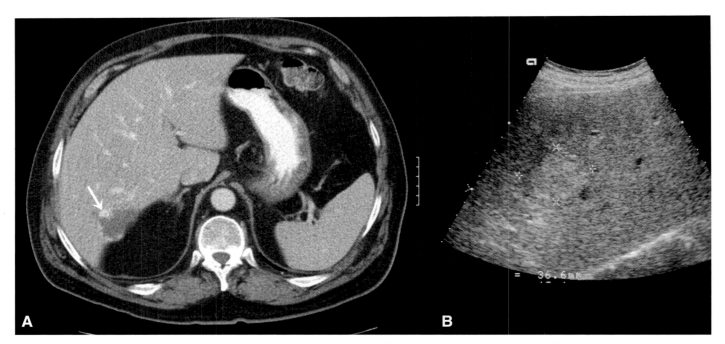

Fig. 10. (A), *Computed tomography of the abdomen shows a cavernous hemangioma within segment 7 of the right lobe of the liver with peripheral enhancement* (arrow). (B), *Corresponding mass (delineated by symbols) on ultrasonography shows hyperechoic features suggestive of cavernous hemangioma.*

for asymptomatic patients. Liver resection is indicated when the diagnosis is in doubt or when severe symptoms develop.

Mesenchymal Tumors

Lipoma

Lipomas are composed entirely of mature fat. They range in size from a few millimeters up to 20 cm. They have characteristic fat attenuation and nonenhancement on contrast CT.[2] There is no apparent risk of malignant transformation, so resection is reserved for symptomatic lesions.

Angiomyolipoma and Other Lipomatous Tumors

Hepatic angiomyolipomas are extremely rare, in contrast to renal angiomyolipomas, of which 40% to 50% occur in patients with tuberous sclerosis.[54,55] Hepatic angiomyolipomas were initially thought to not be associated with tuberous sclerosis,[55] but a few associations have been reported.[56]

These lesions are usually solitary, spherical, soft, and well demarcated.[55] They can range in size from 1 cm to 20 cm in diameter. Microscopically, the tumors are composed of varying proportions of blood vessels, smooth muscle, fat, and hematopoietic tissue.[55] The fat component ranges from less than 10% to more than 50%.[57,58]

Most of the other primary hepatic lipomatous tumors are even rarer. This category includes myelolipomas, composed of hematopoietic cells and fat; angiolipomas, composed of blood vessels and fat; angiomyelolipomas, composed of blood vessels, hematopoietic elements, and fat; and angiomyomyelolipomas, composed of blood vessels, smooth muscle, hematopoietic elements, and fat.

Most of these tumors are asymptomatic at presentation. However, a few patients present with pain from spontaneous intratumoral hemorrhage[59,60] or rupture.[61] There is also one report of a local recurrence of a hepatic angiomyolipoma 6 years after a presumed complete surgical resection.[62]

Because these tumors are typically a mixture of mesenchymal elements and fat, CT usually demonstrates enhancement of the soft-tissue components but not the fat.[2]

Pseudolipoma

Pseudolipoma is a rare encapsulated mass of mature adipose tissue that lies outside the parenchyma of the liver but inside the Glisson capsule. Pseudolipomas are usually asymptomatic, solitary nodules that may be confused with primary or metastatic tumors.

The histologic elements of pseudolipomas are identical to those of twisted peritoneal fat nodules (epiploic appendix) or peritoneal loose bodies.[63] They also may be focally calcified. CT usually reveals a low-density subcapsular mass that may contain calcification.

Leiomyoma

Primary smooth muscle tumors of the liver are rare neoplasms. Hawkins et al.[64] proposed two criteria for making this diagnosis. First, the tumor must be composed of leiomyocytes. Second, a leiomyomatous tumor at some other site may not be present. Patients with leiomyomas, which can reach a large size, are often symptomatic. Most patients with hepatic leiomyomas have been women.

Although these lesions are usually large, they are well circumscribed. The cut surface displays the characteristic distinctive whorled pattern of a leiomyoma. Histologically, interlacing cellular bundles of spindle cells are distributed in a collagenous stroma.[65]

These tumors should be completely resected, because there is no clear-cut way to distinguish benign from malignant smooth muscle tumors in the liver.

Benign Mesothelioma

Benign mesotheliomas, or localized fibrous tumors, of the liver are rare; fewer than 12 cases have been reported. Symptoms include weight loss, general fatigue, abdominal mass, vomiting, and diarrhea. The histologic origin, mesenchymal versus mesothelial, is unknown. The tumors are usually encapsulated and pedunculated, originating mainly in the left lobe.[66] They range in size from 10 cm to more than 30 cm in diameter. Microscopically, these tumors are composed of spindle cells separated by collagen.

The natural history of these tumors is unknown. Most lesions have been resected with no evidence of recurrence.

Mixed Mesenchymal Tumors

Mesenchymal Hamartoma

Mesenchymal hamartomas of the liver are rare benign neoplasms occurring primarily in children younger than 2 years of age and rarely in adults.[67-70] These lesions may be solid, but most are either partially or totally cystic,[71-73] well demarcated or encapsulated, more than 8 cm to 10 cm in diameter, and composed of a variable mixture of abnormal bile ducts, hepatocytes, and immature mesenchyme. There is a marked male predominance, and the right lobe is affected in 80% to 90% of patients.[74] Clinical symptoms, when present, are usually related to a mass effect, producing abdominal distention, respiratory distress, or even vena caval obstruction. Transformation to undifferentiated sarcoma has been reported.[75,76] The typical appearance of hepatic mesenchymal hamartoma on CT or MRI is that of a large, well-demarcated, solid, or multilocular cystic mass. Because the hypervascular solid component enhances on CT, calcification of internal septation may be identified. Although these tumors are primarily benign, total surgical resection is the treatment of choice, although for some patients a conservative procedure, such as wedge resection or enucleation, may be preferable.

Benign Teratoma

Benign teratoma of the liver generally presents as an abdominal mass in children.[77,78] This rare hepatic tumor is composed of several types of mature or immature tissues derived from all three germ layers. Teratomas can become quite large and have the potential for malignant transformation. Therefore, resection usually is recommended.

Neural Tumors

Schwannoma

Schwannoma is a benign nerve sheath tumor composed of neoplastic Schwann cells. Primary schwannomas of the liver are rare and usually are associated with neurofibromatosis.[79,80] However, benign primary hepatic schwannomas not associated with neurofibromatosis have been reported in seven patients.[81-86] Grossly, schwannomas are well demarcated, encapsulated, globular, or ovoid tumors, ranging in size from 4 cm to 30 cm in diameter. Microscopically, the tumors consist predominantly of spindle-shaped cells that proliferate in an interlacing fashion.[81] Patients may become symptomatic from the mass effect of large tumors or intratumoral hemorrhage. Thus, surgical resection may be justified, although malignant transformation of these tumors is not known to occur.

Miscellaneous Tumors

Adrenal Rest Tumor

Adrenal rest tumors of the liver can present either in childhood[87] or in adulthood.[88-90] They sometimes can cause virilization and Cushing syndrome.[87] Histologically, nonfunctional tumors have features identical to those of the healthy adrenal cortex,[88] whereas functional tumors resemble an adrenal cortical tumor.[7] Adrenal rest tumors have a predilection for the right lobe of the liver. Patients usually are cured after resection.

Pancreatic Heterotopia

Nodules of the heterotopic pancreas are typically small and tend to occur in the digestive tract, especially in the antroduodenal region.[91] Because they lack clinical symptoms, they often are found fortuitously. They rarely present as a hepatic mass.[92]

Inflammatory Pseudotumor

Inflammatory pseudotumor of the liver is an unusual acquired mass reported in children and adults, usually with systemic symptoms of fever, malaise, weight loss associated with jaundice, and abdominal pain. There appears to be a male predominance, with a ratio of 8:1. Although infectious and immunologic causes have been suggested, the pathogenesis of this lesion is unknown. Clinical and pathologic features suggest that it may be a complication of a localized infection. However, microorganisms usually are not found on microscopic examination, and cultures from the lesion usually are negative.[93] Published reports indicate that primary sclerosing cholangitis also may be responsible for the development of hepatic pseudotumors.[94,95]

These lesions can be solitary or multiple. They are composed of fibrous tissue with myofibroblasts, and they often are infiltrated by many inflammatory cells, predominantly polyclonal plasma cells.[96] The lesions usually are well circumscribed and may be encapsulated. Occlusive phlebitis may be present within them.[93]

With conservative treatment, these lesions may regress spontaneously.[97-99] Because they often are mistaken clinically and radiologically for a cancer, most reported cases have been treated by operation.[3,100] One patient even presented with markedly increased concentrations of carbohydrate antigen.[3] Some authors advocate operating as the best therapeutic approach for suspected inflammatory hepatic pseudotumor without an early clinical resolution after conservative therapy.[101] However, when a surgical procedure is indicated, it should be limited, yet done with the knowledge that these lesions are prone to recurrence when not totally resected.

Hepatic Splenosis
Hepatic splenosis is the autotransplantation of splenic tissue in the parenchyma or on the surface of the liver after splenic rupture and splenectomy. The lesions usually are found incidentally and generally are asymptomatic. There is one report of diffuse hepatic splenosis mimicking metastatic breast cancer,[102] and there have been two reported cases of isolated hepatic splenosis indistinguishable from FNH or adenoma by standard preoperative studies.[103,104] This diagnosis should be considered in patients with unexplained hepatic neoplasms and a history of splenic trauma.

Peliosis Hepatis
Peliosis hepatis is characterized by blood-filled lacunar spaces in the liver. These lacunae typically are not lined with endothelium. Peliosis hepatis usually has a chronic presentation and is observed most frequently in patients taking androgenic anabolic steroids.[105,106] The condition has been associated with oral contraceptives[107] and other drugs,[108] as well as a variety of other diseases, including human immunodeficiency virus,[109,110] systemic lupus erythematosus,[111] and certain malignancies.[112,113] Although most cases of peliosis hepatis are asymptomatic, this disease can be complicated by acute hepatic failure,

hemorrhagic necrosis of the liver, and intraperitoneal hemorrhage.[114,115] The treatment when symptoms are present includes discontinuation of offending medications, selective hepatic artery embolization, partial hepatectomy, or, occasionally, liver transplantation.

Focal Fatty Change
Focal fatty change presents as a large ill-defined mass due to macrovesicular steatosis that involves multiple contiguous hepatic acini with preservation of the acinar architecture. These lesions may be single or multiple. Their pathogenesis is unknown but has been associated with obesity,[116] alcoholism,[117,118] diabetes mellitus,[119] and chemotherapy.[120] Treatment usually is directed toward correcting the underlying disease, including abstinence from alcohol and control of diabetes. Disappearance of the lesion has been reported after abstinence from alcohol.[121]

CYSTIC LESIONS

Congenital Cysts
Congenital cysts of the liver are dilatations of the biliary tree that are lined with biliary epithelium. Patients with symptoms associated with these cysts present several ways. However, most patients with hepatic cysts are asymptomatic.

Simple Cyst
The majority of patients with simple cysts are asymptomatic. Most of these lesions can be diagnosed reliably with radiographic imaging features and do not require therapeutic intervention. Simple cysts reputedly arise from aberrant development of the intrahepatic bile ducts (Moschcowitz's, von Meyenburg's complex) and usually lack continuity with the biliary ductal system.

Simple cysts can be single or multiple and are distributed randomly throughout the liver. They vary widely in size, from a few millimeters to more than 20 cm in diameter. Histologically, simple cysts are lined with cuboidal epithelia. These lesions contain small clusters of bile ducts surrounded by fibrous portal tracts. As the cysts enlarge, the epithelium flattens and becomes fibrotic.

Approximately 10% of patients with simple cysts are symptomatic. Complications of cysts are uncommon but include hemorrhage, infection, and biliary obstruction. Hemorrhage, the most frequent complication, is usually heralded by sudden acute abdominal pain. Hypotension is unusual unless the cyst is large or hemorrhage is uncontained because of cyst rupture. The indications for treatment are symptoms related to cyst size, complications, growth, or imaging studies that suggest malignancy.

Operative Management

Operative management is elective, and the surgical treatment of choice is complete cyst excision. Several caveats about cyst excision warrant comment. First, simple cysts grow by expansion not by invasion. Consequently, the parenchyma immediately adjacent to the cyst atrophies or attenuates, and the major vasculature and ducts are splayed around the cyst. Second, the interface between the cyst and the surrounding parenchyma and ducts remains discrete. These features allow development of a plane of dissection immediately between the cyst and the liver parenchyma and even between the cyst and the major vessels and bile ducts. When the risk of operating is not excessive, complete excision is advisable.

Cyst decompression during excision should be avoided, because it complicates or even precludes simple local cyst excision, is complicated technically, or is not possible because of earlier decompression. A site of inadvertent entry into the cyst during simple excision should be closed before completing the dissection and removing the cyst. If the cyst wall is densely adherent to major intrahepatic vasculature or bile ducts, the cyst wall should be left adherent to these structures to avoid potential damage. To reduce the risk of recurrence, residual cyst wall epithelium can be ablated by electrocautery, laser, or alcohol. The recurrence rate is related to the amount of residual cyst wall epithelium after excision. Bile-stained contents or cholangiotomies should prompt identification of the exact site of the bile leak and ligation of the severed ductal defect. Roux-en-Y cystenterostomy is rarely indicated for simple cysts, regardless of their size or complications. A total or near-total excision, with intraperitoneal marsupialization, almost always can be performed with less risk of recurrence or complication than can a cystenterostomy.

Externally draining the cyst excision site with a suction catheter prevents any perihepatic accumulation and controls any transient bile leaks. Cyst fenestration can be performed either laparoscopically or by laparotomy. Regardless of the approach, laparoscopy or open laparotomy, wide excision of the superficial cyst wall can reduce recurrence. This operative technique permits continual reabsorption of the cyst secretions by the peritoneum. Infected cysts should be treated as hepatic abscesses, with percutaneous external drainage. If operative drainage is required, a portion of the cyst wall should be excised to facilitate long-term drainage. Omental packing of the excision site is unnecessary.

Percutaneous Aspiration

Percutaneous aspiration alone has limited efficacy. The reaccumulation of fluid in the cyst approaches 100%.

Aspiration may be used as a way to determine if a cyst is the cause of symptoms or as a temporizing measure prior to definitive therapy. Initially, diagnostic cyst aspiration is performed to confirm whether the cyst is symptomatic and to exclude biliary communication. If a simple cyst is confirmed by a nonpurulent, nonbilious aspirate, the cyst contents should be aspirated completely. Although recurrence after aspiration alone is almost certain, symptomatic recurrence is not. If symptoms do recur, repeat aspiration with alcohol ablation or excision can be used.

Alcohol Ablation

If alcohol ablation is chosen as the method of therapy, the cyst is intubated percutaneously and aspirated completely. Percutaneous sclerosis after aspiration and alcohol instillation ablates the secretory epithelial lining of the cyst and reduces recurrence. If blood or bile is encountered when the cyst is first aspirated, the procedure is aborted, because sclerosants may cause irreparable bile duct or vascular injury. If the aspirate is clear, alcohol is injected into the cyst temporarily through a drainage catheter, and the patient's position is altered to ensure exposure of alcohol to the entire epithelial surface of the cyst. The alcohol is then aspirated, and the drainage catheter removed. When the epithelium is ablated successfully, the cyst is obliterated gradually by fibrous contraction. Most simple cysts will respond to aspiration with alcohol ablation. Although several interventions may be necessary in some patients, there are few reported complications.

Polycystic Liver Disease

Unlike simple cysts, polycystic liver disease (PLD) is inherited either as an autosomal recessive trait associated with congenital hepatic fibrosis in infancy or childhood or as an autosomal dominant trait presenting in adulthood. PLD progresses insidiously over the years and is associated with polycystic renal disease and progressive renal insufficiency. However, liver failure due to PLD is uncommon. Indeed, even with marked hepatosplenomegaly and portal hypertension, liver function may be normal. PLD in adults also may be associated with multiple cysts of the pancreas, spleen, ovaries, and lungs.

Symptoms develop late in the natural history of PLD and are related to increased liver volume and adjacent visceral compression. The most common complaints are increasing abdominal girth, chronic abdominal pain, satiety, weight loss, respiratory compromise, physical disability, and descensus. Ascites can be prominent, although other stigmata of chronic liver disease are rare. Physical examination reveals a large nodular liver. Abdominal tenderness is uncommon. Results of liver function tests are commonly normal or only mildly abnormal. The diagnosis of PLD is readily confirmed by ultrasonography or CT, but CT most clearly defines the extent of liver and adjacent organ involvement.

Treatment

Surgical intervention is reserved for selected patients who exhibit greatly impaired clinical performance due to a massively enlarged liver or complications of rupture, infection, or hemorrhage. Choice of treatment is dictated by the extent of liver involvement and by the associated complications. Percutaneous aspiration with alcohol ablation may provide prolonged symptomatic relief for patients with a few dominant cysts. Operative management becomes more formidable for patients with more diffuse hepatic involvement. Cyst fenestration and intraperitoneal marsupialization or resection have been the mainstay of surgical therapy. Resection poses greater risk because of the possibility of biliary ductal injury, vascular compromise, and liver insufficiency caused by cystic distortion of the intrahepatic anatomy. Cyst decompression by fenestration avoids these risks. However, the number and size of cysts and the bulky liver mass often limit decompression technically. Fenestration with intraperitoneal marsupialization has provided temporary symptomatic relief, but long-term reduction in abdominal girth has rarely been documented. Anatomical hepatic resection in combination with cyst fenestration has been used successfully in carefully selected symptomatic patients. Candidates for combined resection and fenestration should have at least two adjacent liver segments relatively free of cystic involvement, near normal liver function, greatly impaired clinical performance due to increased liver mass, and no significant cardiopulmonary compromise. At operation, anatomical resection is preceded by lobar vascular isolation without inflow occlusion. The transection plane is developed by sequential cyst fenestration, and intraseptal vessels and bile ducts are suture ligated. Cholecystectomy is performed to eliminate potential confounding diagnostic problems postoperatively.

Thirty-one patients underwent liver resection and fenestration for PLD at Mayo Clinic between July 1985 and September 1993.[122] Twenty-eight of 29 surviving patients with adequate follow-up have experienced immediate and sustained relief of symptoms and improved quality of life. Mean liver volume was reduced from 9,357 mL preoperatively to 3,567 mL postoperatively. Selected patients who have severe PLD with favorable anatomy benefit from liver resection and fenestration with acceptable operative morbidity and mortality.

Laparoscopic treatment of PLD is evolving. As in open surgical procedures, wide unroofing or fenestration is required for successful results. It may be difficult to reach deeply situated cysts laparoscopically; thus, this approach should be used in patients with predominantly large cysts.[123] Although the early results are encouraging, long-term studies are needed to determine the benefits and indications of laparoscopic fenestration in PLD.

Neoplastic Cysts

Biliary Cystadenoma and Cystadenocarcinoma

Biliary cystadenoma is a rare cystic neoplasm that constitutes only 5% of all intrahepatic cysts of biliary origin. The most frequent symptoms and signs are nonspecific and include abdominal pain, nausea, fullness, increased girth, and palpable mass. Obstructive jaundice[88,124,125] or spontaneous rupture also may occur.[126] There is a female predominance for biliary cystadenoma; 80% of reported cases occur in middle-aged women. There also may be a predilection for the right hepatic lobe.[124]

The appearance of a multiloculated or thick-walled cyst with solid intracystic components identified by abdominal CT or ultrasonography should suggest a cystic neoplasm. Cystadenomas are characterized histologically by moderate to dense cellular-supporting stroma and cuboidal or columnar mucus-producing epithelium with papillary projections. Biliary cystadenoma may undergo malignant transformation.[127-129] The malignant variant, cystadenocarcinoma, shows a similar stromal composition with papillary adenocarcinoma lining the cysts and invading the cyst wall. Hypervascularity of the cyst wall suggests a cystadenocarcinoma. Importantly, a cystadenocarcinoma may involve the cyst wall only focally. Therefore, numerous histologic sections are required to exclude malignancy. Because of the risk of unpredictable malignant progression and the more practical risk of recurrence after partial excision,[130] cystadenomas should be resected completely. Enucleation can be used to excise cystadenomas. Only rarely is anatomical resection required because of size or location.

Regardless of the diagnostic technique, cystadenoma cannot be accurately distinguished from cystadenocarcinoma. Therefore, complete surgical resection is the recommended treatment.

Traumatic Cysts

Traumatic cysts occur after major injury to the liver that causes disruption of intrahepatic bile ducts or formation of a subcapsular hematoma. These rare cysts constitute less than 0.5% of liver cysts. Because traumatic cysts do not have an epithelial lining, they actually represent hepatic pseudocysts. The contained rupture usually presents as a cystic mass filled with old blood or bile. Clinical presentation resembles that of simple cysts of the liver. The indication and treatment options are also similar. Occasionally, these lesions resolve spontaneously. Therefore, a period of observation is the preferred approach unless the severity of symptoms precludes delay. Because the cyst lining is nonsecretory, partial excision is adequate.

NEWER OPERATIVE APPROACHES

Liver Transplantation

Orthotopic liver transplantation is rarely performed for benign hepatic neoplasms. Patients with unresectable benign hepatic neoplasms, severe symptoms, and potentially life-threatening complications, however, have been treated by orthotopic liver transplantation with good long-term outcome.[131-134] Recently, extended ex situ liver resection and subsequent autotransplantation were successfully performed in two patients with benign tumors located at critical sites not amenable to in vivo resection.[135]

Current data on the natural history of PLD suggest that the progression of cystic disease is slow and that patients are provided with prolonged benefits from nontransplant surgical procedures. In a few selected patients, liver transplantation is indicated. For example, candidates for transplantation may include patients with progressive PLD after resection or fenestration, patients with liver failure with or without renal failure, or patients with diffuse PLD without segmental sparing.

Laparoscopy

Recent innovations in laparoscopic techniques and instrumentation make possible resection of cystic and solid lesions of the liver. The earlier experience gained with laparoscopic fenestration of solitary giant hepatic cysts[136-140] has been applied with good early results to the management of patients with PLD[123,137] and benign solid tumors.[136,141,142] Laparoscopic management is suitable for almost all solitary cysts, regardless of size and anatomical location, whereas only anteriorly located dominant cysts in patients with PLD are suitable for this approach.[143] For patients with benign solid neoplasms, only lesions located in the left lobe (segments 2-4) or in the anterior segments of the right lobe (segment 5 or 6) are suitable for laparoscopic resection.[141,143,144] Early reports suggest that laparoscopic management of cystic and solid hepatic lesions may provide similar results to open techniques, with the added benefits of shorter hospitalization and the avoidance of the morbidity of laparotomy. However, larger series with longer follow-up will be required before laparoscopy can be considered the treatment of choice for these rare hepatic lesions.

CONCLUSION

Recent advances in abdominal imaging techniques have contributed immensely to the increased discovery of benign hepatic lesions. Benign hepatic neoplasms often pose diagnostic and therapeutic challenges. Although most cysts can be diagnosed reliably on the basis of radiographic imaging features, some cannot. Benign hepatic lesions can be classified as solid or cystic. Solid tumors can be grouped further according to their epithelial or mesenchymal origin.[1] Only about half the described solid lesions are common enough to assume clinical importance for the practicing surgeon. These include FNH, hepatocellular adenoma, hemangiomas, and bile duct adenomas. Management of these lesions usually depends on the histology, the natural history, and any associated symptoms.

The majority of patients with these benign hepatic lesions are asymptomatic and do not have any complications. Hence, most of these lesions would go undiscovered throughout life. In general, it is safe to observe closely an incidentally found, asymptomatic benign hepatic lesion of small to moderate size, as long as the benignity is certain. Benign neoplasms and cysts requiring surgical intervention are relatively rare. In general, operative management is pursued when there is rapid growth, when malignancy cannot be excluded, when there is a risk of rupture, when hemorrhage or malignant transformation has occurred, or when incapacitating or debilitating symptoms demand intervention.

When clinically indicated, hepatic resection is safe and effective in the management of benign hepatic neoplasms and cysts. The increasing number of reports of successful laparoscopic management of benign solid and cystic lesions of the liver provides evidence that the procedure is feasible and safe.[136,141,143-145] Laparoscopic hepatic surgical procedures may provide similar long-term results to open techniques but with decreased hospitalization and morbidity as well as a faster return to work.[146] Although the total resection of a benign hepatic neoplasm generally is considered curative, the patients still require follow-up. There are documented recurrences after an apparent complete surgical resection.[13,147] Liver transplantation may be an option for patients with unresectable benign hepatic lesions that cause severe symptoms and potentially life-threatening complications.

Appropriate and successful management of these lesions requires the surgeon to be thoroughly familiar with their gross appearances, radiologic characteristics, clinical significance, and natural history.

REFERENCES

1. Ishak KG, Rabin L: Benign tumors of the liver. Med Clin North Am 59:995-1013, 1975
2. Horton KM, Bluemke DA, Hruban RH, Soyer P, Fishman EK: CT and MR imaging of benign hepatic and biliary tumors. Radiographics 19:431-451, 1999
3. Ogawa T, Yokoi H, Kawarada Y: A case of inflammatory pseudo-tumor of the liver causing elevated serum CA19-9 levels. Am J Gastroenterol 93:2551-2555, 1998
4. Yamaguchi M, Kuzume M, Matsumoto T, Matsumiya A, Nakano H, Kumada K: Spontaneous rupture of a nonparasitic liver cyst complicated by intracystic hemorrhage. J Gastroenterol 34:645-648, 1999
5. Dumortier J, Lombard-Bohas C, Valette PJ, Boillot O, Scoazec JY, Berger F, Claudel-Bonvoisin S: Needle tract recurrence of hepatocellular carcinoma after liver transplantation. Gut 47:301, 2000
6. Schotman SN, De Man RA, Stoker J, Zondervan PE, Ijzermans JN: Subcutaneous seeding of hepatocellular carcinoma after percutaneous needle biopsy. Gut 45:626-627, 1999
7. Goodman ZD: Benign tumors of the liver. *In* Neoplasms of the Liver. Edited by K Okuda, KG Ishak. Tokyo, Springer-Verlag, 1987, pp 105-125
8. Nagorney DM: Benign hepatic tumors: focal nodular hyperplasia and hepatocellular adenoma. World J Surg 19:13-18, 1995
9. Iwatsuki S, Todo S, Starzl TE: Excisional therapy for benign hepatic lesions. Surg Gynecol Obstet 171:240-246, 1990
10. Nichols FC III, van Heerden JA, Weiland LH: Benign liver tumors. Surg Clin North Am 69:297-314, 1989
11. Kerlin P, Davis GL, McGill DB, Weiland LH, Adson MA, Sheedy PF II: Hepatic adenoma and focal nodular hyperplasia: clinical, pathologic, and radiologic features. Gastroenterology 84:994-1002, 1983
12. Knowles DM II, Casarella WJ, Johnson PM, Wolff M: The clinical, radiologic, and pathologic characterization of benign hepatic neoplasms: alleged association with oral contraceptives. Medicine (Baltimore) 57:223-237, 1978
13. Klatskin G: Hepatic tumors: possible relationship to use of oral contraceptives. Gastroenterology 73:386-394, 1977
14. Christopherson WM, Mays ET, Barrows G: A clinicopathologic study of steroid-related liver tumors. Am J Surg Pathol 1:31-41, 1977
15. Mays ET, Christopherson WM, Barrows GH: Focal nodular hyperplasia of the liver: possible relationship to oral contraceptives. Am J Clin Pathol 61:735-746, 1974
16. Stauffer JQ, Lapinski MW, Honold DJ, Myers JK: Focal nodular hyperplasia of the liver and intrahepatic hemorrhage in young women on oral contraceptives. Ann Intern Med 83:301-306, 1975
17. Mentha G, Rubbia-Brandt L, Howarth N, Majno P, Morel P, Terrier F: Management of focal nodular hyperplasia and hepatocellular adenoma. Swiss Surg 5:122-125, 1999
18. Mathiew D, Bruneton JN, Drouillard J, Pointreau CC, Vasile N: Hepatic adenomas and focal nodular hyperplasia: dynamic CT study. Radiology 160:53-58, 1986
19. Weimann A, Ringe B, Klempnauer J, Lamesch P, Gratz KF, Prokop M, Maschek H, Tusch G, Pichlmayr R: Benign liver tumors: differential diagnosis and indications for surgery. World J Surg 21:983-990, 1997
20. Shortell CK, Schwartz SI: Hepatic adenoma and focal nodular hyperplasia. Surg Gynecol Obstet 173:426-431, 1991
21. Rogers JV, Mack LA, Freeny PC, Johnson ML, Sones PJ: Hepatic focal nodular hyperplasia: angiography, CT, sonography, and scintigraphy. AJR Am J Roentgenol 137:983-990, 1981
22. Davis DC, Wulfeck D, Donovan MS: Hepatocellular adenoma: case report with Tc-99m SC uptake and radiologic correlation. Clin Nucl Med 21:8-10, 1996
23. Lubbers PR, Ros PR, Goodman ZD, Ishak KG: Accumulation of technetium-99m sulfur colloid by hepatocellular adenoma: scintigraphic-pathologic correlation. AJR Am J Roentgenol 148:1105-1108, 1987
24. Foster JH, Berman MM: The malignant transformation of liver cell adenomas. Arch Surg 129:712-717, 1994
25. Gyorffy EJ, Bredfeldt JE, Black WC: Transformation of hepatic cell adenoma to hepatocellular carcinoma due to oral contraceptive use. Ann Intern Med 110:489-490, 1989
26. Neuberger J, Portmann B, Nunnerley HB, Laws JW, Davis M, Williams R: Oral-contraceptive-associated liver tumours: occurrence of malignancy and difficulties in diagnosis. Lancet 1:273-276, 1980
27. Gonzalez F, Marks C: Hepatic tumors and oral contraceptives: surgical management. J Surg Oncol 29:193-197, 1985
28. Rooks JB, Ory HW, Ishak KG, Strauss LT, Greenspan JR, Hill AP, Tyler CW Jr: Epidemiology of hepatocellular adenoma: the role of oral contraceptive use. JAMA 242:644-648, 1979
29. Mays ET, Christopherson WM, Mahr MM, Williams HC: Hepatic changes in young women ingesting contraceptive steroids: hepatic hemorrhage and primary hepatic tumors. JAMA 235:730-732, 1976
30. Sears HF, Smith G, Powell RD: Hepatic adenoma associated with oral contraceptive use: an unusual clinical presentation. Arch Surg 111:1399-1403, 1976
31. Baum JK: Liver tumors and oral contraceptives (letter to the editor). JAMA 232:1329, 1975
32. Edmondson HA, Reynolds TB, Henderson B, Benton B: Regression of liver cell adenomas associated with oral contraceptives. Ann Intern Med 86:180-182, 1977
33. Edmondson HA, Henderson B, Benton B: Liver-cell adenomas associated with use of oral contraceptives. N Engl J Med 294:470-472, 1976
34. Malt RA, Hershberg RA, Miller WL: Experience with benign tumors of the liver. Surg Gynecol Obstet 130:285-291, 1970
35. Cheng PN, Shin JS, Lin XZ: Hepatic adenoma: an observation from asymptomatic stage to rupture. Hepatogastroenterology 43:245-248, 1996
36. Andersen PH, Packer JT: Hepatic adenoma: observations after estrogen withdrawal. Arch Surg 111:898-900, 1976
37. Sogaard PE: Nodular transformation of the liver, alpha-fetoprotein, and hepatocellular carcinoma. Hum Pathol 12:1052, 1981
38. Nakanuma Y, Ohta G, Sasaki K: Nodular regenerative hyperplasia of the liver associated with polyarteritis nodosa. Arch Pathol Lab Med 108:133-135, 1984
39. Reynolds WJ, Wanless IR: Nodular regenerative hyperplasia of the liver in a patient with rheumatoid vasculitis: a morphometric study suggesting a role for hepatic arteritis in the pathogenesis. J Rheumatol 11:838-842, 1984
40. Wanless IR: Micronodular transformation (nodular regenerative hyperplasia) of the liver: a report of 64 cases among 2,500 autopsies and a new classification of benign hepatocellular nodules. Hepatology 11:787-797, 1990
41. Curry GW, Beattie AD: Pathogenesis of primary hepatocellular carcinoma. Eur J Gastroenterol Hepatol 8:850-855, 1996

42. Iha H, Nakashima Y, Fukukura Y, Tanaka M, Wada Y, Takazawa T, Nakashima O, Kojiro M: Biliary hamartomas simulating multiple hepatic metastasis on imaging findings. Kurume Med J 43:231-235, 1996

43. Hedayati B, Burke D, Shousha S, Allen-Mersh TG: A cystic biliary tumour responding to regional fluorinated pyrimidine infusion. Eur J Surg Oncol 24:451-452, 1998

44. Yaziji N, Martin L, Hillon P, Favre JP, Henninger JF, Piard F: Cholangiocarcinoma arising from biliary micro-hamartomas in a man suffering from hemochromatosis [French]. Ann Pathol 17:346-349, 1997

45. Trastek VF, van Heerden JA, Sheedy PF II, Adson MA: Cavernous hemangiomas of the liver: Resect or observe? Am J Surg 145:49-53, 1983

46. Stayman JW Jr, Polsky HS, Blaum L: Case report: ruptured cavernous hemangioma of the liver. Pa Med 79:62-63, 1976

47. Hochwald SN, Blumgart LH: Giant hepatic hemangioma with Kasabach-Merritt syndrome: Is the appropriate treatment enucleation or liver transplantation? HPB Surg 11:413-419, 2000

48. Akiyoshi K, Mizote H, Tanaka Y, Nakagawa M: Capillary hemangioma of the liver with Kasabach-Merritt syndrome in a neonate: report of a case. Surg Today 30:86-88, 2000

49. Mewes T, Moldenhauer H, Pfeifer J, Papenberg J: The Kasabach-Merritt syndrome: severe bleeding disorder caused by celiac arteriography: reversal by heparin treatment. Am J Gastroenterol 84:965-971, 1989

50. Gedaly R, Pomposelli JJ, Pomfret EA, Lewis WD, Jenkins RL: Cavernous hemangioma of the liver: anatomic resection vs. enucleation. Arch Surg 134:407-411, 1999

51. Stavropoulos M, Vagianos C, Scopa CD, Dragotis C, Androulakis J: Solitary hepatic lymphangioma. A rare benign tumour: a case report. HPB Surg 8:33-36, 1994

52. Sathyavagiswaran L, Sherwin RP: Acute and chronic pericholangiolitis in association with multifocal hepatic lymphangiomatosis. Hum Pathol 20:601-603, 1989

53. Veloso FT, Ribeiro AT, Teixeira AA, Ramalhao J, Saleiro J, Serrao D: Biliary papillomatosis: report of a case with 5-year follow-up. Am J Gastroenterol 78:645-648, 1983

54. Bender BL, Yunis EJ: The pathology of tuberous sclerosis. Pathol Annu 17:339-382, 1982

55. Goodman ZD, Ishak KG: Angiomyolipomas of the liver. Am J Surg Pathol 8:745-750, 1984

56. Hirasaki S, Koide N, Ogawa H, Ujike K, Shinji T, Tsuji T: Tuberous sclerosis associated with multiple hepatic lipomatous tumors and hemorrhagic renal angiomyolipoma. Intern Med 38:345-348, 1999

57. Takayasu K, Shima Y, Muramatsu Y, Moriyama N, Yamada T, Makuuchi M, Hirohashi S: Imaging characteristics of large lipoma and angiomyolipoma of the liver: case reports. Cancer 59:916-921, 1987

58. Roberts JL, Fishman EK, Hartman DS, Sanders R, Goodman Z, Siegelman SS: Lipomatous tumors of the liver: evaluation with CT and US. Radiology 158:613-617, 1986

59. Low VH, Breidahl WH, Robbins PD: Hepatic angiomyolipoma. Abdom Imaging 19:540-542, 1994

60. Fobbe F, Hamm B, Schwarting R: Angiomyolipoma of the liver: CT, MR, and ultrasound imaging. J Comput Assist Tomogr 12:658-659, 1988

61. Guidi G, Catalano O, Rotondo A: Spontaneous rupture of a hepatic angiomyolipoma: CT findings and literature review. Eur Radiol 7:335-337, 1997

62. Croquet V, Pilette C, Aube C, Bouju B, Oberti F, Cervi C, Arnaud JP, Rousselet MC, Boyer J, Cales P: Late recurrence of a hepatic angiomyolipoma. Eur J Gastroenterol Hepatol 12:579-582, 2000

63. Karhunen PJ: Hepatic pseudolipoma. J Clin Pathol 38:877-879, 1985

64. Hawkins EP, Jordan GL, McGavran MH: Primary leiomyoma of the liver: successful treatment by lobectomy and presentation of criteria for diagnosis. Am J Surg Pathol 4:301-304, 1980

65. Herzberg AJ, MacDonald JA, Tucker JA, Humphrey PA, Meyers WC: Primary leiomyoma of the liver. Am J Gastroenterol 85:1642-1645, 1990

66. Lecesne R, Drouillard J, Le Bail B, Saric J, Balabaud C, Laurent F: Localized fibrous tumor of the liver: imaging findings. Eur Radiol 8:36-38, 1998

67. Murray JD, Ricketts RR: Mesenchymal hamartoma of the liver. Am Surg 64:1097-1103, 1998

68. Bilge O, Emre A, Cevikbas U, Acarli K, Alper A, Ariogul O: Liver hamartoma in an adult: report of a rare case. Surg Today 26:513-516, 1996

69. Yamamoto M, Hagihara H, Mogaki M, Iimuro Y, Fujii H, Ainota T, Akahane Y, Matsumoto Y: Adult mesenchymal hamartoma of the liver mimicking bile duct cystadenoma. J Gastroenterol 29:518-524, 1994

70. Chau KY, Ho JW, Wu PC, Yuen WK: Mesenchymal hamartoma of liver in a man: comparison with cases in infants. J Clin Pathol 47:864-866, 1994

71. Das PC, Rao PL, Radhakrishna K: Cystic hamartoma of the liver in children. J Indian Med Assoc 95:517-518, 1997

72. Motiwale SS, Karmarkar SJ, Oak SN, Kalgutkar AD, Deshmukh SS: Cystic mesenchymal hamartoma of the liver: a rare condition. Indian J Cancer 33:157-160, 1996

73. Megremis S, Sfakianaki E, Voludaki A, Chroniaris N: The ultrasonographic appearance of a cystic mesenchymal hamartoma of the liver observed in a middle-aged woman. J Clin Ultrasound 22:338-341, 1994

74. Helal A, Nolan M, Bower R, Mair B, Debich-Spicer D: Pathological case of the month: mesenchymal hamartoma of the liver. Arch Pediatr Adolesc Med 149:315-316, 1995

75. Lauwers GY, Grant LD, Donnelly WH, Meloni AM, Foss RM, Sanberg AA, Langham MR Jr: Hepatic undifferentiated (embryonal) sarcoma arising in a mesenchymal hamartoma. Am J Surg Pathol 21:1248-1254, 1997

76. Gallivan MV, Lack EE, Chun B, Ishak KG: Undifferentiated ("embryonal") sarcoma of the liver: ultrastructure of a case presenting as a primary intracardiac tumor. Pediatr Pathol 1:291-300, 1983

77. Alam K, Maheshwari V, Aziz M, Ghani I: Teratoma of the liver: a case report. Indian J Pathol Microbiol 41:457-459, 1998

78. Witte DP, Kissane JM, Askin FB: Hepatic teratomas in children. Pediatr Pathol 1:81-92, 1983

79. Morikawa Y, Ishihara Y, Matsuura N, Miyamoto H, Kakudo K: Malignant schwannoma of the liver. Dig Dis Sci 40:1279-1282, 1995

80. Lederman SM, Martin EC, Laffey KT, Lefkowitch JH: Hepatic neurofibromatosis, malignant schwannoma, and angiosarcoma in von Recklinghausen's disease. Gastroenterology 92:234-239, 1987

81. Wada Y, Jimi A, Nakashima O, Kojiro M, Kurohiji T, Sai K: Schwannoma of the liver: report of two surgical cases. Pathol Int 48:611-617, 1998

82. Yoshida M, Nakashima Y, Tanaka A, Mori K, Yamaoka Y: Benign schwannoma of the liver: a case report. Nippon Geka Hokan 63:208-214, 1994

83. Hytiroglou P, Linton P, Klion F, Schwartz M, Miller C, Thung SN: Benign schwannoma of the liver. Arch Pathol Lab Med 117:216-218, 1993

84. Heffron TG, Coventry S, Bedendo F, Baker A: Resection of primary schwannoma of the liver not associated with neurofibromatosis. Arch Surg 128:1396-1398, 1993

85. Bekker GM: Neurofibroma of the liver [Russian]. Sov Med 10:120-121, 1982

86. Pereira Filho RA, Souza SA, Oliveira Filho JA: Primary neurilemmal tumour of the liver: case report. Arq Gastroenterol 15:136-138, 1978

87. Wilkins L, Ravitch MM: Adrenocortical tumor arising in the liver of a three year old boy with signs of virilism and Cushing's syndrome: report of a case with cure after partial resection of the right lobe of the liver. Pediatrics 9:671-681, 1952

88. Arai K, Muro H, Suzuki M, Oba N, Ito K, Sasano H: Adrenal rest tumor of the liver: a case report with immunohistochemical investigation of steroidogenesis. Pathol Int 50:244-248, 2000

89. Contreras P, Altieri E, Liberman C, Gac A, Rojas A, Ibarra A, Ravanal M, Seron-Ferre M: Adrenal rest tumor of the liver causing Cushing's syndrome: treatment with ketoconazole preceding an apparent surgical cure. J Clin Endocrinol Metab 60:21-28, 1985

90. Wallace EZ, Leonidas JR, Stanek AE, Avramides A: Endocrine studies in a patient with functioning adrenal rest tumor of the liver. Am J Med 70:1122-1125, 1981

91. Nicolau A, Bruneton JN, Balu C, Aubanel D, Roux P: Radiologic study of aberrant pancreas of gastroduodenal topography: apropos of 11 cases [French]. J Radiol 64:319-324, 1983

92. Mobini J, Krouse TB, Cooper DR: Intrahepatic pancreatic heterotopia: review and report of a case presenting as an abdominal mass. Am J Dig Dis 19:64-70, 1974

93. Horiuchi R, Uchida T, Kojima T, Shikata T: Inflammatory pseudotumor of the liver: clinicopathologic study and review of the literature. Cancer 65:1583-1590, 1990

94. Toda K, Yasuda I, Nishigaki Y, Enya M, Yamada T, Nagura K, Sugihara J, Wakahara T, Tomita E, Moriwaki H: Inflammatory pseudotumor of the liver with primary sclerosing cholangitis. J Gastroenterol 35:304-309, 2000

95. Nonomura A, Minato H, Shimizu K, Kadoya M, Matsui O: Hepatic hilar inflammatory pseudotumor mimicking cholangiocarcinoma with cholangitis and phlebitis: A variant of primary sclerosing cholangitis? Pathol Res Pract 193:519-525, 1997

96. Coffin CM, Watterson J, Priest JR, Dehner LP: Extrapulmonary inflammatory myofibroblastic tumor (inflammatory pseudotumor): a clinicopathologic and immunohistochemical study of 84 cases. Am J Surg Pathol 19:859-872, 1995

97. Young TH, Chao YC, Tang HS: Spontaneous regression of hepatic pseudotumor demonstrated by Ga-67 imaging. Clin Nucl Med 23:624, 1998

98. Zamir D, Jarchowsky J, Singer C, Abumoch S, Groisman G, Ammar M, Weiner P: Inflammatory pseudotumor of the liver: a rare entity and a diagnostic challenge. Am J Gastroenterol 93:1538-1540, 1998

99. Jais P, Berger JF, Vissuzaine C, Paramelle O, Clays-Schouman E, Potet F, Mignon M: Regression of inflammatory pseudotumor of the liver under conservative therapy. Dig Dis Sci 40:752-756, 1995

100. Lacaille F, Fournet JC, Sayegh N, Jaubert F, Revillon Y: Inflammatory pseudotumor of the liver: a rare benign tumor mimicking a malignancy. Liver Transpl Surg 5:83-85, 1999

101. Mangiante GL, Colombari R, Portuese A, Bortolasi L, Marinello P, Colucci G, Montresor E, Serio GE: Inflammatory pseudotumor of the liver: case report and review of the literature. G Chir 18:417-420, 1997

102. Foroudi F, Ahern V, Peduto A: Splenosis mimicking metastases from breast carcinoma. Clin Oncol 11:190-192, 1999

103. D'Angelica M, Fong Y, Blumgart LH: Isolated hepatic splenosis: first reported case. HPB Surg 11:39-42, 1998

104. Gruen DR, Gollub MJ: Intrahepatic splenosis mimicking hepatic adenoma. AJR Am J Roentgenol 168:725-726, 1997

105. Cabasso A: Peliosis hepatis in a young adult bodybuilder. Med Sci Sports Exerc 26:2-4, 1994

106. Ishak KG: Hepatic lesions caused by anabolic and contraceptive steroids. Semin Liver Dis 1:116-128, 1981

107. Staub PG, Leibowitz CB: Peliosis hepatis associated with oral contraceptive use. Australas Radiol 40:172-174, 1996

108. Larrey D, Freneaux E, Berson A, Babany G, Degott C, Valla D, Pessayre D, Benhamou JP: Peliosis hepatis induced by 6-thioguanine administration. Gut 29:1265-1269, 1988

109. Koehler JE, Tappero JW: Bacillary angiomatosis and bacillary peliosis in patients infected with human immunodeficiency virus. Clin Infect Dis 17:612-624, 1993

110. Radin DR, Kanel GC: Peliosis hepatis in a patient with human immunodeficiency virus infection. AJR Am J Roentgenol 156:91-92, 1991

111. Matsumoto T, Yoshimine T, Shimouchi K, Shiotu H, Kuwabara N, Fukuda Y, Hoshi T: The liver in systemic lupus erythematosus: pathologic analysis of 52 cases and review of Japanese Autopsy Registry Data. Hum Pathol 23:1151-1158, 1992

112. Otani M, Ohaki Y, Nakatani Y, Ito E, Shimoyama K, Misugi K: An autopsy case of renal cell carcinoma associated with extensive peliosis hepatis. Acta Pathol Jpn 42:62-68, 1992

113. Bhaskar KV, Joshi K, Banerjee CK, Rao RK, Verma SC: Peliosis hepatis in Hodgkin's disease: an infrequent association. Am J Gastroenterol 85:628-629, 1990

114. Takiff H, Brems JJ, Pockros PJ, Elliott ML: Focal hemorrhagic necrosis of the liver: a rare cause of hemoperitoneum. Dig Dis Sci 37:1910-1914, 1992

115. Hayward SR, Lucas CE, Ledgerwood AM: Recurrent spontaneous intrahepatic hemorrhage from peliosis hepatis. Arch Surg 126:782-783, 1991

116. Andersen T, Christoffersen P, Gluud C: The liver in consecutive patients with morbid obesity: a clinical, morphological, and biochemical study. Int J Obes 8:107-115, 1984

117. Kudo M, Ikekubo K, Yamamoto K, Hino M, Ibuki Y, Tomita S, Komori H, Orino A, Todo A: Focal fatty infiltration of the liver in acute alcoholic liver injury: hot spots with radiocolloid SPECT scan. Am J Gastroenterol 84:948-952, 1989

118. Tang-Barton P, Vas W, Weissman J, Salimi Z, Patel R, Morris L: Focal fatty liver lesions in alcoholic liver disease: a broadened spectrum of CT appearances. Gastrointest Radiol 10:133-137, 1985

119. Grove A, Vyberg B, Vyberg M: Focal fatty change of the liver: a review and a case associated with continuous ambulatory peritoneal dialysis. Virchows Arch A Pathol Anat Histopathol 419:69-75, 1991

120. Foged E, Bjerring P, Kragballe K, Sogaard H, Zachariae H: Histologic changes in the liver during etretinate treatment. J Am Acad Dermatol 11:580-583, 1984

121. Rich HG: Resolution of focal fatty infiltration of the liver. South Med J 89:1024-1027, 1996
122. Que F, Nagorney DM, Gross JB Jr, Torres VE: Liver resection and cyst fenestration in the treatment of severe polycystic liver disease. Gastroenterology 108:487-494, 1995
123. Kabbej M, Sauvanet A, Chauveau D, Farges O, Belghiti J: Laparoscopic fenestration in polycystic liver disease. Br J Surg 83:1697-1701, 1996
124. Sutton CD, White SA, Berry DP, Dennison AR: Intrahepatic biliary cystadenoma causing luminal common bile duct obstruction. Dig Surg 17:297-299, 2000
125. Taketomi A, Tamada R, Takenaka K, Kawano R, Maeda T, Sugimachi K: A case of biliary cystadenoma with obstructive jaundice. Oncol Rep 5:833-835, 1998
126. Chang MS, Chen MC, Chou FF, Sheen-Chen SM, Chen WJ: Spontaneous rupture of hepatobiliary cystadenoma: a case report. Changgeng Yi Xue Za Zhi 18:392-397, 1995
127. Joseph J-M, Martinet O, Prelly M, Fontolliet C, Gillet M, Reis ED: Malignant transformation of a liver cystadenoma. Surg Rounds 23:522-526, 2000
128. Matsuoka Y, Hayashi K, Yano M: Case report: malignant transformation of biliary cystadenoma with mesenchymal stroma: documentation by CT. Clin Radiol 52:318-321, 1997
129. Woods GL: Biliary cystadenocarcinoma: case report of hepatic malignancy originating in benign cystadenoma. Cancer 47:2936-2940, 1981
130. Stoupis C, Ros PR, Dolson DJ: Recurrent biliary cystadenoma: MR imaging appearance. J Magn Reson Imaging 4:99-101, 1994
131. Tepetes K, Selby R, Webb M, Madariaga JR, Iwatsuki S, Starzl TE: Orthotopic liver transplantation for benign hepatic neoplasms. Arch Surg 130:153-156, 1995
132. Egawa H, Berquist W, Garcia-Kennedy R, Cox KL, Concepcion W, So SK, Esquivel CO: Respiratory distress from benign liver tumors: a report of two unusual cases treated with hepatic transplantation. J Pediatr Gastroenterol Nutr 19:114-117, 1994
133. Klompmaker IJ, Sloof MJ, van der Meer J, de Jong GM, de Bruijn KM, Bams JL: Orthotopic liver transplantation in a patient with a giant cavernous hemangioma of the liver and Kasabach-Merritt syndrome. Transplantation 48:149-151, 1989
134. Miller C, Mazzaferro V, Makowla L, ChapChap P, Demetris J, Tzakis A, Esquivel CO, Iwatsuki S, Starzl TE: Orthotopic liver transplantation for massive hepatic lymphangiomatosis. Surgery 103:490-495, 1988
135. Oldhafer KJ, Lang H, Schlitt HJ, Hauss J, Raab R, Klempnauer J, Pichlmayr R: Long-term experience after ex situ liver surgery. Surgery 127:520-527, 2000
136. Katkhouda N, Hurwitz M, Gugenheim J, Mavor E, Mason RJ, Waldrep DJ, Rivera RT, Chandra M, Campos GM, Offerman S, Trussler A, Fabiani P, Mouiel J: Laparoscopic management of benign solid and cystic lesions of the liver. Ann Surg 229:460-466, 1999
137. Hansen P, Bhoyrul S, Legha P, Wetter A, Way LW: Laparoscopic treatment of liver cysts. J Gastrointest Surg 1:53-60, 1997
138. Zacherl J, Imhof M, Fugger R, Fritsch A: Laparoscopic unroofing of symptomatic congenital liver cysts. Surg Endosc 10:813-815, 1996
139. Krahenbuhl L, Baer HU, Renzulli P, Z'Graggen K, Frei E, Buchler MW: Laparoscopic management of nonparasitic symptom-producing solitary hepatic cysts. J Am Coll Surg 183:493-498, 1996
140. Hauser CJ, Poole GV: Laparoscopic fenestration of a giant simple hepatic cyst: case report and technical considerations. Surg Endosc 8:884-886, 1994
141. Samama G, Chiche L, Brefort JL, Le Roux Y: Laparoscopic anatomical hepatic resection: report of four left lobectomies for solid tumors. Surg Endosc 12:76-78, 1998
142. Gugenheim J, Mazza D, Katkhouda N, Goubaux B, Mouiel J: Laparoscopic resection of solid liver tumours. Br J Surg 83:334-335, 1996
143. Katkhouda N, Mavor E: Laparoscopic management of benign liver disease. Surg Clin North Am 80:1203-1211, 2000
144. Cuesta MA, Meijer S, Paul MA, de Brauw LM: Limited laparoscopic liver resection of benign tumors guided by laparoscopic ultrasonography: report of two cases. Surg Laparosc Endosc 5:396-401, 1995
145. Zacherl J, Scheuba C, Imhof M, Jakesz R, Fugger R: Long-term results after laparoscopic unroofing of solitary symptomatic congenital liver cysts. Surg Endosc 14:59-62, 2000
146. Diez J, Decoud J, Gutierrez L, Suhl A, Merello J: Laparoscopic treatment of symptomatic cysts of the liver. Br J Surg 85:25-27, 1998
147. Conter RL, Longmire WP Jr: Recurrent hepatic hemangiomas: possible association with estrogen therapy. Ann Surg 207:115-119, 1988

LIVER DISEASES NECESSITATING LIVER TRANSPLANTATION

Charles B. Rosen, M.D.

Only 30 years ago, liver transplantation was an experimental surgical procedure. Results with animal experimentation were promising, but clinical experience was limited to only a few patients at several centers throughout the world. Successes were rare.

The technical aspects of liver transplantation were developed in animal models in the late 1950s and early 1960s. These techniques were refined further during early clinical procedures in the 1960s and 1970s. Despite technical success, patient survival was poor. Deaths due to rejection or infection were common, and fewer than 30% of patients were alive 1 year after transplantation. The results of liver transplantation dramatically improved with the introduction of cyclosporine in the early 1980s. Cyclosporine, in combination with corticosteroids, provided clinicians with safe and effective immunosuppressive therapy and accounted for a 100% increase in patient survival. With increasing success, liver transplantation gained widespread acceptance.

In 1983, a National Institutes of Health conference paved the way for increasing application of liver transplantation in clinical practice. More surgeons learned to perform liver transplantation, and by 1990 there were nearly 100 liver transplant centers in the United States alone. With this explosion of activity, technical innovations such as venous bypass and development of additional immunosuppressive and antirejection medications led to further improvements in patient outcome. Currently, national patient survival rates are 87.0% at 1 year and 75.1% at 5 years after liver transplantation.[1] Thus, liver transplantation has now emerged as the standard of care for patients with a multitude of acute and chronic end-stage liver diseases.

The Liver Transplant Program at Mayo Clinic began in 1985 with a multidisciplinary team of transplant surgeons, hepatologists, anesthesiologists, pathologists, specialists in critical care and infectious diseases, and allied health professionals. During the past 17 years, more than 1,300 liver transplantations have been performed at Mayo Clinic in Rochester, Minnesota, and results have been outstanding. The program's philosophy is to practice a team approach to patient care with clinical protocols specifically designed to achieve superb results, facilitate clinical research, and provide an outstanding opportunity for medical and surgical education. This "Mayo model of care" has been adopted by many other transplant programs throughout the world and has served as a template for the development of liver transplantation at Mayo Clinic in Jacksonville, Florida, in 1998 and Mayo Clinic in Scottsdale, Arizona, in 1999. This chapter presents the Mayo Clinic approach to liver transplantation, including indications, evaluation of patients, technical aspects of organ procurement and transplantation, maximizing use of cadaver donor organs (including split liver transplantation), and living-donor transplantation.

LIVER DISEASE AND INDICATIONS FOR TRANSPLANTATION

Liver Disease
The aim of liver transplantation is to provide prolonged survival with a satisfactory quality of life for patients with acute or chronic end-stage liver disease. The most common diseases leading to liver transplantation in adults are alcoholic cirrhosis (21.6%), hepatitis C (19.5%), cryptogenic

cirrhosis (12%), primary biliary cirrhosis (10.9%), primary sclerosing cholangitis (9.9%), hepatitis B (6.1%), fulminant hepatic failure (5.4%), autoimmune hepatitis (5%), malignancy (4.6%), metabolic diseases (3.3%), and other conditions (1.7%) (Fig. 1).[2] Recently, more transplantations are being performed for patients with cirrhosis due to hepatitis C or alcohol or both. In pediatric patients, biliary atresia is the most common disease (55%), followed by metabolic diseases (15.4%), other cholestatic diseases (10.7%), fulminant hepatic failure (10.5%), cryptogenic cirrhosis (5.6%), malignancies (1.5%), and autoimmune disease (1.3%) (Fig. 2).[2]

Indications

The indications for liver transplantation are not the liver diseases themselves but the complications of the diseases that threaten patients' lives and their quality of life. These complications include ascites and spontaneous bacterial peritonitis, variceal hemorrhage, encephalopathy, pruritus, hepatorenal syndrome, muscle wasting, growth failure (children), failure to thrive, and development of hepatocellular carcinoma. The development of one or more of these complications in a patient with liver disease is a strong reason to proceed with evaluation for liver transplantation. Several metabolic disorders also are commonly treated with liver transplantation.

Acute fulminant liver failure due to acute viral hepatitis, toxin exposure, or an idiosyncratic drug reaction has a dismal natural history. Affected patients present with an acute illness, and jaundice and severe hepatic synthetic dysfunction develop shortly thereafter. The development of encephalopathy is an ominous sign, because death is

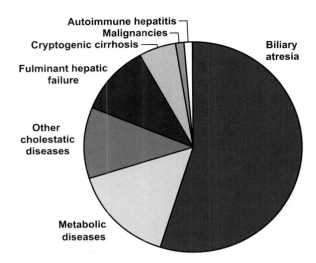

Fig. 2. Diseases necessitating liver transplantation in pediatric patients.

commonly due to cerebral edema. This condition warrants emergency evaluation for liver transplantation.

Hepatocellular Carcinoma

Hepatocellular carcinoma is the most common primary malignant liver tumor and one of the most common malignancies worldwide. Approximately 80% of the tumors arise in the setting of chronic liver disease, especially disease due to hepatitis B, hepatitis C, and alcohol. The incidence of hepatocellular carcinoma is increasing rapidly in association with the increasing incidence of cirrhosis due to hepatitis C. The natural history of small tumors (≤ 3 cm) is poor; few patients live beyond 3 years. At many centers, liver resection in the setting of cirrhosis is associated with high morbidity (20%-40%), high mortality (10%-35%), and a high probability of synchronous or metachronous tumors. Furthermore, many patients have advanced cirrhosis that precludes liver resection.

In the past, liver transplantation was reserved for patients with advanced tumor stage, and results were poor. During the early 1990s, transplantation for patients with incidental tumors (found during examination of explanted livers) had excellent results, and liver transplantation has now emerged as the treatment of choice for patients with early-stage cancer arising in the setting of chronic liver disease. During the 5 years from 1992 to 1997, 27 patients with early-stage hepatocellular carcinoma (one tumor ≤ 5 cm in diameter or up to three tumors all ≤ 3 cm in diameter) underwent chemoembolization followed by orthotopic liver transplantation at Mayo Clinic. Patient survival was 91% at 1 year and 84% at 2 years after transplantation.[3] Transarterial chemoembolization and other ablative procedures may limit progression of disease for

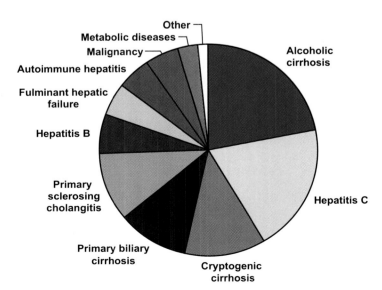

Fig. 1. Diseases necessitating liver transplantation in adults.

patients awaiting transplantation and possibly avoid tumor dissemination during the transplant procedure.

Cholangiocarcinoma

In the past, unresectable hilar cholangiocarcinoma was treated with liver transplantation, but fewer than 20% of patients survived beyond 5 years. An adjuvant therapy protocol developed at Mayo Clinic in the early 1990s includes preoperative radiation with chemosensitization before liver transplantation.[4] Selection criteria include unresectable hilar cholangiocarcinoma that does not extend below the level of the cystic duct, absence of regional lymph node metastasis, and suitability of the patient for transplantation.

Radiation treatment is with 4,000 to 4,500 cGy administered by external beam followed by 2,000 to 3,000 cGy transbiliary catheter radiation with iridium. 5-Fluorouracil therapy is given during radiation therapy and continued up until the time of transplantation. Before transplantation, patients undergo abdominal exploration to rule out regional lymph node metastases, peritoneal metastases, or local extension of disease to adjacent tissues and organs. At exploration, approximately half of patients have locally extensive or metastatic disease precluding subsequent transplantation.

The protocol achieved excellent results. Of the first 14 patients, 12 were alive and disease-free 3 to 8 years after transplantation. Only one tumor recurred (mediastinal lymph node metastasis), and only one patient died (4 months after transplantation from unknown cause). Because of this favorable experience, criteria were broadened, and pancreatoduodenectomy with liver transplantation for locally extensive disease has been successful in several patients.

Portal Hypertension

Variceal hemorrhage and medically refractory ascites are complications of portal hypertension amenable to surgical treatment. Distal splenorenal shunt effectively treats bleeding gastroesophageal varices. This shunt is appropriate for patients with satisfactory hepatic synthetic function, absence of ascites, and hepatopedal portal venous flow. The shunt has an advantage over central shunts in that it is followed by less hepatic encephalopathy. Moreover, it does not substantially affect outcome from a subsequent liver transplantation. It can be left intact during liver transplantation without having an adverse effect on portal venous flow to the transplanted liver.

Central shunts effectively treat variceal hemorrhage and ascites. The major drawbacks are postoperative encephalopathy and worsening of liver function. Central shunts generally require ligation at the time of liver transplantation. The presence of a central shunt considerably increases the technical difficulty of subsequent liver transplantation and adversely affects outcome.

Transjugular intrahepatic portosystemic shunt is an excellent option for patients awaiting liver transplantation. It provides a central shunt with little impact on subsequent liver transplantation. Because the procedure is performed by a vascular radiologist, it avoids a major intra-abdominal open operation in the setting of severe liver disease. The shunt is easily occluded if severe encephalopathy develops. The major drawback is durability; transjugular intrahepatic portosystemic shunt necessitates frequent surveillance and intervention to maintain long-term patency.

Peritoneovenous shunt is a surgical option for the treatment of massive ascites refractory to medical therapy. These shunts are reasonably effective, but durability and risk of infection limit widespread use.

Liver transplantation is the most effective therapy for most patients with variceal hemorrhage or refractory ascites. Thus, we prefer to avoid surgical shunts—and especially central shunts—for potential transplant recipients. Transjugular intrahepatic portosystemic shunt is an excellent bridge to transplantation and a better option than a surgical shunt for most patients with progressive liver disease who are awaiting or potentially in need of liver transplantation.

EVALUATION OF PATIENTS

Evaluation of patients for liver transplantation and the medical management of patients with liver disease greatly affect the outcome of liver transplantation. Most transplant centers, including Mayo Clinic's, rely on a multidisciplinary team to evaluate and manage patients with end-stage liver disease. The evaluation includes a comprehensive medical examination, a psychosocial assessment, and patient education. Patients are initially seen by a transplant hepatologist for a full hepatology consultation. Additional consultations are obtained from the disciplines of transplantation surgery, anesthesiology and critical care, infectious disease, psychiatry, and dentistry. Other medical conditions often warrant additional consultations. A transplant nurse coordinates the evaluation and provides patient education.

The aims of the evaluation are to obtain an accurate diagnosis of the underlying liver disease, optimize medical management of the liver disease, and rule out conditions and diseases in other organ systems that would jeopardize outcome. Ultrasonography is used to screen for mass lesions in the liver and to assess the patency of the portal vein. We prefer computed tomography with an intravenous contrast agent to evaluate for possible portal vein thrombosis detected on ultrasonography. Echocardiography and a cardiac stress test (such as dobutamine stress echocardiography) are done to assess cardiac function and screen for pulmonary hypertension (which is often associated with liver disease). We perform an endoscopic cholangiography and determine the serum level of carbohydrate antigen (CA) 19-9 for all patients with primary sclerosing cholangitis to detect possible cholangiocarcinoma. A metastatic work-up is done for all patients with primary malignancies who are being considered for liver transplantation.

The transplant team closely follows all patients awaiting transplantation. Any change in a patient's medical condition may affect the likelihood of receiving a donor organ or being able to undergo transplantation if an organ became available. All patients are reevaluated every 3 to 6 months and as conditions warrant.

ORGAN ALLOCATION AND ACCEPTANCE

Organ allocation in the United States is administered through the United Network for Organ Sharing (UNOS). Distribution of cadaver donor liver is first "local" within the organ procurement organization, regional (11 UNOS regions), and then national. Allocation is based on medical status (1, 2A, 2B, and 3), blood type, and waiting time. The Child-Turcotte-Pugh score largely determines a patient's medical status. Minimal listing criteria require a Child-Turcotte-Pugh score of 7 or more to be registered on the UNOS list as a status 3 patient. A score of 10 or more is required for status 2B. Patients with lower scores but severe complications or hepatocellular carcinoma (one lesion ≤ 5 cm or up to three lesions with the largest ≤ 3 cm) also qualify for status 2B. Critically ill patients with a Child-Turcotte-Pugh score of 10 or more who require hospitalization in the intensive care unit for a major complication such as ascites, hepatorenal syndrome, variceal hemorrhage, or encephalopathy qualify for status 2A. Patients with acute fulminant liver failure, primary graft failure after transplantation, or hepatic artery thrombosis within 7 days after transplantation are registered as status 1 and benefit from regional sharing.

There is considerable controversy about UNOS organ distribution and allocation policies. UNOS is in the process of developing a new allocation policy based on severity of illness. The Mayo Model for End-Stage Liver Disease (MELD) recently was adopted by UNOS for a new allocation system that will replace the current status 3, 2B, and 2A definitions. The MELD score is based on reliable and quantitative laboratory test results (international normalized ratio for prothrombin time, bilirubin and creatinine levels) and accurately predicts the probability of death within 3 months for adults with chronic liver disease.[5] A similar model is under development for pediatric patients. Patients with acute liver disease, hepatic artery thrombosis within a week of transplantation, and primary graft failure will continue to be registered with an emergency status.

It remains the prerogative of the transplant surgeon to decide whether to accept an organ once it becomes available for an individual patient. The transplant surgeon must assess the donor situation, including the risk of graft failure, disease transmission from the donor (infection, malignancy), and size match. We have found that donor height, rather than weight, is the best predictor of organ size. In general, adults can accommodate a liver from a donor within 20 to 30 cm of their height. This margin is smaller for patients with small cirrhotic livers and an absence of ascites. The margin is larger for patients with large livers (cholestatic liver disease, Budd-Chiari syndrome) or massive ascites.

The criteria for organ acceptance have greatly expanded during the past few years with the ever worsening shortage of donor livers. Marginal organs—those at higher risk for failure or dysfunction—include organs from older donors and donors with infection, hypotension, electrolyte disturbances, high liver enzyme values, and hepatic steatosis. We now use these marginal organs more often for patients who are likely to die before another organ becomes available. We have found that livers from older donors function well after transplantation, although they do have less regenerative capacity. Indeed, many marginal organs work well, especially if preservation time and implantation time (warm ischemia) are both kept to a minimum.

Organs from high-risk donors (donors at higher risk for transmission of disease), such as those with hepatitis B or hepatitis C, can be used for similarly infected recipients. Older donors have a higher risk of harboring a malignancy that could be transplanted to the recipient. Donors with a history of high-risk behavior may transmit hepatitis or human immunodeficiency virus even if results of screening serologic tests are negative. Organs from high-risk donors may be used in situations that warrant the increased risk of disease transmission.

ABDOMINAL ORGAN PROCUREMENT IN CADAVER DONORS

Procurement of the liver is most often done in conjunction with procurement of the kidney and pancreas. All abdominal organs are removed after an in situ arterial flush with a cold organ preservation solution (ViaSpan, Barr Laboratories, Pomona, NY). As depicted in Figure 3, the solution is administered through the distal aorta with

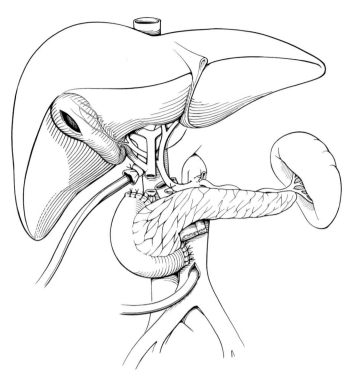

Fig. 3. Abdominal organ procurement with aortic and portal venous flush.

occlusion of the proximal aorta superior to the celiac trunk. The liver is separately infused through the portal or inferior mesenteric veins. The donor is exsanguinated through a cannula in the infrarenal inferior vena cava or, preferably, by dividing the inferior vena cava at its junction with the right atrium. Many transplant programs prefer the "rapid flush technique" with en bloc removal of the abdominal organs and separation on a back table. This technique is quick and effective, especially in hemodynamically unstable donors, and avoids potential injury to vascular structures before perfusion. We favor the alternative, which is to dissect out the abdominal organs before perfusion. Pre-perfusion dissection takes longer, but it avoids a prolonged back table dissection and potential rewarming of the organs. The dissection also enables direct portal vein cannulation, which is beneficial for both the liver and the pancreas in a combined procurement.

Abdominal multiorgan procurement is performed through a midline incision with a sternotomy. An additional supraumbilical transverse incision enables retraction of the abdominal wall flaps with towel clips and affords the best possible exposure. The liver is examined by bimanual palpation to check for mass lesions and trauma. The hilus and gastrohepatic omentum are palpated to check for replaced hepatic arteries in case a rapid flush becomes necessary. The abdomen is thoroughly examined for

organ injury (trauma victims) and unknown abnormalities (especially malignancies in older donors). In the absence of a thoracic organ procurement team, the lungs also are examined carefully for malignancy.

The right colon, small bowel, and mesentery are completely mobilized and reflected superiorly to expose the distal abdominal aorta. The aorta is encircled just above its bifurcation in preparation for later ligation and cannulation. The inferior mesenteric artery is divided, the left renal vein is exposed, and the superior mesenteric artery is exposed posteriorly and encircled with a vessel loop. The viscera are replaced, and the head of the pancreas and duodenum are retracted inferiorly to facilitate dissection of the common hepatic artery.

The gastrohepatic omentum is opened, and the right gastric artery is divided just distal to the proper hepatic artery. If present, a replaced left hepatic artery arising from the left gastric artery is dissected free from the lesser gastric curve, dividing the gastric branches. The common hepatic artery is exposed along the superior aspect of the pancreas from the gastroduodenal artery to the splenic artery. Often, a small branch to the pancreas close to the celiac trunk requires division. The proximal splenic artery is encircled with a vessel loop. The left gastric artery is divided close to its origin in the absence of a replaced left hepatic artery. Division of the celiac plexus and diaphragmatic crura exposes the celiac trunk and supraceliac abdominal aorta.

The gastroduodenal artery is divided only after celiac stenosis is ruled out. Division of this artery affords anterior exposure of the portal vein. The common bile duct is encircled to the right of the portal vein. The bile duct is sharply divided and suture ligation is done distally. Bleeding from the pericholedochal vessels often necessitates suture ligation. The gallbladder is opened, and the gallbladder and bile duct are flushed free of bile with irrigation fluid. The tissue posterior and lateral to the portal vein is divided, and a check is done for a replaced right hepatic artery arising from the superior mesenteric artery. If present, this artery is dissected free from the posterior head of the pancreas down to its takeoff from the superior mesenteric artery. The tissues between the portal vein and the common and proper hepatic arteries are divided, as is the coronary vein. The portal vein is encircled with a heavy tie in preparation for cannulation. If a delay is necessary because of procurement efforts with the thoracic organs, the liver is mobilized by taking down the bare area and retroperitoneal attachments, encircling the infrahepatic cava, and dividing the right adrenal vein.

After dissection of the liver, the pancreas is prepared for removal by dividing the gastrocolic omentum and short gastric vessels, mobilizing the spleen and pancreas, and dividing the inferior mesenteric vein. The superior border of the pancreas is dissected free to the vessel loop encircling the splenic vein. The encircled superior mesenteric artery is dissected free, and the tissues between the celiac trunk and superior mesenteric artery are divided on the anterior aspect of the aorta (which avoids injury to the renal arteries). The stomach and duodenum are infused with antibiotic solution before division of the duodenum with a stapler just distal to the pylorus. The proximal jejunum also is divided with a stapler. The transverse mesocolon is dissected free from the pancreas, dividing the middle colic vessels. The jejunal mesentery is divided to the root of the mesentery. The superior mesenteric artery and vein can be separately divided between ligatures or together after application of a 30-mm linear vascular stapler. Division of the mesenteric root enables removal of the entire small bowel and colon from the abdominal cavity. Furthermore, division of the superior mesenteric vessels avoids unnecessary perfusion of the small bowel and colon.

After administration of a large intravenous dose of heparin, the distal aorta is ligated and cannulated with cystotubing flushed with cold preservation solution. A second set of tubing is prepared for cannulation of the portal vein. In coordination with the thoracic organ procurement team, the supraceliac aorta is occluded, the aortic flush is begun, and the intrapericardial cava is cut at its junction with the right atrium to allow exsanguination. The portal vein is cannulated through a transverse venotomy. The venotomy is made so as to leave an adequate length of vein for both the pancreas and the liver grafts, usually at the level of the coronary vein. The abdominal organs are covered with saline slush and flushed with 2 to 4 L through the aorta and 1 to 2 L through the portal vein.

The thoracic organs, liver, pancreas, and kidneys are removed in order. The inferior vena cava is divided below the liver, and care is taken to avoid injury to the right renal vein. The splenic artery is divided, and the entire celiac trunk and common hepatic artery are taken with the liver. If present, a replaced right hepatic artery is taken with the proximal superior mesenteric artery; this artery is divided just distal to the origin of the replaced right hepatic artery. The liver is examined on the back table, the bile duct is flushed free of bile, and the phrenic veins along the suprahepatic cava are ligated to prepare the liver for implantation. A small wedge biopsy is taken from the inferior edge of the liver, and the liver is bagged in triplicate and placed on ice for transport to the transplant center. The donor iliac vessels are taken, one side for the liver and the other for the pancreas, to provide interposition grafts if necessary. Mesenteric lymph nodes are also taken for tissue typing and lymphocytotoxic crossmatch tests. If there is any concern about the appearance of the liver, arrangements are made for an experienced liver pathologist to examine the biopsy by frozen section in the transplant center. We generally accept donor livers with up to 30% macrovesicular steatosis.

LIVER TRANSPLANTATION: RECIPIENT OPERATION

The recipient operation involves hepatectomy, implantation of the donor liver, reperfusion, and biliary reconstruction. The operation is coordinated with the donor operation so as to minimize ex vivo preservation time. Generally, a preservation time less than 12 hours is satisfactory. Shorter times are safer for marginal organs. The recipient is brought to the operating room after arrival of the donor liver and examination of the biopsy specimen (if necessary). The patient is placed in the supine position with 90° extension of both upper extremities. Vascular access is obtained after the induction of general anesthesia. We favor insertion of a Swan-Ganz catheter through a right internal jugular line, placement of a large-bore catheter in each antecubital vein, and insertion of two radial artery catheters for monitoring and blood draws. Insertion of a Foley catheter and placement of both lower and upper body forced-air warmers (Bair Huggers, Augustine Medical, Inc., Eden Prairie, MN) complete the patient preparation. Autotransfusion and a rapid infusion pump are routinely available for all transplants.

Hepatectomy

A bilateral subcostal incision is made well below the costal margin and extended in the midline to the xiphoid. The round ligament is divided between ligatures, because there is usually recanalization of the umbilical vein in patients with cirrhosis. The falciform ligament is divided, and retraction is achieved with the rib retractor (Stieber) and the retractor holding device (Iron Intern, Automated Medical Products Corp., Sewaren, NJ) (Fig. 4). This system enables a surgeon to perform the operation with one assistant. After examination of the abdomen, the viscera are retracted inferiorly and the liver superiorly to facilitate dissection of the portal vein, hepatic artery, and bile duct. We favor dividing vascular tissue after ligation in continuity. Neural, lymphatic, and connective tissue are divided with cautery. The cystic duct, common hepatic duct, and branches of the hepatic artery are divided, and the portal vein is dissected free from the pancreas to the hilum of the liver. A clip is applied to the cystic duct stump, and a long tie is left on the distal common hepatic duct for later identification.

The left triangular ligament is divided, and the left lateral portion of the liver is mobilized by dividing its attachments to the diaphragm. This is then reflected to the vascular clamp above the anastomosis. The interposition graft is brought through the transverse mesocolon and lesser sac, anterior to the pancreas, with care taken to avoid twisting the graft.

The right liver is mobilized by dividing the right triangular ligament, the bare area on the diaphragm, and the retroperitoneal attachments with cautery. The retrohepatic inferior vena cava is mobilized at the discretion of the surgeon. Mobilization of the inferior vena cava is helpful when there is a large caudate lobe, which encircles the cava. Caval mobilization is also necessary when transplantation is performed with retrohepatic cava replacement. The right adrenal vein is divided between ties, and the infrahepatic cava is encircled. The posterior aspect of the retrohepatic cava is then dissected free from the retroperitoneum up to the diaphragm.

We favor caval-sparing hepatectomy for most liver transplant procedures. Caval-sparing hepatectomy avoids occlusion of the cava and provides better venous return to the heart and renal vein outflow than can be achieved with venous bypass. The spontaneous portosystemic collateral vessels present with chronic liver disease afford satisfactory mesenteric decompression during the anhepatic phase of the operation, and we have rarely encountered problems with visceral edema. This technique also avoids potential complications and the cost of venous bypass and shortens the anhepatic period.

The portal vein is divided between heavy ties in the hilum of the liver to begin the anhepatic phase of the operation. The liver is dissected free from the retrohepatic cava by oversewing and dividing the caudate and larger inferior hepatic venous tributaries to the cava. The right hepatic vein is encircled and divided after application of a 15- or 30-mm linear vascular stapler parallel to the inferior vena cava. The common trunk of the left and middle hepatic veins is occluded with a Klintmalm clamp, and the veins are divided at the level of the parenchyma. A cuff is fashioned by dividing the tissue between the orifices of the left and middle hepatic veins.

Implantation and Reperfusion

The donor liver is brought up to the operative field. The donor infrahepatic vena cava is oversewn with 3-0 polypropylene, and the suture is left untied so that the cava can serve as a vent during reperfusion. The donor suprahepatic cava is trimmed as short as possible, and the liver is placed in the orthotopic position and covered with laparotomy pads containing saline slush. The donor suprahepatic cava is sewn to the common trunk of the recipient left and middle hepatic veins with running 3-0 or 4-0 polypropylene suture in an everting end-to-end fashion. The liver is flushed free of preservation solution with

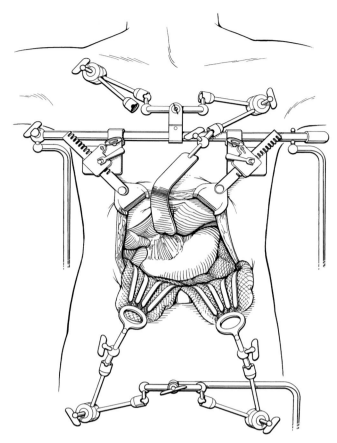

Fig. 4. Exposure procedure for liver transplantation with Stieber rib retractor and Iron Intern.

right, and the gastrohepatic omentum is divided between ligatures. The caudate lobe of the liver then is retracted anteriorly to enable division of its peritoneal attachment to the retrohepatic inferior vena cava.

We prefer to prepare for arterial reconstruction before beginning the anhepatic phase of the operation. The recipient common hepatic artery is dissected free along the superior border of the pancreas, dividing and often excising the overlying lymphatic tissue. A large coronary vein or varices frequently lie within these tissues and require suture ligation. The gastroduodenal artery is temporarily left intact.

If the recipient common hepatic artery does not appear satisfactory, donor iliac artery is used as an interposition graft between the infrarenal aorta and the donor common hepatic artery. Dividing the ligament of Treitz and retracting the duodenum and viscera to the right expose the infrarenal aorta. The aorta is encircled with umbilical tape and occluded with a Satinsky clamp. The donor proximal iliac artery is sewn to the aorta in an end-to-side fashion with 5-0 polypropylene. The aortic clamp is removed, and the interposition graft is occluded with a

500 mL of saline with added glycine (glycine rinse solution) through the portal vein, and the effluent is allowed to escape through the infrahepatic cava suture line. The arterial anastomosis may be done at this time if the recipient artery is readily available and the anastomosis can be done without undue prolongation of the anhepatic time. The arterial anastomosis should be done before reperfusion if there is a potential problem with portal flow or the portal anastomosis. The recipient gastroduodenal artery is divided between ligatures, and the common hepatic artery is divided and occluded with a small vascular clamp. The donor artery is trimmed to appropriate length and sewn to the recipient artery in an end-to-end fashion with running 6-0 or 7-0 polypropylene suture, incorporating a small "growth factor" with each tie. Alternatively, the donor artery can be sewn to an interposition graft already in place.

The recipient portal vein is occluded with a vascular clamp, divided below the ligature, and flushed to assess portal flow and remove clot that may have formed behind the ligature. The donor vessel is trimmed to appropriate length, and the two vessels are sewn together in an end-to-end fashion with running 6-0 polypropylene suture. Anterior and posterior stay sutures, retracted to the right and left, respectively, afford excellent exposure for both suture lines. A 10-mm to 15-mm "growth factor" is incorporated with each tie. The anastomoses are depicted in Figure 5.

In coordination with anesthesia, the liver is reperfused by releasing the portal vein clamp. Several hundred milliliters of blood is allowed to escape through the infrahepatic cava suture line. The suture line is then tied as the Klintmalm clamp is removed. The anastomoses are inspected for hemostasis. If not already done, the arterial anastomosis is

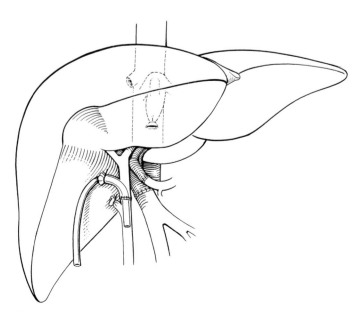

Fig. 5. Liver implantation after caval-sparing hepatectomy.

performed with a small vascular clamp on the donor artery to prevent back bleeding.

Caval Replacement and Venous Bypass

Caval replacement may have advantages over the caval-sparing technique for patients with Budd-Chiari syndrome and caval involvement, hepatocellular carcinoma adjacent to the inferior vena cava, and cholangiocarcinoma with a small or absent caudate liver between the tumor and the inferior vena cava and for patients with prior caval replacement who are having retransplantation. In general, we favor venous bypass for all caval replacement operations in adults. Pediatric patients tolerate cava occlusion well and do not require venous bypass.

After mobilization of the liver and retrohepatic inferior vena cava, the bypass tubing is connected to a pump (Biomedicus, Medtronic Inc., Minneapolis, MN) and flushed with saline. The left femoral vein is cannulated with a 17F femoral *arterial* cannula. The portal vein is cannulated with a 9F Gott shunt. Venous return is through a 12F antecubital catheter. Typically, this arrangement allows for flow of 1.5 to 2.0 L/min throughout the anhepatic phase of the operation.

The liver is removed after occlusion of the inferior vena cava above and below the liver. The upper cava cuff is fashioned from the orifices of the left, middle, and right hepatic veins in addition to the cava itself. The suprahepatic cava anastomosis is performed first. The anterior suture line of the infrahepatic cava anastomosis is left untied, and a stump of tubing is inserted to serve as a vent during reperfusion. The portal cannula is clamped and withdrawn just before the portal anastomosis. After reperfusion, the femoral cannula is removed and bleeding from the puncture site is controlled with a large stitch through the skin and subcutaneous tissue.

Portal Vein Thrombosis

Portal vein thrombosis is usually detected before transplantation with Doppler ultrasonography. We prefer computed tomography with an intravenous contrast agent to assess the mesenteric venous system when portal vein thrombosis is suspected from ultrasonography. If the confluence of the superior mesenteric vein and splenic vein is patent, portal venous flow can almost always be achieved with portal endophlebectomy. The occluded portal vein is opened with a transverse venotomy. A plane of dissection is developed circumferentially in the media of the vein wall down to the confluence of the superior mesenteric and splenic veins such that the thrombus can be extracted.

When the thrombus extends to the superior mesenteric vein, donor iliac vein may be used as an interposition graft between the recipient superior mesenteric vein and the donor portal vein. The recipient superior mesenteric vein is exposed in the root of the small bowel mesentery. The middle colic vein can be used as a guide and also divided to enhance exposure. The interposition graft is sewn to the anterior aspect of the superior mesenteric vein in an end-to-side fashion. On occasion, we have also used interposition grafts to the recipient splenic and inferior mesenteric veins to obtain portal venous inflow to the donor liver.

Biliary Reconstruction

Biliary reconstruction is most often accomplished with a duct-to-duct anastomosis. Patients with primary sclerosing cholangitis, cholangiocarcinoma, or biliary atresia require a Roux-en-Y choledochojejunostomy. A choledochojejunostomy also may be necessary when a size mismatch is large or there is a problem with approximation of the donor and recipient ducts.

A duct-to-duct anastomosis is performed after trimming of both ducts to avoid redundancy. Bleeding from the pericholedochal vessels is controlled with fine sutures. We have had the most success with an end-to-end anastomosis using running 5-0 polyglactic acid suture. We prefer leaving a biliary tube in place to obtain a cholangiogram during the immediate postoperative period. Traditional T tubes caused frequent problems with bile leaks at the duct exit site, especially after removal. We now use a firm 4F or 5F ureteral catheter threaded through the donor cystic duct stump (Fig. 6). The tube is secured with a hemorrhoid rubber band and an absorbable suture ligature to prevent leakage from the duct after tube removal. The tube also can be placed in the recipient cystic duct stump, distal to the anastomosis. In either location, the tube enables monitoring of bile output and postoperative cholangiography. The tube is left in place for 3 weeks or longer if there is a need to reassess the bile ducts. Complications from this tube have been exceedingly rare.[6]

Choledochojejunostomy requires fashioning of a Roux-en-Y jejunal limb. We prefer a short limb, 20 to 30 cm, which is often amenable to endoscopic cholangiography. The jejunojejunostomy is performed with a two-layer hand-sewn technique. In our experience, stapled anastomoses have had problems with delayed (5-7 days) postoperative bleeding. The choledochojejunostomy is performed over a 7F tube with running 5-0 polyglactic acid suture. The tube is inserted in the bowel with a 10F angiocatheter, creating a tunnel through the bowel wall (Fig. 7). The exit site is imbricated in a Witzel fashion. This tube also enables monitoring of bile output and postoperative cholangiography. As with the cystic duct tubes, complications have been exceedingly rare.

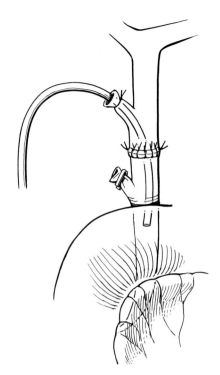

Fig. 6. Choledochocholedochostomy with biliary tube in donor cystic duct stump.

Postoperative and Long-term Care

All patients are taken directly to the intensive care unit after completion of the operation. Most patients can be extubated within several hours. All are observed in the intensive care unit for graft function and bleeding. Ultrasonography is done on the first and seventh postoperative days to confirm patency of all vessels with flows in the normal directions. Cholangiography is also done during the first week to assess the biliary anastomosis.

Immunosuppressive therapy is rapidly changing because of the emergence of more effective medications. Currently, most centers use a calcineurin inhibitor (cyclosporine or tacrolimus), corticosteroids, and often an additional agent such as azathioprine or mycophenolate mofetil. Acute rejection episodes are confirmed by liver biopsy and treated with corticosteroid bolus therapy. Graft function is monitored with laboratory tests, and dysfunction is assessed with ultrasonography, cholangiography, and biopsy as necessary. We prefer to obtain a liver biopsy specimen from all patients 1 week after transplantation in order to detect and treat early rejection. We attribute our low gram-negative bacterial and fungal infection rates to use of oral selective bowel decontamination and avoidance of antibiotics with anaerobic activity.[7]

A typical hospital stay is 7 to 14 days, depending on development of complications and the patient's condition

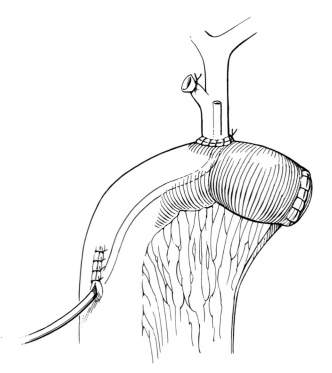

Fig. 7. Roux-en-Y choledochojejunostomy with biliary tube.

before transplantation. Most patients stay close to the transplant center for several weeks after dismissal to enable close observation and adjustment of immunosuppressive medication. A transplant nurse coordinator facilitates long-term care, including monitoring of laboratory tests and immunosuppression. We attempt to taper the dose of corticosteroids such that the therapy can be discontinued after 6 months and to achieve maintenance immunosuppression with a single agent, tacrolimus. Our multidisciplinary team approach to patient care has enabled us to achieve superb patient and graft survival rates. The 1-year and 5-year patient survival rates were 90% and 81%, respectively, for more than 1,000 patients who had liver transplantation at Mayo Clinic in Rochester, Minnesota, from 1985-2000 (Fig. 8). Although we now perform transplantation in patients with more advanced disease and worse medical conditions (due to prolonged waiting time) and patients with more technically challenging situations, patient survival increased to 92.9% at 1 year during 1996-2000 (Fig. 9).

SPLIT LIVER TRANSPLANTATION

Split liver transplantation—use of a single cadaver donor liver for two patients—evolved from experiences with graft reduction and left lateral liver transplantation from live adult donors for pediatric patients. The anatomy of the liver enables its division with preservation of arterial and portal venous inflow, biliary output, and venous outflow for each split graft. Split liver transplantation most often is used for pediatric patients requiring small grafts. The left lateral portion of the liver is an excellent graft for many pediatric patients, and the remaining right liver can be used for another patient, often a small adult. Most split grafts are done by dividing the donor liver through segment 4 with dissection of the left liver vessels along the undersurface of segment 4. An appropriate portion of segment 4 is included on the left graft to match the size of the left graft recipient. The remaining portion of segment 4 remains with the right liver but atrophies because of devascularization. It is also possible to divide a donor liver to the right of the middle hepatic vein, as is done with right liver procurement in a living donor. This type of split may be performed to enable transplantation in two patients of similar size.

Split liver grafts can be prepared before perfusion—in situ, or after perfusion and removal of the whole liver—ex vivo. The procedure was initially done ex vivo so as not to interfere with procurement of other organs. The whole organ is taken back to the transplant center, and the split is performed on a sterile back table. The ex vivo technique avoids prolongation of the procurement operation at a host donor hospital and possible blood loss and damage to other organs.

Many centers now perform the procedure in situ, and anecdotal experience suggests better subsequent graft function with the in situ technique. The technique does avoid possible prolongation of graft preservation time and facilitates use of the liver grafts in separate transplant centers.

When splitting a liver for a pediatric patient and a small adult, we generally prefer the ex vivo technique. The whole liver is brought back to the transplant center. A cholangiogram is obtained through the donor bile duct

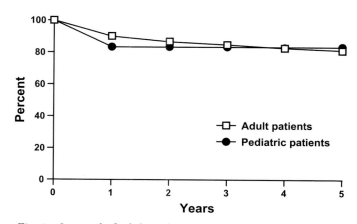

Fig. 8. Survival of adult and pediatric patients after liver transplantation at Mayo Clinic, Rochester, Minnesota, 1985-2000.

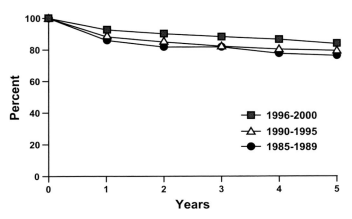

Fig. 9. Increasing survival of adult patients after liver transplantation at Mayo Clinic, Rochester, Minnesota, 1985-2000.

to rule out an anatomical abnormality (such as a right duct draining into the left duct) that precludes safe division of the liver. The liver is placed dorsal side up in cold preservation solution. The left hepatic vein orifice is examined, checking for a large inferior left hepatic vein that could preclude splitting of the liver. The proper hepatic artery is dissected free from surrounding tissue up to and past its bifurcation. The decision whether to proceed with the split then is made based on the venous, arterial, and biliary anatomy.

It is usually best to divide the right hepatic artery; because it is larger than the left, it facilitates the arterial anastomosis in the recipient. The left portal vein is encircled and divided along the undersurface of the left medial liver, segment 4. There are usually several branches to the caudate that are divided between ties. The stump on the right is oversewn. The bile duct is divided sharply; it is usually adherent to the liver capsule. The extrahepatic duct is included with the right liver because its blood supply is usually from the right hepatic artery. The left hepatic vein is excised from the suprahepatic inferior vena cava, including a small rim of cava, and the cava is closed in a longitudinal fashion. The capsule of the liver is scored and the parenchyma is divided along the plane from the left hepatic vein to the inferior aspect of segment 4. We prefer to divide the liver with an ultrasonic surgical aspirator (Cavitron, Valley Lab. Inc., Boulder, CO), individually tying larger bile ducts and blood vessels. The caudate lobe is kept with the right liver graft, although it is usually devascularized during dissection of the left portal vein. The procedure results in a right liver graft (segments 5-8) with the entire retrohepatic cava, main portal vein, extrahepatic bile duct, and right hepatic artery and in a smaller left liver graft (segments 2, 3, and a variable portion of 4) with the left hepatic vein, left portal vein, left bile duct, and common and proper hepatic artery.

The right split liver graft is implanted as if it were a whole organ. Caval-sparing hepatectomy with an anastomosis to the left-middle hepatic vein trunk and caval replacement are both possible. Implantation of the left split liver graft does require caval-sparing hepatectomy, and the short left hepatic bile duct requires reconstruction with a Roux-en-Y hepaticojejunostomy.

Split liver grafts do afford a modest increase in the number of organs available for transplantation. The procedure is as safe as graft size reduction for the primary recipient. There is a modest increase in risk for biliary complications in the secondary recipient, but that patient benefits from receiving a transplant sooner than might be possible with a whole organ graft.

LIVING-DONOR LIVER TRANSPLANTATION

Living-donor liver transplantation began with use of the left lateral portion of the liver from adult donors to children in the early 1990s. This procedure has proved to be safe for donors and effective for pediatric patients. Widespread application of this procedure, in addition to split liver transplantation, has helped reduce the number of deaths among pediatric patients on the waiting list. Adult-to-adult liver transplantation evolved from success with pediatric experiences, especially in Japan, where cadaver organ donation is problematic. Most adult-to-adult living-donor liver transplants are now right liver grafts.[8]

Advantages of living-donor liver transplantation include an opportunity for transplantation in a timely manner, a reduction in waiting time and pretransplantation morbidity and mortality, use of a healthy donor liver with minimal preservation time, increased availability of cadaver donor livers for patients unable to receive a living-donor liver, and a realistic opportunity for foreign national patients and patients with special circumstances to undergo transplantation. The disadvantages include a 0.5% to 1.0% risk of donor death, donor morbidity and discomfort, increased cost (compared with cadaver-donor transplantation) because of donor evaluation and care, and the potential for coercion of donors.

Early results with adult-to-adult living-donor liver transplantation in which left liver grafts were used were less satisfactory than those with right liver grafts. Left liver grafts were associated with more biliary complications in the recipient, presumably due to the blood supply of the left duct often coming from the right hepatic artery. Currently, most adult-to-adult transplantations are done with right liver grafts (Fig. 10 and 11). Right liver grafts provide the recipient more mass (necessary to accommodate the high portal venous flow associated with portal hypertension) and larger vessels for vascular anastomoses.

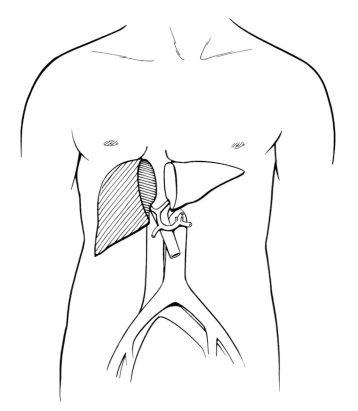

Fig. 10.   Procurement of right liver lobe from a living donor.

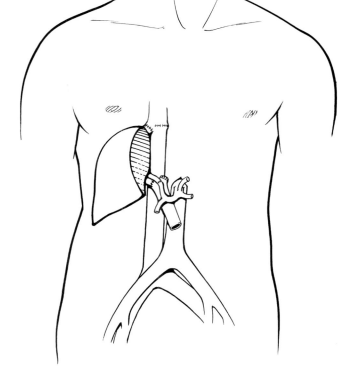

Fig. 11.   Implantation of right liver lobe into a living recipient.

Furthermore, the right liver lies in a natural position in the recipient (Fig. 11).

Need

The waiting list for cadaver donor livers has increased dramatically during the past 10 years, but the number of available organs has reached a plateau of 4,500 to 5,000 livers per year in the United States. The number of available organs has not increased despite many initiatives to increase organ donation (education of health care professionals and the public, legislative action, expansion of the donor pool with transplantation of marginal organs and organs from high-risk donors, and split liver transplantation). Patient waiting times continue to increase, and patients must become more ill to receive a cadaver-donor liver. More than 1,500 Americans die each year while awaiting liver transplantation. Furthermore, more than 4 million Americans are infected with the hepatitis C virus, and cirrhosis, liver failure, or hepatocellular carcinoma will develop in 30% to 40% within the next 5 to 10 years. Clearly, the need for transplantation is increasing and the availability of cadaver donor organs is limited.

Living-Donor Evaluation

The possibility of living-donor liver transplantation is discussed with all patients who are evaluated for liver transplantation or are awaiting transplantation. Patients likely to benefit from living donor liver transplantation are encouraged to explore this possibility with family members and close personal friends. Potential donors are encouraged by the patient to contact a living donor coordinator at the transplant center. The coordinator, who is not involved with the recipient's care, then initiates evaluation of the donor. The evaluation is done in a stepwise fashion: 1) identification and preliminary assessment, 2) comprehensive medical evaluation, 3) comprehensive psychosocial assessment to ensure donor altruism and absence of coercion, and 4) morphologic work-up to assess the suitability of the potential donor's liver for the intended recipient.

Potential donors are provided with information about liver donation, including that the risk of death is 0.5% to 1.0%. They are assured that all possible effort will be made to protect their privacy regarding medical and social issues and their decision whether or not to proceed with donation. The coordinator obtains a brief medical history. The transplant team reviews the information and decides whether the potential donor should proceed with the comprehensive medical evaluation.

The medical evaluation involves a thorough history, physical examination, and tests designed to identify any conditions likely to increase operative risk. This evaluation includes screening tests for malignancies, a cardiac stress test such as dobutamine stress echocardiography, and blood tests. A psychiatrist and social worker with expertise in transplantation see potential donors to assess family and social support and the potential donor's ability to tolerate stress.

The morphologic work-up includes a volumetric assessment of the liver with either magnetic resonance imaging or computed tomography. The potential graft size is estimated to determine the graft-to-recipient body weight ratio and the proportion of liver to be left after procurement. In general, the minimal graft-to-recipient body weight ratio is 0.8%, and the hepatic resection should not exceed 70% of the donor liver mass. Computed tomography or magnetic resonance imaging also details the hepatic venous anatomy. A percutaneous liver biopsy is done to rule out steatosis or subclinical liver disease precluding liver donation. Hepatic angiography is performed as the final study to obtain a detailed assessment of the arterial supply to the liver, including anatomical variations that could preclude donation. The biliary anatomy is not delineated before the procurement operation because of the risks associated with endoscopic or percutaneous cholangiography. Furthermore, it is unlikely that biliary anatomical variations would preclude use of the liver; multiple bile ducts can be separately sewn to a Roux-en-Y jejunal limb during the recipient operation.

Living-Donor Operation

The donor operation is performed in a large operating room to accommodate fluoroscopy, a back table, an ultrasonic dissector, and a cell saver. We use an epidural catheter to provide postoperative analgesia. A cell saver for intraoperative blood salvage is used to reduce the chance for nonautologous blood transfusion. Excellent exposure is achieved with a bilateral subcostal incision extended in the midline to the xiphoid, the standard liver transplant incision. Retraction is achieved with a rib retractor (Stieber) and retractor holding device (Iron Intern). Mobilization is limited to the right liver and division of the falciform and round ligaments.

The cystic duct is cannulated to obtain an operative cholangiogram. Cholangiography is performed with fluoroscopic guidance. Occlusion of the distal common bile duct during infusion of a contrast agent affords excellent visualization of the intrahepatic ducts. Several views are obtained to visualize the origin of the right duct(s). The gallbladder is then removed. The cystic duct is retracted anteriorly, and the right hepatic artery is dissected free from the bile duct to the liver. The right portal vein is isolated, and the right bile duct(s) is encircled.

The right liver is completely mobilized by dividing the right triangular ligament, bare area, and retroperitoneal attachments. The small inferior hepatic and caudate veins on the right are divided between ties. Large veins (≥ 5 mm) are preserved. The right hepatic vein is encircled with a vessel loop.

The right hepatic artery and portal vein are temporarily occluded to identify the plane of demarcation on the surface of the liver. Intrahepatic anatomy also may be further delineated with intraoperative ultrasonography. The liver is divided just to the right of the middle hepatic vein, from the gallbladder fossa to the vena cava. The liver capsule is scored with cautery. The parenchyma is divided with the vasculature intact. We favor use of the ultrasonic dissector and individual ligation of larger vessels and bile ducts. Often there are larger tributaries to the middle hepatic vein from segments 5 and 7 that are oversewn. These vessels are usually visible on preoperative imaging studies. The right bile duct(s) is divided during the course of the parenchymal division.

Heparin (2,000 U) is administered intravenously. The liver surfaces are carefully inspected for bile leaks and hemostasis. The right hepatic artery is divided after ligation, and the right portal vein is divided after application of a stapler at its origin. The donor cava is controlled with a side-biting clamp, and the right hepatic vein is divided, with a small rim of cava taken as a cuff. If present, a large (> 5 mm) inferior right hepatic or caudate vein also is taken with a small rim of cava. The right liver graft is passed off the operative field to the back table, where it is flushed with cold preservation solution. The graft is then bagged in triplicate in cold solution and placed on ice to await implantation.

The donor caval venotomy is oversewn. The vessels, bile ducts, and liver surface are carefully inspected for viability, leaks, and hemostasis. The falciform ligament is reapproximated to the diaphragm to prevent torsion of the remaining liver, and the incision is closed after placement of a single drain.

Recipient Operation

Recipient hepatectomy for living-donor liver transplantation is similar to that for cadaver-donor transplantation. However, the short donor artery and portal vein require high dissection of both the artery and the portal vein in the recipient. It is best to preserve the bifurcation of the portal vein and as much as possible of the right hepatic artery. Caval-sparing hepatectomy is necessary, and complete mobilization of the inferior vena cava facilitates the hepatic venous anastomosis. We generally dissect the liver from the retrohepatic inferior vena cava up to the major hepatic veins. The common trunk of the left and middle hepatic veins is divided after application of a 30-mm linear vascular stapler. The inferior vena cava is partially occluded with a side-biting clamp extending above and below the right hepatic vein. The right hepatic vein is divided, and a stump of vein is left on the cava. The venotomy can be extended on to the cava above or below the vein to accommodate the donor right hepatic vein.

Implantation of a right liver graft involves an end-to-side anastomosis of the donor right hepatic vein to the recipient inferior vena cava, usually incorporating the recipient right hepatic vein stump. The liver is usually small enough so that the posterior suture line can be sewn with the liver reflected to the left and the anterior suture line sewn with the liver reflected to the right. The anterior suture line is left untied to vent the liver during reperfusion. Any additional inferior or caudate veins are implanted in the recipient cava, with application of an additional side-biting caval clamp and a longitudinal venotomy.

The donor right portal vein is flushed with glycine rinse solution and sewn to the recipient portal vein in an end-to-end fashion incorporating a 10- to 15-mm "growth factor" with each tie. Rarely, there may be separate donor right anterior and posterior portal veins that can be sewn individually to the recipient portal vein bifurcation. Cadaver-donor iliac veins are also kept available for venous interposition grafts.

The arterial anastomosis, usually between the donor right hepatic artery and the recipient proper hepatic artery, can be done before or after reperfusion. We favor sewing the anastomosis before reperfusion; this avoids applying a small vascular clamp to the donor artery to prevent back bleeding after reperfusion. Mobilization of the common hepatic artery and division of the gastroduodenal artery provide additional length to the recipient proper hepatic artery. The anastomosis is usually done with running 7-0 polypropylene suture, incorporating a small growth factor with each tie. If it is not possible to use the recipient artery, donor or recipient gonadal and saphenous veins or cadaver donor iliac artery can be used as interposition grafts.

In coordination with anesthesia, the liver is reperfused by releasing the portal and hepatic artery clamps. Venous blood is vented through the anterior hepatic vein suture line before removal of the side-biting caval clamp.

Biliary reconstruction most often requires a Roux-en-Y jejunal limb, especially if there are multiple donor ducts. Smaller ducts require use of interrupted resorbable sutures. We prefer intubation with internal tubes such as segments of 5F pediatric feeding tubes or 2.5F pediatric umbilical catheters. A longer length of the tube is left in the bowel to enable endoscopic retrieval if necessary.

Postoperative Management

Management of living-donor liver recipients is similar to that of cadaver donor recipients. There is an increased risk for arterial thrombosis because the vessels are smaller, and we favor anticoagulation with low-molecular-weight heparin during the first week after transplantation. The recipients also have smaller grafts and may have temporary graft dysfunction. As with split liver transplantation, biliary complications arise more frequently than with whole organ grafts.

Living donors must recover from a major operation. Previously healthy, they endure incision discomfort, minor complications associated with major abdominal operations, and work-related issues such as potential loss of income. Donors must also deal with guilt associated with their decision to donate. They have confounding responsibilities—to themselves, their spouses and dependents, and the recipient. Furthermore, they have strong commitments to the recipient and must be prepared to deal with an adverse recipient outcome such as a major complication, graft loss requiring retransplantation, or death.

Living-donor liver transplantation is done only because of the shortage of cadaver donor organs. The goals of the procedure are to minimize donor risk, achieve results comparable to those with cadaver-donor transplantation, enable more patients to undergo transplantation, avoid patient death and morbidity while awaiting transplantation, and provide an opportunity for donors to give someone the gift of life.

REFERENCES

1. 2001 Annual Report of the U.S. Scientific Registry for Transplant Recipients and the Organ Procurement and Transplantation Network: Transplant data: 1991-2000. U.S. Department of Health and Human Services, Health Resources and Services Administration, Office of Special Programs, Division of Transplantation, Rockville, Maryland, United Network for Organ Sharing, Richmond, Virginia

2. Wiesner RH: Current indications, contraindications, and timing for liver transplantation. *In* Transplantation of the Liver. Edited by RW Busuttil, GB Klintmalm. Philadelphia, WB Saunders Company, 1996, pp 71-84

3. Harnois DM, Steers J, Andrews JC, Rubin JC, Pitot HC, Burgart L, Wiesner RH, Gores GJ: Preoperative hepatic artery chemoembolization followed by orthotopic liver transplantation for hepatocellular carcinoma. Liver Transpl Surg 5:192-199, 1999

4. De Vreede I, Steers JL, Burch PA, Rosen CB, Gunderson LL, Haddock MG, Burgart L, Gores GJ: Prolonged disease-free survival after orthotopic liver transplantation plus adjuvant chemoirradiation for cholangiocarcinoma. Liver Transpl 6:309-316, 2000

5. Kamath PS, Wiesner RH, Malinchoc M, Kremers W, Therneau TM, Kosberg CL, D'Amico G, Dickson ER, Kim WR: A model to predict survival in patients with end-stage liver disease. Hepatology 33:464-470, 2001

6. Steers JL, Marsman W, Rodriquez L, Krom RAF, Wiesner RH: An improved technique of biliary drainage following orthotopic liver transplantation with choledochocholedochostomy (abstract). Liver Transpl Surg 1:450, 1995

7. Wiesner RH, Hermans PE, Rakela J, Washington JA II, Perkins JD, DiCecco S, Krom R: Selective bowel decontamination to decrease gram-negative aerobic bacterial and *Candida* colonization and prevent infection after orthotopic liver transplantation. Transplantation 45:570-574, 1988

8. Marcos A: Right lobe living donor liver transplantation: a review. Liver Transpl 6:3-20, 2000

Chapter 15

BILIARY STONE DISEASE

Shaheen Zakaria, M.D.
Salman Zaheer, M.D.
John H. Donohue, M.D.

Biliary calculus disease is one of the most common disorders affecting the gastrointestinal tract. With the advent of laparoscopic cholecystectomy, management of this disease has evolved at an unprecedented rate. Numerous other options, including endoscopic papillotomy, dissolution therapy, and extracorporeal shock wave lithotripsy, provide nonsurgical alternatives for selected patients with gallstones.

HISTORICAL OVERVIEW

By the 18th century, pain and fluctuating jaundice were recognized as typical symptoms of gallstone disease. The first cholecystostomy, performed by John S. Bobbs in a patient with hydrops of the gallbladder, was described in the *Transactions of the Indiana State Society* in 1868. Carl Langenbuch performed the first cholecystectomy on July 15, 1882. The first cholecystectomy in the United States was performed in 1886 by Justus Ohage. Four years later, Ludwig Courvoisier successfully removed a stone from the common bile duct. In the 1980s, nonoperative management of biliary stone disease by oral and contact dissolution agents and lithotripsy was introduced. Mouret, in Lyon, revolutionized the management of cholelithiasis after the first report of laparoscopic cholecystectomy in 1984.[1]

Diagnostic techniques were developed in parallel with therapeutic advances. In 1924, Warren Cole and Ewarts Graham obtained the first cholecystogram in humans. Operative cholangiography was described by Mirizzi in 1932, and cholescintigraphy, high-resolution oral cholecystography, and percutaneous transhepatic and endoscopic retrograde cholangiography have been developed since 1950.[1] In the past 2 decades, advances have been made in ultrasonography, computed tomography, and various choledochoscopic techniques.

BILIARY ANATOMY

The liver, gallbladder, and extrahepatic bile ducts are derived from the caudal portion of the foregut.[2] The gallbladder is a pear-shaped organ with a bulbous fundus at the distal end, followed by the body, which tapers into a narrow neck, and the diverticulum-like Hartmann pouch. The fundus and the caudal surface of the gallbladder are covered by visceral peritoneum reflected from the liver. The rest of the organ is bound to the right inferior fossa of the liver by connective tissue and blood vessels.[3] The cystic duct has the spiral valves of Heister, which can make catheterization difficult. The cystic duct is usually 2 to 4 cm long, but the length varies enormously. It curves medially and caudally in the hepatoduodenal ligament, normally entering the lateral aspect of the supraduodenal portion of the common hepatic duct at an acute angle to form the common bile duct.

The left medial and lateral segmental ducts join to form the left hepatic duct that runs caudally to the medial segment of the left liver in a horizontal direction to join the right hepatic duct. The right hepatic duct is usually formed from the union of the right posterior and right anterior segmental ducts, just within the parenchyma of the liver. The confluence of the right and left hepatic ducts most commonly occurs extrahepatically, anterior to the portal venous bifurcation. Anomalies of the right ductal system, particularly the right posterior duct, which may join the left hepatic duct or enter the common hepatic duct separately, are common. The common hepatic duct descends in the hepatoduodenal ligament and is joined by the cystic duct to form the common bile duct. The common bile duct is approximately 8 cm in length with an internal diameter varying from 4 to 6 mm. The common bile duct is divided into four segments: supraduodenal, retroduodenal, intrapancreatic, and intraduodenal. The distal end of the common bile duct is encircled by the sphincter of Oddi, which regulates the flow of bile into the duodenum.[2]

The gallbladder receives arterial blood from the cystic artery, normally a branch of the right hepatic artery. The cystic artery is usually found within the triangle of Calot, defined as the area bordered by the cystic duct, the common hepatic duct, and the inferior border of the liver. The cystic vein empties into the portal vein. Lymphatics from the gallbladder drain to the cystic duct lymph node located near the neck of the gallbladder. The retroduodenal, common hepatic, and right hepatic arteries supply the extrahepatic biliary ducts. Their branches form a plexus on the duct that includes two axial vessels at the medial (3 o'clock) and lateral (9 o'clock) aspects of the duct. The venous drainage from the extrahepatic bile duct is to the portal vein. Lymph nodes lying posterior to the common hepatic and common bile duct receive lymphatic drainage, which then passes to the common hepatic, celiac, retroduodenal, retropancreatic, and para-aortic nodal groups.[3] The gallbladder and biliary tree are supplied by the autonomic nervous system. The hepatic branches of the vagal nerve provide parasympathetic innervation, and the celiac plexus supplies the sympathetic neural component.[4]

Variations in the anatomy are important for the surgeon, and detailed descriptions can be attained from a major hepatobiliary surgical text.[5]

GALLSTONES

Ten percent of the U.S. population harbor gallstones, and approximately 500,000 cholecystectomies are done annually in the United States. The prevalence of gallstone disease in white women ranges from 5% to 15% in those younger than 50 years and is approximately 25% in older women. The prevalence ranges from 4% to 10% in white men younger than 50 years and from 10% to 15% in older men.[6] The prevalence is higher in Latinos and Native Americans.

Predisposing factors for gallstone formation are older age, female sex, pregnancy, ethnicity, family history, obesity, rapid weight loss, ileal disease and other intestinal conditions that impair bile salt reabsorption, total parenteral nutrition, exogenous estrogen use, and, probably, diabetes mellitus.

Classification of Gallstones
Gallstones are biochemically and pathophysiologically classified into cholesterol and pigmented stones.

Cholesterol Stones
Approximately 75% of gallstones are cholesterol stones.[7] Cholesterol gallstones form when the cholesterol concentration in the bile exceeds the ability of bile to retain it in solution (Fig. 1). Crystal nuclei form and grow to form stones. Lithogenic bile most commonly results from increased biliary cholesterol content, which accompanies increasing age and higher serum estrogen levels. Some ethnic groups have decreased bile acid synthesis or a combination of high biliary cholesterol and decreased bile salts. Several interrelated factors also contribute to stone formation. Cholesterol hypersecretion induces gallbladder hypomotility and increased mucin production, accelerating the formation of cholesterol crystals and gallstones.[8] Infection is not an etiologic factor for cholesterol gallstones.

Pigmented Stones
A quarter of gallstones are pigmented stones.[7] Their major component is calcium hydrogen bilirubinate. They develop as a result of increased β-glucuronidase activity and a higher concentration of unconjugated bilirubin. Eighty percent of pigmented stones are *black pigment stones* that

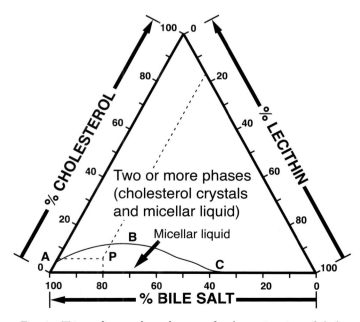

Fig. 1. Tricoordinate phase diagram for determination of cholesterol saturation index. Gallstones form when tricoordinate points (P) lie above the line A B C. (From Small DM: Gallstones. N Engl J Med 279:588-593, 1968. By permission of the Massachusetts Medical Society.)

contain calcium hydrogen bilirubinate, calcium phosphate, and calcium carbonate in a mucin glycoprotein matrix. The pigment is chemically degraded and polymerized during its retention in the gallbladder. Because of the polymerization of bilirubin, these stones are insoluble in all solvents. Clinical conditions that increase unconjugated bilirubin secretion or impair the secretion of bile salts result in the precipitation of calcium bilirubinate and cause the formation of black pigment stones.[9] These conditions include chronic liver disease, chronic hemolysis, administration of total parenteral nutrition, and Crohn's disease. Black pigment stones are formed exclusively in the gallbladder in a sterile environment.

The pathogenesis of *brown pigment stones* is the enzymatic hydrolysis of biliary lipids by bacterial enzymes that produce bile supersaturated with the calcium salts of unconjugated bilirubin, saturated long-chain fatty acids, and deconjugated bile acids. The calcium bilirubinate in these stones can be resolubilized. Brown pigment stones constitute 20% of all pigmented stones and develop from clinical conditions that produce an infected obstruction of the common bile duct, including stones and strictures.[9]

Biliary Sludge
Biliary sludge is the thick mixture of gallbladder mucoprotein and tiny entrapped cholesterol crystals. It may be an intermediate step in gallstone formation. In most patients, sludge disappears spontaneously; however, in 8% asymptomatic gallstones develop and in 13% symptomatic gallstones requiring cholecystectomy develop.[10]

Clinical Presentations of Gallstones

Asymptomatic Gallstones
In many patients with gallstones, symptoms never develop. Comfort and associates[11] studied 112 patients at Mayo Clinic between 1925 and 1934. These patients had asymptomatic gallstones discovered during laparotomy for unrelated abdominal conditions. With biliary colic, with or without jaundice, used as the end point, symptoms developed in 19% of patients during 10 to 20 years of follow-up, and the average annual incidence was 1.4%. Acute cholecystitis, gallstone pancreatitis, and other complications occur at rates of 1% to 2% per year in asymptomatic patients.[12] Because of this, cholecystectomy is generally reserved for patients who have gallstone symptoms or complications. Patients being considered for cardiac or lung transplantation are routinely screened for gallstones. Patients considered candidates for laparoscopic cholecystectomy should have the operation electively, before they are placed on the active

waiting list for transplantation. They tolerate elective cholecystectomy much better than immunosuppressed patients who have had transplantation and in whom complications of gallstone disease develop.[13]

Biliary "Colic"
Biliary colic is a misnomer in that, typically, biliary symptoms have the gradual onset of a steady right upper quadrant or epigastric pain, not a colicky pain. This occurs when a stone is impacted in the cystic duct or at the Hartmann pouch (Fig. 2 A). Episodes of biliary pain typically develop after meals and are often associated with nausea and sometimes vomiting. The pain lasts for minutes to hours and may radiate to the back or to the tip of the right scapula. The physical findings during an episode of biliary pain are not impressive. The pain resolves spontaneously in most patients and diminishes with parenteral analgesics.

Some patients with cholelithiasis complain of vague abdominal discomfort, localized either in the right upper quadrant or in the epigastrium. They may be unable to specify the relation between the meals and the pain. Symptoms not likely to be related to gallstones include heartburn, eructation, and increased flatulence.

Chronic Cholecystitis
Chronic cholecystitis is a pathologic diagnosis. *Primary* chronic cholecystitis lacks an initial acute inflammatory phase and is characterized by a thin-walled gallbladder with intact villous mucosa. The inflammatory cell infiltrate is primarily lymphocytes.

Secondary chronic cholecystitis develops after one or more bouts of acute cholecystitis. The acute inflammatory changes of the gallbladder wall, which may include edema, leukocyte infiltration, and mucosal necrosis, all resolve over 3 to 4 weeks. These findings are replaced by granuloma formation after 1 week, and fibroblast proliferation and collagen formation occur by 2 to 3 weeks. Occasionally, buried mucosal crypts (Rokitansky-Aschoff sinuses) occur within the gallbladder muscularis. The gallbladder mucosa becomes attenuated in chronic cholecystitis with loss of the usual villous appearance, and the muscular layer becomes fibrotic and thickened (Fig. 2 B).

Acute Calculus Cholecystitis
Obstruction of the cystic duct or Hartmann pouch by a stone may initiate acute cholecystitis (Fig. 2 C). The persistence and severity of pain serve to distinguish biliary colic from acute cholecystitis clinically. Biliary colic rarely lasts for more than a few hours, whereas acute cholecystitis often lasts for several days without treatment. The duration and degree of obstruction are probably the two

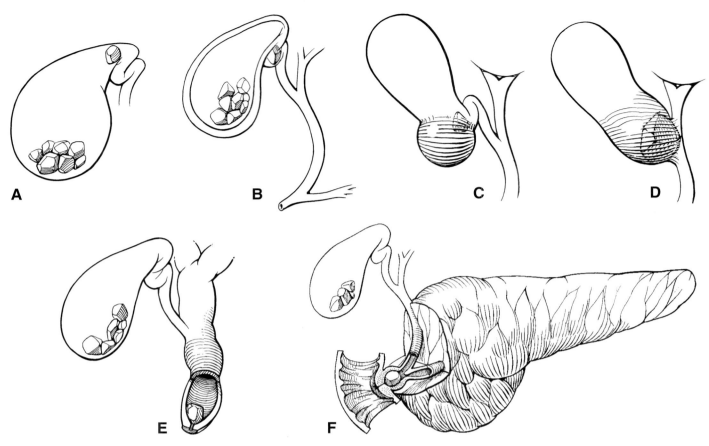

Fig. 2. Clinical presentations of cholelithiasis. (A), Gallstone obstructing cystic duct causes pain. (B), Chronic cholecystitis due to obstruction of cystic duct. (C), Acute cholecystitis. (D), Mirizzi syndrome. (E), Choledocholithiasis. (F), Pancreatitis due to choledocholithiasis.

variables that determine the extent of inflammation and the progression of disease. In more than 90% of patients with acute cholecystitis, the obstruction of bile outflow is relieved spontaneously and the inflammation subsides. In approximately 5%, the blockage persists with distention and inflammation of the gallbladder, which in turn produce vascular compromise with ischemia and necrosis of the gallbladder.

The role of bacteria in the pathogenesis of acute cholecystitis is unclear. Gut flora can be cultured from the bile or gallbladder wall in 50% to 75% of patients with acute cholecystitis.[14] The initiating factor in acute cholecystitis is ductal obstruction, whereas infection is a secondary event. Another important factor in the pathogenesis of acute cholecystitis may be erosion of the mucosa by a stone. The loss of mucosal integrity allows bile salts access to deeper tissue planes with solubilization of cell membrane lipids. Lecithin, pancreatic enzymes, and prostaglandins also may add to the gallbladder inflammation. Hydrops of the gallbladder results from obstruction of the cystic duct by a stone with chronic distention of the gallbladder but no acute inflammation. This suggests that acute

cholecystitis is not an inevitable consequence of long-standing gallbladder outflow obstruction.

The usual presenting symptom of acute cholecystitis is pain, usually localized tenderness in the right upper quadrant, often with radiation toward the tip of the scapula. Between 60% and 75% of patients report a history of one or more similar episodes. Diaphragmatic irritation can lead to referred pain in the right shoulder. Nausea and vomiting occur in 60% to 70% of patients.

Acute cholecystitis results in a fever in 80% of patients. Elderly and immunocompromised patients (e.g., those receiving steroids) may not mount a febrile response. The most reliable clinical finding is tenderness in the right upper quadrant or the epigastrium or both. Rebound and referred tenderness are generally indicative of more advanced disease. In 33% of patients, the examiner may palpate a mass in the right upper quadrant, usually the omentum overlying the inflamed gallbladder. Jaundice occurs in 10% of patients without common ductal disease. Hyperbilirubinemia in these patients may be the result of obstruction of the bile duct from choledochal sphincter spasm induced by the inflammatory process or, rarely, entry of bile pigments into the circulation by way of the damaged gallbladder mucosa. However, concomitant choledocholithiasis most often causes jaundice. Common duct stones are present in 10% to 15% of patients with acute cholecystitis.

Abnormal laboratory findings include leukocytosis in 85% of patients, increased total serum bilirubin level in 50%, and increased serum amylase level in 33%.

Emphysematous Cholecystitis

Emphysematous cholecystitis, a potentially lethal complication, develops in about 1% of patients with acute cholecystitis. It is more common in the elderly and in patients with diabetes. The radiographic demonstration of gas within the gallbladder wall occurs as a result of gas-producing bacteria. *Clostridium perfringens* is the most commonly cultured organism. Gangrene and perforation of the gallbladder are common sequelae, warranting emergency cholecystectomy.

Mirizzi Syndrome

Mirizzi syndrome refers to a benign mechanical obstruction of the common hepatic duct by a large stone impacted at the neck of the gallbladder or cystic duct (Fig. 2 *D*). This rare entity was found in 0.5% of 2,000 biliary operations performed at Mayo Clinic during 10 years.[15] McSherry et al.[16] proposed a classification system based on the presence or absence of a cholecystocholedochal fistula. Type I Mirizzi syndrome is the acute variant with external compression by a stone, without a fistula. Type II is a chronic condition in which a cholecystocholedochal fistula has occurred as a result of stone erosion.

The clinical presentation of Mirizzi syndrome mimics that of acute cholecystitis with hyperbilirubinemia. Ultrasonographic features suggestive of the diagnosis include an abnormally thickened gallbladder, large gallstones, and diffuse proximal bile duct dilatation. If Mirizzi syndrome is suspected preoperatively, endoscopic cholangiography can better define the biliary anatomy and demonstrate a small eccentric bile duct stricture adjacent to the stone. Some patients require urgent cholecystectomy for complicated acute cholecystitis. When the hepatic ductal compression has been caused by acute inflammation, the common hepatic duct almost always returns to normal diameter after the offending stone has been removed. During the operative dissection, care must be taken to avoid creating a defect in the common hepatic duct. An open cholecystectomy is a better option if the diagnosis is known preoperatively. The gallbladder should be mobilized from the fundus toward the common bile duct. When the inflammation is too severe to excise the gallbladder completely, the gallbladder can be opened and impacted stones

removed. If copious bile returns with removal of stone, Mirizzi syndrome is confirmed. In type I Mirizzi syndrome, the gallbladder can be removed completely or partially. In type II Mirizzi syndrome, complete removal of the gallbladder leads to a lateral defect of the common hepatic duct or complete duct transection. A cuff of the gallbladder can be saved for flap closure of the hepaticodochotomy or, alternatively, a hepaticoduodenostomy, a Roux-en-Y hepaticojejunostomy, or a jejunal serosal patch can be used to close the defect in the common hepatic duct. An operative cholangiogram is imperative to ensure integrity of the biliary tree and to document ductal stones. Common bile duct exploration should be undertaken only when safe. In other patients, an endoscopic sphincterotomy should be performed postoperatively.[15,17,18]

Gallstone Ileus

Gallstone ileus is a mechanical obstruction of the intestine by a gallstone. The erosion of a gallstone through the wall of the gallbladder into adjacent intestine or colon occurs by two mechanisms. Pressure necrosis of the gallbladder wall results from a large gallstone or from acute cholecystitis by way of acute inflammation and necrosis. The duodenum, jejunum, or the hepatic flexure of the colon may become adherent to the gallbladder. The duodenum is the most frequent site of fistula formation, followed by hepatic flexure of colon and, least often, the jejunum. The cholecystoenteric fistula may close spontaneously or remain patent. A large stone entering the small bowel becomes impacted in the narrowest part of the intestine, namely, the distal ileum. A classic presentation of gallstone ileus includes a history of episodes of partial small bowel obstruction as the stone passes toward the narrower distal small intestine (tumbling obstruction). Plain abdominal radiographs often show air in the biliary tree, distended loops of obstructed small intestine, and a radiopaque gallstone in the right lower quadrant. Ultrasonography may show residual gallstones or dilatation of the biliary tree or both.

The treatment of gallstone ileus necessitates relief of the intestinal obstruction, usually with an enterotomy and removal of the impacted stone. Definitive correction of the biliary-enteric fistula at the same procedure is not advocated in most patients.[19] The mortality associated with concurrent surgical treatment of intestinal obstruction and the cholecystenteric fistula is higher than that with relief of intestinal obstruction alone (16.9% and 11.7%, respectively).[20] The fistula closes spontaneously in many patients. A persistent cholecystenteric fistula is suggestive of additional stones within the gallbladder or common duct. Only symptomatic patients should have an elective cholecystectomy and fistula closure at a later date.

Diagnosis of Gallstones

Three diagnostic tests are established for the preoperative evaluation of cholelithiasis: real-time ultrasonography, cholescintigraphy, and oral cholecystography. Abdominal ultrasonography is the preferred test for evaluating patients with suspected cholelithiasis and cholecystitis. Real-time ultrasonography provides information about the presence of gallstones, the size of the gallbladder, the thickness of the gallbladder wall, the presence of pericholecystic fluid collection, ductal size, and the presence of ductal stones (Fig. 3). Only 1% to 1.5% of the examinations are nondiagnostic; the sensitivity is 90% to 98%, and the specificity is 70% to 98%.[21] Ultrasonography also can evaluate the liver, pancreas, and right kidney, detecting some nonbiliary causes of right upper quadrant pain. Additional advantages include the absence of radiation exposure and no requirement for normal digestive and hepatic function.

Radionuclides attached to iminodiacetic acid compounds are rapidly extracted from the bloodstream by the liver and excreted into bile to provide a direct image of the gallbladder and biliary tract. The major value of biliary radioscintigraphy is to determine the patency of the cystic duct. Normally, the scan outlines the functional liver and extrahepatic biliary tract, including the gallbladder. Later images show the radionuclide flowing into the upper small intestine. In acute calculus cholecystitis, for which cholescintigraphy has nearly 100% sensitivity, the gallbladder is not visualized because of cystic duct obstruction (Fig. 4). Complete hepatic or common bile duct obstruction can be detected, but the resolution is insufficient to differentiate stones from tumor or other lesions. In a usual clinical setting of right upper quadrant tenderness, fever, and leukocytosis, gallstones on ultrasonography confirm the diagnosis of acute cholecystitis.[21] Biliary scintigraphy may be useful for establishing a precise diagnosis in patients with acalculous cholecystitis, atypical symptoms, or confounding diagnoses.

When the ultrasonographic examination is inconclusive, oral cholecystography may play a role in the evaluation for suspected gallbladder disease. Oral cholecystography relies on the excretion of a halogenated compound by the liver into bile. The gallbladder is visualized after the reabsorption of water and solutes results in concentration of the contrast medium. Although the accuracy of oral cholecystography has been reported to be as high as 95%, several important conditions preclude satisfactory examination, including acute illness, poor patient compliance, inability to absorb the tablets, and jaundice (total bilirubin > 2 mg/dL) or hepatic dysfunction. Oral cholecystography provides data about gallbladder function, cystic duct patency, and gallstone composition and numbers. This constitutes important information for patients undergoing gallstone dissolution or extracorporeal shock wave lithotripsy.

Management of Gallstones

Surgical Management

Surgical management remains the best means of intervention for most patients with symptomatic cholelithiasis. Medical therapies are considered second-line therapy and are used in patients unfit for any surgical intervention.

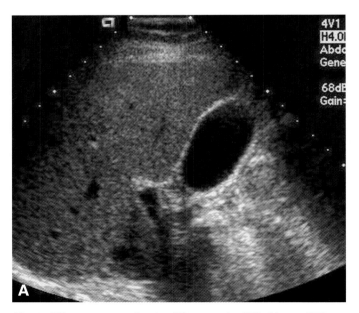
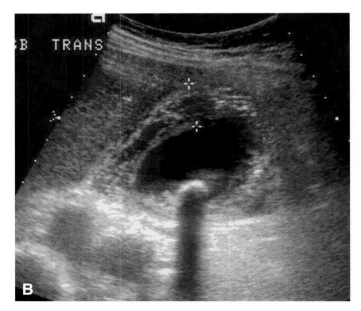

Fig. 3. Ultrasonograms showing (A) *normal gallbladder and* (B) *acute cholecystitis with a gallstone and a thickened, irregular gallbladder wall.*

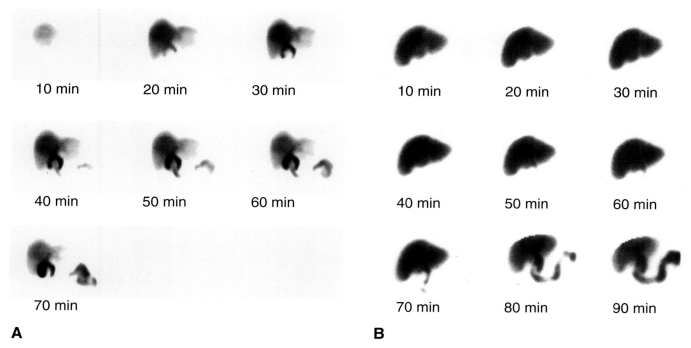

10 min   20 min   30 min   10 min   20 min   30 min

40 min   50 min   60 min   40 min   50 min   60 min

70 min   70 min   80 min   90 min

A   **B**

Fig. 4. Hepatoiminodiacetic acid scans showing (A) normal biliary excretion and gallbladder filling and (B) the absence of gallbladder uptake as a result of acute cholecystitis.

Cholecystostomy

Cholecystostomy, or drainage of the gallbladder to the exterior with a tube, is most commonly indicated for patients with acute cholecystitis who are too ill to tolerate general anesthesia and cholecystectomy. It also may be used in moribund patients for the treatment of acute empyema or hydrops of the gallbladder. Occasionally, it is used for decompression of the biliary tract in a patient with cholangitis; however, endoscopic or transhepatic drainage is more reliable and safer.

Cholecystostomy is usually accomplished percutaneously by using radiologic (ultrasonography) guidance or, infrequently, with an open technique. The open technique is used rarely, such as when the inflammatory changes in the hepatoduodenal ligament do not permit safe cholecystectomy or when acute decompensation occurs intraoperatively.

With the *percutaneous technique* (Fig. 5 A), the patient receives antibiotics (third-generation cephalosporin), and the procedure is performed with the patient under local anesthesia. With ultrasonographic or computed tomographic guidance, a 22-gauge needle is advanced through the caudal edge of the liver into the gallbladder. After appropriate intraluminal positioning is confirmed by the aspiration of bile, a 10F or 12F catheter is inserted into the gallbladder over a guidewire. The catheter has a self-retention mechanism (e.g., pigtail configuration) that prevents dislodgment.

The catheter is anchored to the skin and connected to a drainage bag. Although this is usually an effective procedure, the patient must be observed carefully. If clinical improvement does not occur, further treatment may be needed for gangrenous cholecystitis or cholangitis.

In the *open cholecystostomy technique* (Fig. 5 B), local anesthesia is preferred, and a small right subcostal incision is used. The gallbladder is freed of adhesions, and the surrounding area is packed off with laparotomy pads to prevent spillage of infected bile. A large-caliber aspiration needle attached to a syringe or a trocar with a suction attachment is inserted into the fundus of the gallbladder. The gallbladder contents are aspirated. A limited (1.5 cm) incision is made at the aspiration site, and the interior of the gallbladder is examined digitally. All stones are removed with a forceps. Any stone impacted at the neck of the gallbladder or within the proximal cystic duct usually can be freed by external manual compression or with an intraluminal scoop or biliary grasping instrument plus external manipulation. After all accessible stones are removed, a Malecot or Foley catheter is placed within the gallbladder. The tube is anchored to the gallbladder with a purse-string absorbable suture and brought out through the abdomen wall with a separate limited incision in the right upper quadrant.

The operative mortality rate of emergency open cholecystostomy may be as high as 20% to 25% in patients

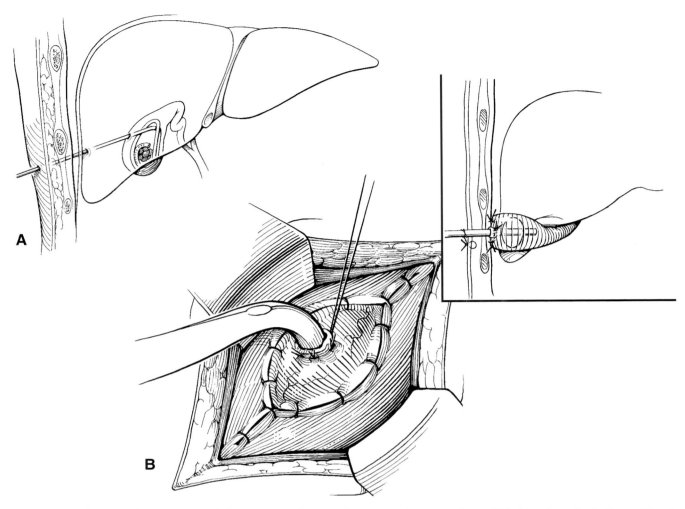

Fig. 5. (A), *Technique of percutaneous cholecystostomy, showing drainage catheter entering gallbladder through the liver.* (B), *Open cholecystostomy tube placement with catheter secured with purse-string sutures and the gallbladder secured to the abdominal wall* (inset).

receiving a general anesthetic. An open cholecystostomy performed with the patient under local anesthesia is associated with a mortality rate of 10%, and percutaneous cholecystostomy has a mortality rate of approximately 1.5%.[22,23] It is important to keep patients under observation and plan a cholecystectomy at a later date.

Open Cholecystectomy
Cholecystectomy, usually for symptomatic gallstones, is one of the mainstays of general surgical practice. Traditionally, this procedure has been performed through an open upper abdominal incision and abdominal exploration, which necessitates several days of postoperative hospitalization and 4 to 6 weeks of convalescence. The rapid popularization and widespread acceptance of laparoscopic cholecystectomy have relegated open cholecystectomy to patients untreatable laparoscopically because of lack of access or complicated biliary disease.

The indications for open cholecystectomy are as follows:
Symptomatic gallstones in patients with uncorrected coagulopathy
Calcified gallbladder wall (porcelain gallbladder) (laparoscopic cholecystectomy can be tried first, unless there is known, or a high suspicion of, gallbladder cancer)
Large (≥ 3 cm) gallstones that predispose the patient to carcinoma of the gallbladder should be treated prophylactically with cholecystectomy[24] (laparoscopic cholecystectomy can be tried first, unless there is known, or a high suspicion of, gallbladder cancer)
Intra-abdominal adhesions or technical difficulties preventing proper delineation of biliary anatomy by laparoscopy
Complications during laparoscopic cholecystectomy (e.g., ductal injury or leak, bleeding, bowel injury)
Unexpected findings during laparoscopic cholecystectomy (e.g., cholecystenteric fistula, malignancy)

Patients with severe chronic lung disease unable to withstand pneumoperitoneum. Such patients are rare and laparoscopic cholecystectomy usually can be accomplished with lower-pressure insufflation

Open cholecystectomy is typically performed with the patient under general anesthesia, but regional anesthesia can be used in selected patients. The patient is positioned supine on the operating table, and prophylactic antibiotics (third-generation cephalosporin) are given when anesthesia is induced. Prophylaxis for deep venous thrombophlebitis should be used in patients at increased risk for this complication. After the abdomen and lower chest are prepared and draped, a right subcostal (Kocher), upper midline, or transverse right upper quadrant incision can be used for exposure. Once the abdominal cavity is entered, full exploration is undertaken. The hepatic flexure of the colon is retracted inferiorly and held with moist laparotomy pads. An automatic retractor system can be used to lift the abdominal wall cephalad and to the patient's right, and a second retractor is placed to hold the liver in the cephalad direction. Adhesions between omentum or viscera and the gallbladder are divided sharply. The fundus and infundibulum of the gallbladder are held with Kelly clamps and retracted laterally.

A longitudinal incision is made in the peritoneum forming the anterior leaf of the hepatoduodenal ligament, and the cystic duct is identified where it arises from the gallbladder infundibulum. Blunt dissection in this area with a Kitner or sponge stick facilitates identification of the cystic duct. The cystic duct is dissected circumferentially and ligated close to the gallbladder with absorbable suture. When indicated, cholangiography is used to facilitate making a small cystic ductotomy and cannulating the duct. Fluoroscopic cholangiography is superior to static imaging. Once cholangiography is completed, the catheter is removed and the cystic duct is ligated with an absorbable suture and divided distally. The cystic artery usually lies cephalad to the cystic duct. It is isolated, ligated, and divided. Both the cystic duct and the cystic artery have considerable variation in anatomy. It is critical to ligate both of these structures close to the gallbladder to avoid injury to major ducts and the proper or right hepatic artery.

The gallbladder is dissected from the liver bed by scoring the parietal peritoneum near the gallbladder-liver junction with electrocautery and peeling the gallbladder away from the liver, leaving Glisson's capsule on the gallbladder fossa and not perforating the gallbladder. The gallbladder fossa is irrigated with saline and examined for hemostasis. The abdominal wound is closed in a standard fashion.

For patients in whom the neck of the gallbladder, the cystic duct, and the cystic artery are involved by dense inflammatory changes, the gallbladder should be excised from the fundus toward the infundibulum (retrograde dissection) to lessen the risk of bile duct injury.

Postoperative care includes narcotic analgesia, early ambulation, chest physiotherapy, deep-breathing exercises, and early institution of a general diet with the return of bowel function. The average duration of hospitalization is 2 to 5 days, but it is prolonged in patients with advanced or severe acute cholecystitis.

The mortality rate from open cholecystectomy has remained relatively constant between 1.5% and 2%.[25] Biliary fistulas occur in 0.6% of patients, and ductal injuries occur in about 0.16%.[26] The incidence of retained common bile duct stones depends on the number of stones present or whether any are cleared from the common bile duct (see below).

Laparoscopic Cholecystectomy

In 1987, Dubois developed a technique for laparoscopic cholecystectomy.[27] The first clinical series in the United States was reported by Reddick and Olsen in 1989.[28] The first peer-reviewed report in the United States, presented by Zucker and colleagues before The Society for Surgery of the Alimentary Tract in 1990, confirmed the safety and efficacy of the procedure.[29] A National Institutes of Health Consensus Conference held in 1992 concluded that laparoscopic cholecystectomy was the "treatment of choice" for most patients with symptomatic gallstones.[30]

All patients with symptomatic gallstones who can tolerate general anesthesia and have transabdominal access to the right upper quadrant without concurrent pathologic conditions not amenable to laparoscopic intervention are considered candidates for laparoscopic cholecystectomy. Patients with uncorrectable coagulopathy, usually from underlying liver disease, do poorly when treated with any operative procedure, especially laparoscopic techniques in which the limited access impedes hemostatic procedures. The most common factor preventing laparoscopic cholecystectomy is the presence of dense or diffuse intra-abdominal adhesions. Multiple previous incisions may not pose any problem, and an exploratory laparoscopy should be considered before proceeding with laparotomy. Dense inflammatory changes often limit transperitoneal access to the right upper quadrant or prevent proper delineation of the biliary anatomy. In both instances, open cholecystectomy is indicated. Organ enlargement, most commonly distended bowel, and the near-term uterus also may impair the laparoscopic approach to the gallbladder. Although laparoscopy in the first trimester of pregnancy has no specific risk, elective operation should be avoided. Laparoscopic cholecystectomy is possible, and preferably performed, in the second trimester.

After preoperative evaluation of the biliary tract disease and overall patient status, the procedure should be conducted electively, when possible. The patient is placed supine. A single dose of parenteral prophylactic antibiotic (third-generation cephalosporin) is administered just before the operation. Nasogastric or orogastric and urinary bladder catheters are optional. Prophylaxis for deep venous thrombophlebitis is used only in patients at increased risk.

The first assistant and scrub nurse stand to the patient's right. A set of sterile laparotomy instruments should be available in case urgent conversion to an open procedure is necessary. An electrocautery unit and suction irrigation equipment complete the technical array (Fig. 6).

The patient is positioned in a moderate Trendelenburg position (approximately 20° head down) while the first trocar or pneumoperitoneum is introduced. Either an open or a closed technique can be used for initiating pneumoperitoneum with a small incision in the region of the umbilicus.

The patient is then placed in reverse Trendelenburg position, with the right side rotated 20° anteriorly to aid exposure of the right upper quadrant. After placement of the laparoscope, the remaining cannulas are placed under video control: a 10-mm trocar in the epigastrium (primary

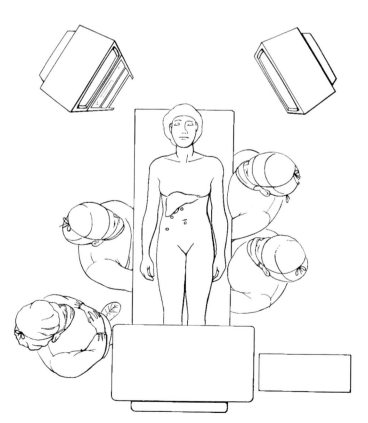

Fig. 6. Patient positioning for laparoscopic cholecystectomy with four instrument port sites and sites marked.

surgical port) and two 5-mm trocars, one near the anterior axillary line several centimeters below the costal margin and the other 2 to 4 cm below the right costal margin near the midclavicular line or more laterally, especially if operative cholangiography is performed. Occasionally, a fifth instrument port may be needed to retract a ptotic or enlarged left lateral sector of the liver.

A brief abdominal inspection should be performed before starting the cholecystectomy. A ratcheted grasper is placed through the lateral subcostal port for cephalad traction of the gallbladder fundus, and a second grasper is placed through the medial subcostal port for retraction of Hartmann's pouch.

The surgeon can readily proceed without an assistant by manipulating the midclavicular port with the left hand to provide countertraction on the gallbladder. Adhesions to the gallbladder are best taken down with careful blunt dissection, because an adherent duodenum can be inadvertently perforated with electrocautery or scissors. Adhesions to the liver should be cauterized or lysed sharply, because stripping of Glisson's capsule can cause troublesome bleeding. Any blood in the field will absorb a great deal of light and darken the operative field considerably.

Dissection is begun on the lateral surface of the gallbladder, where the risk of injury to the bile duct or of encountering major blood vessels is minimal. The gallbladder is retracted medially and the peritoneum alone is incised initially. The dissection can then be deepened, with care taken to avoid division of any structure that is not transparent when surrounded by a laparoscopic instrument. During this portion of the procedure, a ductal structure, usually the cystic duct, will become visible at the medial aspect of the field. After the lateral peritoneum is opened, the gallbladder is retracted laterally and slightly caudad, and only the peritoneum is incised on the medial surface of the gallbladder. The dissection is deepened, with the surgeon staying on the wall of the gallbladder to avoid injury to structures in the hepatoduodenal ligament. The cystic artery is normally isolated during this portion of the dissection. Before it is clipped and divided, its course onto the gallbladder wall should be confirmed so as to avoid hepatic arterial injuries. More caudally and posteriorly, the junction of the gallbladder and cystic duct will become apparent, and a large window usually can be opened by cleaning the tissue away from the gallbladder, thoroughly isolating the cystic duct. Lateral and caudad retraction on the gallbladder during this dissection orients the cystic duct at a right angle to the hepatoduodenal ligament, providing a larger margin of safety against injury to the common duct. Identification of the cystic duct-common hepatic duct confluence is not warranted. This maneuver is impossible when the two ducts are fused or the cystic duct crosses posterior to the hepatic duct, both common anatomical variants.

The debate regarding routine versus selective operative cholangiography continues without resolution. There are indisputable reasons for operative cholangiography, including unclear anatomy during the operation, suspicion of common duct stones based on clinical, laboratory, or intraoperative (large cystic duct) findings, concerns about an intraoperative ductal injury, and surgical training to ensure that operative cholangiography can be performed when needed.

A cholangiogram is obtained by placing a clip at the junction of the gallbladder and the cystic duct and making a limited incision in the wall of the proximal cystic duct with microscissors. The lack of return of bile through the ductotomy implies distal obstruction. Visible stone debris found in the cystic duct should be extracted or milked back from the common duct by gentle compression of the distal cystic duct when there is not prompt backflow of bile from the ductotomy. A cholangiogram catheter is placed through the medial 5-mm subcostal port and placed within the cystic duct. Various fine-gauge catheters are available. A beaded catheter placed with a specialized clamp to secure the catheter in position, a balloon-tip catheter that holds the catheter in place atraumatically, and catheters that can be secured with a surgical clip placed gently on the catheter itself are all options for cholangiography.

Operative cholangiography is best performed with a portable fluoroscopy unit, preferably a high-resolution digital system. A sterilely covered C arm can be manipulated by the surgeon while injecting radiographic contrast material and viewing the fluoroscopic images. Radiopaque instruments must be removed or repositioned during cholangiography. Hard copies of selected images should be made for a permanent record. After completion of cholangiography, the cystic duct is occluded by placing two titanium clips on the distally dissected portion of the duct. The cystic artery should also be occluded with two clips and both structures divided with scissors. In patients with known residual common duct stones or a wide or friable cystic duct, a ligature also should be placed for a more secure closure.

The gallbladder then is removed from the undersurface of the liver, usually with cautery dissection. It is important to stay next to the gallbladder wall; dissection in an improper plane leads to unnecessary bleeding from the liver, possible bile leak from the gallbladder fossa, or perforation of the gallbladder with spillage of bile and stones. Before the gallbladder fundus is detached from its bed, the gallbladder fossa and gallbladder hilum are inspected for hemostasis and secure clip placement.

The gallbladder is freed from its final attachments, and if only small stones are present the gallbladder can be removed easily through the epigastric port. If large stones are present, the epigastric incision will need to be enlarged or the camera can be moved to the epigastric port and the gallbladder removed through a larger incision at the umbilicus port site. Because the abdominal wall is thinner at the umbilicus, enlargement of the incision is easier. The gallbladder is partially delivered through the incision and opened, and bile is aspirated before removal. If multiple stones are present, they may be extracted with a forceps before delivery of the gallbladder or the incision may be enlarged. Friable gallbladders and specimens filled with stones should be placed in a specimen bag before extraction to avoid stone spillage.

After the gallbladder is removed, the camera is replaced in the umbilical port, the liver is retracted cephalad, and the operative field is irrigated with saline to remove blood clots and debris. The cephalad cannulas are removed under laparoscopic visualization. After release of the pneumoperitoneum, fascial sutures (0- or 1-gauge absorbable suture material) are placed at the 10-mm cannula sites and the skin of all four incisions is closed with absorbable subcuticular sutures. If a nasogastric or orogastric tube and Foley catheter were placed, they are removed before the patient leaves the operating room.[24,31]

Patients are offered oral intake, as tolerated, the day of operation and are usually dismissed within 24 hours if they are comfortable, ambulatory, tolerating a regular diet, and urinating normally. Patients are advised to gradually return to normal activities as tolerated; the mean recovery time is 7 to 10 days.

The outcome of more than 100,000 laparoscopic cholecystectomies, including our experience at Mayo Clinic between July 1990 and December 1991, is summarized in Tables 1 and 2.[32] Proceeding to laparotomy for technical considerations or intraoperative complications should not be regarded as a complication. The most feared complication of any cholecystectomy is injury to the major extrahepatic biliary tree. The incidence of this complication increased with the advent of laparoscopic cholecystectomy, but it has declined with greater surgeon experience.[33] Although the mortality with laparoscopic cholecystectomy is less than that with open cholecystectomy, the younger median age of patients and the less complex nature of the gallstone disease treated laparoscopically explain much of this discrepancy. The number of cholecystectomies performed in the United States has increased substantially (about 30%).[34,35] This increase may explain the comparable mortality of the two procedures.

Table 1.—Results of Laparoscopic Cholecystectomy

Country, year of report	No. of patients	Conversion to laparotomy, %	Complications, %	Duct injuries, %	Mortality, %	Mean no. of hospital days
Europe, 1991	1,236	3.6	1.6	0.3	0	3
United States, 1991	1,518	4.7	5.1	0.5	0.07	1.2
United States, 1992	1,983	4.5	2.1	0.3	0.10	NS
International, 1992	2,671	3.7	NS	0.2	0.11	NS
Canada, 1992	2,201	4.3	6.4	0.1	0	1
Belgium, 1992	3,244	6.5	6.4	0.5	0.20	NS
Switzerland, 1992	1,091	8.1	2.8	0.5	0	NS
France, 1992	2,955	4.8	3.4	0.6	0.20	NS
France, Belgium, 1992	6,091	5.3	4.6	0.2	0.20	NS
United States, 1993	77,604	NS	2.0	0.6	0.04	NS
United States, 1993	9,597	NS	2.5	0.3	0.04	NS
Switzerland, 1994	3,722	7.0	4.8	0.6	0.08	4.4
Mexico, 1994	2,399	4.1	8.9	0.3	0.12	NS
Mayo Clinic, 1991	542	5.0	NS	0	0	1

NS, not stated.
From Donohue.[24] By permission of Current Medicine.

Early Versus Delayed Cholecystectomy
Traditionally, the standard practice for patients with acute cholecystitis was to admit them to the hospital for intravenous treatment with fluids and antibiotics. An elective cholecystectomy was performed 6 to 10 weeks later, allowing time for the inflammatory process to settle. This traditional approach has been challenged by several studies.[36,37] These studies demonstrated similar morbidity and mortality patterns for early cholecystectomy, in addition to the reduced hospitalization costs and fewer recurrent episodes of acute cholecystitis. In this era of laparoscopic cholecystectomy, an initial attempt to remove the inflamed gallbladder laparoscopically should be considered within 72 hours of the onset of symptoms. Delay beyond this time leads to a substantially higher incidence of conversion to open cholecystectomy. In the setting of acute inflammation, this procedure should be undertaken only by experienced surgeons. The conversion rate to open cholecystectomy in this situation is 20% to 30%, whereas it is 3% to 5% in an elective setting.[37]

Medical Management

Medical Dissolution
The hypothesis that altered hepatic secretion of cholesterol is the primary pathogenesis of cholesterol gallstones has prompted numerous attempts at gallstone dissolution. Chenodeoxycholic acid was first used to reduce bile

lithogenicity, but currently ursodeoxycholic acid is used for stone dissolution because it is a safer and a more effective drug. The incidence of complete stone resolution depends heavily on several factors. Patient selection criteria may be divided into superoptimal, optimal, and acceptable (Table 3).[38]

With use of an optimal dose of bile acids for 2 years, bile acid therapy (BAT) completely dissolves gallstones in 90% of patients who have superoptimal criteria, but only 3% of patients meet these guidelines. The cure rate with BAT when criteria are optimal is approximately 60% (15% of patients with gallstones). When the selection criteria are acceptable, the cure rate decreases to 40%. Among patients with symptomatic cholelithiasis, 70% are ineligible for BAT because of a nonfunctioning gallbladder on oral cholecystography, stone size more than 20 mm in diameter, calcified gallstones, severe biliary symptoms, or complications and other exclusions. Within 2 months of discontinuing BAT after complete dissolution of gallstones, bile becomes saturated with cholesterol. Recurrent gallstones develop in 50% of treated patients (10% per year for 5 years, with few recurrences thereafter).[38]

Limited information is available about the outcome of BAT for noncholesterol, calcium bilirubinate stones. Some investigators have demonstrated stone solubilization with a combination of a mucolytic agent, a chelating agent, and a strong detergent.

BAT is a costly regimen and should be reserved for fragile patients who are not candidates for invasive treatments.

Table 2.—Bile Duct, Vascular, and Bowel Injuries During 77,604 Laparoscopic Cholecystectomies

Injury site	No. of patients	No. of patients requiring laparotomy
Bile duct		
Common bile duct	271	239
Common hepatic duct	38	38
Right hepatic duct	8	7
Aberrant duct	48	25
Cystic duct	94	38
Total	459 (0.59%)	347
Blood vessels		
Retroperitoneal		
Aorta	13	12
Inferior vena cava	5	3
Iliac artery	11	10
Iliac veins	7	6
Subtotal	36 (0.05%)	31
Porta hepatis vasculature		
Hepatic artery	44	36
Cystic artery	73	63
Portal vein	5	4
Subtotal	122 (0.16%)	103
Other intra-abdominal vessels	35 (0.05%)	24
Total vascular injuries	193 (0.25%)	158
Bowel		
Small intestine	57	42
Colon	35	26
Duodenum	12	12
Stomach	5	5
Total	109 (0.14%)	85

From Deziel et al.[32] By permission of Excerpta Medica.

Contact Dissolution

Instilling potent organic solvents directly into the gallbladder through a percutaneous cholecystostomy catheter can dissolve some gallstones. Mono-octanoin and methyl-*tert*-butyl ether are the two best-studied solvents. Neither agent is suitable for oral ingestion. High-risk patients with symptomatic stones and those who refuse operation are potential candidates for contact dissolution. In the high-risk patient with acute cholecystitis, a percutaneous cholecystostomy catheter can be placed for gallbladder decompression until the acute inflammation settles, after which dissolution can be performed, only if the cystic duct is patent (Fig. 7).[39] Patients most likely to respond to contact dissolution are similar to those with favorable criteria for BAT. Only noncalcified, cholesterol stones can be solubilized. Computed tomography with thin sections of the gallbladder is done to rule out calcification. Unlike BAT, multiple large stones may be effectively treated with contact dissolution. Complete dissolution with methyl-*tert*-butyl ether can occur within 12 hours. The experience with this technique is limited, but 30% of patients have stone recurrence at 2 years of treatment and 60% within 5 years. Documented side effects include transient abdominal pain, nausea, emesis, duodenitis, and complications related to catheter placement.

Biliary Lithotripsy

Extracorporeal shock wave lithotripsy (ESWL) was first developed in the early 1980s by Dornier, a German aircraft

Table 3.—Selection Criteria for Bile Acid Therapy (BAT) and Extracorporeal Shock Wave Lithotripsy (ESWL)

	BAT	ESWL
Superoptimal	Stones ≤ 5 mm in diameter	
	Cholesterol stones	
	Functioning gallbladder	
	Nonobese patient	
	Mild biliary symptoms	
	No liver disease	
Optimal	Stones ≤ 10 mm in diameter	Single stone ≤ 20 mm in diameter
	Cholesterol stones	Radiolucent stone
	Functioning gallbladder	Functioning gallbladder
	Nonobese patient	
	Mild biliary symptoms	
Acceptable	Stones ≤ 20 mm in diameter	Stones ≤ 30 mm in diameter
	Minimal stone calcification	Three or fewer stones
	Functioning gallbladder	Functioning gallbladder
		Calcified rim < 3 mm

From Strasberg and Clavien.[38] By permission of the American Association for the Study of Liver Diseases.

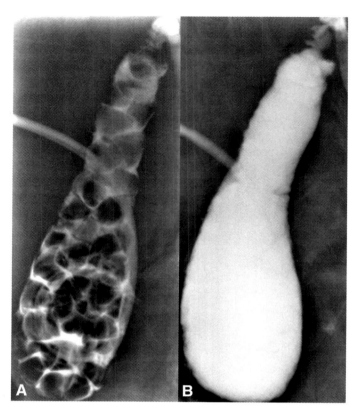

Fig. 7. Percutaneous cholangiograms obtained before (A) *and after* (B) *contact dissolution treatment with methyl-*tert-*butyl ether.*

manufacturer, after the successful use of this device in the treatment of kidney stones. After the equipment was modified to fragment gallstones, Sackmann and associates[40] reported the first successful management of gallstones in 1988. The incidence of success depends on selection criteria (Table 3). Only 7% of patients with symptomatic gallstones are optimal candidates for ESWL, but cure rates of 95% have been achieved. For patients with acceptable criteria, 16% with symptomatic gallstones can be treated, and the primary success rate is 80%.[38] About 75% of patients are ineligible for ESWL because they have more than three gallstones, stones more than 30 mm in diameter, a nonfunctional gallbladder, or a densely calcified stone. The results of combination therapy with ESWL and litholytic medications are better. The recurrence rates of gallstones after ESWL are 7% at 1 year, 13% at 3 years, and 31% at 5 years.[41] Sixty percent of patients with recurrence have symptomatic gallstone disease. Complications include biliary colic, acute cholecystitis, cholangitis, and pancreatitis.

Potential advantages of ESWL include avoidance of surgical intervention and a high rate of acceptance by the patients. Because laparoscopic cholecystectomy is associated with short hospital stay and fast recovery time

and it eliminates the recurrence of gallstones and the development of gallbladder malignancy, the use of biliary lithotripsy is extremely limited.

CHOLEDOCHOLITHIASIS

Common duct stones are found in 8% to 16% of patients who have cholelithiasis (Fig. 2 *E* and *F*). The incidence of common duct stones increases with age. Of all patients who undergo cholecystectomy, 1% to 2% have symptomatic retained stones that will necessitate further intervention.[42]

Classification and Pathogenesis of Choledocholithiasis

Common bile duct stones are classified according to their location, the timing of formation, and their composition. *Primary* bile duct stones form de novo within the bile ducts and are usually composed of calcium bilirubinate (brown pigment stones). They form as a result of biliary stasis and infection. Clinical settings associated with primary duct stones are posttraumatic biliary stricture, a narrowed biliary enteric anastomosis, stenosis or dysfunction of the sphincter of Oddi, sclerosing cholangitis, and Asian cholangiohepatitis. In addition to stone extraction, the cause of bile stasis must be alleviated to prevent primary stone recurrence. Bile duct stones detected after a 2-year symptom-free period following cholecystectomy are also classified as primary duct stones. *Secondary* bile duct stones are usually cholesterol stones, formed in the gallbladder, that have passed into the choledochus by way of the cystic duct or a cholecystocholedochal fistula. Complete removal of secondary choledocholithiasis alone is usually adequate therapy for this condition.

Clinical Presentation of Choledocholithiasis

Asymptomatic Stones

Stones may be chronically present in the common bile duct without causing problems. Because of the uncertainty about the natural history of common duct stones and the severity of potential complications, documentation is an indication for their removal.

Intermittent Jaundice

Patients with common bile duct stones typically present with intermittent pain and obstructive jaundice (icterus, pruritus, dark-colored urine, and acholic stools). This symptom complex arises from a nonimpacted stone causing intermittent obstruction. Clinical examination during symptoms will reveal signs of obstructive jaundice. Laboratory results reveal mild hyperbilirubinemia and an increased serum alkaline phosphatase level.

Cholangitis

When a stone in the common bile duct becomes impacted, causing complete obstruction (Fig. 2 *E*), the patient more frequently experiences pain in the right upper quadrant accompanied by fever and jaundice (Charcot's triad). Occasionally, these symptoms are accompanied by septic shock and neurologic signs of confusion or coma (Reynold's pentad), signaling the presence of suppurative cholangitis, a condition in which infected bile is under pressure within the biliary tree. The patient will have all the signs of septic shock and obstructive jaundice. Investigations reveal leukocytosis, hyperbilirubinemia, and increased levels of alkaline phosphatase, serum glutamic-oxalacetic transaminase, and serum glutamic-pyruvic transaminase. This condition necessitates immediate resuscitation, broad-spectrum parenteral antibiotics (i.e., levofloxacin and metronidazole), and emergency decompression of the ductal system to prevent death. About 15% of patients with cholangitis will meet the criteria for emergency treatment.[43,44] The remaining patients respond to fluid resuscitation and intravenous antibiotics, which allow timely diagnostic intervention and management.

Biliary Pancreatitis

Acute pancreatitis develops in about 4% to 8% of patients with cholelithiasis.[45] Biliary pancreatitis results from choledocholithiasis, producing obstruction and spasm of the ampullary sphincter mechanism, which result in the reflux of bile into the pancreatic duct (Fig. 2 *F*). Patients present with severe epigastric pain, nausea, and vomiting. There may be accompanying abdominal distention, ileus, and tenderness in the epigastrium. The pancreatitis is mild and self-limiting in 75% of patients. Biliary pancreatitis may progress to a fulminant illness characterized by local pancreatic and peripancreatic necrosis, along with multiple-system organ failure in the remaining 25%, although only 3% to 5% have severe complications of this condition.[46,47] Serum amylase or lipase levels are used to secure the diagnosis of pancreatitis. The diagnosis of biliary pancreatitis is supported by increased levels of bilirubin, alkaline phosphatase, and serum glutamic-pyruvic transaminase. Patients may be assessed for severity of disease using the criteria proposed by Ranson (Table 4).[48]

Patients with mild pancreatitis have zero to two Ranson criteria, whereas those with severe pancreatitis meet three or more criteria. Patients in the first category require only bowel rest and adequate parenteral fluids, whereas the remaining patients require more intensive care.

In 1988, Kelly and Wagner[46] reported a prospective, randomized trial that compared early operation with conventional therapy (i.e., letting the acute inflammation

Table 4.—Ranson Criteria: Clinical and Biochemical Variables Correlating With the Severity of Acute Pancreatitis

At admission or diagnosis
  Age > 55 years
  Leukocyte count > 16,000/mm^3
  Blood glucose > 200 mg/100 mL
  Serum lactate dehydrogenase > 350 IU/L
  Serum glutamic-oxalacetic transaminase > 250 Sigma Frankel units
During initial 48 hours
  Hematocrit value decreases more than 10%
  Blood urea nitrogen increases more than 5 mg/100 mL
  Serum calcium level is less than 8 mg/100 mL
  Arterial PO$_2$ is less than 60 mm Hg
  Base deficit more than 4 mEq/L
  Estimated fluid sequestration more than 6 L

From Ranson.[48] By permission of the American College of Gastroenterology.

resolve and doing an elective cholecystectomy at a later date) in 165 patients with biliary pancreatitis. In patients with severe pancreatitis, the mortality rate was 48% in those randomized to early operation and 11% in controls. For patients with mild disease, the timing of operation did not appear to affect outcome. Mortality was 3% for early operation and 0% for delayed operation. A prospective, randomized trial of urgent endoscopic retrograde cholangiography (ERC) and papillotomy versus standard conservative treatment was reported by Neoptolemos et al.[49] The 121 patients with gallstone pancreatitis were stratified according to severity; they underwent ERC and, if stones were present in the common bile duct, papillotomy. The morbidity, mortality, and duration of hospitalization were considerably less in patients with severe biliary pancreatitis who underwent urgent ERC and papillotomy.

On the basis of these studies, patients with mild biliary pancreatitis should be managed conservatively until clinical resolution of the pancreatitis, but they should undergo laparoscopic cholecystectomy with intraoperative cholangiography shortly thereafter, preferably during the same hospitalization. Most of them already have passed their stones and will not need common duct manipulation. Patients with severe biliary pancreatitis should have urgent ERC and, if stones are present, papillotomy and stone extraction. A laparoscopic or open cholecystectomy should be undertaken later as dictated by the clinical situation.

Diagnosis of Choledocholithiasis

The diagnosis of choledocholithiasis is based on a patient's clinical findings, biochemical tests, biliary ultrasonography, and cholangiography.

Ultrasonography of the gallbladder and common bile duct is a simple, safe, and cost-effective way to diagnose biliary outlet obstruction. A common bile duct diameter more than 1 cm in association with jaundice has a positive predictive value for choledocholithiasis of 90% to 100%. Ultrasonography is not reliable, however, for direct visualization of common bile duct stones.

Precise delineation of the intrahepatic and extrahepatic biliary tree, localization of anatomical abnormalities, and information about the size, location, and number of stones can best be achieved with ERC (Fig. 8). The ability to provide therapeutic intervention makes ERC superior to ultrasonography and percutaneous transhepatic cholangiography. Specific indications for percutaneous transhepatic cholangiography include failure of ERC to visualize the common bile duct, lack of endoscopic access because of previous operation (gastrectomy with Roux-en-Y or Billroth II anastomosis), or unavailability of a skilled endoscopist to perform ERC.

Management of Choledocholithiasis

Our management of choledocholithiasis is considered in relation to various clinical scenarios (Fig. 9).

Suspected Choledocholithiasis

Patients thought to have choledocholithiasis on the basis of clinical presentation, biochemical profile, and ultrasonography are candidates for ERC or laparoscopic stone extraction. If stones are documented on ERC, endoscopic papillotomy and stone extraction are undertaken. An elective laparoscopic cholecystectomy then follows. For unfit or elderly patients, successful endoscopic clearance of the common bile duct is often sufficient therapy and cholecystectomy is not mandatory.[50] For patients in whom ERC is unsuccessful or in an institution where laparoscopic removal is preferred, laparoscopic cholecystectomy with intraoperative cholangiography is performed. If this shows stones, common bile duct exploration, either laparoscopically or by an open surgical method, is undertaken, depending on the expertise available.

Choledocholithiasis Discovered During Laparoscopic Cholecystectomy and Intraoperative Cholangiography

In about 7% of patients who undergo elective cholecystectomy, unsuspected common bile duct stones are found on routine intraoperative cholangiography. In many institutions, postoperative ERC, endoscopic papillotomy, and stone extraction is the procedure of choice. The success rate of ERC stone removal is 85% to 90% (up to 95% in some institutions); thus, it is a valid option in the postoperative setting.[51] Patients who have stones less than 2 mm in

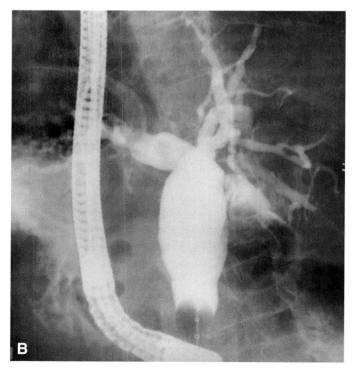

Fig. 8. Endoscopic retrograde cholangiograms showing (A) *multiple common duct stones and* (B) *completion film after sphincterotomy and endoscopic stone extraction.*

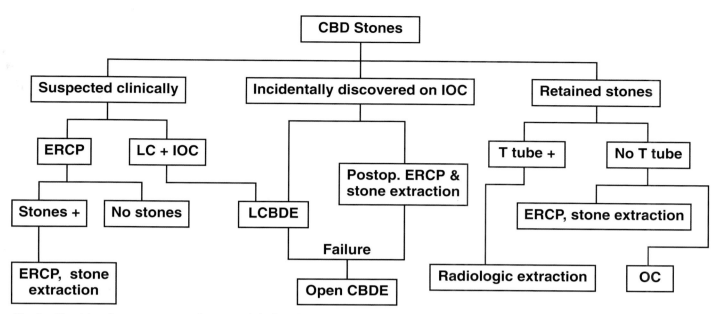

Fig. 9. Algorithm for management of common bile duct (CBD) stones. ERCP, endoscopic retrograde cholangiopancreatography; IOC, intra-operative cholangiography; LC, laparoscopic cholecystectomy; LCBDE, laparoscopic common bile duct exploration; OC, open cholecystectomy.

diameter can be observed, unless symptoms develop, because most small stones pass spontaneously. Patients with multiple, large (> 2 cm) common bile duct stones or a large dilated common bile duct require open choledocholithotomy and choledochoenterostomy. Patients with a known periampullary duodenal diverticulum (e.g., on intraoperative cholangiography) or previous gastric resection with Billroth II anastomoses will not generally be candidates for endoscopic retrograde cholangiopancreatography. If feasible, a laparoscopic common bile duct exploration should be undertaken in these patients (Fig. 10).

Retained Common Bile Duct Stones
The incidence of retained stones is a function of the number of stones found at exploration of the common bile duct. If no stones are present, the incidence is only 1% to 2%, but it approaches 80% when five or more stones have been extracted.[13] These usually represent stones missed in the intrahepatic biliary tree. In addition to operation, other methods are now available for the treatment of such patients. The selection of therapy is based on local expertise and the presence or absence of a T tube placed during a previous choledochotomy.

For patients with retained common bile duct stones and a T tube, radiologic extraction is the usual method of stone retrieval. This is an outpatient procedure performed 4 to 8 weeks postoperatively, after a good T-tube tract has formed. The T tube is removed and a Dormia basket is passed into the mature T-tube tract. The basket is manipulated under fluoroscopic guidance to remove

stones. The success rate ranges from 80% to 97%. Dissolution therapy and fragmentation with ESWL are other options but have lower success rates.

For patients with retained common bile duct stones and no T tube in place, endoscopic retrograde cholangiopancreatography with endoscopic sphincterotomy and stone extraction is the procedure of choice. About 5% of

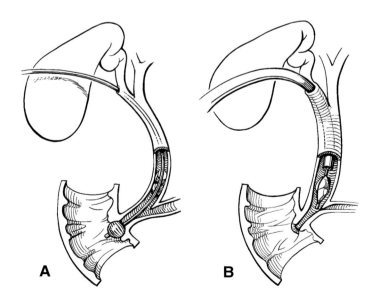

Fig. 10. Management of choledocholithiasis with laparoscopic transcystic duct approach to the common bile duct. (A), Balloon catheter removal of stones. (B), Removal with flexible choledo-choscopy with wire basket snare.

patients with retained common bile duct stones require an operation because of the inability to remove the stones nonsurgically.[51] Reoperation should be planned approximately 3 months after the initial operation, whenever possible, to allow the inflammatory process to regress. The simplest procedure is to reexplore the common bile duct, remove the stones, and place a T tube. If the common bile duct is quite large or common bile duct stones develop after initial choledochotomy, a biliary enteric anastomosis should be performed to reduce the risk of further primary choledocholithiasis formation. Side-to-side or end-to-side choledochoduodenostomy and Roux-en-Y choledochojejunostomy are operative options. In a patient with a thin-walled, small common bile duct, transduodenal sphincteroplasty is the operation of choice.[13]

Open Common Bile Duct Exploration

The indications for open common bile duct exploration were well delineated above.

The initial positioning, incision, and exposure are the same as those for an open cholecystectomy. A complete Kocher maneuver is necessary to mobilize the duodenum and allow palpation of the intrapancreatic portion of the common bile duct and the major papillae. The parietal peritoneum that holds the second and third portions of the duodenum is sharply incised, allowing for finger dissection posterior to the duodenum and the pancreas. The common bile duct is identified in the hepatoduodenal ligament by clearance of its anterior and lateral surface. Following the cystic duct or its stump distally to its junction with the common hepatic duct facilitates identification. Fine-needle aspiration of bile from the common bile duct ensures correct identification. Operative cholangiography is performed. The duct is opened longitudinally cephalad to the duodenum with a No. 15 scalpel blade and Potts scissors. After this, a biliary Fogarty catheter is passed through the ampulla into the duodenum. On inflation of the balloon, the catheter can be palpated through the duodenal wall and is gently withdrawn against the ampulla. The balloon is deflated and then gently reinflated as it is pulled back into the bile duct. The balloon is then brought back to the choledochotomy site while inflation pressure is maintained. Stones are removed and a similar procedure is repeated for the proximal biliary tree.

The next step in stone retrieval is irrigation of the biliary tree. External compression, stone forceps, and scoops can gently be used for fixed stones. Care must be taken to avoid injury to the ductal wall, ductal mucosa, and the ampulla. Choledochoscopy, either rigid or flexible, provides the opportunity for directly visualizing common bile duct stones that might otherwise be overlooked. Wire baskets can be passed through the working channel of the choledochoscope for stone extraction (Fig. 11 *A*).

After successful removal of all ductal stones, a latex T tube is positioned in the common bile duct. The T tube is sized to fit comfortably in the duct. The arms of the T tube should be short and beveled to aid in easy removal. The back wall of the T tube is also removed to facilitate its insertion and removal. The tube should be brought out at the lower extremity of the choledochotomy, which is closed snugly around the tube with absorbable sutures (Fig. 11 *B*). The tube is brought out through a separate lateral stab incision in as direct a route as possible. This provides easier instrumentation in instances of retained stones. The tube is irrigated to check for bile leaks and to ensure a watertight closure. A completion cholangiogram through the T tube confirms clearance of the common bile duct. A closed-suction catheter is placed in the subhepatic space. The T tube is attached to a drainage bag, and the abdominal incision is closed in the usual fashion.

Routine postoperative care is generally the same as that for open cholecystectomy. The T tube is left in situ for 3 to 6 weeks to allow a tract to form around it. The T tube is clamped to ensure free drainage into the duodenum. A T-tube cholangiogram is obtained under antibiotic cover. The T tube can be safely removed if there is free flow of contrast medium into the duodenum without evidence of ductal leakage or retained calculi.

Laparoscopic Common Bile Duct Exploration

The indications for laparoscopic exploration of the common bile duct are the same as those for open exploration, and the choice is institution- and expertise-dependent.

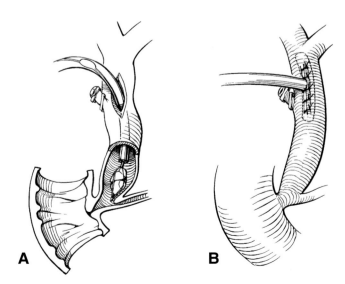

Fig. 11. Open or laparoscopic common bile duct exploration. (A), *Stone extraction with a basket.* (B), *Closure of choledochotomy over a T tube.*

The laparoscopic exploration techniques can be applied through a transcystic or a transductal approach. It is often more helpful to insert one or more cannulas to assist in exposure and operative dissection and, in some cases, to perform suturing and knot tying. Laparoscopic exploration of the bile ducts should be performed before complete dissection of the gallbladder from the liver bed to ease exposure of the common bile duct.

The opening made in the cystic duct is enlarged. A 4F Fogarty balloon catheter is introduced through one of the cannulas and then guided into the common bile duct under fluoroscopic guidance. The tip of the catheter is then passed through the ampulla, and the balloon is inflated. The balloon is withdrawn until resistance of the ampulla is felt and then slowly deflated as it crosses the ampulla. The balloon is inflated once again and then pulled through the common bile duct and out of the cystic duct. Stones are withdrawn from the cystic duct just ahead of the balloon tip. Alternatively, a Segura-type basket and flexible choledochoscope also can be used for removal of stones under direct vision. In addition, an electrohydraulic lithotriptor can be used to fragment an impacted or a large common bile duct stone. This technique must be done under direct vision. The cystic duct remnant is closed with surgical clips or ligature after completion of stone retraction. A T tube is not placed.

If the cystic duct lumen is small or has a long and tortuous course inserting low into the common bile duct or the stone is large, it may prove safer and easier to explore the common bile duct with choledochotomy. The midportion is identified and the anterior surface freed from the surrounding structures. An opening is made over the anterior surface large enough to introduce the necessary devices for stone extraction. A T tube is inserted at the end of the procedure.

Retained stones are the most frequent complication of common bile duct exploration; their incidence is about 5%.[52] Management of these retained stones was outlined above. Postoperative pancreatitis, bile leakage from the choledochotomy site, bile duct injury, dislodgment of the T tube, and common bile duct stricture are less common complications.

Biliary leakage and bile duct injury declare themselves with pain and fever, with or without abnormal results of liver function tests and jaundice. Other manifestations include bile in the subhepatic drain or biliary ascites. Computed tomography of the abdomen reveals intra-abdominal fluid collection. Minor collections can be treated by percutaneous drainage under radiologic guidance. If the patient improves, no further action is needed; however, in the presence of a major leak, jaundice, cholangitis, or any suspicion of iatrogenic bile duct trauma, ERC is mandatory.

If ERC demonstrates bile leakage, endoscopic management involves nasobiliary drain placement or endoscopic stenting. A subhepatic drain should be left in situ until the bile leak is controlled and stops. If ERC confirms a ductal injury, a period of drainage (usually by percutaneous transhepatic route) with appropriate antibiotics should precede surgical intervention. Partial injuries and common bile duct strictures may declare themselves months to years afterward.

The overall mortality rate after supraduodenal choledochotomy for benign biliary tract disease is 1% to 3%.[53,54] Age (older than 70 years), heart disease, and cholangitis are the three most important variables that affect operative mortality.

CONCLUSION

Gallstone disease is a common surgical problem. A general surgeon should be well aware of the diagnostic options and management guidelines. In this era of widespread availability of ultrasonography and laparoscopy, diagnostic and management guidelines for uncomplicated gallstones are clear-cut. The presence of common bile duct stones adds a layer of complexity to the diagnosis and management alternatives. Although diagnostic strategies remain noncontroversial, the management of common bile duct stones continues to be institution- and expertise-dependent.

REFERENCES

1. Beal JM: Historical perspective of gallstone disease. Surg Gynecol Obstet 158:181-189, 1984
2. Frierson HF Jr: The gross anatomy and histology of the gallbladder, extrahepatic bile ducts, Vaterian system, and minor papilla. Am J Surg Pathol 13:146-162, 1989
3. Benson EA, Page RE: A practical reappraisal of the anatomy of the extrahepatic bile ducts and arteries. Br J Surg 63:853-860, 1976
4. Toouli J: Biliary tract. In An Illustrated Guide to Gastrointestinal Motility. Second edition. Edited by D Kumar, D Wingate. Edinburgh, Churchill Livingstone, 1993, pp 393-409
5. Smadja C, Blumgart LH: The biliary tract and the anatomy of biliary exposure. In Surgery of the Liver and Biliary Tract. Vol 1. Edited by LH Blumgart. Edinburgh, Churchill Livingstone, 1988, pp 11-22
6. Diehl AK: Epidemiology and natural history of gallstone disease. Gastroenterol Clin North Am 20:1-19, 1991
7. Carey MC: Pathogenesis of gallstones. Am J Surg 165:410-419, 1993
8. Johnston DE, Kaplan MM: Pathogenesis and treatment of gallstones. N Engl J Med 328:412-421, 1993
9. Donovan JM, Carey MC: Physical-chemical basis of gallstone formation. Gastroenterol Clin North Am 20:47-66, 1991
10. Lee SP, Maher K, Nicholls JF: Origin and fate of biliary sludge. Gastroenterology 94:170-176, 1988
11. Comfort MW, Gray HK, Wilson JM: The silent gallstone: a ten to twenty year follow-up study of 112 cases. Ann Surg 128:931-937, 1948
12. Friedman GD: Natural history of asymptomatic and symptomatic gallstones. Am J Surg 165:399-404, 1993
13. Gupta D, Sakorafas GH, McGregor CG, Harmsen WS, Farnell MB: Management of biliary tract disease in heart and lung transplant patients. Surgery 128:641-649, 2000
14. Lou MA, Mandal AK, Alexander JL, Thadepalli H: Bacteriology of the human biliary tract and the duodenum. Arch Surg 112:965-967, 1977
15. Bower TC, Nagorney DM: Mirizzi syndrome. HPB Surg 1:67-74, 1988
16. McSherry CK, Ferstenberg H, Virshup M: The Mirizzi syndrome: suggested classification and surgical therapy. Surg Gastroenterol 1:219, 1982
17. Dewar G, Chung SC, Li AK: Operative strategy in Mirizzi syndrome. Surg Gynecol Obstet 171:157-159, 1990
18. Baer HU, Matthews JB, Schweizer WP, Gertsch P, Blumgart LH: Management of the Mirizzi syndrome and the surgical implications of cholecystocholedochal fistula. Br J Surg 77:743-745, 1990
19. Day EA, Marks C: Gallstone ileus: review of the literature and presentation of thirty-four new cases. Am J Surg 129:552-558, 1975
20. Reisner RM, Cohen JR: Gallstone ileus: a review of 1001 reported cases. Am Surg 60:441-446, 1994
21. Health and Policy Committee: How to study the gallbladder. Ann Intern Med 109:752-754, 1988
22. Spain DA, Bibbo C, Ecker T, Nosher JL, Brolin RE: Operative tube versus percutaneous cholecystostomy for acute cholecystitis. Am J Surg 166:28-31, 1993
23. Klimberg S, Hawkins I, Vogel SB: Percutaneous cholecystostomy for acute cholecystitis in high-risk patients. Am J Surg 153:125-129, 1987
24. Donohue JH: Laparoscopic cholecystectomy. In Gastroenterology and Hepatology: the Comprehensive Visual Reference. Vol 6: Gallbladder and Bile Ducts. Edited by NF LaRusso. Philadelphia, Churchill Livingstone, 1997, pp 4.1-4.16
25. Morgenstern L, Wong L, Berci G: Twelve hundred open cholecystectomies before the laparoscopic era: a standard for comparison. Arch Surg 127:400-403, 1992
26. Roslyn JJ, Binns GS, Hughes EF, Saunders-Kirkwood K, Zinner MJ, Cates JA: Open cholecystectomy: a contemporary analysis of 42,474 patients. Ann Surg 218:129-137, 1993
27. Dubois F, Icard P, Berthelot G, Levard H: Coelioscopic cholecystectomy: preliminary report of 36 cases. Ann Surg 211:60-62, 1990
28. Reddick EJ, Olsen DO: Laparoscopic laser cholecystectomy: a comparison with mini-lap cholecystectomy. Surg Endosc 3:131-133, 1989
29. Zucker KA, Bailey RW, Gadacz TR, Imbembo AL: Laparoscopic guided cholecystectomy. Am J Surg 161:36-42, 1991
30. National Institutes of Health Consensus Development Conference Statement on Gallstones and Laparoscopic Cholecystectomy. Am J Surg 165:390-398, 1993
31. Donohue JH, Grant CS, Farnell MB, van Heerden JA: Laparoscopic cholecystectomy: operative technique. Mayo Clin Proc 67:441-448, 1992
32. Deziel DJ, Millikan KW, Economou SG, Doolas A, Ko ST, Airan MC: Complications of laparoscopic cholecystectomy: a national survey of 4,292 hospitals and an analysis of 77,604 cases. Am J Surg 165:9-14, 1993
33. Woods MS, Traverso LW, Kozarek RA, Tsao J, Rossi RL, Gough D, Donohue JH: Characteristics of biliary tract complications during laparoscopic cholecystectomy: a multi-institutional study. Am J Surg 167:27-33, 1994
34. Steiner CA, Bass EB, Talamini MA, Pitt HA, Steinberg EP: Surgical rates and operative mortality for open and laparoscopic cholecystectomy in Maryland. N Engl J Med 330:403-408, 1994
35. Legorreta AP, Silber JH, Costantino GN, Kobylinski RW, Zatz SL: Increased cholecystectomy rate after the introduction of laparoscopic cholecystectomy. JAMA 270:1429-1432, 1993
36. Van der Linden W, Edlund G: Early versus delayed cholecystectomy: the effect of a change in management. Br J Surg 68:753-757, 1981
37. Norrby S, Herlin P, Holmin T, Sjodahl R, Tagesson C: Early or delayed cholecystectomy in acute cholecystitis? A clinical trial. Br J Surg 70:163-165, 1983
38. Strasberg SM, Clavien PA: Cholecystolithiasis: lithotherapy for the 1990s. Hepatology 16:820-839, 1992
39. Thistle JL, May GR, Bender CE, Williams HJ, LeRoy AJ, Nelson PE, Peine CJ, Petersen BT, McCullough JE: Dissolution of cholesterol gallbladder stones by methyl tert-butyl ether administered by percutaneous transhepatic catheter. N Engl J Med 320:633-639, 1989
40. Sackmann M, Delius M, Sauerbruch T, Holl J, Weber W, Ippisch E, Hagelauer U, Wess O, Hepp W, Brendel W: Shock-wave lithotripsy of gallbladder stones: the first 175 patients. N Engl J Med 318:393-397, 1988
41. Sackmann M, Niller H, Klueppelberg U, von Ritter C, Pauletzki J, Holl J, Berr F, Neubrand M, Sauerbruch T, Paumgartner G: Gallstone recurrence after shock-wave therapy. Gastroenterology 106:225-230, 1994

42. Giurgiu DIN, Roslyn JJ: Calculous biliary disease. *In* Surgery: Scientific Principles and Practice. Second edition. Edited by LJ Greenfield, M Mulholland, KT Oldham, et al. Philadelphia, Lippincott-Raven Publishers, 1997, pp 1033-1056

43. Boey JH, Way LW: Acute cholangitis. Ann Surg 191:264-270, 1980

44. Thompson JE Jr, Tompkins RK, Longmire WP Jr: Factors in management of acute cholangitis. Ann Surg 195:137-145, 1982

45. Armstrong CP, Taylor TV, Jeacock J, Lucas S: The biliary tract in patients with acute gallstone pancreatitis. Br J Surg 72:551-555, 1985

46. Kelly TR, Wagner DS: Gallstone pancreatitis: a prospective randomized trial of the timing of surgery. Surgery 104:600-605, 1988

47. Tsiotos GG, Luque-de Leon E, Soreide JA, Bannon MP, Zietlow SP, Baerga-Varela Y, Sarr MG: Management of necrotizing pancreatitis by repeated operative necrosectomy using a zipper technique. Am J Surg 175:91-98, 1998

48. Ranson JH: Etiological and prognostic factors in human acute pancreatitis: a review. Am J Gastroenterol 77:633-638, 1982

49. Neoptolemos JP, Carr-Locke DL, London NJ, Bailey IA, James D, Fossard DP: Controlled trial of urgent endoscopic retrograde cholangiopancreatography and endoscopic sphincterotomy versus conservative treatment for acute pancreatitis due to gallstones. Lancet 2:979-983, 1988

50. Hill J, Martin DF, Tweedle DE: Risks of leaving the gallbladder in situ after endoscopic sphincterotomy for bile duct stones. Br J Surg 78:554-557, 1991

51. Gadacz TR: Reoperation versus alternatives in retained biliary calculi. Surg Clin North Am 71:93-108, 1991

52. Martindale RG, Gadacz TR: Treatment of common duct stones. *In* Shackelford's Surgery of the Alimentary Tract. Vol III. Fourth edition. Edited by GD Zuidema. Philadelphia, WB Saunders Company, 1996, p 289

53. Larraz-Mora E, Mayol J, Martinez-Sarmiento J, Alvarez-Bartolom M, Larroque-Derlon M, Fernandez-Represa JA: Open biliary tract surgery: multivariate analysis of factors affecting mortality. Dig Surg 16:204-208, 1999

54. O'Sullivan ST, Hehir DJ, O'Sullivan GC, Kirwan WO: Open common bile duct exploration—end of an epoch? Ir J Med Sci 165:32-34, 1996

Chapter 16

BENIGN BILIARY STRICTURES

Grettel K. Wentling, M.D.
Juan M. Sarmiento, M.D.
J. Kirk Martin, Jr., M.D.
David M. Nagorney, M.D.

Almost a century has passed since William J. Mayo, M.D., described seven patients who had operative loss of continuity of the common bile duct. Three patients were treated with end-to-end anastomosis of the divided duct, and "...after the plan so successfully used by Halsted," one patient underwent choledochoduodenostomy. Dr. Mayo summarized the Mayo Clinic experience in 1905 by writing, "First, the common duct may be united end to end, by through-and-through catgut sutures...Second, the common, and in certain cases the hepatic, duct may be implanted into the duodenum, provided a peritoneal covered portion of the intestine be chosen for the purpose."[1] Although the operative approach has changed, the basic surgical principles remain the same.

Benign biliary strictures comprise various disorders causing mechanical obstruction to the normal flow of bile. This obstruction can result from external compression of the ducts or from congenital, ischemic, infective, or inflammatory conditions. Although the causes of benign biliary strictures are heterogeneous, all result clinically in one final common pathway—namely, mechanical biliary obstruction with possible cholestatic hepatocellular injury.

This chapter reviews the major advances in surgical treatment of benign extrahepatic biliary strictures. The past decade witnessed an explosion in the field of endoscopic and radiologic interventional techniques for palliation or definitive treatment of biliary strictures. Because an in-depth discussion of these treatments is beyond the scope of this chapter, the reader is referred to major texts in endoscopic gastroenterology and interventional radiology for review of the nonoperative approaches.

ANATOMY AND VASCULAR SUPPLY OF THE BILIARY TREE

A sound understanding of the anatomy and vascular supply of the biliary tree is essential to any surgeon, because failure to recognize anomalous or aberrant anatomy can have disastrous consequences. The extrahepatic biliary system within the hepatoduodenal ligament is the most lateral structure in this area. The common hepatic duct is formed by the union of the main right and left hepatic ducts as they exit the liver. The left hepatic duct has a longer extrahepatic course and, therefore, is more surgically accessible for biliary reconstruction (Hepp-Couinaud technique). The length of the common hepatic duct is variable because it depends on the point at which it is joined by the cystic duct; its average length is approximately 4 cm. The cystic duct usually enters the common hepatic duct on its right lateral border. Variations in the junction of the cystic and common hepatic ducts are not unusual and need to be recognized. For example, the cystic duct may be long and tortuous, may pass behind the common hepatic duct to enter posteriorly or on its left lateral border, may be extremely short or absent, or may share a long common wall with the common bile duct. In addition, an accessory hepatic duct may enter either the cystic or common hepatic duct (Fig. 1).

The common bile duct, normally 3 to 4 mm in diameter, has been subdivided into four anatomical regions: the supraduodenal, retroduodenal, intrapancreatic, and intraduodenal portions. The supraduodenal region is in the right lateral margin of the hepatoduodenal ligament, anterior to the portal vein and lateral to the proper hepatic artery. The retroduodenal common bile duct descends

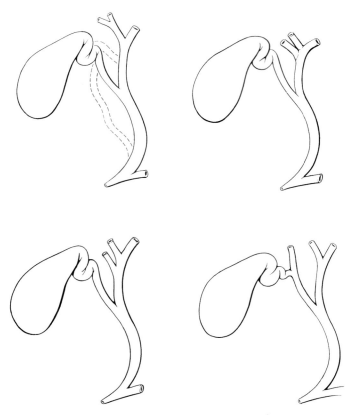

Fig. 1. Cystic duct and right hepatic duct anomalies.

behind the first portion of the duodenum, where it either grooves or enters the pancreatic head to become the intrapancreatic portion. It then enters the wall of the duodenum (the intraduodenal portion of the duct) where it travels a short distance before forming the papilla of Vater. The common bile duct and pancreatic duct may join each other in one of three ways: 1) they form a common duct of 1 to 8 mm in length (60%)—an ampulla; 2) they open in the duodenum contiguously as a double-barrel structure (38%); or 3) they open separately in the duodenum (2%).[2] Periampullary diverticula (so-called peri-vaterian diverticula) are also common in this region and can distort the normal anatomy.

The anatomical variations of importance to the surgeon occur primarily in the supraduodenal bile duct. These anomalies involve mainly the right and left hepatic ducts and the variation with which the cystic duct joins the common hepatic duct. The most common of these variations are shown in Figure 1.

Knowledge of the vascular supply to the extrahepatic biliary system is important, because focal ischemia of the bile duct is responsible for or contributes to a large proportion of benign bile duct strictures. Proximally (hepatic aspect), the extrahepatic bile duct is supplied by branches of the right (mainly) and left hepatic arteries, whereas

distally, it is supplied by branches from the gastroduodenal and pancreaticoduodenal arteries. The duct also has a rich anastomotic arterial network that coalesces laterally into two axial arteries within the wall of the bile duct at the 3-o'clock and 9-o'clock positions. Unfortunately, approximately 20% of patients lack a true anastomotic network between the proximal and distal arterial supply of the common bile duct, resulting in functional end arteries.[3] Strictures after operation or injury may be more prone to occur in these patients because of a relative ductal ischemia.

Clinically important variations in the anatomy of the cystic and hepatic arteries also occur frequently. The most common of these is the replaced right hepatic artery, in which the right hepatic artery, which usually arises from the proper hepatic artery in the hepatoduodenal ligament, arises from the superior mesenteric artery and usually passes posterior to the head and neck of the pancreas and lies posterior to the bile duct and portal vein in the hepatoduodenal ligament. Much less frequently, the common hepatic artery can arise from the superior mesenteric artery (the so-called replaced common hepatic artery). The left hepatic artery can (10%-20%) arise from the left gastric artery (as a truly replaced or an accessory left hepatic artery). Other variations include the right hepatic artery passing anterior to the bile duct and a curved right hepatic artery ("caterpillar hump"). An anomalous cystic artery may arise from the duodenal, left hepatic, or common hepatic artery. Accessory cystic arteries are also common.

PATHOPHYSIOLOGY OF BILE DUCT INJURIES AND STRICTURES

Chronic partial or complete obstruction of the major intrahepatic and extrahepatic bile ducts leads to increased intraductal pressure, disrupting the tight junctions that form the barrier between the sinusoids and canaliculi. Such disruption allows bile with its accumulated toxins and bacteria to reflux into the hepatic parenchyma, inducing a local inflammatory process. As this process progresses, collagen and other extracellular membrane proteins are deposited around the bile ducts and ductules, ultimately causing fibrosis and scarring (so-called biliary cirrhosis).[4,5] If the obstruction is relieved early, this process is reversible, but the return to normal hepatic function may occur slowly.

Chronic complete biliary obstruction may lead to atrophy of the affected liver segment or lobe, with compensatory hypertrophy of the remaining nonobstructed liver parenchyma (the so-called atrophy-hypertrophy complex). An atrophy-hypertrophy complex usually is associated with a hepatic arterial or portal venous injury ipsilateral with the atrophy. Rotational deformity of the hypertrophied segment can cause anatomical displacement of the extrahepatic duct, which may make access and subsequent repair difficult. Bile is normally sterile, but stones in the duct or manipulation of a totally or partially obstructed duct can lead to bacterial colonization (bacteriobilia). Finally, bile and debris can collect in the dilated, obstructed ducts and lead to recurrent bouts of cholangitis. Recurrent episodes of cholangitis often necessitate drainage either percutaneously or endoscopically before definitive repair.

Biliary obstruction clinically causes jaundice, with increased levels of serum bilirubin and alkaline phosphatase. Total serum bilirubin levels usually correlate with the degree of obstruction, reaching a plateau of 20 to 30 mg/dL in the presence of complete biliary obstruction, when the urinary excretion equals the daily production rate. When serum bilirubin levels exceed 30 mg/dL, biliary cirrhosis or some other associated hepatopathy should be suspected, and these portend a worse prognosis. Increases in the serum alkaline phosphatase level do not correlate as well with the degree of obstruction, although this enzyme remains a useful clinical marker of cholestasis. Levels of the cytoplasmic enzymes, aspartate transaminase and alanine transaminase, usually are increased only mildly in the presence of early mechanical obstruction of the biliary tree, but they become markedly increased in long-standing obstruction, reflecting a chronic injury to the affected liver parenchyma. Serum albumin concentrations also may be low in chronic biliary obstruction, reflecting both hepatic dysfunction and the maldigestion caused by the absence of bile in the intestinal lumen.

Renal Injury

Patients with severe obstructive jaundice are at increased risk for acute renal failure. The pathogenesis is multifactorial and has been subject to extensive research. Abnormalities in renal structure and function, including cellular degeneration, decrease in renal blood flow, and diminished urinary concentrating ability, are all associated with obstructive jaundice. In addition, patients have impaired circulatory homeostasis, with exaggerated responses to blood loss and with decreased effective blood volume as blood is sequestered in the splanchnic circulation. Obstructive jaundice also compromises the integrity of the gastrointestinal mucosal barrier against enteric pathogens and their toxins (e.g., endotoxins), predisposing to bacteremia and sepsis. These factors, in combination with the additional stress of operation, can compromise renal function and lead to acute renal failure. An increase in the serum creatinine level in patients with biliary obstruction should prompt rapid intervention to relieve the obstruction and avert uremia and renal failure.

Systemic Toxicity

Cholangitis due to bacteriobilia and increased biliary pressure can cause life-threatening sepsis. Absorption of endotoxins from infected bile and the subsequent endotoxemia can precipitate the systemic inflammatory response syndrome. Bile salts have an anti-endotoxin effect, and in their absence the protective (and trophic) effects of biliary secretions on gastrointestinal mucosa are lost, leading to breakdown of the intestinal mucosal barrier with increased absorption of endotoxin and other enterotoxins.[6] The phagocytic function of Kupffer cells is also depressed, allowing exodus of endotoxin into the systemic circulation from the portal circulation.[7] A systemic inflammatory response ensues, mediated by the release of proinflammatory cytokines such as tumor necrosis factor-α and interleukin-1 and -6. The systemic effects of endotoxin have been researched extensively and include, among others, fever, endothelial cell injury, complement activation, intravascular coagulation, and injury to specific organ systems such as the kidney and lung. Left untreated, multiorgan system dysfunction and death can ensue.

Classification of Bile Duct Injuries and Strictures

Benign biliary strictures are typically classified into five types, originally proposed by Bismuth,[8] based on the site of the extrahepatic biliary stricture (Fig. 2). This classification system is well recognized, is widely used, and standardizes the nomenclature for interpretation and comparative research. This classification provides a useful structure for therapeutic decision making, whether surgical, endoscopic, or radiologic. Strasberg et al.[9] expanded the Bismuth classification and incorporated acute injury with extrahepatic biliary fistulas. This classification is particularly appropriate for laparoscopic injuries and is detailed below.

CAUSES OF BENIGN BILIARY STRICTURES

External Compression

Mirizzi Syndrome

Mirizzi syndrome, first described by Mirizzi in 1948,[10] consists of impaction of a gallstone(s) in Hartmann's pouch of the gallbladder or in the cystic duct. Pericholecystic inflammation causes partial or complete obstruction of the common hepatic duct (Mirizzi type 1). Sometimes, the stone erodes through the gallbladder neck or cystic duct into the adjacent hepatic duct, resulting in a cholecystocholedochal fistula (Mirizzi type 2) with various degrees of obstruction of the bile duct. Mirizzi syndrome should be suspected in patients with a

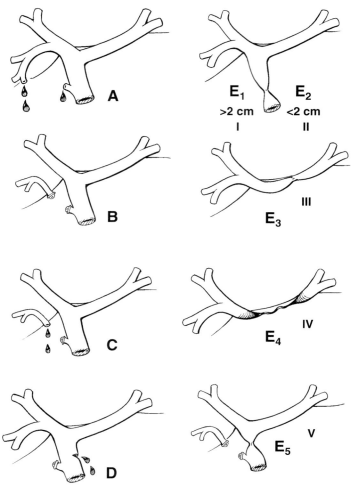

Fig. 2. Classification of injuries and strictures of the bile duct, proposed by Bismuth[8] and expanded by Strasberg et al.[9] Note that the letters A to E5 are the Strasberg nomenclature, and the Roman numerals I through V in the E injuries are the original Bismuth nomenclature. (From Murr et al.[23] By permission of Mayo Foundation.)

defect in the wall of the common hepatic duct.[11] In the presence of a fistula, partial cholecystectomy with stone extraction and construction of a cholecystocholedochojejunostomy or cholecystocholedochoduodenostomy should be performed. Although cholecystectomy should *not* be performed in the infirm elderly patient if a cholecystocholedochal fistula is present, cholecystectomy and hepaticojejunostomy is preferred in younger or fit patients.[11]

Duodenal Diverticula

Duodenal diverticula are usually asymptomatic but may occasionally cause biliary obstruction and cholangitis in addition to their more common complications of duodenal obstruction, bleeding due to ulceration, or pancreatitis.[12] Duodenal diverticula are most commonly located near the ampulla of Vater[13] and are termed perivaterian diverticula. They can be either extraluminal or intraluminal; intraluminal diverticula are thought by some anatomists to be the remnants of a duodenal web. Extraluminal diverticula are far more common. Both types rarely occur before the age of 40 years. Patients with peri-vaterian duodenal diverticula have a much greater incidence of gallstones and choledocholithiasis than patients without such diverticula, presumably related to relative biliary stasis. It is usually through this process that peri-vaterian diverticula lead to recurrent pancreatitis, cholangitis, common bile duct obstruction, and jaundice.[12] All these complications are indications for operative intervention.

Duodenal diverticulum is diagnosed with upper endoscopy or a barium study. Treatment is diverticulectomy by duodenotomy. Care must be taken to avoid compromise of the ampulla, and biliary sphincterotomy or sphincteroplasty may be necessary to ensure adequate biliary drainage.

Inflammation

Duodenal Ulcer

In very rare cases, transmural inflammation from penetrating duodenal ulcers may affect the head of the pancreas and distal common bile duct.[14] Over time, fibrosis in the region may lead to stricture formation or a choledochoduodenal fistula, or it may masquerade as a pancreatic or duodenal cancer with distal bile duct obstruction. This complication of chronic duodenal ulcer disease should be suspected in a patient with a long history of symptomatic duodenal ulcers who presents with jaundice or cholangitis.[14,15]

Upper gastrointestinal endoscopy and ERCP are indicated to evaluate the gastroduodenal region and the bile duct, respectively. Current histamine$_2$ (H$_2$)-receptor

long-standing history of symptomatic cholelithiasis who present with jaundice and cholecystitis. Preoperative diagnosis with delineation of the anatomy is imperative to avoid further intraoperative damage to the biliary tree and to avoid approaching the obstruction as a malignancy. Either percutaneous transhepatic cholangiography (PTC) or endoscopic retrograde cholangiopancreatography (ERCP) will define the site and length of ductal narrowing. Typically, an eccentric smooth compression of the duct is evident cholangiographically, which differs from the annular, irregular, concentric appearance of malignant strictures. Computed tomography (CT) may help to support the diagnosis of a benign inflammatory condition versus a malignant neoplasm.

Treatment of Mirizzi syndrome consists of cholecystectomy and, if possible, repair or reconstruction of the blockers, proton pump inhibitors, and *Helicobacter pylori* surveillance (and treatment if necessary) may facilitate healing and avert the need for operative management. Rarely, a benign diagnosis may not be possible, and radical resection or biliary bypass for suspected malignancy may be indicated.

Chronic Pancreatitis

Chronic pancreatitis is associated with inflammation and scarring of the intrapancreatic common bile duct, leading to extrinsic stricture of the biliary tree. These strictures are typically long and smooth (involving the entire intrapancreatic portion of the common bile duct) and may or may not be associated with dilatation of the proximal bile ducts. However, numerous configurations of benign strictures have been recognized and classified. Although the exact incidence of common bile duct stricture in chronic pancreatitis is unknown, a literature review supports an estimate of nearly 6%.[16]

Patients with benign biliary strictures due to chronic pancreatitis are frequently asymptomatic. Increases in liver enzyme and, less commonly, serum bilirubin levels suggest the presence of a biliary stricture, because chronic pancreatitis alone usually does not result in increased levels of serum bilirubin or alkaline phosphatase. Intermittent or chronic abdominal pain related to the underlying pancreatitis also may be present. Jaundice, when present, is usually mild, but cholangitis is rare. Differentiating a benign from a malignant distal bile duct stricture in patients with chronic pancreatitis can be challenging clinically. Although imaging of the pancreas with CT and endoscopic ultrasonography and endoscopic brushings and biopsy can confirm malignancy, false-negative findings are not uncommon and warrant careful counsel with the patient.

Choledochoduodenostomy and, more commonly, choledochojejunostomy are the preferred treatments for benign biliary strictures due to chronic pancreatitis. Because duodenal stenosis may complicate chronic pancreatitis, choledochoduodenostomy, although simpler and faster than choledochojejunostomy, should be reserved for the patient with a supple, uninvolved duodenum. In patients with a pancreatic mass on CT or in whom the biopsy is equivocal or cannot exclude malignancy, pancreatoduodenectomy is an alternative treatment. Sphincteroplasty has not been successful and is contraindicated in the long-term management of biliary obstruction from chronic pancreatitis, because the intrapancreatic biliary stricture is usually long (3-4 cm) and extends proximal to the sphincter complex. Experience is limited regarding balloon dilation and stenting. Patients with a short life expectancy or who are otherwise not surgical candidates may benefit from endoscopic intervention, but long-term success is unlikely given the natural history of chronic pancreatitis and the current functional durability of any endoscopic stent.

Iatrogenic Stricture: Intraoperative Injuries

Most benign biliary strictures today are caused by intraoperative bile duct injuries during laparoscopic cholecystectomy. Although laparoscopic cholecystectomy compared with open cholecystectomy offers many real and potential advantages, including shorter hospital stay, cosmetically appealing smaller incisions, and faster return to normal activity, it unfortunately also has at least a twofold higher (and possibly even greater) risk of injury to the biliary tree. These injuries can have disastrous consequences.[9,17,18] The frequency of injury to the duct is less than 1% for open cholecystectomies.[18,19] The reported incidence for laparoscopic cholecystectomy ranges from 0% to 7%, although the true incidence probably lies somewhere between.[20-22] Despite increasing experience with laparoscopic cholecystectomy, injuries continue to occur.[23]

The causes of biliary injury during laparoscopic cholecystectomy are multifactorial. Initially, surgeon inexperience played a major role in the higher incidence of biliary injury—the so-called learning curve effect,[21] but biliary injuries occur even in experienced hands. Initially, injuries were likely related to limited or naïve laparoscopic skills and inadequate laparoscopic hardware. Currently, however, misdirected gallbladder retraction, inflammation, and scarring—all of which obscure the region—also play a part. Precise, clear visualization of the structures in the hepatoduodenal ligament is absolutely necessary for safe dissection in this area.[24] Both ductal and vascular structures need to be identified clearly; if such visualization is not possible, a surgeon's pride should never get in the way of converting to an open procedure. As experience grows, surgeons are always trying to perform more and more difficult cases laparoscopically—and thus one needs constantly to remember the tenet of safe laparoscopic cholecystectomy.

Anatomical variations in the ductal and arterial anatomy of the biliary tree are common. The surgeon must be cognizant of the variability and define the salient anatomy unequivocally at operation. Most patients with laparoscopic biliary injuries have a "classic injury" or a similar variation. In the classic injury, the common duct is mistaken for the cystic duct with transection and devascularization of a segment of both the common and the hepatic ducts, often in association with a right hepatic arterial injury.[25] In this classic pattern of injury, a portion of the biliary tree is actually removed or devascularized, making subsequent repair a challenge.

Another variation on the common injury is misidentification of the common bile duct for the cystic duct, but in this case the proximal clips are correctly placed on the cystic duct; however, the entry of the common hepatic duct with the cystic duct-common bile duct junction is not appreciated. Therefore, the common duct is ligated distally, the cystic duct is actually transected, and the gallbladder is removed. This approach leaves a wide open common hepatic duct, allowing for biliary decompression into the peritoneal cavity. A second variation involves correct identification of the cystic duct, but the common bile or hepatic duct is "tented" and subsequently clipped, transected, or removed with placement of the distal clips. A third variation on the classic pattern of biliary injury occurs when an aberrant right hepatic duct is mistaken for the cystic duct and is either ligated and divided or not appreciated and transected (Fig. 2).

A major contributing factor to inadvertent injury to the biliary system during laparoscopic cholecystectomy is attempted control of intraoperative bleeding, which obscures the view.[26] Overaggressive or poorly visualized use of the cautery hook may cause thermal injury to the duct which results in delayed stricture formation. Excess fat, inflammation, or fibrosis in the region of Calot's triangle, as with blood, also can obscure the anatomy and make dissection hazardous. Excessive ductal traction also has been implicated as a factor in biliary injury. During laparoscopic cholecystectomy, traction on the gallbladder should be both anterior and lateral. Cephalad traction causes tenting of the bile duct upward toward the hilum, which makes it more easily mistaken for the cystic duct. Maintenance of anterolateral traction on the infundibulum opens up Calot's triangle, allowing safer dissection. Finally, one reason for biliary ductal injury during laparoscopy is the use of monopolar cautery near the bile duct in conjunction with dissection and the potential for devascularization of the duct.[27]

Many biliary injuries are recognized during operation; of those initially unrecognized, most usually are diagnosed within a few days to weeks. Complaints of ongoing abdominal pain, fever, or jaundice should alert the surgeon to a potential biliary injury and prompt immediate investigation to determine its presence. When an injury is recognized at the time of operation, operative repair should be considered only if the surgeon is experienced with the repair dictated by the specific injury. The best chance for a successful outcome is during the first repair; also, most lawsuits result from inappropriate initial management with failure to alert the patient and family adequately and immediately of the potentially serious nature of the injury. If true expertise and experience in complicated biliary operation is unavailable, the injury should be drained and the patient transferred immediately (within 12-24 hours) to a center with an experienced hepatobiliary surgeon. Transfer should *not* be delayed.

Any patient with a biliary tract injury requires cholangiography to determine the site and extent of injury *before* operative repair. Either PTC or ERCP can be used to image the biliary tract. The major caveat of imaging, regardless of method, is complete visualization of both the biliary system *proximal* (hepatic side) to the injury and the injury. "Bilomas" are drained percutaneously. Stents may be placed during ERCP or PTC for biliary decompression. Importantly, all segments should be drained. Although magnetic resonance cholangiography also can define biliary tract injuries, it lacks the interventional capability of ERCP or PTC.[28] Its role for benign strictures is yet undefined.

In 1995, Strasberg et al.[9] proposed a revised classification system for biliary injuries that incorporated the Bismuth stricture schema with a wider range of injuries (leaks, fistulas), particularly those noted after the clinical introduction of laparoscopic cholecystectomy (Fig. 2). Injuries are classified as types A to E, and type E is subdivided into E1 through E5 according to the Bismuth classification. Type A injuries are bile leaks from a minor duct still in continuity with the common bile duct. These typically occur from the cystic duct or liver bed and are the most common type after laparoscopic cholecystectomy. Type B injuries consist of segmental occlusion of the biliary tree, such as an occlusive clip injury on an aberrant right hepatic duct. When the aberrant duct is transected but not occluded, it is termed a type C injury. Type C injuries result in intraperitoneal bile collections, whereas type B injuries are asymptomatic or present with the early or even late findings of pain or cholangitis. Lateral injury to extrahepatic bile ducts is classified as type D. Types E1 through E5 involve circumferential injury to the major bile ducts according to the Bismuth classification (Fig. 2).

Iatrogenic bile duct injuries may be divided into four groups based on their management:
1. Simple leaks: These may be either from the gallbladder bed (ducts of Luschka) or from the cystic duct stump. After the site and extent of injury are defined with cholangiography, a stent should be placed either to traverse the leak point (cystic duct leak) if possible or to decompress the bile duct and decrease the intraductal pressure, allowing the leak to seal. Bile fluid collections also should be drained percutaneously.
2. Incomplete duct lacerations: If detected at the time of operation, these can be repaired primarily over a T tube, provided there has not been an extensive cautery injury or devascularization of the duct. If detected late, a stent may be tried for several months. Alternatively, and especially if the patient is young and a good

surgical candidate, Roux-en-Y choledochojejunostomy is usually the best option.

3. Duct transections: Unfortunately, these devastating injuries (commonly the classic pattern of injury) take place all too often relative to other types of injury and typically involve the hilar bile ducts, leading to a serious injury. The surgical management of these problems is discussed thoroughly in the following pages.

4. Late postoperative strictures: The treatment of this problem is discussed below. Of note is the recent introduction of endoscopic techniques, such as balloon dilation and stenting, to the therapeutic interventions.

This discussion of intraoperative biliary injuries has focused on those occurring during laparoscopic cholecystectomy, but injury can occur, of course, during other major intra-abdominal procedures. These include but are not limited to hepatic resection, liver transplantation, and pancreatic operation.

Miscellaneous

A host of other causes for biliary obstruction exist, including traumatic injury (both blunt and penetrating), anastomotic strictures, radiation-induced fibrosis, primary sclerosing cholangitis, and the extremely rare benign biliary tumor (e.g., adenoma, leiomyoma, and papillomatosis). Rarely, a primary benign biliary stricture at the hepatic ductal bifurcation mimics a hilar cholangiocarcinoma. Preoperative differentiation of these strictures from cholangiocarcinomas is usually impossible, and treatment involves resection.

DIAGNOSIS OF BENIGN BILIARY STRICTURES

A relevant history and physical examination should initiate the evaluation. Any history of recent or distant biliary tract operation, symptomatic or asymptomatic cholelithiasis, or pancreatitis should be noted. Available intraoperative cholangiograms and postoperative notes should be reviewed. Physical findings of jaundice, abdominal pain, fever, rigors, and bilious drainage from recent incisions may be present. A hypertrophied liver or palpable gallbladder also may be evident. Laboratory evaluation should include determination of liver enzyme, bilirubin, and serum albumin values and prothrombin time. Tumor markers (carbohydrate antigen 19-9, carcinoembryonic antigen) may be helpful for distinguishing benign from malignant strictures in the clinical setting of delayed presentations years or even a decade or more after cholecystectomy; if results are negative, however, they are of little usefulness.

ERCP provides direct visualization of the extrahepatic and intrahepatic biliary tree for definition of the site and extent of injury or stricture. The complication rate with ERCP varies from 2% to 7%,[29] and pancreatitis is the most common complication. ERCP also allows for retrograde endobiliary stenting or nasobiliary drainage. Cholangiography also can be performed percutaneously through a transhepatic route (PTC). Like ERCP, PTC also is associated with the risk of hemorrhage, hemobilia, or bile leak. ERCP is best used for distal biliary strictures and an incomplete biliary obstruction. In contrast, PTC should be the primary imaging method for patients with markedly increased serum bilirubin (≥ 15 mg/dL), for patients with suspected complete obstruction, or for hilar injuries. Proximal strictures are more appropriate for PTC, because the most important information required by the operating surgeon should be the proximal (hepatic) extent of the injury, especially if the stricture occurs less than 2 cm distal to the hepatic duct confluence or occurs intrahepatically. Although both PTC and ERCP allow for brush biopsies of the stricture, neither cytologic nor biopsy evaluation, because of low sensitivity, warrants routine use and neither is pertinent in acute injuries.

Abdominal ultrasonography should be used initially to determine the presence of intrahepatic and extrahepatic ductal dilatation or perihepatic fluid collections. Ultrasonography-guided drainage of fluid collections should be performed before direct cholangiography. Identification of ductal dilatation with ultrasonography favors PTC for definition of the ductal system. Additionally, ultrasonography with Doppler images can be used to recognize any major injury to the periductal hepatic artery or portal vein. Ultrasonographic quality is often limited, however, by overlying bowel gas and obesity. Moreover, characterizing the injury is difficult, and static spot images are not equivalent to real-time ultrasonographic images, even if well defined. For these reasons, most surgeons favor abdominal CT as the best imaging method. CT offers the advantages of complete abdominal visualization and clear anatomical details. The intrahepatic and extrahepatic ducts, regional vasculature, hepatic parenchyma, ascites, and other related intra-abdominal organs such as the pancreas and duodenum can be defined clearly. Moreover, most surgeons are much more familiar with interpreting a CT scan than an ultrasonogram. CT-guided drainage is equivalent to that for ultrasonography. Importantly, if the drainage of perihepatic collections contains bile, cholangiography through drainage catheters can define the site and extent of injury and may obviate PTC or ERCP.

OPERATIVE TREATMENT OF BENIGN BILIARY STRICTURES

Most benign postoperative biliary strictures are treated most effectively and durably by surgically establishing unobstructed bilioenteric continuity. Although limited success has been reported with transhepatic or endoscopic balloon dilation and stenting,[30-32] most literature suggests that a bilioenteric anastomosis tailored to the patient's level of injury or stricture and performed by an experienced hepatobiliary surgeon offers the best chance of long-term patency.

The four cornerstones of biliary reconstructive surgery are as follows:[33]

1. Adequate but not excessive exposure (dissection) of the duct(s) proximal to the stricture, with careful avoidance of circumferential dissection of the duct, especially on its lateral and posterior aspects
2. Anastomosis of bowel to a well-vascularized, uninflamed duct of adequate size
3. Apposition of biliary mucosa to intestinal mucosa to minimize the risk of recurrent stricture
4. Construction of a tension-free anastomosis

Dr. William J. Mayo realized the importance of a tension-free anastomosis, describing "...the second portion of the duodenum should be loosened and drawn to the right and held by fixation sutures, preventing tension on the duct suture line."[1] We, however, have come to favor a Roux-en-Y hepaticojejunostomy technique with use of interrupted 4-0 absorbable sutures. Regardless of duct size, the Roux limb of jejunum is the most versatile, mobile, and reliable conduit for restoration of bile flow. The details of the anastomosis are shown below. Because the suture material is absorbable, knots can be either intraluminal or extraluminal. Some surgeons alternate dyed and undyed suture to facilitate orderly suture placement and tying. A spring or other type of suture holder that organizes each suture can be used to keep them separated as they are placed.[33] Running absorbable suture also may be used, a technique preferable in dilated ducts (> 1 cm). Although running suture may narrow the anastomosis if pulled taut, gentle tension with separate anterior and posterior running suture should prevent this problem. "Serosal" external sutures may be used to secure the anastomosis without tension to the periductal tissues, provided the suture placement avoids devascularization of the bile duct.

Either a T tube or a straight tube (10F) can be placed to splint the anastomosis and decompress the proximal ducts. With distal biliary strictures, a small 10F T tube can be inserted into the proximal duct above the anastomosis with a long lower limb extending across the anastomosis. Another technique involves inserting a small 7F catheter into the jejunal Roux-en-Y limb retrograde across the anastomosis. Concern exists regarding duct size, especially for anastomoses in patients with small friable ducts, an inflamed subhepatic space, or recurrent strictures or in those who are immunosuppressed. We tend not to use intraoperatively placed transhepatic tubes, as do some groups. If the need for repeat postoperative cholangiography or repeat interventional access (e.g., multiple retained intrahepatic stones or strictures) is anticipated, a transhepatic drain can be placed intraoperatively in retrograde fashion. In patients with indwelling transhepatic drains, the anastomosis is constructed around the drain, which is then left in situ for postoperative drainage and splinting.

Postoperative cholangiograms are obtained 5 to 7 days postoperatively. An intraperitoneal drain, usually left in Morison's pouch, is removed after cholangiography and a successful trial of stent clamping. Cholangiography is repeated before stent removal for progressive laboratory evidence of cholestasis or cholangitis or because of concern of ischemia. Importantly, we believe that the benefits of short-term access to the biliary tree exceed any potential disadvantage related to the stent, especially in high-risk anastomoses. Intrabiliary tubes (T tubes, straight tubes, or intraoperatively placed transhepatic tubes) are removed in 6 weeks if cholangiography shows good flow, no leak, and a decompressed intrahepatic ductal system. We do not support the concept that chronic transhepatic "stenting" of a proximal anastomosis is of benefit in a well-performed, technically satisfactory biliary-enteric anastomosis.

Bismuth Type I Injuries

End-to-End Anastomosis

This technique is rarely, if ever, indicated. An end-to-end anastomosis is viable only when the duct proximal and distal to a very short (< 1 cm) *acute* injury can be safely brought together without tension. There must be little loss of the bile duct length or periductal devascularization; this situation is extremely unusual in the pathogenesis of most biliary ductal injuries. Careful but limited dissection of the proximal and distal portions of the injured duct without excessive devascularization is mandatory. The duodenum should be mobilized to reduce tension, and the anastomosis constructed with absorbable suture in a single layer over a T tube (Fig. 3). Permanent suture probably should not be used because it can serve as a later nidus for stone formation. Basically, this approach is applicable only to acute sharp transections or limited ductal clipping. It should not be used for other acute injuries or postoperative strictures. This repair is notorious for its high rate of stricture recurrence.[34,35] This technique is most successful if there is little discrepancy in size between the proximal and distal duct. This situation is very rare, and we advise against this type of repair.

Choledochoduodenostomy

This procedure is ideally suited for bile duct injuries involving the more distal common bile duct. Again, the

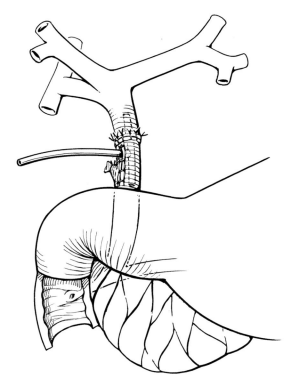

Fig. 3. Primary end-to-end anastomosis over a T tube.

duodenum should be mobilized to increase exposure and to decrease tension on the anastomosis. The anastomosis can be constructed either side-to-side (most commonly, Fig. 4) or end-to-side. Occasionally, dissection behind the duodenum is necessary to expose adequate length. Also, for benign intrapancreatic biliary strictures (an uncommon situation), use of the more posterior aspect of the proximal duodenum minimizes the distance between duct and duodenum. Among his conclusions in a 1926 review of the Mayo Clinic experience, E. Starr Judd, M.D., stated, "Anastomosis of the stump of the common duct...to an opening in the duodenum over a tube is the most satisfactory operation."[36] His astute observation holds true today in selected patients.

Hepaticojejunostomy or Choledochojejunostomy
An anastomosis to a Roux-en-Y jejunal limb is the preferred method for repairing proximal strictures because it permits a tension-free anastomosis to a limb of jejunum. The choledochojejunostomy is constructed end-to-side or side-to-side to a 45- to 60-cm retrocolic or antecolic limb of jejunum (Fig. 5).

Bismuth Type II and III Injuries
In general, the more proximal the bile duct injury or stricture, the more difficult and challenging the surgical reconstruction. If the right and left ductal confluence is fully

intact, two basic surgical options exist. One option is to drain the proximal ducts through a single anastomosis to the proximal common hepatic duct. The size of the anastomosis depends on the diameter of the common hepatic duct. The second option is to drain the proximal ducts through a wide anastomosis of the proximal common hepatic duct and distal left main duct after incising the anterior common hepatic duct and left duct wall longitudinally (Hepp-Couinaud procedure) (Fig. 6). The second method is our preferred approach but requires maintenance of continuity of the right and left ductal systems through an intact hilar confluence. The results of this approach are illustrated in Figure 7, showing a Bismuth type III injury after laparoscopic cholecystectomy, for which a Hepp-Couinaud procedure was performed.

Exposure of the Left Duct (Hepp-Couinaud Approach)
The left hepatic duct has a longer extrahepatic course than the right hepatic duct. Consequently, it is more accessible and amenable to a longer anastomosis. After the hilar plate is incised at the base of segment 4 of the liver, the left duct is exposed. A longitudinal incision is made in its anteroinferior aspect. A side-to-side bilioenteric anastomosis is constructed to a 45- to 60-cm Roux-en-Y jejunal limb. Rarely, a secure anastomosis cannot be constructed between the jejunal limb and the bile duct; alternatively, the jejunum can be sutured to the Glisson capsule and the liver parenchyma as a hepaticoenterostomy. The risk of postoperative complications and the long-term failure rate, however, are high, and this approach should be avoided unless no direct mucosa-to-mucosal bilioenteric anastomosis is possible.

The mucosal graft technique proposed by Sir Rodney Smith may be a better alternative in this unusual clinical situation.[37] Briefly, the serosa and the muscularis of the jejunum are incised to allow the mucosa to protrude. The mucosa is punctured, a small transhepatic tube is maneuvered intraluminally, and the mucosa is tied to the tube with an absorbable suture. The tube is pulled back into the liver until the jejunal mucosa abuts the proximal hepatic duct and then is secured to the liver capsule to maintain apposition of the biliary and jejunal mucosa. This "sutureless" anastomosis has proven durable and far more reliable than portoenterostomy; nevertheless, the need for this type of biliary drainage procedure should be rare.

Ligamentum Teres (Segment 3) Approach
Occasionally, the left hepatic duct is inaccessible or too scarred for an anastomosis. In this situation, a ligamentum teres (round ligament) approach is used for repair. The dissection plane is initiated within the umbilical fissure at the superior portion of the ligamentum teres and carried

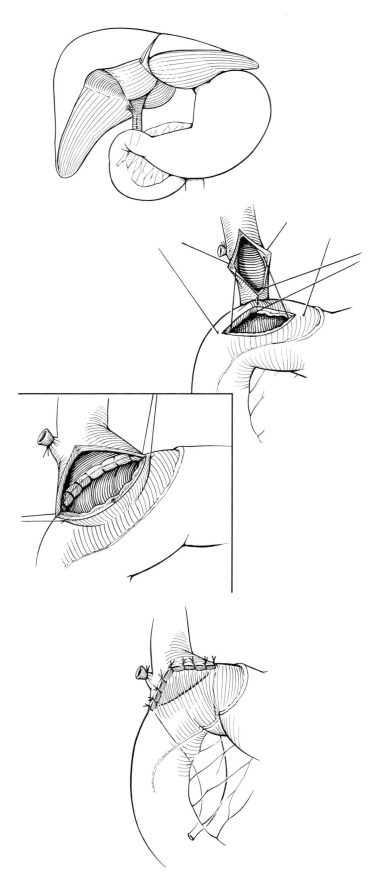

Fig. 4. Side-to-side choledochoduodenostomy.

into the hepatic parenchyma to the junction of ducts from segments 3 and 4 (4B). At this point, the left system can be identified inferior to the left branch of the portal vein; in an obstructed biliary tree, adequate length and diameter of duct are usually available to construct a cholangioenterostomy. Alternatively, the wedge approach can be used by taking a wedge of hepatic parenchyma about 1 cm to the left of the umbilical tissues where a branch of the ductal system is usually readily found (Fig. 8). Both this technique and the segment 3 approach are aided by use of intraoperative ultrasonography. This technique is used primarily in the clinical setting of hilar malignancies. Although patency of the ductal confluence is preferable, drainage of the left lobe alone is usually adequate for palliation provided the right ducts are not infected.

Longmire Procedure
This technique, first described in 1948 by Longmire and Sanford,[38] rests on the premise that extrahepatic biliary obstruction causes generalized intrahepatic ductal dilatation. This procedure is most commonly used for malignant obstruction of the hepatic duct (e.g., advanced carcinoma of the gallbladder). The left lobe of the liver is first mobilized, and a Roux limb of jejunum is prepared. The left lateral sector of the liver is resected to expose a peripheral intrahepatic duct for the anastomosis. Intraoperative ultrasonography facilitates identification of the duct and defines the extent of resection. This technique is rarely used, because the small peripheral intrahepatic ducts are delicate and more prone to late stricture. Consequently, long-term outcome is often poor.

Bismuth Type IV Injuries
These injuries are the most challenging strictures to repair because of the proximal location and variant anatomy. The surgical options for these proximal biliary strictures are classified as single or double biliary-enteric anastomoses.

Single Biliary-Enteric Anastomoses: Construction of a New Common Hepatic Duct
After the hilar plate is entered and the right and left hepatic ducts are mobilized (taking care to avoid unnecessary dissection, which may lead to ischemia), the medial walls of the ducts proximal to the stricture are incised. The two lobar hepatic ducts are apposed with suture along adjacent walls to create a "new" common hepatic duct. This single orifice is anastomosed to a Roux limb of jejunum to form a biliary-enteric anastomosis. This procedure requires both a long extrahepatic left lobar duct and extensive experience in biliary operations.[33]

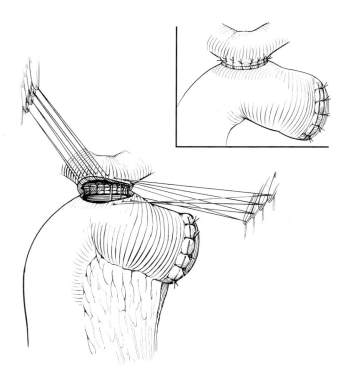

Fig. 5. End-to-side hepaticojejunostomy.

Double Biliary-Enteric Anastomoses

A double hepaticojejunostomy may be necessary to reconstruct the biliary tree in Bismuth type IV injuries (i.e., when the right and left hepatic ducts are separated). Adequate duct length with viable mucosa and tension-free techniques are mandatory. In patients in whom one lobar duct is suitable for anastomosis but the other duct is of poor quality or in a poor location, a single hepaticojejunostomy can be combined with another drainage procedure (e.g., either a technique such as a segment 3 approach or, in the presence of lobar atrophy or lobar intrahepatic stones or abscess, a hepatic lobectomy).

Bismuth Type V Injuries

Sectoral duct injuries pose difficulties in repair through a hilar approach. Hilar scarring and duct retraction are the major contributing factors. The right lateral sector is injured most frequently. This duct can be accessed through the recessus dextra of Gans if present or by a transparenchymal ultrasonographically localized approach to expose the duct for reconstruction. The Longmire procedure has little applicability with today's image-guided dissection.

Use of the Gallbladder

In some instances, the gallbladder can be used as a conduit for definitive biliary drainage. Importantly, the cystic duct must be patent and enter the common bile duct 5 to 10 mm above the most proximal extent of the stricture. The

long-term outcome (mean, 8 years of follow-up) of these anastomoses was shown to be successful in biliary decompression in 85% of cases.[39] Loop or Roux-en-Y cholecystojejunostomy was the procedure most commonly used, but cholecystoduodenostomy or cholecystogastrostomy was also used. This operative strategy should be kept in mind when the gallbladder is present and the primary obstructive process is benign and distal.

OUTCOMES

Interpretation of the current data on bile duct strictures and injuries is confounded by multiple causes, the types and timing of repair, technical approaches, and, most importantly, the duration of follow-up. Generalized recommendations, even for a specific type of injury, are difficult because of the low overall frequency of injuries and the absence of controlled trials comparing treatment options. Despite these confounding factors, several findings are supported by the collective published data. Patients who undergo repair by experienced hepatobiliary surgeons at the time of initial injury or for the initial repair have better long-term outcomes than those who

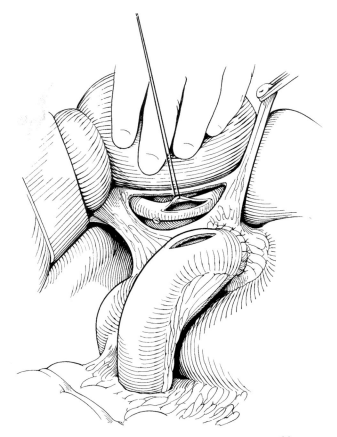

Fig. 6. Hepp-Couinaud procedure. (From Murr et al.[23] By permission of Mayo Foundation.)

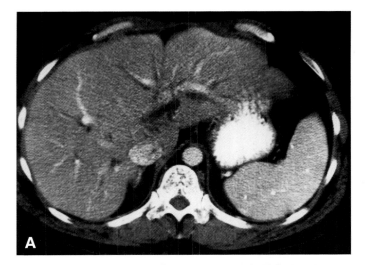

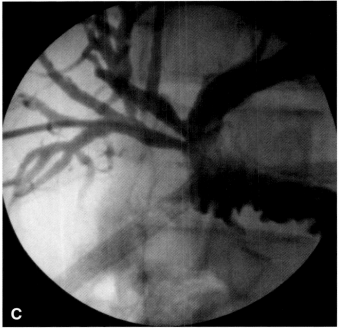

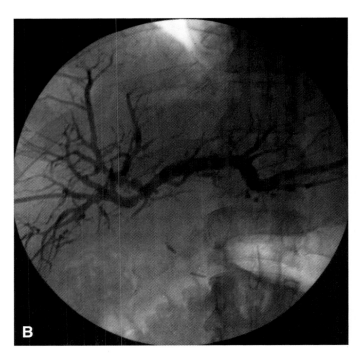

Fig. 7. A patient with bile duct injury after laparoscopic chole-cystectomy. (A), Computed tomogram shows intrahepatic biliary dilatation. (B), Percutaneous cholangiogram. Note that both hepatic ducts communicate but no common hepatic duct is visualized (Bismuth type III). (C), Cholangiogram obtained after operative repair (Hepp-Couinaud procedure) with free flow of contrast agent into the jejunal limb.

undergo delayed or revised repair.[40] These operations can be difficult and time-consuming and involve special techniques that are best addressed by a multidisciplinary approach to the diagnosis and timing of therapy. Consequently, any complex biliary injury recognized at the time of operation by a surgeon with minimal experience in complex biliary reconstruction should not be repaired at that time. Instead, the patient should be stabilized and transferred as soon as possible (within 24 hours) to an institution with hepatobiliary expertise. The patient's best chance of a favorable long-term outcome is the initial repair.

Table 1 shows the outcome of several recent series of bile duct repairs for injuries associated with laparoscopic cholecystectomy. Success should accompany 85% or more of the repairs. We prefer immediate repair in fresh bile duct injuries, even on the same day (the time needed to transfer the patients to us from a local unit) or within 24 to 48 hours with concurrent medical conditions permitting. It is not necessarily our preferred practice to place percutaneous transhepatic stents and delay the early reconstruction, because scarring other than that elicited by the primary biliary abnormality is minimal and the anatomy is unchanged from the description of the primary surgeon.[23] Alternatively, if transfer has been delayed (1 week or more) or recognition of the injury was delayed, control of intra-abdominal infection, bile leaks, or collections is necessary before attempting repair. Definitive repair must be deferred until the patient's generalized condition and perihepatic inflammation and sepsis are controlled. Finally,

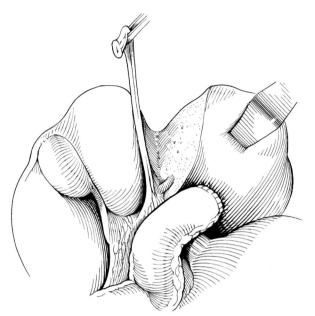

Fig. 8. Segment 3 approach (with wedge resection).

repair of some injuries should be deferred because the size of the bile ducts proximal to the stricture or injury are simply too small (≤ 2-3 mm) for repair, especially if biliary-enteric anastomosis is required.

CONCLUSION

Biliary tract injuries and strictures are probably more common than suggested in the literature. Certainly, there is a need for a unified system both to report and to assess long-term outcomes. Because of the complex nature of biliary injuries, patients should be treated with a multidisciplinary approach that combines the techniques of interventional radiology, gastroenterology, and surgery. Referring these patients to major centers of excellence that perform a high volume of hepatobiliary procedures ensures optimal care and facilitates long-term evaluation with regard to type of injury and procedure performed.

Table 1.—Surgical Outcomes of Bile Duct Repair After Laparoscopy-Induced Bile Duct Injury

Institution	No. of patients	Operative mortality, %	Success rate, %	Mean follow-up, mo
Johns Hopkins[41]	52	0	92	33
Cleveland Clinic[42]	34	0	91	36
University of Pennsylvania[43]	32	3	83	12
University of Alabama[27]	27	4	81	30
Mayo Clinic, Rochester[23]	59	2	88	44

REFERENCES

1. Mayo WJ: Some remarks on cases involving operative loss of continuity of the common bile duct, with the report of a case of anastomosis between the hepatic duct and the duodenum. Ann Surg 42:90-96, 1905
2. Avisse C, Flament J-B, Delattre J-F: Ampulla of Vater: anatomic, embryologic, and surgical aspects. Surg Clin North Am 80:201-212, 2000
3. Nagorney DM, van Heerden JA: Surgical anatomy of the liver and biliary tree. *In* Liver Cancer. Edited by JC Bottino, RW Opfell, FM Muggia. Boston, Martinus Nijhoff Publishing, 1985, pp 87-98
4. Maher JJ, McGuire RF: Extracellular matrix gene expression increases preferentially in rat lipocytes and sinusoidal endothelial cells during hepatic fibrosis in vivo. J Clin Invest 86:1641-1648, 1990
5. Friedman SL: Molecular mechanisms of hepatic fibrosis and principles of therapy. J Gastroenterol 32:424-430, 1997
6. Bailey ME: Endotoxin, bile salts and renal function in obstructive jaundice. Br J Surg 63:774-778, 1976
7. Clements WD, Halliday MI, McCaigue MD, Barclay RG, Rowlands BJ: Effects of extrahepatic obstructive jaundice on Kupffer cell clearance capacity. Arch Surg 128:200-204, 1993
8. Bismuth H: Postoperative strictures of the bile duct. Clin Surg Int 5:209-218, 1982
9. Strasberg SM, Hertl M, Soper NJ: An analysis of the problem of biliary injury during laparoscopic cholecystectomy. J Am Coll Surg 180:101-125, 1995
10. Mirizzi PL: Sindrome del conducto hepatico. G Int Chir 8:731, 1948
11. Bower TC, Nagorney DM: Mirizzi syndrome. HPB Surg 1:67-74, 1988

12. Mackenzie ME, Davies WT, Farnell MB, Weaver AL, Ilstrup DM: Risk of recurrent biliary tract disease after cholecystectomy in patients with duodenal diverticula. Arch Surg 131:1083-1085, 1996

13. Lotveit T, Skar V, Osnes M: Juxtapapillary duodenal diverticula. Endoscopy 20 Suppl 1:175-178, 1988

14. Kim CH, Farrugia G, Farnell MB: High-grade obstruction of the proximal extrahepatic bile duct: an unusual complication of duodenal ulcer disease. Am J Gastroenterol 86:1826-1828, 1991

15. Sarr MG, Shepard AJ, Zuidema GD: Choledochoduodenal fistula: an unusual complication of duodenal ulcer disease. Am J Surg 141:736-740, 1981

16. Stahl TJ, Allen MO, Ansel HJ, Vennes JA: Partial biliary obstruction caused by chronic pancreatitis: an appraisal of indications for surgical biliary drainage. Ann Surg 207:26-32, 1988

17. McMahon AJ, Fullarton G, Baxter JN, O'Dwyer PJ: Bile duct injury and bile leakage in laparoscopic cholecystectomy. Br J Surg 82:307-313, 1995

18. Deziel DJ, Millikan KW, Economou SG, Doolas A, Ko ST, Airan MC: Complications of laparoscopic cholecystectomy: a national survey of 4,292 hospitals and an analysis of 77,604 cases. Am J Surg 165:9-14, 1993

19. Woods MS, Traverso LW, Kozarek RA, Tsao J, Rossi RL, Gough D, Donohue JH: Characteristics of biliary tract complications during laparoscopic cholecystectomy: a multi-institutional study. Am J Surg 167:27-33, 1994

20. Donohue JH, Farnell MB, Grant CS, van Heerden JA, Wahlstrom HE, Sarr MG, Weaver AL, Ilstrup DM: Laparoscopic cholecystectomy: early Mayo Clinic experience. Mayo Clin Proc 67:449-455, 1992

21. The Southern Surgeons Club: A prospective analysis of 1,518 laparoscopic cholecystectomies. N Engl J Med 324:1073-1078, 1991

22. Zucker KA, Bailey RW, Gadacz TR, Imbembo AL: Laparoscopic guided cholecystectomy. Am J Surg 161:36-42, 1991

23. Murr MM, Gigot JF, Nagorney DM, Harmsen WS, Ilstrup DM, Farnell MB: Long-term results of biliary reconstruction after laparoscopic bile duct injuries. Arch Surg 134:604-609, 1999

24. Donohue JH, Grant CS, Farnell MB, van Heerden JA: Laparoscopic cholecystectomy: operative technique. Mayo Clin Proc 67:441-448, 1992

25. Davidoff AM, Branum GD, Meyers WC: Clinical features and mechanisms of major laparoscopic biliary injury. Semin Ultrasound CT MR 14:338-345, 1993

26. Rossi RL, Schirmer WJ, Braasch JW, Sanders LB, Munson JL: Laparoscopic bile duct injuries: risk factors, recognition, and repair. Arch Surg 127:596-601, 1992

27. Mirza DF, Narsimhan KL, Ferraz Neto BH, Mayer AD, McMaster P, Buckels JA: Bile duct injury following laparoscopic cholecystectomy: referral pattern and management. Br J Surg 84:786-790, 1997

28. Coakley FV, Schwartz LH, Blumgart LH, Fong Y, Jarnagin WR, Panicek DM: Complex postcholecystectomy biliary disorders: preliminary experience with evaluation by means of breath-hold MR cholangiography. Radiology 209:141-146, 1998

29. Vennes JA: Technique of ERCP. In Gastroenterologic Endoscopy. Edited by MV Sirvik JR. Philadelphia, WB Saunders Company, 1987, pp 562-580

30. Mueller PR, van Sonnenberg E, Ferrucci JT Jr, Weyman PJ, Butch RJ, Malt RA, Burhenne HJ: Biliary stricture dilatation: multicenter review of clinical management in 73 patients. Radiology 160:17-22, 1986

31. Coons HG: Self-expanding stainless steel biliary stents. Radiology 170:979-983, 1989

32. Pitt HA, Miyamoto T, Parapatis SK, Tompkins RK, Longmire WP Jr: Factors influencing outcome in patients with postoperative biliary strictures. Am J Surg 144:14-21, 1982

33. Sarmiento JM: Hepaticojejunostomy. Op Tech Gen Surg 3:295-303, 2000

34. Andren-Sandberg A, Johansson S, Bengmark S: Accidental lesions of the common bile duct at cholecystectomy. II. Results of treatment. Ann Surg 201:452-455, 1985

35. Csendes A, Diaz JC, Burdiles P, Maluenda F: Late results of immediate primary end to end repair in accidental section of the common bile duct. Surg Gynecol Obstet 168:125-130, 1989

36. Judd ES: Stricture of the common bile duct. Ann Surg 84:404-410, 1926

37. Smith R: Hepaticojejunostomy with transhepatic intubation: a technique for very high strictures of the hepatic ducts. Br J Surg 51:186-194, 1964

38. Longmire WP Jr, Sanford MC: Intrahepatic cholangiojejunostomy with partial hepatectomy for biliary obstruction. Surgery 24:264-276, 1948

39. Oishi AJ, Sarr MG, Nagorney DM, Traynor MD, Mucha P Jr: Long-term outcome of cholecystoenterostomy as a definitive biliary drainage procedure for benign disease. World J Surg 19:616-619, 1995

40. Blumgart LH, Kelley CJ, Benjamin IS: Benign bile duct stricture following cholecystectomy: critical factors in management. Br J Surg 71:836-843, 1984

41. Lillemoe KD, Martin SA, Cameron JL, Yeo CJ, Talamini MA, Kaushal S, Coleman J, Venbrux AC, Savader SJ, Osterman FA, Pitt HA: Major bile duct injuries during laparoscopic cholecystectomy: follow-up after combined surgical and radiologic management. Ann Surg 225:459-468, 1997

42. Walsh RM, Henderson JM, Vogt DP, Mayes JT, Grundfest-Broniatowski S, Gagner M, Ponsky JL, Hermann RE: Trends in bile duct injuries from laparoscopic cholecystectomy. J Gastrointest Surg 2:458-462, 1998

43. Bauer TW, Morris JB, Lowenstein A, Wolferth C, Rosato FE, Rosato EF: The consequences of a major bile duct injury during laparoscopic cholecystectomy. J Gastrointest Surg 2:61-66, 1998

Chapter 17

CANCER OF THE GALLBLADDER

John H. Donohue, M.D.

Carcinoma of the gallbladder is a highly lethal disease rarely diagnosed at an early stage. Gallbladder cancer was diagnosed in an estimated 6,900 patients in the United States in 2000, and 3,400 of them will die from this malignancy.[1] For most patients who present with advanced-stage disease, surgical treatment can provide only palliation. Surgical resection is the only potentially curative treatment for less extensive tumors. This chapter emphasizes the Mayo Clinic approach to the surgical treatment of patients with carcinoma of the gallbladder diagnosed preoperatively or discovered incidentally during cholecystectomy.

BASIC FOCUSED PATHOPHYSIOLOGY AND MOLECULAR BIOLOGY

Etiology

Many factors have been associated with carcinoma of the gallbladder, most of which are the result of chronic inflammation of the gallbladder mucosa. The most common etiologic factor is gallstones, but a malignancy of the gallbladder will develop in only a tiny fraction of patients (about 1%) with cholelithiasis, and as many as 25% of patients with carcinoma do not have documented stones.[2] Single large stones (diameter ≥ 3.0 cm) have been associated more than smaller gallstones with an increased risk of cancer.[3] A recent prospective study[4] found that increases in the number and size of gallstones in patients with gallbladder cancer are merely functions of long-standing gallstone disease in older patients.

An anomalous junction of the pancreatic and common bile duct has been recognized for decades as a risk factor for biliary tract carcinoma.[5] Patients who have this anatomical variant and in whom choledochal cysts develop are known to be especially prone to malignant degeneration, hypothesized to occur due to chronic reflux of pancreatic secretions alone or in combination with bile stasis. Gallbladder cancer may develop in patients with an anomalous junction of the pancreatic and common bile ducts, either with[6] or without[7] choledochal cysts.

Other types of chronic gallbladder inflammation known to increase the risk of gallbladder cancer include chronic typhoid carrier status[8] and porcelain gallbladder. In the latter pathologic condition, chronic irritation of the gallbladder results in calcification of the mucosa that is often accompanied by adenomatous and squamous metaplastic changes. Patients with mucosal calcifications have a 10% to 25% risk of cancer.[9] Thus, after a diagnosis of porcelain gallbladder, especially when mucosal calcification is involved, cholecystectomy should be performed. In the absence of mucosal calcification, segmental calcification of the wall of the gallbladder appears to have only a minimal association with neoplastic degeneration.[10]

Several known carcinogens have been associated with carcinoma of the gallbladder. Rubber-product workers have an increased risk, and animal studies also have implicated nitrosamines and methylcholanthrene as carcinogens that result in gallbladder cancer.[11]

Polypoid lesions of the gallbladder are common, but most represent cholesterol or hyperplastic polyps. Adenomatous gallbladder polyps increase the risk of carcinoma but do not become a major risk until the polyp reaches a larger diameter (>1 cm).[12] Any large (>1 cm) polypoid mass of the gallbladder mucosa or one that serial ultrasonographic evaluations show is growing should be treated with cholecystectomy.

Genetic factors also may contribute to the risk of gallbladder cancer. Women have 3 times the risk of malignancy of men, most likely because of their higher incidence of gallstones and higher concentrations of estrogen.[13] The incidence of gallbladder cancer varies widely around the world, with the highest rates reported in Israel, Mexico, Bolivia, Chile, and Japan.[14] In the United States, the southwestern states, especially New Mexico,[15] have the highest incidence of this cancer, largely as a function of the increased prevalence among Hispanics[16] and Native Americans.[17] Interactions among genetic and environmental factors are likely to affect the development of carcinoma of the gallbladder, but exact correlations are not known.

Natural History

Although many carcinomas of the gallbladder are assumed to arise from a dysplastic mucosal abnormality, with an in situ carcinoma phase,[12] these findings of disease progression usually are not apparent at diagnosis. In some cancers, the tumor appears to arise from normal gallbladder mucosa.[18] In cancers of the biliary tree, three gross types of tumor growth have been categorized: papillary, nodular, and sclerosing. More often, papillary cancers are lower grade, have less-invasive characteristics, and carry a more favorable prognosis.[19] In contrast, sclerosing tumors are high-grade lesions that infiltrate the full thickness of the gallbladder and adjacent organs early in development and portend a poor prognosis. The characteristics of nodular cancers are intermediate between those of papillary and sclerosing carcinomas.[20]

The more biologically aggressive the cancer, the sooner it enters a vertical growth phase and invades the lamina propria, muscularis propria, and serosal layers of the gallbladder wall. Invasion of these layers provides access to the lymphatic and venous systems along the cystic duct and through the bed of the gallbladder into the liver. Lymphatic drainage of the gallbladder is to the hepatoduodenal ligament, with subsequent flow to the retropancreatic, celiac, superior mesenteric, and para-aortic lymph node groups. Venous drainage usually is into the substance of the adjacent liver and only rarely through the portal vein within the liver. These factors explain the pattern of lymphatic and vascular metastases described by Fahim et al.[21]

After the tumor growth has breached the serosal covering or the hepatic attachments of the gallbladder, the tumor can invade adjacent organs, most commonly the liver. On the free serosal surface, the duodenum, structures of the hepatoduodenal ligament, and the transverse colon are the typical sites of direct involvement. Rupture of the free peritoneal surface and peritoneal dissemination often occur in patients with advanced-stage gallbladder carcinoma. Peritoneal seeding and hepatic metastases are the most common sites of distant metastatic disease. Pulmonary and osseous metastases occur less frequently.

Prognostic Factors

The stage of the tumor at presentation is the primary determinant of eventual patient outcome. Although some authors still use the Nevin classification[22] for gallbladder cancer, most currently report their data using the TNM cancer staging system of the American Joint Commission on Cancer (AJCC)[23] (Table 1). The recommendations for curative surgical procedures depend on accurate tumor staging (see below). The probability of patient survival can be determined by tumor staging. Figure 1 shows survival curves for patients with different stages of gallbladder carcinoma. In addition to the extent of the cancer, the performance status of the patient is a significant predictor of outcome, let alone suitability for a major surgical procedure. The Eastern Cooperative Oncology Group (ECOG) classification developed by Zubrod et al.[24] is used most often to grade the performance status of patients (Table 2).

Pathology

Most carcinomas of the gallbladder are adenocarcinomas. Histologic variants, including papillary, nodular, and sclerosing adenocarcinomas, have been well characterized and may correlate with outcome (see above). Metaplasia occurs not infrequently, resulting in adenosquamous, squamous, and carcinosarcoma cancers. True sarcomas, carcinoid tumors, and small-cell cancers have been reported, but all are exceedingly rare.[25]

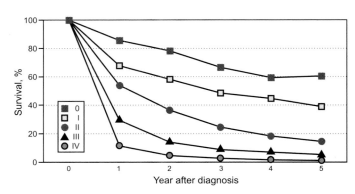

Fig. 1. *Cumulative survival of patients with gallbladder cancer by AJCC stage (all forms of treatment included). Roman numerals signify stage of disease. (From Donohue et al.[50] By permission of the American Cancer Society.)*

Table 1.—TNM Staging for Carcinoma of the Gall-bladder

Primary tumor (T)
  TX   Primary tumor cannot be assessed
  T0   No evidence of primary tumor
  Tis   Carcinoma in situ
  T1   Tumor invades lamina propria or muscle layer
        T1a   Tumor invades lamina propria
        T1b   Tumor invades muscle layer
  T2   Tumor invades the perimuscular connective tissue; no extension beyond serosa or into liver
  T3   Tumor perforates the serosa (visceral peritoneum) and/or directly invades the liver and/or one other adjacent organ or structure, such as the stomach, duodenum, colon, pancreas, omentum, or extrahepatic bile ducts
  T4   Tumor invades main portal vein or hepatic artery or invades multiple extrahepatic organs or structures
Regional lymph nodes (N)
  NX   Regional lymph nodes cannot be assessed
  N0   No regional lymph node metastasis
  N1   Regional lymph node metastasis (hilar lymph nodes [i.e., within the hepatoduodenal ligament], plus celiac, periduodenal, peripancreatic, and superior mesenteric lymph nodes)
Distant metastases (M)
  MX   Distant metastasis cannot be assessed
  M0   No distant metastasis
  M1   Distant metastasis

Stage grouping

Stage	T	N	M
0	Tis	N0	M0
IA	T1	N0	M0
IB	T2	N0	M0
IIA	T3	N0	M0
IIB	T1-T3	N1	M0
III	T4	Any N	M0
IV	Any T	N2	M0
	Any T	Any N	M1

From American Joint Committee on Cancer.[23] By permission of the American Joint Committee on Cancer.

DIAGNOSIS AND IMAGING

Clinical Presentation

Patients with gallbladder cancer have no pathognomonic symptoms. There are also no symptoms or signs to separate patients with gallbladder cancer who have symptoms of biliary colic or acute inflammation from those with only gallstones, unless more advanced disease is present. Nausea, anorexia, and weight loss are common in patients with carcinoma of the gallbladder. Generally, the loss of weight is a poor prognostic sign. Jaundice indicates extrahepatic biliary obstruction or extensive hepatic metastases. Occult or occasionally clinical gastrointestinal hemorrhage may occur as a result of hemobilia or direct invasion of an adjacent portion of the gastrointestinal tract. Gastrointestinal tract obstruction, usually of the proximal duodenum or transverse colon, may occur with locally advanced tumors, with or without distant metastasis. Peritoneal seeding may lead to intestinal obstruction or the development of ascites, which are both ominous clinical findings.[2]

Similarly, no findings on physical examination can distinguish early-stage cancer of the gallbladder from symptomatic gallstones. A gallbladder carcinoma large enough to be palpable in the right upper quadrant feels no different than any other malignancy involving the liver. As in all patients who have aggressive gastrointestinal carcinomas, supraclavicular adenopathy should be sought on physical examination. Signs of peritoneal dissemination, including palpable metastases, ascites, nodules in the pelvic cul-de-sac palpable per rectum (Blumer's shelf), or a Sister Mary Joseph's node, are indicative of a poor prognosis. (Sister Mary Joseph was Dr. William J. Mayo's scrub nurse. She sometimes noted a hard nodule just under the umbilicus while preparing the abdomen for operation in patients with gastrointestinal malignancies. The nodule almost always proved to be a metastasis.)

Table 2.—Eastern Cooperative Oncology Group Performance Status Scale

Grade
  0   Fully active; able to carry on all activities without restriction
  1   Restricted in physically strenuous activity, but ambulatory and able to carry out work of a light or sedentary nature (e.g., light housework, office work)
  2   Ambulatory and capable of all self-care but unable to carry out any work activities; up and about more than 50% of waking hours
  3   Capable of limited self-care only; confined to bed or chair more than 50% of waking hours
  4   Completely disabled; cannot carry on any self-care; totally confined to bed or chair

Data from Zubrod et al.[24]

Laboratory Evaluation

As in patients with cholelithiasis, abnormal serum levels of the enzymes alkaline phosphatase, aspartate aminotransferase, and alanine aminotransferase are common in patients with carcinoma of the gallbladder, but an increased concentration of bilirubin is present much less frequently, except with locally advanced or metastatic disease. Tumor markers are nonspecific for gallbladder cancer, but both carcinoembryonic antigen and carbohydrate antigen 19-9 may be increased in patients with carcinoma of the gallbladder. Carbohydrate antigen 19-9 is more likely to be increased, as it is with other malignancies and inflammatory conditions of the biliary tract and pancreas.

Imaging

Many cancers of the gallbladder are diagnosed only during cholecystectomy. Ultrasonography of the biliary tract is the most sensitive preoperative imaging tool. A large gallbladder polyp (>1 cm) or asymmetric thickening of the gallbladder wall is suggestive of gallbladder carcinoma, but neither is a specific finding for this disease. Overall, ultrasonography is diagnostic in only 30% of patients.[26] In patients suspected of having gallbladder cancer on ultrasound examination or whose disease is found during cholecystectomy, evaluation of the entire abdomen with spiral computed tomography or magnetic resonance imaging is indicated. In many patients with advanced disease, these tests reveal gross invasion of the liver, involvement of adjacent extrahepatic structures, the cause of any biliary obstruction, and the presence of regional adenopathy and some distant metastases (hepatic metastases are more apparent than peritoneal seeding).

In two 1993 reports,[27,28] the diagnosis of cancer with preoperative imaging (e.g., ultrasonography, computed tomography) was possible before exploration in only 35% to 40% of patients. However, these articles did not include current state-of-the-art imaging studies. Earlier recommendations for evaluation of gallbladder cancer included visceral angiography and cholangiography, but these tests are seldom indicated, given the resolution of current high-quality computed tomography and magnetic resonance imaging studies. When a major surgical procedure with curative intent is being considered, chest radiographs also should be obtained preoperatively.

INDICATIONS FOR OPERATION

Operative resection is the only effective treatment for carcinoma of the gallbladder. A curative procedure should be considered in patients who have tumors that can be excised completely with clear margins and who are suitable candidates for an operation. Most gallbladder cancers have metastasized before diagnosis, and evidence of the spread of disease should be sought on preoperative studies and diagnostic laparoscopy before exploratory laparotomy. Incomplete resection provides no survival benefit to patients and should not be undertaken knowingly unless it can be expected to be palliative.

In patients with possible gallbladder cancer indicated on preoperative imaging, the definitive operation should be performed with a laparotomy rather than as a laparoscopic procedure. Similarly, if evidence of localized gallbladder carcinoma is discovered during laparoscopic cholecystectomy, the operation should be converted to an open procedure for several reasons. First, staging of the cancer is more accurate with lymphadenectomy and complete intraoperative assessment of the abdomen. Second, as reported by several authors,[29-31] disseminated tumor spread may occur after laparoscopic cholecystectomy due to bile spillage and transection of the tumor during laparoscopic manipulation. Indeed, tumor recurrence at the sites of laparoscopic ports is common after a laparoscopic cholecystectomy in patients with gallbladder carcinoma. For some patients, unnecessary violation of the tumor during laparoscopic cholecystectomy prevents a curative operation. Third, an operation of the appropriate magnitude can be achieved immediately after conversion to laparotomy, rather than as a second procedure when only laparoscopic cholecystectomy is pursued.

Patients found incidentally to have in situ gallbladder cancer (stage 0) at cholecystectomy do not require further operative treatment. Several series[2,32,33] have shown excellent survival for these patients. Similarly, reports[34,35] have shown that patients with T1 carcinoma of the gallbladder also can be treated adequately with a simple cholecystectomy. However, multiple histologic sections of the T1 tumor should be evaluated to assess for penetration of the cancer transmurally and to determine whether tumor transgression occurred during the gallbladder excision.[34] If either condition is present, more radical surgical procedures with curative intent should be considered. All patients with T1 cancers who are not reexplored should have baseline computed tomography of the abdomen to assess for regional adenopathy or other sites of residual tumor. All patients with clinical gallbladder cancers of stage IB to stage IIB should be assessed for potential resectability. Patients with distant metastases (M1) or with radiographic or clinical evidence of para-aortic nodal metastases are classified stage IV and are not considered candidates for curative operations. Patients with T4 cancer (stage III) are generally unresectable because of locally advanced cancer, although curative surgery is feasible in some, especially when the surgeon is able to perform vascular reconstruction.

Palliative cholecystectomy benefits patients with gall-bladder cancer who have acute cholecystitis or symptomatic cholelithiasis. Patients with jaundice caused by unresectable carcinoma of the gallbladder generally are managed best by percutaneous transhepatic biliary drainage catheters or an endoscopically placed biliary stent. In patients whose tumors are found to be unresectable at laparotomy, a Roux-en-Y jejunal limb may be anastomosed to the confluence of the left and right hepatic ducts, but this site usually is not accessible. A biliary bypass, using the segment III round-ligament approach, is another technical option; however, nonsurgical biliary drainage is still the simplest, most effective method of palliation. Patients with gastric outlet or colonic obstruction should be treated with an operative bypass procedure.

CONDUCT OF THE OPERATION

Preoperative Preparation

Treatment options that should be discussed preoperatively with patients who have a clinically resectable carcinoma of the gallbladder include radical cholecystectomy (subsegmental resections of segments IVB and V adjacent to the gallbladder fossa and a regional lymphadenectomy), with or without resection of adherent structures such as the common bile duct, duodenum, and colon; on occasion, a major hepatectomy may be necessary. Patients who have had a laparoscopic cholecystectomy should be told that the port site incisions also must be excised. Patients are given a mechanical bowel preparation, prophylaxis to avert deep venous thrombophlebitis, and perioperative intravenous antibiotics (usually a first-generation cephalosporin).

Diagnostic Laparoscopy

A diagnostic laparoscopy, with the patient supine, should be performed in all patients with gallbladder cancer, because occult peritoneal and hepatic metastases are often not evident on noninvasive imaging, which would preclude celiotomy. This procedure is of value, even in patients who recently have had a laparoscopic cholecystectomy for presumably benign symptomatic gallbladder disease, because the original surgeon may not have assessed for metastatic disease.

The laparoscope is best inserted at the umbilicus. If the patient has had a laparoscopic cholecystectomy, the previous port site should be excised and the cannula placed under direct vision using the Hassan technique. One or two cannulae are placed in the upper abdomen under direct vision. Old port sites should be used and excised when practical. Special attention should be paid to the surface of the liver and to the visceral and parietal peritoneal surfaces

in the abdomen and pelvis. If ascites is present, a sample should be sent for cytologic evaluation and inspection should be conducted for peritoneal seeding. Any abnormalities should undergo biopsy and be evaluated by frozen section histologic analysis. If no findings are present to indicate unresectability of the tumor, the surgeon should proceed to open exploration for potential resection.

Incision and Exposure

A bilateral subcostal incision gives excellent access for radical cholecystectomy (Fig. 2). Most of the three rostral cannula sites from the laparoscopic cholecystectomy can be included in a single incision. During the procedure, all three incision sites should be excised because of potential tumor seeding at these locations from the initial operation.[36,37] To provide rostral exposure, a self-retaining retractor is placed on both costal margins after the round and falciform ligaments of the liver are divided. A thorough abdominal exploration evaluates for hepatic, peritoneal, and distant nodal metastases. The extent of

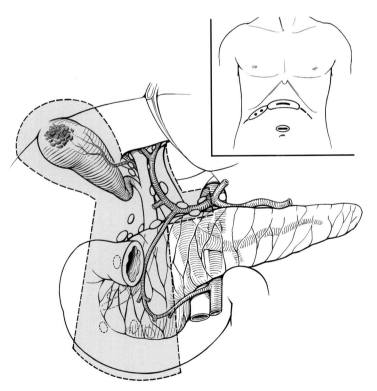

Fig. 2. The patient has undergone a previous attempt at laparoscopic cholecystectomy, at which time an invasive gallbladder cancer was diagnosed. The inset (upper right) *shows the typical bilateral subcostal incision used for radical cholecystectomy, including excision of the laparoscopic port sites. The umbilical port site is excised separately. The main drawing shows the extent of the cholecystectomy and gallbladder bed resection of parts of segments 4B and 5, and the extent of the regional lymphadenectomy of a radical cholecystectomy.*

the primary tumor and its adherence to or invasion of adjacent organs also are investigated. The hepatic flexure of the colon is mobilized, allowing placement of a second self-retaining retractor to hold the transverse colon caudally. A generous Kocher maneuver close to the posterior aspect of the pancreas leaves the retropancreatic nodes behind in the retroperitoneum (Fig. 3). Partial division of the right hepatic triangular and cardinal ligaments also may help expose the caudal portion of the liver.

Radical Cholecystectomy; Hepatic Resection

If there is no gross invasion of the liver parenchyma, a 2-cm margin of normal liver parenchyma should be resected with the gallbladder or with the gallbladder fossa if a cholecystectomy has been performed previously (Fig. 3). After scoring the lines of resection with electrocautery, the surgeon should divide the parenchyma with cautery or an ultrasonic dissector. If gross invasion of the adjacent liver is present near the gallbladder fundus, a wider margin of parenchyma from segment 4B and segment 5 should be

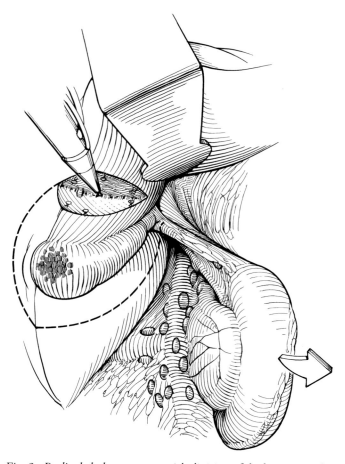

Fig. 3. Radical cholecystectomy with division of the liver parenchyma using an ultrasonic dissector. The duodenum has been mobilized (arrow)*, leaving the retroduodenal and retropancreatic lymph nodes posteriorly in the retroperitoneum for later dissection.*

included. If the carcinoma invades the liver near the neck of the gallbladder, an extended right hepatectomy (portion segment 4B, segments 5-8) should achieve adequate pathologic margins.

Radical Cholecystectomy; Regional Lymphadenectomy

The pattern of lymphatic spread in gallbladder cancer has been well detailed.[21,38,39] The pericholecystic lymph node is usually the first site of regional tumor metastasis. Other lymph nodes in the hepatoduodenal ligament also are involved, followed by metastases to the retroduodenal, retropancreatic, hepatic artery, celiac, superior mesenteric, and finally the para-aortic nodal groups.

Because of the possible occurrence of nodal metastases in patients with carcinoma of the gallbladder, a regional lymphadenectomy is an integral part of the radical surgical management considered potentially curative. Lymph nodes within the shaded area in Figure 2 should be included in the dissection. The hepatoduodenal ligament should be skeletonized during this procedure to expose fully the common bile duct, proper hepatic artery, and portal vein and to clear them circumferentially of adherent lymphatic channels and nerves. The soft tissue behind the head of the pancreas and behind the encircling duodenum also is resected so that the anterior surfaces of the inferior vena cava and aorta can be observed. The nodal tissue along the common hepatic artery to its origin at the celiac axis also is included with the other specimens. Although some Japanese authors[40] have recommended a formal para-aortic nodal dissection or even a concomitant pancreatoduodenectomy, this extensive resection is not a proven means of improving patient outcome.

To remove all nodal tissue with the retroperitoneal tissue, the lymphadenectomy requires mobilization of the pancreatic head, immediately posterior to the duodenum and pancreatic parenchyma (Fig. 3). At the caudad end of the suprapancreatic common bile duct, prominent lymph nodes are in continuity with the retroduodenal and retropancreatic nodal groups. Other lymph nodes are posterior to the portal vein. These nodes should be removed together by incising the retroperitoneal tissues, exposing the inferior vena cava and aorta at the inferomedial and inferolateral aspects of the dissection, and mobilizing these tissues cephalad toward the pericholedochal nodes. The lymph nodes of the hepatoduodenal ligament should be removed separately from the retroduodenal and retropancreatic lymph nodes.

The portal lymph node dissection is easier to start along the right lateral side of the hepatoduodenal ligament, exposing the full length of the lateral side of the suprapancreatic common bile duct and common hepatic duct. At the inferolateral aspect of the hepatoduodenal ligament, one or more small branches of the portal vein usually must be controlled with ligation or cautery. It may be easier to divide the lymphatics posterior to the portal vein and remove the nodal specimen from the lateral hepatoduodenal ligament separately; however, all the lateral nodes usually can be pushed posteriorly and toward the left for removal from the hepatoduodenal ligament as a single specimen (Fig. 4). The peritoneum overlying the anterior surface of the hepatoduodenal ligament is incised rostrally at the base of the liver and caudally at the cephalad border of the first portion of the duodenum. The extrahepatic bile ducts, the main and proximal left and right portal veins, and the proper hepatic artery and its branches are dissected and freed by removing the relatively sparse but tenacious fibroareolar tissue, which includes some lymphatics, nodes, and the autonomic nerves to the liver. After the anterior surface of the hepatoduodenal ligament has been cleared, the previously dissected nodes from the lateral and posterior side of this structure also can be detached after dividing the tissue at the medial edge of the hepatoduodenal ligament. The latter generally are easiest to expose by pushing them toward the midline with the fingers of the left hand in the epiploic foramen.

The last portion of the lymphadenectomy involves skeletonization of the common hepatic artery, including the lymph nodes that lie anteriorly and posteriorly to this vessel. This specimen usually includes some adjacent suprapancreatic lymph nodes. Small arterial and venous vessels are encountered during this dissection, the control of which is essential for a thorough nodal dissection. The regional lymph node dissection is completed by removing the fibroareolar tissue and nodes to the right and anterior to the celiac trunk. Figure 4 shows this portion of the operation completed before removal of the lymph nodes from the hepatoduodenal ligament.

A drain is not required routinely. However, if a bile leak from the site of the hepatic resection or skeletonization of the extrahepatic bile duct is a concern, a closed suction drain should be left near the gastroepiploic foramen in the right subhepatic space.

Operative Considerations in Laparoscopic Cholecystectomy

Because laparoscopic ports are often the site of recurrence after a gallbladder carcinoma is resected by laparoscopic cholecystectomy, they should be excised during an open curative resection.[30,31,36,37] The upper three previous laparoscopic incisions usually can be encompassed in the subcostal incision, with a full-thickness excision from the skin to the peritoneum. The periumbilical port site should be excised separately. The omentum and other tissues adherent to the gallbladder bed should be excised en bloc

with the adjacent liver tissue. In all other respects, the radical cholecystectomy procedure is conducted as described above.

Extended Resections

Locally advanced disease may be evidenced by tumor adherence to adjacent organs. The involved structures typically include the common hepatic and common bile ducts, omentum, duodenum, transverse colon, and loops of small bowel. Because benign fibrous adhesions cannot be distinguished from transmural tumor growing into an adjacent structure, the involved structure(s) should be removed en bloc during any curative surgical procedure. Evidence of distal metastases, especially peritoneal seeding and extensive distal nodal metastases, should be sought carefully before proceeding with radical resection. Figure 5 demonstrates removal of a portion of adherent duodenum during a radical cholecystectomy. A limited duodenal resection may be closed primarily. To avoid tension on the biliary enteric anastomosis, removal of a segment of the extrahepatic bile duct usually necessitates reconstruction

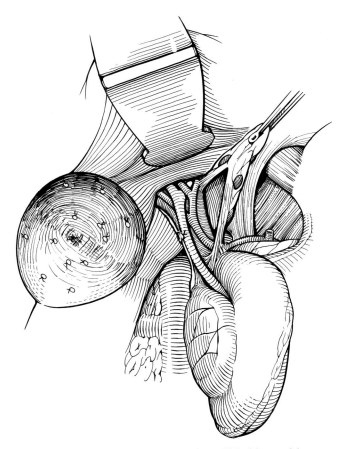

Fig. 4. Radical cholecystectomy. The gallbladder and liver surrounding the gallbladder have been resected, and the hepatoduodenal lymph nodes have been freed from all surfaces but the anteromedial side of the portal triad.

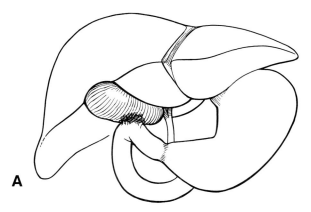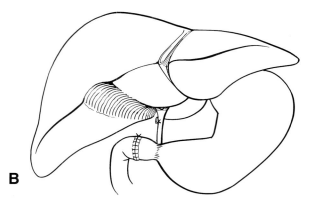

Fig. 5. (A), *Gallbladder cancer adherent to the duodenum.* (B), *The gallbladder, adjacent portions of the liver, adherent portion of the duodenum, and regional lymph nodes have been resected. The defect in the duodenum has been repaired by a transverse closure using sutures.*

with a Roux-en-Y hepaticojejunostomy. Pancreaticoduodenectomy has been recommended for locally advanced gallbladder cancer by some Japanese surgeons,[41-43] but it is not recommended by Western authors except in exceptional cases of gallbladder cancer.

Postoperative Care

No special treatment is required after radical cholecystectomy. If a nasogastric tube is used, it usually can be removed by the morning after the operation. When evidence of normal gastrointestinal function (i.e., hunger, flatus) returns, a diet is restarted, then advanced to a full diet as rapidly as tolerated. Immediate postoperative parenteral or epidural narcotics are followed by oral analgesics after resumption of a diet.

Most patients can be discharged 5 to 7 days after their operation, unless they required an extrahepatic bile duct resection. Full recovery to preoperative activities generally takes 4 to 6 weeks. Although several authors have evaluated the efficacy of adjuvant radiation therapy with and without fluorouracil radiosensitization,[44-46] no controlled data exist to justify its routine use. Radiation therapy with chemosensitization should be considered for localized sites of known or suspected microscopic residual disease. Because diffuse peritoneal, hepatic, or other sites of distant metastasis are not uncommon with advanced-stage gallbladder cancer, radiation therapy will have only a limited impact on patient survival. No effective adjuvant or neoadjuvant chemotherapy regimen for carcinoma of the gallbladder has been reported.[47]

Surgical Outcomes

Because survival traditionally has been so poor (5-year survival about 5%) for all patients with gallbladder cancer, some surgeons[48] question the need for any operation more radical than cholecystectomy. Not surprisingly, the best results occur in those patients with in situ (stage 0) gallbladder carcinoma discovered incidentally. Most patients with this stage of tumor are cured, although 5-year survival is still well below 100%, mostly due to deaths unrelated to cancer.[49,50] Although even Tis gallbladder cancer has recurred diffusely after laparoscopic cholecystectomy, no detectable decline in survival has been noted since the advent of routine laparoscopic cholecystectomy.[50] Even with limited invasion of the gallbladder wall in stage IA or T1 cancer, patient survival declines considerably. More advanced primary tumor stage or nodal metastases have an even greater negative impact on patient survival, even with more radical resections. Although Japanese surgeons claim improved survival with major hepatectomy and pancreaticoduodenectomy, no controlled data exist to support these radical operations. Table 3 reviews 5-year survival by stage from several reported series in the United States,[50,51] Europe,[54,56] and Japan.[43,52,53,55] For most patients with gallbladder cancer, metastatic disease at diagnosis negates any benefit of aggressive surgery on improving survival.

CONCLUSION

Carcinoma of the gallbladder is an aggressive and usually fatal illness that occurs predominantly in older women with gallstones. Its nonspecific symptoms often indicate advanced-stage disease. If the diagnosis is suspected preoperatively (an uncommon scenario), metastatic disease should be excluded with standard imaging studies and preceliotomy laparoscopic staging. In patients with localized disease only, an extirpative operation should be performed by an open celiotomy. When gallbladder cancer is encountered unexpectedly during a laparoscopic cholecystectomy, the procedure should be converted to an open operation before mobilization of the gallbladder. If the diagnosis is only made postoperatively, another operation should be undertaken, as appropriate, by tumor stage. Simple cholecystectomy is adequate for

Table 3.—Five-Year Survival by Stage of Gallbladder Cancer

Gallbladder cancer stage	Reference															
	Gagner[51] (1991)		Matsumoto[52] (1992)		Onoyama[53] (1995)		Ruckert[54] (1996)		Tsukada[55] (1996)		Benoist[56] (1998)		Donohue[50] (1998)		Todoroki[43] (1999)	
	Patients		Patients		Patients		Patients		Patients		Patients		Patients		Patients	
	No.	%	No.	%	No.	%	No.	%	No.	%	No.	%	No.	%	No.	%
0	NA	NA	NA	NA	NA	NA	NA	NA	NA	NA	NA	NA	60	60	NA	NA
I	NA	40	4	100	28	79	6	33	15	91	36	44	169	39	13	100
II	NA	9	9	90	11	64	10	33	24	85	24	24	179	15	19	78
III	NA	7	8	38	12	44	12	8	28	40	13	13	240	5	7	69
IV	NA	1	27	19	14	8	53	2	39	19	9	0	822	1	96	11

NA, not available.

stage 0 and stage IA cancer. For more advanced cancers, the operation of choice is a radical cholecystectomy, including partial hepatectomy and regional lymphadenectomy, with en bloc resection of structures adherent to the gallbladder. The presence of distant metastases (e.g., hepatic metastases, peritoneal seeding, or gross nodal involvement beyond the hepatoduodenal ligament) indicates nonresectable disease. Postoperative therapy with external beam radiation with 5-fluorouracil chemosensitization should be considered in selected cases, although no controlled data support the efficacy of this approach for this malignancy. The overall poor results of the surgical treatment of gallbladder cancer emphasize the need for better techniques and adjuvant therapies.

REFERENCES

1. Greenlee RT, Murray T, Bolden S, Wingo PA: Cancer statistics, 2000. CA Cancer J Clin 50:7-33, 2000
2. Piehler JM, Crichlow RW: Primary carcinoma of the gallbladder. Surg Gynecol Obstet 147:929-942, 1978
3. Diehl AK: Gallstone size and the risk of gallbladder cancer. JAMA 250:2323-2326, 1983
4. Csendes A, Becerra M, Rojas J, Medina E: Number and size of stones in patients with asymptomatic and symptomatic gallstones and gallbladder carcinoma: a prospective study of 592 cases. J Gastrointest Surg 4:481-485, 2000
5. Babbitt DP: Congenital choledochal cysts: new etiological concept based on anomalous relationships of the common bile duct and pancreatic bulb [French]. Ann Radiol 12:231-240, 1969
6. Kimura K, Ohto M, Saisho H, Unozawa T, Tsuchiya Y, Morita M, Ebara M, Matsutani S, Okuda K: Association of gallbladder carcinoma and anomalous pancreaticobiliary ductal union. Gastroenterology 89:1258-1265, 1985
7. Tanaka K, Nishimura A, Yamada K, Ishibe R, Ishizaki N, Yoshimine M, Hamada N, Taira A: Cancer of the gallbladder associated with anomalous junction of the pancreatobiliary duct system without bile duct dilatation. Br J Surg 80:622-624, 1993
8. Welton JC, Marr JS, Friedman SM: Association between hepatobiliary cancer and typhoid carrier state. Lancet 1:791-794, 1979
9. Berk RN, Armbuster TG, Saltzstein SL: Carcinoma in the porcelain gallbladder. Radiology 106:29-31, 1973
10. Stephen AE, Berger DL: Carcinoma in the porcelain gallbladder: a relationship revisited. Surgery 129:699-703, 2001
11. Fortner JG: The experimental induction of primary carcinoma of the gallbladder. Cancer 8:689-700, 1955
12. Kozuka S, Tsubone N, Yasui A, Hachisuka K: Relation of adenoma to carcinoma in the gallbladder. Cancer 50:2226-2234, 1982
13. Paraskevopoulos JA, Dennison AR, Johnson AG: Primary carcinoma of the gallbladder. HPB Surg 4:277-289, 1991
14. Pitt HA, Dooley WC, Yeo CJ, Cameron JL: Malignancies of the biliary tree. Curr Probl Surg 32:1-90, 1995
15. Lowenfels AB, Lindstrom CG, Conway MJ, Hastings PR: Gallstones and risk of gallbladder cancer. J Natl Cancer Inst 75:77-80, 1985
16. Menck HR, Mack TM: Incidence of biliary tract cancer in Los Angeles. Natl Cancer Inst Monogr 62:95-99, 1982
17. Black WC, Key CR, Carmany TB, Herman D: Carcinoma of the gallbladder in a population of Southwestern American Indians. Cancer 39:1267-1279, 1977
18. Yamamoto M, Nakajo S, Tahara E: Histogenesis of well-differentiated adenocarcinoma of the gallbladder. Pathol Res Pract 184:279-286, 1989
19. Ouchi K, Owada Y, Matsuno S, Sato T: Prognostic factors in the surgical treatment of gallbladder carcinoma. Surgery 101:731-737, 1987
20. Sumiyoshi K, Nagai E, Chijiiwa K, Nakayama F: Pathology of carcinoma of the gallbladder. World J Surg 15:315-321, 1991

21. Fahim RB, McDonald JR, Richards JC, Ferris DO: Carcinoma of the gallbladder: a study of its mode of spread. Ann Surg 156:114-124, 1962

22. Nevin JE, Moran TJ, Kay S, King R: Carcinoma of the gallbladder: staging, treatment, and prognosis. Cancer 37:141-148, 1976

23. American Joint Committee on Cancer: AJCC Cancer Staging Manual. Sixth edition. Edited by FL Greene, DL Page, ID Fleming, AG Fritz, CM Balch, DG Haller, M Morrow. New York, Springer-Verlag, 2002, pp 139-144

24. Zubrod CG, Schneiderman M, Frei E III, Brindley C, Gold GL, Shnider B, Oviedo R, Gorman J, Jones R Jr, Jonsson U, Colsky J, Chalmers T, Ferguson B, Dederick M, Holland J, Selawry O, Regelson W, Lasagna L, Owens AH Jr: Appraisal of methods for the study of chemotherapy of cancer in man: comparative therapeutic trial of nitrogen mustard and triethylene thiophosphoramide. J Chron Dis 11:7-33, 1960

25. Rosai J (editor): Ackerman's Surgical Pathology. Vol 1. Eighth edition. St Louis, Mosby-Year Book, 1996, pp 943-968

26. Tsuchiya Y: Early carcinoma of the gallbladder: macroscopic features and US findings. Radiology 179:171-175, 1991

27. Ouchi K, Suzuki M, Saijo S, Ito K, Matsuno S: Do recent advances in diagnosis and operative management improve the outcome of gallbladder carcinoma? Surgery 113:324-329, 1993

28. Ohtani T, Shirai Y, Tsukada K, Hatakeyama K, Muto T: Carcinoma of the gallbladder: CT evaluation of lymphatic spread. Radiology 189:875-880, 1993

29. Fong Y, Brennan MF, Turnbull A, Colt DG, Blumgart LH: Gallbladder cancer discovered during laparoscopic surgery: potential for iatrogenic tumor dissemination. Arch Surg 128:1054-1056, 1993

30. Wibbenmeyer LA, Wade TP, Chen RC, Meyer RC, Turgeon RP, Andrus CH: Laparoscopic cholecystectomy can disseminate in situ carcinoma of the gallbladder. J Am Coll Surg 181:504-510, 1995

31. Yoshida T, Matsumoto T, Sasaki A, Morii Y, Ishio T, Bandoh T, Kitano S: Laparoscopic cholecystectomy in the treatment of patients with gallbladder cancer. J Am Coll Surg 191:158-163, 2000

32. Bivins BA, Meeker WR Jr, Weiss DL, Griffen WO Jr: Carcinoma in situ of the gallbladder: a dilemma. South Med J 68:297-300, 1975

33. Cubertafond P, Gainant A, Cucchiaro G: Surgical treatment of 724 carcinomas of the gallbladder: results of the French Surgical Association Survey. Ann Surg 219:275-280, 1994

34. Shirai Y, Yoshida K, Tsukada K, Muto T: Inapparent carcinoma of the gallbladder: an appraisal of a radical second operation after simple cholecystectomy. Ann Surg 215:326-331, 1992

35. Yamagushi K, Chijiiwa K, Saiki S, Nishihara K, Takashima M, Kawakami K, Tanaka M: Retrospective analysis of 70 operations for gallbladder carcinoma. Br J Surg 84:200-204, 1997

36. Fong Y, Heffernan N, Blumgart LH: Gallbladder carcinoma discovered during laparoscopic cholecystectomy: aggressive reresection is beneficial. Cancer 83:423-427, 1998

37. Suzuki K, Kimura T, Ogawa H: Long-term prognosis of gallbladder cancer diagnosed after laparoscopic cholecystectomy. Surg Endosc 14:712-716, 2000

38. Shirai Y, Yoshida K, Tsukada K, Ohtani T, Muto T: Identification of the regional lymphatic system of the gallbladder by vital staining. Br J Surg 79:659-662, 1992

39. Shimada H, Endo I, Togo S, Nakano A, Izumi T, Nakagawara G: The role of lymph node dissection in the treatment of gallbladder carcinoma. Cancer 79:892-899, 1997

40. Shinkai H, Kimura W, Sata N, Muto T, Nagai H: A case of gallbladder cancer with para-aortic lymph node metastasis who has survived more than seven years after the primary extended radical operation. Hepatogastroenterology 43:1370-1376, 1996

41. Nakamura S, Nishiyama R, Yokoi Y, Serizawa A, Nishiwaki Y, Konno H, Babba S, Muro H: Hepatopancreatoduodenectomy for advanced gallbladder carcinoma. Arch Surg 129:625-629, 1994

42. Shirai Y, Ohtani T, Tsukada K, Hatakeyama K: Combined pancreaticoduodenectomy and hepatectomy for patients with locally advanced gallbladder carcinoma: long term results. Cancer 80:1904-1909, 1997

43. Todoroki T, Kawamoto T, Takahashi H, Takada Y, Koike N, Otsuka M, Fukao K: Treatment of gallbladder cancer by radical resection. Br J Surg 86:622-627, 1999

44. Buskirk SJ, Gunderson LL, Adson MA, Martinez A, May GR, McIlrath DC, Nagorney DM, Edmundson GK, Bender CE, Martin JK Jr: Analysis of failure following curative irradiation of gallbladder and extrahepatic bile duct carcinoma. Int J Radiat Oncol Biol Phys 10:2013-2023, 1984

45. Bosset JF, Mantion G, Gillet M, Pelissier E, Boulenger M, Maingon P, Corbion O, Schraub S: Primary carcinoma of the gallbladder: adjuvant postoperative external irradiation. Cancer 64:1843-1847, 1989

46. Todoroki T: Radiation therapy for primary gallbladder cancer. Hepatogastroenterology 44:1229-1239, 1997

47. Todoroki T: Chemotherapy for gallbladder carcinoma: a surgeon's perspective. Hepatogastroenterology 47:948-955, 2000

48. Wanebo HJ, Castle WN, Fechner RE: Is carcinoma of the gallbladder a curable lesion? Ann Surg 195:624-631, 1982

49. Donohue JH, Nagorney DM, Grant CS, Tsushima K, Ilstrup DM, Adson MA: Carcinoma of the gallbladder: Does radical resection improve outcome? Arch Surg 125:237-241, 1990

50. Donohue JH, Stewart AK, Menck HR: The National Cancer Data Base report on carcinoma of the gallbladder, 1989-1995. Cancer 83:2618-2628, 1998

51. Gagner M, Rosse RL: Radical operations for carcinoma of the gallbladder: present status in North America. World J Surg 15:344-347, 1991

52. Matsumoto Y, Fujii H, Aoyama H, Yamamoto M, Sugahara K, Suda K: Surgical treatment of primary carcinoma of the gallbladder based on the histologic analysis of 48 surgical specimens. Am J Surg 163:239-245, 1992

53. Onoyama H, Yamamoto M, Tseng A, Ajiki T, Saitoh Y: Extended cholecystectomy for carcinoma of the gallbladder. World J Surg 19:758-763, 1995

54. Ruckert JC, Ruckert RI, Gellert K, Hecker K, Muller JM: Surgery for carcinoma of the gallbladder. Hepatogastroenterology 43:527-533, 1996

55. Tsukada K, Hatakeyama K, Kurosaki I, Uchida K, Shirai Y, Muto T, Yoshida K: Outcome of radical surgery for carcinoma of the gallbladder according to the TNM stage. Surgery 120:816-821, 1996

56. Benoist S, Panis Y, Fagniez PL: Long-term results after curative resection for carcinoma of the gallbladder. French University Association for Surgical Research. Am J Surg 175:118-122, 1998

Chapter 18

Pancreatic and Periampullary Carcinoma

Glenroy Heywood, M.D.
Michael B. Farnell, M.D.

Neoplasms that originate from the tissues of the pancreatic head and periampullary region are often considered collectively because they are similar with regard to clinical presentation, histologic findings, and surgical management.[1-5] A pragmatic definition of periampullary tumors includes all neoplasms arising at or within 2 cm of the papilla of Vater. Periampullary neoplasms may originate from the ampulla of Vater, bile duct, duodenum, or head of the pancreas, and although this distinction has very important implications with regard to prognosis, in clinical practice this distinction can prove difficult to determine preoperatively. The patient presenting with obstructive jaundice and a 3-cm low-density mass in the head of the gland most assuredly harbors a pancreatic head carcinoma. However, when the lesion is much smaller, as is often the case, it may be virtually impossible to determine the site of origin on preoperative imaging, at operation, and even at pathologic examination (gross and histologic) of the resected specimen. The therapeutic nihilist may consider the outcome for resected pancreatic carcinoma dismal (recent evidence suggests it may be improving[6-10]), but patients with periampullary cancers, when resected, clearly have a better prognosis and should not be denied operation because of such misguided pessimism.

Pancreatic and periampullary malignancies constitute 5% of all gastrointestinal cancers, and the vast majority (80%-90%) are pancreatic ductal adenocarcinoma. In 1998, pancreatic cancer was the fourth-leading cause of cancer-related deaths in the United States, totaling some 28,900 deaths.[11]

Pancreatoduodenectomy (Whipple procedure) is currently the procedure of choice for potentially curative invasive adenocarcinoma of the head of the pancreas and periampullary area. Whipple first described one-stage pancreatectomy in 1941.[12] Since then, other surgeons have made several modifications to this procedure. In 1946, Waugh and Clagett,[13] from Mayo Clinic, described their modification of the one-stage procedure; this is still used today. Other milestones in the evolution of pancreatoduodenectomy include the regional pancreatectomy introduced by Fortner in 1973[14] and pylorus-preserving pancreatoduodenectomy described by Traverso and Longmire in 1978[15] (Fig. 1).

Major concerns regarding operation for pancreatic and periampullary cancer have been the complexity of the procedure and the associated high morbidity and mortality rates from operation. In the 1960s, most surgeons reported operative mortality rates of 20% to 40%.[16,17] These in combination with dismal long-term survival[18] led to questioning of whether the treatment was worse than the disease. In the contemporary era, considerable advances in diagnostic methods, patient selection, postoperative care, and expertise in many facets of pancreatic surgery have contributed to a dramatic improvement in the safety of the operation. Indeed, several recently published series have shown a substantial decrease in operative mortality rates to consistently less than 5%.[6,7,19,20] Moreover, some of these series have shown improvement in long-term survival after resection for ductal carcinoma of the pancreatic head.[6-10] Although review of our experience failed to confirm improving long-term survival,[21] we recognize that surgical resection offers the only chance for cure, and we therefore approach patients aggressively, recommending resection to fit candidates with locoregional

271

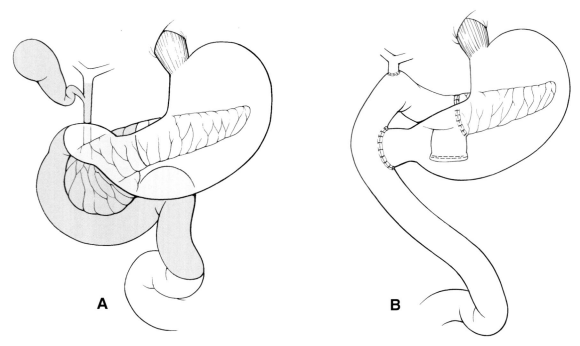

Fig. 1. (A), *Extent of resection* (shaded area) *with pylorus-preserving pancreatoduodenectomy.* (B), *The completed reconstruction after pylorus-preserving pancreatoduodenectomy. An end-to-side mucosa-to-mucosa pancreaticojejunostomy is performed. An end-to-side hepaticojejunostomy is performed approximately 4 to 6 cm distal to the pancreaticojejunostomy. Finally, an antecolic end-to-side duodenojejunostomy is fashioned.*

disease. At Mayo Clinic, the goals of surgical therapy for pancreatic and periampullary cancer outlined by Waugh and Clagett[13] have not changed in more than a half century: there should be a reasonable chance of cure, the operative mortality rate should not outweigh the chance for cure, and the patient should be left in as normal a condition as possible. Fundamental to our current approach to carcinoma of the pancreatic head and periampullary region are the following principles: 1) the least invasive and most cost-effective diagnostic methods should be used, 2) laparotomy should be performed with therapeutic rather than diagnostic intent, 3) resection offers the only potential for cure, and 4) operation offers the best palliation for patients with good performance status and a clinically resectable pancreatic or periampullary lesion.

CLINICOPATHOLOGY

Pathology

The great majority of pancreatic and periampullary cancers belong to the adenocarcinoma group, although other rare benign and malignant neoplasms affect the periampullary region. Functioning and nonfunctioning islet cell tumors and cystic neoplasms are addressed in Chapters 19 and 22, respectively. This chapter is limited to adenocarcinoma, but the reader should recognize that sarcomas, lymphomas, carcinoids, schwannomas, and metastatic tumors may occur and mimic pancreatic head and periampullary adenocarcinoma in clinical presentation. Periampullary villous tumors of the duodenum are addressed in Chapter 25. Among resected periampullary adenocarcinomas, 50% to 70% are cancer of the pancreatic head, 15% to 25% are ampullary cancer, 5% to 10% are biliary cancer, and 10% are duodenal cancer.[22] Of importance, ampullary, biliary, and duodenal neoplasms are more often resectable and have a better prognosis when resected for cure; thus, a "resectable" pancreatic neoplasm should be approached aggressively so as not to deny the patient a chance for cure.

Accurate anatomical and histologic classification of periampullary cancers can be very difficult. Not uncommonly, the original clinical diagnosis is changed after careful pathologic review of the resected specimen. The location of the main tumor mass, as determined by inspection of the resected specimen and the presence and anatomical location of any component of carcinoma in situ, can facilitate accurate classification within any of the four categories—pancreatic, biliary, ampullary, and duodenal. Nevertheless, despite these maneuvers, some periampullary cancers evade an unequivocal anatomical classification.[23,24]

Staging

Two staging systems for pancreatic cancer have evolved during the past 15 years. Japanese patients are staged according to the staging system of the Japanese Pancreas Society.[25] This system is probably more precise for defining the local tumor growth and the involvement of various structures adjacent to the pancreas, but it is a complicated system and not used widely in Western countries.

Western patients are staged according to the Union Internationale Contra Cancrum (UICC) TNM staging system.[26] This system is based on the size and extent of the primary tumor (T), the status of the regional lymph nodes (N), and the presence of metastatic disease (M). This system considers lymph node metastases as the most important prognostic factor and is simple to apply. We use the TNM system for staging pancreatic and periampullary adenocarcinoma (Table 1). TNM staging for nonpancreatic periampullary tumors is similar.[27]

Tumor

Extension of a primary pancreatic or periampullary tumor to adjacent tissues is an advanced T stage of disease and portends a poorer prognosis with an increased rate of invasion of lymphatic, venous, and perineural structures.[28] When any nonpancreatic periampullary cancer invades the pancreatic parenchyma, the prognosis worsens, and the frequency of lymphatic involvement increases.[29,30] Invasion of ampullary cancers into the duodenal wall does not have the same adverse implication as does pancreatic invasion.[31] Pancreatic invasion or origin from the pancreatic parenchyma portends a poor prognosis.[32]

Lymph Nodes and Neural Spread

Lymph Node Metastases

Pancreatic cancers present with nodal metastases in 56% to 79% of patients,[21,33-35] duodenal carcinoma in 36% to 47%,[36] ampullary cancers in 30% to 50%,[23] and bile duct cancers in 56% to 69%.[37-39] Invasion of the pancreas by a nonpancreatic periampullary cancer substantially increases the frequency of lymph node metastases, including metastases in the para-aortic area.[32]

Ampullary tumors are less prone to nodal metastases. Most frequently, these cancers metastasize to peripancreatic nodes (N1 nodes)[40] and seldom to celiac nodes or nodes to the left of the superior mesenteric artery (N2 nodes).[41] In contrast, nodal involvement of pancreatic cancer more frequently involves both N1 and N2 nodal groups (Fig. 2).

Duodenal tumors seem to be inherently biologically different from pancreatic cancers because, even though the frequency of nodal metastasis is 36% to 47%, the 5-year

Table 1.—TNM Staging of Pancreatic Carcinoma

Primary tumor (T)

TX	Primary tumor cannot be assessed
T0	No evidence of primary tumor
Tis	In situ carcinoma
T1	Tumor limited to the pancreas and is 2 cm or less in greatest dimension
T2	Tumor limited to the pancreas and is more than 2 cm in greatest dimension
T3	Tumor extends directly to any of the following: duodenum, bile duct, or peripancreatic tissues
T4	Tumor extends directly to any of the following: stomach, spleen, colon, or adjacent blood vessels

Regional lymph nodes (N)

NX	Regional lymph nodes cannot be assessed
N0	No regional lymph node metastasis
N1	Regional lymph node metastasis
	pN1a Metastasis in a single regional lymph node
	pN1b Metastasis in multiple regional lymph nodes

Distant metastases (M)

MX	Presence of distant metastasis cannot be assessed
M0	No distant metastasis
M1	Distant metastasis

Stage grouping

Stage	T	N	M
0	Tis	N0	M0
I	T1-2	N0	M0
II	T3	N0	M0
III	Any T	N1	M0
IVA	T4	Any N	M0
IVB	Any T	Any N	M1

From Fleming et al.[27] By permission of the American Joint Committee on Cancer.

survival rate approaches 40% to 50%.[36] In contrast, the presence of positive lymph nodes in patients with pancreatic cancer is associated with a 5-year survival of only 5%.[21,42] These observations support an aggressive posture with regard to resection of duodenal and ampullary cancers, even in the presence of positive lymph nodes.[36,43]

Perineural Invasion

Perineural invasion, particularly intrapancreatic, generally portends a poor prognosis. Because involvement of the mesenteric neural plexus is usually extensive, it is difficult to achieve a negative retroperitoneal margin even with radical resection.[44,45] Cameron et al.[46] found no correlation between neural invasion and survival, but Mayo

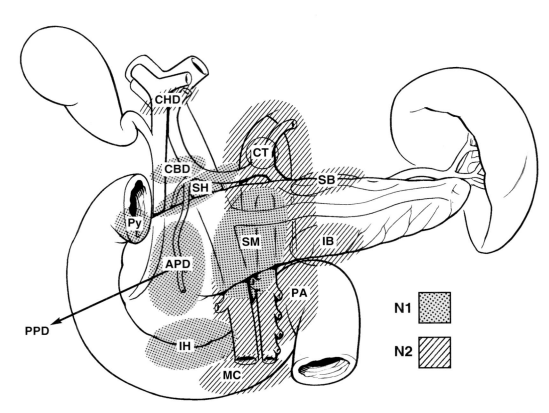

Fig. 2. Peripancreatic and regional lymph node groups. Peripancreatic node groups (N1): superior pancreas (SH), lymph nodes superior to the head and body of the pancreas; inferior pancreas (IH), lymph nodes inferior to the head and body of the pancreas; anterior pancreas, anterior pancreaticoduodenal (APD), pyloric (Py), and proximal superior mesenteric (SM) lymph nodes; posterior pancreas: posterior pancreaticoduodenal (PPD), common bile duct (CBD) or pericholedochal, and proximal superior mesenteric (SM) nodes; splenic: hilum of the spleen and tail of the pancreas. Regional node groups (N2): hepatic artery; infrapyloric (for tumors of the head only); subpyloric (for tumors of the head only); celiac (CT) (for tumors of the head only); distal superior mesenteric, retroperitoneal, and lateral aortic (PA); common hepatic duct (CHD); superior body of pancreas (SB); inferior body of pancreas (IB); middle colic (MC).

Clinic investigators[21] and other groups[47,48] have reported decreased survival rates for patients with nerve plexus invasion. Most patients with pancreatic cancer have perineural invasion,[49] which may contribute to the high rate of retroperitoneal recurrence. In contrast, local recurrence is less common in resected ampullary carcinoma, in which perineural invasion occurs in only 5% to 17%.[50] When perineural invasion is present with nonpancreatic periampullary cancers, the prognosis is similar to that with pancreatic cancer.

Biomolecular Markers
A wide array of serum tumor markers is available for the screening and diagnosis of pancreatic cancer and periampullary cancer. These markers include carcinoembryonic antigen, carbohydrate antigen (CA) 19-9, CA 125, CA 50, CA 242, CAM 17.1, Span-1, Dupan-2, and elastase-1. None of these available markers are sufficiently accurate and reliable for the diagnosis of pancreatic and periampullary cancer.

The tumor-associated antigen CA 19-9 assay is the most specific and sensitive of these common tumor assays,[51,52] and CA 19-9 has become the predominant tumor marker for the diagnosis of adenocarcinoma of the pancreas. CA 19-9 is a Lewis blood group-related mucin; therefore, the serum CA 19-9 value is not expected to be increased in patients who are negative for Lewis blood group.[53] The maximal achievable sensitivity of the CA 19-9 assay is 95% because about 5% of the general population is negative for the Lewis blood type.[54] The serum CA 19-9 level correlates with tumor burden and thus is often normal in patients with small tumors.[52] CA 19-9 has not proved to be useful as an independent and reliable marker for diagnosing pancreatic cancer. However, distinct and sustained increases postoperatively have been useful as a good predictor of recurrence.[55-57] An increased serum CA 19-9 value postoperatively does not necessarily confirm the presence of recurrent disease, because transient increases can occur.[58] Currently, no reproducible parameters for CA 19-9 increases accurately define recurrence. There are reports that increases in these tumor markers provide independent, objective prognostic information.[59] We do not routinely use tumor markers in our clinical decision making because of their low sensitivity, specificity, and accuracy.

DIAGNOSIS

Clinical Evaluation

The symptoms and physical findings caused by pancreatic and periampullary neoplasms are usually nonspecific and vague.[60] Nonetheless, evaluation of the patient with a presumed adenocarcinoma of the pancreas or periampullary region necessitates a careful history and a thorough physical examination, especially in the young patient.[61] Information is sought to determine clinically the extent of disease, identifying important medical comorbidities and assessing performance status to determine whether the patient is a candidate for operation. Periampullary neoplasms usually present with extrahepatic biliary obstruction, but there may be subtle differences in the timing of onset of jaundice relative to cancer-related constitutional symptoms. Jaundice, pain, and weight loss are the most common symptoms in patients with cancer of the pancreatic head; however, jaundice usually manifests late because obstruction of the bile duct or ampullary region generally occurs with a more advanced local progression. Tumors of the body and tail do not obstruct the bile duct, hence patients do not present with early jaundice; instead, they usually present with abdominal or back pain. Tumors that are strategically located close to the pancreatic duct, particularly lesions of the uncinate process of the pancreas, may obstruct the pancreatic duct before obstructing the bile duct, resulting in steatorrhea before the onset of jaundice. Also, constitutional symptoms of abdominal pain, malaise, vomiting, early satiety, anorexia, or weight loss may precede the onset of jaundice. Patients also may present with other symptoms such as back pain, an ominous predictor of unresectability and of poor survival.[62] Almost all patients with adenocarcinoma of the body and tail of the pancreas present with abdominal or back pain,[63] often more severe than the pain associated with tumors of the pancreatic head.[64] Pain as a predominant symptom in cancer of the body of the pancreas was first described by Chauffard in 1908.[65]

Glucose intolerance may develop 6 to 12 months before onset of jaundice in as many as 10% of patients with pancreatic cancer. Therefore, the diagnosis of pancreatic cancer should be strongly entertained when adult-onset diabetes develops in a nonobese patient with a negative family history of diabetes. This disease process may be related to release of islet-associated pancreatic peptide, a diabetogenic hormone.

Jaundice is the most common early symptom in patients with adenocarcinoma located in the distal bile duct or ampulla, and it usually precedes other constitutional symptoms. Clinical jaundice in carcinoma of the ampulla of Vater may be intermittent and associated with cholangitis, because these tumors may undergo repeated necrosis and sloughing, allowing temporary resolution of jaundice and cholangitis. Occult gastrointestinal bleeding from the ulcerated tumor may cause anemia in up to a third of patients. The clinical triad of intermittent painless jaundice, anemia, and a palpable gallbladder is relatively specific for ampullary cancer but it occurs in less than 10% of patients. Silver-colored stools due to the combination of steatorrhea and blood is thought to be pathognomonic of ampullary cancer, but it is a rare presentation.

The clinical presentation of duodenal adenocarcinoma is similar to that of adenocarcinoma elsewhere in the intestinal tract in that it may present with anemia from occult gastrointestinal blood loss, melena, and eventual obstruction. Patients with familial adenomatous polyposis and Gardner syndrome are at particularly high risk for development of duodenal or periampullary cancer.[66-70] Therefore, this association has implications with regard to surveillance for future development of ampullary or duodenal neoplasm.

The physical examination should be directed to identify any subtle evidence of advanced or metastatic disease, such as ascites, left supraclavicular adenopathy (Virchow's node), periumbilical nodules (Sister Mary Joseph's nodules), a palpable liver mass, or a palpable pelvic shelf on rectal examination (Blumer's shelf). A palpable gallbladder (Courvoisier's sign) suggests a malignant obstruction of the common bile duct until proved otherwise.

Laboratory Evaluation

We obtain selective laboratory tests to screen for evidence of organ system dysfunction, coagulation abnormalities, and gastrointestinal blood loss and to assess nutritional status. Liver function tests may reveal the pattern of obstructive jaundice but are of little prognostic value.

Computed Tomography

We rely heavily on high-quality, multiphase, thin-section, helical computed tomography (CT) with oral and intravenous contrast agents. The thin cuts through the pancreas and periampullary region are crucial for both diagnosis and staging of pancreatic and periampullary cancer. Notwithstanding the excellent images obtained with contrast-enhanced spiral CT, it is not highly accurate for the identification of peripancreatic nodal metastases,[71] nor is it very accurate for the identification of peritoneal metastases or hepatic metastases less than 1 cm in size.[72,73]

Peripancreatic and upper abdominal lymphadenopathy may be noted, but it is often the result of obstructive jaundice. Therefore, we would still offer operation to the patient who otherwise meets the criteria for resection.

Our approach is tailored by the clinical presentation and the presence or absence of an obvious mass on abdominal CT. Three scenarios will be addressed: 1) obvious mass with or without obstructive jaundice, 2) obstructive jaundice without a mass, and 3) pancreatic duct stricture with no mass or jaundice.

Obvious Pancreatic Mass With or Without Obstructive Jaundice

In patients in whom a mass is visualized, the size of the mass and its relationship to other peripancreatic structures can be determined, thus allowing assessment of local resectability. Although the average size of resected pancreatic head tumors is 3.1 cm in the Mayo Clinic experience,[21] we do not deny patients resection on the basis of the size of the tumor alone. Preservation of fat planes around the major peripancreatic vascular structures such as the celiac axis, hepatic arteries, superior mesenteric artery, and superior mesenteric-portal venous structures suggests a lack of direct tumor invasion and is consistent with resectability (Fig. 3).[74]

Isolated involvement of the superior mesenteric-portal vein confluence has historically been a contraindication for resection in patients with adenocarcinoma of the pancreas. We do not consider superior mesenteric vein or portal vein involvement an absolute contraindication to resection unless there is circumferential encasement or occlusion. Several groups[75-77] have reported that patients who require segmental resection of the superior mesenteric vein or superior mesenteric-portal vein confluence

have a median survival similar to that of patients who undergo standard pancreatoduodenectomy and no substantial difference in mortality.[78,79] Tumor invasion of the superior mesenteric vein or superior mesenteric-portal vein confluence appears to be a function of tumor location rather than an indicator of biologic aggressiveness.[76]

Abdominal CT accurately predicts adherence of pancreas to the superior mesenteric-portal vein confluence in 84% of patients, as confirmed by the surgeon at operation.[80] Adherence may be the result of a peritumoral inflammatory reaction, but histologic confirmation of vessel invasion is present in the majority of cases. Accordingly, when vein and pancreas are not easily separated, tumor invasion should be assumed and venous resection considered if it is the only obstacle to an otherwise margin-negative resection.

Obstructive Jaundice Without a Pancreatic Mass

It is not unusual for patients to present with obstructive jaundice in the absence of an obvious pancreatic mass. Ampullary or duodenal carcinoma should be excluded by endoscopic examination. The presence of both bile duct and pancreatic duct dilation on abdominal CT is virtually diagnostic of a periampullary neoplasm, and further invasive attempts at imaging are not required before operation.

In the absence of both a pancreatic mass and an abdominal CT double-duct sign, further investigation is, however, warranted. In this setting, we prefer endoscopic retrograde cholangiopancreatography (ERCP) to exclude a potentially benign cause. Recently, in such patients we have used endoscopic ultrasonography for diagnosis (and even biopsy on occasion), although its precise role is still being determined. Percutaneous transhepatic cholangiography, albeit rarely used, may be

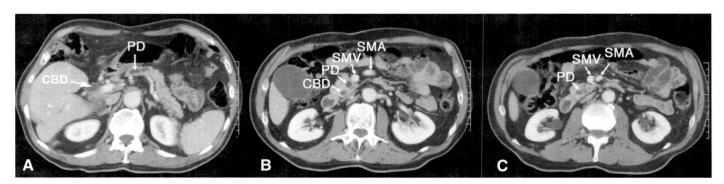

Fig. 3. Computed tomograms (section thickness, 1.5 mm) obtained at the time of intravenous contrast enhancement. (A), Dilation of both the common bile duct (CBD) and the pancreatic duct (PD), "double-duct" sign. Although there is no obvious mass in the head of the pancreas, the presence of the double-duct sign is virtually diagnostic of a periampullary neoplasm. At resection, this proved to be an invasive grade 4, 2 x 1.5 x 0.5 cm, signet ring cell carcinoma at the ampulla. (B), Note normal fat plane around the superior mesenteric vein (SMV) and superior mesenteric artery (SMA), suggesting a lack of direct tumor invasion, which is consistent with resectability. (C), Dilation of the PD in the immediate supra-ampullary area suggests the presence of a neoplasm at or just proximal to the ampulla.

indicated if the proximal extent of the biliary obstruction remains unclear. The role of magnetic resonance cholangiopancreatography in this clinical setting has yet to be fully defined but holds promise.

Pancreatic Duct Stricture, No Mass or Jaundice
In the absence of obstructive jaundice, an unexplained stricture of the pancreatic duct, without clinical or radiologic evidence of chronic pancreatitis, is presumed to harbor malignancy, and resection is advocated. These tumors are usually small and thus amenable to potentially curative resection. We do acknowledge that some of these presumed malignant strictures will prove benign.[81]

Endoscopic Retrograde Cholangiopancreatography and Stents
Because helical abdominal CT, our initial imaging method of choice, is relatively sensitive for defining both biliary obstruction and small pancreatic tumors, we do not routinely use ERCP or percutaneous transhepatic cholangiography for preoperative evaluation. However, as noted above, ERCP is our diagnostic method of choice in the jaundiced patient with a history of gallstone disease but without CT evidence of a pancreatic or periampullary mass.

We actively discourage the insertion of endobiliary stents in patients who are candidates for resection, because sphincterotomy and stent placement have intrinsic complications such as perforation, bleeding, or pancreatitis[82,83] and may increase the incidence of postoperative pancreatic fistulas.[84] These complications may not only delay and complicate definitive operation but, if necrotizing post-ERCP pancreatitis develops, also render it impossible.[83] Preoperative biliary drainage increases the risk of wound or intra-abdominal infective morbidity and death after pancreatoduodenectomy.[85] Therefore, we use biliary stents with a high degree of selectivity, reserving their use to ameliorate severe pruritus when a considerable delay in scheduling the operation is necessary or if the serum bilirubin value is more than 30 mg/dL, suggesting biliary cirrhosis; if the serum bilirubin value does not decrease to less than 5 mg/dL after biliary decompression, major pancreatectomy may be contraindicated.

Magnetic Resonance Imaging and Magnetic Resonance Cholangiopancreatography
The role of magnetic resonance imaging (MRI) in the diagnosis and staging of pancreatic and periampullary cancer is still unclear. Several studies have reported no discernible advantage of MRI over CT for identifying tumor resectability.[86-88] The new technique of ultrafast MRI was reported by Trede et al.[89] to be superior to classic CT for both staging and determination of resectability. However, ultrafast MRI has to be compared with state-of-the-art spiral CT to clearly define its role in the preoperative evaluation and staging of pancreatic and periampullary cancer.

Magnetic resonance cholangiopancreatography (MRCP), which is noninvasive, is gaining widespread use in the diagnostic evaluation of pancreatic and biliary obstruction and may replace diagnostic ERCP.[90] It also may avoid the use of invasive procedures in the early postoperative setting for assessing the integrity and patency of pancreatic and biliary enteric anastomoses. Real-time volume rendering of MRCP has been reported to be helpful for displaying the residual biliary tract, the anastomotic site, and the enteric tract in surgical biliary-enteric anastomoses.[91] Secretin MRCP shows pancreatic secretion into the reconstructed jejunum, confirming the patency of the anastomosis.

The clinical role of MRI and MRCP in the evaluation of pancreaticobiliary malignancy is evolving and may gradually replace the diagnostic use of the invasive direct imaging procedures of ERCP and percutaneous transhepatic cholangiography. MRCP has been shown to play a valuable role in evaluating patients in whom ERCP failed.[92] We are currently evaluating the accuracy of MRI with MRCP for assessing pancreatic and biliary disease.

Positron Emission Tomography
Positron emission tomography is a new imaging technique that capitalizes on the increased metabolism of glucose by cancer cells as the basis of imaging.[93] A report by Nakamoto et al.[94] suggested that positron emission tomography was more reliable than CT or ultrasonography for detecting liver metastases from pancreatic cancer. Other studies also have suggested that it may be more accurate than CT for diagnosing lymph node metastases[95] and differentiating chronic pancreatitis from pancreatic cancer.[96] The widespread use of this imaging method is still limited by its high cost; thus, its role in evaluating periampullary cancer is yet to be determined.

Angiography
We rarely use angiography in the preoperative staging and assessment of the resectability of pancreatic cancer. Proponents of its use suggest that it is useful both to visualize vascular invasion and to define critical anomalies of the celiac and superior mesenteric arteries.[97,98] However, apart from complete occlusion of the hepatic artery or portal vein, narrowing of these structures is not specific for tumor invasion and may be a false-positive sign. Explanations for false-positive findings include spasm of the superior mesenteric artery mimicking tumor encasement,[99]

"notching" in the vicinity of the superior mesenteric-portal venous junction (a normal variant), and coiling of the hepatic artery causing indentation of the portal vein.[100] The absence of angiographic abnormalities excludes neither the diagnosis of pancreatic cancer nor the presence of vascular invasion.

The experienced pancreatic surgeon should be prepared to recognize and deal with any vascular anomalies encountered intraoperatively. However, preoperative angiography may be helpful when helical abdominal CT shows arterial collaterals through and around the head of the pancreas. This finding is suggestive of celiac artery stenosis or occlusion, and performing a concomitant hepatic artery bypass after pancreatic resection will prevent postoperative hepatic ischemia.

Intraoperative vascular assessment may be difficult in patients with preoperative radiation-induced fibrosis or adhesions from recent exploration or palliative biliary bypass; therefore, preoperative visceral angiography may help identify vascular structures and reduce the risk of iatrogenic arterial injury.

Endoscopic Ultrasonography

Endoscopic ultrasonography allows for close scrutiny of the pancreas, its ductal anatomy, the portal vein, and the superior mesenteric artery and vein. There is increasing interest in its application for the local staging (T and N) and tissue confirmation of pancreatic and periampullary adenocarcinoma.[101,102] Limitations to the routine use of endoscopic ultrasonography include the expense, need for conscious sedation, limited assessment of the liver, and the importance of its operator dependence.

The role of endoscopic ultrasonography in our practice is evolving. Currently, we do not reject patients for operation solely on the findings of this test if the lesion appears otherwise resectable on abdominal CT. Currently, endoscopic ultrasonography with biopsy is recommended to establish tissue diagnosis in nonoperative candidates, in patients suspected of having pancreatic lymphoma, and in patients with a suspected pancreatic or periampullary mass that cannot be confirmed by abdominal CT or ERCP.

Laparoscopy

High-resolution, contrast-enhanced spiral CT misses small hepatic or peritoneal metastases in 5% to 10% of patients whose tumor appears resectable.[72,73] When preoperative staging laparoscopy identifies unsuspected peritoneal or superficial liver metastases,[103,104] laparotomy can be avoided and palliation achieved endoscopically. We do not use staging laparoscopy routinely given the low yield for unsuspected peritoneal or hepatic

metastasis. Rather, we perform limited laparoscopy as the preliminary step at operation in patients for whom a palliative procedure may not be required. These patients include those with preoperatively placed endobiliary stents, proximal lesions without biliary or duodenal obstruction, and pancreatic body or tail lesions.[105] Suspicious peritoneal or hepatic lesions are biopsied, and the operation terminated if metastatic disease is confirmed. If laparoscopy is negative, we proceed directly to exploration with the patient under the same anesthetic.

We also do not embrace "extended" laparoscopy and laparoscopic ultrasonography for the determination of nodal or vascular involvement, for the following reasons: 1) operative palliation is superior for patients with locally irresectable disease, 2) lymphadenopathy within the confines of the standard operative field is not a contraindication to operation, 3) when abdominal CT suggests adherence to the portal vein-superior mesenteric vein confluence, we are prepared to perform en bloc resection of the confluence, if necessary. This decision, in our hands, is best determined surgically.

Indication for Preoperative or Intraoperative Biopsy

Our decision relative to operation is primarily based on the patient's clinical presentation and radiographic findings. We, therefore, do not require preoperative histologic confirmation of malignancy before resection in a good-risk patient with obstructive jaundice and a presumed pancreatic or periampullary mass. Malignancy cannot be definitely excluded by a negative biopsy result, and the need for tissue confirmation before resection may deny operation to patients with small tumors who may potentially derive the most benefit. In addition, fine-needle aspiration biopsy is associated with the risk, albeit small, of needle tract complications such as hemorrhage,[83,106] needle tract seeding,[107,108] or tumor dissemination (very controversial). Post-biopsy pancreatitis occasionally occurs.[109] Histologic confirmation of malignancy is reserved for patients who are candidates for neoadjuvant protocols or those who are not operative candidates and are being considered for palliative chemoradiation therapy. Currently, preoperative or intraoperative biopsy has no role in the routine evaluation of a good-risk patient with a clinically resectable pancreatic mass. For patients with a duodenal or ampullary mass that is easily and safely accessed, endoscopy or intraoperative biopsy may be used. Endoscopic biopsy, however, may provide false-negative results. Benignity of a duodenal or ampullary mass can be ascertained only after complete excision. The approach to ampullary villous lesions is discussed in more detail in Chapter 25.

INDICATION FOR OPERATION

Simply stated, the indication for operation in fit candidates is the clinical diagnosis of a localized pancreatic or periampullary malignancy. Achieving a clinical diagnosis of a pancreatic head or periampullary malignancy may be straightforward or complex (as discussed in the imaging and staging sections of this chapter). Tissue confirmation is not mandatory, and if sought and required it may both complicate operation and deny surgical therapy to patients who potentially can most benefit. In our experience, when the clinical diagnosis of pancreatic head or periampullary malignancy is made and resection is undertaken, a benign pathologic process is present in approximately 5% of patients.[81] Given the relative safety of pancreatoduodenectomy in the current era (operative mortality < 4%), the observation that patients experience a good quality of life after pancreatoduodenectomy,[110] and that operation achieves relief of symptoms, this approach, in our opinion, is appropriate.

Surgical resection benefits only patients with locoregional disease. Appropriate preoperative imaging should be undertaken to exclude systemic metastases. There should be no radiologic evidence of encasement of the superior mesenteric, celiac, or hepatic arteries and no radiologic evidence of occlusion of the superior mesenteric-portal vein confluence. If the surgeon is prepared to perform venous resection and reconstruction, segmental venous involvement (without occlusion and collateral formation) is not a contraindication to operation. Nodal metastases within the standard operative field (N1 or peripancreatic nodes) do not preclude resection.

The candidate for resection should have a good performance status and the physiologic reserve to withstand the stress of a major abdominal procedure. Assessing the physiologic status of the patient may be straightforward in the young, fit patient or more rigorous in patients with comorbidities necessitating targeted assessment of major organ system function and attendant operative risk. Chronologic age alone should not be an absolute contraindication to pancreatoduodenectomy.[111,112]

CONDUCT OF THE OPERATION

Potentially Curative Resection

Our preferred procedure for pancreatic head and periampullary malignancy is the pylorus-preserving pancreatoduodenectomy.[113] Otherwise identical to standard pancreatoduodenectomy, it differs in preserving the entire stomach, pylorus, and a proximal segment of duodenum. Given that pyloric and perigastric nodes are not removed if the pylorus is preserved, some surgeons favor standard pancreatoduodenectomy (with distal gastrectomy) for carcinoma of the head of the pancreas.[114] Although it is somewhat less radical relative to the amount of nodal tissue removed, long-term survival has not been shown to be influenced by pyloric preservation.[115] Similarly, total pancreatectomy has no added advantage over segmental pancreatectomy.[116,117]

Pylorus-preserving pancreatoduodenectomy is initiated with a right subcostal incision or an upper midline incision if the costal margin is vertically oriented. The liver and peritoneal surfaces are then carefully inspected and palpated to exclude the presence of metastases. A wide Kocher maneuver is performed to confirm that the tumor does not invade the retroperitoneum or the superior mesenteric artery. The tissue along the posterior and medial aspect of this artery is palpated to exclude gross tumor extension. We rely heavily on the preoperative abdominal CT for assessing this important tumor-vessel relationship; however, occasionally it may be false-negative, and in such patients achieving a negative margin in the region of the uncinate process may well be problematic. The incision is extended as a bilateral subcostal incision if exploration reveals no tumor dissemination outside the field of resection (Fig. 4).

The right colon is then mobilized by first releasing the hepatic flexure inferiorly, and the Kocher maneuver is continued to the right lateral aspect of the superior mesenteric vein (Fig. 5). The greater omentum is freed from the right half of the transverse mesocolon, allowing entrance into the lesser sac, thus exposing the entire anterior surface of the pancreas (Fig. 6). The anterior and lateral aspect of the superior mesenteric vein is exposed by dividing the gastrocolic venous trunk (Fig. 7 A). At this point, we assess the relationship of the neck of the pancreas to the superior mesenteric-portal vein confluence. This is accomplished by carefully insinuating a blunt clamp between the anterior surface of the superior mesenteric-portal vein confluence and the posterior surface of the pancreas (Fig. 7 B). The gastrohepatic ligament is then divided, the right gastric and gastroduodenal arteries are ligated and divided, and the suprapancreatic portal vein exposed (Fig. 8 A-C). This step allows further development of a continuous tumor-free plane between the anterior surface of the superior mesenteric vein and portal vein and the posterior surface of the pancreas (Fig. 8 D). The presence of a tumor-free plane is relative confirmation of resectability. This plane often can be developed despite fixation of the tumor to the posterior-lateral wall of the superior mesenteric vein or portal vein.

Posterolateral adherence usually is not revealed until after the duodenal and pancreatic transection, by which point the surgeon already has committed to pancreatoduodenectomy. This highlights the importance for pancreatic

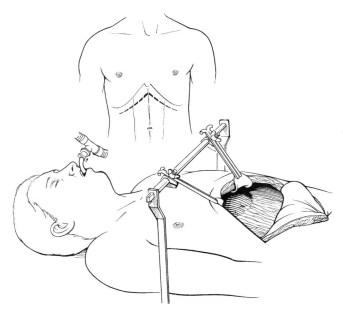

Fig. 4. The abdomen is opened through a bilateral subcostal incision, except in patients who have a narrow, vertically oriented costal arch, in which case a vertical midline upper abdominal incision is used. Fixed-abdominal retractors are used to achieve adequate exposure. (From Farnell MB: Pylorus-preserving pancreatoduodenectomy. Operative Tech Gen Surg 3:31-44, 2001. By permission of Mayo Foundation.)

lateral venorrhaphy, primary end-to-end anastomosis, or an interposition graft. We have used externally reinforced polytetrafluoroethylene grafts in this location with satisfactory results.[117,118]

With resectability confirmed, the gallbladder is removed from its bed, with mobilization and transection of the common hepatic bile duct cephalad to its junction with the cystic duct. The ligament of Treitz is mobilized, and the jejunum is divided 8 to 10 cm distal to the ligament of Treitz with its mesentery sequentially ligated and divided back to the fourth portion of the duodenum (Fig. 9). The now mobilized duodenum and jejunum then are passed beneath the superior mesenteric vessels into the supramesocolic compartment. The right gastroepiploic artery is divided and the skeletonized duodenum is prepared for transection 3 cm distal to the pylorus (Fig. 10). The neck of the pancreas is now transected anterior to the portal vein and reflected laterally, allowing visualization of small venous tributaries (Fig. 11 A and B). The portal-superior mesenteric vein is teased from the portal vein groove, and the venous branches to the uncinate process are ligated in continuity and divided. The inferiorly located highest jejunal vein requires ligation and division to adequately mobilize the superior mesenteric-portal vein confluence (Fig. 11 C). These maneuvers allow the portal vein to be retracted medially so as to expose the anterior aspect of the superior mesenteric artery. The specimen is retracted to the right, now remaining fixed only by the retroperitoneal soft tissue around the superior mesenteric artery and its arterial branches. This soft tissue along the anterior and

surgeons to have a technical strategy for the management of this situation. If venous resection is required, it is reserved as the last step in the extirpative portion of the procedure. Depending on the extent of the venous resection, we reconstruct the superior mesenteric-portal vein confluence with

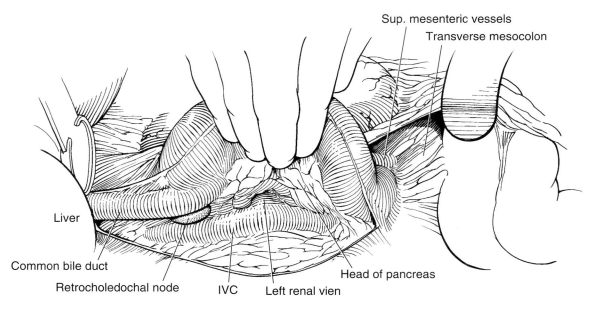

Fig. 5. The right colon is mobilized by first releasing the hepatic flexure inferiorly, and a Kocher maneuver is performed to elevate the duodenum and the head of the pancreas. IVC, inferior vena cava; Sup., superior. (From Farnell MB: Pylorus-preserving pancreatoduodenectomy. Operative Tech Gen Surg 3:31-44, 2001. By permission of Mayo Foundation.)

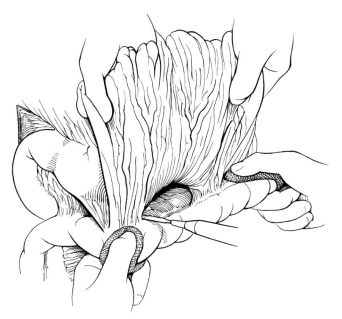

Fig. 6. The greater omentum is freed from the right half of the transverse colon in an avascular manner, allowing entrance into the lesser sac. (From Farnell MB: Pylorus-preserving pancreatoduodenectomy. Operative Tech Gen Surg 3:31-44, 2001. By permission of Mayo Foundation.)

right lateral walls of the superior mesenteric artery is the retroperitoneal margin, an area that may account for a high rate of local recurrence.

The superior mesenteric artery is skeletonized, and the arterial branches coursing into the uncinate process are serially clamped, divided, and ligated, thus achieving a maximal margin and ensuring complete removal of the uncinate process of the pancreas. One should take special care in isolating and ligating the inferior pancreaticoduodenal artery (Fig. 11 *D*).

Before submission of specimens to the pathology laboratory, margins are harvested from the specimen, and these should include the bile duct, pancreatic neck, and uncinate process. Positive resection margins on the bile duct, pancreatic neck, or uncinate process mandate further resection, if feasible, until clear.

Reconstruction is also done in an orderly and stepwise fashion. The transected jejunal limb is brought through a small incision in the transverse mesocolon to the right of the middle colic vessels or under the superior mesenteric vessels. Our preference for pancreatic anastomosis is a two-layer, end-to-side, duct-to-mucosa pancreatojejunostomy. A free-floating silicone catheter is used to facilitate accurate

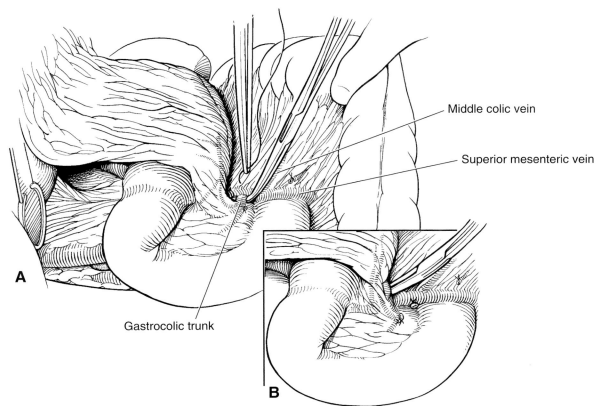

Middle colic vein

Superior mesenteric vein

Gastrocolic trunk

Fig. 7. (A), The anterior and lateral aspect of the superior mesenteric vein is exposed by dividing the gastrocolic venous trunk. (B), The relationship of the neck of the pancreas to the superior mesenteric-portal vein confluence is assessed by carefully insinuating a blunt clamp between the posterior surface of the pancreas and the vein. (From Farnell MB: Pylorus-preserving pancreatoduodenectomy. Operative Tech Gen Surg 3:31-44, 2001. By permission of Mayo Foundation.)

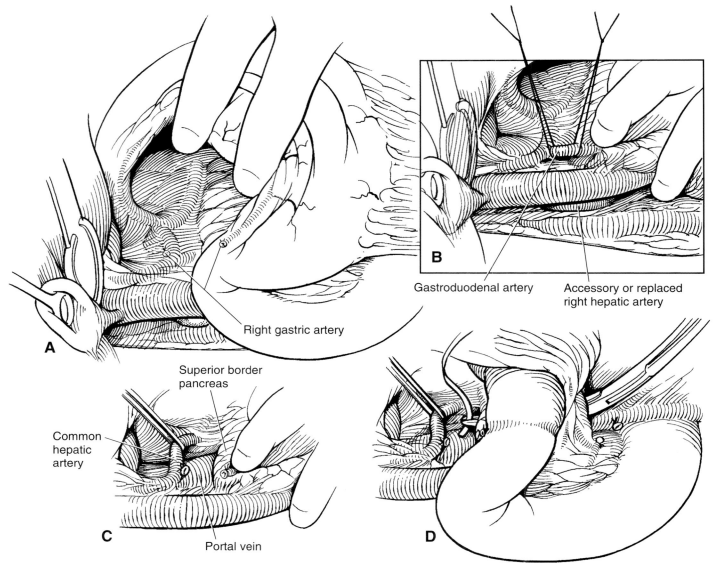

Fig. 8. (A), *Exposure and ligation of the right gastric artery.* (B), *Exposure and ligation of the gastroduodenal artery. A replaced or accessory right hepatic artery, if present, may be palpated running posterior and lateral to the common bile duct.* (C), *The portal vein is exposed by retracting the common hepatic artery cephalad, thus allowing the development of a plane between the superior border of the pancreas inferiorly and the common hepatic artery superiorly.* (D), *A blunt clamp is used to pass a tape around the neck of the pancreas.* (*From Farnell MB: Pylorus-preserving pancreatoduodenectomy. Operative Tech Gen Surg 3:31-44, 2001. By permission of Mayo Foundation.*)

suture placement, thereby ensuring patency of the anastomosis (Fig. 12 A-C). Both dunking pancreatojejunostomy and pancreatogastrostomy are acceptable alternatives.

An end-to-side hepaticojejunostomy is performed 4 to 6 cm distal to the pancreatic anastomosis with a single layer of interrupted or continuous absorbable sutures (Fig. 12 D).

We previously placed intraluminal "venting" tubes to augment "decompression" of the jejunal limb. These externally draining tubes usually traversed the hepaticojejunostomy or the jejunal limb and had their intraluminal tip located near the biliary or pancreatic anastomosis. We no longer use them routinely, because recent analysis of our

experience showed that intraluminal venting drains offered no distinct advantage but rather added an additional source of morbidity.[119]

The jejunum is secured at the point where it traverses the mesocolon, and an antecolic end-to-side duodenojejunostomy is fashioned (Fig. 12 E). The opening at the ligament of Treitz is then closed. Intraperitoneal drains are placed routinely in the subhepatic area and adjacent to the pancreatic anastomosis (Fig. 12 F).

Feeding jejunostomy and gastrostomy tubes are used selectively because most patients are able to resume oral intake within a short time postoperatively. However, if

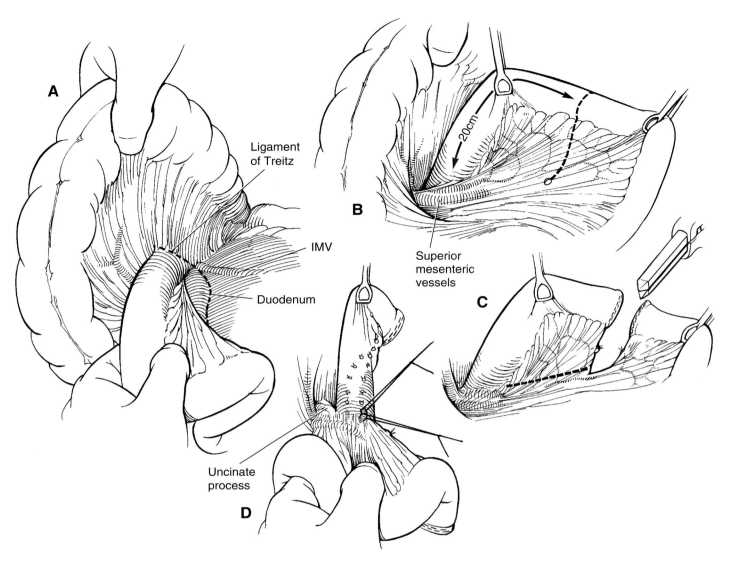

Fig. 9. (A), *Mobilization of the ligament of Treitz. IMV, inferior mesenteric vein.* (B) *and* (C), *The jejunum is mobilized, stapled, and transected approximately 20 cm beyond the ligament of Treitz.* (D), *The proximal jejunal branches are serially clamped, divided, and ligated proximally to the fourth portion of the duodenum to a point at which the uncinate process of the pancreas becomes visible. (From Farnell MB: Pylorus-preserving pancreatoduodenectomy. Operative Tech Gen Surg 3:31-44, 2001. By permission of Mayo Foundation.)*

postoperative complications preclude oral intake, then parenteral nutritional support is implemented until resolution and resumption of feeding.

Extended Lymphadenectomy

The presence of lymph node metastases has a considerable impact on tumor recurrence and long-term survival in patients who undergo potentially curative resection for ductal adenocarcinoma of the head of the pancreas.[21,46,120] In an effort to eradicate regional nodal disease before the development of distant metastases, several groups have advocated extended lymphadenectomy (as first described in 1973 by Fortner[14] as the "regional pancreatectomy") in patients

undergoing radical pancreatoduodenectomy.[121-123] Japanese surgeons have adopted this approach aggressively and have reported improvement in survival rates compared with the standard Whipple operation.[124,125] These results have been difficult to interpret because of differences in the staging systems and the use of historic controls instead of prospective randomization. However, a recent prospective randomized trial suggested a trend toward longer survival in a selected subgroup of node-positive patients treated with an extended lymphadenectomy with no substantial increase in morbidity or mortality.[126]

At Mayo Clinic, we have instituted a prospective trial comparing standard pancreatoduodenectomy with

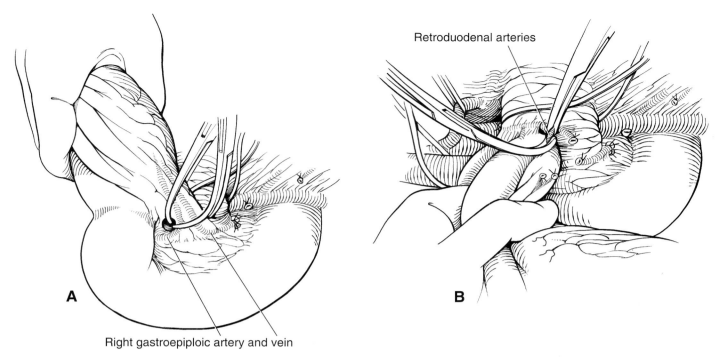

Retroduodenal arteries

A

B

Right gastroepiploic artery and vein

Fig. 10. Duodenal skeletonization. (A), The inferior aspect of the duodenum is freed by clamping, dividing, and ligating the right gastroepiploic artery and vein. (B), Retraction of the stomach directly anteriorly and placement of the duodenum on traction, facilitating the division and ligation of the retroduodenal arteries. (From Farnell MB: Pylorus-preserving pancreatoduodenectomy. Operative Tech Gen Surg 3:31-44, 2001. By permission of Mayo Foundation.)

pancreatoduodenectomy and harvest of the celiac, superior mesenteric artery, hepatic artery, common bile duct, and para-aortic nodes in patients with ductal carcinoma of the proximal pancreas. To date, we have learned that extended lymphadenectomy can be performed safely. Impact on survival is yet to be determined.

As a means to ensure reliable evaluation of the safety and potential efficacy of this procedure, extended lymphadenectomy should be performed only in the confines of an appropriately sanctioned, randomized trial at centers that are very experienced in pancreatic operation and have low operative morbidity and mortality rates.

Alternatives to Pancreatoduodenectomy
Pancreatoduodenectomy remains the treatment of choice for invasive periampullary adenocarcinoma. However, in the treatment of some ampullary or periampullary duodenal cancers, a more conservative approach of local excision can be advocated in selected patients. This approach is usually reserved only for early-stage cancer (carcinoma in situ, pTis) or for patients who are unfit for radical operation.

Although ampullectomy has been performed for more than a century, its role in the treatment of selected ampullary or periampullary duodenal cancers is still controversial despite improved T staging with the use of endoscopic ultrasonography.[127,128] This controversy is due in part to variations

in the surgical techniques of ampullectomy, which range from simple excision of the ampullary tumor and contiguous duodenal mucosa to wide resection of the tumor, including the papilla and adjacent duodenal, ductal, and pancreatic tissue.[129-131] Ampullectomy may be indicated in high-risk patients with low-risk stage (pTis and pT1 N0 M0), well-differentiated (grade 1-2) cancers.[132,133] Similarly, early duodenal cancers not involving the papilla may be treated by transduodenal excision or partial duodenectomy.

It is important to remember that final tumor staging is possible only after definitive histopathologic examination of the resected specimen and, most importantly, 6% to 10% of early T1 ampullary cancers or carcinoma in situ lesions harbor lymph node metastases.[133] Regardless of the criteria for selecting patients, the overall survival is less, and local recurrence rates exceed those for pancreatoduodenectomy.[134]

Operative Palliation
Operative palliation is reserved for patients with good performance status who have either metastatic or locally irresectable disease at the time of planned resection with curative intent.[135] A Roux-en-Y hepaticojejunostomy is our procedure of choice for palliation of biliary obstruction.[136] However, choledochoduodenostomy or cholecystojejunostomy may on occasion be better alternatives if body habitus, edema, or induration of the mesocolon or

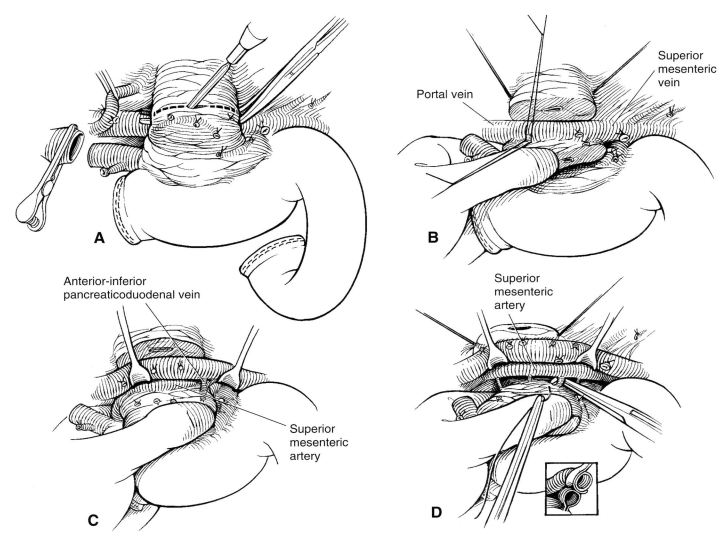

Fig. 11. (A), *Hemostatic sutures are placed on the inferior and superior borders of the pancreas before dividing the neck of the pancreas with cautery over a right-angle clamp.* (B), *The divided head of the pancreas is reflected laterally, allowing visualization of small venous tributaries from both the portal vein and the superior mesenteric vein. These are carefully ligated in continuity and divided.* (C), *Retracting the superior mesenteric-portal vein confluence to the patient's left exposes the superior mesenteric artery. A large venous trunk is typically encountered on the posterior aspect of the superior mesenteric vein, the highest jejunal vein that is ligated in continuity and divided.* (D), *The specimen is retracted to the right, now remaining fixed only by the retroperitoneal soft tissue around the superior mesenteric artery and its arterial branches to the uncinate process of the pancreas. These are carefully clamped, divided, and suture ligated. The arterial branches originating from the posterolateral aspect of the superior mesenteric artery are very friable and easily avulsed and may cause troublesome hemorrhage* (inset). *(From Farnell MB: Pylorus-preserving pancreatoduodenectomy. Operative Tech Gen Surg 3:31-44, 2001. By permission of Mayo Foundation.)*

the hepatoduodenal ligament from prolonged obstructive jaundice makes construction of a hepaticojejunostomy difficult. If a cholecystojejunostomy is contemplated, then cholangiography should be performed to confirm both patency of the cystic duct and its entry into the common bile duct well proximal to the tumor.

Duodenal obstruction eventually occurs in 15% to 30% of patients with unresectable cancer of the head of the pancreas.[137-141] Our current practice is to perform concomitant retrocolic prophylactic gastrojejunostomy at the time of surgical palliation for biliary obstruction. This approach obviates reoperation for subsequent duodenal obstruction and does not increase the operative mortality.[141] Patients with unresectable duodenal or ampullary adenocarcinoma are managed in a similar fashion with biliary or gastroenteric bypass.

Nonoperative Palliation

Symptomatic patients who are not candidates for operation are offered the most efficacious and cost-effective

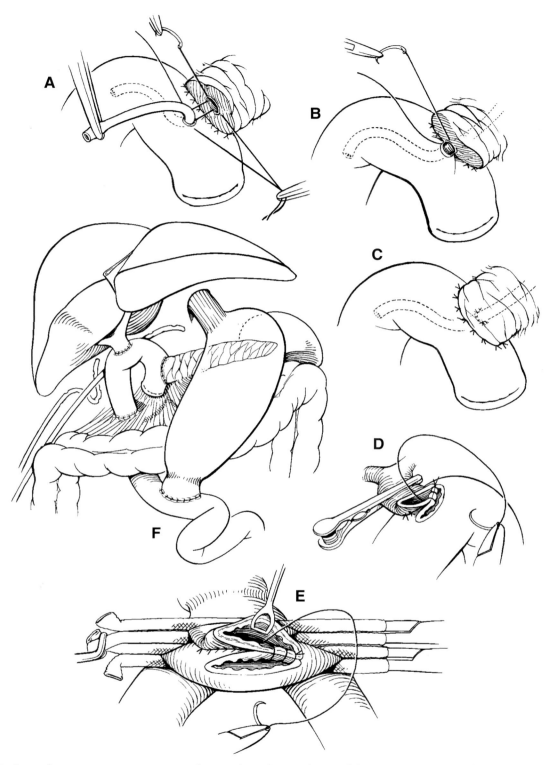

Fig. 12. (A), *End-to-side pancreaticojejunostomy. The capsule and parenchyma of the pancreas are sutured to the seromuscular layer of the jejunum with interrupted 3-0 or 4-0 nonabsorbable sutures. A small full-thickness opening is made into the jejunum with an insulated-tip cautery. A silicone catheter of a diameter somewhat smaller than the pancreatic duct is placed in the jejunal opening and helps to direct the placement of sutures. (B), The silicone catheter is then advanced into the pancreatic duct to facilitate placement of the anterior row of sutures. (C), Completed anterior row of the anastomosis. (D), An end-to-side hepaticojejunostomy is performed 4 to 6 cm distal to the pancreatic anastomosis with a single layer of interrupted or continuous absorbable sutures. (E), An antecolic end-to-side duodeno-jejunostomy is fashioned with a single layer of running 3-0 absorbable suture. (F), Completed reconstruction and drain placement. (From Farnell MB: Pylorus-preserving pancreatoduodenectomy. Operative Tech Gen Surg 3:31-44, 2001. By permission of Mayo Foundation.)*

means of nonoperative palliation. Histologic confirmation of malignancy is obtained to confirm the diagnosis and to allow palliative radiation or chemotherapy, if indicated. Endoscopically placed biliary stents are preferred over percutaneous transhepatic stents, which have the inherent risk of hemorrhage, hemobilia, and bile leak. Percutaneous endoscopic gastrostomy can be used to provide symptomatic relief of duodenal obstruction in patients in whom the risk of operation is prohibitive or those in the terminal stages of the disease. A separate tube for enteral feeding can be introduced through the gastrostomy and advanced endoscopically distal to the duodenal obstruction. Recently, endoscopic expandable metal stents have been used in the treatment of malignant duodenal obstruction.[142-145] A recent retrospective analysis of our limited experience with this new method suggests that it is as efficacious as operation with fewer hospital days and less cost.[146] Randomized trials are needed to confirm these findings.

Postoperative Management
A good outcome after pancreatoduodenectomy is also dependent on meticulous perioperative care. Postoperative admission to the intensive care unit is, however, not necessary or routine, and invasive monitoring and laboratory analysis are used selectively. Prophylactic antacid therapy is instituted, and a short course of perioperative antibiotic coverage (< 24 hours) is used unless stent placement has resulted in preoperative cholangitis. In that instance, a therapeutic course of antibiotic coverage is administered. Postoperative administration of octreotide is not used prophylactically but is reserved for patients with established pancreatic fistula.[147] Our success with the use of octreotide, however, has been disappointing.[146]

Use of nasogastric tubes is usually discontinued within 24 to 48 hours, and intraperitoneal drains are removed when the volume is less than 30 mL per 24 hours. Drain fluid is not routinely checked for amylase. However, if the output is high, we measure the amylase content and maintain the drain in place until the amylase normalizes.

SURGICAL OUTCOME
The incidence of postoperative complications remains high despite the marked reduction in mortality. We reviewed the incidence and management of complications after pancreatoduodenectomy in 279 patients at our institution.[148] Postoperative complications occurred in 46% of patients and included delayed gastric emptying (23%), pancreatojejunal anastomotic leak (17%), intra-abdominal sepsis (10%), biliary-enteric anastomotic leak (9%), gastrointestinal tract bleeding (5%),

intra-abdominal hemorrhage (3%), pancreatitis (1%), urinary tract infection (2%), and pulmonary dysfunction or infection (7%).

Morbidity

Delayed Gastric Emptying
Delayed gastric emptying, defined as the inability to tolerate full oral intake by the 14th postoperative day, was present in 23% of patients and prolonged their duration of hospitalization (28 vs. 13 days; $P < 0.05$). The incidence of delayed gastric emptying was higher in patients with pancreatojejunal anastomotic leak than in those without leak (54% vs. 17%; $P < 0.05$). However, there was no increase in operative mortality in patients with delayed gastric emptying. As a corollary, if delayed gastric emptying develops postoperatively, an occult pancreatojejunal anastomotic leakage should be excluded with appropriate imaging. The incidence of delayed gastric emptying was not increased in patients with pylorus-preserving operation or truncal vagotomy (27% vs. 23%, respectively). All patients except one were managed successfully with prolonged nasogastric suction. One patient required revision of the gastrojejunostomy. All patients were tolerating adequate oral intake at the time of dismissal from the hospital.

Pancreatic Anastomotic Leak
Pancreatic anastomotic leak was defined as recovery of fluid from peripancreatic drains with an amylase level 5 times greater than normal or as leakage demonstrated radiologically. Anastomotic leak was detected in 48 patients and prolonged the duration of hospitalization (30 vs. 13 days; $P < 0.05$). Leaks were more common in patients with a soft pancreas (28% vs. 9%) and those with a high median intraoperative blood loss (1,150 vs. 970 mL). The incidence of pancreatic anastomotic leak was not associated with the type of pancreatic anastomotic technique (intussuscepting end-to-end vs. end-to-side) or the use of T-tube jejunal limb decompression.[149]

Most of the leaks were managed with continued drainage by the intraoperatively placed peripancreatic drains (36 patients, 80%). Two patients required percutaneous placement of a drain and were successfully managed with the addition of a somatostatin analogue. Only nine patients (19%) required reoperation specifically for uncontrolled pancreatic leak. Of these, five patients required completion pancreatectomy, three patients were successfully treated with operative drainage and closure of the site of leak, and one patient underwent peripancreatic drainage. Two of the five patients who required completion pancreatectomy died postoperatively. Although the overall perioperative mortality was greater in patients with a pancreatic anastomotic leak (8% vs. 2%), it did not achieve statistical significance ($P = 0.07$). Nineteen patients were dismissed home with a peripancreatic drain in place. All anastomotic leaks eventually closed without sequelae.

Intra-abdominal Abscess or Sepsis

Twenty-nine (10%) patients had a clinical picture and a radiologically defined intra-abdominal fluid collection consistent with an abscess. Their duration of hospitalization was increased (30 vs. 15 days; $P < 0.05$), as was the postoperative mortality (17%). The incidence of intra-abdominal abscess was clearly associated with pancreatojejunostomy leak. The frequency of intra-abdominal abscess was 42% in the presence of a pancreatic anastomotic leak and only 2% in the absence of a leak. Intra-abdominal abscess was not associated with preoperative biliary decompression, the duration of operation, or the preoperative serum albumin level. Patients were treated with antibiotics in combination with continued drainage by the initial operative drains (4%), percutaneous drainage (4%), and reoperation (2%).

Biliary Leak

Biliary-enteric anastomotic leak, as evidenced by bile in the drains, occurred in 24 patients (9%) and prolonged their hospitalization (24 vs. 13 days; $P < 0.05$). Bile leaks were not associated with the size of bile duct, technique of anastomosis, preoperative or perioperative biliary drainage, or the preoperative bilirubin level. Although most bile leaks were easily controlled with conservative management, the operative mortality was increased in this group of patients but was primarily related to other associated conditions. Most biliary leaks closed spontaneously with conservative management, and only three patients required reoperation for closure or for uncontrolled biliary leak. The biliary leak eventually closed in the 10 patients who were dismissed home with a drain in place.

Hemorrhage

Gastrointestinal Tract Bleeding

Upper gastrointestinal tract bleeding occurred in 14 patients (5%) and increased the duration of their hospitalization (31 vs. 13 days; $P < 0.05$) but not the mortality rate. The frequency of bleeding with conventional pancreatoduodenectomy was similar to that with pylorus-preserving resection (5% vs. 4%). Most patients (11 of 14) were managed conservatively with supportive care and interventional endoscopic treatment. However, three of these patients eventually required reoperation to control bleeding either at the pancreatic remnant (two patients) or at the gastrojejunostomy (one patient).

Intra-abdominal Bleeding

Intra-abdominal hemorrhage (> 1,000 mL) occurred in eight patients (3%) early postoperatively. Semi-emergency reoperation for control of bleeding was necessary in four of the eight patients. Bleeding was usually arterial from the bed of the resected pancreatic head or from portal venous branches. Although postoperative bleeding was not associated with increased intraoperative blood loss, the overall operative mortality rate was increased in patients with intra-abdominal hemorrhage (30% vs. 2%).

Miscellaneous Complications

Small bowel obstruction developed in two patients and required reoperation before dismissal. Acute necrotizing pancreatitis occurred in one patient, who required completion pancreatectomy. Wound infection developed in 7% of patients. Medical complications that prolonged the duration of hospitalization included pulmonary failure or pneumonia (7%), myocardial infarction (1%), hepatic failure (2%), and renal failure (2%). We take an aggressive early approach to the management of complications, selectively using both nonoperative and operative therapeutic options. Most complications were tolerated and managed nonoperatively. Overall, reoperation was required in only 24 (9%) of the 279 patients.

Mortality

The postoperative mortality rate after pancreatoduodenectomy for pancreatic head and periampullary cancers varies greatly but has recently decreased to less than 4% at centers experienced in pancreatic surgery (Tables 2-5).

ADJUVANT THERAPY

Adjuvant external beam radiotherapy with the radiosensitizer 5-fluorouracil is the standard therapy offered to patients with pancreatic and periampullary cancer who undergo potentially curative resection or margin-positive resection.[161,162] A recent prospective randomized trial conducted by the European Organization for Research and Treatment of Cancer showed little benefit to this standard treatment.[163] However, this trial may have been underpowered, and the course of chemotherapy was much shorter than standardly given. We, therefore, await the results from larger trials before changing our practice. In addition, we believe that all patients who undergo resection of ductal carcinoma of the pancreas should be considered for adjuvant radiation and chemotherapy.[161,164,165]

Palliative chemoradiation therapy is offered to patients who have locally advanced disease without distant metastases; this provides an expected 3- to 6-month survival advantage.[166] Patients with metastatic disease outside the peripancreatic region have an expected survival of approximately 6 months and usually do not benefit from palliative chemoradiation therapy.

LONG-TERM FOLLOW-UP

The overall 5-year survival is greater for duodenal and ampullary cancers, intermediate for bile duct cancer, and least for pancreatic cancer (Tables 2-5). Ductal adenocarcinoma of the pancreas remains a lethal disease for most patients. Historically, the 5-year survival has been less than 10% after curative resection.[167-169]

Recently, several centers with special expertise in pancreatic surgery have reported improved 5-year actuarial survival in excess of 20% after potentially curative resection.[46,100,170,171] This result prompted us to review critically the clinicopathologic characteristics of the 186 consecutive patients who underwent resection for ductal adenocarcinoma of the pancreatic head from 1981 to 1991.[21] After careful review of the histologic specimen by both a Mayo Clinic pathologist and an external pathologist, 12 patients were discovered to have nonductal pancreatic cancer and were excluded; 174 patients remained for analysis. The operative mortality rate was 3% and the 5-year overall actuarial survival was 7% (Fig. 13). Sixteen percent (28 patients) had macroscopically incomplete resection, and 56% (98 patients) had positive lymph nodes. Five-year survival was greater for patients with node-negative disease than for those with node-positive disease (14% vs. 1%, $P < 0.001$) (Fig. 14). Survival was 23% in the subset of patients with negative nodes and no perineural or duodenal invasion. Stage also significantly affected survival; 5-year survival rates were 14% for stage I, 0% for stage II, and 1% for stage III disease (Fig. 15). When patients were stratified according to tumor size only, the 5-year survival rate was 20% for patients with a tumor size 2 cm or less and a dismal 1% for patients with tumors more than 3 cm (Fig. 16).

Historically, adenocarcinoma of the body and tail of the pancreas has been considered a disease with a poor prognosis and very few long-term survivors.[138,172]

Table 2.—Outcome After Pancreatoduodenectomy for Adenocarcinoma of the Pancreas

Reference	No. of patients	Operative mortality, %	Operative morbidity, %	Median survival, mo	5-Year survival, %
Benassai et al., 2000[7]	75	5	24	17	18.7
Yeo et al., 1998[42]	148	NR	NR	12	15
Zerbi et al., 1998[150]	101	4	43	16	8
Sperti et al., 1996[151]	113	15	NR	NR	12
Wade et al., 1995[152]	252	8	37	15	9
Yeo et al., 1995[153]	201	5	NR	18	26
Nitecki et al., 1995[21]*	174	3	33	17.5	7

NR, not reported.
*From Mayo Clinic.

Table 3.—Outcome After Pancreatoduodenectomy for Adenocarcinoma of the Distal Common Bile Duct

Reference	No. of patients	Operative mortality, %	Operative morbidity, %	Median survival, mo	5-Year survival, %
Takao et al., 1999[154]	58	NR	NR	NR	32
Yeo et al., 1998[42]	30	NR	NR	22	27
Zerbi et al., 1998[150]	27	4	44	22	13
Wade et al., 1997[155]	30	11	NR	22	22
Nakeeb et al., 1996[156]	73	1	33	NR	30
Nagorney et al., 1993[157]*	22	5	24	NR	43

NR, not reported.
*From Mayo Clinic.

Table 4.—Outcome After Pancreatoduodenectomy for Ampullary Adenocarcinoma

Reference	No. of patients	Operative mortality, %	Operative morbidity, %	Median survival, mo	5-Year survival, %
Beger et al., 1999[132]	88	3	25	NR	42
Roberts et al., 1999[158]	32	9	59	NR	46
Su et al., 1999[120]	13	15	48	38	33
Klempnauer et al., 1998[31]	94	10	26	NR	38
Yeo et al., 1998[42]	46	NR	NR	49	39
Dorandeu et al., 1997[159]	42	7	22	NR	44
Monson et al., 1991[23]*	104	5.7	NR	34	34

NR, not reported.
*From Mayo Clinic.

Table 5.—Outcome After Pancreatoduodenectomy for Adenocarcinoma of the Duodenum

Reference	No. of patients	Operative mortality, %	Operative morbidity, %	Median survival, mo	5-Year survival, %
Bakaeen et al., 2000[36]*	50	1	64	NR	54
Ohigashi et al., 1998[160]	24	0	NR	NR	57
Sohn et al., 1998[111]	35	3	57	NR	67
Yeo et al., 1998[42]	17	NR	NR	NR	59

NR, not reported.
*From Mayo Clinic.

However, recently several institutions have reported 5-year survival rates of about 20% after curative resection.[173,174] A careful review of all patients at Mayo Clinic who underwent potentially curative distal pancreatectomy for ductal adenocarcinoma of the body and tail of the pancreas during a 25-year period failed to confirm improving long-term survival.[175] The median overall survival was 10 months, and disease-free survival rates were 15% at 2 years and 8% at 5 years. These results are not substantially different for those reported after resection for pancreatic head carcinoma. The operative mortality rate was zero.

Primary adenocarcinoma of the duodenum has a better prognosis than pancreatic cancer and in general has slightly better survival rates than primary ampullary adenocarcinoma after pancreatoduodenectomy (Tables 2-5). Most recent series,[42,111,160] including ours,[30] report 5-year survival rates ranging from approximately 30% to more than 60% and operative mortality rates of 5% or less. Metastasis to lymph nodes, advanced tumor stage, and positive resection margins are associated with decreased survival after resection.[30] Despite positive lymph nodes, pancreatoduodenectomy may still offer cure if complete tumor resection with negative margins is achieved.[30,43,176]

The prognosis of ampullary adenocarcinoma, like that of duodenal cancer, is more favorable after resection, especially when compared with ductal pancreatic cancer. Five-year survival rates approach 50% (Table 4), even when metastases are present in regional nodes.[177]

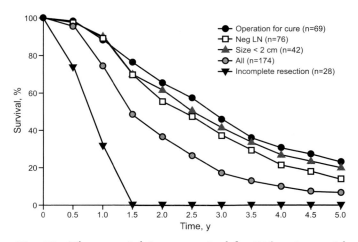

Fig. 13. The actuarial 5-year survival for 174 patients with resected adenocarcinoma of the pancreatic head according to various factors. LN, lymph nodes; Neg, negative. (From Nitecki et al.[21] By permission of Lippincott Williams & Wilkins.)

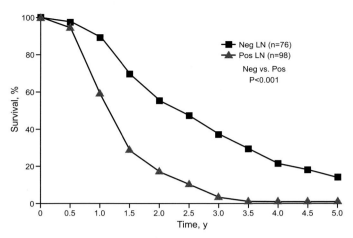
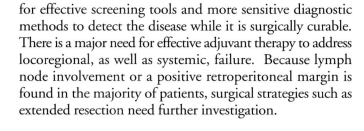

Fig. 14. Actuarial 5-year survival for 174 patients with resected adenocarcinoma of the pancreatic head according to lymph node (LN) involvement. Neg, negative; Pos, positive. (From Nitecki et al.[21] By permission of Lippincott Williams & Wilkins.)

Adenocarcinoma of the distal common bile duct represents approximately 5% of all periampullary cancers. There is a paucity of accurate survival data for distal bile duct cancer because of its rarity and because previous reports have included it among survival data for either periampullary cancer or all bile duct cancer.[157,178-180] Recent series,[38,154,156] including our own, examining outcome of treatment for distal bile duct cancer report 5-year survival ranging from 30% to as high as 54%.[181]

Although surgical resection is the only curative strategy for the treatment of pancreatic and periampullary cancers, the overall survival in many patients undergoing curative resection remains discouraging. This result underscores the need for effective screening tools and more sensitive diagnostic methods to detect the disease while it is surgically curable. There is a major need for effective adjuvant therapy to address locoregional, as well as systemic, failure. Because lymph node involvement or a positive retroperitoneal margin is found in the majority of patients, surgical strategies such as extended resection need further investigation.

CONCLUSION

Considerable progress has been made in the diagnosis, preoperative staging, patient selection, and safety of the operations for pancreatic and periampullary cancers. Although these cancers share similar major characteristics, they differ in outcome after curative resection. The overall survival after pancreatoduodenectomy is greatest for patients with ampullary and duodenal adenocarcinoma, intermediate for patients with distal bile duct cancer, and least for patients with pancreatic cancer. Because surgical resection is the only chance for cure, we strongly advocate operation for patients with locoregional disease who are good surgical candidates.

Fundamental to our surgical approach is the efficient use of the least invasive and most effective radiologic methods to diagnose and stage the disease and select patients for operation. We believe that laparotomy should be performed with therapeutic rather than diagnostic intent and that operation offers the best palliation for patients with good performance status who have locally unresectable disease or occult metastases at the time of exploration.

Despite the decreasing operative mortality, the operative morbidity remains significant. However, with the availability of interventional radiologic procedures, most

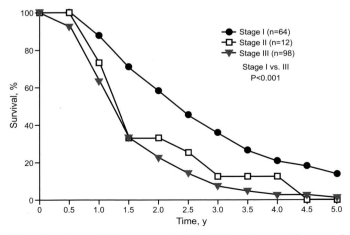
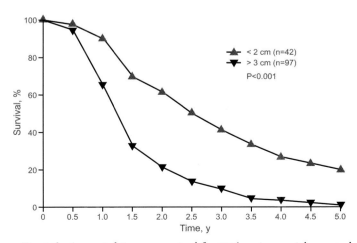

Fig. 15. Actuarial 5-year survival for 174 patients with resected adenocarcinoma of the pancreatic head according to pathologic stage. (From Nitecki et al.[21] By permission of Lippincott Williams & Wilkins.)

Fig. 16. Actuarial 5-year survival for 174 patients with resected adenocarcinoma of the pancreatic head according to tumor size. (From Nitecki et al.[21] By permission of Lippincott Williams & Wilkins.)

of these complications can be managed nonoperatively and conservatively. The overall quality of life after pancreatoduodenectomy is good, but there is a need for better disease-specific quality-of-life assessment for patients with periampullary carcinoma.

Adjuvant external beam radiotherapy in combination with 5-fluorouracil is the standard therapy offered to patients who undergo potentially curative or margin-positive resection. Whether neoadjuvant chemoradiation or extended lymphadenectomy will improve survival is yet to be determined. Undoubtedly, the quest for methods to provide earlier diagnosis and more effective approaches for the management of locally advanced disease will continue and will, it is hoped, lead to improved outcome for patients with pancreatic and periampullary cancer.

REFERENCES

1. Farnell MB, Nagorney DM, Sarr MG: The Mayo Clinic approach to the surgical treatment of adenocarcinoma of the pancreas. Surg Clin North Am 81:611-623, 2001
2. Sarmiento JM, Nagorney DM, Sarr MG, Farnell MB: Periampullary cancers: Are there differences? Surg Clin North Am 81:543-555, 2001
3. Murr MM, Sarr MG, Oishi AJ, van Heerden JA: Pancreatic cancer. CA Cancer J Clin 44:304-318, 1994
4. Farley DRF, Michael B, Donohue JH, Thompson GB, van Heerden JA, Grant CS, Sarr MG: The surgical management of pancreatic cancer: the Mayo Clinic approach. Probl Gen Surg 14:109-116, 1997
5. Farley DR, Sarr MG: Management of the apparent periampullary malignancy: preoperative evaluation and operative treatment. *In* Surgery for Gastrointestinal Cancer: a Multidisciplinary Approach. Edited by HJ Wanebo. Philadelphia, Lippincott-Raven Publishers, 1997, pp 383-392
6. Yeo CJ: The Johns Hopkins experience with pancreaticoduodenectomy with or without extended retroperitoneal lymphadenectomy for periampullary adenocarcinoma. J Gastrointest Surg 4:231-232, 2000
7. Benassai G, Mastrorilli M, Quarto G, Cappiello A, Giani U, Mosella G: Survival after pancreaticoduodenectomy for ductal adenocarcinoma of the head of the pancreas. Chir Ital 52:263-270, 2000
8. Yeo CJ, Cameron JL: Improving results of pancreaticoduodenectomy for pancreatic cancer. World J Surg 23:907-912, 1999
9. Millikan KW, Deziel DJ, Silverstein JC, Kanjo TM, Christein JD, Doolas A, Prinz RA: Prognostic factors associated with resectable adenocarcinoma of the head of the pancreas. Am Surg 65:618-623, 1999
10. Tsiotos GG, Farnell MB, Sarr MG: Are the results of pancreatectomy for pancreatic cancer improving? World J Surg 23:913-919, 1999
11. Parker SL, Davis KJ, Wingo PA, Ries LA, Heath CW Jr: Cancer statistics by race and ethnicity. CA Cancer J Clin 48:31-48, 1998
12. Whipple AO: Rationale of radical surgery for cancer of pancreas and ampullary region. Ann Surg 114:612-615, 1941
13. Waugh JM, Clagett OT: Resection of duodenum and head of pancreas for carcinoma: analysis of 30 cases. Surgery 20:224-232, 1946
14. Fortner JG: Regional resection of cancer of the pancreas: a new surgical approach. Surgery 73:307-320, 1973
15. Traverso LW, Longmire WP Jr: Preservation of the pylorus in pancreaticoduodenectomy. Surg Gynecol Obstet 146:959-962, 1978
16. Lansing PB, Blalock JB, Ochsner JL: Pancreatoduodenectomy: a retrospective review 1949 to 1969. Am Surg 38:79-86, 1972
17. Morris PJ, Nardi GL: Pancreaticoduodenal cancer: experience from 1951 to 1960 with a look ahead and behind. Arch Surg 92:834-837, 1966
18. Gudjonsson B: Cancer of the pancreas: 50 years of surgery. Cancer 60:2284-2303, 1987
19. Schwarz RE, Keny H, Ellenhorn JD: A mortality-free decade of pancreatoduodenectomy: Is quality independent of quantity? Am Surg 65:949-954, 1999
20. Rios G, Conrad A, Cole D, Adams D, Leveen M, O'Brien P, Baron P: Trends in indications and outcomes in the Whipple procedure over a 40-year period. Am Surg 65:889-893, 1999
21. Nitecki SS, Sarr MG, Colby TV, van Heerden JA: Long-term survival after resection for ductal adenocarcinoma of the pancreas: Is it really improving? Ann Surg 221:59-66, 1995

22. Yeo CJ, Cameron JL, Sohn TA, Lillemoe KD, Pitt HA, Talamini MA, Hruban RH, Ord SE, Sauter PK, Coleman J, Zahurak ML, Grochow LB, Abrams RA: Six hundred fifty consecutive pancreaticoduodenectomies in the 1990s: pathology, complications, and outcomes. Ann Surg 226:248-257, 1997

23. Monson JR, Donohue JH, McEntee GP, McIlrath DC, van Heerden JA, Shorter RG, Nagorney DM, Ilstrup DM: Radical resection for carcinoma of the ampulla of Vater. Arch Surg 126:353-357, 1991

24. Andersen HB, Baden H, Brahe NE, Burcharth F: Pancreaticoduodenectomy for periampullary adenocarcinoma. J Am Coll Surg 179:545-552, 1994

25. Japan Pancreas Society Classification of Pancreatic Carcinoma. Tokyo, Kanehara Press, 1996

26. Sobin LH, Wittekind C: TNM Classification of Malignant Tumours. Fifth edition. New York, J Wiley, 1997

27. Fleming ID, Cooper JS, Henson DE, Hutter RVP, Kennedy BJ, Murphy GP, O'Sullivan B, Sobin LH, Yarbro JW: AJCC Cancer Staging Manual. Fifth edition. Philadelphia, Lippincott-Raven, 1997

28. Yamaguchi K, Enjoji M: Carcinoma of the ampulla of Vater: a clinicopathologic study and pathologic staging of 109 cases of carcinoma and 5 cases of adenoma. Cancer 59:506-515, 1987

29. Harada N, Treitschke F, Imaizumi T, et al: Pancreatic invasion is a prognostic indicator after radical resection for carcinoma of the ampulla of Vater. J Hepatobiliary Pancreat Surg 4:215, 1997

30. Willett CG, Warshaw AL, Convery K, Compton CC: Patterns of failure after pancreaticoduodenectomy for ampullary carcinoma. Surg Gynecol Obstet 176:33-38, 1993

31. Klempnauer J, Ridder GJ, Maschek H, Pichlmayr R: Carcinoma of the ampulla of Vater: determinants of long-term survival in 94 resected patients. HPB Surg 11:1-11, 1998

32. Kayahara M, Nagakawa T, Ueno K, Ohta T, Takeda T, Miyazaki I: Lymphatic flow in carcinoma of the distal bile duct based on a clinicopathologic study. Cancer 72:2112-2117, 1993

33. Delcore R, Rodriguez FJ, Forster J, Hermreck AS, Thomas JH: Significance of lymph node metastases in patients with pancreatic cancer undergoing curative resection. Am J Surg 172:463-468, 1996

34. Nagakawa T, Kobayashi H, Ueno K, Ohta T, Kayahara M, Miyazaki I: Clinical study of lymphatic flow to the paraaortic lymph nodes in carcinoma of the head of the pancreas. Cancer 73:1155-1162, 1994

35. Nakao A, Harada A, Nonami T, Kaneko T, Murakami H, Inoue S, Takeuchi Y, Takagi H: Lymph node metastases in carcinoma of the head of the pancreas region. Br J Surg 82:399-402, 1995

36. Bakaeen FG, Murr MM, Sarr MG, Thompson GB, Farnell MB, Nagorney DM, Farley DR, van Heerden JA, Wiersema LM, Schleck CD, Donohue JH: What prognostic factors are important in duodenal adenocarcinoma? Arch Surg 135:635-641, 2000

37. Bortolasi L, Burgart LJ, Tsiotos GG, Luque-De Leon E, Sarr MG: Adenocarcinoma of the distal bile duct: a clinicopathologic outcome analysis after curative resection. Dig Surg 17:36-41, 2000

38. Kurosaki I, Tsukada K, Hatakeyama K, Muto T: The mode of lymphatic spread in carcinoma of the bile duct. Am J Surg 172:239-243, 1996

39. Yoshida T, Shibata K, Yokoyama H, Morii Y, Matsumoto T, Sasaki A, Kitano S: Patterns of lymph node metastasis in carcinoma of the distal bile duct. Hepatogastroenterology 46:1595-1598, 1999

40. Shirai Y, Ohtani T, Tsukada K, Hatakeyama K: Patterns of lymphatic spread of carcinoma of the ampulla of Vater. Br J Surg 84:1012-1016, 1997

41. Kayahara M, Nagakawa T, Ueno K, Ohta T, Tsukioka Y, Miyazaki I: Surgical strategy for carcinoma of the pancreas head area based on clinicopathologic analysis of nodal involvement and plexus invasion. Surgery 117:616-623, 1995

42. Yeo CJ, Sohn TA, Cameron JL, Hruban RH, Lillemoe KD, Pitt HA: Periampullary adenocarcinoma: analysis of 5-year survivors. Ann Surg 227:821-831, 1998

43. Pickleman J, Koelsch M, Chejfec G: Node-positive duodenal carcinoma is curable. Arch Surg 132:241-244, 1997

44. Kayahara M, Nagakawa T, Konishi I, Ueno K, Ohta T, Miyazaki I: Clinicopathological study of pancreatic carcinoma with particular reference to the invasion of the extrapancreatic neural plexus. Int J Pancreatol 10:105-111, 1991

45. Nagakawa T, Mori K, Nakano T, Kadoya M, Kobayashi H, Akiyama T, Kayahara M, Ohta T, Ueno K, Higashino Y: Perineural invasion of carcinoma of the pancreas and biliary tract. Br J Surg 80:619-621, 1993

46. Cameron JL, Crist DW, Sitzmann JV, Hruban RH, Boitnott JK, Seidler AJ, Coleman J: Factors influencing survival after pancreaticoduodenectomy for pancreatic cancer. Am J Surg 161:120-124, 1991

47. Takahashi T, Ishikura H, Motohara T, Okushiba S, Dohke M, Katoh H: Perineural invasion by ductal adenocarcinoma of the pancreas. J Surg Oncol 65:164-170, 1997

48. Nakao A, Harada A, Nonami T, Kaneko T, Takagi H: Clinical significance of carcinoma invasion of the extrapancreatic nerve plexus in pancreatic cancer. Pancreas 12:357-361, 1996

49. Ozaki H, Kinoshita T, Kosuge T, Egawa S, Kishi K: Effectiveness of multimodality treatment for resectable pancreatic cancer. Int J Pancreatol 7:195-200, 1990

50. Nakai T, Koh K, Kawabe T, Son E, Yoshikawa H, Yasutomi M: Importance of microperineural invasion as a prognostic factor in ampullary carcinoma. Br J Surg 84:1399-1401, 1997

51. Gupta MK, Arciaga R, Bocci L, Tubbs R, Bukowski R, Deodhar SD: Measurement of a monoclonal-antibody-defined antigen (CA19-9) in the sera of patients with malignant and nonmalignant diseases: comparison with carcinoembryonic antigen. Cancer 56:277-283, 1985

52. Steinberg WM, Gelfand R, Anderson KK, Glenn J, Kurtzman SH, Sindelar WF, Toskes PP: Comparison of the sensitivity and specificity of the CA 19-9 and carcinoembryonic antigen assays in detecting cancer of the pancreas. Gastroenterology 90:343-349, 1986

53. Ritts RE, Pitt HA: CA 19-9 in pancreatic cancer. Surg Oncol Clin N Am 7:93-101, 1998

54. Steinberg W: The clinical utility of the CA 19-9 tumor-associated antigen. Am J Gastroenterol 85:350-355, 1990

55. Montgomery RC, Hoffman JP, Riley LB, Rogatko A, Ridge JA, Eisenberg BL: Prediction of recurrence and survival by post-resection CA 19-9 values in patients with adenocarcinoma of the pancreas. Ann Surg Oncol 4:551-556, 1997

56. Willett CG, Daly WJ, Warshaw AL: CA 19-9 is an index of response to neoadjunctive chemoradiation therapy in pancreatic cancer. Am J Surg 172:350-352, 1996

57. van den Bosch RP, van Eijck CH, Mulder PG, Jeekel J: Serum CA 19-9 determination in the management of pancreatic cancer. Hepatogastroenterology 43:710-713, 1996

58. Pohl AL: Surveillance of cancer patients with tumor markers. J Tumor Marker Oncol 2:1-14, 1987

59. Takeuchi M, Kondo S, Sugiura H, Katoh H: Pre-operative predictors of short-term survival after pancreatic cancer resection. Hepatogastroenterology 45:2399-2403, 1998

60. Tsiotos GG, Sarr MG: Diagnosis and clinical staging of pancreatic cancer. *In* Surgical Diseases of the Pancreas. Third edition. Edited by JM Howard, Y Idezuki, I Ihse, RA Prinz. Baltimore, Williams & Wilkins, 1998, pp 497-513

61. Ivy EJ, Sarr MG, Reiman HM: Nonendocrine cancer of the pancreas in patients under age forty years. Surgery 108:481-487, 1990

62. Kelsen DP, Portenoy R, Thaler H, Tao Y, Brennan M: Pain as a predictor of outcome in patients with operable pancreatic carcinoma. Surgery 122:53-59, 1997

63. Andren-Sandberg A, Wagner M, Tihanyi T, Lofgren P, Friess H: Technical aspects of left-sided pancreatic resection for cancer. Dig Surg 16:305-312, 1999

64. Grahm AL, Andren-Sandberg A: Prospective evaluation of pain in exocrine pancreatic cancer. Digestion 58:542-549, 1997

65. Chauffard A: Le cancer du corps du pancreéas. Bull Acad Med 60:242-255, 1908

66. Jagelman DG, DeCosse JJ, Bussey HJ: Upper gastrointestinal cancer in familial adenomatous polyposis. Lancet 1:1149-1151, 1988

67. Sarre RG, Frost AG, Jagelman DG, Petras RE, Sivak MV, McGannon E: Gastric and duodenal polyps in familial adenomatous polyposis: a prospective study of the nature and prevalence of upper gastrointestinal polyps. Gut 28:306-314, 1987

68. Iwama T, Mishima Y, Utsunomiya J: The impact of familial adenomatous polyposis on the tumorigenesis and mortality at the several organs: its rational treatment. Ann Surg 217:101-108, 1993

69. Offerhaus GJ, Giardiello FM, Krush AJ, Booker SV, Tersmette AC, Kelley NC, Hamilton SR: The risk of upper gastrointestinal cancer in familial adenomatous polyposis. Gastroenterology 102:1980-1982, 1992

70. Spigelman AD, Williams CB, Talbot IC, Domizio P, Phillips RK: Upper gastrointestinal cancer in patients with familial adenomatous polyposis. Lancet 2:783-785, 1989

71. Taoka H, Hauptmann E, Traverso LW, Barnett MJ, Sarr MG, Reber HA: How accurate is helical computed tomography for clinical staging of pancreatic cancer? Am J Surg 177:428-432, 1999

72. Andersen HB, Effersoe H, Tjalve E, Burcharth F: CT for assessment of pancreatic and periampullary cancer. Acta Radiol 34:569-572, 1993

73. Ross CB, Sharp KW, Kaufman AJ, Andrews T, Williams LF: Efficacy of computerized tomography in the preoperative staging of pancreatic carcinoma. Am Surg 54:221-226, 1988

74. Fuhrman GM, Charnsangavej C, Abbruzzese JL, Cleary KR, Martin RG, Fenoglio CJ, Evans DB: Thin-section contrast-enhanced computed tomography accurately predicts the resectability of malignant pancreatic neoplasms. Am J Surg 167:104-111, 1994

75. Takahashi S, Ogata Y, Aiura K, Kitajima M, Hiramatsu K: Combined resection of the portal vein for pancreatic cancer: preoperative diagnosis of invasion by portography and prognosis. Hepatogastroenterology 47:545-549, 2000

76. Harrison LE, Brennan MF: Portal vein resection for pancreatic adenocarcinoma. Surg Oncol Clin N Am 7:165-181, 1998

77. Fuhrman GM, Leach SD, Staley CA, Cusack JC, Charnsangavej C, Cleary KR, El-Naggar AK, Fenoglio CJ, Lee JE, Evans DB: Rationale for en bloc vein resection in the treatment of pancreatic adenocarcinoma adherent to the superior mesenteric-portal vein confluence. Pancreatic Tumor Study Group. Ann Surg 223:154-162, 1996

78. Leach SD, Lee JE, Charnsangavej C, Cleary KR, Lowy AM, Fenoglio CJ, Pisters PW, Evans DB: Survival following pancreaticoduodenectomy with resection of the superior mesenteric-portal vein confluence for adenocarcinoma of the pancreatic head. Br J Surg 85:611-617, 1998

79. Harrison LE, Brennan MF: Portal vein involvement in pancreatic cancer: A sign of unresectability? Adv Surg 31:375-394, 1997

80. Bold RJ, Charnsangavej C, Cleary KR, Jennings M, Madray A, Leach SD, Abbruzzese JL, Pisters PW, Lee JE, Evans DB: Major vascular resection as part of pancreaticoduodenectomy for cancer: radiologic, intraoperative, and pathologic analysis. J Gastrointest Surg 3:233-243, 1999

81. Smith CD, Behrns KE, van Heerden JA, Sarr MG: Radical pancreatoduodenectomy for misdiagnosed pancreatic mass. Br J Surg 81:585-589, 1994

82. Masci E, Toti G, Mariani A, Curioni S, Lomazzi A, Dinelli M, Minoli G, Crosta C, Comin U, Fertitta A, Prada A, Passoni GR, Testoni PA: Complications of diagnostic and therapeutic ERCP: a prospective multicenter study. Am J Gastroenterol 96:417-423, 2001

83. Temudom T, Sarr MG, Douglas MG, Farnell MB: An argument against routine percutaneous biopsy, ERCP, or biliary stent placement in patients with clinically resectable periampullary masses: a surgical perspective. Pancreas 11:283-288, 1995

84. Sohn TA, Yeo CJ, Cameron JL, Pitt HA, Lillemoe KD: Do preoperative biliary stents increase postpancreaticoduodenectomy complications? J Gastrointest Surg 4:258-267, 2000

85. Povoski SP, Karpeh MS Jr, Conlon KC, Blumgart LH, Brennan MF: Preoperative biliary drainage: impact on intraoperative bile cultures and infectious morbidity and mortality after pancreaticoduodenectomy. J Gastrointest Surg 3:496-505, 1999

86. Megibow AJ, Zhou XH, Rotterdam H, Francis IR, Zerhouni EA, Balfe DM, Weinreb JC, Aisen A, Kuhlman J, Heiken JP: Pancreatic adenocarcinoma: CT versus MR imaging in the evaluation of resectability—report of the Radiology Diagnostic Oncology Group. Radiology 195:327-332, 1995

87. Muller MF, Meyenberger C, Bertschinger P, Schaer R, Marincek B: Pancreatic tumors: evaluation with endoscopic US, CT, and MR imaging. Radiology 190:745-751, 1994

88. Warshaw AL, Gu ZY, Wittenberg J, Waltman AC: Preoperative staging and assessment of resectability of pancreatic cancer. Arch Surg 125:230-233, 1990

89. Trede M, Rumstadt B, Wendl K, Gaa J, Tesdal K, Lehmann KJ, Meier-Willersen HJ, Pescatore P, Schmoll J: Ultrafast magnetic resonance imaging improves the staging of pancreatic tumors. Ann Surg 226:393-405, 1997

90. Gaa J, Wendl K, Tesdal IK, Meier-Willersen HJ, Lehmann KJ, Bohm C, Mockel R, Richter A, Trede M, Georgi M: Combined use of MRI and MR cholangiopancreatography and contrast enhanced dual phase 3-D MR angiography in diagnosis of pancreatic tumors: initial clinical results [German]. Rofo Fortschr Geb Rontgenstr Neuen Bildgeb Verfahr 170:528-533, 1999

91. Sho M, Nakajima Y, Kanehiro H, Hisanaga M, Nishio K, Nagao M, Tatekawa Y, Ikeda N, Kanokogi H, Yamada T, Hirohashi S,

Hirohashi R, Uchida H, Nakano H: A new evaluation of pancreatic function after pancreatoduodenectomy using secretin magnetic resonance cholangiopancreatography. Am J Surg 176:279-282, 1998

92. Takehara Y: MR pancreatography: technique and applications. Top Magn Reson Imaging 8:290-301, 1996

93. Weber WA, Schwaiger M, Avril N: Quantitative assessment of tumor metabolism using FDG-PET imaging. Nucl Med Biol 27:683-687, 2000

94. Nakamoto Y, Higashi T, Sakahara H, Tamaki N, Kogire M, Imamura M, Konishi J: Contribution of PET in the detection of liver metastases from pancreatic tumours. Clin Radiol 54:248-252, 1999

95. Bares R, Klever P, Hauptmann S, Hellwig D, Fass J, Cremerius U, Schumpelick V, Mittermayer C, Bull U: F-18 fluorodeoxyglucose PET in vivo evaluation of pancreatic glucose metabolism for detection of pancreatic cancer. Radiology 192:79-86, 1994

96. Rajput A, Stellato TA, Faulhaber PF, Vesselle HJ, Miraldi F: The role of fluorodeoxyglucose and positron emission tomography in the evaluation of pancreatic disease. Surgery 124:793-797, 1998

97. Biehl TR, Traverso LW, Hauptmann E, Ryan JA Jr: Preoperative visceral angiography alters intraoperative strategy during the Whipple procedure. Am J Surg 165:607-612, 1993

98. Rong GH, Sindelar WF: Aberrant peripancreatic arterial anatomy: considerations in performing pancreatectomy for malignant neoplasms. Am Surg 53:726-729, 1987

99. Dooley WC, Cameron JL, Pitt HA, Lillemoe KD, Yue NC, Venbrux AC: Is preoperative angiography useful in patients with periampullary tumors? Ann Surg 211:649-654, 1990

100. Trede M, Schwall G, Saeger HD: Survival after pancreatoduodenectomy: 118 consecutive resections without an operative mortality. Ann Surg 211:447-458, 1990

101. Caletti G, Fusaroli P: Endoscopic ultrasonography. Endoscopy 33:158-166, 2001

102. Ahmad NA, Lewis JD, Ginsberg GG, Rosato EF, Morris JB, Kochman ML: EUS in preoperative staging of pancreatic cancer. Gastrointest Endosc 52:463-468, 2000

103. Conlon KC, Brennan MF: Laparoscopy for staging abdominal malignancies. Adv Surg 34:331-350, 2000

104. Fernandez-del Castillo C, Warshaw AL: Laparoscopy for staging in pancreatic carcinoma. Surg Oncol 2 Suppl 1:25-29, 1993

105. Luque-de Leon E, Tsiotos GG, Balsiger B, Barnwell J, Burgart LJ, Sarr MG: Staging laparoscopy for pancreatic cancer should be used to select the best means of palliation and not only to maximize the resectability rate. J Gastrointest Surg 3:111-117, 1999

106. Di Stasi M, Lencioni R, Solmi L, Magnolfi F, Caturelli E, De Sio I, Salmi A, Buscarini L: Ultrasound-guided fine needle biopsy of pancreatic masses: results of a multicenter study. Am J Gastroenterol 93:1329-1333, 1998

107. Bergenfeldt M, Genell S, Lindholm K, Ekberg O, Aspelin P: Needle-tract seeding after percutaneous fine-needle biopsy of pancreatic carcinoma: case report. Acta Chir Scand 154:77-79, 1988

108. Ferrucci JT, Wittenberg J, Margolies MN, Carey RW: Malignant seeding of the tract after thin-needle aspiration biopsy. Radiology 130:345-346, 1979

109. Beazley RM: Needle biopsy diagnosis of pancreatic cancer. Cancer 47 Suppl:1685-1687, 1981

110. McLeod RS: Quality of life, nutritional status and gastrointestinal hormone profile following the Whipple procedure. Ann Oncol 10 Suppl 4:281-284, 1999

111. Sohn TA, Lillemoe KD, Cameron JL, Pitt HA, Kaufman HS, Hruban RH, Yeo CJ: Adenocarcinoma of the duodenum: factors influencing long-term survival. J Gastrointest Surg 2:79-87, 1998

112. Spencer MP, Sarr MG, Nagorney DM: Radical pancreatectomy for pancreatic cancer in the elderly: Is it safe and justified? Ann Surg 212:140-143, 1990

113. Sakorafas GH, Friess H, Balsiger BM, Buchler MW, Sarr MG: Problems of reconstruction during pancreatoduodenectomy. Dig Surg 18:363-369, 2001

114. Jones L, Russell C, Mosca F, Boggi U, Sutton R, Slavin J, Hartley M, Neoptolemos JP: Standard Kausch-Whipple pancreatoduodenectomy. Dig Surg 16:297-304, 1999

115. Mosca F, Giulianotti PC, Balestracci T, Di Candio G, Pietrabissa A, Sbrana F, Rossi G: Long-term survival in pancreatic cancer: pylorus-preserving versus Whipple pancreatoduodenectomy. Surgery 122:553-566, 1997

116. Sarr MG, Behrns KE, van Heerden JA: Total pancreatectomy: an objective analysis of its use in pancreatic cancer. Hepatogastroenterology 40:418-421, 1993

117. Farley DR, Sarr MG, Van Heerden JA: Pancreatic resection for ductal adenocarcinoma: total pancreatectomy versus partial pancreatectomy. Semin Surg Oncol 11:124-131, 1995

118. Sarmiento JM, Que FG, Thompson GB, Farnell MB: Survival analysis of patients with portal vein resection during pancreaticoduodenectomy for pancreatic cancer. A case-control study (abstract #2462). SSAT Abstracts 2001 Digestive Disease Weekly. Retrieved November 11, 2002, from the World Wide Web: http://www.ssat.com/cgi-bin/2001_abstracts.cgi

119. Sakorafas GH, Farnell MB, Nagorney DM, Farley DR, Que FG, Donohue JH, Thompson GG, Sarr MG: Management of peripancreatic vasculature during pancreatoduodenectomy: tips to avoid severe haemorrhage. Eur J Surg Oncol 25:524-528, 1999

120. Su CH, Shyr YM, Lui WY, P'Eng FK: Factors affecting morbidity, mortality and survival after pancreaticoduodenectomy for carcinoma of the ampulla of Vater. Hepatogastroenterology 46:1973-1979, 1999

121. Pedrazzoli S, Michelassi F: Extent of lymphadenectomy in the surgical treatment of adenocarcinoma of the head of the pancreas. J Gastrointest Surg 4:229-230, 2000

122. Imamura M, Hosotani R, Kogire M: Rationale of the so-called extended resection for pancreatic invasive ductal carcinoma. Digestion 60 Suppl 1:126-129, 1999

123. Iacono C, Facci E, Bortolasi L, Zamboni G, Scarpa A, Talamini G, Prati G, Nifosi F, Serio G: Intermediate results of extended pancreaticoduodenectomy: Verona experience. J Hepatobiliary Pancreat Surg 6:74-78, 1999

124. Ishikawa O: What constitutes curative pancreatectomy for adenocarcinoma of the pancreas? Hepatogastroenterology 40:414-417, 1993

125. Nagakawa T, Konishi I, Ueno K, Ohta T, Akiyama T, Kanno M, Kayahara M, Miyazaki I: The results and problems of extensive radical surgery for carcinoma of the head of the pancreas. Jpn J Surg 21:262-267, 1991

126. Pedrazzoli S, DiCarlo V, Dionigi R, Mosca F, Pederzoli P, Pasquali C, Kloppel G, Dhaene K, Michelassi F: Standard versus extended lymphadenectomy associated with pancreatoduodenectomy in the surgical treatment of adenocarcinoma of the head of the pancreas: a multicenter, prospective, randomized study. Lymphadenectomy Study Group. Ann Surg 228:508-517, 1998

127. Quirk DM, Rattner DW, Fernandez-del Castillo C, Warshaw AL, Brugge WR: The use of endoscopic ultrasonography to reduce the cost of treating ampullary tumors. Gastrointest Endosc 46:334-337, 1997

128. Rattner DW, Fernandez-del Castillo C, Brugge WR, Warshaw AL: Defining the criteria for local resection of ampullary neoplasms. Arch Surg 131:366-371, 1996

129. Farouk M, Niotis M, Branum GD, Cotton PB, Meyers WC: Indications for and the technique of local resection of tumors of the papilla of Vater. Arch Surg 126:650-652, 1991

130. Gertsch P, Matthews JB, Lerut J, Baer HU, Blumgart LH: The technique of papilloduodenectomy. Surg Gynecol Obstet 170:254-256, 1990

131. Gray G, Browder W: Villous tumors of the ampulla of Vater: local resection versus pancreatoduodenectomy. South Med J 82:917-920, 1989

132. Beger HG, Treitschke F, Gansauge F, Harada N, Hiki N, Mattfeldt T: Tumor of the ampulla of Vater: experience with local or radical resection in 171 consecutively treated patients. Arch Surg 134:526-532, 1999

133. Klein P, Reingruber B, Kastl S, Dworak O, Hohenberger W: Is local excision of pT1-ampullary carcinomas justified? Eur J Surg Oncol 22:366-371, 1996

134. Farnell MB, Sakorafas GH, Sarr MG, Rowland CM, Tsiotos GG, Farley DR, Nagorney DM: Villous tumors of the duodenum: reappraisal of local vs. extended resection. J Gastrointest Surg 4:13-21, 2000

135. Gough DB, Sarr MG: Bypass procedures: surgical treatment of pancreatic cancer. In The Pancreas. Vol 2. Edited by HG Beger, AL Warshaw, MW Büchler, DL Carr-Locke, JP Neoptolemos, C Russell, MG Sarr. Oxford, Blackwell Science, 1998, pp 1062-1070

136. Sarr MG: Palliation of jaundice: gastrointestinal obstruction. J Gastrointest Surg 3:343-344, 1999

137. Sarr MG, Gladen HE, Beart RW Jr, van Heerden JA: Role of gastroenterostomy in patients with unresectable carcinoma of the pancreas. Surg Gynecol Obstet 152:597-600, 1981

138. Yeo CJ: Pancreatic cancer: 1998 update. J Am Coll Surg 187:429-442, 1998

139. Schwarz A, Beger HG: Biliary and gastric bypass or stenting in nonresectable periampullary cancer: analysis on the basis of controlled trials. Int J Pancreatol 27:51-58, 2000

140. Lillemoe KD, Cameron JL, Hardacre JM, Sohn TA, Sauter PK, Coleman J, Pitt HA, Yeo CJ: Is prophylactic gastrojejunostomy indicated for unresectable periampullary cancer? A prospective randomized trial. Ann Surg 230:322-328, 1999

141. Sarr MG, Cameron JL: Surgical management of unresectable carcinoma of the pancreas. Surgery 91:123-133, 1982

142. Das A, Sivak MV Jr: Endoscopic palliation for inoperable pancreatic cancer. Cancer Control 7:452-457, 2000

143. Jung GS, Song HY, Kang SG, Huh JD, Park SJ, Koo JY, Cho YD: Malignant gastroduodenal obstructions: treatment by means of a covered expandable metallic stent—initial experience. Radiology 216:758-763, 2000

144. Soetikno RM, Carr-Locke DL: Expandable metal stents for gastric-outlet, duodenal, and small intestinal obstruction. Gastrointest Endosc Clin N Am 9:447-458, 1999

145. Venu RP, Pastika BJ, Kini M, Chua D, Christian R, Schlais J, Brown RD: Self-expandable metal stents for malignant gastric outlet obstruction: a modified technique. Endoscopy 30:553-558, 1998

146. Cullen JJ, Sarr MG, Ilstrup DM: Pancreatic anastomotic leak after pancreaticoduodenectomy: incidence, significance, and management. Am J Surg 168:295-298, 1994

147. Lowy AM, Lee JE, Pisters PW, Davidson BS, Fenoglio CJ, Stanford P, Jinnah R, Evans DB: Prospective, randomized trial of octreotide to prevent pancreatic fistula after pancreaticoduodenectomy for malignant disease. Ann Surg 226:632-641, 1997

148. Miedema BW, Sarr MG, van Heerden JA, Nagorney DM, McIlrath DC, Ilstrup D: Complications following pancreaticoduodenectomy: current management. Arch Surg 127:945-949, 1992

149. Fallick JS, Farley DR, Farnell MB, Ilstrup DM, Rowland CM: Venting intraluminal drains in pancreaticoduodenectomy. J Gastrointest Surg 3:156-161, 1999

150. Zerbi A, Balzano G, Leone BE, Angeli E, Veronesi P, Di Carlo V: Clinical presentation, diagnosis and survival of resected distal bile duct cancer. Dig Surg 15:410-416, 1998

151. Sperti C, Pasquali C, Piccoli A, Pedrazzoli S: Survival after resection for ductal adenocarcinoma of the pancreas. Br J Surg 83:625-631, 1996

152. Wade TP, el-Ghazzawy AG, Virgo KS, Johnson FE: The Whipple resection for cancer in U.S. Department of Veterans Affairs Hospitals. Ann Surg 221:241-248, 1995

153. Yeo CJ, Cameron JL, Lillemoe KD, Sitzmann JV, Hruban RH, Goodman SN, Dooley WC, Coleman J, Pitt HA: Pancreaticoduodenectomy for cancer of the head of the pancreas: 201 patients. Ann Surg 221:721-731, 1995

154. Takao S, Shinchi H, Uchikura K, Kubo M, Aikou T: Liver metastases after curative resection in patients with distal bile duct cancer. Br J Surg 86:327-331, 1999

155. Wade TP, Prasad CN, Virgo KS, Johnson FE: Experience with distal bile duct cancers in U.S. Veterans Affairs hospitals: 1987-1991. J Surg Oncol 64:242-245, 1997

156. Nakeeb A, Pitt HA, Sohn TA, Coleman J, Abrams RA, Piantadosi S, Hruban RH, Lillemoe KD, Yeo CJ, Cameron JL: Cholangiocarcinoma: a spectrum of intrahepatic, perihilar, and distal tumors. Ann Surg 224:463-473, 1996

157. Nagorney DM, Donohue JH, Farnell MB, Schleck CD, Ilstrup DM: Outcomes after curative resections of cholangiocarcinoma. Arch Surg 128:871-877, 1993

158. Roberts RH, Krige JE, Bornman PC, Terblanche J: Pancreaticoduodenectomy of ampullary carcinoma. Am Surg 65:1043-1048, 1999

159. Dorandeu A, Raoul JL, Siriser F, Leclercq-Rioux N, Gosselin M, Martin ED, Ramee MP, Launois B: Carcinoma of the ampulla of Vater: prognostic factors after curative surgery: a series of 45 cases. Gut 40:350-355, 1997

160. Ohigashi H, Ishikawa O, Tamura S, Imaoka S, Sasaki Y, Kameyama M, Kabuto T, Furukawa H, Hiratsuka M, Fujita M, Hashimoto T, Hosomi N, Kuroda C: Pancreatic invasion as the prognostic indicator of duodenal adenocarcinoma treated by pancreatoduodenectomy plus extended lymphadenectomy. Surgery 124:510-515, 1998

161. Gastrointestinal Tumor Study Group: Further evidence of effective adjuvant combined radiation and chemotherapy following curative resection of pancreatic cancer. Cancer 59:2006-2010, 1987

162. Kalser MH, Ellenberg SS: Pancreatic cancer: adjuvant combined radiation and chemotherapy following curative resection. Arch Surg 120:899-903, 1985

163. Klinkenbijl JH, Jeekel J, Sahmoud T, van Pel R, Couvreur ML, Veenhof CH, Arnaud JP, Gonzalez DG, de Wit LT, Hennipman A, Wils J: Adjuvant radiotherapy and 5-fluorouracil after curative resection of cancer of the pancreas and periampullary region: phase III trial of the EORTC gastrointestinal tract cancer cooperative group. Ann Surg 230:776-782, 1999
164. Foo ML, Gunderson LL: Adjuvant postoperative radiation therapy +/- 5-FU in resected carcinoma of the pancreas. Hepatogastroenterology 45:613-623, 1998
165. Foo ML, Gunderson LL, Nagorney DM, McIlrath DC, van Heerden JA, Robinow JS, Kvols LK, Garton GR, Martenson JA, Cha SS: Patterns of failure in grossly resected pancreatic ductal adenocarcinoma treated with adjuvant irradiation +/- 5 fluorouracil. Int J Radiat Oncol Biol Phys 26:483-489, 1993
166. Moertel CG, Frytak S, Hahn RG, O'Connell MJ, Reitemeier RJ, Rubin J, Schutt AJ, Weiland LH, Childs DS, Holbrook MA, Lavin PT, Livstone E, Spiro H, Knowlton A, Kalser M, Barkin J, Lessner H, Mann-Kaplan R, Ramming K, Douglas HO Jr, Thomas P, Nave H, Bateman J, Lokich J, Brooks J, Chaffey J, Corson JM, Zamcheck N, Novak JW: Therapy of locally unresectable pancreatic carcinoma: a randomized comparison of high dose (6000 rads) radiation alone, moderate dose radiation (4000 rads + 5-fluorouracil), and high dose radiation + 5-fluorouracil. The Gastrointestinal Tumor Study Group. Cancer 48:1705-1710, 1981
167. Grace PA, Pitt HA, Tompkins RK, DenBesten L, Longmire WP Jr: Decreased morbidity and mortality after pancreatoduodenectomy. Am J Surg 151:141-149, 1986
168. Warshaw AL, Swanson RS: Pancreatic cancer in 1998. Possibilities and probabilities. Ann Surg 208:541-553, 1988
169. Piorkowski RJ, Blievernicht SW, Lawrence W Jr, Madariaga J, Horsley JS III, Neifeld JP, Terz JJ: Pancreatic and periampullary carcinoma: experience with 200 patients over a 12 year period. Am J Surg 143:189-193, 1982
170. Cameron JL, Pitt HA, Yeo CJ, Lillemoe KD, Kaufman HS, Coleman J: One hundred and forty-five consecutive pancreaticoduodenectomies without mortality. Ann Surg 217:430-435, 1993
171. Warshaw AL, Fernandez-del Castillo C: Pancreatic carcinoma. N Engl J Med 326:455-465, 1992
172. Saltzman A, Horvitz A, Dyckman J: Survival for 25 years following partial pancreatectomy for carcinoma of the body of the pancreas. Mt Sinai J Med 54:427-428, 1987
173. Sperti C, Pasquali C, Pedrazzoli S: Ductal adenocarcinoma of the body and tail of the pancreas. J Am Coll Surg 185:255-259, 1997
174. Brennan MF, Moccia RD, Klimstra D: Management of adenocarcinoma of the body and tail of the pancreas. Ann Surg 223:506-511, 1996
175. Dalton RR, Sarr MG, van Heerden JA, Colby TV: Carcinoma of the body and tail of the pancreas: Is curative resection justified? Surgery 111:489-494, 1992
176. Ryder NM, Ko CY, Hines OJ, Gloor B, Reber HA: Primary duodenal adenocarcinoma: a 40-year experience. Arch Surg 135:1070-1074, 2000
177. Shirai Y, Tsukada K, Ohtani T, Hatakeyama K: Carcinoma of the ampulla of Vater: Is radical lymphadenectomy beneficial to patients with nodal disease? J Surg Oncol 61:190-194, 1996
178. Warren KW, Choe DS, Plaza J, Relihan M: Results of radical resection for periampullary cancer. Ann Surg 181:534-540, 1975
179. Tarazi RY, Hermann RE, Vogt DP, Hoerr SO, Esselstyn CB Jr, Cooperman AM, Steiger E, Grundfest S: Results of surgical treatment of periampullary tumors: a thirty-five-year experience. Surgery 100:716-723, 1986
180. Tompkins RK, Thomas D, Wile A, Longmire WP Jr: Prognostic factors in bile duct carcinoma: analysis of 96 cases. Ann Surg 194:447-457, 1981
181. Fong Y, Blumgart LH, Lin E, Fortner JG, Brennan MF: Outcome of treatment for distal bile duct cancer. Br J Surg 83:1712-1715, 1996

Chapter 19

ISLET CELL TUMORS

Geoffrey B. Thompson, M.D.

Islet cell neoplasms have been an important part of the surgical heritage at Mayo Clinic. Drs. W. J. Mayo, J. T. Priestley, O. H. Beahrs, M. A. Adson, W. H. ReMine, D. C. McIlrath, A. J. Edis, J. A. van Heerden, D. M. Nagorney, and C. S. Grant have all been or remain well recognized in the field. It is within this intellectual environment that the author has received unselfish support, guidance, and friendship, making one young surgeon's vision a reality. Nowhere is the team approach more apparent than in the management of these fascinating and not infrequently elusive hormonal factories. Without the able support of our endocrinologists, radiologists, and pathologists, our surgical successes would be few. Mayo Clinic physicians and surgeons have never functioned in isolation. Much of our success also stems from the ongoing work of investigators outside Mayo Clinic whose ideas and talents have been shared in the operating rooms, conference rooms, hotel lobbies, and even golf courses around the globe. To them, we and our patients owe a debt of gratitude.

It was in 1869 that a German medical student, Paul Langerhans (1847-1888), first described the pancreatic islets that bear his name. Nearly 60 years later, in 1927, came the first report of a patient with hypoglycemia associated with a tumor of the islet cells. Wilder and associates[1] reported an islet cell carcinoma in an orthopedic surgeon who had spells of unconsciousness and blood sugar levels of 25 mg/dL during the attack. William J. Mayo, M.D. (see Fig. 3, Chapter 1, page 2), during an exploratory operation on the patient, found a tumor of the pancreas with metastases to the liver, lymph nodes, and mesentery. An extract prepared from the tumor displayed insulin-like activity when injected into a rabbit. It was, however, left to Roscoe Graham, M.D. (Toronto, 1929), to perform the first curative operation for a benign insulinoma. In 1944, James T. Priestley, M.D. (see Fig. 14, Chapter 1, page 9), a Mayo Clinic surgeon, performed the first successful total pancreatectomy; the patient had an occult insulinoma. Since 1927, more than 350 patients have had operation for insulinoma at Mayo Clinic,[2] and most of the procedures have been successful.

A. G. E. Pearse first proposed the concept of amine precursor uptake and decarboxylation, in 1966. He noted that endocrine cells throughout the body had similar cytochemical and ultrastructural characteristics. These cells shared the ability to take up amine precursors, decarboxylate them, and finally produce various bioactive peptides and amines. He postulated that these cells all were of neuroectodermal origin stemming from the neural crest. It is now known that at least some of these cells have an endodermal origin.[2]

In 1954, Wermer reported a family in which five members had evidence of involvement of one or more endocrine glands (pituitary, parathyroid, and pancreas). The autosomal dominant syndrome was called Wermer syndrome but is now referred to as multiple endocrine neoplasia type I (MEN I).[2] Larsson, Chandrasekharappa, and others[3-5] are responsible for identification and positional cloning of the gene in MEN I (menin). The MEN I locus has been mapped to chromosome 11q13. The menin gene is a tumor suppressor gene in which both alleles are inactivated in tumor cells either by deletion of the gene or by mutations of the active portion. Germline mutations are able to be identified in 90% of affected families with MEN I. Somatic mutations in the menin gene also have been described in sporadic endocrine tumors.

The advent of radioimmunoassay and immunocytochemistry led to identification and characterization of many islet cell syndromes. Today, less than 20% of all islet cell tumors are classified as nonfunctioning (Fig. 1). All islet cell tumors vary with regard to their hormone production, demographics, size, location, malignant potential, and prognosis. The morbidity associated with these tumors more often than not relates to the hormonal sequelae and less often to the tumor burden itself.

There is striking histologic similarity among islet cell tumors, most all of which are often composed of very uniform cells within a vascular stroma (starry-sky appearance). These cells coalesce to form trabecular, acinar, or solid patterns. Anaplastic and unusual forms with clear cells, oncocytes, or mucin production can make it difficult to identify few islet cell malignancies on routine microscopy (hematoxylin-eosin). Immunocytochemistry for neuroendocrine tumor markers (neuron-specific enolase, chromogranin A, and synaptophysin) can be of help if the results are positive. Immunostains for a peptide profile (e.g., insulin, gastrin, glucagon, somatostatin, human pancreatic polypeptide) do not necessarily correlate with the tumor's clinical behavior. Insulinomas may stain only sparsely for insulin or not at all, indicating a very efficient manufacturing and delivery process. However,

a clinically "nonfunctioning" tumor may stain strongly for several peptides because of the cell's relative inability to release the peptide in concentrations large enough to elicit symptoms. Hormonal patterns, both clinical and immunocytochemical, may change with tumor recurrence and progression of disease over time. Multihormonal production by islet cell tumors also can occur (e.g., insulin and gastrin, gastrin and adrenocorticotropic hormone).[2]

This chapter discusses insulinomas, gastrinomas, glucagonomas, vasoactive intestinal polypeptide tumors, somatostatinomas, and islet cell carcinomas.

INSULINOMA

Background
Insulinomas are the most common of the islet cell tumors, yet they remain a rarity. The incidence in persons of northern European descent is 4 cases per 1 million patient-years. Sixty percent of patients are women with a median age at presentation of 47 years (range, 8-83 years). Virtually all tumors are intrapancreatic. Approximately 90% are solitary and 10% multiple. The tumors are malignant in 6% of cases, and 8% are associated with MEN I. Initial operation is curative in 88%, and long-term survival is normal. Recurrence rates of 7% (sporadic) and 21% (MEN I) have been reported at 20 years.[6]

Clinical Presentation
In a retrospective analysis of 60 patients with insulinoma, 85% had various combinations of diplopia, blurred vision, palpitations, sweating, and weakness, 80% had confusion or abnormal behavior, 53% had amnesia or coma, and 12% had generalized seizures.[6] Symptoms of hypoglycemia (Table 1) begin at plasma glucose concentrations of less than 55 mg/dL, and central nervous system function is impaired at 50 mg/dL or less. The symptoms of hypoglycemia are divided into two overlapping groups: 1) autonomic symptoms, which include sweating, trembling, anxiety, nausea, palpitations, hunger, and tingling, and 2) neuroglycopenic symptoms, which are more specific of insulinoma, including confusion, dizziness, tiredness, headache, difficulty speaking and thinking, inability to concentrate, and weakness.

Although classically associated with fasting and exercise, symptoms do occur postprandially in patients with insulinoma, and in particular in patients with adult nesidioblastosis.[7] Symptoms of hypoglycemia are nonspecific; thus, it is important to obtain plasma glucose measurements during symptoms to eliminate the possibility of a problem other than a hypoglycemic disorder. A normal plasma glucose concentration obtained during

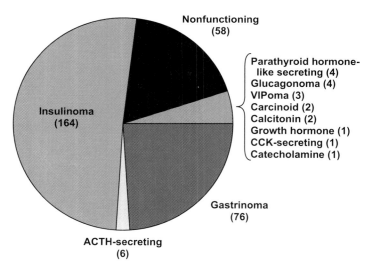

Fig. 1. Distribution of islet cell tumors in 322 patients treated at Mayo Clinic from 1960-1986. ACTH, adrenocorticotropic hormone; CCK, cholecystokinin; VIP, vasoactive intestinal polypeptide. (From van Heerden JA, Thompson GB: The surgical approach to islet cell tumors of the pancreas. In Surgery of the Pancreas. Second edition. Edited by M Trede, DC Carter. New York, Churchill Livingstone, 1997, pp 589-606. By permission of Pearson Professional.)

Table 1.—Signs and Symptoms Associated With Endogenous Hyperinsulinism

Autonomic (less specific)	Neuroglycopenic (specific)
Sweating	Confusion
Anxiety	Abnormal behavior
Trembling	Dizziness
Nausea	Difficulty speaking
Hunger	Headache
Palpitations	Weakness
Tingling sensation	Inability to concentrate

symptoms virtually rules out the possibility of an insulinoma. Symptoms of hypoglycemia associated with a plasma glucose value less than 50 mg/dL, relief of symptoms with the administration of glucose, and correction of the hypoglycemic state (Whipple's triad) prompt the need for further evaluation.

Clinical Evaluation

Localizing studies should never, or almost never, be performed to establish the diagnosis of endogenous hyperinsulinism because false-positive and false-negative imaging studies occur. The exception to this rule is discussed below in "Adult Nesidioblastosis." Hyperinsulinism should be confirmed biochemically, and factitious hypoglycemia should be excluded before localizing studies are performed because false-positive and false-negative localizing studies may lead to poor surgical outcomes. Factitious hypoglycemia most often is found in female health care workers and in persons who have relatives with diabetes. A clinical "pearl," according to F. J. Service, M.D., is that when insulinoma is suspected, the physician must be wary of the patient who travels a long distance alone for evaluation. Virtually all patients with true insulinoma recognize the need for having a companion nearby at all times.

A *supervised* 72-hour fast forms the basis for diagnosis of endogenous hyperinsulinism. The results of the fast are positive (hypoglycemia) within 12 hours in 35%, within 24 hours in 75%, within 48 hours in 92%, and at 72 hours in 99%. Insulinomas can be present when the result of a 72-hour fast is negative, but this is exceedingly rare.[6] A positive fast result (Table 2), consisting of fasting hypoglycemia (plasma glucose ≤ 45 mg/dL), concomitant hyperinsulinemia (plasma insulin ≥ 3 μIU/mL), plasma C-peptide levels measured by immunochemiluminetric (ICMA) assay of 200 or more pmol/L, and plasma proinsulin levels by ICMA of 5 or more pmol/L, confirms the endogenous (versus factitious) nature of hyperinsulinemia. For accurate diagnosis, it is critical that the patient has

neuroglycopenia at the time the fast is ended. Assays for both first- and second-generation sulfonylurea drugs must be done on plasma obtained at completion of the fast, thus ruling out a factitious cause in patients with increases in both plasma insulin and C-peptide levels. A C-peptide level of 200 pmol/L or more obviates measurement of insulin antibodies, which would rarely be positive in cases of factitious hypoglycemia because of the widespread use of recombinant human insulin preparations.[6]

Other useful measurements are the "insulin surrogates," which can be measured quickly at the end of the fast; positive results strongly suggest a hyperinsulinemic state as opposed to less common causes of hypoglycemia (e.g., glycogen storage disorders). Plasma β-hydroxybutyrate concentrations tend to be especially low in patients with insulinoma because of the antiketogenic effect of insulin (< 2.7 mmol/L). Also, the intravenous administration of 1 mg of glucagon increases the peak plasma glucose concentration by 25 mg/dL or more within 30 minutes at the end of the fast. This phenomenon is due to glucagon counteracting the glycogenic and anti-glycogenolytic effects of insulin.[6] Glycated hemoglobin levels of less than 4.1% (normal, 4.0%-7.0%) strongly support the diagnosis of insulinoma.

Occasionally, a witnessed hypoglycemic event may occur. If so, these end-of-fast laboratory studies can be done immediately; if results are confirmatory, the prolonged supervised fast can be avoided.

Localization

Once the diagnosis is confirmed, reasonable attempts at preoperative localization should be undertaken. Localization helps in planning operation, educating the patient, and relieving both surgeon and patient anxiety. Only the rare insulinoma is extrapancreatic, 90% of tumors are solitary,

Table 2.—Diagnostic Criteria for Insulinoma at Termination of a 72-Hour Fast

Factor	Concentration
Plasma glucose	≤ 45 mg/dL
Plasma insulin (ICMA)	≥ 3 μIU/mL
Plasma C-peptide (ICMA)	≥ 200 pmol/L
Plasma proinsulin (ICMA)	≥ 5 pmol/L
Plasma sulfonylureas (1st- and 2nd-generation)	Negative
β-Hydroxybutyrate	< 2.7 mmol/L
Change in glucose with 1 mg intravenous glucagon	≥ 25 mg/dL at 30 minutes

ICMA, immunochemiluminometric assay.

and nearly all are demonstrable intraoperatively by an experienced surgeon aided by real-time intraoperative ultrasonography. Eighty percent of insulinomas are less than 2 cm in diameter. Most importantly, the surgeon should recognize that, unlike past understanding of insulinomas, the tumors are equally distributed through the gland; there is no predilection to the body or tail region.

Our localizing protocol has evolved over the years and continues to evolve (Fig. 2). In a series of 119 patients treated surgically at Mayo Clinic since the introduction of intraoperative ultrasonography, only 3 failures occurred with or without preoperative localization: in only 1 patient was no tumor found, and the other 2 patients had diffuse disease associated with MEN I and adult nesidioblastosis.[7] Accordingly, preoperative localization is not mandatory when the operation is performed by an experienced surgeon and ultrasonographer. However, the three patients may have benefited by preoperative use of selective arterial calcium injection and hepatic vein sampling for insulin (modified Imamura test) (Fig. 3).[8,9] With this technique, two catheters are placed through a groin approach. The femoral venous catheter is threaded and wedged into the right hepatic vein. The femoral artery catheter is used to sequentially cannulate the splenic,

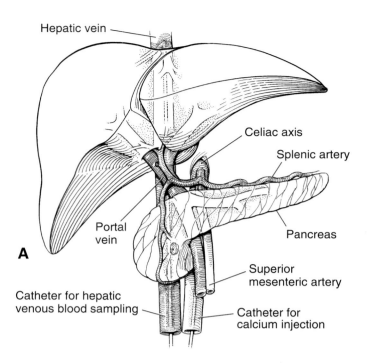

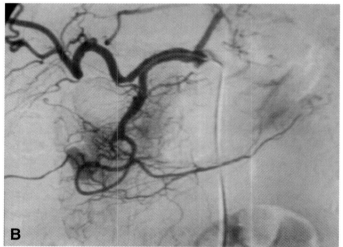

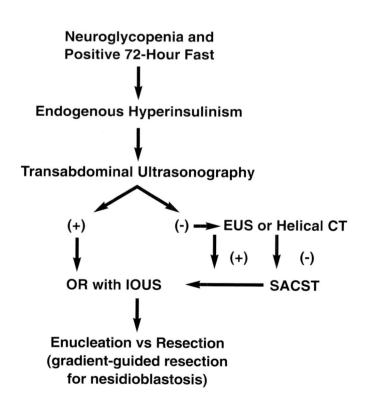

Fig. 2. Algorithm for localization and treatment of benign insulinoma. CT, computed tomography; EUS, endoscopic ultrasonography; IOUS, intraoperative ultrasonography; OR, operating room; SACST, selective arterial calcium stimulation testing.

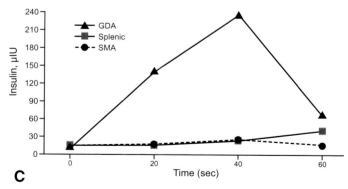

Fig. 3. Selective arterial calcium stimulation testing (A). Angiographic image (B) and venous sampling (C) data confirm presence of insulinoma in head of pancreas. GDA, gastroduodenal artery; SMA, superior mesenteric artery.

gastroduodenal, and superior mesenteric arteries that supply the various regions of the pancreas. Although there is considerable overlap, the body and tail of the pancreas are supplied predominantly from the splenic artery, the head of the gland by the gastroduodenal artery, and the uncinate process by the branches of the superior mesenteric artery. Calcium is a potent secretagogue for insulin from abnormal β cells. A step-up in any one of the arterial distributions of twofold to threefold or more within the first 90 seconds is highly accurate for regionalizing an insulinoma or abnormal β-cell function. Step-ups in multiple arterial distributions suggest nesidioblastosis or multiple adenomas, as in MEN I and adult nesidioblastosis. This information can be particularly useful in the rare patient in whom no tumor is found at operation because it allows for gradient-guided (not blind) resections. When hepatic metastases are suspected, intra-arterial calcium injection of the hepatic artery can be confirmatory. In recent reports, the sensitivity of this technique for detecting insulinomas has been as high as 94%.[10] A tumor blush is found on the angiographic phase of the selective arterial calcium injection study in 50% to 60% of patients with insulinoma.[11,12]

Our approach, therefore, continues to include transabdominal real-time ultrasonography.[12-14] By today's standards, it is noninvasive and relatively inexpensive. In experienced hands, sensitivity can be as high as 60%, which negates the need for any further studies before operation. For patients in whom transabdominal ultrasonography is negative, we perform endoscopic ultrasonography[15,16] instead of spiral computed tomography.[15,17,18] Like transabdominal ultrasonography, endoscopic ultrasonography is very much observer-dependent, but in experienced hands its sensitivity has been reported as high as 90%.[15,16] Pedunculated tumors and tumors in the tail of the pancreas remain a challenge for the endoscopic ultrasonographer, but a well-performed negative test of the head of the gland almost certainly ensures the finding of an insulinoma in the distal body or tail at surgical exploration. Endoscopic ultrasonography is not only expensive but also not totally innocuous; it is uncomfortable, requires sedation, and has a risk of perforation if there is underlying abnormality (e.g., esophageal stricture) in the upper gastrointestinal tract. Helical computed tomography (triple-phase) has imaged some insulinomas not previously seen on conventional computed tomography. Good sensitivity data are not readily available, but the sensitivity of computed tomography probably lies somewhere between that of transabdominal ultrasonography and endoscopic ultrasonography.

Somatostatin-receptor scintigraphy has been notoriously unreliable for insulinomas.[19] We will often perform selective arterial calcium injection[10] when ultrasonography and computed tomography are negative, primarily because of our increasing awareness of adult nesidioblastosis and the recognition that a positive test result aids in performing an appropriate gradient-guided resection if the tumor remains truly occult at exploration. The best sensitivities and non-Medicare charges relative to ultrasonography reported to date for various localizing studies are outlined in Table 3.

Operative Treatments
Surgical removal of insulinoma is the only curative form of treatment. Frequent meals, diazoxide, calcium channel blockers, and octreotide offer limited palliation and are not without side effects or ongoing hypoglycemic episodes.[6]

The night before operation, patients are given a 10% intravenous glucose infusion at approximately 80 mL/h. At 4 AM, use of all glucose-containing fluids is stopped, and glucose levels are determined hourly. A syringe with 50% dextrose is kept near the bedside for incremental dosing if the patient becomes symptomatic or if the plasma glucose concentration decreases to less than 60 mg/dL. The operation is the first on the operating schedule to avoid prolonged periods of hypoglycemia. Withholding glucose allows demonstration of glucose rebound in most patients after successful tumor removal. At operation, an indwelling radial arterial catheter is placed such that the patient's arms

Table 3.—Best Sensitivities for Localization of Insulinoma

Method	Sensitivity, %	Non-Medicare charges*
Selective arterial calcium stimulation	> 90	15x
Selective angiography	50-60	10x
Endoscopic ultrasonography	> 90	9x
Somatostatin receptor scintigraphy	60	9x
Helical computed tomography (triple-phase)	82†	5x
Intraoperative real-time ultrasonography	90	3x
Transabdominal ultrasonography	60	1x
Palpation and intraoperative ultrasonography	98	

*Charges relative to ultrasonography.
†Sensitivity likely ranges between that of ultrasonography and endoscopic ultrasonography. Figure cited is for dual-phase studies.

can be tucked and plasma glucose determinations can be checked frequently. Typically, a glucose rebound of 20 mg/dL or more occurs during the first 20 to 30 minutes after a successful procedure. This result, however, may be delayed for up to several hours, and false-positive results can occur. Although this rebound is reassuring, intraoperative glucose monitoring is not absolutely essential.[20]

Laparotomy is performed through a transverse epigastric or upper midline incision, depending on the patient's body habitus. After thorough exploration for metastatic disease, the gastrocolic omentum is freed from the transverse colon, entering the lesser sac. The duodenum is widely mobilized. Mobilization of the hepatic flexure of the colon is also useful for exposing the uncinate process. If necessary, lateral venous tributaries to the superior mesenteric vein can be divided for better exposure of a generous uncinate process. The right gastroepiploic vessels also should be divided to facilitate complete exposure of the head of the gland. Finally, the avascular plane along the inferior border of the pancreatic body is incised, allowing for bimanual and bidigital palpation of the body, tail, neck, uncinate process, and head of the pancreas. Insulinomas are firmer than the surrounding normal pancreas and vary from gray to tan to plum-purple. If the insulinoma is not readily apparent, the spleen should be mobilized from its lateral attachments, allowing for complete delivery of the body and tail for inspection and palpation. The superior mesenteric vein and gastroduodenal artery should be exposed. They are useful landmarks and reference points for intraoperative ultrasonography. Whether or not the tumor is readily apparent, intraoperative ultrasonography (Fig. 4) is performed to look for additional tumors or suspicious adenopathy, to assess the proximity of the insulinoma to the pancreatic and bile ducts, and to examine the liver for possible metastases. Intraoperative ultrasonography also can be used to localize and biopsy (by fine-needle aspiration) suspicious pancreatic and liver lesions.[10,14,21,22]

Enucleations can be safely performed in most instances and are the preferred operation for insulinomas located to the right of the superior mesenteric vein. Enucleations are performed with an endarterectomy spatula, fine clips, and bipolar cautery to maintain a bloodless field and to avoid major ductal disruption (Fig. 5). Enucleation sites are left open (not closed), and all sites are drained with closed-suction catheters. Pancreatoduodenectomy is rarely needed but can be done safely when necessary to avoid or treat major ductal injury; when required, a pyloric-preserving procedure is preferred. Tumors in the body, tail, and neck of the gland not amenable to enucleation or with resultant major ductal injury after enucleation can be treated with splenic-preserving distal pancreatectomy (Fig. 6) in some but not all patients.[23] The spleen can be

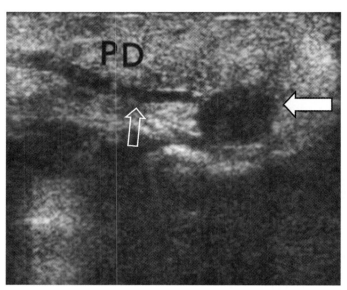

Fig. 4. *Intraoperative sonogram shows hypoechoic insulinoma in head of pancreas* (white arrow). *PD, pancreatic duct* (open arrow).

preserved in thin people by complete separation of the splenic artery and vein from the overlying pancreas. The tedious portion of the dissection is related to the venous tributaries from the body and tail of the pancreas to the splenic vein; this is particularly difficult in older, obese patients in whom the vein is almost always intrapancreatic.[24] Another option is to maintain blood flow to the spleen through the short gastric vessels by dividing the splenic artery and vein away from the splenic hilum. This maneuver usually is effective when the spleen size is normal. Large spleens will likely atrophy, failing to maintain adequate organ function long term. A potential complication associated with this approach is late splenic abscess.

Intravenous-push injection of 70 to 140 units of secretin can demonstrate major ductal disruption after

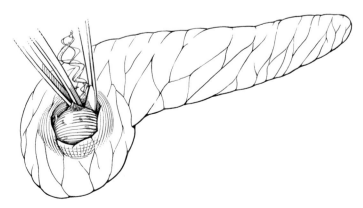

Fig. 5. *Enucleation of an insulinoma from the pancreatic head with use of an endarterectomy spatula and bipolar cautery.*

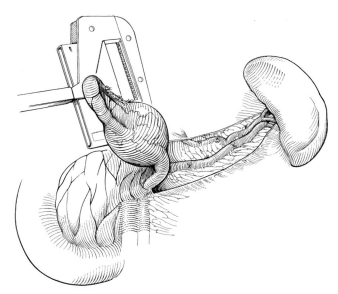

Fig. 6. Splenic-preserving distal pancreatectomy with an automatic stapling device for insulinoma in pancreatic body and tail. Note individual ligation of small venous and arterial tributaries to and from splenic vessels.

enucleation. Secretin causes the pancreatic duct to dilate, which facilitates viewing its entire course with intraoperative ultrasonography after enucleation. Major ductal injuries in the head can be treated with a tiny silicone stent, fine absorbable sutures, and external drainage or, when technically feasible, by internal drainage into a defunctionalized 45-cm Roux-en-Y limb.[23]

Laparoscopic operation for insulinoma has been successful in a handful of patients with the aid of laparoscopic ultrasonography. Five such patients have been treated in this way at Mayo Clinic. The ideal patient seems to be one with a pedunculated tumor or a tumor in the tail of the pancreas visible to the naked eye or by laparoscopic intraoperative ultrasonography. Limited mobilization and the use of automatic stapling devices facilitate such an approach. Large studies comparing complication rates with those of standard open operation remain to be published.[25-29]

If no tumor is found, blind distal resection should not be performed.[30] Insulinomas are *equally distributed throughout the gland*, and most missed islet cell tumors are ultimately found in the head or uncinate process of the gland. Reoperations after unsuccessful blind distal resections increase both the risk of subsequent or operative morbidity (fistulas, abscess, and pseudocyst formation) and the risk of development of diabetes mellitus and its attendant complications. If completion pancreatectomy becomes necessary, cure will be ensured, but premature death from the apancreatic state also can occur; thus, the treatment may be worse than the disease.[30] If good data on selective arterial calcium infusion are available, a gradient-guided

resection can be performed, particularly if the step-up occurs in the distribution of the splenic artery alone. If preoperative data suggest diffuse disease, an extended distal pancreatectomy to the right of the superior mesenteric vein should be done.

Rebound hyperglycemia is expected and may last for several days. Insulin should not be administered unless plasma glucose concentrations exceed 250 mg/dL. Few patients have development of diabetes mellitus in long-term follow-up after successful removal of an insulinoma, but it is not always clear whether this is related to the operative resection or the patient's own natural history.

Our overall operative morbidity rate for patients with insulinomas was 21%, and pancreatic complications occurred in 12%. Most of these complications (fistula, abscess, and pseudocyst) are successfully managed nonoperatively with drainage.[31]

MEN I With Hyperinsulinism

Hyperinsulinism is second in frequency to Zollinger-Ellison syndrome (ZES) in terms of functioning pancreatic islet cell syndromes in patients with MEN I. Hyperinsulinism occurs in about 20% of patients with MEN I. In about 20% of these patients, the insulin-producing tumor is solitary. However, because of the diffuse nature of the islet cell process in these patients (adenomatosis, dysplastic islets, and nesidioblastosis), helical (spiral) computed tomography is probably all that is necessary preoperatively to rule out obvious malignant tumors or metastases. Endoscopic ultrasonography can, however, provide valuable information with regard to tumors in the head and uncinate process of the gland (Fig. 7). An 80% to 85% distal subtotal pancreatectomy with enucleation of additional remnant adenomas is required to achieve long-term euglycemia in these patients.[32] Patients with concomitant hypergastrinemia need additional procedures (see "ZES in MEN I," below). Patients who have MEN I with hyperinsulinism need to be informed of the potential 20% recurrence rate over time. Currently, routine genetic testing for menin is not performed. Hyperparathyroidism and hyperprolactinemia, in general, do not pose immediate life-threatening risks to the patient. It is hoped that, in the future, specific mutations for patients at risk for the highly malignant islet cell tumors will be identified, leading to earlier intervention. Death from islet cell tumor is the most common tumor-specific cause of death in patients with MEN I.

Adult Nesidioblastosis

Although rare and found in the glands of asymptomatic patients, β cells budding from exocrine ducts (nesidioblastosis) (Fig. 8) can be a cause of endogenous hyperinsulinism in adults. Often, there are also increased numbers of

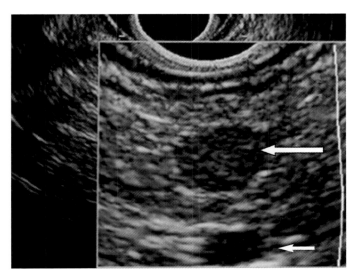

Fig. 7. Endoscopic ultrasonogram, showing otherwise occult islet cell tumor in head of pancreas (large arrow). *Portal vein* (small arrow).

dysplastic islets. The clinical picture is usually that of postprandial hypoglycemia with a negative 72-hour fast. When symptoms of neuroglycopenia are severe, selective arterial calcium stimulation testing should be performed. We have operated on 11 consecutive adult patients with this clinical scenario. With follow-up as long as 5 years, 80% of patients have benefited from gradient-guided distal pancreatectomy. These results are somewhat analogous to the results of extended distal pancreatectomy for nesidioblastosis in the pediatric age group.[7,33]

Malignant Insulinoma

Insulin-producing islet cell carcinomas account for less than 10% of all insulinomas. Prognosis depends on the stage of the disease.[34-36] Patients with hepatic metastases fare worse than those with localized disease or regional lymphadenopathy alone. Formal pancreatic resection (distal pancreatectomy or pancreatoduodenectomy) and extended regional lymphadenectomies are the procedures of choice for localized disease and in selected patients with advanced disease who have uncontrolled hormonal sequelae.[37] Solitary liver metastases should be treated with hepatic resection.[38] Multiple liver metastases can be treated with surgical debulking,[38] hepatic artery embolization, chemoembolization, systemic chemotherapy, cryotherapy, and thermal ablation techniques, providing prolonged symptomatic relief and extended survival in select patients. Thermal ablation or radiofrequency ablation often can be performed percutaneously. Diazoxide has limited usefulness because of side effects. The depot form of octreotide may provide more convenient symptom relief without the need for multiple daily injections.[39-44]

GASTRINOMA

Background

The syndrome of gastrointestinal ulceration, gastric hypersecretion, and diarrhea arising in the presence of a non-β islet cell tumor of the pancreas was first described by Zollinger and Ellison in 1955.[45] These pancreatic tumors were presumed to elaborate an acid secretagogue, initially uncharacterized, that led to the virulent peptic ulcer diathesis. Unless the target organ was removed in its entirety (total gastrectomy), patients frequently experienced gastrointestinal hemorrhage, perforation, obstruction, and recurrent marginal ulceration after seemingly adequate "peptic ulcer" operations. A lack of effective antisecretory agents coupled with the inability to readily localize the majority of gastrinomas originally mandated the need for total gastrectomy, an often life-saving operation.

With the discovery of gastrin and the development and widespread availability of radioimmunoassay in the 1970s, the diagnosis of ZES was simplified. The diagnosis requires a high level of suspicion. Recurrent ulcers (*Helicobacter pylori*-negative), multiple ulcers in ectopic locations (distal duodenum, jejunum, and esophagus), chronic diarrhea, failed ulcer operations, ulcers at a young age, prominent gastric folds or a family history of ulcers, hypercalcemia, or pituitary tumors (MEN I) raise the possibility of ZES. It should be emphasized that ZES is responsible for only 0.1% of all peptic ulcers.

Gastrinomas are the second most common islet cell tumor. However, as will be discussed, most gastrinomas are extrapancreatic and are focused within the wall of the duodenum. The estimated annual incidence of gastrinoma is 2 to 4 per 1 million population. These tumors may appear at any age, but their incidence is greatest between ages 40 and

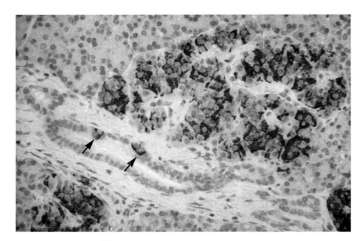

Fig. 8. Nesidioblastosis in a patient with endogenous hyperinsulinism. Note β cells (insulin immunostain-positive cells) budding off exocrine duct (arrows).

60 years. The male:female ratio is 3:2. Gastrinomas occur predominantly in the duodenum and pancreas and may appear sporadically (75%) or as part of the MEN I syndrome (25%). Sporadic tumors are typically single, although those associated with MEN I are frequently multiple. All gastrinomas are potentially malignant, and sites of metastases include peripancreatic lymph nodes, liver, and bone.

Because of the high level of suspicion, many patients who have ZES today present with rather typical peptic ulcer symptoms or chronic diarrhea alone (10%). The accompanying diarrhea or steatorrhea results from gastric hypersecretion in combination with inactivation of pancreatic enzymes by high concentrations of hydrochloric acid within the proximal duodenum. Occasional patients still present with bleeding or perforation.

Diagnosis

Classically, a patient with ZES has a serum gastrin concentration more than 500 pg/mL with a 1-hour basal acid output of more than 15 mEq/h (intact stomach) when antisecretory medication has not been given for at least 3 to 5 days. Similarly, a fasting gastric pH more than 3.0 without medication virtually rules out ZES. Caution must be exercised in withholding antisecretory medications because if active, deep ulcers are present, bleeding or perforation may ensue. Other causes of hypergastrinemia include the use of proton pump inhibitors, atrophic gastritis, renal failure, gastric outlet obstruction, antral G-cell hyperplasia, and postgastrectomy retained antrum. The secretin provocative or stimulation test is the most specific test for diagnosing ZES. Unfortunately, secretin is no longer manufactured. After a baseline serum gastrin concentration is determined, a standard secretin bolus is administered intravenously. An idiosyncratic increase in the serum gastrin concentration by more than 200 pg/mL is diagnostic in the setting of hyperchlorhydria. The secretin provocative test can be performed with the patient receiving proton pump inhibitors. This provocative test is the diagnostic procedure of choice, especially when the basal serum gastrin concentration is in the range of 200 to 500 pg/mL (Table 4). Alternative provocative tests include a test meal or calcium infusion test. Patients with ZES have an increase in fasting gastrin levels of less than 50%, whereas all others with hypergastrinemia have an increase of more than 50% (without proton pump inhibitors). An increase of more than 395 pg/mL, with calcium infusion, in serum gastrin level over pre-infusion gastrin levels is considered positive for ZES.

Cimetidine, a histamine$_2$-receptor antagonist, was first introduced in 1977 as an effective antisecretory medication for patients with ZES. Requirements for very large doses, tachyphylaxis, antiandrogenic properties, intolerance, and

noncompliance were frequent. Ranitidine and famotidine had far fewer antiandrogenic side effects, but the other issues remained. In the past decade, the new class of proton pump inhibitors (now available for intravenous use) has given physicians the ability to shut down gastric acid secretion completely, with easy dosing, no tachyphylaxis, and few side effects. Today, ulcer complications and related deaths are virtually unheard of. The need for total gastrectomy for ZES currently is a clinical rarity.

Localization and Treatment

The illusion of wellness with antisecretory medication, coupled with low surgical cure rates in the past, led many physicians to consider ZES solely a medical disorder. Actually, all gastrinomas have malignant potential, and 30% to 40% have already metastasized to lymph nodes or liver at the time of diagnosis. Although many patients, especially those with MEN I, can live for many years with this malignant process, many will die prematurely with this cancer. During the past decade, it has become apparent that the duodenum and not the pancreas is the most common site for primary gastrinomas.[46] Between 70% and 90% of tumors in patients with sporadic ZES and more than 90% of tumors in patients with MEN I are duodenal in origin. These tiny microcarcinoids are frequently less than 1 cm in size, are submucosal, and have a propensity to spread to regional lymph nodes, whereas pancreatic primary tumors often spread hematogenously to the liver.

Extraduodenal and extrapancreatic primary sites have been described in lymph nodes (controversial), jejunum, stomach, liver, biliary tree, omentum, and gonads. Some 80% to 90% of gastrinomas arise within the so-called gastrinoma triangle bounded by the duodenum, pancreatic

Table 4.—Diagnosis of Zollinger-Ellison Syndrome*

Factor	Value
Hypergastrinemia	> 500 pg/mL[†]
Hyperchlorhydria	Gastric pH < 3.0 or basal acid output > 15 mEq/h (intact stomach)
Secretin provocative test	> 200 pg/mL increase from basal serum gastrin concentration with infusion of intravenous secretin

*Studies performed only after patients have not been receiving antisecretory drugs for 3 to 5 days (not necessary for secretin provocative test).
[†]For equivocal gastrins (e.g., < 500 but > 200 pg/mL), perform secretin provocative test. If secretin is unavailable, consider a meal test.

head, and extrahepatic biliary tree. With excellent control of the ulcer diathesis and a better understanding of tumor location and spread, successful localization of gastrinomas is now common at major endocrine centers. Preoperative localization is possible in approximately two-thirds of patients (Table 5 and Fig. 9).[47,48] This observation should not deter one from surgical exploration because the tumors, especially duodenal, are often small but frequently localized to a limited anatomical region.

Helical (spiral) computed tomography may demonstrate a pancreatic primary or enlarged lymph nodes, but more importantly, this method is very good at ruling out hepatic metastases; magnetic resonance imaging is even better for detecting metastases from islet cell carcinomas. Endoscopic ultrasonography is becoming a highly sensitive method for imaging the pancreas, particularly the difficult to examine pancreatic head. Somatostatin receptor scintigraphy[47-49] is much more useful for evaluation of gastrinoma than insulinoma, probably due to differences in the subtype of somatostatin receptor expressed on the cell surface. Somatostatin receptor scintigraphy is useful and probably more accurate than computed tomography for imaging hepatic metastases and metastases at other distant sites (e.g., bone) and also may demonstrate enlarged peripancreatic lymph nodes in association with a small duodenal gastrinoma or a pancreatic primary tumor itself. The Imamura test (selective arterial secretin injection with hepatic vein sampling for gastrin) also can be helpful for regionalizing gastrinomas.

Most surgeons agree that patients with diffuse hepatic metastases are best treated with proton pump inhibitors. If more than 90% of the tumor burden in the liver can be resected safely, debulking procedures may offer prolonged palliation and perhaps survival. Chemotherapy with streptozotocin and doxorubicin, long-acting depot octreotide, angiographic chemoembolization, and selective use of cryoablation and thermoablation techniques for hepatic metastases offer patients with these slow-growing malignancies a chance at meaningful palliation and survival. For patients with stable diffuse disease confined to the liver alone, orthotopic hepatic transplantation is a consideration in selected patients. Apparent solitary metastasis should be resected, especially if no other primary tumor is found, because it may be the rare but well-described hepatic or biliary primary tumor.[50] Magnetic resonance imaging[51] is more sensitive than computed tomography for detecting metastatic hepatic disease from an islet cell primary tumor, but this method tends to be more time-consuming and is less readily available. Somatostatin receptor scintigraphy can detect tumors in 70% to 80% of patients with ZES. In patients with

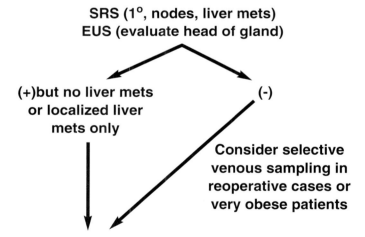

ZOLLINGER-ELLISON SYNDROMES
(↑gastrin, hyperchlorhydria
⊕ secretin stimulation test)

SRS (1°, nodes, liver mets)
EUS (evaluate head of gland)

(+)but no liver mets
or localized liver
mets only

(-)

Consider selective
venous sampling in
reoperative cases or
very obese patients

O.R. with IOUS (examine ovaries for occult 1°)

Fig. 9. Algorithm for localization and treatment of gastrinoma. Helical computed tomography is used for large primary pancreatic tumors. At operation (O.R.) with intraoperative ultrasonography (IOUS), the options are 1) duodenotomy and full-thickness excision of primary tumor and lymphadenectomy, 2) enucleation and lymphadenectomy for a small pancreatic primary tumor, 3) Whipple or distal pancreatectomy for a large pancreatic primary tumor, and 4) resection of localized liver metastases (consider cryoablation or radiofrequency ablation and cholecystectomy). EUS, endoscopic ultrasonography; mets, metastasis; SRS, somatostatin receptor scintigraphy; 1°, primary tumor.

Table 5.—Sensitivities of Tests for Localization of Gastrinoma

Test	Sensitivity, %
Helical computed tomography	?*
Somatostatin receptor scintigraphy	70-80†
Endoscopic ultrasonography	‡
Selective arterial secretin stimulation	> 90§
Intraoperative ultrasonography, palpation with exploratory duodenotomy	80-90

*Good for ruling out liver metastases and large pancreatic head primary tumors.
†Often demonstrates enlarged peripancreatic nodes—an excellent indication of a duodenal primary tumor.
‡Excellent for ruling out a pancreatic head primary tumor.
§Regionalization more so than localization. Helpful in reoperative setting.

sporadic ZES without diffuse hepatic metastases, we treat the patient with proton pump inhibitors for 2 to 3 weeks to allow time for active ulcers to heal. Often with the first dose of medication, diarrhea and pain subside.

At operation, exploration is performed with intravenous infusion of proton pump inhibitors. A thorough exploration outside the gastrinoma triangle to include the liver, omentum, stomach, and ovaries should be performed first. Regional nodes should be excised after the lesser sac is entered and the duodenum is widely mobilized. Intraoperative ultrasonography and bidigital palpation of the entire pancreas and duodenum should follow. Duodenal transillumination through a gastroscope may demonstrate a small duodenal primary tumor. All suspicious nodules should undergo biopsy or be excised. If a primary tumor is not detected, the duodenum should be opened, and an exploratory duodenotomy with excision of suspicious nodules should be performed (Fig. 9 and 10). There is no advantage for adding a highly selective vagotomy. Rapid intraoperative gastrin assays may prove useful when they become readily available. Blind resection such as with a pancreatoduodenectomy is not recommended. Selective arterial secretin injection with hepatic vein sampling for gastrin should be reserved for patients who have previously undergone operation and in whom reoperation is contemplated.

Today, gastrinomas can be located and removed in 90% of patients with sporadic ZES. Nearly 60% of patients will appear cured in the immediate postoperative period, and 30% will remain eugastrinemic, as demonstrated by basal and stimulated gastrin levels determined while patients are not taking medications long-term.[52-55] The presence of hepatic metastases portends a less favorable prognosis. Aggressive surgical treatment of sporadic ZES clearly delays or reduces the risk of development of hepatic metastases. Postoperatively, patients should have basal serum gastrin concentrations checked every 6 to 12 months or sooner, should symptoms occur. Helical computed tomography, somatostatin receptor scintigraphy, and endoscopic ultrasonography should be used selectively if serum gastrin concentrations are increasing. Selected patients with localized recurrences can be rendered eugastrinemic with reoperation.[56]

ZES in MEN I

Some 20% of patients with ZES are in MEN I kindreds, and 50% of patients with MEN I have hypergastrinemia. The pancreas in MEN I is characterized by dysplastic islet cells throughout the gland, adenomatosis, and nesidioblastosis. Duodenal microcarcinoids tend to be multifocal.[57] The nature of ZES in MEN I tends to be more indolent than its sporadic counterpart.[58] Symptoms are often well controlled with medication and subtotal parathyroidectomy. Nonetheless, the highest cause-specific mortality in patients with MEN I is from pancreaticoduodenal tumors.[59] Although cure rates are less frequent than in sporadic disease, eugastrinemia has been achieved in selected patients with MEN I.[57] Thompson

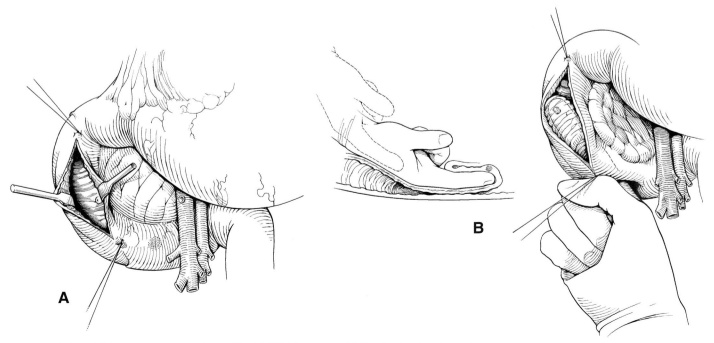

Fig. 10. (A) *and* (B), *Operation popularized by N. W. Thompson, M.D., for duodenal gastrinomas.*

(Fig. 11) advocates a distal pancreatectomy, enucleation of pancreatic head tumors, removal of duodenal primary tumors, and regional lymphadenectomy. Regional lymphadenectomy includes the nodes along the duodenum, pancreas, hepatoduodenal ligament, and arterial branches to the level of the celiac axis. Other investigators have omitted the distal pancreatectomy, and still others advocate pancreatoduodenectomy or pancreatic-sparing duodenectomies with pancreatic enucleations because duodenal tumors are the principal source of gastrin. In experienced hands, morbidity from these procedures has been acceptable. Only long-term follow-up will determine whether such procedures alter the natural history of this disease and improve quality of life.[60] If specific mutations in the MEN I gene can be found to correlate with aggressive pancreaticoduodenal disease, appropriate prophylactic operation or perhaps even gene therapy may become a possibility.[5]

GLUCAGONOMA

Glucagonomas are very rare tumors. A patient with a malignant islet cell tumor and signs and symptoms compatible with what we would now call the glucagonoma syndrome was first described in 1942.[2] McGavran et al.[61] described a similar patient in the 1960s in whom ultrastructural analysis of the causal neoplasm showed a glucagon-secreting α-cell tumor. The classic syndrome as we know it today, however, was not fully appreciated until Mallinson and colleagues[62] described nine patients with the glucagonoma syndrome (Table 6) in 1974. Glucagonomas rank far below gastrinomas and insulinomas in terms of frequency. Female patients appear to outnumber men with a frequency of 2-3:1. The mean age at diagnosis is 52 years (range, 20-73 years). Glucagonoma associated with the MEN I syndrome is rare. Unlike their gastrin- and insulin-secreting counterparts, glucagonomas tend to be large. More than 80% of glucagonomas are malignant, and more than half have evidence of metastatic disease at diagnosis. Multiplicity of primary tumors is rare, and metastases are often found, as one might expect, in the liver and regional lymph nodes. Close to 90% of these tumors are found within the body and tail of the pancreas, a distribution that coincides with the normal α-cell distribution within the gland. Glucagonomas show no specific histologic characteristics, other than those shared by other endocrine tumors. Mitotic figures and nuclear atypia are rare. Immunostaining tends to be positive for glucagon-containing granules, but these cells also may stain for other peptides, most frequently pancreatic polypeptide. Electron microscopy typically reveals

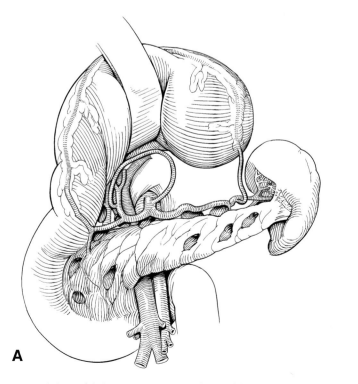
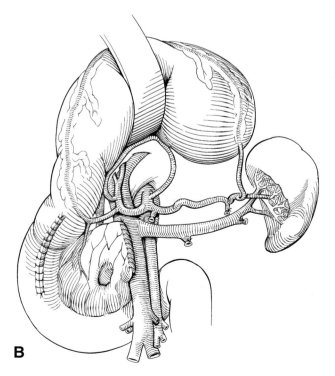

Fig. 11. (A) *and* (B), *Operation popularized by N. W. Thompson, M.D., for patients with multiple endocrine neoplasia type I and Zollinger-Ellison syndrome includes a distal pancreatectomy, enucleation of islet cell tumor in the remaining gland, exploratory duodenotomy for microcarcinoids, and lymphadenectomy.*

Table 6.—Glucagonoma Syndrome

Manifestations	Physiologic effects of glucagon
Glucose intolerance (80%)	↑ Gluconeogenesis
Necrolytic migratory erythema (67%)	↑ Glycogenolysis
Normochromic, normocytic anemia (85%)	↑ Ketogenesis
	↓ Glycolysis
Stomatitis, glossitis, vulvovaginitis	↓ Lipogenesis
Deep venous thrombosis	↑ Lipolysis
Neuropathy	Hypoaminoacidemia
Diarrhea	↓ Erythropoiesis

variable numbers of secretory granules; the cells of benign tumors are fully granulated, whereas those of malignant tumors have few such granules.

Glucagon is stored and released by the pancreas in response to hypoglycemia or stress. It is a potent stimulator of gluconeogenesis, glycogenolysis, and ketogenesis. Glucagon also inhibits glycolysis and lipogenesis. The exaggeration of these effects leads to the biochemical and clinical features of the glucagonoma syndrome.

The most common manifestation of the glucagonoma syndrome is some degree of glucose intolerance, occurring in more than 80% of patients. Because the glucose intolerance is rarely of great clinical significance, the condition often goes undiagnosed for many years until the effects of metastatic disease become apparent or until development of the pathognomonic necrotizing rash so characteristic of the glucagonoma syndrome. This necrolytic migratory erythema (Fig. 12) occurs in two-thirds of patients with glucagonoma syndrome. The association of this rash with the clinical finding of glucose intolerance strongly suggests the presence of a glucagonoma. The rash begins most

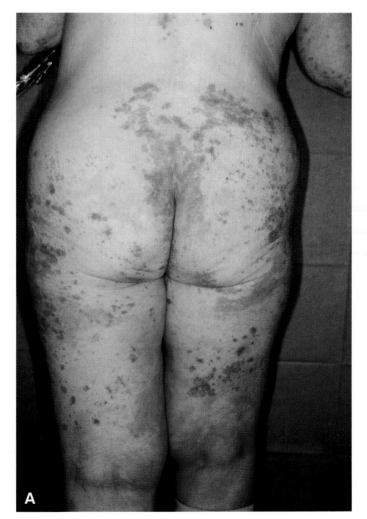
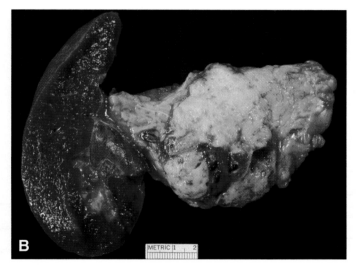
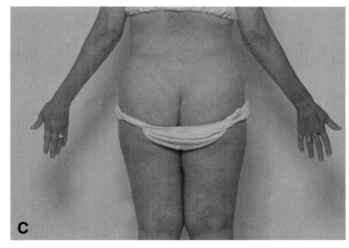

Fig. 12. Necrolytic migratory erythema (A) *in a patient with a malignant glucagonoma* (B). *Complete resolution 6 months after distal pancreatectomy* (C).

frequently in the intertriginous areas and in the skin around the mouth, vagina, and anus. Eventually it can involve the trunk, thighs, extremities, and face. The rash begins as erythematous patches that spread annularly or serpiginously to become confluent. The erythematous plaques become raised and develop central bullae that slough, leaving necrotic centers and serous crusts. Healing takes place in 2 to 3 weeks, leaving hyperpigmented sites. The process is chronic, recurrent, and migratory. The rash is attributed to the hypoaminoacidemia that results from the profound catabolic effects of glucagon. Interestingly, intravenous administration of amino acids ameliorates the dermatitis, as does octreotide, by reducing systemic glucagon levels.

A normochromic, normocytic anemia occurs in about 85% of patients with the glucagonoma syndrome and may be related to glucagon's ability to depress erythropoiesis. Stomatitis, glossitis, chronic vulvovaginitis, and neuropathy also occur with this syndrome. Weight loss can be severe and may be explained by excessive lipolysis and gluconeogenesis. Both muscle and visceral protein stores are substantially diminished. Deep venous thrombosis and thromboembolism are also common in patients with the glucagonoma syndrome. The exact cause of this hypercoagulable state is not clear, but fatal pulmonary embolism is a common cause of death. Long-term anticoagulation therapy or venous filters are commonly required to prevent such lethal events. Diarrhea occurs in a small number of patients. Glucagonomas, like many functional endocrine tumors, produce and secrete other peptides, some of which may enhance intestinal mobility.

Because most of the clinical findings in patients with the glucagonoma syndrome are nonspecific, it is not until the cutaneous manifestations appear that the diagnosis is even considered. This delay probably is responsible for the high rate of metastatic spread and attainment of large tumor size before clinical detection. Although a skin biopsy may be diagnostic, the finding of hyperglucagonemia is usually confirmatory. Normal serum glucagon concentrations range from 25 to 250 pg/mL. Although serum glucagon concentrations can be increased in patients with renal failure, cirrhosis, hepatic failure, or severe stress, the values rarely exceed 500 pg/mL. In patients with the glucagonoma syndrome, serum concentrations often exceed 1,000 pg/mL. A secretin challenge test yields a paradoxical increase in glucagon secretion in patients with the glucagonoma syndrome, but this test is rarely, if ever, necessary. Because glucagonomas are usually very large and solitary, helical computed tomography is a very accurate and sensitive method for localizing these tumors. Somatostatin receptor scintigraphy, angiography, and venous sampling can be helpful for localizing small tumors not detected by computed tomography, but these tests are rarely required.

Surgical removal of the primary tumor, before it has metastasized, offers the only chance for cure. However, for the reasons previously discussed, the surgical cure rate is low, with only 30% of patients being cured. With surgical removal, the clinical manifestations rapidly abate, unless an extensive pancreatic resection leaves the patient with persistently abnormal glucose metabolism from reduction of the β-cell mass. As with other endocrine tumors of the pancreas, small solitary tumors can sometimes be enucleated, although more often than not, given their large size and location, distal pancreatectomy or near-total pancreatectomy is required. Even if there is metastatic tumor, radical excision or debulking should be strongly considered because of the tumor's slow growth and the profoundly debilitating effects of excess glucagon secretion. Debulking may result in prolonged clinical remission.

Considerable symptom improvement also has been achieved with the use of the long-acting somatostatin analogue and depot octreotide. Other treatments, including systemic chemotherapy with streptozotocin, 5-fluorouracil, dacarbazine, doxorubicin, and chlorozotocin, given singly or in various combinations, have response rates up to 70%. Hepatic artery embolization followed by systemic chemotherapy for the treatment of functioning hepatic metastases also has been used with variable degrees of success.[63,64]

Before any operation for glucagonoma, it is important to bring patients into an optimal state of health. The preoperative use of additional parenteral nutrition, octreotide, anticoagulants, and venous filters may greatly improve the underlying catabolic state and lessen the risk of fatal perioperative embolic complications.[2]

VIPoma SYNDROME

The VIPoma syndrome (Verner-Morrison syndrome) (Table 7) is very rare. Only a few hundred patients have been reported in the literature.[2,65-67] This syndrome is characterized by the combination of watery diarrhea, hypokalemia, and achlorhydria, sometimes referred to as the WDHA syndrome. In fact, patients are rarely achlorhydric but rather hypochlorhydric, suggesting the term WDHH syndrome. Verner and Morrison first described this syndrome in 1958.[65] It was not until 1970, however, that vasoactive intestinal peptide (VIP) was first isolated from bovine intestine. VIP causes smooth muscle relaxation, stimulation of small intestinal secretion, and inhibition of gastric acid secretion. There is still significant controversy as to whether VIP acts alone or in combination with other substances to produce the clinical manifestations of this syndrome. Plasma concentrations of histidine isoleucine, a potent stimulator of small intestinal secretion, are increased in patients with the VIPoma

Table 7.—VIPoma Syndrome

Manifestations	Physiologic effects
Watery diarrhea (profuse, secretory)	Smooth muscle relaxation
Hypokalemia	Stimulation of intestinal secretion
Hypochlorhydria	Inhibition of gastric acid secretion
Metabolic acidosis	
Severe electrolyte imbalance	
Arrhythmia	
Renal failure	

syndrome. Prostaglandin E also has been suggested as the primary secretagogue in these patients.

The VIPoma syndrome typically occurs in middle-aged adults, although 10% of patients are younger than 10 years. Of the tumors, 85% are located in the pancreas, and 15% are associated with ganglioneuromas. About 75% of VIPomas are located in the body and tail of the pancreas, 50% are malignant, and more than half of these have metastasized to the liver or regional nodes at diagnosis. In contrast, 90% of the neural tumors are benign. Approximately 4% of patients with VIPoma syndrome have MEN I. The vast majority of the tumors are solitary, ranging in size from 2 to 6 cm. Islet cell hyperplasia and nesidioblastosis have been described in association with VIPoma syndrome.

VIP is distributed widely throughout the gastrointestinal tract and the nervous system. In the pancreas, VIP is found in conjunction with the nerve cells and the pancreatic D1 cells. VIP has several potential physiologic roles. It may facilitate peristalsis, stimulate pancreatic fluid and bicarbonate secretion, and inhibit solute absorption while stimulating water and ion secretion by the intestine.

The pathophysiologic effects of increased plasma concentrations of VIP and other peptides give rise to the VIPoma syndrome. The predominant symptom is a profuse secretory diarrhea; more than 70% of patients produce 3 liters or more of stool per day. Diarrhea, which is typically episodic and usually explosive, has been described as thin and tea-colored. Abdominal cramping, weakness, and hypotension result, along with severe electrolyte imbalance and metabolic acidosis. Patients are usually hypochlorhydric. Other findings less commonly present include flushing, glucose intolerance, hypophosphatemia, hypercalcemia, and nephrolithiasis. Death usually results from dehydration and severe electrolyte abnormalities, which may lead to cardiac rhythm disturbances or renal failure. The VIPoma syndrome is diagnosed by confirming the presence of secretory diarrhea. Stool cultures should be performed to rule out infectious causes, and a 48- to 72-hour fast should be instituted to rule out osmotic causes such as lactose intolerance. ZES is characterized by low gastric pH and by an ulcer diathesis, in contrast to the situation affecting patients with the VIPoma syndrome. Nasogastric suction ablates the diarrhea in ZES but has no effect on the diarrhea of VIPoma. The somatostatinoma syndrome typically yields steatorrhea, and the carcinoid syndrome is characterized by increased urinary concentrations of 5-hydroxyindoleacetic acid. The best diagnostic test, however, is measurement of the fasting serum VIP concentration; with VIPoma, mean concentrations of 1,000 pg/mL are typical. VIP secretion may be episodic, and thus repeated measurements may be necessary. Helical computed tomography is the most reliable localizing method; angiography and venous sampling are less sensitive. Endoscopic ultrasonography, intraoperative ultrasonography, and somatostatin receptor scintigraphy may play a role for small tumors but usually prove unnecessary.

The treatment of choice for VIPoma syndrome is surgical removal of the offending tumor. Small solitary tumors can be treated with enucleation or distal pancreatectomy. However, because 75% of the tumors are located in the body and tail of the pancreas, blind distal pancreatectomies can be considered with tumors too small to localize. Before adopting this approach, however, both adrenal glands and the abdominal midline should be carefully examined from the diaphragm to the bladder for ganglioneuromas. Like glucagonomas, metastatic tumors respond to near-total debulking, even if this maneuver is only palliative. Preoperative stabilization of the patient is extremely important and includes adequate hydration with correction of electrolyte and acid-base abnormalities. Prednisone may help to control the diarrhea by a poorly understood mechanism. Indomethacin, because of its inhibition of prostaglandin synthesis, also may be of benefit in decreasing stool volume. Octreotide has proved to be the most promising agent for management; in more than 70% of patients it decreases circulating VIP concentrations, decreases stool volume, and reverses many of the metabolic and electrolyte abnormalities. Chemotherapy may be of some benefit. Streptozotocin produces a 50% response rate, and when it is used in combination with 5-fluorouracil the response rate may be increased further. Intra-arterial infusion of streptozotocin also may be of some benefit. More recently, interferon alfa has been used in the management of these patients.[68]

SOMATOSTATINOMA SYNDROME[2,69,70]

Ganda and Larsson first described patients with somatostatinomas in 1977. The syndrome (Table 8) is characterized by steatorrhea, diabetes mellitus, hypochlorhydria, and cholelithiasis. Somatostatin, when first identified, was shown to inhibit growth hormone secretion (thus its name). Since then, somatostatin has been localized not only to the hypothalamus but also to many other sites, including the pancreatic D cells, stomach, duodenum, and small intestine. It is generally known to be a global inhibitor of the release of many diverse gastrointestinal regulatory peptide hormones.

Very few patients with somatostatinomas have been described. The mean age at onset is 51 years, and the sex distribution is equal. The tumors tend to be large and solitary. Two-thirds occur in the pancreas and generally are found in the pancreatic head. Other primary sites include the duodenum, ampulla of Vater, and the small bowel. Ampullary lesions are more common in von Recklinghausen's neurofibromatosis and histologically display characteristic psammoma bodies. Unfortunately, like glucagonomas, most of these tumors are malignant. Rarely, they may be associated with other familial endocrinopathies.

All of the clinical findings in the somatostatinoma syndrome can be explained on the basis of global inhibition of peptide secretion due to somatostatin excess. Diabetes mellitus is caused by suppression of insulin secretion. Steatorrhea is caused by decreased pancreatic exocrine secretion and impaired fat absorption. Gallstones are common and are probably due to the suppression of cholecystokinin secretion and perhaps to the inhibition of biliary tract motility by somatostatin. This constellation of symptoms, along with increased circulating somatostatin levels, confirms the diagnosis. Tolbutamide may be used to provoke somatostatin release in patients with equivocal findings. Because of the large size of these tumors, computed tomography

Table 8.—Somatostatinoma Syndrome

Manifestations	Physiologic effects of somatostatin
Steatorrhea	Suppression of insulin secretion
Diabetes mellitus	↓ Pancreatic exocrine secretion
Hypochlorhydria	Suppression of cholecystokinin
Cholelithiasis	↓ Biliary motility
	↓ Gastrin

and ultrasonography are sensitive imaging methods to localize the anatomical site of the tumor. The surgical management is similar to that described for glucagonomas and VIPomas. However, with the predominance of somatostatinomas in the head of the pancreas, a pyloric-preserving pancreatoduodenectomy may be necessary. Again, debulking a large primary tumor or debulking hepatic metastases may provide effective palliation of symptoms for prolonged periods. Chemotherapy has achieved variable response rates in patients with advanced disease. Obviously, this is one tumor in which octreotide is contraindicated.

ISLET CELL CARCINOMAS

Islet cell carcinoma of the pancreas, although rare, is important to recognize because of higher resectability rates and better survival than its ductal counterpart.[34-36] Between 1985 and 1993, 64 patients with islet cell carcinoma were treated at Mayo Clinic (Fig. 13): 47% had functioning tumors, and 53% had nonfunctioning tumors (i.e., their clinical presentation was not that of hormonal excess).

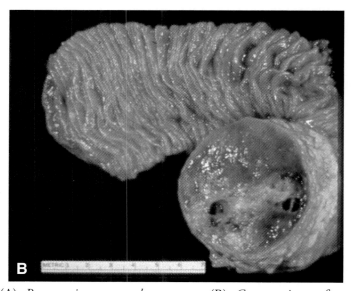

Fig. 13. Nonfunctioning islet cell carcinoma in head of pancreas. (A), *Preoperative computed tomogram.* (B), *Gross specimen after pyloric-preserving pancreatoduodenectomy.*

Gastrinoma, glucagonoma, and insulinoma were the most common functioning tumors. Potentially curative resections were performed in 26%, palliative procedures in 55%, and exploratory celiotomy alone in 19%. Symptomatic improvement was achieved with operation in 96% of patients (mean duration, 22 months). Survival rates were 66% at 3 years and 49% at 5 years. In patients undergoing curative resection, the disease-free survival rate at 3 years was 53%. The presence of diffuse hepatic metastases was a predictor of poor survival at 3 years, and there was no statistically significant difference in survival between functioning and nonfunctioning groups. Although curative resection for islet cell carcinomas is rare, meaningful palliation can be achieved in many patients with acceptable morbidity and rare perioperative mortality.[71] Liver transplantation has been successful in selected patients with diffuse hepatic metastases after surgical control of extrahepatic disease.[72]

THE MEN I PANCREAS

Much has already been said regarding the MEN I pancreas (Fig. 14), particularly with regard to patients with hyperinsulinism and hypergastrinemia. The question often arises, though, how best to follow patients with MEN I for the development of potentially malignant islet

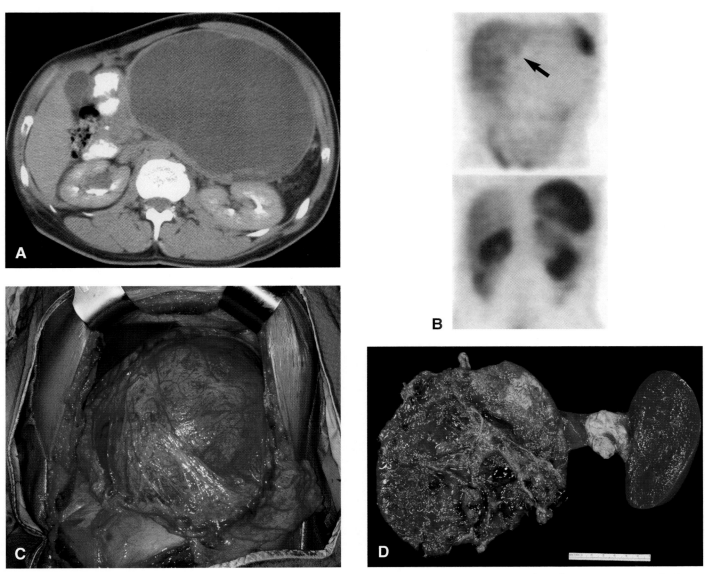

Fig. 14. Patient with multiple endocrine neoplasia type I and mild hypoglycemia. (A), Massive cystic islet cell tumor, pancreatic body, on helical computed tomography. (B), Somatostatin receptor scintigraphy faintly shows tumor (upper, arrow) and shows additional islet cell tumor (lower) not seen on computed tomography. (C), Intraoperative view of 25-cm islet cell tumor (note omental varices from compression of splenic vein). (D), Gross specimen showing additional islet cell tumors in pancreatic tail.

cell tumors (Fig. 15). Family history is certainly important, and if the family history suggests aggressive islet cell tumors, screening should be thorough and more frequent. In patients with MEN I, islet cell tumors develop in nearly 70%, and 50% will have evidence of hypergastrinemia. Although the tumors tend to be more indolent in MEN I than in sporadic cases, death from islet cell tumor is the most common disease-specific cause of death in patients with MEN I, and metastases do not necessarily correlate with tumor size. Surveillance should include endoscopic ultrasonography, somatostatin receptor scintigraphy (for non-insulinoma islet cell tumors), and serial measurements of plasma gastrin and human pancreatic polypeptide levels.[73] Other hormones should be screened for when clinically indicated. It has been suggested that very high concentrations of pancreatic polypeptide are associated with radiographically visible tumors and that hypergastrinemia is a clue to the presence of multiple duodenal microcarcinoids. Endoscopic ultrasonography and somatostatin receptor scintigraphy are the best methods for staging pancreatic disease and for surveillance. Positron emission tomography is probably less sensitive than somatostatin receptor scintigraphy because of the slow growth associated with islet cell tumors. Once disease is apparent, we recommend surgical exploration with the operations described for the MEN I pancreas for hyperinsulinism and hypergastrinemia. In the absence of hypergastrinemia, it is probably not necessary to perform routine exploratory duodenotomy. Surveillance for duodenopancreatic tumors should begin during the early teens.

In a recent report from Marburg, Germany,[59] an aggressive surgical approach appeared justified for pancreaticoduodenal tumors in patients with MEN I because symptom-free long-term survival could be demonstrated. In a genetic analysis in the same report, MEN I gene mutations in exons 3-8 seem to be associated with milder behavior, as opposed to those truncating mutations in exons 2, 9, and 10. These findings may have more important implications as screening programs become available.[74] Once genetic testing becomes routine, initial genetic counseling will be imperative.

VERY RARE ISLET CELL TUMORS

Other tumors have been described with production of parathyroid hormone-related peptides, adrenocorticotropic hormone, corticotropin-releasing factor, serotonin, cholecystokinin, neurotensin, gastrointestinal inhibitory peptide, growth hormone-releasing hormone, and melanocyte-stimulating hormone. Pure pancreatic polypeptide tumors have been described with a high malignant potential. These should be treated with surgical resection when technically

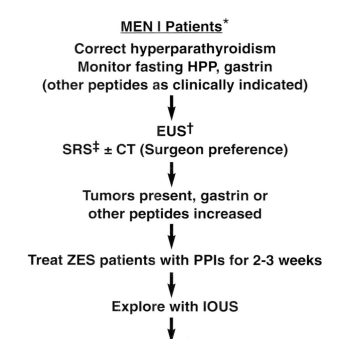

MEN I Patients*
Correct hyperparathyroidism
Monitor fasting HPP, gastrin
(other peptides as clinically indicated)

↓

EUS†
SRS‡ ± CT (Surgeon preference)

↓

**Tumors present, gastrin or
other peptides increased**

↓

Treat ZES patients with PPIs for 2-3 weeks

↓

Explore with IOUS

↓

    A. Consider Ann Arbor operation
or   **(duodenotomy for ZES patients)**
    B. Whipple procedure (+) distal enucleations
or   **(malignant periampullary tumors)**
    C. Pancreas-sparing duodenectomy (for ZES)
    plus enucleations
    D. Extended distal pancreatectomy for
    hyperinsulinism

*Fig. 15. Algorithm for evaluation and management of multiple endocrine neoplasia type I (MEN I) pancreas. CT, computed tomography; HPP, human pancreatic polypeptide; IOUS, intraoperative ultrasonography; PPI, proton pump inhibitors; ZES, Zollinger-Ellison syndrome. *Begin surveillance between 15 and 20 years of age in asymptomatic patients. †Endoscopic ultrasonography, primarily to examine the head and uncinate process. ‡Somatostatin receptor scintigraphy, to look for locoregional and distant metastases.*

feasible. The management of symptomatic hepatic metastases is similar to that for other advanced neuroendocrine tumors. More often, pancreatic polypeptide serves as a marker for other functional endocrine tumors and is often cosecreted with the principal hormone. Adrenocorticotropic hormone-secreting tumors can be a cause of Cushing's syndrome (ectopic syndrome) and are usually widely metastatic at diagnosis. Treatment, therefore, has focused on end-organ ablation, namely, bilateral adrenalectomy (laparoscopic or open). Islet cell tumors also have been associated with von Hippel-Lindau disease and should be considered when solid or partially cystic pancreatic tumors are noted in family members. Treatment is similar to that for other islet cell tumors with an emphasis on organ preservation.[2]

REFERENCES

1. Wilder RM, Allan FN, Power MH, Robertson HE: Carcinoma of the islands of the pancreas: hyperinsulinism and hypoglycemia. JAMA 89:348-355, 1927

2. van Heerden JA, Thompson GB: Islet cell tumors of the pancreas. *In* Surgery of the Pancreas. Edited by M Trede, DC Carter. Edinburgh, Churchill Livingstone, 1993, pp 545-561

3. Larsson C, Skogseid B, Oberg K, Nakamura Y, Nordenskjold M: Multiple endocrine neoplasia type 1 gene maps to chromosome 11 and is lost in insulinoma. Nature 332:85-87, 1988

4. Chandrasekharappa SC, Guru SC, Manickam P, Olufemi SE, Collins FS, Emmert-Buck MR, Debelenko LV, Zhuang Z, Lubensky IA, Liotta LA, Crabtree JS, Wang Y, Roe BA, Weisemann J, Boguski MS, Agarwal SK, Kester MB, Kim YS, Heppner C, Dong Q, Spiegel AM, Burns AL, Marx SJ: Positional cloning of the gene for multiple endocrine neoplasia-type 1. Science 276:404-407, 1997

5. Bartsch D, Kopp I, Bergenfelz A, Rieder H, Munch K, Jager K, Deiss Y, Schudy A, Barth P, Arnold R, Rothmund M, Simon B: MEN1 gene mutations in 12 MEN1 families and their associated tumors. Eur J Endocrinol 139:416-420, 1998

6. Service FJ: Hypoglycemic disorders. N Engl J Med 332:1144-1152, 1995

7. Service FJ, Natt N, Thompson GB, Grant CS, van Heerden JA, Andrews JC, Lorenz E, Terzic A, Lloyd RV: Noninsulinoma pancreatogenous hypoglycemia: a novel syndrome of hyperinsulinemic hypoglycemia in adults independent of mutations in Kir6.2 and SUR1 genes. J Clin Endocrinol Metab 84:1582-1589, 1999

8. Aoki T, Sakon M, Ohzato H, Kishimoto S, Oshima S, Yamada T, Higaki N, Nakamori S, Gotoh M, Ishikawa O, Ohigashi H, Imaoka S, Hasuike Y, Shibata K, Monden M: Evaluation of preoperative and intraoperative arterial stimulation and venous sampling for diagnosis and surgical resection of insulinoma. Surgery 126:968-973, 1999

9. Doppman JL: Preoperative diagnosis of a small endocrine tumor of the pancreas. AJR Am J Roentgenol 168:1376-1377, 1997

10. Brown CK, Bartlett DL, Doppman JL, Gorden P, Libutti SK, Fraker DL, Shawker TH, Skarulis MC, Alexander HR: Intra-arterial calcium stimulation and intraoperative ultrasonography in the localization and resection of insulinomas. Surgery 122:1189-1193, 1997

11. Boukhman MP, Karam JM, Shaver J, Siperstein AE, DeLorimier AA, Clark OH: Localization of insulinomas. Arch Surg 134:818-822, 1999

12. Galiber AK, Reading CC, Charboneau JW, Sheedy PF II, James EM, Gorman B, Grant CS, van Heerden JA, Telander RL: Localization of pancreatic insulinoma: comparison of pre- and intraoperative US with CT and angiography. Radiology 166:405-408, 1988

13. Gorman B, Charboneau JW: Sonographic detection on insulinoma. Endocrinologist 2:29-32, 1992

14. Gorman B, Charboneau JW, James EM, Reading CC, Grant CS, Van Heerden JA, Telander RL, Service FJ: Benign pancreatic insulinoma: preoperative and intraoperative sonographic localization. AJR Am J Roentgenol 147:929-934, 1987

15. Muller MF, Meyenberger C, Bertschinger P, Schaer R, Marincek B: Pancreatic tumors: evaluation with endoscopic US, CT, and MR imaging. Radiology 190:745-751, 1994

16. Thompson GB (Guest reviewer): Endocrine surgery: localization of pancreatic neuroendocrine tumors. Curr Surg 50:41-46, 1993

17. King CM, Reznek RH, Bomanji J, Ur E, Britton KE, Grossman AB, Besser GM: Imaging neuroendocrine tumours with radio-labelled somatostatin analogues and X-ray computed tomography: a comparative study. Clin Radiol 48:386-391, 1993

18. Rossi P, Baert A, Passariello R, Simonetti G, Pavone P, Tempesta P: CT of functioning tumors of the pancreas. AJR Am J Roentgenol 144:57-60, 1985

19. Meko JB, Doherty GM, Siegel BA, Norton JA: Evaluation of somatostatin-receptor scintigraphy for detecting neuroendocrine tumors. Surgery 120:975-983, 1996

20. Tutt GO Jr, Edis AJ, Service FJ, van Heerden JA: Plasma glucose monitoring during operation for insulinoma: a critical reappraisal. Surgery 88:351-356, 1980

21. Grant CS, Norton JA, Thompson NW: Insulinoma and gastrinoma. Expert opinions regarding diagnosis, localization, and surgical management. *In* Hepatobiliary and Pancreatic Tumours. Edited by G Serio, C Huguet, RCN Williamson. Edinburgh, Graffham Press, 1994, p 37

22. Grant CS, van Heerden J, Charboneau JW, James EM, Reading CC: Insulinoma: the value of intraoperative ultrasonography. Arch Surg 123:843-848, 1988

23. Thompson GB: Insulinoma. *In* Endocrine Surgery. Edited by RA Prinz, ED Staren. Georgetown, Landes Bioscience, 2000, pp 222-228

24. Kimura W, Inoue T, Futakawa N, Shinkai H, Han I, Muto T: Spleen-preserving distal pancreatectomy with conservation of the splenic artery and vein. Surgery 120:885-890, 1996

25. Collins R, Schlinkert RT, Roust L: Laparoscopic resection of an insulinoma. J Laparoendosc Adv Surg Tech A 9:429-431, 1999

26. Cuschieri SA, Jakimowicz JJ: Laparoscopic pancreatic resections. Semin Laparosc Surg 5:168-179, 1998

27. Dexter SP, Martin IG, Leindler L, Fowler R, McMahon MJ: Laparoscopic enucleation of a solitary pancreatic insulinoma. Surg Endosc 13:406-408, 1999

28. Vezakis A, Davides D, Larvin M, McMahon MJ: Laparoscopic surgery combined with preservation of the spleen for distal pancreatic tumors. Surg Endosc 13:26-29, 1999

29. Gagner M, Pomp A, Herrera MF: Early experience with laparoscopic resections of islet cell tumors. Surgery 120:1051-1054, 1996

30. Thompson GB, Service FJ, van Heerden JA, Carney JA, Charboneau JW, O'Brien PC, Grant CS: Reoperative insulinomas, 1927 to 1992: an institutional experience. Surgery 114:1196-1204, 1993

31. Grant CS: Surgical aspects of hyperinsulinemic hypoglycemia. Endocrinol Metab Clin North Am 28:533-554, 1999

32. O'Riordain DS, O'Brien T, van Heerden JA, Service FJ, Grant CS: Surgical management of insulinoma associated with multiple endocrine neoplasia type I. World J Surg 18:488-493, 1994

33. Thompson GB, Service FJ, Andrews JC, Lloyd RV, Natt N, van Heerden JA, Grant CS: Noninsulinoma pancreatogenous hypoglycemia syndrome: an update in 10 surgically treated patients. Surgery 128:937-944, 2000

34. Grant CS: Surgical management of malignant islet cell tumors. World J Surg 17:498-503, 1993

35. Thompson GB, van Heerden JA, Grant CS, Carney JA, Ilstrup DM: Islet cell carcinomas of the pancreas: a twenty-year experience. Surgery 104:1011-1017, 1988

36. Lo CY, van Heerden JA, Thompson GB, Grant CS, Soreide JA, Harmsen WS: Islet cell carcinoma of the pancreas. World J Surg 20:878-883, 1996

37. Phan GQ, Yeo CJ, Hruban RH, Lillemoe KD, Pitt HA, Cameron JL: Surgical experience with pancreatic and peripancreatic neuroendocrine tumors: review of 125 patients. J Gastrointest Surg 2:472-482, 1998

38. Que FG, Nagorney DM, Batts KP, Linz LJ, Kvols LK: Hepatic resection for metastatic neuroendocrine carcinomas. Am J Surg 169:36-42, 1995

39. Bilchik AJ, Sarantou T, Foshag LJ, Giuliano AE, Ramming KP: Cryosurgical palliation of metastatic neuroendocrine tumors resistant to conventional therapy. Surgery 122:1040-1047, 1997

40. Huang YH, Lee CH, Wu JC, Wang YJ, Chang FY, Lee SD: Functional pancreatic islet cell tumors with liver metastasis: the role of cytoreductive surgery and transcatheter arterial chemoembolization: a report of five cases. Zhonghua Yi Xue Za Zhi (Taipei) 61:748-754, 1998

41. Moertel CG, Lavin PT, Hahn RG: Phase II trial of doxorubicin therapy for advanced islet cell carcinoma. Cancer Treat Rep 66:1567-1569, 1982

42. Moertel CG, Lefkopoulo M, Lipsitz S, Hahn RG, Klaassen D: Streptozocin-doxorubicin, streptozocin-fluorouracil or chlorozotocin in the treatment of advanced islet-cell carcinoma. N Engl J Med 326:519-523, 1992

43. Siperstein AE, Rogers SJ, Hansen PD, Gitomirsky A: Laparoscopic thermal ablation of hepatic neuroendocrine tumor metastases. Surgery 122:1147-1154, 1997

44. Wymenga AN, Eriksson B, Salmela PI, Jacobsen MB, Van Cutsem EJ, Fiasse RH, Valimaki MJ, Renstrup J, de Vries EG, Obert KE: Efficacy and safety of prolonged-release lanreotide in patients with gastrointestinal neuroendocrine tumors and hormone-related symptoms. J Clin Oncol 17:1111, 1999

45. Zollinger RM, Ellison EH: Primary peptic ulcerations of the jejunum associated with islet cell tumors of the pancreas. Ann Surg 142:709-723, 1955

46. Thompson NW, Vinik AI, Eckhauser FE: Microgastrinomas of the duodenum: a cause of failed operations for the Zollinger-Ellison syndrome. Ann Surg 209:396-404, 1989

47. Alexander HR, Fraker DL, Norton JA, Bartlett DL, Tio L, Benjamin SB, Doppman JL, Goebel SU, Serrano J, Gibril F, Jensen RT: Prospective study of somatostatin receptor scintigraphy and its effect on operative outcome in patients with Zollinger-Ellison syndrome. Ann Surg 228:228-238, 1998

48. Ruszniewski P, Amouyal P, Amouyal G, Grange JD, Mignon M, Bouche O, Bernades P: Localization of gastrinomas by endoscopic ultrasonography in patients with Zollinger-Ellison syndrome. Surgery 117:629-635, 1995

49. Scott BA, Gatenby RA: Imaging advances in the diagnosis of endocrine neoplasia. Curr Opin Oncol 10:37-42, 1998

50. Norton JA, Doherty GM, Fraker DL, Alexander HR, Doppman JL, Venzon DJ, Gibril F, Jensen RT: Surgical treatment of localized gastrinoma within the liver: a prospective study. Surgery 124:1145-1152, 1998

51. Kelekis NL, Semelka RC: MRI of pancreatic tumors. Eur Radiol 7:875-886, 1997

52. Alexander HR, Bartlett DL, Venzon DJ, Libutti SK, Doppman JL, Fraker DL, Norton JA, Gibril F, Jensen RT: Analysis of factors associated with long-term (five or more years) cure in patients undergoing operation for Zollinger-Ellison syndrome. Surgery 124:1160-1166, 1998

53. Norton JA, Doppman JL, Jensen RT: Curative resection in Zollinger-Ellison syndrome: results of a 10-year prospective study. Ann Surg 215:8-18, 1992

54. Norton JA, Fraker DL, Alexander HR, Venzon DJ, Doppman JL, Serrano J, Goebel SU, Peghini PL, Roy PK, Gibril F, Jensen RT: Surgery to cure the Zollinger-Ellison syndrome. N Engl J Med 341:635-644, 1999

55. Farley DR, van Heerden JA, Grant CS, Thompson GB: Extrapancreatic gastrinomas: surgical experience. Arch Surg 129:506-511, 1994

56. Jaskowiak NT, Fraker DL, Alexander HR, Norton JA, Doppman JL, Jensen RT: Is reoperation for gastrinoma excision indicated in Zollinger-Ellison syndrome? Surgery 120:1055-1062, 1996

57. Thompson NW: Current concepts in the surgical management of multiple endocrine neoplasia type 1 pancreatic-duodenal disease: results in the treatment of 40 patients with Zollinger-Ellison syndrome, hypoglycaemia or both. J Intern Med 243:495-500, 1998

58. van Heerden JA, Thompson GB: The Zollinger-Ellison syndrome in patients with multiple endocrine neoplasia type I (MEN-I). Probl Gen Surg 7:550-563, 1990

59. Bartsch DK, Langer P, Wild A, Schilling T, Celik I, Rothmund M, Nies C: Pancreaticoduodenal endocrine tumors in multiple endocrine neoplasia type 1: Surgery or surveillance? Surgery 128:958-966, 2000

60. MacFarlane MP, Fraker DL, Alexander HR, Norton JA, Lubensky I, Jensen RT: Prospective study of surgical resection of duodenal and pancreatic gastrinomas in multiple endocrine neoplasia type 1. Surgery 118:973-979, 1995

61. McGavran MH, Unger RH, Recant L, Polk HC, Kilo C, Levin ME: A glucagon-secreting alpha-cell carcinoma of the pancreas. N Engl J Med 274:1408-1413, 1966

62. Mallinson CN, Bloom SR, Warin AP, Salmon PR, Cox B: A glucagonoma syndrome. Lancet 2:1-5, 1974

63. Kvols LK, Buck M: Chemotherapy of metastatic carcinoid and islet cell tumors: a review. Am J Med 82:77-83, 1987

64. Kvols LK, Buck M, Moertel CG, Schutt AJ, Rubin J, O'Connell MJ, Hahn RG: Treatment of metastatic islet cell carcinoma with a somatostatin analogue (SMS 201-995). Ann Intern Med 107:162-168, 1987

65. Verner JV, Morrison AB: Islet cell tumor and a syndrome of refractory watery diarrhea and hypokalemia. Am J Med 25:374-380, 1958

66. Soga J, Yakuwa Y: VIPoma/diarrheogenic syndrome: a statistical evaluation of 241 reported cases. J Exp Clin Cancer Res 17:389-400, 1998

67. Hengst K, Nashan B, Avenhaus W, Ullerich H, Schlitt HJ, Flemming P, Pichlmayr R, Domschke W: Metastatic pancreatic VIPoma: deteriorating clinical course and successful treatment by liver transplantation. Z Gastroenterol 36:239-245, 1998

68. Oberg K, Norheim I, Lind E, Alm G, Lundqvist G, Wide L, Jonsdottir B, Magnusson A, Wilander E: Treatment of malignant carcinoid tumors with human leukocyte interferon: long-term results. Cancer Treat Rep 70:1297-1304, 1986

69. Larsson LI, Hirsch MA, Holst JJ, Ingemansson S, Kuhl C, Jensen SL, Lundqvist G, Rehfeld JF, Schwartz TW: Pancreatic somatostatinoma: clinical features and physiological implications. Lancet 1:666-668, 1977

70. Soga J, Yakuwa Y: Somatostatinoma/inhibitory syndrome: a statistical evaluation of 173 reported cases as compared to other pancreatic endocrinomas. J Exp Clin Cancer Res 18:13-22, 1999

71. Phan GQ, Yeo CJ, Cameron JL, Maher MM, Hruban RH, Udelsman R: Pancreaticoduodenectomy for selected periampullary neuroendocrine tumors: fifty patients. Surgery 122:989-996, 1997

72. Dousset B, Houssin D, Soubrane O, Boillot O, Baudin F, Chapuis Y: Metastatic endocrine tumors: Is there a place for liver transplantation? Liver Transpl Surg 1:111-117, 1995

73. Mutch MG, Frisella MM, De Benedetti MK, Doherty GM, Norton JA, Wells SA Jr, Lairmore TC: Pancreatic polypeptide is a useful plasma marker for radiographically evident pancreatic islet cell tumors in patients with multiple endocrine neoplasia type 1. Surgery 122:1012-1019, 1997

74. Wang EH, Ebrahimi SA, Wu AY, Kashefi C, Passaro E Jr, Sawicki MP: Mutation of the MENIN gene in sporadic pancreatic endocrine tumors. Cancer Res 58:4417-4420, 1998

ACUTE AND CHRONIC PANCREATITIS

Nicholas J. Zyromski, M.D.
Michael L. Kendrick, M.D.
Michael G. Sarr, M.D.

Although the pancreas is (at least in the authors' opinions) the most interesting and fascinating organ of the gastrointestinal tract, it also is an unforgiving opponent when injured by acute or chronic inflammation. Most gastrointestinal surgeons regale "war stories" related to their experiences (usually abundant) with the injured pancreas. This chapter emphasizes operative intervention in the management of both acute and chronic pancreatitis. However, the prudent gastrointestinal physician or surgeon frequently benefits the patient most with a conservative, nonoperative approach.

ACUTE PANCREATITIS

Acute pancreatitis is an acute inflammatory process of the pancreatic parenchyma with variable involvement of regional tissues or remote organ systems. Acute pancreatitis spans a broad clinical spectrum from a mild, self-limiting condition to a rapidly fatal, overwhelming local and systemic process with sepsis and multisystem organ failure. Acute pancreatitis is classified clinically as mild (associated with minimal or no organ dysfunction and an uneventful recovery), moderate (involving a less rapidly resolving local and systemic illness with concurrent, but limited organ dysfunction), or severe (associated with local complications, such as pancreatic or peripancreatic necrosis, infection or abscess, and systemic toxicity), manifesting as multiple organ dysfunction or failure and the sepsis syndrome either with or without bacterial or (recently) fungal infection.

Etiopathogenesis of Acute Pancreatitis

Etiology

Alcohol and gallstone disease are implicated as the causal factors in up to 85% of patients with acute pancreatitis (Table 1). The most common cause varies with the geographic locale—if in the inner city, then alcohol; if rural, then gallstones. Endoscopic retrograde cholangiopancreatography (ERCP) has become an increasingly important causal factor in acute pancreatitis, especially in communities with aggressive endoscopists, occurring in up to 5% of patients undergoing ERCP, especially when any intervention, such as endoscopic sphincterotomy or placement of stents, accompanies the ERCP.[1] Other, less common factors include hyperlipidemia, trauma, ischemia,[2,3] and pancreas divisum. Despite growing insight into this disease, the cause remains idiopathic in 5% to 10% of patients. An impressive list of medications is associated with acute pancreatitis, but few, such as antiretroviral (human immunodeficiency virus) medications and azathioprine, have solid clinical evidence of cause and effect.[4] Hereditary pancreatitis[5] is a rare autosomal dominant condition in which two now well-characterized molecular mutations in the trypsinogen gene result in failure of the normal protective inactivation of prematurely activated cationic trypsin within acinar cells.

Pathogenesis

The current thinking is that, virtually irrespective of the cause, acute pancreatitis results from a primary cell death

Table 1.—Causes of Acute Pancreatitis

Common	Unusual
Alcohol	Hereditary pancreatitis
Gallstone (choledocholithiasis)	Hyperlipidemia
ERCP and endoscopic	Viral infection
sphincterotomy	Medications*
Idiopathic	Ischemia
	Periampullary diverticula
	Sphincter of Oddi dysfunction
	? Pancreas divisum
	Postoperative
	Jamaican scorpion bite

ERCP, endoscopic retrograde cholangiopancreatography.

*Most commonly, azathioprine, antiretroviral (human immunodeficiency virus) drugs, birth control pills (by inducing hyperlipidemia), and valproic acid, but not corticosteroids.

of the acinar cell. Acute pancreatitis thus appears to be initiated by a final common pathway or closely interrelated pathways involving a primary inhibition of exocrine enzyme secretion from the acinar cell (or, less commonly, a primary intracellular activation of trypsin from its inactive precursor trypsinogen, such as hereditary pancreatitis). This disruption of stimulus-receptor coupling leads to buildup of zymogen granules (intracellular organelles that store the digestive enzymes synthesized by the acinar cell), which appear to fuse intracellularly with lysosomes. Because lysosomes contain acid hydrolases, they have the ability to activate the intracellular proteases synthesized as inactive *pro*enzyme precursors, such as trypsinogen, which are normally activated only extracellularly in the duodenum by the mucosally derived enzyme enterokinase. This theory of "colocalization," while still controversial as to the cellular origin of the signal(s) leading to the intracellular activation of proenzymes, nevertheless appears to explain several of the different experimental models of mild to severe acute pancreatitis in animals and also in humans. Thus, the older, classic proposed pathogenetic explanations involving reflux of bile into the pancreatic duct, activation of the digestive enzymes in the pancreatic duct or in the parenchyma, or primary "rupture" of the pancreatic duct with intraparenchymal "extravasation" of pancreatic juice are now thought of as "ancient history." The current thinking is that acute pancreatitis, regardless of cause, occurs through a primary acinar cell injury with premature intracellular activation of digestive enzymes. Liberation of these activated enzymes (such as proteases, lipases, amylases, phosphatases, elastases) into the parenchyma then results in "autodigestion" of the pancreas and surrounding tissues.

Diagnosis of Acute Pancreatitis

Clinical Presentation

A thorough history and physical examination are often sufficient to suspect the diagnosis of acute pancreatitis in most patients, but the diagnosis still remains one of exclusion. In the setting of a recent binge of drinking (the patient often presents on a Sunday or Monday morning) or in a known alcoholic with a history of acute pancreatitis, acute pancreatitis is a likely explanation. A clinical pearl is that the first episode of acute alcoholic pancreatitis almost never occurs after the age of 30 years; patients susceptible to alcohol-induced acute pancreatitis commonly are affected early in the course of their alcohol abuse, usually in their late teens or early 20s. Similarly, in someone older than 50 years who presents with acute onset of epigastric pain without any known predisposing factor and in whom an ulcer is excluded, acute pancreatitis is most likely to be of biliary and not alcohol origin.

Textbooks frequently describe pathognomonic findings such as Grey Turner sign (ecchymosis in the flanks) and Cullen sign (periumbilical ecchymosis). One of the authors (M.G.S.) has spent 11 clinical years in a busy inner-city hospital with a very high admission rate of acute pancreatitis and 17 years at Mayo Clinic in Rochester, Minnesota, and has seen this too-often-referred-to spectrum of cutaneous coagulopathy only once. More commonly, when a patient presents with acute (crescendo) onset of epigastric pain with no other obvious cause (after excluding an intra-abdominal catastrophe—see below), and an increased serum amylase (or lipase) value, acute pancreatitis should be considered.

As stated above, acute pancreatitis must remain, however, a diagnosis of exclusion. Other abdominal catastrophes can present as acute epigastric pain: perforated gastric or duodenal ulcers, acute intestinal infarction, perforated diverticulitis, closed loop intestinal obstruction or infarction, and others. Usually, however, the onset of pain with acute pancreatitis is a bit more gradual (crescendo) than in the other conditions and often there are prodromal symptoms. Nevertheless, these other possibilities must be at least entertained and ruled out, at a minimum, with abdominal radiography with the intent of looking for free air. Other investigations (computed tomography, ultrasonography, or even visceral angiography) may be warranted. On occasion, despite the strong suspicion of acute pancreatitis, even the wary clinician-surgeon will make the objective diagnosis only at the time of exploratory celiotomy because of the inability to exclude a life-threatening abdominal catastrophe.

Laboratory Investigations

Increased serum amylase and lipase values are common findings (90%-95% sensitive) early in acute pancreatitis but lend no information about prognosis or severity; thus, they are of limited benefit beyond their initial use in diagnosis given their rapid return to normal. An increased serum amylase or lipase value is by no means pathognomonic of acute pancreatitis but does clearly support its clinical diagnosis. The serum lipase value is reported to be more sensitive and specific than the amylase value, but our experience at Mayo Clinic does not support this relationship. We have found that an increased serum lipase value is much less specific, and thus we strongly favor serum amylase measurements to help support the diagnosis of acute pancreatitis. A serum amylase level more than 1,000 U/L (normal in our laboratory, < 115 U/L) occurs in 90% of patients with biliary pancreatitis and may help differentiate biliary from alcohol-induced pancreatitis. However, beware of the chronic alcoholic with recurrent "acute" pancreatitis in whom the serum amylase value may be only mildly increased or even normal. The most reliable predictor of a biliary origin for acute pancreatitis is an alanine transaminase level 150 IU/L or more (normal, < 18 IU/L), which has a positive predictive value of 95%.

Serum trypsinogen, phospholipase A_2, and the activation peptides (trypsinogen activation peptide and carboxypeptidase activation peptide) seem to correlate with the severity of acute pancreatitis and may help in recognition of the presence of necrotizing pancreatitis. However, clinically useful assays are not readily available currently, and they are of little use in diagnosis.

Imaging
Abdominal radiographic findings, although imperative in the evaluation, are nonspecific in acute pancreatitis; but, as stated above, they may assist in excluding diagnoses with similar presentations. Abnormal intestinal gas patterns common in acute pancreatitis include diffuse ileus or a focal "ileus" of the duodenum (E sign), the jejunum (sentinel loop sign), or the colon (colon cutoff sign). However, these findings are *not* pathognomonic. Ultrasonography is useful for evaluating the biliary system when the diagnosis of biliary pancreatitis is entertained, but it should not be relied on for the diagnosis or staging of acute pancreatitis; the overlying bowel gas precludes adequate pancreatic imaging in as many as 40% of patients. Nevertheless, in the appropriate clinical setting, when the pancreas can be imaged and shows diffuse pancreatic enlargement or peripancreatic edema (fluid), the ultrasonographic findings may be enough to confirm the diagnosis of acute pancreatitis and thereby dictate management.

Computed tomography is an important adjunct in evaluating the inflamed pancreas and may be indicated in patients with severe epigastric pain of uncertain origin. However, it should not be considered imperative in the *diagnosis* of acute pancreatitis; rather, it is more important

for defining the presence and extent of complications in patients with established acute pancreatitis, such as fluid collections, necrosis, and infection (see "Complications of Acute Pancreatitis," page 325). Common findings of computed tomography in the acute setting include pancreatic enlargement (swelling, edema), pancreatic or peripancreatic fluid collections, and areas of nonenhancement of the pancreatic parenchyma by the intravenous contrast agent. Indeed, with necrotizing pancreatitis, the necrosis (and thereby lack of perfusion to the necrotic regions) is already established by the time the patient presents with abdominal pain.[6]

Management of Acute Pancreatitis
The management of patients with acute pancreatitis is usually noninterventional and mandates consideration of the cause, severity, and presence of complications (Tables 2 and 3). Patients with mild disease (usually an "edematous" pancreatitis) are generally managed successfully by eliminating oral intake, by giving intravenous hydration, and by providing appropriate parenteral analgesia once the diagnosis is secure. With these conservative measures, most patients with mild acute pancreatitis have a self-limited course and prompt resolution of symptoms. They rarely have long-term sequelae. In patients with vomiting or gastric distention, nasogastric decompression may provide symptomatic relief but does not alter the course or severity of the disease. Because of the self-limiting nature of mild acute pancreatitis, antibiotic prophylaxis is not warranted. If a biliary origin is suspected or proved, a same-admission cholecystectomy should be undertaken once the pain has resolved, provided there is no severe intraperitoneal inflammatory reaction. This approach will prevent the possibility of recurrent acute pancreatitis caused by the passage of another gallstone through the papilla of Vater, which occurs in as many as 30% of patients during the ensuing 3 months.

Moderate to severe pancreatitis develops in approximately 10% of patients with acute pancreatitis and requires a more aggressive, intensive therapy. Prompt restoration

Table 2.—Indications for Operative Intervention in Severe Acute Pancreatitis

Absolute	Relative
Infected necrosis	Sterile necrosis with deteriorating, recalci-
Colonic necrosis	trant organ failure
	Sterile necrosis without improvement 6 to
	12 weeks after onset of disease
	Nonresolving intestinal obstruction

Table 3.—Management of Complications in Acute Pancreatitis

Complication	Initial management
Acute fluid collections	Observation unless symptomatic
Pseudocysts	Surgical or endoscopic internal drainage*
Sterile necrosis	Maximal ICU therapy[†]
Infected necrosis	Necrosectomy and drainage
Pancreatic abscess	Radiologic percutaneous drainage[‡]

*In symptomatic or enlarging pseudocysts, otherwise observation only.

[†]Surgical intervention in patients with prolonged or worsening organ failure despite maximal intensive care unit (ICU) therapy.

[‡]Surgical drainage for inaccessible or extensive multiloculated collections.

of circulatory volume and arterial oxygen tension is needed, and organ-specific intensive care and monitoring are mandatory. Severe acute pancreatitis is complicated by the systemic inflammatory response syndrome, sepsis, or organ failure, which is typically precipitated by necrosis or infected necrosis of the pancreas.

Many seemingly rational management approaches have been evaluated in patients with severe pancreatitis in an attempt to halt progression of the inflammatory process. Antacids or antisecretory acid inhibitors (the theory is to decrease secretin release and decrease pancreatic exocrine secretion), intravenous peptides that inhibit pancreatic exocrine secretion (somatostatin, calcitonin), antiproteases to combat active trypsin and other proteases, and even peritoneal lavage in an attempt to remove active intraperitoneal "toxins" have all been studied. Unfortunately, none of these approaches has shown any merit. We believe strongly, however, that prophylactic antibiotics with good penetration of pancreatic tissue (usually imipenem) are indicated in patients with necrotizing pancreatitis. In several large, prospective, randomized trials, appropriate antibiotics reduced the incidence of infected necrosis.[7] In several of these studies, failure of prophylactic antibiotics to improve overall mortality consistently may have resulted from the increased mortality associated with fungal superinfection, which occurs in a small percentage (5%-10%) of patients with acute necrotizing pancreatitis.[8] Concomitant use of oral antifungal prophylaxis in patients receiving prolonged, broad-spectrum antibiotics seems prudent, but this treatment approach remains to be substantiated.

The role of cytokine manipulation in ameliorating or abating the systemic sequelae of acute pancreatitis is currently an area of intense research. The development of systemic illness from pancreatitis is believed to occur because the pancreatic injury attracts inflammatory cells (such as macrophages, leukocytes, monocytes), which release a barrage of cytokines into the portal system. This cytokine cascade is then amplified by the liver and lungs with systemic release of greater magnitudes of these and other inflammatory agents. This cytokine cascade results in distant organ effects in the lungs, kidneys, gut, and liver with establishment of the programmed sepsis syndrome, at this stage independent of any actual "infection." The predominant role of interleukin-1 and tumor necrosis factor-α in inducing both local and systemic effects, such as tissue injury or apoptosis, fever, hypotension, cachexia, and shock, has been described. Platelet-activation factor mediates many of the systemic manifestations of acute pancreatitis early in the cascade. Initial clinical trials of the platelet-activation factor antagonist lexipafant (British Biotech, Annapolis, Maryland) suggested that the agent reduces organ failure, although a subsequent very large, prospective, randomized, multicenter trial proved disappointing (as yet unpublished data). Currently, no inflammatory antagonists (or of recent interest, proinhibitory interleukins) are of proven benefit clinically in patients with severe acute pancreatitis.

Another consideration is nutritional support. Although parenteral or enteral nutrition is not indicated for patients with mild pancreatitis, early *enteral* feeding delivered beyond the ligament of Treitz actually may reduce development of certain complications and also may decrease mortality in patients with severe pancreatitis.[9] In experimental studies, superinfection of areas of pancreatic and peripancreatic necrosis has been shown to derive from the gut flora. Acute pancreatitis disrupts the gut mucosal barrier, allowing bacterial translocation in animals. Although never directly demonstrated in humans, strong evidence suggests that pancreatitis alters the gut "barrier" in humans with entry not of bacteria but of gut-derived systemic inflammatory mediators and endotoxins into the lymphatic system and thereby into the systemic circulation. Experimental evidence (and some clinical studies) strongly suggest that early enteral feeding not only provides nutritional support but also helps maintain the gut barrier. Other intuitive advantages of enteral over parenteral nutrition include reduced cost and avoidance of central intravenous catheter-related complications.

Thus, early management of moderate or severe acute pancreatitis remains primarily supportive, the only active interventions being early use of prophylactic antibiotics and antifungal agents and provision of nutritional support, initially through a parenteral route but with early conversion to an enteral route.

Severity Scoring of Acute Pancreatitis

Many surgeons, including ourselves, found little use for clinical scoring systems in patients with acute pancreatitis before 1995, because no specific treatments or interventions were available. Now, with the benefit of prophylactic antibiotics and the interest in establishment of early enteral nutrition, scoring systems to identify patients with severe disease early in its course now have new meaning. Multifactor systems such as the original Ranson criteria[10] and the more simplified Glasgow criteria use multiple clinical, biochemical, and hematologic indices and are able to predict severity and outcome in patients with acute pancreatitis with reasonable accuracy; however, these scoring systems require 48 hours of assessment before accurate and complete categorization.

Conversely, the Acute Physiology and Chronic Health Evaluation (the APACHE II score)[11] allows immediate stratification of patients on admission, can be done daily to evaluate disease progression and therapeutic response, and is even more predictive of the severity and outcome of acute pancreatitis. Tremendous interest has been devoted to finding a single serum factor predictive of disease severity. Indicators that provide a reasonable ability to discriminate mild from severe acute pancreatitis include interleukins-6 and -8 and polymorphonuclear elastase, all of which peak in the first 24 hours of the disease. However, few hospitals have the ability to perform the assays rapidly and easily. C-reactive protein is an excellent discriminator of disease severity 48 hours after the onset of symptoms and has an accuracy similar to that of the multifactor systems.

Complications of Acute Pancreatitis

In most patients, acute pancreatitis is mild and associated with an uncomplicated, self-limited course. In up to 25% of patients, however, the disease is associated with local or systemic complications such as fluid collections, necrosis, infection, or organ failure. General management approaches are outlined in Table 3.

Peripancreatic Fluid Collections

Acute peripancreatic fluid collections, the most common complication of acute pancreatitis, occur in up to 50% of patients. These collections (Fig. 1) occur early in the course of acute pancreatitis and, unlike pseudocysts, lack a fibrous wall. The fluid is typically serous, emanating from the pancreatic or peripancreatic inflammatory process, but also may contain pancreatic secretions if pancreatic ductal disruption is present. Most of these collections regress spontaneously without intervention and need no treatment, especially no percutaneous drainage.

Pseudocysts develop in up to 10% of patients with acute pancreatitis and are defined as collections of pancreatic

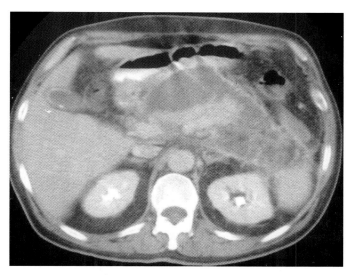

Fig. 1. Computed tomogram of an acute fluid collection complicating acute pancreatitis.

enzyme-rich secretions with a thickened, fibrous, nonepithelialized wall that usually includes the surrounding viscera (Fig. 2). Pseudocysts result from persistence of acute fluid collections caused by failure of a ductal disruption to close by cicatrization, thus forming a defined tract from a pancreatic duct into or through the pancreatic parenchyma.[12] Persistence of this communication results in accumulation of pancreatic secretions, inciting a chronic inflammatory process that induces development of a thickened fibrinous wall of granulation tissue. Pancreatic ductal disruptions most commonly are found at the genu of the pancreatic duct at the junction of the neck with the head of the gland (50%), followed by the body (30%) and tail

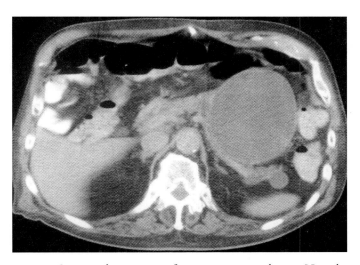

Fig. 2. Computed tomogram of a pancreatic pseudocyst. Note the lack of associated pancreatic parenchymal necrosis and the minimal debris within the cystic collection. (Contrast this with Fig. 3.)

(20%). Pseudocysts most frequently occur anteriorly in the lesser sac. Pancreatic pseudocysts are persistent acute fluid collections and imply an ongoing communication with the pancreatic ductal system. Pancreatic pseudocysts should be carefully distinguished from areas of cystic necrosis, which also may contain extravasated exocrine secretions into the area of necrosis because of a disrupted pancreatic duct in the area of parenchymal necrosis (see "Pancreatic Necrosis," below). Classically, however, a pancreatic pseudocyst is a rounded, cystic area associated with minimal parenchymal or peripancreatic necrosis (although the ductal disruption obviously originated from an area of focal necrosis). Treatment of pseudocysts is different from that of cystic degeneration of areas of pancreatic parenchymal necrosis.[13]

Pancreatic Necrosis

Necrotizing pancreatitis occurs in approximately 5% of patients with acute pancreatitis and should be suspected in patients in whom initial fluid resuscitation fails or in those requiring prolonged hospitalization or intensive medical management. The necrosis may be pancreatic or peripancreatic or both. Extrapancreatic necrosis alone with a viable pancreas (a poorly appreciated variant) has been noted in about 20% of patients and portends a better prognosis.[14] The necrosis may be minimal or may involve the entire gland and surrounding retroperitoneal fat; the extent of necrosis has been shown to correlate directly with organ failure and subsequent outcome. Necrotizing pancreatitis may be suspected from the clinical course, but objective confirmation relies on dynamic, contrast-enhanced computed tomography. This imaging technique begins by defining images through the pancreas initially with only an oral contrast agent. Then, a rapid intravenous infusion of contrast agent is given, and computed tomography cuts through the pancreas are obtained during the parenchymal phase of the intravenous contrast agent (Fig. 3). This technique of imaging is sensitive and specific for parenchymal enhancement (viable, perfused pancreas) and for nonenhanced, hence nonperfused, pancreas (necrosis).[6] In contrast, the presence of peripancreatic necrosis is less well imaged. However, stranding and "inflammatory" reaction in the right or left retroperitoneal paracolic gutter or extending into the base of the small bowel mesentery or retroperitoneally behind (posterior to) the small bowel mesentery should raise suspicion of considerable peripancreatic necrosis (Fig. 4).

Infection

Superinfection of pancreatic necrosis (so-called infected necrosis) occurs in 30% to 70% of patients with necrotizing pancreatitis and may very well depend on the extent of necrosis and the severity of the systemic manifestations. Infection is a time-dependent complication of necrotizing pancreatitis. The best estimates of when superinfection occurs suggest that seeding of the necrosis occurs in 24% of patients in the first week, in 36% by 2 weeks, and in 71% by 3 weeks after the onset of necrotizing acute pancreatitis.[15] The computed tomographic finding of extraluminal gas within areas of necrosis is pathognomonic of infection (Fig. 5); however, it is not present in all patients with infected necrosis. Percutaneous fine-needle aspiration

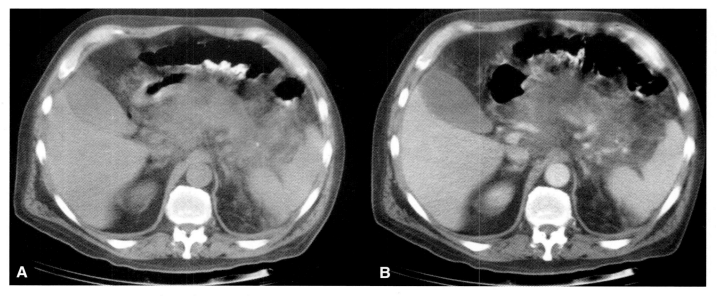

Fig. 3. Dynamic contrast-enhanced computed tomograms of necrotizing pancreatitis. Note the areas of pancreatic parenchyma (A) that fail to enhance after an intravenous contrast agent is given (B).

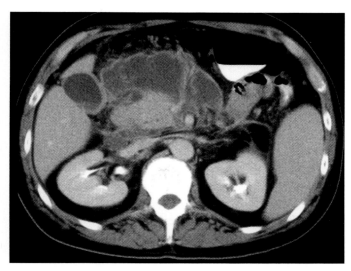

Fig. 4. Dynamic contrast-enhanced computed tomogram from a patient with peripancreatic necrosis but without recognizable pancreatic parenchymal necrosis. The pancreas appears to enhance normally. (From Sakorafas et al.[14] By permission of the Journal of the American College of Surgeons.)

with subsequent Gram stain and culture of the aspirate is a safe and reliable preoperative test for infected necrosis. A monomicrobial isolate is cultured in 75% of patients with infected pancreatic necrosis; polymicrobial and mixed bacterial-fungal infections are less common. Gram-negative aerobic bacteria have been the most common isolates, with

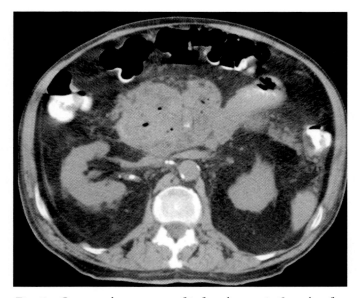

Fig. 5. Computed tomogram of infected necrosis 6 weeks after onset of necrotizing pancreatitis. Note presence of extraluminal gas within areas of pancreatic and peripancreatic necrosis. (From Tsiotos GG, Sarr MG: Management of fluid collections and necrosis in acute pancreatitis. Curr Gastroenterol Rep 1:139-144, 1999. By permission of Current Science.)

Escherichia coli, Klebsiella, Proteus, and Enterobacter predominating in most reports. Multiple routes of bacterial superinfection have been implicated, but colonic translocation seems to be the predominant route.[9] Recently, fungal infection has been found with increasing frequency in patients with infected necrotizing pancreatitis, probably as a function of treatment with broad-spectrum prophylactic antibiotics. Fungal infection portends a more complicated course with increased mortality.[8]

Pancreatic abscess is a late (and rare) complication of necrotizing pancreatitis, occurring in less than 4% of patients with necrotizing pancreatitis. It is differentiated from infected necrosis by the presence of purulent exudate (pus) and positive bacterial or fungal cultures but with little or no necrosis (Fig. 6). This definition, in essence, represents an "infected" pseudocyst. Note that the definition we have chosen to use is based on a multidisciplinary symposium held in Atlanta in 1992, which attempted to develop acceptable criteria for complications of acute pancreatitis.[16] This definition of pancreatic abscess differs from that in much of the past literature, which referred to infected necrosis as "pancreatic abscesses." Not all surgical pancreatologists (including the authors) accept this definition of pancreatic abscess, but we have used it in an attempt to comply with the Atlanta convention. The morbidity and mortality associated with pancreatic abscess are substantially less than with infected pancreatic necrosis, provided the abscess is treated with appropriate interventional or surgical management.

Surgery for Acute Pancreatitis
As alluded to (See "Management of Acute Pancreatitis," page 323), operative intervention has no role in the early

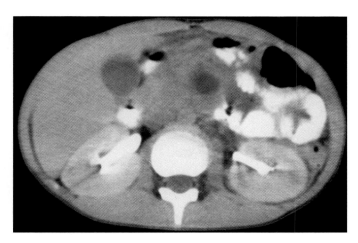

Fig. 6. Computed tomogram of a pancreatic abscess, defined by the Atlanta convention as a localized area of extravasated exocrine secretion that becomes infected (in essence an "infected" pseudocyst) but in the absence of extensive necrosis.

stages of acute pancreatitis (Table 2). Operation should be reserved for the *complications* of acute pancreatitis. Indeed, the role of operative intervention has become more clearly defined in recent years. In necrotizing pancreatitis, the pendulum has swung from early surgical intervention (within the first week or two) with aggressive pancreatic resection to delayed and selective operative intervention with resection limited to the necrotic material with the goal of preserving all viable tissue. This approach of "necrosectomy" (as opposed to simple peripancreatic drainage, which was ineffective in "draining or evacuating" the necrotic tissue) has improved overall mortality from a rate of 70% of patients at risk in the past to the current rates of 10% to 20%.[17,18] Infected necrosis is an absolute indication for operative debridement, which reduces mortality. Management of sterile pancreatic necrosis remains an area of controversy. Patients with documented sterile necrosis should be managed nonoperatively with prophylactic antibiotics and nutritional support for 10 days to 3 weeks; the patient's clinical status, APACHE II score, and serial imaging with computed tomography, if indicated, should be used to monitor the course of disease and the response to therapy. For patients with sterile necrosis and persistent, worsening organ failure despite maximal intensive care, most experienced centers advocate necrosectomy, but this practice is based on little or no objective data and is a well-meaning intervention of desperation.

Infected Necrosis

In patients with confirmed infected necrosis, operative "necrosectomy" is indicated. Although there have been anecdotal reports of successful percutaneous, laparoscopic, or endoscopic "internal" transgastric drainage,[19] these successes have been largely in patients with *localized* infected necrosis in whom repeated interventions have been done by very talented practitioners. Most patients with infected necrosis have more extensive and multiple areas of necrosis and are not candidates for endoscopic or percutaneous approaches. In patients with infected necrosis, necrosectomy is usually advocated at the time bacterial infection is confirmed. In some patients, culture results of a fine-needle aspirate are positive in a clinically stable or improving patient. Immediate necrosectomy may not be warranted in such patients, especially within the first 3 weeks from the onset of the pancreatitis; treatment with the culture-directed antibiotic of choice and a delay to allow full demarcation of necrosis may be prudent.[15] This approach is controversial and remains to be substantiated; however, we have been pleased with recent results of this approach. When infection of pancreatic necrosis is recognized during the second and third weeks of the disease and the patient deteriorates despite maximal aggressive medical support, immediate necrosectomy is indicated.

Nonresolving Sterile Necrosis

Most surgeons avoid operation during the first 2 to 3 months of sterile necrosis. However, if there appears to be no steady clinical improvement, if the patient does not seem to be thriving, and especially if the sterile necrosis is preventing the ability to eat because of a mass effect mechanically blocking either the gastric outlet or the fourth portion of the duodenum (the necrotizing process from the body of the pancreas often extends through the left mesocolon to involve and obstruct the small bowel at the ligament of Treitz), then an "elective" necrosectomy may be warranted. We prefer to wait 6 to 8 weeks after the onset of acute pancreatitis before contemplating this approach. In contrast, others intervene as early as 3 weeks after onset of acute pancreatitis.[20]

Necrosectomy: Techniques

The rationale for operative necrosectomy is that removal of the necrotic or infected material removes the septic stimulus responsible for ongoing organ failure.[21] The goal of necrosectomy is careful, meticulous, and total operative debridement of all necrotic or infected material. A recent computed tomogram is invaluable for guiding the surgeon to ensure complete debridement of all necrotic material and collections. Necrosectomy is generally performed with blunt finger dissection of necrotic tissue to minimize injury to major vessels and viable pancreas.[22] The doughy or puttylike texture of the necrotic pancreatic parenchyma and peripancreatic fat is easily appreciated by palpation. Necrotic debris that is adherent and cannot be gently teased free should be left in place and removed in successive debridements to avoid potential hemorrhage. Likewise, "bridges" of tissue passing through the area of necrosis that do not come out with the necrotic bolus should be left intact, because they usually are viable larger blood vessels that have not thrombosed or become necrotic. Finger-fracturing these bridges may cause hemorrhage that can be very difficult to control.

The method of necrosectomy varies little among experienced centers, but subsequent drainage and management of ongoing exudation and extravasation of pancreatic exocrine secretions differ considerably (Table 4). Surgical options include necrosectomy followed by 1) open packing with marsupialization of the pancreatic bed, in essence creating a laparostomy[23]; 2) wide peripancreatic drainage with multiple temporary, "stuffed" Penrose-type drains removed 5 to 10 days postoperatively[24]; 3) placement of an infusion catheter and multiple drainage catheters in the peripancreatic region to allow continuous, high-volume (2 L/h) peripancreatic lavage for 2 to 4 weeks postoperatively[17]; and 4) planned reoperations at 2-day intervals for repeated necrosectomy or debridement with delayed primary

Table 4.—Types of Pancreatic Necrosectomy to Control Ongoing Peripancreatic Exudation or Pancreatic Fistula

Open marsupialization of pancreatic bed with repeated open packing
Closed one-stage necrosectomy followed by wide peripancreatic drainage with temporary "stuffed" passive drains and closed suction drains
Necrosectomy with closed postoperative peripancreatic lavage
Necrosectomy with planned repeated exploration(s) for debridement with delayed primary closure over closed suction drains

wound closure over multiple soft closed suction drains after all necrotic material has been debrided.[25,26] Although no randomized, controlled trials have compared these methods, each method has similar rates of complications and mortality. We prefer an initial necrosectomy followed by planned reoperative necrosectomy as indicated until the necrotic process has been arrested and further necrosis is no longer identified.[26]

Other operative considerations should include treating the inciting cause if possible, provision of early enteral nutritional support, and patient comfort. For instance, if the cause of the pancreatitis is gallstone-related, attempts at cholecystectomy and, if necessary, choledocholithotomy are warranted, provided they can be undertaken safely. Strong consideration should be given to a feeding jejunostomy; we prefer the smaller-diameter needle catheter jejunostomy[27] that can be converted to a larger-diameter jejunostomy by interventional techniques if prolonged enteral feeding is required.[28] Finally, for necrosis involving the head of the pancreas (and thus the periduodenal region) in patients who are extremely ill or in the elderly, a formal tube gastrostomy is much better tolerated than prolonged nasogastric intubation.

Pancreatic abscess, according to the Atlanta classification (infected cystic structure with minimal necrosis), may be managed with percutaneous drainage. Operative management is largely reserved for areas that are inaccessible using percutaneous techniques, areas with extensive loculation precluding adequate percutaneous drainage, or when other conditions require open intervention (such as cholangitis or intestinal obstruction).

Special Situations

Pancreatic Pseudocysts
Use of the term "pancreatic pseudocyst" has led to much confusion. By accepted definition, a pancreatic pseudocyst has no formal epithelial wall and contains pancreatic exocrine secretions in direct communication with the pancreatic "ductal system." The Atlanta conference attempted to define peripancreatic cystic collections into a meaningful classification, because not all fluid collections in and around the pancreas in patients with pancreatic abnormality are really "pancreatic pseudocysts," and their true nature often determines their appropriate treatment and prognosis.

Peripancreatic acute fluid collections occur during an episode of acute pancreatitis. They usually are inflammatory reactions to the pancreatic inflammation, do not have a high amylase activity (signifying a lack of communication with the pancreatic ductal system), and resolve. They tend to have an irregular shape. No interventional treatment is necessary or indicated.

Pancreatic pseudocysts are (originally) acute fluid collections caused by disruptions of the pancreatic ductal system with extravasation of exocrine secretions. They have not resolved because, by the definition of the Atlanta classification, they have persisted for at least 6 weeks after the onset of acute pancreatitis. These fluid collections also occur in chronic pancreatitis and often do not follow a defined exacerbation of the chronic pancreatitis. Pancreatic pseudocysts are usually round and well defined; they are not associated with extensive pancreatic and peripancreatic necrosis (see next paragraph) and usually contain very little debris within the fluid-filled cystic cavity.

Difficulties arise in the terminology of peripancreatic fluidlike collections that occur in conjunction with acute necrotizing pancreatitis.[12] These fluidlike or cystlike areas of liquefaction necrosis are not acute fluid collections and are not true pancreatic pseudocysts despite the fact that they might communicate with the pancreatic duct as a result of pancreatic parenchymal necrosis with ductal disruption. These cystlike areas of liquefaction necrosis are not well defined, tend not to be round, and contain a heterogeneous intracystic material containing both liquid and solid or semisolid necrotic matter. If they are composed only of peripancreatic fat necrosis, the amylase activity will be low; if they contain areas of pancreatic parenchymal necrosis (and virtually always associated peripancreatic fat necrosis), the fluid may or may not contain an increased amylase activity, depending on whether the pancreatic ductal necrosis has sealed itself. It is important to differentiate these areas of liquefaction necrosis from true pancreatic pseudocysts, because their appropriate treatment and prognosis vary greatly.

Pseudocyst formation is a common complication of both acute (5%-10%) and chronic (20%-40%) pancreatitis. Up to 80% of peripancreatic fluid collections developing during episodes of acute pancreatitis resolve spontaneously. In contrast, pseudocysts forming as sequelae of chronic pancreatitis frequently are associated with proximal pancreatic ductal abnormalities (stenosis, disruption) and have a much lower rate of spontaneous resolution. Several studies have found that pseudocysts persisting for more than 6 weeks have a decreased frequency of spontaneous resolution; however, some do resolve, and many never lead to serious complications. Indeed, a study by Vitas and Sarr[13] showed that serious complications develop in only 10% to 12%, a finding thus questioning the classic surgical dictum that all pseudocysts persisting for more than 6 weeks after acute pancreatitis necessitate operative drainage because of the very high frequency of serious complications.

Asymptomatic patients with pseudocysts can be managed expectantly and followed with serial abdominal computed tomography. Size of the pseudocyst alone does not mandate intervention—some asymptomatic patients with large pseudocysts who have been followed conservatively have not had an increased frequency of complications. Treatment is indicated for complications (bleeding or free peritoneal rupture), extensive symptoms (abdominal pain, gastrointestinal tract obstruction, insidious weight loss, nausea and vomiting), or an enlarging pseudocyst. Some authors also advocate treatment of all perisplenic pseudocysts persisting for more than 6 weeks, because the rate of hemorrhage associated with pseudocysts in this location is high, although this approach remains controversial.

The primary *nonsurgical options* for treatment of a pancreatic pseudocyst are computed tomography- or ultrasonography-guided percutaneous external drainage and endoscopic internal drainage. Simple needle aspiration of a pseudocyst, unless done for diagnosis, should not be performed because of its association with an extremely high rate of recurrence. Percutaneous drainage with large-caliber, pigtail catheters can be performed safely with computed tomography or ultrasonography guidance. This approach should not be undertaken if there is evidence of considerable abnormality of the proximal pancreatic duct (stricture, disruption) because of the high risk of a persistent pancreatic-cutaneous fistula. Endoscopic cystenterostomy has been performed with increasing frequency in recent years. For this approach to be successful, patients must have appropriate anatomy: the pseudocyst must closely abut (≤ 1 cm) and adhere to the stomach or duodenum, allowing a cystenterostomy to be created through the bulging portion of the cyst. Chronic pseudocysts with their slow development are usually thick-walled and adherent; acute pseudocysts have thinner walls and are at greater risk for intraperitoneal spillage of cyst contents. Endoscopic drainage is technically challenging, but reasonable success has been obtained in appropriately selected patients.

Usually internal pigtail stents are placed into the cyst and routed to the organ of entry. Recent case reports have detailed several new, minimally invasive methods of pseudocyst drainage, including transpapillary cyst drainage (with a stent placed across the ductal disruption with a guidewire), percutaneous internal drainage with endoscopic guidance, and laparoendoscopic internal drainage. The usefulness of these methods remains to be validated by long-term follow-up. The goal of all these methods is to drain the pseudocyst into the gut (allowing the pancreatic ductal disruption to heal) or to maintain a permanent new site of entry of pancreatic exocrine secretions.

Pseudocysts are treated objectively by internal drainage, external drainage, or resection.[13] General principles of *operative management* of pseudocysts include complete evacuation of the cystic contents, biopsy of the cyst wall to exclude a pancreatic cystic neoplasm masquerading as a pseudocyst,[12] and, if possible or necessary, treatment of the underlying pancreatic ductal abnormality. Pseudocysts arising insidiously in patients with chronic pancreatitis generally can be treated at the time of diagnosis if symptomatic, whereas those arising during or after episodes of acute pancreatitis should be followed for at least 4 to 6 weeks to ensure adequate maturation of the pseudocyst wall (to better hold sutures).

If intervention is required before the cyst wall has matured adequately, simple external drainage is usually the best choice. External drainage usually is reserved for patients with infected pseudocysts, complications (hemorrhage, free peritoneal rupture), or pseudocysts with immature walls. Pancreatic fistulas may develop in as many as 30% of patients after external drainage.

Resection is a useful option for treatment of intrapancreatic pseudocysts in the tail of the gland, those not amenable to internal drainage, and those associated with substantial hemorrhage. Some consideration should be given to preoperative angiography with transcatheter thrombosis of pseudoaneurysms associated with hemorrhage from a pseudocyst. This approach offers definitive treatment of the pseudocyst and the ductal and arterial abnormalities.

Internal drainage, however, is the operative treatment of choice. Cystogastrostomy, cystoduodenostomy, or Roux-en-Y cystojejunostomy are used in an attempt to create a permanent internal fistula between the pseudocyst and gastrointestinal tract.[13] Cystogastrostomy is useful for treating cysts in the lesser sac; these usually originate from the genu of the pancreatic duct and thus tend to abut the distal body and proximal antrum of the stomach. Division of the gastrocolic ligament may allow inspection of the posterior aspect of the stomach and pseudocyst to ensure adequate fusion; however, usually this is unnecessary, because the fixation between the stomach and the inflammatory pseudocyst can be appreciated. Anterior gastrotomy then exposes the lumen of the stomach, and the cyst is entered by way of a posterior gastrotomy. It is probably wise to aspirate the pseudocyst transgastrically before creating an anterior gastrotomy to ensure appropriate placement of the gastrotomy incision. After complete evacuation of cystic contents and biopsy of the cyst wall, a long cystogastrostomy extending from the edges of the defect is constructed with a hemostatic closure "reefing" the common wall of stomach and cyst. Large pseudocysts in the lesser sac may be better treated with Roux-en-Y cystojejunostomy to ensure adequate drainage. Roux-en-Y cystojejunostomy is the most versatile method of internal drainage. The Roux limb of jejunum additionally may be used to decompress the pancreatic duct proximally or distally in patients with chronic pancreatitis and ductal stricture or, in addition, to drain an obstructed bile duct. The wise surgeon orients the Roux limb from the patient's left to right, bringing the Roux limb to the left of the middle colic vessels, not to the right. This approach allows the mesentery of the Roux limb to be away from the superior mesenteric vein (rather than overlying it) should another resective procedure on the pancreatic head be required in the future.

Pseudocysts arising from the head of the pancreas or uncinate process and abutting the duodenum may be drained by way of cystoduodenostomy, taking care to avoid the intrapancreatic common bile duct, ampulla, and gastroduodenal artery.

Many options are available for treatment of pancreatic pseudocysts. Percutaneous drainage with computed tomographic guidance may be useful for simple pseudocysts without proximal ductal obstruction. Endoscopic internal drainage is technically demanding but may be the procedure of choice in selected patients. External surgical drainage is indicated for treating complicated pseudocysts or those with immature walls. Internal surgical drainage is the treatment of choice for most patients; a cystenterostomy is created through the stomach, duodenum, or a Roux-en-Y limb of jejunum. Surgical drainage should include evacuation of the cystic contents, treatment of ductal abnormalities, and biopsy of the cyst wall to exclude cystic neoplasm.[13]

Colonic Necrosis

Rarely (about 2%), colonic necrosis involving the left transverse colon is noted at necrosectomy, or occasionally it is the indication for operative intervention.[29] This complication seems to be due to thrombosis of either the middle colic vessels or the local colonic mesenteric arcade as the necrotizing process extends through the transverse

mesocolon. Obviously, this problem requires segmental colectomy, proximal colonic diversion, and closure (or exteriorization) of the distal colon with restoration of colonic continuity at a later date, after the pancreatic process has been resolved. Colonic necrosis also may occur after operative necrosectomy, sometimes necessitating colectomy and proximal diversion. In contrast, colonic fistulas that become evident on sinography through a peripancreatic drain or when fecal-stained matter is noted in a drain in an otherwise asymptomatic patient usually heal spontaneously and do not necessitate aggressive intervention.

Pancreatic Fistulas

Necrosectomy of areas of pancreatic parenchymal necrosis often leads to prolonged drainage of pancreatic juice from disrupted pancreatic ducts which is "controlled" by the peripancreatic drains.[29] Pancreatic ascites is extremely rare.[30] These external pancreatic fistulas usually close spontaneously provided no proximal ductal obstruction exists and the fistula does not arise from an isolated pancreatic remnant. The latter may occur after complete necrosis of the neck of the pancreas with separation of the distal duct from continuity with the duodenum. These fistulas may erode into other structures.[31] Duodenal necrosis also can manifest as a pancreatic fistula.[32] In general, however, with patience, adequate drainage, and, if necessary, an endoscopic sphincterotomy and possibly a temporary pancreatic ductal stent, the fistulas slowly close over 2 to 6 months. We have had little success with octreotide treatment. Although we use it, we discontinue its use if there is no dramatic and immediate (within 48 hours) decrease in the volume of output. For persistent, low-output (< 300 mL a day) fistulas, we usually start to inch out the drain a centimeter or two every week beginning 3 months after necrosectomy. For persistent fistulas that fail to close or for high-output fistulas, we favor reoperation with drainage of the now well-formed fistulous tract into a Roux-en-Y jejunal limb as an onlay procedure.

Intra-abdominal Hemorrhage

Hemorrhage after necrosectomy may occur from development of a pseudoaneurysm of an intrapancreatic or peripancreatic artery or from involvement of a vessel from either extension of the necrotizing process or pressure erosion by a drain.[33] If the hemorrhage is arterial and brisk, consideration should be given to managing the bleeding with angiographic embolization rather than reoperation. This approach is especially prudent if the bleeding occurs after 1 week or more postoperatively, when safe exposure and control of the bleeding site would be very difficult (or even impossible).

Severe Gallstone Pancreatitis

Although most patients have a rapid improvement that allows a safe, same-admission cholecystectomy, a highly selected group with very severe pancreatitis has deterioration within the first 24 to 48 hours and will benefit from emergency endoscopic sphincterotomy. If a stone is impacted at the ampulla and is extracted by sphincterotomy, mortality and morbidity seem to improve. Indications for emergency ERCP and sphincterotomy include a decompensating clinical course within the first 72 hours of onset, documented or highly suspected choledocholithiasis, and persistently increased or increasing serum liver transaminase and bilirubin values.

Outcomes of Acute Pancreatitis

In patients who die early in the course of severe acute pancreatitis, the cause is almost exclusively from the systemic inflammatory response and multiple organ failure in the setting of necrotizing pancreatitis and not from infection per se.[34,35] The incidence of early organ failure directly correlates with the extent of necrosis. Later deaths (> 2 weeks after onset of pancreatitis) are related to the presence of infected necrosis. Obesity is independently associated with an increased risk of complications, and a body mass index more than 30 is a predictor of a poor outcome. Outcome is improved with prolonged intensive care management in all patients with severe pancreatitis, reserving necrosectomy for those with a recalcitrant clinical course or infected necrosis.

Long-term complications after operative management of severe necrotizing pancreatitis include wound hernias (about 20%) and pancreatic insufficiency (Table 5). The extent of pancreatic endocrine and exocrine insufficiency also correlates with the extent of pancreatic parenchymal necrosis.[36] Endocrine insufficiency usually develops during the initial hospitalization. In contrast, exocrine insufficiency may improve over time (probably due to resolution of the acute inflammation) or may develop or progress after dismissal (likely related to scarring and fibrosis of the pancreatic parenchyma).

CHRONIC PANCREATITIS

Chronic pancreatitis is defined by the Cambridge International Workshop on Pancreatitis as "continuing inflammatory disease of the pancreas characterized by irreversible morphologic change and typically causing pain and/or permanent loss of function."[37] The disease usually is characterized by recurrent attacks of severe abdominal pain with progressive fibrosis of the gland ultimately leading to exocrine and endocrine insufficiency. Chronic pancreatitis also may become evident in a previously

Table 5.—Morbidity After Operation for Acute Necrotizing Pancreatitis

Condition	%
Fistula	35
Pancreaticocutaneous	14
Intestinal	6
Colonic	11
Duodenal	7
Gastric	3
Hemorrhage	18
Abscess	13
Pseudocysts	2

Modified from Tsiotos et al.[26] By permission of Excerpta Medica.

"asymptomatic" patient who presents with onset of symptoms of pancreatic insufficiency (without pain).

Etiopathogenesis of Chronic Pancreatitis

Etiology

In the Western world, the principal cause of chronic pancreatitis is alcohol abuse, accounting for 60% to 70% of all patients. Mechanical ductal obstruction from various causes (posttraumatic, necrotizing acute pancreatitis, pancreas divisum) is the cause in a small number of patients. Cystic fibrosis and hyperparathyroidism are rare causes of chronic pancreatitis. Worldwide, tropical (nutritional) chronic pancreatitis is prevalent, primarily in the poorest parts of Africa and India. This disease is poorly understood and may be due to protein malnutrition or ingestion of toxic substances. In the United States, the cause is idiopathic in 15% to 30% of patients. Increasing evidence suggests that there are two subgroups (early and late onset) of idiopathic chronic pancreatitis and that the pain patterns and natural history of this disease differ substantially from those of alcoholic chronic pancreatitis. Hereditary pancreatitis leading to chronic pancreatitis (see page 321) is a rare form of disease caused by autosomal point mutations of the trypsinogen gene; these mutations lead to an inhibition of intracellular trypsin inactivation and autodigestion at times of unusual pancreatic stress (Table 6). Gallstones almost never are the cause of chronic pancreatitis involving the entire gland. However, a previous episode of gallstone-induced acute pancreatitis may cause a pancreatic ductal stricture that may then lead to chronic pancreatitis involving the pancreatic parenchyma distal to the stricture (so-called postobstructive chronic pancreatitis).

Table 6.—Causes of Chronic Pancreatitis

Chronic alcohol abuse
Mechanical ductal disruption
    Biliary
    Traumatic/stricture
    Pseudocyst
Pancreas divisum
Cystic fibrosis
Hyperparathyroidism
Tropical (nutritional)
Hereditary pancreatitis
Idiopathic

Pathogenesis

The pathogenesis of chronic pancreatitis remains poorly understood, although several mechanisms have been proposed. The ductal obstruction theory suggests that increased protein secretion in pancreatic juice forms protein plugs that obstruct the smaller ducts and ultimately cause pancreatic calcification. Lithostatin (formerly called pancreatic-stone protein) is a protein found in high concentrations in pancreatic juice which appears to inhibit calcium precipitation in vitro. Its involvement in the pathogenesis of chronic pancreatitis remains highly controversial. Another theory proposes toxic metabolite and free radical formation as the initial event leading to fibrosis. The most well-accepted pathogenesis is the necrosis-fibrosis hypothesis, which suggests that focal necrosis from repeated bouts of acute inflammation leads to fibrosis and scarring, with subsequent stricture and obstruction of the pancreatic ducts.

Special consideration should be given to the cause of pain in chronic pancreatitis, because this symptom is the primary indication for surgical consultation and operative intervention in most patients.[38] The precise cause of pain remains poorly understood. Increased intraductal and intraparenchymal pressures have been well documented in patients with chronic pancreatitis, and internal drainage alone provides satisfactory pain relief in 70% to 80% of patients with a dilated main pancreatic duct. The relatively high recurrence of pain after operative ductal drainage (40%-50% at 5 years) and the lack of pain with some strictures and obstructions associated with increased ductal pressure confound this hypothesis. Increased pressure (both ductal and parenchymal) somehow likely contributes to the pain of chronic pancreatitis. Indeed, some investigators have suggested that the pain may be a type of compartment syndrome.[39] The rigid, fibrotic pancreatic capsule prevents changes in parenchymal volume, thereby increasing parenchymal pressure. Histologic evidence has shown the presence of chronic perineural inflammation and fibrosis of chronic pancreatitis, and recent evidence has shown that levels of nerve growth factor and its receptor Trk-A correlate with the extent of fibrosis and intensity of pain in chronic pancreatitis, supporting the idea that neural changes may be involved in the pathogenesis of pain. A subjective concept is that the head of the gland represents the "pacemaker" of pain, and thus proximal resection (pancreatoduodenectomy) will relieve the pain.[40]

Clinical Presentation of Chronic Pancreatitis

Patients most commonly present with a history of repeated episodes of acute pancreatitis that gradually (over 10-15 years) develops into a more chronic, epigastric pain syndrome. The usual patient is a 35- to 45-year-old chronic alcoholic with a long history of alcohol abuse; alcoholic chronic pancreatitis in a patient younger than 30 years would be unusual, because progression of the disease usually takes 1 to 2 decades. The pain is typically of a boring quality and often radiates through to the mid back. This often debilitating pain may be exacerbated by food and is usually described to be worse at night. Signs of exocrine (steatorrhea) or endocrine (hyperglycemia) pancreatic insufficiency are often absent at initial presentation, but they usually develop within 3 to 10 years. Because chronic pancreatitis is a progressive, indolent disease, and because the pancreatic insufficiency appears to develop as a result of mechanical destruction of the parenchyma (rather than an immunologic or autoimmune type process), low (but still measurable) endogenous plasma insulin concentrations typically prevent the onset of a brittle diabetes mellitus.

Other presentations may involve mechanical complications of the fibrotic reaction or an associated pancreatic pseudocyst. Involvement of the second portion of the duodenum may lead to a mechanical obstruction retarding gastric emptying. Similarly, the intrapancreatic portion of the common bile duct can become extrinsically compressed, leading most commonly to a "subclinical" extrahepatic biliary obstruction (dilated bile duct and increased serum alkaline phosphatase level with a normal serum bilirubin value) or, more rarely, a true mechanical obstructive jaundice. A related but unusual presentation is sinistral, or "left-sided," portal hypertension with gastric varices related to thrombosis or external compression or obstruction of the splenic vein; the presenting sign usually is bleeding gastric varices.[41]

The most unusual presentation is nonpainful pancreatic exocrine insufficiency. Patients, often elderly women, present with abdominal cramping, weight loss, and steatorrhea without a history of abdominal pain.

Diagnosis of Chronic Pancreatitis

The variable course of pain, exocrine and endocrine insufficiency, and complicating factors, as well as the difficulty in obtaining tissue for histologic evaluation, can make the diagnosis of chronic pancreatitis challenging. Clinical features provide the strongest clues, but the physician must maintain a high degree of clinical suspicion. Increased values of serum pancreatic enzymes (amylase, lipase), which are the hallmark of acute pancreatitis during attacks, are often unimpressive in chronic pancreatitis, and normal levels do not exclude the diagnosis of chronic pancreatitis. Goals of diagnosing chronic pancreatitis should include establishment of cause (with family testing when indicated), exclusion of pancreatic carcinoma, detailing local complications, and staging the severity of functional impairment. Imaging studies include plain abdominal radiography, in which the presence of diffuse pancreatic calcification confirms the diagnosis. Computed tomography also shows pancreatic calcification (Fig. 7) but also delineates pancreatic ductal dilatation (Fig. 8), glandular atrophy, and extrapancreatic manifestations such as biliary obstruction, splenic vein thrombosis with splenomegaly, perihilar splenic varices, and, if advanced, gastric varices. Sometimes the pancreas looks remarkably normal on computed tomography.

The standard for diagnosis of chronic pancreatitis today is endoscopic retrograde cholangiopancreatography (ERCP) or magnetic resonance cholangiopancreatography (MRCP) for evaluation of the ductal system. ERCP may show areas of pancreatic ductal stenosis or obstruction, but equally prevalent are more subtle findings of blunting of the secondary and tertiary branches of the pancreatic ductal tree. When the bile duct is involved by the chronic inflammation, the intrapancreatic portion usually is involved with a long tapering stricture without a focal mass-like effect. Such a long tapered stricture involving the entire intrapancreatic

portion of the bile duct should strongly suggest chronic pancreatitis as opposed to a pancreatic neoplasm. Newer imaging methods such as endoscopic ultrasonography and MRCP are promising. Some gastroenterologists (and surgeons) believe that endoscopic ultrasonography may prove to be a sensitive diagnostic test for chronic pancreatitis, not only by imaging a dilated pancreatic duct but also, even more so, by documenting parenchymal abnormalities of chronic fibrosis. MRCP, which is a noninvasive means of visualizing the pancreatic and biliary ducts, promises to replace eventually the invasive diagnostic ERCP.

Evaluation of exocrine pancreatic function includes stool analysis for lipid content (3-day collection for 24-hour fecal fat analysis) and pancreatic enzymes (fecal elastase and chymotrypsin), direct measurement of pancreatic enzyme secretion (Lundh test or secretin-caerulein test), or indirect measurement of exocrine function (pancreolauryl urinary excretion test or other labeled oral fats to be ingested then measured in the serum or breath). Endocrine insufficiency is determined by measurement of fasting serum glucose, glucose tolerance testing, or measurement of serum insulin and C-peptide concentrations. The presence of pancreatic endocrine insufficiency corroborates the diagnosis of chronic pancreatitis but in itself is insufficient to establish the diagnosis of chronic pancreatitis.

Management of Chronic Pancreatitis

Medical Therapy

The primary approach to the management of chronic pancreatitis should be medical. Medical treatment of chronic pancreatitis includes avoidance of precipitating factors (especially alcohol), pain control, oral pancreatic

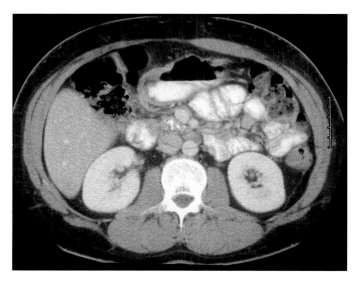

Fig. 7. Computed tomogram of chronic, calcific pancreatitis.

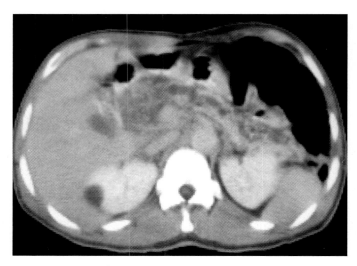

Fig. 8. Computed tomogram of chronic pancreatitis with dilated pancreatic duct.

enzyme replacement, and treatment of maldigestion and hyperglycemia. Although pain relief should always first be attempted with nonnarcotic analgesics, many patients ultimately require narcotic analgesia. Before narcotic therapy is instituted, strong consideration should be given to performing a celiac plexus block (also called a chemical splanchnicectomy).[42] Narcotic abuse is only too prevalent in patients with long-standing chronic pancreatitis and presents an especially difficult challenge in their management; evaluation of the severity of pancreatic pain is very difficult with the confounding factor of narcotic addiction.

There have been sporadic reports of endoscopic intervention with pancreatic ductal sphincterotomy, stenting of the main pancreatic duct, and transampullary extraction of stones from the main pancreatic duct, often in conjunction with lithotripsy. These treatments require advanced endoscopic expertise and may provide temporary pain relief. However, objective evidence of long-lasting effects is scarce, but encouraging. Whether these approaches will provide durable pain relief in this progressive disease remains unknown. All of these nonoperative approaches are temporizing with the hope that the disease will burn itself out with disappearance of the pain (the burnout phenomenon). Burnout often develops with the appearance of pancreatic insufficiency, but it may take years to develop after the initial presentation of chronic pain, especially in the absence of any endocrine or exocrine insufficiency.

Surgical Therapy

Surgical therapy should be considered as palliation of the complications of chronic pancreatitis.[43] The primary indication for operative intervention in chronic pancreatitis is pain refractory to all medical management. Other indications include extrapancreatic complications: obstruction of the gastrointestinal tract or biliary tree, pseudocyst, and hemorrhage.[44] Recently, suspicion of malignancy has become a more frequent indication for operation because of increasingly sophisticated imaging techniques and the documented risk of cancer in chronic pancreatitis of about 1% per year. The overall aim in all operative procedures should be twofold: to relieve the disabling pain of the acute complication and to preserve pancreatic function.

The surgical management of chronic pancreatitis traditionally has been divided into large duct (> 7 mm) and small duct (< 5 mm) disease, with drainage procedures applied to the former and pancreatic resection to the latter.[45] During the past 2 decades, a clearer understanding of the pathophysiology of pancreatic pain, improved imaging techniques, and demonstrated greater safety of pancreaticoduodenectomy have led to considerable

changes in the operative management of chronic pancreatitis. During the past 3 decades, a trend has evolved toward resectional procedures, specifically toward more proximal resection.[46]

Drainage

In 1958, Puestow and Gillesby[47] first reported excellent pain relief in patients with chronic pancreatitis after operative "filleting" of the pancreatic duct and invagination of the gland into a Roux-en-Y limb of jejunum. Splenectomy with a limited distal pancreatectomy was included in their procedure. Two years later, Partington and Rochelle[48] described the lateral pancreaticojejunostomy (with splenic preservation) that is widely used today in patients with large duct disease involving the body and tail of the gland (Fig. 9). The procedure involves opening the length of the main pancreatic duct, with anastomosis to a Roux-en-Y limb of jejunum. An important technical consideration in the procedure is opening adequate ductal length to ensure drainage of the entire gland. Most pancreatic surgeons suggest opening the entire length of the pancreatic duct and removing stone material from primary and secondary ducts, whenever possible. Some largely academic debate persists regarding the best method of anastomosis: two-layer versus a one-layer, full-thickness technique. Although most texts show the Roux limb passing into the lesser sac through the mesocolon to the patient's right of the middle colic vessels, we suggest bringing the Roux limb to the patient's left of the middle colic vessels. Should the patient require reoperation for recurrent pancreatic pain, the probable procedure offered will involve a proximal pancreatic resection (see "Resection," below). The Roux limb lying to the right of middle colic vessels will necessitate its takedown to expose the head of the gland and, if necessary, the superior mesenteric vein; positioning the Roux limb as we suggest avoids this problem.[49]

Immediate results with this treatment have been good (70%-80% pain relief) in patients with ductal dilatation. Progression of disease, continued substance abuse, and other poorly understood factors attenuate these effects in the long run.[50] In many patients (40%-50%) initially treated with drainage alone, recurrent pain will ultimately develop and may require further operative intervention. Drainage procedures also have been studied in patients with small duct disease. Results in that situation, although still controversial, generally have been poor. Currently, most pancreatic surgeons agree that the indication for ductal drainage alone without any parenchymal resection should be restricted to patients with main pancreatic duct dilatation and without evidence of an inflammatory mass in the head of the gland.

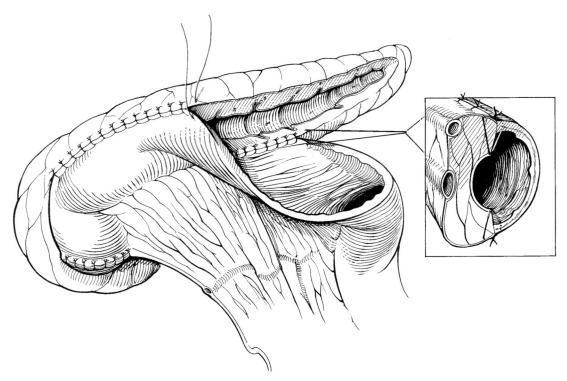

Fig. 9. Partington-Rochelle lateral pancreaticojejunostomy. (From Sakorafas and Sarr.[49] By permission of Mayo Foundation.)

Resection

Historically, patients with chronic pancreatitis were treated with distal pancreatic resection unless there was biliary or gastric obstruction or clear evidence of a mass in the head of the gland. Apparently, the prevailing concept was that pain was proportional to the amount of involved parenchyma. In addition, operative mortality and morbidity were less after distal than after proximal resections. Poor results over time led to more extended distally based resections (60% of gland to 80% to 95%) and even total pancreatectomy.[38] Continued disappointing results with these resections (up to 33% of patients did not obtain any pain relief after total pancreatectomy) and, in addition, the added morbidity of surgically inducing or hastening pancreatic insufficiency in a largely alcoholic population led to acceptance of the hypothesis (generally attributed to Longmire) that the "pacemaker" of pain in chronic pancreatitis is in the head of the gland. Since 1985, the demonstrated trend at Mayo Clinic has been toward proximal resection.[46]

Distal pancreatectomy still remains a viable option, but only for highly selected patients with disease confined exclusively to the distal half of the gland, such as after traumatic ductal disruption or other causes of postobstructive localized pancreatitis.[51] Total pancreatectomy is almost never indicated for treatment of this disease, because the marked endocrine abnormalities are very difficult to manage, particularly in this group of generally noncompliant patients.[52]

Pancreaticoduodenectomy traditionally has been applied to patients with chronic pancreatitis involving the head of the gland (this procedure is described in Chapter 18). The pylorus-preserving modification of this operation has become the preferred method of proximal pancreatic resection at Mayo Clinic. Recent review of our experience with pancreaticoduodenectomy in patients with small duct, head-dominant disease found good results (complete or partial pain relief) in 89% of patients (median follow-up, 6.6 years).[53] Operative morbidity and mortality rates were 32% and 3%, respectively. In general, patients undergoing pancreaticoduodenectomy for chronic pancreatitis have an increased incidence of pancreatic exocrine and endocrine insufficiency postoperatively.

Two modifications of the classic pancreaticoduodenectomy have become accepted recently for treatment of chronic pancreatitis. Beger first described a duodenum-preserving resection of the pancreatic head (now referred to as the Beger procedure) in 1980, and Beger and colleagues recently reported the results for more than 500 patients with chronic pancreatitis.[54] Results in terms of pain relief and improvement of the quality of life were impressive: 91% of patients were considered pain-free or experienced minimal pain after a mean observation period of 14 years. This procedure involves development of the plane between the neck of the pancreas and the superior mesenteric vein with division of the pancreas at the neck of the gland. The head of the gland is then rotated laterally to the patient's right, and the head and uncinate process are subtotally excised in a nonanatomical fashion, being careful to leave a button of pancreatic parenchyma along the second and third portions of the duodenum and maintaining continuity of the superior pancreatoduodenal arterial arcade. A Roux-en-Y limb of jejunum is anastomosed separately to the remnant gland of body and tail and to the button of parenchyma along the duodenum (Fig. 10). The operation allows decompression of the ductal network in the head of the gland and of the intrapancreatic bile duct (if necessary). Preservation of the duodenum, with its important hormonal milieu, and avoidance of the need for a biliary-enteric anastomosis are suggested by proponents of this operation to be major advantages over pancreaticoduodenectomy.

Frey and Amikura[55] reported a technique of local nonanatomical resection of the pancreatic head in combination with longitudinal pancreaticojejunostomy, now referred to as the Frey procedure (Fig. 11). This procedure involves removing the central portion of the head of the gland and filleting the main pancreatic duct with anastomosis to a Roux limb of jejunum. This offers decompression and resection of the head of the gland and provides drainage of the remainder of the body and tail of the gland. The procedure is a technically simpler and less time-consuming operation than pancreaticoduodenectomy or duodenal-preserving pancreatic head resection. In addition, it preserves more

pancreatic parenchyma, theoretically reducing the rate of operatively induced exocrine and endocrine insufficiency. In the initial series reported by Frey and Amikura, pain relief was excellent or improved in 87% of patients during a 37-month follow-up. The frequency of endocrine and exocrine insufficiency was similar to that in patients undergoing longitudinal pancreaticojejunostomy. This procedure should be beneficial in patients with a dilated main duct and enlarged, fibrotic, calcific head. Recently, prospective, randomized trials in small groups of patients have compared the Beger and Frey operations and the Beger procedure and pancreaticoduodenectomy.[56,57] After short-term follow-up (24 and 6 months), all three procedures compared favorably in terms of safety, pain relief, and quality of life. Any of the three operations may be considered for treatment of disease involving the pancreatic head, depending on local experience. Recently, we have become more interested in these duodenal-preserving head resections, and our experience with a small number of such resections (n = 11) has been encouraging.[45]

Nerve Ablation

The pancreas is a highly innervated visceral organ with afferent sympathetic fibers passing through the celiac plexus to form the splanchnic nerves (T5-T12) along their course to the spinal cord and thalamus. Celiac plexus block with chemical agents (phenol, ethanol, corticosteroids) has been very successful for palliating the pain of pancreatic carcinoma and for providing temporary relief in some patients with chronic

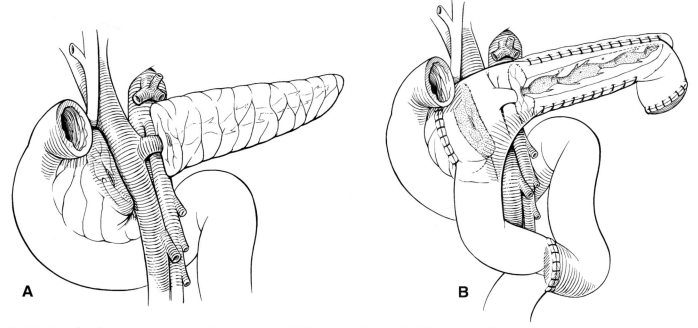

A   **B**

Fig. 10. Duodenal-preserving resection of pancreatic head (Beger procedure). (A), Transection of pancreatic neck with resection of portion of head of gland. (B), Roux limb anastomosis to remnant body and tail and to rim of pancreas along duodenum.

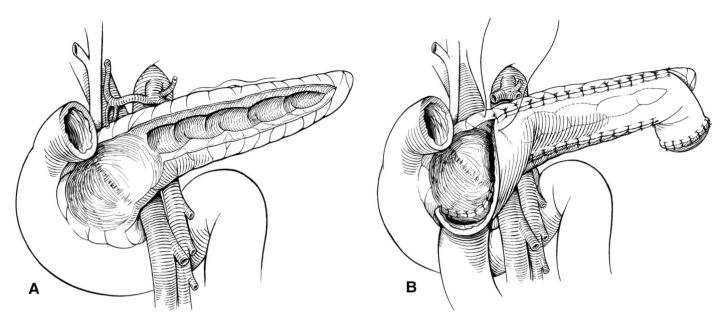

Fig. 11. Frey procedure. (A), *Filleting of pancreatic duct and coring out of head of the gland.* (B), *Roux-en-Y drainage of both the "filleted" duct and the cored-out head.*

pancreatitis.[42] However, long-term results with this technique and surgical denervation applied to patients with chronic pancreatitis have been unpredictable and generally poor.

Advances in endoscopic surgical techniques have rekindled an interest in minimally invasive denervation, especially thoracoscopic splanchnicectomy.[58] Several small series have shown good short-term pain relief after bilateral thoracoscopic splanchnicectomy. Preoperative differentiation of visceral from somatic pain with differential epidural analgesia may offer a useful tool for selection of patients. Historically disappointing results of thoracic splanchnicectomy by way of open thoracotomy emphasize the fact that longer follow-up and larger numbers of patients are needed to assess the efficacy of this approach.

CONCLUSION

Chronic pancreatitis remains a challenge to manage because of the variable progression of the disease, the high proportion of patients with alcohol and narcotic dependency, and the variable degree of glandular involvement. Patients with chronic pancreatitis come to the surgeon's attention because of complications of the disease, either as organ complications or pain that is unmanageable with conventional medical means. The wide variety of surgical options allows surgical therapy to be tailored to each patient's disease process. The goals of all surgical therapies, however, remain similar: to provide resolution of pain and organ complications and preserve as much pancreatic function as possible.

REFERENCES

1. Fung AS, Tsiotos GG, Sarr MG: ERCP-induced acute necrotizing pancreatitis: Is it a more severe disease? Pancreas 15:217-221, 1997
2. Sakorafas GH, Tsiotos GG, Sarr MG: Ischemia/reperfusion-induced pancreatitis. Dig Surg 17:3-14, 2000
3. Sakorafas GH, Tsiotos GG, Bower TC, Sarr MG: Ischemic necrotizing pancreatitis: two case reports and review of the literature. Int J Pancreatol 24:117-121, 1998
4. Runzi M, Layer P: Drug-associated pancreatitis: facts and fiction. Pancreas 13:100-109, 1996
5. Miller AR, Nagorney DM, Sarr MG: The surgical spectrum of hereditary pancreatitis in adults. Ann Surg 215:39-43, 1992
6. Johnson CD, Stephens DH, Sarr MG: CT of acute pancreatitis: correlation between lack of contrast enhancement and pancreatic necrosis. AJR Am J Roentgenol 156:93-95, 1991
7. Pederzoli P, Bassi C, Vesentini S, Campedelli A: A randomized multicenter clinical trial of antibiotic prophylaxis of septic complications in acute necrotizing pancreatitis with imipenem. Surg Gynecol Obstet 176:480-483, 1993
8. Grewe M, Tsiotos GG, Luque de-Leon E, Sarr MG: Fungal infection in acute necrotizing pancreatitis. J Am Coll Surg 188:408-414, 1999
9. Lehocky P, Sarr MG: Early enterol feeding in severe acute pancreatitis: Can it prevent secondary pancreatic (super) infection? Dig Surg 17:571-577, 2000
10. Ranson JH, Rifkind KM, Roses DF, Fink SD, Eng K, Spencer FC: Prognostic signs and the role of operative management in acute pancreatitis. Surg Gynecol Obstet 139:69-81, 1974
11. Knaus WA, Draper EA, Wagner DP, Zimmerman JE: APACHE II: a severity of disease classification system. Crit Care Med 13:818-829, 1985
12. Yeo CJ, Sarr MG: Cystic and pseudocystic diseases of the pancreas. Curr Probl Surg 31:165-243, 1994
13. Vitas GJ, Sarr MG: Selected management of pancreatic pseudocysts: operative versus expectant management. Surgery 111:123-130, 1992
14. Sakorafas GH, Tsiotos GG, Sarr MG: Extrapancreatic necrotizing pancreatitis with viable pancreas: a previously under-appreciated entity. J Am Coll Surg 188:643-648, 1999
15. Mier J, Leon EL, Castillo A, Robledo F, Blanco R: Early versus late necrosectomy in severe necrotizing pancreatitis. Am J Surg 173:71-75, 1997
16. Bradley EL III: A clinically based classification system for acute pancreatitis: summary of the International Symposium on Acute Pancreatitis, Atlanta, GA, September 11 through 13, 1992. Arch Surg 128:586-590, 1993
17. Beger HG, Buchler M, Bittner R, Block S, Nevalainen T, Roscher R: Necrosectomy and postoperative local lavage in necrotizing pancreatitis. Br J Surg 75:207-212, 1988
18. Pemberton JH, Nagorney DM, Becker JM, Ilstrup D, Dozois RR, Remine WH: Controlled open lesser sac drainage for pancreatic abscess. Ann Surg 203:600-604, 1986
19. Baron TH, Thaggard WG, Morgan DE, Stanley RJ: Endoscopic therapy for organized pancreatic necrosis. Gastroenterology 111:755-764, 1996
20. Rattner DW, Legermate DA, Lee MJ, Mueller PR, Warshaw AL: Early surgical debridement of symptomatic pancreatic necrosis is beneficial irrespective of infection. Am J Surg 163:105-109, 1992
21. Sarr MG: Surgical approach #2 to severe necrotizing pancreatitis. Curr Opin Crit Care 5:162-163, 1999
22. Sarr MG: Planned reoperative necrosectomy/debridement for necrotizing acute pancreatitis with delayed primary closure. Dig Surg 11:252-256, 1994
23. Davidson ED, Bradley EL III: "Marsupialization" in the treatment of pancreatic abscess. Surgery 89:252-256, 1981
24. Fernandez-del Castillo C, Rattner DW, Makary MA, Mostafavi A, McGrath D, Warshaw AL: Debridement and closed packing for the treatment of necrotizing pancreatitis. Ann Surg 228:676-684, 1998
25. Sarr MG, Nagorney DM, Mucha P Jr, Farnell MB, Johnson CD: Acute necrotizing pancreatitis: management by planned, staged pancreatic necrosectomy/debridement and delayed primary wound closure over drains. Br J Surg 78:576-581, 1991
26. Tsiotos GG, Luque-de Leon E, Soreide JA, Bannon MP, Zietlow SP, Baerga-Varela Y, Sarr MG: Management of necrotizing pancreatitis by repeated operative necrosectomy using a zipper technique. Am J Surg 175:91-98, 1998
27. Sarr MG: Appropriate use, complications and advantages demonstrated in 500 consecutive needle catheter jejunostomies. Br J Surg 86:557-561, 1999
28. Walters AM, Bender CE, Sarr MG: Percutaneous conversion of needle catheter jejunostomy to large bore jejunostomy for long term use. Surg Gynecol Obstet 173:397-398, 1991
29. Tsiotos GG, Smith CD, Sarr MG: Incidence and management of pancreatic and enteric fistulas after surgical management of severe necrotizing pancreatitis. Arch Surg 130:48-52, 1995
30. Johst P, Tsiotos GG, Sarr MG: Pancreatic ascites: a rare complication of necrotizing pancreatitis: a case report and review of the literature. Int J Pancreatol 22:151-154, 1997
31. Sakorafas GH, Sarr MG, Farnell MB: Pancreaticobiliary fistula: an unusual complication of necrotising pancreatitis. Eur J Surg 167:151-153, 2001
32. Sakorafas GH, Tsiotos GG, Sarr MG: Experience with duodenal necrosis: a rare complication of acute necrotizing pancreatitis. Int J Pancreatol 25:147-149, 1999
33. Tsiotos GG, Munoz Juarez MM, Sarr MG: Intraabdominal hemorrhage complicating surgical management of necrotizing pancreatitis. Pancreas 12:126-130, 1996
34. Sarr MG, Tsiotos GG: Necrosectomy for acute necrotizing pancreatitis. In Mastery of Surgery. Vol 2. Fourth edition. Edited by RJ Baker, JE Fischer. Philadelphia, Lippincott Williams & Wilkins, 2001, pp 1281-1287
35. Libsch K, Sarr MG: Necrotizing pancreatitis. In The Practice of General Surgery. Edited by KI Bland. Philadelphia, WB Saunders, 2002, pp 731-737
36. Tsiotos GG, Luque-de Leon E, Sarr MG: Long-term outcome of necrotizing pancreatitis treated by necrosectomy. Br J Surg 85:1650-1653, 1998
37. Sarner M, Cotton PB: Classification of pancreatitis. Gut 25:756-759, 1984
38. Sarr MG, Sakorafas GH: Incapacitating pain of chronic pancreatitis: a surgical perspective of what is known and what needs to be known. Gastrointest Endosc 49:S85-S89, 1999
39. Karanjia ND, Widdison AL, Leung F, Alvarez C, Lutrin FJ, Reber HA: Compartment syndrome in experimental chronic obstructive pancreatitis: effect of decompressing the main pancreatic duct. Br J Surg 81:259-264, 1994
40. Wong GY, Sakorafas GH, Tsiotos GG, Sarr MG: Palliation of pain in chronic pancreatitis: use of neural blocks and neurotomy. Surg Clin North Am 79:873-893, 1999

41. Sakorafas GH, Sarr MG, Farley DR, Farnell MB: The significance of sinistral portal hypertension complicating chronic pancreatitis. Am J Surg 179:129-133, 2000

42. Wong GY, Wiersema MJ, Sarr MG: Palliation of pain in adenocarcinoma of the pancreas. *In* Atlas of Clinical Oncology: Pancreatic Cancer. Edited by JL Cameron. Hamilton, Ontario, BC Decker, 2001, pp 231-246

43. Sakorafas GH, Farnell MB, Nagorney DM, Sarr MG: Surgical management of chronic pancreatitis at the Mayo clinic. Surg Clin North Am 81:457-465, 2001

44. Sakorafas GH, Sarr MG, Farley DR, Que FG, Andrews JC, Farnell MB: Hemosuccus pancreaticus complicating chronic pancreatitis: an obscure cause of upper gastrointestinal bleeding. Langenbecks Arch Surg 385:124-128, 2000

45. Sakorafas GH, Farnell MB, Farley DR, Rowland CM, Sarr MG: Long-term results after surgery for chronic pancreatitis. Int J Pancreatol 27:131-142, 2000

46. Sakorafas GH, Sarr MG: Changing trends in operations for chronic pancreatitis: a 22-year experience. Eur J Surg 166:633-637, 2000

47. Puestow CB, Gillesby WJ: Retrograde surgical drainage of pancreas for chronic relapsing pancreatitis. Arch Surg 76:898-907, 1958

48. Partington PF, Rochelle REL: Modified Puestow procedure for retrograde drainage of the pancreatic duct. Ann Surg 152:1037-1043, 1960

49. Sakorafas GH, Sarr MG: Tricks in the technique of lateral pancreaticojejunostomy. Eur J Surg 166:498-500, 2000

50. Mannell A, Adson MA, McIlrath DC, Ilstrup DM: Surgical management of chronic pancreatitis: long-term results in 141 patients. Br J Surg 75:467-472, 1988

51. Sakorafas GH, Sarr MG, Rowland CM, Farnell MB: Post-obstructive chronic pancreatitis: results with distal resection. Arch Surg 136:643-648, 2001

52. Stone WM, Sarr MG, Nagorney DM, McIlrath DC: Chronic pancreatitis: results of Whipple's resection and total pancreatectomy. Arch Surg 123:815-819, 1988

53. Sakorafas GH, Farnell MB, Nagorney DM, Sarr MG, Rowland CM: Pancreatoduodenectomy for chronic pancreatitis: long-term results in 105 patients. Arch Surg 135:517-523, 2000

54. Buchler MW, Friess H, Bittner R, Roscher R, Krautzberger W, Muller MW, Malfertheiner P, Berger HG: Duodenum-preserving pancreatic head resection: long-term results. J Gastrointest Surg 1:13-19, 1997

55. Frey CF, Amikura K: Local resection of the head of the pancreas combined with longitudinal pancreaticojejunostomy in the management of patients with chronic pancreatitis. Ann Surg 220:492-504, 1994

56. Buchler MW, Friess H, Muller MW, Wheatley AM, Beger HG: Randomized trial of duodenum-preserving pancreatic head resection versus pylorus-preserving Whipple in chronic pancreatitis. Am J Surg 169:65-69, 1995

57. Izbicki JR, Bloechle C, Knoefel WT, Kuechler T, Binmoeller KF, Broelsch CE: Duodenum-preserving resection of the head of the pancreas in chronic pancreatitis: a prospective, randomized trial. Ann Surg 221;350-358, 1995

58. Bradley EL III, Reynhout JA, Peer GL: Thoracoscopic splanchnicectomy for "small duct" chronic pancreatitis: case selection by differential epidural analgesia. J Gastrointest Surg 2:88-94, 1998

Chapter 21

PANCREAS TRANSPLANTATION AFTER COMPLICATIONS OF DIABETES MELLITUS

Mikel Prieto, M.D.
Scott L. Nyberg, M.D.
Mark D. Stegall, M.D.

BACKGROUND AND HISTORICAL CONSIDERATIONS

Type 1 diabetes mellitus is a major epidemiologic problem in the United States. The prevalence in the US population is estimated to be more than 1 million with about 30,000 new cases per year.[1] The annual direct and indirect costs of diabetes are believed to exceed 90 billion dollars.[1]

In recent years, major strides have been made in the medical treatment of patients with type 1 diabetes mellitus. These advances include intensive insulin therapy regimens, insulin pump devices, and strict control of hypertension and hypercholesterolemia.[2] However, a continuous insulin delivery device, coupled with a glucose-sensing device or an artificial pancreas, has not yet become available despite intensive research. Patients continue to require multiple insulin injections and blood glucose measurements to achieve usually imperfect and sometimes erratic control of their blood glucose. Many diabetic patients typically exhibit wide deviations in plasma glucose levels, which in the long term may be responsible for development of the secondary complications of diabetes.

Pancreas transplantation for the management of diabetes initially was considered in the 1960s during the early era of transplantation. At the time, diabetic patients were not considered candidates for kidney transplantation alone because of concerns that persistent diabetes might damage the transplanted kidney. A group of surgeons at the University of Minnesota led by Lillehei and Kelly performed the first combined transplantations of a kidney and a pancreaticoduodenal graft.[3] These early attempts were fraught with complications and high mortality, and the procedure was almost abandoned in the early 1970s. Pancreas transplantation remained an experimental procedure into the early 1980s. Before that time, it was performed at a few centers, but morbidity and mortality rates were high. In the 1980s, technical modifications eventually improved the success rate and limited complications. The introduction of more effective immunosuppressive agents (i.e., cyclosporine in the 1980s and tacrolimus in the 1990s) improved patient and graft survival to levels similar to those of kidney transplantation alone.[4-7] By 2001, the number of patients receiving pancreas transplants had increased to more than 1,300 per year in the United States.[7]

PANCREAS TRANSPLANTATION: INDICATIONS AND OUTCOMES

Diabetes mellitus is the most common cause of renal failure in the United States, and end-stage diabetic nephropathy is the most common indication for pancreas transplantation. Thus, most pancreas transplantations are performed in conjunction with kidney transplantation (Table 1) (simultaneous pancreas-kidney transplantation [SPK]). Alternatively, a living-donor kidney may be transplanted first, followed later by a cadaveric pancreas transplant when a donor becomes available (pancreas after kidney transplantation [PAK]). Some nonuremic diabetics might receive a pancreas transplant because of hypoglycemic unawareness or brittle diabetes (pancreas transplantation alone [PTA]). Of 1,319 pancreas transplants in 2001, 884 were SPKs, 304 were PAKs, and 131 were PTAs (Table 1). In recent years, the 1-year survival rate for pancreas grafts is approximately

Table 1.—Pancreas Transplantation in the United States

| Year | Type of transplantation, no. of patients | | | |
	SPK	PAK	PTA	Total
1999	934	220	121	1,275
2000	912	299	122	1,333
2001	884	304	131	1,319

PAK, pancreas after kidney transplantation; PTA, pancreas transplantation alone (see also Table 2); SPK, simultaneous pancreas-kidney transplantation.
Data from Scientific Registry of Transplant Recipients: Transplant Statistics: Annual Report: Reference Tables. Retrieved June 24, 2003, from the World Wide Web: http://www.ustransplant.org/annual_reports/ar02/refTables100/ar02_table_108_dh.htm.

92% for patients with SPK and 80% for those with PAK or PTA.[7]

At Mayo Clinic, Rochester, Minnesota, the overall approach to pancreas transplantation differs somewhat from the national approach. Our group favors living-donor kidney transplantation whenever possible, even in patients who might otherwise receive a pancreas transplant. Most of our pancreas transplants are PAK and PTA rather than SPK (Table 2).

DIABETES AND END-STAGE RENAL DISEASE

Diabetic patients with advanced renal insufficiency who are already undergoing dialysis or will require dialysis soon are the primary candidates for a pancreas transplant. Usually, these patients also are being considered for a kidney transplant. The evaluations for pancreas and kidney transplantation should be made concurrently.

If the patient has a suitable living kidney donor, we recommend living-donor kidney transplantation before pancreas transplantation, for several reasons. First, the long-term graft survival of a living-donor kidney (88% at 3 years) is greater than that of a cadaveric kidney allograft (78% at 3 years).[8] Second, in most instances, the recipient can undergo transplantation without having to undergo a period of dialysis (waiting times for a combined cadaver kidney-pancreas transplant are 3-5 years in most regions). Finally, maximizing the use of living-donor kidneys allows cadaveric kidneys to be allocated to recipients without a living donor. After the patient has received the kidney transplant and has recovered (usually 2-3 months), he or she is placed on the waiting list for a cadaveric PAK. Patients who do not have a living kidney donor are placed on a waiting list for SPK.

Patients with diabetes and renal failure routinely have extensive comorbid factors, such as severe peripheral vascular disease, coronary artery disease, obesity, neuropathy, and gastropathy. A pancreas transplant may add prohibitive risk to some patients. In these cases, a kidney transplant alone, especially from a living donor, may be a more reasonable option. Age is another consideration. In general, patients older than 55 years are less likely to receive pancreas allografts in conjunction with a kidney transplant.

PREOPERATIVE EVALUATION AND PREPARATION

The evaluation of a patient for kidney or pancreas transplantation should include a thorough history and physical examination, including an evaluation of renal function and cardiac status. The standard assessment of ischemic cardiac disease at our institution is dobutamine echocardiography. Most diabetic patients being evaluated for kidney or pancreas transplantation undergo this test. Patients with a positive result or with any signs or symptoms of ischemia undergo coronary angiography. When indicated, coronary angioplasty or bypass is performed before transplantation.

PANCREAS TRANSPLANTATION FOR NONUREMIC DIABETIC PATIENTS

Some patients are referred for pancreas transplantation because of quality-of-life issues associated with brittle diabetes. These patients undergo a thorough physical and laboratory evaluation, including measurement of their renal function. These patients are given a class of powerful immunosuppressive drugs called calcineurin inhibitors (e.g., cyclosporine, tacrolimus). These drugs are nephrotoxic and cause a decrease in renal function. For patients with moderate to advanced renal disease,

Table 2.—Pancreas Transplantation at Mayo Clinic, Rochester, Minnesota

| Year | Type of transplantation, no. of patients | | | |
	SPK	PAK	PTA	Total
2000	6	13	6	25
2001	4	30	14	48
2002	6	18	16	40

PAK, pancreas after kidney transplantation; PTA, pancreas transplantation alone; SPK, simultaneous pancreas-kidney transplantation.

nephrotoxicity may mean a premature progression to end-stage renal disease and dialysis. With this consideration in mind, we can separate candidates for a preemptive pancreas transplantation into three groups by their glomerular filtration rate (GFR): 1) more than 70 mL/min, 2) less than 35 mL/min, and 3) 35 mL/min to 70 mL/min.

Patients who have near-normal renal function (GFR > 70 mL/min) are good candidates for a preemptive pancreas transplant. They have less risk of postoperative renal dysfunction.

Patients with advanced renal dysfunction (GFR < 35 mL/min) are poor candidates for a preemptive pancreas transplant, because end-stage renal failure is likely to develop prematurely after transplantation. Most of these patients are placed on the waiting list for a combined kidney-pancreas transplant, or they are considered for a living-donor kidney transplant in preparation for a pancreas transplant.

The treatment of patients who have moderate renal dysfunction (GFR between 35 mL/min and 70 mL/min) is still controversial. They usually have normal or slightly increased serum creatinine levels and no clinical signs of uremia. When these patients receive a solitary pancreas transplant, they are at risk for progressive renal failure due to calcineurin-inhibitor nephrotoxicity. These patients have two options. If they have a living kidney donor, their first option is to receive a pancreas transplant with the understanding that they probably will also need a kidney transplant soon. In this situation, the living donor is a "backup" donor if the renal function of the patient deteriorates after transplantation. A second alternative for these patients is to wait until their renal function deteriorates enough to require a combined kidney-pancreas transplant or a living-donor kidney transplant followed by a pancreas transplant. All these decisions must be individualized for each patient and may vary greatly according to the specific circumstances.

ISLET TRANSPLANTATION

Pancreatic islet transplantation is an emerging treatment for nonuremic diabetic patients. It has been performed in humans since the 1970s, but in the past it was associated with a low success rate and negligible long-term insulin independence. However, a report of successful islet transplantation in seven consecutive patients has renewed enthusiasm about this procedure.[9] Several transplant centers in North America and Europe have started or plan to start an islet transplantation program as an option for nonuremic diabetic patients.

A major benefit of islet transplantation may be the ability to reverse diabetes successfully with less morbidity than pancreas transplantation. Corticosteroid-free immunosuppression and refinements in the isolation techniques seem to be the keys to successful islet transplantation. Islet transplantation undoubtedly will have an important role in the treatment of diabetes mellitus in the future.

BENEFITS OF PANCREAS TRANSPLANTATION

No prospective randomized trials have assessed the efficacy of pancreas transplantation on the secondary complications of diabetes. However, numerous single-center studies show that a successful pancreas transplantation leads to extremely good glycemic control with average glycosylated hemoglobin of 5% to 6%.[10] The presence of glucagon in the pancreas provides counterregulatory control, preventing hypoglycemia.

Several studies suggest that pancreas transplantation improves diabetic neuropathy. One study showed that nerve and muscle action potentials improved or remained stable in patients after successful pancreas transplantation, whereas these potentials continued to decrease in diabetic recipients whose pancreas transplants failed early after the procedure.[11] In a recent long-term study at Mayo Clinic, Rochester, Minnesota, nerve conduction improved in recipients of pancreas transplants, but the muscle strength of these patients remained low, possibly due to poor conditioning or myopathy.[12]

Pancreas transplantation has been reported to stabilize the progression of retinopathy, but the studies generally have been poorly controlled. One study of nonuremic pancreas transplant recipients showed apparent stabilization of retinopathy. In patients with successful pancreas transplants 5 years after transplantation, only 30% progressed to a more severe stage of retinopathy, whereas progression occurred in 55% of patients whose transplants failed.[13]

Pancreas transplantation clearly appears to prevent recurrence of diabetic nephropathy in the transplanted kidney. In almost all diabetic patients who receive only a kidney transplant, the lesions of diabetic nephropathy recur within 2 years of transplantation.[14] Yet, combining a pancreas transplant with a kidney graft will prevent these lesions. Recurrent diabetic nephropathy can destroy a transplanted kidney in patients with poor glycemic control, but the process may take more than a decade.

With diabetes as the leading cause of kidney failure, the preemptive use of pancreas transplantation might prevent development of kidney failure in native kidneys.[15] However, few data exist on the progression of kidney dysfunction in nonuremic patients. One study suggested that pancreas transplantation can reverse the lesions of diabetic nephropathy in native kidneys (e.g., decreased tubular basement membrane, decreased mesangial matrix volume), but glycemic control for longer than 5 years was necessary before detectable changes occurred.[16] As previously stated, the use of nephrotoxic immunosuppressive agents such as tacrolimus and cyclosporine in pancreas transplant recipients who are nonuremic usually leads to deterioration in native renal function. Indeed, in some patients with decreased renal function, PTA can lead to renal failure in the first few months after transplantation.

SURGICAL TECHNIQUE

Pancreas Recovery Procedure

The cadaveric donor pancreas procedure usually is performed during a multiorgan donor-recovery procedure by an experienced multiorgan transplant team. Pancreatic grafts usually are offered first within the local Organ Procurement Organization but frequently are shipped around the country to different transplant centers. Thus, a fairly standardized procedure has been developed. The entire multiorgan recovery procedure is not described in detail here. However, a few important points that relate directly to the pancreatic graft recovery are emphasized.

The pancreas is recovered as a whole organ with the duodenum and the spleen attached. The portal vein usually is transected at its midpoint. In the past, some liver transplant teams have taken the entire portal vein along with the liver graft, but this is unnecessary and frequently makes the pancreatic graft unusable.

The splenic artery is transected at its origin from the celiac trunk, and the superior mesenteric artery (SMA) is taken at its origin from the aorta. In the presence of a right-replaced hepatic artery, the SMA can be transected immediately distal to where this vessel takes off, so that the proximal SMA remains attached to the hepatic graft. In some cases, the liver transplant team does not have to take the SMA together with the right-replaced hepatic artery. Then the replaced hepatic artery can be transected at its origin from the SMA. The dissection of the pancreas can be completed either before or after the en bloc flushing of the abdominal organs with a cold preservation solution. To avoid overflushing the pancreas, which can result in edema, a vessel loop is placed around the origin of the SMA and the splenic arteries and is tightened after a liter of solution has been infused. A nasogastric tube is placed just distal to the pylorus, and the duodenum is flushed with an antibiotic solution. Then the duodenum is stapled just distal to the pylorus (proximal staple line) and distal to the ligament of Treitz (distal staple line). The root of the mesentery usually is transected with a vascular stapler. The pancreas is placed in a well-marked container, covered with solution, and double-bagged. In addition

to the pancreas, the iliac artery and vein of the donor (common, external, and internal iliac arteries and veins) are procured and placed in this container. The arterial iliac bifurcation is used during the bench-work procedure described below. The veins are saved for a possible lengthening of the graft's portal vein, which is rarely necessary. The pancreas then can be shipped to the recipient's transplant center for transplantation.

Bench-work Procedure

The bench-work procedure is performed before transplantation at the receiving transplant center where the procedure will be performed. The donor pancreas should be thoroughly inspected before the procedure is started. This careful inspection avoids last-minute surprises that might make the procedure technically impossible. The pancreas should be kept cold in a basin filled with preservation solution and ice. The goals of the bench-work procedure are to inspect the pancreas and identify any abnormalities or injuries, to remove the spleen, to remove excess duodenum and oversew the stapled ends of the duodenum, to inspect and tie off any small venous or arterial branches, and to anastomose an iliac arterial Y graft to the donor splenic and SMA arteries (Fig. 1).

The bench-work procedure starts with a careful inspection of the pancreas. The duodenum is examined for any evidence of trauma occurring either at the time of the initial injury or during the recovery procedure. The quality of the pancreas also is assessed. A fatty pancreas can be associated with a poorer outcome. Some centers routinely discard those organs. The portal vein and the splenic and SMAs are inspected. Excess adipose tissue usually attached to the pancreas is removed. The integrity of the vascular ligatures around the inferior mesenteric vein, distal common bile duct, and other important structures is ascertained.

A splenectomy is performed on suitable donor organs, care being taken to avoid any injury to the tail of the pancreas. This usually is done with double ligations of the main distal splenic artery and vein. After removal of the spleen, the ligament of Treitz is separated from the uncinate process of the pancreas, and the dissection is carried proximally to separate the fourth portion of the duodenum from the pancreas. The length of the duodenal segment that is left attached to the pancreas may depend on how densely attached the duodenum is to the pancreatic head. In general, shorter segments are preferred for bladder-drained grafts, because they lessen the amount of duodenal secretion into the bladder. After dissection, the distal duodenum is closed with a stapler, unless the bladder anastomosis will be performed with a stapler technique. In this case, the distal duodenum is left open until after completion of the bladder anastomosis. Both stapled ends of the duodenum, proximal and distal, are oversewn with a permanent suture such as polypropylene or silk. Before oversewing the proximal end of the duodenum, the surgeon should ascertain that there is no gastric remnant and that the transection was done distal to the pylorus.

Finally, the vascular structures are examined. To maximize the length of the portal vein, it is dissected proximally to the confluence of the splenic and superior mesenteric veins (Fig. 1). In addition, the transected end of the splenic artery and the SMA are dissected in preparation for placement of a Y graft of bifurcated iliac artery (Fig. 2 A). As explained above, during the organ procurement procedure, the donor iliac arteries from the aortic bifurcation to the inguinal ligament, including the internal iliac artery to the trifurcation, are obtained. The Y graft, consisting of common iliac, internal iliac, and external iliac arteries, is cleaned to remove all perivascular connective tissue. The integrity of the graft is confirmed. The Y graft is trimmed to size, usually with a short limb of the external iliac artery anastomosed end to end to the SMA and with a longer segment of the internal iliac artery anastomosed end to end to the splenic artery. These anastomoses are performed with 6-0 or 7-0 polypropylene suture. The length and positioning of the Y graft may help prevent postoperative arterial thrombosis. In general, the shorter the limbs of the graft, the less likely it will twist or kink.

Pancreatic Transplant Procedure

The transplantation is performed with the pancreas either as a solitary graft or in combination with a kidney transplant. The procedure itself is essentially the same, whether or not the kidney is transplanted simultaneously. At our institution, the pancreatic graft is placed preferentially in the right iliac fossa. For this reason, diabetic patients who undergo kidney transplantation with plans for a later pancreas transplantation usually have the kidney transplant attached to the left iliac vessels.

The transplant procedure starts with a midline incision that extends from about 3 cm above the umbilicus to the pubis. This incision is made down to the fascia, and the abdomen is entered through the midline. The cecum and right colon are mobilized medially and superiorly to expose the proximal right common iliac artery and vein, then a self-retaining retractor is placed. First, the common and external iliac arteries are dissected and looped with vascular loops. Then the common and external iliac veins are dissected similarly. In most cases, ligation and division of all the posterior branches of the iliac vein is necessary to bring the vein anteriorly and lateral to the iliac artery. Full mobilization of the iliac vein minimizes the difficulty of the portal-to-iliac anastomosis and the potential kinking and thrombosis of the vessels at the anastomosis. After immobilization, the pancreas can be brought onto the table and an end-to-side anastomosis can be performed between the portal vein and the iliac vein with a 5-0 or 6-0 polypropylene running suture. Similarly, the proximal end of the Y graft of donor common iliac artery is anastomosed to the midportion of the common iliac artery at a site proximal to the portal venous anastomosis with a 6-0 running polypropylene suture (Fig. 2 B).

After completion of these anastomoses, the vascular clamps are removed from the iliac vessels and the pancreas is reperfused. There is usually some bleeding from small peripancreatic vessels and the mesenteric staple line. Hemostasis is obtained readily, then the duodenal anastomosis is performed to divert pancreatic exocrine and duodenal secretions.

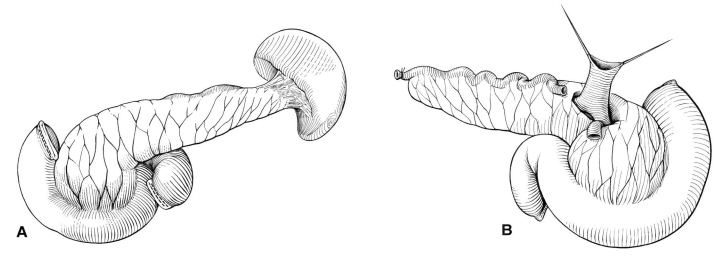

A   **B**

Fig. 1. (A), *Pancreas allograft with spleen attached after procurement but before the bench-work procedure.* (B), *Pancreas allograft after removal of spleen. Sutures are on the lengthened portal vein. The isolated splenic artery and celiac artery are identifiable.*

Pancreatic Exocrine Secretions

Whether bladder or enteric drainage is the best way to treat exocrine secretions after pancreas transplantation is still controversial. Both techniques are described briefly.

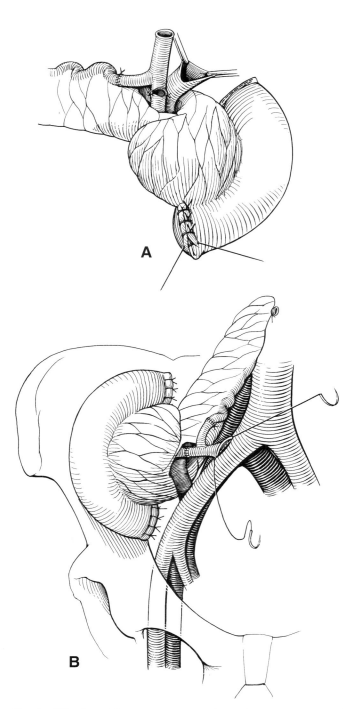

Fig. 2. (A), *Arterial reconstruction with an iliac arterial Y graft sewn to the splenic artery and the superior mesenteric artery.* (B), *Donor iliac arterial anastomosis to the common iliac artery of the recipient.*

Bladder Drainage

After the pancreas is placed in the right lower quadrant with its vessels anastomosed to the iliac vessels and the pancreatic tail placed in the right paracolic gutter, the duodenum is placed close to the bladder. This anastomosis can be hand sewn or stapled.

Hand-sewn Bladder Anastomosis

The anastomosis of the duodenum to the bladder (Fig. 3 *A*) is performed with a two-layer technique similar to a hand-sewn, bowel-to-bowel anastomosis. First, a posterior outer layer is placed with permanent nonabsorbable sutures such as polypropylene. The bladder and the duodenum are then opened and a full-thickness inner layer is placed with an absorbable suture such as a 4-0 polydioxanone suture. After completion of the posterior and inner layers, the anterior row of the external layer is completed.

Stapled Bladder Anastomosis

An end-to-end anastomosis (EEA) stapler is used to complete the bladder anastomosis. An anterior cystotomy is performed, and the EEA stapler, with the anvil removed, is passed through the distal open end of the duodenum to the midportion (Fig. 3 *B*). The tip of the EEA stapler is then passed through the duodenal wall and the posterior bladder wall. The anvil is placed inside the bladder through the anterior cystotomy and secured to the tip of the EEA stapler, which is then closed and fired. The stapled opening between the duodenum and the bladder usually is oversewn with a running layer of polydioxanone suture. The anterior cystotomy is closed in two layers with absorbable sutures. Stapling across the distal duodenum and oversewing the staple line complete the procedure.

Enteric Drainage

Enteric drainage has become the diversion technique of choice at many large transplant centers. This can be done with a simple side-to-side configuration (Fig. 4 *A*) or with creation of a Roux-en-Y limb to isolate the anastomosis from enteric contents (Fig. 4 *B*). The anastomosis between the duodenum and the recipient's distal ileum usually is performed as a standard two-layer side-to-side hand-sewn anastomosis with an internal absorbable layer and a permanent outer layer. Most surgeons place this anastomosis in the proximal ileum upstream from the ileocecal valve to prevent large amounts of pancreatic juice from emptying into the colon.

POSTOPERATIVE MANAGEMENT

In addition to the routine postoperative management of any patient with a major abdominal operation, patients with pancreas transplants present specific challenges. All these patients are diabetic, and many also have extensive coronary artery disease and other comorbidities. Careful monitoring of hemodynamic and cardiovascular factors immediately after the procedure is important. In these patients, extreme swings in systolic and diastolic blood pressure and heart rate should be avoided because they can induce myocardial ischemia. In addition, hypotension in the immediate postoperative period has been associated with graft thrombosis. Pancreatic grafts, particularly in nonuremic diabetics, are at higher risk for vascular thrombosis. These patients usually are given aspirin and subcutaneous or intravenous heparin infusion. Bladder-drained grafts do not require a nasogastric tube. Many of these patients have a return of bowel function within a few days after transplantation. Patients typically are hospitalized 5 to 7 days after pancreas transplantation.

Immunosuppression

Historically, pancreas transplants have had a greater rate of rejection than other organs. In addition, monitoring for rejection can be more difficult. For these reasons, especially in preemptive pancreas transplantations, most transplant centers use a combination of calcineurin-based maintenance immunosuppression protocols and antilymphocytic induction therapy.[17] Our current protocol includes antithymocyte rabbit immunoglobulin (Thymoglobulin) induction for 7 to 10 days, in addition to tacrolimus, mycophenolate mofetil, and prednisone.[18] This regimen has reduced the acute rejection rate of PTA and PAK in our patients to less than 10%, and immunologic graft loss is rare (Fig. 5).

Monitoring for Rejection

In SPK when the pancreas and the kidney are derived from the same donor, serum creatinine is a relatively reliable marker for rejection of either organ. However, markers for rejection in PAK and PTA are somewhat lacking. In our experience, biochemical markers, such as serum lipase and amylase or urinary amylase (in a bladder-drained pancreas), are helpful in monitoring patients for rejection. However, we also use protocol pancreas allograft biopsies to monitor for rejection. These biopsies are performed percutaneously with ultrasound guidance at 3 weeks and 3 months after transplantation. In a recent study from our institution, 10% of patients without biochemical abnormalities showed rejection on biopsy at these points.[18] Conversely, biopsies can help confirm rejection suggested by biochemical abnormalities. In the same study, we found that one-third of patients with biochemical evidence of

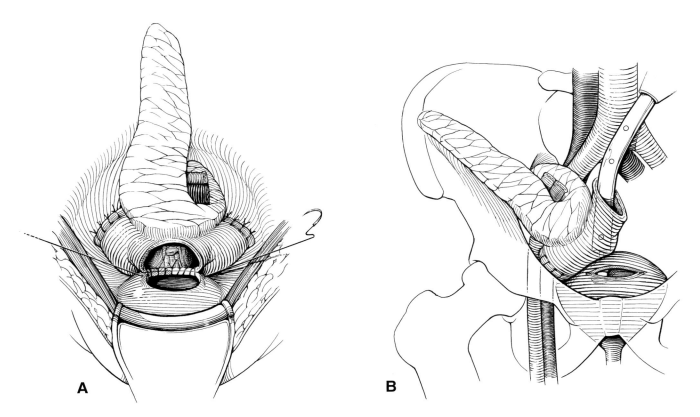

Fig. 3. Bladder drainage of exocrine secretions. (A), *Hand-sewn duodenocystostomy.* (B), *Stapled anastomosis.*

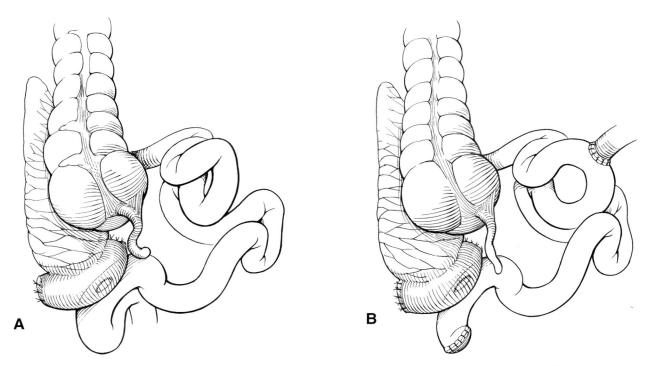

Fig. 4. Enteric drainage of the exocrine pancreas. (A), A side-to-side duodenal-ileal anastomosis. (B), A duodenal-ileal Roux-en-Y anastomosis.

rejection had a normal pancreas biopsy. Rarely, graft pain, malaise, and fever are associated with rejection. Hyperglycemia in the early posttransplantation period usually is caused by the diabetogenic effects of drugs,

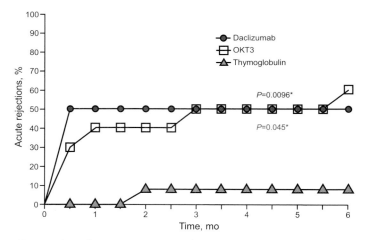

Fig. 5. Actual rejection rates in solitary pancreas transplantation (PAK + PTA) during the first 6 months after transplantation at Mayo Clinic, Rochester, Minnesota, using three different antibody induction regimens (daclizumab, n=6; OKT3, n=10; and Thymoglobulin, n=13). Significance determined by the χ^2 test. OKT3, muromonab-3; PAK, pancreas after kidney transplantation; PTA, pancreas transplantation alone. (From Stegall et al.[18] By permission of Lippincott Williams & Wilkins.)

such as corticosteroids and tacrolimus, and rarely indicates rejection. However, hyperglycemia that occurs months after transplantation may indicate advanced, irreversible, chronic rejection.

After dismissal from the hospital, patients are monitored closely as outpatients by transplant physicians and coordinators. Frequent blood tests and visits to the transplant center are routine during the first month.

Postoperative Complications

Allograft Rejection

Rejection of a pancreas transplant usually is manifested by moderate increases in serum amylase and serum lipase and by a sharp decline in urine amylase in bladder-drained grafts. The urine amylase is collected and reported as a timed collection in international units per hour (usually for 8-12 hours). This is done because the enzyme is secreted directly into the bladder and not cleared through the kidney. Therefore, normal variations in urine volume falsely affect the amylase concentration in the urine. The rate of rejection for pancreas transplants has decreased progressively since the introduction of stronger maintenance immunosuppression and induction therapy. At our institution, for example, the rate of pancreas allograft rejection is less than 10%, which compares well to the rates for kidney transplants. The treatment for these rejection episodes usually includes a monoclonal or poly-clonal antibody against activated lymphocytes such as OKT3 or Thymoglobulin. A change in fasting serum glucose usually indicates an unfavorable prognosis. By the time hyperglycemia ensues, most islets in the graft have been destroyed.

Thrombosis

Graft thrombosis is the most common cause of early post-operative graft loss. Thrombosis is relatively rare in SPK recipients, probably due to the mild coagulopathy associated with uremia. However, the rate of graft thrombosis in PAK and PTA recipients is higher, ranging from 2% to 10%. The postoperative edema that sometimes occurs in the pancreas, usually because of factors associated with the donor operation or the preservation time, may be a contributing factor. Enteric drainage grafts also have been associated with a higher rate of graft thrombosis than bladder-drainage grafts. This may be due to increased mobility of the head of the pancreas causing a twisting or rotating motion in the vascular pedicle.

Pancreatic graft thrombosis usually is manifested by a sudden increase in serum glucose. The diagnosis is confirmed by ultrasonography consistent with no perfusion of the gland. Affected patients require a graft pancreatectomy. Salvaging the graft by thrombectomy is seldom possible.

Graft Pancreatitis

The complication of graft pancreatitis can occur early or late in the posttransplantation course. The pathogenesis differs in these two situations. In the immediate post-transplantation period, graft pancreatitis usually is due to a preservation or reperfusion injury. A major postoperative increase in pancreatic serum enzymes often occurs in the first few days. Close monitoring of the serum chemistry values usually shows progressive normalization. Postoperative graft pancreatitis that occurs later usually is caused by the reflux of urine into the pancreatic duct (reflux pancreatitis) or by a urinary tract infection in bladder-drained grafts. Reflux pancreatitis is treated initially by placement of a Foley catheter to decompress the urinary tract. Reflux pancreatitis can be differentiated from acute allograft rejection with a percutaneous biopsy guided by computed tomography. Patients with a neurogenic bladder and major voiding difficulties are particularly prone to reflux pancreatitis and ultimately may require conversion of the transplant from bladder to enteric drainage.

Postoperative Bleeding

To prevent graft thrombosis, especially in nonuremic patients, many centers use anticoagulation therapy with intravenous heparin infusion. These patients are at risk for postoperative bleeding, requiring blood transfusions and reexploration. Unlike thrombosis, though, this complication rarely is associated with graft loss or increased morbidity. The bleeding site rarely is the vascular anastomosis itself. Instead, bleeding usually emanates from small venous branches in the body and tail of the pancreas.

Another site of hemorrhage can be the bladder or the enteric anastomosis. This complication is manifested by gross hematuria in bladder-drainage grafts or by bleeding in the lower gastrointestinal tract in enteric-drainage grafts. This complication usually is treated conservatively with blood transfusions, close hemodynamic monitoring, and continuous bladder irrigation. These episodes tend to be self-limiting and usually require no surgical intervention. When bleeding persists or causes hemodynamic instability, bladder-drainage grafts require cystoscopy and fulguration, and enteric-drainage grafts may require laparotomy and takedown of the enteric anastomosis.

Bladder or Enteric Anastomotic Breakdown

Anastomotic breakdown is more difficult to manage in patients with enteric-drainage grafts because of the extensive intraperitoneal contamination usually associated with it. Small-bladder anastomotic leaks can be treated conservatively by continuous bladder decompression with a Foley catheter. If an operation is required, the surgical procedure may be limited to oversewing the perforation in cases of small leaks with little intra-abdominal contamination. Larger leaks may require takedown of the anastomosis and conversion from bladder-to-enteric or enteric-to-bladder drainage. Patients with extensive contamination, sepsis, or duodenal necrosis may require a transplant pancreatectomy and withdrawal of immunosuppression.

Metabolic Acidosis

Metabolic acidosis typically occurs in patients with bladder-drained pancreatic grafts. The large amount of bicarbonate-rich pancreatic fluid secreted into the bladder causes dehydration and metabolic acidosis. This condition is observed more frequently in patients with moderate or extensive renal dysfunction. In these patients, the acid-base regulatory mechanisms of the kidney are impaired and, therefore, cannot compensate for the bicarbonate loss. This complication usually occurs a few weeks to months after transplantation and usually resolves within the first year. Severe symptoms and multiple rehospitalizations may indicate the need for conversion from bladder to enteric drainage.

Urethritis and Cystitis

Urethritis and cystitis are rare complications associated with bladder-drainage grafts. In most patients, the pancreatic enzymes secreted into the bladder are inactive and cause no symptoms, despite their high concentration in urine. However, a small subset of patients may have acute or chronic chemically induced inflammation of the distal urinary tract. This complication is treated initially conservatively with Foley catheterization. In recurring or severe cases, it may require conversion from bladder drainage to enteric drainage.

CONCLUSION

A successful whole-organ pancreas transplant reproducibly elicits euglycemia in patients with diabetes mellitus. In recent years, advances in immunosuppression and surgical technique have improved graft survival greatly. Pancreas transplantation is indicated in most type 1 diabetic patients with end-stage renal failure who require a kidney transplant. Increasingly, pancreas transplantation after a kidney transplantation is being used with as much success as an SPK. Although controversies about immunosuppression and surgical technique remain, these procedures have become an accepted treatment option for such patients. In addition, pancreas or islet transplantation should be considered as a therapeutic option for nonuremic diabetic patients who have brittle diabetes, impaired quality of life, or early secondary complications.

REFERENCES

1. American Diabetes Association: Standards of medical care for patients with diabetes mellitus. Diabetes Care 17:616-623, 1994

2. The Diabetes Control and Complications Trial Research Group: The effect of intensive treatment of diabetes on the development and progression of long-term complications in insulin-dependent diabetes mellitus. N Engl J Med 329:977-986, 1993

3. Kelly WD, Lillehei RC, Merkel FK, Idezuki Y, Goetz FC: Allotransplantation of the pancreas and duodenum along with the kidney in diabetic nephropathy. Surgery 61:827-837, 1967

4. Gruessner RW, Sutherland DE, Najarian JS, Dunn DL, Gruessner AC: Solitary pancreas transplantation for nonuremic patients with labile insulin-dependent diabetes mellitus. Transplantation 64:1572-1577, 1997

5. Bartlet ST, Schweitzer EJ, Johnson LB, Kuo PC, Papadimitriou JC, Drachenberg CB, Klassen DK, Hoehn-Saric EW, Weir MR, Imbembo AL: Equivalent success of simultaneous pancreas kidney and solitary pancreas transplantation: a prospective trial of tacrolimus immunosuppression with percutaneous biopsy. Ann Surg 224:440-449, 1996

6. Gruessner RW, Burke GW, Stratta R, Sollinger H, Benedetti E, Marsh C, Stock P, Boudreaux JP, Martin M, Drangstveit MB, Sutherland DE, Gruessner A: A multicenter analysis of the first experience with FK506 for induction and rescue therapy after pancreas transplantation. Transplantation 61:261-273, 1996

7. Gruessner AC, Sutherland DE: Analyses of pancreas transplant outcomes for United States cases reported to the United Network for Organ Sharing (UNOS) and non-US cases reported to the International Pancreas Transplant Registry (IPTR). Clin Transpl 1999, pp 51-69

8. Scientific Registry of Transplant Recipients. Retrieved June 24, 2003, from the World Wide Web: http://www.ustransplant.org/tables/KI200211-10CL.HTML

9. Shapiro AM, Lakey JR, Ryan EA, Korbutt GS, Toth E, Warnock GL, Kneteman NM, Rajotte RV: Islet transplantation in seven patients with type 1 diabetes mellitus using a glucocorticoid-free immunosuppressive regimen. N Engl J Med 343:230-238, 2000

10. Stegall MD, Simon M, Wachs ME, Chan L, Nolan C, Kam I: Mycophenolate mofetil decreases rejection in simultaneous pancreas-kidney transplantation when combined with tacrolimus or cyclosporine. Transplantation 64:1695-1700, 1997

11. Kennedy WR, Navarro X, Goetz FC, Sutherland DE, Najarian JS: Effects of pancreatic transplantation on diabetic neuropathy. N Engl J Med 322:1031-1037, 1990

12. Dyck PJ, Velosa JA, Pach JM, Sterioff S, Larson TS, Norell JE, O'Brien PC, Dyck PJB: Increased weakness after pancreas and kidney transplantation. Transplantation 72:1403-1408, 2001

13. Ramsay RC, Goetz FC, Sutherland DE, Mauer SM, Robison LL, Cantrill HL, Knobloch WH, Najarian JS: Progression of diabetic retinopathy after pancreas transplantation for insulin-dependent diabetes mellitus. N Engl J Med 318:208-214, 1988

14. Bilous RW, Mauer SM, Sutherland DE, Najarian JS, Goetz FC, Steffes MW: The effects of pancreas transplantation on the glomerular structure of renal allografts in patients with insulin-dependent diabetes. N Engl J Med 321:80-85, 1989

15. Stegall MD, Larson TS, Kudva YC, Grande JP, Nyberg SL, Prieto M, Velosa JA, Rizza RA: Pancreas transplantation for the prevention of diabetic nephropathy. Mayo Clin Proc 75:49-56, 2000

16. Fioretto P, Steffes MW, Sutherland DE, Goetz FC, Mauer M: Reversal of lesions of diabetic nephropathy after pancreas transplantation. N Engl J Med 339:69-75, 1998

17. Stegall MD, Kim DY, Larson TS: Immunosuppression in pancreas transplantation. Graft 4:500-507, 2001

18. Stegall MD, Kim DY, Prieto M, Cohen AJ, Griffin MD, Schwab TR, Nyberg SL, Velosa JA, Gloor JM, Innocenti F, Bohorquez H, Dean PG, Carpenter HA, Leontovich ON, Sterioff S, Larson TS: Thymoglobulin induction decreases rejection in solitary pancreas transplantation. Transplantation 72:1671-1675, 2001

CYSTIC TUMORS OF THE PANCREAS

Glenroy Heywood, M.D.
Jon A. van Heerden, M.D.

Cystic tumors of the pancreas have been recognized and broadly categorized for more than a century. However, during the past decade, interest in these primary cystic neoplasms has increased, for many reasons. First, improvements in, and the availability of newer methods of, pancreatic imaging, such as computed tomography, ultrasonography, and magnetic resonance imaging, have increased our recognition of this often asymptomatic entity. Second, in 1978, Compagno and Oertel[1,2] made an important contribution to our understanding of the association of the histopathologic features and natural history or malignant potential of these cystic neoplasms. They clearly differentiated the benign serous cystadenoma from the potentially or overtly malignant mucinous cystadenoma and cystadenocarcinoma. Third, this distinction has highlighted the importance of preoperative radiologic and histopathologic differentiation of these two entities from inflammatory pancreatic pseudocysts, because there is a radical difference in their respective management. In many patients, cystic neoplasms have been incorrectly diagnosed and treated as pancreatic pseudocysts and occasionally managed by "cyst"-enteric drainage. Finally, there has been a momentum toward surgical resection of pancreatic lesions because of the decreased morbidity and mortality after pancreatic resection and the optimistic reports of improvement in long-term survival.

HISTOPATHOLOGIC CLASSIFICATION

Primary cystic neoplasms of the pancreas are lesions of epithelial and other origins. But epithelial neoplasms by far make up the majority (90%) of these cystic tumors.[3]

Compagno and Oertel[1,2] revolutionized our understanding of these neoplasms in 1978 when they defined the cell type of the epithelial lining and outlined the differences in tumor biology, natural history, and malignant potential of cystic neoplasms based on the differentiation of serous from mucinous lesions. Because of this seminal work, the vast majority of primary cystic neoplasms of the pancreas are now classified into either of two groups: serous or mucinous cystic neoplasms. This classification is tremendously important because serous neoplasms are uniformly benign[2] and mucinous neoplasms have a latent or overt risk of malignancy (Table 1).[1] Our group[4] recently described a novel histopathologic classification of mucinous cystic neoplasms into three types: mucinous cystadenoma, noninvasive proliferative cystic neoplasm, and invasive mucinous

Table 1.—Primary Cystic Neoplasms of the Pancreas

Serous cystadenoma*
Mucinous cystadenoma and cystadenocarcinoma spectrum*
Intraductal papillary mucinous neoplasms*
Acinar cell cystadenocarcinoma
Cystic teratoma
Cystic islet cell neoplasm
Cystic choriocarcinoma
Angiomatous neoplasms
    Angiomas
    Lymphangiomas
    Hemangioendotheliomas

*Most common.

cystadenocarcinoma. This categorization seems to predict long-term outcome after complete operative resection.

Serous Cystadenoma

The gross appearance of serous cystic neoplasms is typically that of a honeycombed cluster of small cysts with diameters of less than 2 cm (Fig. 1 A).[5] These neoplasms vary in size from a few centimeters to as large as 25 cm (mean size, 6-10 cm). The cyst wall is usually thin, is almost translucent, and separates easily from the surrounding structures. These features are due to the lack of inflammatory or fibrous reaction, which, in contrast, is so typical in pancreatic pseudocysts.[5] The fluid content in the cysts is usually clear, lacks mucin, and is of low viscosity. There is no obvious anatomical predilection, but serous cystadenomas tend to occur more frequently in the head of the pancreas, in contrast to mucinous cystadenomas, which are often found in the body and tail.[6]

The cysts are lined by a low cuboidal, bland-appearing, glycogen-rich epithelium (Fig. 1 B).[6] The epithelium is discontinuous in 40% of specimens.[7] Electron microscopic and immunohistochemical studies have suggested that the cell of origin of serous cystadenomas is the centroacinar cell[8] and not the pancreatic mucin-producing ductal cells, thought to be the origin of mucinous cystic neoplasms.[9] Hence, their epithelium does not produce mucin, one of the distinguishing features. The lack of characteristic cellular features of atypia or dysplasia in the epithelium[6] supports the benign nature of these neoplasms.

The fibrous stroma separating the cystic areas is relatively vascular and may calcify, giving rise to the characteristic sunburst, radial, or stellate scar pattern on computed tomography (Fig. 1 C).[6,10] When present, this finding is diagnostic.

The lining epithelial cells stain richly for glycogen, but specific stains for mucin, chromogranin, neuropeptides, endocrine peptides, and carcinoembryonic antigen are characteristically negative.[2,11] In analyses of the cystic fluid, concentrations of other markers such as carbohydrate antigens 19-9, 72-4, 15.3, and 125 are usually low.[12,13]

Mucinous Cystadenoma

Mucinous cystic neoplasms, in contrast, exhibit a more varied and heterogeneous spectrum, ranging from the benign cystadenoma with an underlying but yet true potential for malignant transformation to the uncommon cystadenocarcinoma with tissue invasion and aggressive metastatic potential.[1]

Grossly, mucinous cystic neoplasms are often different from their microcystic serous counterpart. These neoplasms typically consist of large cysts with septa, peripheral calcification, and sometimes a solid component (Fig. 2 A).[14] They are characterized by a macrocystic appearance with less than six cysts, each usually larger than 2 cm in diameter and a tumor diameter of up to 25 cm (mean, 8-10

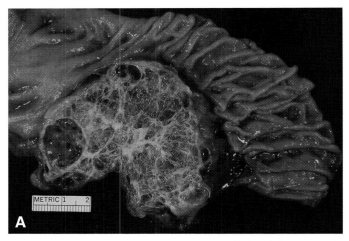

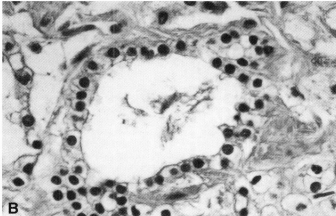

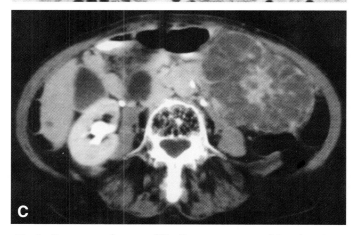

Fig. 1. Serous cystadenoma. (A), Gross appearance. Note the microcystic honeycombed appearance. (B), Cyst lined with low cuboidal epithelium and separated by a vascular fibrous stroma. (C), Computed tomography scan with calcification of the intercystic stroma, showing a characteristic sunburst, radial, or central stellate scar. (B from Pyke et al.[6] By permission of Lippincott Williams & Wilkins.)

cm).[5] Infrequently, the neoplasm has only one macrocyst. Individual cysts typically contain thin or thick papillary fronds or septa that, when present on computed tomography, ultrasonography, or magnetic resonance imaging, are diagnostic. In the absence of malignant transformation and invasion, the surrounding tissues usually lack any inflammatory reaction. The intracystic fluid is thicker and more viscous than in serous cystadenomas and it contains mucus. Although there is no anatomical predilection, these neoplasms more commonly occur in the body and tail of the pancreas.[7]

The cysts are lined by a tall columnar epithelium that produces mucin (Fig. 2 B). The histopathologic spectrum varies from a uniform layer of mucinous cells, as found in benign mucinous cystadenoma, to a more proliferative subtype composed of various degrees of atypia, dysplasia, papillary epithelial infolding, and even carcinoma in situ but without tissue invasion.[4] In contrast, the invasive variant (mucinous cystadenocarcinoma) may contain both benign and proliferative epithelium but with areas of frank stromal invasion. This invasive variant is relatively rare. Mucinous tumors are notorious for having discontinuous

areas of atypia, dysplasia, carcinoma in situ, and frankly invasive carcinoma within the same neoplasm.[7]

The lining epithelium stains for mucin and for specific stains such as carcinoembryonic antigen, serotonin, and somatostatin, thus supporting a possible origin from ductal or stem cells.[15] Cystic fluid concentrations of carbohydrate antigen 19-9, 72-4, 15.3, and 125 and viscosity are usually increased.[12,15]

Intraductal Papillary Mucinous Tumor
Intraductal papillary mucinous tumors, often described as intraductal papillary neoplasms[16] or mucinous ductal ectasia,[17] have attracted considerable attention since the report in 1982 by Ohhashi et al.,[18] who proposed that they constitute an entity that is clinically distinct from mucinous cystic neoplasms.

Grossly, there is ectasia of the main pancreatic duct or branch ducts (Fig. 3). Ectatic branch ducts sometimes appear as a grapelike cluster of mucin-filled structures around the main pancreatic duct.[19] Ductal dilatation varies from a generalized dilatation of the main pancreatic duct throughout all or part of its extent to a more segmental dilatation of the pancreatic ducts involving a major segment of the gland. The dilated ducts are usually filled with mucin or with grossly visible papillary neoplasms ranging from 0.7 to 7.5 cm.[19,20] It is unclear whether the ductal dilatation is due to partial obstruction from mucin or to the abnormal dysplastic ductal epithelium.

Microscopically (Fig. 4), the epithelial lining, either in the main pancreatic duct or in branch ducts, is flat, micropapillary, or grossly papillary and may involve segments of simple tall columnar cells with other areas representing the spectrum of changes from mucinous hyperplasia to severe dysplasia to frank carcinoma.[19] In situ or invasive cancer is present at diagnosis in 30% to 50% of patients.[19,21]

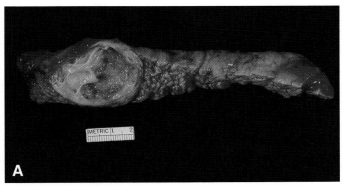

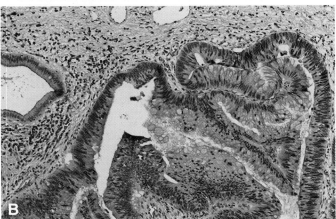

Fig. 2. Mucinous cystadenoma. (A), Gross features. In this specimen from a Whipple procedure, the macrocystic adenoma of the head of the pancreas has been cut across to show the presence of a large cyst. (B), Cysts lined with tall mucin-containing columnar epithelium.

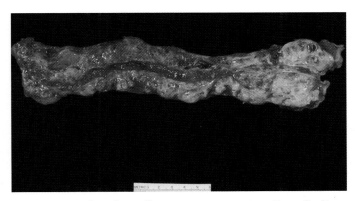

Fig. 3. Intraductal papillary mucinous tumor. Gross findings. The main pancreatic duct is diffusely ectatic, and the pancreatic parenchyma is atrophied in association with chronic pancreatitis.

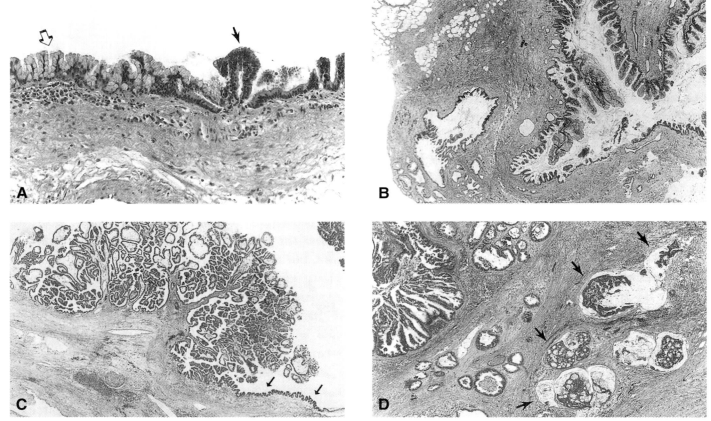

Fig. 4. Intraductal papillary mucinous tumor. Microscopic findings. (A), *Micropapillary dysplasia* (closed arrow) *can be distinguished from nonneoplastic micropapillary hyperplasia* (open arrow) *by the increased nuclear:cytoplasmic ratio, hyperchromasia, and tightly packed nuclei in micropapillary dysplasia.* (B), *Dysplasia frequently extends from the main pancreatic duct into branch ducts.* (C), *Grossly visible papillomas arise from zones of flat or micropapillary dysplasia* (arrows). (D), *Invasive adenocarcinoma component* (arrows), *in this case showing colloid carcinoma-like growth. (From Loftus et al.[19] By permission of the American Gastroenterological Association.)*

Immunohistochemical analyses of *p53* and *Ki-67* showed that tissue expression of the oncogenes was considerably greater in malignant intraductal papillary mucinous tumor than in the benign counterpart.[22] In another study,[23] point mutations were detected in the K-*ras* oncogene and in the *p53* tumor suppressor gene in pancreatic juice. These findings suggest that alterations of K-*ras* and *p53* genes are common in the development of intraductal papillary mucinous tumor, and genetic analysis of these in pancreatic juice may be a useful tool in diagnosis and management of this disease.[23,24]

DIAGNOSIS AND IMAGING

Cystic neoplasms of the pancreas are a diagnostic challenge for the clinician and the pathologist. As a result, many cases have been misdiagnosed. In a report from Massachusetts General Hospital,[25] as many as one-third of all pancreatic cystic neoplasms and 40% of mucinous tumors referred to that institution were previously misdiagnosed as

pancreatic pseudocysts; as a result, many were treated inappropriately. General guidelines (Table 2) may assist in the initial screening of a patient with a peripancreatic cystic mass. Patients with pancreatic pseudocysts are usually male, tend to be younger (<50 years), and usually give a clear history of acute or chronic pancreatitis due to alcohol abuse or trauma. Diagnostic imaging usually shows a single cyst with a thick wall and without multiple loculations. Frequently there are associated pancreatic and retroperitoneal inflammatory changes. The concentration of amylase in both serum and cyst is usually increased. In contrast, patients with cystic neoplasms are generally older (>50 years) and female and lack a recent history of pancreatic abnormality. Diagnostic imaging often shows multiple cysts without pancreatic or peripancreatic inflammatory changes. The concentration of amylase in serum and cyst fluid is usually normal in patients with cystic neoplasms.

Most cystic neoplasms are found during diagnostic imaging for an unrelated complaint. Unlike many other

Table 2.—Guidelines for the Differentiation of Cystic Neoplasms From Pancreatic Pseudocysts

Characteristic	Cystic neoplasm	Pseudocyst
Age	Older	Younger
Sex	Male < female	Male > female
Pancreatic event	Absent	Present
Imaging	Multiple cysts without adjacent inflammation	Single cyst with peripancreatic inflammation
Endoscopic retrograde pancreatography	Normal	Ductal changes, communication with cyst (>70%)
Serum amylase value	Normal	Increased (50%-70%)
Cyst fluid amylase value	Normal	Increased
Gross appearance	Thin wall, not adherent to adjacent structures, clear cyst fluid	Thick wall, adherent to adjacent structures, cyst fluid dirty

pancreatic disorders, no symptoms or signs are pathogno-monic of cystic neoplasms. When symptoms are present, they usually are related to the effects of the pancreatic mass. There may be a vague feeling of epigastric or left upper abdominal fullness and early satiety.[6] Although many of the tumors are very large, they rarely cause duodenal obstruction or obstructive jaundice from bile duct obstruction. Because they do not invade the retroperitoneum, back pain is unlikely and infrequent.

The clinician needs to maintain a suspicion that a cystic neoplasm is present, especially in a patient with a large pancreatic mass without duodenal obstruction, jaundice, pain, or a history of acute or chronic pancreatic disease. Exceptions are patients with intraductal papillary mucinous tumor, who may have a different presentation. The majority of these patients present with epigastric or back pain, acute or chronic pancreatitis, and pancreatic insufficiency.[19] Because most peripancreatic masses are not neoplastic, an objective diagnosis of cystic neoplasms relies strongly on diagnostic imaging that shows a cystic pancreatic mass and on the appropriate clinical presentation.

After a peripancreatic cystic lesion is discovered, three important and logical diagnostic steps follow: first, confirmation of the intrapancreatic origin of the cyst; second, ruling out the diagnosis of a pseudocyst; and third, identification of cystic neoplasms that will necessitate resection because of existing or potential malignancy.

Computed Tomography and Ultrasonography

The initial challenge for the surgeon is the preoperative differentiation of true cystic neoplasms from pancreatic pseudocysts. This often can be accomplished with reasonable certainty using computed tomography and ultrasonography.[5] However, these methods are less reliable for the differentiation of complex, multiloculated pseudocysts, cystic islet cell tumors, or other rare cystic neoplasms.

Endoscopic ultrasonography makes it possible to demonstrate the pancreatic parenchyma in more detail than is possible with conventional transabdominal ultrasonography. Endoscopic ultrasonography also can differentiate cystic and solid pancreatic tumors and detect localized cystic lesions or papillary projections in the cystic lesions.[26]

Pancreatic pseudocysts usually are single without multiple loculations. The wall is usually thick and is rarely calcified. There is often associated peripancreatic and retroperitoneal inflammation. The presence of a peculiar solid component within the wall of a cyst is virtually pathognomonic of a cystic neoplasm and should help in the differentiation from pseudocyst.

Serous neoplasms, as mentioned earlier, are typically multicystic (Fig. 5 A) and usually consist of cysts less than 2 cm.[5] Central calcification is present in about 20% of serous cystadenomas that give rise to a "sunburst" or stellate central scar on computed tomography.[6,10]

Mucinous cystic neoplasms are usually composed of fewer than six cysts with sizes generally more than 2 cm (Fig. 5 B), hence the older term "macro-cystic."[5] On computed tomography, 20% of mucinous cystadenomas have some calcification,[7] which tends to be patchy and peripheral. When the calcification is eggshell in appearance, there is an increased likelihood of a mucinous cystadenocarcinoma.[7] Size of the cyst is of no discriminating value, and computed tomography and ultrasonography are unable to differentiate benign from malignant mucinous cystadenoma in the absence of metastatic disease.

Computed tomography and ultrasonography are very accurate for delineating the markedly dilated pancreatic duct in intraductal papillary mucinous tumor.[19] These studies usually show diffusely dilated ducts with filling defects suggestive of mucin, segmental cystic lesions, and associated macrocystic lesions independent of the ductal system.[19,27,28] Intraductal ultrasonography[29] is a new

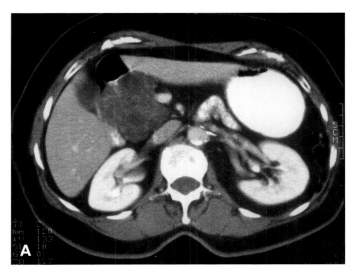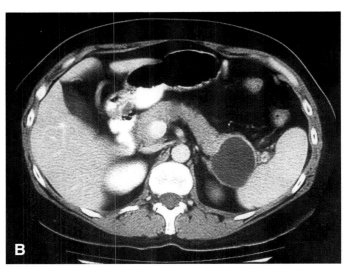

Fig. 5. (A), *Serous cystadenoma. Computed tomography scan showing enhancement of the septa separating the cysts.* (B), *Mucinous cystadenoma. Computed tomography scan showing a hypodense lesion in the tail of the pancreas surrounded by a thick vascularized capsule.*

method that allows more detailed diagnosis of pancreatic tumors and is relatively precise in the diagnosis of cystic lesions. With the duodenoscope, the ultrasonographic microprobe is inserted into the main pancreatic duct through the papilla of Vater. This probe provides clear pictures of the internal architecture and demographics of the pancreas. Intraductal ultrasonography can visualize the duct epithelium clearly. The ultrasonographic findings suggestive of malignancy are irregular wall thickness, mural nodules, mucous echoes, and solid tumors with a mixed echogenic pattern.[30] There is great optimism that this method will be very useful for differentiating benign from malignant mucin-producing pancreatic tumors. However, this technology is still in its infancy, and further studies will be required to define its role clearly. Generally, if the diagnosis remains uncertain after computed tomography and ultrasonography, endoscopic retrograde cholangiopancreatography or magnetic resonance cholangiopancreatography may be recommended.

Endoscopic Retrograde Pancreatography and Magnetic Resonance Pancreatography

Endoscopic retrograde pancreatography and magnetic resonance pancreatography offer little additional benefit in the evaluation of serous or mucinous neoplasms, primarily because there is usually no communication with the pancreatic ductal system.[14] These studies may be helpful for differentiating cystic neoplasms from pancreatic pseudocysts that may have ductal communication. Endoscopic retrograde pancreatography was considered the imaging standard for the diagnosis of intraductal papillary mucinous tumor, revealing a segmental or diffusely dilated ductal system and intraductal filling defects due to mucinous

concretions of duct-associated neoplastic lesions (Fig. 6 *A*).[31] Mucin oozing from the papilla of Vater at the time of duodenoscopy is relatively specific for intraductal papillary mucinous tumor.[20] Although this capability is lost with magnetic resonance pancreatography, it has the benefit of good ductal delineation without the invasive risks (Fig. 6 *B*). Intraductal papillary mucinous tumor may represent two clinically distinct subtypes: main duct tumors and branch duct tumors.[32] Main duct tumors are found more frequently in the body or tail of the pancreas and branch duct tumors in the head of the pancreas, especially in the uncinate process. Endoscopic retrograde pancreatography and magnetic resonance pancreatography can distinguish these two subtypes.

Angiography

Angiography has little additional discriminative value. However, it may show enhancement of the vascular stroma separating the microcystic areas in serous cystadenoma, but at least 30% of mucinous cystic neoplasms are hypervascular and show a similar stromal vascular enhancement.[7]

Laparoscopy

Since its inception, laparoscopy has gained widespread application in both diagnosis and staging of many pancreatic diseases. Schachter et al.[33] reported their experience with laparoscopy and laparoscopic ultrasonography for the management of pancreatic cystic lesions. In 15 patients, information obtained from laparoscopic ultrasonography contributed new data in eight patients (53%) when compared with conventional imaging. Unfortunately, the authors did not state whether this additional information changed the preoperative diagnosis obtained

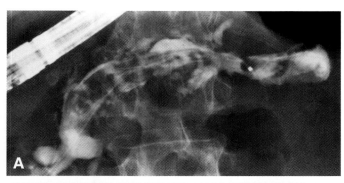
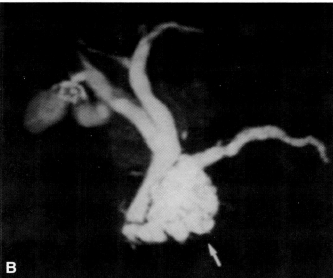

Fig. 6. Intraductal papillary mucinous tumor. (A), Representative endoscopic retrograde pancreatography scan showing diffuse dilatation of the main pancreatic duct with numerous intraluminal filling defects. (B), Three-dimensional magnetic resonance pancreatography scan showing the entire dilated side branch (arrow) *with the main pancreatic duct. (B from Sai J: MRCP: Early Diagnosis of Pancreatobiliary Diseases. Tokyo, Springer-Verlag, 2000, p 105. By permission of Springer-Verlag Tokyo.)*

nature of serous cystadenoma, its exceedingly rare incidence of malignant transformation,[34] and the formidable morbidity and mortality rates of pancreatic resection.[35-37] This therapeutic philosophy has changed currently to a more aggressive surgical approach, primarily a result of the decline in the mortality rate after major pancreatic operation,[38-40] the increasing reports of complications of serous cystadenoma,[41] the rare possibility of malignant transformation (seven reported patients with malignant serous cystadenocarcinoma),[42] the rare, but real, complications from preoperative diagnostic procedures,[7,25] and, most importantly, the inability for confident differentiation of benign serous from premalignant mucinous neoplasms.

When resection is contemplated, the following factors are considered: the clinical presentation and symptoms, the certainty of a preoperative diagnosis of serous cystadenoma versus a mucinous neoplasm, the safety of pancreatic resection, the experience of the surgeon, and the potential consequences of nonresective treatment.

Conservative management is justified for a well-documented asymptomatic serous cystadenoma without duct or vascular obstruction.[43] This approach is, however, reserved for the frail, elderly patient with substantial comorbidity who is a poor surgical risk.[6] If this nonresectional management is adopted, the patient should be followed at least annually with computed tomography or ultrasonography because complications develop unpredictably in some tumors.[43] Most importantly, both the patient and the surgeon must be cognizant of the small risk for misdiagnosis of a mucinous for a serous neoplasm.

Although conservative management is acceptable, conservative operation such as enucleation, cystenterostomy, external drainage, or percutaneous intracystic sclerosis is usually not suggested. Again, with the exception of the symptomatic high-risk patient, consideration may be given to bypass-type procedures without formal resection. In our practice, simple cyst enucleation and local cyst resection have been associated with an extremely high risk of pancreatic leak and fistulas.[6]

Mucinous Cystic Neoplasm
In contrast to serous cystadenomas, mucinous cystic neoplasms have a latent or overt potential for malignant transformation.[1] Therefore, appropriate management necessitates complete resection, even when the patient is asymptomatic and regardless of whether the lesion is located in the proximal or distal pancreas. This resection is often relatively straightforward because of the preponderance of lesions in the body or tail of the pancreas amenable to distal pancreatectomy. However, extensive resection of neighboring organs and, if necessary (albeit rarely), the portal vein is justified because the 5-year

with conventional imaging. They reported a sensitivity of 78%, with two false-positive examinations. This approach of laparoscopy, biopsy of the cyst wall, and analysis of tumor markers in cyst fluid needs further evaluation to determine its role in the diagnostic algorithm of pancreatic cystic lesions.

INDICATION FOR OPERATION AND CONDUCT OF OPERATION

Serous Cystadenoma
Historically, the prevailing therapeutic philosophy for serous cystadenoma was that of judicious observation. This conservative approach was based on the indolent

survival rate may surpass 50%, which far exceeds that of ductal adenocarcinoma after complete resection.[44] As an example, in one series,[45] four patients with presumably mucinous cystadenocarcinoma and vascular involvement (one with gastroduodenal, two with portal vein encasement) were alive at a median follow-up of 4 years after complete resection.

Intraductal Papillary Mucinous Tumor

Intraductal papillary mucinous tumors also manifest a high latent or overt malignant potential. In all likelihood, all of the pancreatic duct epithelium is at risk, except for the unusual patient with localized segmental disease.[19] Therefore, total pancreatectomy is often advocated. However, because total pancreatectomy might not be an appropriate consideration in some patients, a lesser pancreatectomy must be considered. Many groups, especially from Japan, have sought to stratify patients according to whether the predominant area of involvement is the main duct or branch duct.[32,46,47] This clinical differentiation of intraductal papillary mucinous tumors involving the main duct and branch duct may have prognostic and therapeutic importance. In some series,[46,48,49] the rates of malignancy were higher for main duct tumors than for branch duct tumors. They recommended distal pancreatectomy for most main duct tumors and total pancreatectomy on occasion, depending on the degree of diffuse ductal dilatation or when a cancer-free margin cannot be achieved.[32] Pancreatoduodenectomy is recommended for branch duct tumors, which occur most frequently in the pancreatic head. Further studies will be needed to determine whether these are truly two distinct subtypes on which to base management decisions. Nevertheless, these neoplasms should be resected to remove all the adenomatous or malignant mucosa to prevent recurrence in the pancreatic remnant. The extent of resection can be facilitated by intraoperative frozen-section examination of the resection margin and possibly by pancreatoscopy.

Cystic Neoplasm Discovered Incidentally at Operation

A very difficult management scenario is the appropriate treatment when a cystic neoplasm of the pancreas is found incidentally during celiotomy for another cause. The dilemma is the need for gross differentiation of serous from mucinous neoplasms without the benefit of preoperative imaging. Intraoperative ultrasonography may offer some assistance. Management is governed by the "5-S rule" (symptoms, site, safety, surgeon, and spread). The factors discussed earlier in regard to the management of patients without symptoms must be applied. The site of the pancreatic lesion will affect the surgical decision; for instance, if the tumor is located in the body and tail, then a distal pancreatectomy, which is associated with low morbidity and mortality, is acceptable without attempts at histologic differentiation. Tumors in the proximal pancreas pose a much more difficult problem, and the safety of resection and experience of the surgeon become most important because of the potentially high morbidity and mortality rates associated with proximal pancreatectomy. Any diagnostic maneuver that could spread tumor cells should not be attempted. An open biopsy could potentially spill tumor cells, and the discontinuous epithelium could lead to a misdiagnosis of benignity. Transduodenal needle biopsy and aspiration of cyst content for amylase, mucin, or quick assay of tumor markers may be indicated. Rapid intraoperative immunocytochemical staining, using antibodies against carbohydrate antigen 19-9, carcinoembryonic antigen, and other related antigens, may become a useful adjunct in this clinical situation if this analysis becomes readily available.[50] If cyst fluid analysis reveals mucin or mucinous epithelium, then a diagnosis of mucinous cystic neoplasm can be made confidently, thus warranting simultaneous or delayed resection. If the cyst fluid analysis does not show mucin or a mucinous epithelium, then repeat intraoperative biopsies, more extensive analysis of markers, and radiologic imaging should be obtained.

ADJUVANT THERAPY

The role of adjuvant chemotherapy or radiation in the treatment of epithelial cystic neoplasms of the pancreas is as yet undefined. The indication for such therapy is likely related to the histologic classifications.

Serous cystadenomas are usually benign and require no further therapy, except for the extremely rare malignant serous cystadenocarcinoma, for which adjuvant therapy could be considered. Mucinous cystic neoplasms have a more varied and heterogeneous spectrum, and thus the selection of patients for adjuvant treatment is more difficult. However, our recent detailed clinicopathologic classification appears to correlate with outcome and may help in selection of the high-risk patient for whom adjuvant chemotherapy or radiation therapy is indicated. The benign mucinous and proliferative mucinous neoplasms likely will not require further therapy, because none of the 77 patients in our series[4] had recurrent disease with up to 30 years of follow-up. There was only one 5-year survivor in the group of patients with the malignant variant of invasive mucinous cystadenocarcinoma. Therefore, adjuvant chemotherapy and radiation therapy should strongly be considered for this group despite a curative resection and also for patients in whom the surgical margin is unclear or involved. Two reports[51,52] suggest a possible benefit of 5-fluorouracil and external beam radiation therapy for mucinous cystadenocarcinoma.

The appropriate management of intraductal papillary mucinous tumor is unclear, as is any role for adjuvant therapy. Because it is a mucinous neoplasm, the recommendation concerning adjuvant treatment is probably similar to that for mucinous cystic neoplasms. Several reports have suggested that main duct tumors have higher rates of malignancy than branch duct tumors.[46,48,49] But most importantly, main duct tumors with stromal invasion appear to have a more aggressive course[32] and probably should be considered for adjuvant therapy.

SURGICAL OUTCOMES AND LONG-TERM FOLLOW-UP

Serous Cystic Neoplasm
Nearly all serous cystadenomas are benign tumors,[2] and thus operative excision should provide cure for all patients, except for the rare patient with the malignant variant of cystadenocarcinoma, which has been documented histologically in only seven patients.[42,53-57]

Morbidity and Mortality Rates
In our series reported in 1992,[6] the operative morbidity rate was 38%. Six patients had pancreatic fistulas, two of whom had undergone enucleation. Both of these patients required reoperative management of the fistulas. Other complications necessitating reoperation included bile leaks, gastric stasis, pancreatic pseudocyst formation, and postoperative pancreatitis. The operative mortality rate was 10%; one patient had pulmonary embolus, two patients had superior mesenteric artery occlusion, and one patient had an undetermined cause of death.

Survival
Patients will have an excellent prognosis because their disease-specific mortality should be almost zero, except for the rare patient with cystadenocarcinoma. The median survival in our series was 16 years; the survival rate was 90% at 2 years, 81% at 5 years, and 64% at 10 years.

The accompanying operative morbidity and mortality rates for this generally benign neoplasm make the concept of preoperative diagnosis of serous cystadenoma very important. Conservative management is wholly justified for a well-documented serous cystadenoma. However, the potential consequences of nonresective treatment must be considered and include a very small risk of malignant transformation,[42] hemorrhage, chronic pancreatitis, recurrent acute pancreatitis,[6] or slow progressive enlargement with the eventual development of obstructive symptoms. Therefore, patients should be followed with annual ultrasonography.

Mucinous Cystic Neoplasm
We suggest and support a very aggressive surgical approach for mucinous cystic neoplasms. The prevailing understanding was that mucinous cystadenomas are biologically benign and have a favorable prognosis after complete resection.[34] Mucinous cystadenocarcinoma is considered to be less aggressive from a malignant standpoint than the more common ductal adenocarcinoma.[44] Previous work, including data from our institution, reported 5-year survival rates of 60% to 70% after complete resection of mucinous cystadenocarcinomas.[34] Reported recurrence rates after resection of cystadenocarcinomas vary widely and are unpredictable.

We recently reclassified these neoplasms as mucinous cystadenomas, noninvasive proliferative mucinous cystic neoplasms, or invasive cystadenocarcinomas according to specific histologic criteria.[4] Tumors were designated as mucinous cystadenomas if they contained a single layer of uniform cuboidal or columnar mucin-containing cells with no dysplasia (Fig. 7). Neoplasms were classified as noninvasive proliferative mucinous cystic neoplasms (Fig. 8) if areas of epithelium consisted of multiple cell layers (three or more) or microscopic or gross polypoid formations with or without low- or high-grade dysplasia but without objective evidence of invasion. This group also included neoplasms with gross intracystic polyp formation but without tissue invasion. Lesions with invasion were classified as invasive mucinous cystadenocarcinomas (Fig. 9). Invasion was documented by one or more of the following features: infiltrating irregular dysplastic glands with stromal desmoplasia, irregular nest of cells, single cell invasion, or invasion of the vascular space. We applied this classification to all patients who underwent

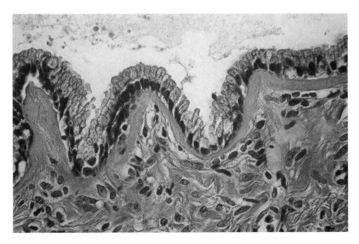

Fig. 7. Mucinous cystadenoma of the pancreas, histologic features. Monotonously regular, single layer of benign-appearing mucinous epithelial cells. (From Sarr et al.[4] By permission of Lippincott Williams & Wilkins.)

curative resection for cystic mucinous neoplasms at Mayo Clinic in Rochester, Minnesota, from 1940-1997. Results are outlined in the following paragraphs.

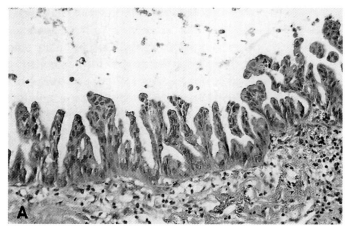

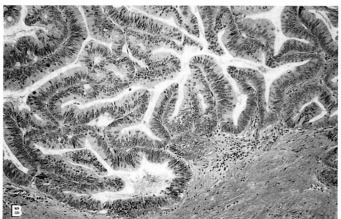

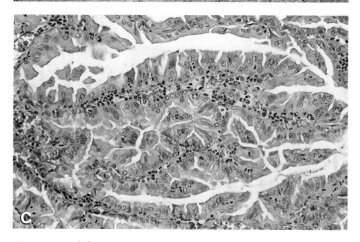

Fig. 8. Proliferative mucinous cystic neoplasms of the pancreas, spectrum of histologic changes. (A), Irregular papillary epithelial growth. Epithelial cells heaped up; nuclei mildly atypical. (B), Papillary epithelial fronds with low-grade nuclear dysplasia. (C), High-grade nuclear dysplasia and papillary or polypoid intracystic growth. (From Sarr et al.[4] By permission of Lippincott Williams & Wilkins.)

1. Mucinous cystadenoma (54 patients): Considerable postoperative morbidity occurred in six patients and included reoperation for drainage of an intraoperative abscess in two, operative drainage of a pancreatic pseudocyst in two, and pancreaticocutaneous fistula in two. There was one operative mortality (2%) related to postoperative fistula and hemorrhage 2 months after cyst enucleation. There were no recurrences in this group after a mean follow-up of 11 years (range, 2-31 years). The 5-year survival rate was 89%; of the six intervening deaths, one was operative, and five were due to unrelated causes. There was no disease-specific death among the 26 patients followed for more than 10 years.

2. Noninvasive proliferative cystic neoplasms (23 patients): Considerable morbidity occurred in one patient in whom an intra-abdominal abscess developed. There was one operative mortality (4%) related to multiple system organ failure after completion proximal pancreatectomy. There has been no recurrence in this group of patients after a follow-up of 8 years (range, 2-25 years). There was no disease-specific death among the patients followed for more than 10 years.

3. Mucinous cystadenocarcinoma (7 patients): There was one operative death (14%) after pancreatoduodenectomy but no serious postoperative morbidity. Only one patient survived longer than 5 years without evidence of recurrent carcinoma. This patient had only a single microscopic focus of stromal invasion. According to this proposed histologic classification, benign cystadenomas and noninvasive proliferative mucinous cystic neoplasms

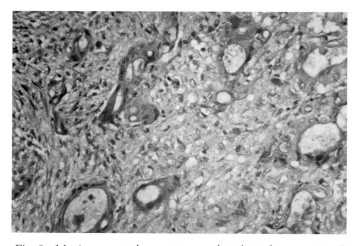

Fig. 9. Mucinous cystadenocarcinoma, histologic features. Small irregular glands and single cells with high-grade nuclear dysplasia invading the stroma and eliciting a desmoplastic stromal response (i.e., proliferating fibroblast surrounding infiltrating malignant epithelium). (From Sarr et al.[4] By permission of Lippincott Williams & Wilkins.)

do not recur after complete resection and probably do not need follow-up as aggressive as would be expected for invasive mucinous cystadenocarcinomas.

4. Intraductal papillary mucinous tumors: There have been many reports about this tumor since it was first described in 1982.[16,27,58] However, many issues, such as diagnosis, prognosis, and selection of the most appropriate surgical management, remain unclear. Similar to mucinous cystic neoplasms, prognosis is strongly associated with the presence of stromal invasion. In our series,[19] 4 of the 15 patients (27%) had obvious invasive carcinoma at operation, and 3 died; none of the 11 patients without invasion died of recurrence. Other groups have reported similar survival for patients with invasive intraductal papillary mucinous tumors.[28] Intraductal ultrasonography[29] is an emerging technology that so far has shown promise for the detection of carcinoma in situ and small tumors and for assessing the intraductal spread of tumor, parenchymal invasion, and the presence of intraductal mural nodules. This method may greatly improve our ability to diagnose, treat, and follow these patients.

CONCLUSION

After a peripancreatic cystic lesion is discovered, the clinician should 1) confirm the intrapancreatic origin of the cyst, 2) rule out the diagnosis of a pseudocyst, and 3) identify cystic neoplasms that will require resection because of existing or potential malignancy. Most cystic neoplasms of the pancreas can be recognized and differentiated from one another and from other benign cystic disorders of the pancreas on the basis of clinical presentation and an objective imaging test. The biologic characteristics of each subset of cystic neoplasms are distinctly different, and these are reflected in the differences in their management.

Serous cystadenomas are the most common type of cystic neoplasm of the pancreas and are universally benign, except for the extremely rare serous cystadenocarcinoma. Surgical resection is advocated for good-risk patients because benignity can be determined reliably only by histologic examination after pancreatic resection. However, conservative management is justified for a well-documented serous cystadenoma that is asymptomatic without ductal or vascular obstruction in a frail, elderly patient with considerable comorbidity who is a poor surgical risk.

Mucinous cystic neoplasms have a latent or overt potential for malignant transformation; therefore, complete resection is considered the appropriate management. With complete resection and adequate histopathologic examination based on our novel classification scheme, absence of tissue invasion predicts a curative operation. In contrast, a histologic diagnosis of invasive cystadenocarcinoma portends a dismal prognosis, similar to ductal adenocarcinoma of the pancreas.

Intraductal papillary mucinous tumor manifests a high latent or overt malignant potential. However, its management remains somewhat uncertain because the entire ductal epithelium may be at risk. The procedure of choice is complete surgical excision of the involved epithelium. Total pancreatectomy is required for diffuse tumor involving the entire duct, but it should be tailored to the individual patient. Pancreatoduodenectomy is reasonable for segmental lesions involving only the proximal pancreatic duct and, similarly, a distal pancreatectomy is reasonable for lesions involving only the distal gland. Segmental pancreatectomy recently was suggested as a reasonable surgical procedure for localized lesions, but long-term follow-up is required to determine the adequacy of this procedure.

The role of neoadjuvant or adjuvant chemotherapy or radiation in the treatment of epithelial cystic neoplasms of the pancreas is as yet undefined. Mucinous cystic neoplasms and intraductal papillary mucinous tumors with invasion should be considered for adjuvant chemotherapy and radiation therapy despite a curative resection.

Emerging technologies such as intraductal ultrasonography and immunohistochemical analysis for oncogenes or tumor suppressor genes may greatly improve our ability to diagnose, treat, and follow patients with cystic neoplasms of the pancreas.

REFERENCES

1. Compagno J, Oertel JE: Mucinous cystic neoplasms of the pancreas with overt and latent malignancy (cystadenocarcinoma and cystadenoma): a clinicopathologic study of 41 cases. Am J Clin Pathol 69:573-580, 1978

2. Compagno J, Oertel JE: Microcystic adenomas of the pancreas (glycogen-rich cystadenomas): a clinicopathologic study of 34 cases. Am J Clin Pathol 69:289-298, 1978

3. Fernandez-del Castillo C, Warshaw AL: Cystic tumors of the pancreas. Surg Clin North Am 75:1001-1016, 1995

4. Sarr MG, Carpenter HA, Prabhakar LP, Orchard TF, Hughes S, van Heerden JA, DiMagno EP: Clinical and pathologic correlation of 84 mucinous cystic neoplasms of the pancreas: Can one reliably differentiate benign from malignant (or premalignant) neoplasms? Ann Surg 231:205-212, 2000

5. Johnson CD, Stephens DH, Charboneau JW, Carpenter HA, Welch TJ: Cystic pancreatic tumors: CT and sonographic assessment. AJR Am J Roentgenol 151:1133-1138, 1988

6. Pyke CM, van Heerden JA, Colby TV, Sarr MG, Weaver AL: The spectrum of serous cystadenoma of the pancreas: clinical, pathologic, and surgical aspects. Ann Surg 215:132-139, 1992

7. Warshaw AL, Compton CC, Lewandrowski K, Cardenosa G, Mueller PR: Cystic tumors of the pancreas: new clinical, radiologic, and pathologic observations in 67 patients. Ann Surg 212:432-443, 1990

8. Alpert LC, Truong LD, Bossart MI, Spjut HJ: Microcystic adenoma (serous cystadenoma) of the pancreas: a study of 14 cases with immunohistochemical and electron-microscopic correlation. Am J Surg Pathol 12:251-263, 1988

9. Albores-Saavedra J, Gould EW, Angeles-Angeles A, Henson DE: Cystic tumors of the pancreas. Pathol Annu 25:19-50, 1990

10. Ghahremani GG, Meyers MA, Port RB: Calcified primary tumors of the gastrointestinal tract. Gastrointest Radiol 2:331-339, 1978

11. Levy M, Levy P, Hammel P, Zins M, Vilgrain V, Amouyal G, Amouyal P, Molas G, Flejou JF, Voitot H: Diagnosis of cystadenomas and cystadenocarcinomas of the pancreas: study of 35 cases [French]. Gastroenterol Clin Biol 19:189-196, 1995

12. Lewandrowski KB, Southern JF, Pins MR, Compton CC, Warshaw AL: Cyst fluid analysis in the differential diagnosis of pancreatic cysts: a comparison of pseudocysts, serous cystadenomas, mucinous cystic neoplasms, and mucinous cystadenocarcinoma. Ann Surg 217:41-47, 1993

13. Hammel P, Levy P, Voitot H, Levy M, Vilgrain V, Zins M, Flejou JF, Molas G, Ruszniewski P, Bernades P: Preoperative cyst fluid analysis is useful for the differential diagnosis of cystic lesions of the pancreas. Gastroenterology 108:1230-1235, 1995

14. Yeo CJ, Sarr MG: Cystic and pseudocystic diseases of the pancreas. Curr Probl Surg 31:165-243, 1994

15. Albores-Saavedra J, Angeles-Angeles A, Nadji M, Henson DE, Alvarez L: Mucinous cystadenocarcinoma of the pancreas: morphologic and immunocytochemical observations. Am J Surg Pathol 11:11-20, 1987

16. Conley CR, Scheithauer BW, van Heerden JA, Weiland LH: Diffuse intraductal papillary adenocarcinoma of the pancreas. Ann Surg 205:246-249, 1987

17. Agostini S, Choux R, Payan MJ, Sastre B, Sahel J, Clement JP: Mucinous pancreatic duct ectasia in the body of the pancreas. Radiology 170:815-816, 1989

18. Ohhashi K, Murakimi Y, Maruyama M, Takekoshi T, Ohta H, Ohhashi I: Four cases of mucous secreting pancreatic cancer [Japanese]. Prog Dig Endosc 20:348-351, 1982

19. Loftus EV Jr, Olivares-Pakzad BA, Batts KP, Adkins MC, Stephens DH, Sarr MG, DiMagno EP: Intraductal papillary-mucinous tumors of the pancreas: clinicopathologic features, outcome, and nomenclature. Members of the Pancreas Clinic, and Pancreatic Surgeons of Mayo Clinic. Gastroenterology 110:1909-1918, 1996

20. Rickaert F, Cremer M, Deviere J, Tavares L, Lambilliotte JP, Schroder S, Wurbs D, Kloppel G: Intraductal mucin-hypersecreting neoplasms of the pancreas: a clinicopathologic study of eight patients. Gastroenterology 101:512-519, 1991

21. Kloppel G: Clinicopathologic view of intraductal papillary-mucinous tumor of the pancreas. Hepatogastroenterology 45:1981-1985, 1998

22. Islam HK, Fujioka Y, Tomidokoro T, Sugiura H, Takahashi T, Kondo S, Katoh H: Immunohistochemical analysis of expression of molecular biologic factors in intraductal papillary-mucinous tumors of pancreas—diagnostic and biologic significance. Hepatogastroenterology 46:2599-2605, 1999

23. Kaino M, Kondoh S, Okita S, Hatano S, Shiraishi K, Kaino S, Okita K: Detection of K-ras and p53 gene mutations in pancreatic juice for the diagnosis of intraductal papillary mucinous tumors. Pancreas 18:294-299, 1999

24. Kondo G: Study on effects of mouth guard on ventilation [Japanese]. Kokubyo Gakkai Zasshi 64:326-347, 1997

25. Warshaw AL, Rutledge PL: Cystic tumors mistaken for pancreatic pseudocysts. Ann Surg 205:393-398, 1987

26. Kobayashi G, Fujita N, Lee S, Kimura K, Watanabe H, Mochizuki F: Correlation between ultrasonographic findings and pathological diagnosis of mucin producing tumor of the pancreas [Japanese]. Nippon Shokakibyo Gakkai Zasshi 87:235-242, 1990

27. Morohoshi T, Kanda M, Asanuma K, Kloppel G: Intraductal papillary neoplasms of the pancreas: a clinicopathologic study of six patients. Cancer 64:1329-1335, 1989

28. Nagai E, Ueki T, Chijiiwa K, Tanaka M, Tsuneyoshi M: Intraductal papillary mucinous neoplasms of the pancreas associated with so-called "mucinous ductal ectasia": histochemical and immunohistochemical analysis of 29 cases. Am J Surg Pathol 19:576-589, 1995

29. Furukawa T, Oohashi K, Yamao K, Naitoh Y, Hirooka Y, Taki T, Itoh A, Hayakawa S, Watanabe Y, Goto H, Hayakawa T: Intraductal ultrasonography of the pancreas: development and clinical potential. Endoscopy 29:561-569, 1997

30. Inui K, Nakazawa S, Yoshino J, Yamachika H, Kanemaki N, Wakabayashi T, Okushima K, Taki N, Nakamura Y, Takashima T, Hattori T, Miyoshi H: Mucin-producing tumor of the pancreas—intraluminal ultrasonography. Hepatogastroenterology 45:1996-2000, 1998

31. Dabezies MA, Campana T, Friedman AC: ERCP in the diagnosis of ductectatic mucinous cystadenocarcinoma of the pancreas. Gastrointest Endosc 36:410-411, 1990

32. Kobari M, Egawa S, Shibuya K, Shimamura H, Sunamura M, Takeda K, Matsuno S, Furukawa T: Intraductal papillary mucinous tumors of the pancreas comprise 2 clinical subtypes: differences in clinical characteristics and surgical management. Arch Surg 134:1131-1136, 1999

33. Schachter PP, Avni Y, Gvirz G, Rosen A, Czerniak A: The impact of laparoscopy and laparoscopic ultrasound on the management of pancreatic cystic lesions. Arch Surg 135:260-264, 2000

34. Hodgkinson DJ, ReMine WH, Weiland LH: Pancreatic cystadenoma: a clinicopathologic study of 45 cases. Arch Surg 113:512-519, 1978

35. Morris PJ, Nardi GL: Pancreaticoduodenal cancer: experience from 1951 to 1960 with a look ahead and behind. Arch Surg 92:834-837, 1966
36. Lansing PB, Blalock JB, Ochsner JL: Pancreatoduodenectomy: a retrospective review 1949 to 1969. Am Surg 38:79-86, 1972
37. Gilsdorf RB, Spanos P: Factors influencing morbidity and mortality in pancreaticoduodenectomy. Ann Surg 177:332-337, 1973
38. Trede M, Schwall G, Saeger HD: Survival after pancreatoduodenectomy: 118 consecutive resections without an operative mortality. Ann Surg 211:447-458, 1990
39. Cameron JL, Pitt HA, Yeo CJ, Lillemoe KD, Kaufman HS, Coleman J: One hundred and forty-five consecutive pancreaticoduodenectomies without mortality. Ann Surg 217:430-435, 1993
40. Fernandez-del Castillo C, Rattner DW, Warshaw AL: Standards for pancreatic resection in the 1990s. Arch Surg 130:295-299, 1995
41. Sarles H, Cambon P, Choux R, Payan MJ, Odaira S, Laugier R, Sahel J: Chronic obstructive pancreatitis due to tiny (0.6 to 8 mm) benign tumors obstructing pancreatic ducts: report of three cases. Pancreas 3:232-237, 1988
42. George DH, Murphy F, Michalski R, Ulmer BG: Serous cystadenocarcinoma of the pancreas: A new entity? Am J Surg Pathol 13:61-66, 1989
43. Le Borgne J: Cystic tumours of the pancreas. Br J Surg 85:577-579, 1998
44. Ridder GJ, Maschek H, Klempnauer J: Favourable prognosis of cystadeno- over adenocarcinoma of the pancreas after curative resection. Eur J Surg Oncol 22:232-236, 1996
45. Siech M, Schmidt-Rohlfing B, Mattfeldt T, Beger HG: Radical surgery in cystadenoma of the pancreas—long-term experiences with 35 patients [German]. Langenbecks Arch Chir Suppl Kongressbd 115:1341-1343, 1998
46. Yamada M, Kozuka S, Yamao K, Nakazawa S, Naitoh Y, Tsukamoto Y: Mucin-producing tumor of the pancreas. Cancer 68:159-168, 1991
47. Kawarada Y, Yano T, Yamamoto T, Yokoi H, Imai T, Ogura Y, Mizumoto R: Intraductal mucin-producing tumors of the pancreas. Am J Gastroenterol 87:634-638, 1992
48. Itoh S, Ishiguchi T, Ishigaki T, Sakuma S, Maruyama K, Senda K: Mucin-producing pancreatic tumor: CT findings and histopathologic correlation. Radiology 183:81-86, 1992
49. Obara T, Magushi H, Saitoh Y, Itoh A, Arisato S, Ashida T, Nishino N, Ura H, Namiki M: Mucin-producing tumor of the pancreas: natural history and serial pancreatogram changes. Am J Gastroenterol 88:564-569, 1993
50. Nomoto S, Nakao A, Ichihara T, Takagi H: Intraoperative quick immunoperoxidase staining: a useful adjunct to routine pathological diagnosis in pancreatic carcinoma. Hepatogastroenterology 42:717-723, 1995
51. Doberstein C, Kirchner R, Gordon L, Silberman AW, Morgenstern L, Shapiro S: Cystic neoplasms of the pancreas. Mt Sinai J Med 57:102-105, 1990
52. Wood D, Silberman AW, Heifetz L, Memsic L, Shabot MM: Cystadenocarcinoma of the pancreas: neo-adjuvant therapy and CEA monitoring. J Surg Oncol 43:56-60, 1990
53. Yoshimi N, Sugie S, Tanaka T, Aijin W, Bunai Y, Tatematsu A, Okada T, Mori H: A rare case of serous cystadenocarcinoma of the pancreas. Cancer 69:2449-2453, 1992
54. Widmaier U, Mattfeldt T, Siech M, Beger HG: Serous cystadenocarcinoma of the pancreas. Int J Pancreatol 20:135-139, 1996
55. Siech M, Tripp K, Schmidt-Rohlfing B, Mattfeldt T, Widmaier U, Gansauge F, Gorich J, Beger HG: Cystic tumours of the pancreas: diagnostic accuracy, pathologic observations and surgical consequences. Langenbecks Arch Surg 383:56-61, 1998
56. Eriguchi N, Aoyagi S, Nakayama T, Hara M, Miyazaki T, Kutami R, Jimi A: Serous cystadenocarcinoma of the pancreas with liver metastases. J Hepatobiliary Pancreat Surg 5:467-470, 1998
57. Horvath KD, Chabot JA: An aggressive resectional approach to cystic neoplasms of the pancreas. Am J Surg 178:269-274, 1999
58. Sessa F, Solcia E, Capella C, Bonato M, Scarpa A, Zamboni G, Pellegata NS, Ranzani GN, Rickaert F, Kloppel G: Intraductal papillary-mucinous tumours represent a distinct group of pancreatic neoplasms: an investigation of tumour cell differentiation and K-ras, p53 and c-erbB-2 abnormalities in 26 patients. Virchows Arch 425:357-367, 1994

THROMBOCYTOPENIA AND OTHER HEMATOLOGIC DISORDERS

James M. Swain, M.D.
Richard T. Schlinkert, M.D.

Reports on the anatomy and function of the spleen date to 200 A.D. McClusky et al.[1,2] elegantly detailed the history of our knowledge and suppositions about splenic function in health and illness. Indeed, the spleen has been thought to be the origin of laughter, a minister of the soul, and an organ for crushing food.

In 1926, William J. Mayo, M.D.,[3] described the spleen as part of the reticuloendothelial system. Its function was similar to that of the Kupffer cells of the liver, and the cells of the spleen functioned by phagocytosis. He found splenomegaly to be related at times to the inability of splenic cells to deliver microorganisms or toxins to the liver for destruction and detoxification. Dr. Mayo also reported that removal of an injured spleen seemed to cause no long-term sequelae.[3]

Much has been learned in the past 75 years about splenic function in health and disease. Certainly, many questions remain and investigation continues on the cellular elements and molecular processes of splenic tissue.

Multiple congenital and acquired disorders either contribute to or are a direct cause of pathologic conditions of the spleen. Postsplenectomy sepsis and its associated high rate of mortality increase the risks associated with splenectomy. The risk of postsplenectomy sepsis is low: 0.18 cases per 100 person-years in one Mayo study.[4] However, the risk is greater for children and for patients with malignancies or who are immunocompromised or in ongoing chemotherapy or radiation therapy. Postsplenectomy sepsis may be devastating and rapidly fatal.

In this chapter, we describe thrombocytopenia and other hematologic disorders that can contribute to pathologic conditions of the spleen. The indications for splenectomy, techniques of the procedure, and expected outcomes are reviewed. Splenic trauma is covered in Chapter 44.

ANATOMY AND PHYSIOLOGY

The spleen is derived from mesoderm and has vascular architecture as early as 9 weeks' gestation. The spleen can be quite variable in size, depending on the presence or absence of pathologic states. The mean adult weight of a normal spleen is approximately 160 g, and the average splenic dimensions are 11 cm in length, 7 cm in width, and 3 cm to 4 cm in thickness. The spleen is covered by a fibrous capsule that can be quite thin. The spleen is in close anatomical association with the stomach, left hemidiaphragm, left kidney, left adrenal, splenic flexure of the colon, and pancreas. The major splenic attachments include the gastrosplenic, splenophrenic, splenorenal, and splenocolic ligaments. Minor attachments include the pancreaticosplenic ligament, presplenic fold, and phrenicocolic ligaments. The spleen rests on, but is not attached to, the phrenicocolic ligament. The splenic hilar vessels course through the splenorenal ligament. An accessory spleen is present in 10% to 25% of patients, usually in the gastrosplenic ligament near the splenic hilum.[5-8] Accessory splenic tissue also may be found at distant sites within the abdomen.

The splenic arterial blood supply consists of the splenic artery with a variable contribution from the left gastroepiploic artery. The short gastric vessels also can provide blood to the spleen. The branching arterial supply enters the spleen, which is separated into 2 or 3 lobes with

2 to 10 segments. Splenic lobes are separated by relatively avascular planes.

The arteries divide and end in the marginal zone between white pulp and red pulp. The blood passes directly into sinusoids within the red pulp and eventually drains into splenic veins (closed circulation). Alternatively, the blood enters the splenic sinusoids and passes through slitlike openings with eventual collection in the venous system (open circulation). The spleen consists of 75% to 85% red pulp and 20% white pulp that is divided into three parts. The periarterial lymphatic sheaths contain T lymphocytes and dendritic antigen-containing cells. The lymphoid nodules, also called malpighian corpuscles, contain B lymphocytes. The marginal zone is the third part. Other cells, such as macrophages and plasma cells, may be observed in all zones.

The lymphatics of the spleen are trabecular and subcapsular in location and drain to splenic hilar lymph nodes.

The functions of the spleen involve immunologic, filtrative, and pitting processes. Two of the major immunologic functions of the spleen are antibody production by B cells and phagocytosis by macrophages. In humans, the spleen is the largest producer of IgM.

The spleen acts as a filter to remove old or damaged red blood cells and encapsulated microorganisms. Specific pathologic states can lead to exaggerated destruction of red blood cells and platelets, which are reviewed in subsequent sections.

Pitting is the process of removing intraerythrocytic inclusions. The presence of these inclusions (e.g., Howell-Jolly bodies, Heinz bodies) in the peripheral blood can signify a decrease in or absence of splenic function. The spleen rarely acts as a site of extramedullary hematopoiesis.

PATHOLOGIC CONDITIONS

Certain pathologic states may lead to splenomegaly, hypersplenism (excess destruction of blood cells by the spleen), or both. Other pathologic conditions of the spleen include platelet disorders, congenital and acquired hemolytic anemias, myeloproliferative disorders, lymphomas, primary neoplasms, cysts and abscesses, torsion, hemangiomas, splenic malignancy, and sinistral portal hypertension.

Platelet Disorders

Immune thrombocytopenic purpura (ITP) is the most common nontraumatic indication for splenectomy. ITP is a diagnosis of exclusion. The peripheral smear is normal except for thrombocytopenia. The bone marrow shows normal to increased concentrations of megakaryocytes. Diagnosis should exclude offending medications and infection with the human immunodeficiency virus

(HIV). Testing for HIV is usually required only if risk factors are present.

Platelet function in ITP is normal. An IgG autoantibody has been named as a possible mediator of platelet destruction. The spleen is a major site of antiplatelet antibody production, as well as the major site of platelet destruction. ITP tends to be self-limited in children. Treatment is reserved for children with platelet counts of approximately 30 to 50 x $10^9/\mu L$. ITP in adults is more commonly a chronic disease. The preferred therapy is glucocorticoids. Few patients will have complete remission of ITP with glucocorticoids alone. High-dose intravenous γ-globulin can stop platelet destruction. Patients who do not respond to glucocorticoids or γ-globulin or who relapse after treatment are candidates for splenectomy. Patients with ITP have a normal or slightly enlarged spleen amenable to laparoscopic splenectomy.

Other causes of immune-mediated thrombocytopenia include drugs, pregnancy, HIV, and systemic lupus erythematosus. Treatment for pregnant patients should be withheld until platelet counts fall below 50 x $10^9/\mu L$, or until there are clinical signs of bleeding. Glucocorticoids are the preferred treatment. When splenectomy becomes necessary in pregnant patients, the second trimester is the preferred time. Patients with HIV-induced thrombocytopenia or systemic lupus erythematosus also may respond to splenectomy when medical measures fail.

Thrombotic thrombocytopenic purpura presents with the pentad of fever, thrombocytopenia, hemolytic anemia, renal disease, and central nervous system dysfunction. Plasmapheresis is the preferred treatment.

Congenital Hemolytic Anemias

Hereditary spherocytosis is the most common hemolytic anemia for which splenectomy is advised. It is transmitted as an autosomal dominant trait that results in a deficiency of the membrane structural protein spectrin. This defect leads to increased rigidity of the red blood cells and to a subsequent decrease in their ability to pass through the splenic circulation. The red blood cells become trapped and destroyed. Over time, this process leads to increased turnover in the red blood cells, splenomegaly, and anemia. This type of anemia can be treated successfully with splenectomy, but the procedure should be delayed until after age 10 if possible.

Spectrin is also defective in elliptocytosis, where it is present in a dimeric instead of a tetrameric form. Elliptocytosis usually causes mild hematologic changes that often require no therapy. However, when more than 90% of the red blood cells are affected, clinically significant anemia may be present. Splenectomy will not reverse the congenital defect but will greatly improve anemia and decrease the need for repeated transfusions.

β-Thalassemia is a disorder characterized by the decreased production of the β-globin chain leading to defective hemoglobin synthesis. With normal α-globin chain production, accumulation of intracellular material can lead to structural deformation in the red blood cells. Eventually, destruction of red blood cells, splenomegaly, and anemia can be severe. Splenectomy is reserved for patients with severe symptoms or an increasing need for blood transfusions. Caution should be exercised when conducting splenectomies in this patient population because of the increased severity of postoperative infections.

Patients with autoimmune hemolytic anemia test positive to the Coombs' antiglobulin test. Failure of medical therapy or the continued need for high-dose corticosteroid therapy should prompt consideration of splenectomy.

Autoimmune hemolytic anemia caused by IgG warm-reactive antibodies is mediated by macrophages. Splenic macrophages attach to the Fc portion of the IgG-tagged erythrocytes. This leads to erythrocyte sequestration and destruction in the spleen, for which splenectomy can be beneficial. Conversely, the cold-reactive antibody (IgM-labeled) erythrocytes can undergo immediate intravascular complement-induced destruction peripherally or can be sequestered and removed from circulation predominantly by the liver. Splenectomy usually is not recommended in this patient population.

Lymphomas

Hodgkin's disease is a malignant disorder of the lymphatic system characterized histologically by the Reed-Sternberg cell. It presents with regional lymphadenopathy and is found more commonly above the diaphragm. Staging laparotomy may document the extent of disease below the diaphragm and is reserved for patients who might be candidates for radiotherapy alone. Some centers have treatment plans that combine radiotherapy and chemotherapy protocols for all patients with lymphoma except those with the most limited stage of this disease, which reduces the need for laparotomy to stage the disease.

Non-Hodgkin's lymphoma is the sixth most common cause of cancer-related death in the United States. Its pathogenesis is unclear. Splenectomy is not usually required in this patient population. However, it may aid diagnosis and treatment of splenic-predominant disease, alleviate symptomatic splenomegaly, treat cytopenias, or enhance the effectiveness of chemotherapy.

Chronic Myeloid Disorders

Chronic myeloid disorders represent a collection of neoplastic disease states of stem-cell origin. The presence or absence of the Philadelphia chromosome (*BCR-ABL* translocation) is paramount to the initial classification of these disorders. The presence of the *BCR-ABL* translocation indicates chronic myelocytic leukemia. Philadelphia chromosome-negative disorders are further classified by the appearance of the bone marrow and the clinical manifestation of the disorder. The *BCR-ABL* negative disorders are classified either as myeloproliferative syndrome or as chronic myeloproliferative disorder. The chronic form may be further classified as classic (e.g., polycythemia vera, primary thrombocytosis, agnogenic myeloid metaplasia) or atypical.

Most cases of chronic myeloid disorders are managed medically. Splenectomy may be indicated in select patients with agnogenic myeloid metaplasia who manifest symptoms of splenomegaly, refractory thrombocytopenia, hypercatabolic symptoms, and forward-flow portal hypertension. Disseminated intravascular coagulation should be excluded preoperatively and treated if present.

Abscesses and Cysts

Splenic abscesses are rare. The predominant organisms include *Staphylococcus*, *Salmonella*, *Escherichia coli*, and *Enterococcus*. These abscesses can be found in patients in intensive care units and in immunocompromised patients (e.g., those with acquired immunodeficiency syndrome or those who have undergone organ transplantation or chemotherapy). Patients present with unexplained fever, a left pleural effusion, or left upper quadrant pain, or all three. Treatment may be attempted with open or percutaneous drainage, but most of these abscesses eventually require splenectomy.

Splenic cysts are classified as parasitic and nonparasitic. Parasitic cysts, such as hydatid cysts, may occur in the spleen alone or in conjunction with liver involvement. Splenectomy has been the treatment of choice, but splenic conservation is increasingly used. Partial cystectomy with omentoplasty and drainage or cyst enucleation and marsupialization have yielded good results. As with hydatid cysts of the liver, spillage of cyst contents should be avoided.

Nonparasitic splenic cysts can be primary or secondary to previous trauma (pseudocysts). They usually can be observed if they have a smooth wall and are not septated. Treatment is reserved for patients with symptoms or for pseudocysts larger than 8 cm to 10 cm in diameter. Surgical unroofing of the cyst, which may be done laparoscopically, is usually curative. Alternatively, percutaneous aspiration and sclerosis of the cyst may be done in select cases, but multiple procedures may be required.

Torsion

In some patients, the spleen is attached only by the hilar vessels. This leads to a mobile or wandering spleen that may torse, leading to severe abdominal pain and, at times, splenic infarction. Patients present with abdominal pain and frequently a right lower-quadrant mass (the torsed spleen). Splenectomy is required if the spleen has infarcted. Otherwise, splenopexy is preferred.

Hemangiomas
Hemangiomas may be identified as incidental radiologic findings or as massive lesions with hemorrhage. They have little or no risk of malignant transformation. A recent review from our institution[9] suggests that small (< 4 cm) asymptomatic lesions may be observed safely with interval scans to assess whether they are enlarging. Large or symptomatic lesions should be removed.

Primary Splenic Malignancy
Nonlymphomatous primary splenic malignancies are extremely rare. Splenectomy is indicated for resectable lesions.

Sinistral Portal Hypertension
Splenic vein occlusion may lead to left-sided (sinistral) portal hypertension with gastric varices. The role of splenectomy in the asymptomatic patient is unclear. Treatment for symptomatic disease is splenectomy. Preoperative splenic artery embolization has been advocated by some authors.[10] We have treated this condition with good results in one patient by laparoscopic splenectomy using preoperative splenic artery embolization.[11] Other authors have treated complications of portal hypertension with laparoscopic gastroesophageal devascularization and splenectomy without preoperative embolization.[12]

IMAGING STUDIES
Many imaging techniques are available for evaluation of the spleen. Computed tomography has the advantage of showing precise anatomical and certain physiologic characteristics. Intravenous contrast can be used to help delineate cysts, abscesses, and other intrasplenic lesions from normal parenchyma. Computed tomography also can show other intra-abdominal abnormalities such as lymphadenopathy.

Magnetic resonance imaging can be used to help define vascular characteristics of certain splenic masses (e.g., hemangiomas). Gadolinium enhancement can increase the diagnostic capabilities of magnetic resonance imaging. New software packages allow better images of the upper abdominal structures with less respiratory motion artifact.

Ultrasonography is an inexpensive, noninvasive, painless, and readily available imaging technique. It can give quick and relatively accurate anatomical information.

Radionuclide scintigraphy can show anatomical features of the spleen and some of its physiologic properties.

Technetium ^{99m}Tc sulfur colloid is taken up by macrophages and can be used to determine phagocytic activity within the spleen.

DIAGNOSIS
Evaluation of hematologic disorders should proceed systematically. A detailed history is essential. Complete blood cell counts will help identify quantitative changes in the circulating blood elements. A peripheral smear is essential in evaluating most hematologic disorders. Bone marrow aspirate and biopsy further characterize disorders and frequently lead to definitive diagnosis. Cytogenetic testing may be required, as in the case of patients with chronic myeloid disorders.

SPLENECTOMY

Preoperative Preparation
All patients undergoing splenectomy are immunized against *Haemophilus influenzae* pneumonia. Patients at increased risk of exposure to meningococcus also are immunized against this organism. Ideally, patients should receive these vaccines well before the operation.

The platelet function in patients with ITP is normal. We generally use glucocorticoids to maintain adequate platelet counts preoperatively. Laparoscopic splenectomy seems safe with platelet counts of 10 x 10^9/μL to 20 x 10^9/μL and has been reported with even smaller counts. Although patients may have peri-incisional bruising, extensive bleeding is uncommon. If necessary, γ-globulin may be used preoperatively. Platelet transfusions are a last resort. For other disease states, coagulopathy should be reversed completely if possible preoperatively.

Laparoscopic Splenectomy
The operating room setup is shown in Figure 1. The patient is placed in the right lateral semidecubitus position and rolled slightly posterior from full vertical to allow access to the midline should conversion to an open procedure become necessary. The arms are positioned away from the operative field. The right leg is straight, and the left leg is bent to keep the left thigh from inhibiting the movement of instruments.

Pneumoperitoneum is established using a Veress needle (Fig. 1 inset, port 1). The initial incision is made over the rib margin. This site draws inferiorly as the abdomen expands. A 5-mm trocar is inserted and a 5-mm camera is introduced. The main camera site is placed at a 10-mm port (Fig. 1 inset, port 2), slightly superior to the umbilicus and generally toward the lateral edge of posterior to the spleen. The lateral folds of the splenore-nal ligament (Fig. 4) and of the splenophrenic ligament (Fig. 5) are divided. The filmy tissues between these ligaments and the posterior aspect of the splenic hilar vessels are separated using gentle blunt dissection or ultra-sonic oscillation. After this maneuver, the spleen should be freed completely from surrounding tissue, and the hilum should be mobilized circumferentially.

We prefer transection of the splenic hilum with staplers. To protect against the unlikely event of an arteriovenous fistula, and to further secure vascular inflow, the splenic artery is ligated (Fig. 6) before transection of the splenic hilum. This is performed with silk suture using an extra-corporeal tie. If the splenic artery cannot be identified, then this step is omitted. The spleen is lifted toward the left hemidiaphragm, and the hilum is transected with an endo-scopic stapler (Fig. 7), taking care not to injure the tail of the pancreas. The spleen is placed in a plastic bag and removed after morcellation. Port sites are not enlarged to remove the specimen, because doing so might increase postoperative discomfort.

Pneumoperitoneum is reestablished and hemostasis is checked. The left upper quadrant is irrigated in an effort to prevent left shoulder pain postoperatively. The staple lines are inspected. The trocars are removed under direct vision. The fascia of the 10-mm and 12-mm trocar sites is closed with a fascial closure device, unless the patient is quite thin. All port sites are infiltrated with .25% bupiv-acaine. No drains are used.

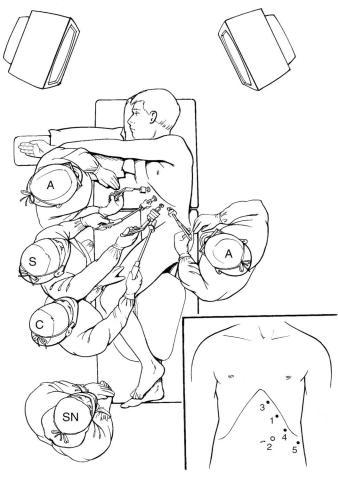

Fig. 1. Operating room setup for laparoscopic splenectomy. A, assis-tants (may use just one assistant); S, surgeon; C, camera operator; SN, scrub nurse. Inset, Port sites for laparoscopic splenectomy. 3 and 5, 5-mm ports for assistants; 1, 5-mm port for surgeon's left hand; 4, 12-mm port for surgeon's right hand; 2, camera port.

the rectus sheath. The placement of this port should allow visualization of the splenic hilum between ports 1 and 4 (Fig. 1 inset). Port 3 is generally placed next and is a 5-mm site used for retraction. Adhesions between the splenic flexure of the colon and the abdominal wall are common. These are taken down, which allows place-ment of port 4 (12 mm) and port 5 (5 mm). The omen-tum and transverse mesocolon are examined for accessory spleens. Likewise, throughout the dissection, accessory splenic tissue is removed. Virtually all dissection is per-formed using ultrasonic shears. Dissection is started at the inferior pole of the spleen. The splenocolic ligament is divided (Fig. 2). Dissection is then carried medial to the spleen and anterior to the pancreas. The gastro-splenic ligament is divided, including the short gastric ves-sels (Fig. 3). This dissection should be carried superior to the spleen, dividing the superior portion of the splenophrenic ligament. Dissection is then performed

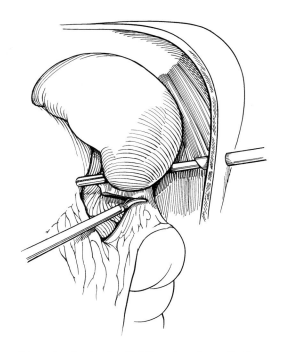

Fig. 2. Dissection begins by dividing the splenocolic ligament.

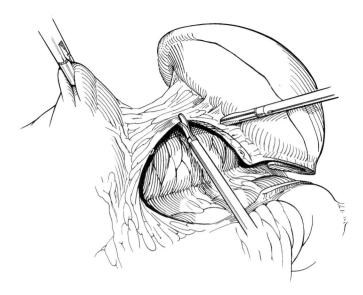

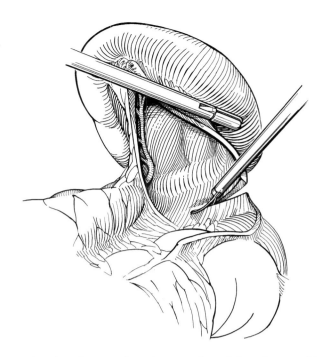

Fig. 3. The lesser sac is entered and the gastrosplenic ligament is divided.

Fig. 4. The spleen is reflected anteriorly and the splenorenal ligament is divided.

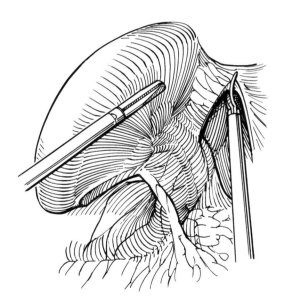

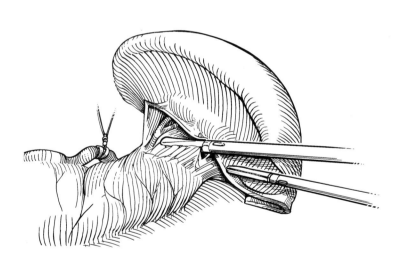

Fig. 5. The splenophrenic ligament is divided. This dissection connects with the anterior dissection superior to the splenic hilum.

Fig. 6. If possible, the splenic artery is ligated.

Technical success rates for laparoscopic splenectomy should be greater than 95% for patients with a spleen of normal size. Short-term and long-term cure rates for ITP have been shown to be equivalent with open or laparoscopic techniques, but laparoscopic splenectomy is associated with less pain and shorter hospitalization.[5,13-15] Approximately 75% of Mayo Clinic patients are dismissed the day after their operation. Therefore, laparoscopic splenectomy is the preferred procedure for patients requiring splenectomy for treatment of ITP.[16] Equivalent rates of success should be observed for other disease states when the patient's spleen is of normal size and vascularity.

Splenomegaly poses unique challenges for the laparoscopic surgeon. Reports on laparoscopic splenectomy for splenomegaly contain few patients. Furthermore, the definition of massive splenomegaly differs. Even large spleens and hypervascular spleens (e.g., in patients with sinistral portal hypertension) may be approached laparoscopically.[17]

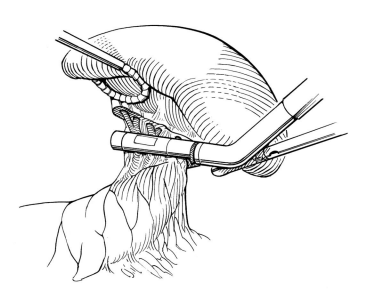

Fig. 7. The tail of the pancreas is protected and the hilar vessels are transected with a linear stapler.

For large spleens, the patient is positioned with the left side elevated about 60°. This position allows easier identification of the splenic hilum without having to lift the heavy spleen. Dissection using the so-called hanged spleen technique initially spares the splenophrenic ligament. After division of the splenocolic and gastrosplenic ligaments, dissection is carried posterior to the splenic hilar vessels. When these ligaments are freed, they are divided with a stapler. If possible, the splenic artery is ligated again before stapling. If the specimen is small enough, it may be placed in a bag for removal. If the spleen is too large to fit into a bag, a counterincision may be required.

When a counterincision is required, the hand-assisted technique may allow the splenectomy to be performed safely with greater ease.[18] Hand-assisted splenectomy is not optimal for smaller spleens.

Open Splenectomy

Ideally, the spleen may be approached through an upper midline incision. It also may be approached through a left subcostal incision. A complete exploration is conducted. The spleen is mobilized by dividing the splenorenal and splenophrenic ligaments. Dissection is carried bluntly posterior to the tail of the pancreas to allow the spleen to be removed from the abdominal cavity. Sponges are placed in the left upper quadrant behind the spleen to keep it elevated and to provide hemostasis on raw surfaces. The splenocolic and gastrosplenic ligaments are divided, and the hilar vessels are divided between clamps and doubly ligated. Suture ligation may be beneficial, particularly for enlarged vessels. No drainage is used afterward.

Dissection for splenomegaly is similar to that for an open splenectomy. Frequently, the enlarged spleen may be mobilized easily into the incision. However, in certain cases the spleen adheres densely to the diaphragm, and these adhesions may be highly vascular. In this situation, the hilum should be controlled first if possible. The technical aspects of splenectomy for splenomegaly may be complex. Many patients have advanced hematologic disease and severe physiologic and immune-related problems. Their perioperative care may be complicated, and a greater rate of perioperative mortality may follow these operations. These procedures should be performed at centers prepared to offer this type of care.

Results

In 1916, Dr. William J. Mayo reported his experience with 135 splenectomies.[19] All cases involved splenomegaly. The operative mortality rate was 8.5%, which is remarkable considering the advanced nature of many of the disease processes and the early state of surgery and blood transfusions in that era. In a subsequent report, Dr. Mayo detailed 417 splenectomies with 10.3% mortality.[20] In that report, mortality was analyzed with respect to disease states. As might be expected, mortality was highest with disease states such as hepatic cirrhosis (32%) and lowest when splenectomy was performed for abnormalities of the red blood cells (5%).

Dr. Mayo emphasized two surgical dictums:
1) See what you are doing
2) Leave a dry field

Failure to follow these principles was cited as the cause of some of the patient deaths in that series. Unlike in the early 1900s, many splenectomies are performed now on patients who have a spleen of normal size. ITP is the most common nontraumatic indication for splenectomy. A spleen of normal size and the lack of hypervascularity should lead to good surgical results.

Laparoscopic techniques have revolutionized splenectomy for ITP. In a review from our institution, 27 patients with ITP underwent attempted laparoscopic splenectomy.[5] The laparoscopic success rate was 96%, with only one conversion to open splenectomy. This conversion was necessary to deal with an unsuspected pancreatic neoplasm. There were no conversions for technical failures. There were no postoperative deaths, and there was only one complication, postoperative pancreatitis, which resolved with conservative therapy. These patients had no need for transfusions due to surgical bleeding, and only one patient received a red blood cell transfusion for preoperative anemia. One patient was given a platelet transfusion early in our experience; however, this treatment is unnecessary in most cases. Mean postoperative stay was 1.5 days.

Accessory spleens were found in 11% of patients. Ninety-two percent of patients responded to splenectomy. Two additional patients subsequently relapsed (mean follow-up, 23 months). At 3 years, there was an 81.5% probability of having a successful outcome (Fig. 8).

These patient outcomes support laparoscopic splenectomy as the procedure of choice for patients who require surgery for ITP.

Costs related to laparoscopic splenectomy also have been analyzed at our institution. In a study of 24 patients, 72% of hospital charges for laparoscopic splenectomy were intraoperative charges (Fig. 9).[21] Preoperative and postoperative hospital charges were 9% and 19%, respectively. Overall hospital charges and intraoperative charges decreased significantly during the period of the study (Fig. 10). Overall charges decreased an average of $233 per patient. This study shows how the cost of this new procedure decreases as surgeons become more adept with the technology. Decreased operative time (Fig. 11) and more judicious use of disposable instruments were the most likely reasons for cost reductions.

The optimum management of the patient undergoing splenectomy for splenomegaly is unclear. Certainly, large spleens (≥ 2.5 kg, in our experience) have been removed laparoscopically. About 30% of patients in our early experience who underwent laparoscopic splenectomy with splenomegaly required conversion to an open procedure. These conversions were all urgent because of bleeding from the splenic veins, and the patients often required a blood transfusion. Hand-assisted techniques may provide better control for these procedures.

In many cases, a large spleen prevents adequate exposure of the splenic hilum. Hilar adenopathy, as observed

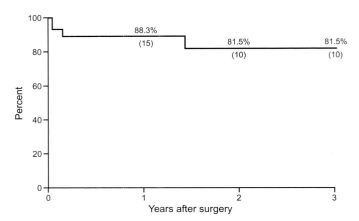

Fig. 8. *Actuarial probability of success (good or excellent results) with use of laparoscopic splenectomy for immune thrombocytopenic purpura, analyzed by Kaplan-Meier method. ( ) = number of patients still at risk. (From Harold et al.[5] By permission of Mayo Foundation for Medical Education and Research.)*

in lymphoma and leukemia, further impairs visibility. Laparoscopic splenectomy for massive splenomegaly (> 3 kg) may violate the dictum "see what you are doing," a lesson learned years ago by Dr. William J. Mayo (see page 371) that is now being relearned by laparoscopic surgeons. Even if the massive spleen is disconnected successfully, it still must be removed. A large counterincision negates some of the benefits of laparoscopic splenectomy, and cutting the spleen into smaller fragments for removal in a bag offends many. Improvements in technique eventually may allow use of laparoscopic splenectomy for massive splenomegaly, but for now we prefer open techniques coupled with modern postoperative analgesia therapy.

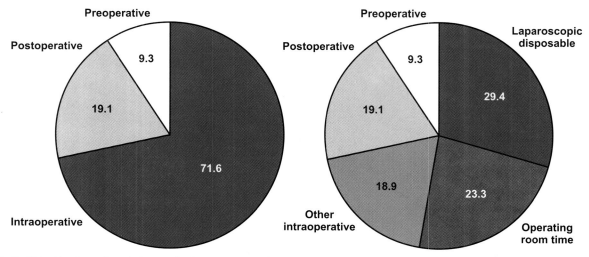

Fig. 9. Left, *Distribution of total charges for laparoscopic splenectomy. Numbers are percentage of total.* Right, *Detail of intraoperative costs. (From Schlinkert et al.[21] By permission of The Society for Surgery of the Alimentary Tract.)*

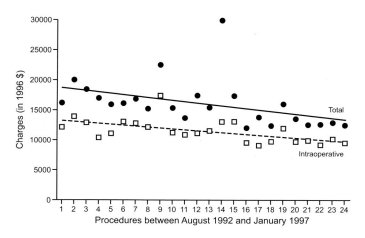

Fig. 10. Summary of total (●) and intraoperative (□) charges over time (P = 0.042, P = 0.004). (From Schlinkert et al.²¹ By permission of The Society for Surgery of the Alimentary Tract.)

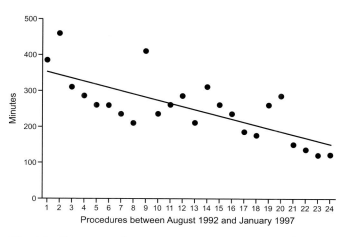

Fig. 11. Summary of operating room times per procedure (P < 0.001). (From Schlinkert et al.²¹ By permission of The Society for Surgery of the Alimentary Tract.)

REFERENCES

1. McClusky DA III, Skandalakis LJ, Colborn GL, Skandalakis JE: Tribute to a triad: history of splenic anatomy, physiology, and surgery: part 1. World J Surg 23:311-325, 1999
2. McClusky DA III, Skandalakis LJ, Colborn GL, Skandalakis JE: Tribute to a triad: history of splenic anatomy, physiology, and surgery: part 2. World J Surg 23:514-526, 1999
3. Mayo WJ: The enlarged spleen. Calif West Med 30:382-386, 1929
4. Schwartz PE, Sterioff S, Mucha P, Melton LJ III, Offord KP: Postsplenectomy sepsis and mortality in adults. JAMA 248:2279-2283, 1982
5. Harold KL, Schlinkert RT, Mann DK, Reeder CB, Noel P, Fitch TR, Braich TA, Camoriano JK: Long-term results of laparoscopic splenectomy for immune thrombocytopenic purpura. Mayo Clin Proc 74:37-39, 1999
6. Katkhouda N, Hurwitz MB, Rivera RT, Chandra M, Waldrep DJ, Gugenheim J, Mouiel J: Laparoscopic splenectomy: outcome and efficacy in 103 consecutive patients. Ann Surg 228:568-578, 1998
7. Halpert B, Györkey F: Lesions observed in accessory spleens of 311 patients. Am J Clin Pathol 32:165-168, 1959
8. Wadham BM, Adams PB, Johnson MA: Incidence and location of accessory spleens (letter). N Engl J Med 304:1111, 1981
9. Willcox TM, Speer RW, Schlinkert RT, Sarr MG: Hemangioma of the spleen: presentation, diagnosis, and management. J Gastrointest Surg 4:611-613, 2000
10. Hiatt JR, Gomes AS, Machleder HI: Massive splenomegaly. Superior results with a combined endovascular and operative approach. Arch Surg 125:1363-1367, 1990
11. Jaroszewski DE, Schlinkert RT, Gray RJ: Laparoscopic splenectomy for the treatment of gastric varices secondary to sinistral portal hypertension. Surg Endosc 14:87, 2000
12. Hashizume M, Tanoue K, Morita M, Ohta M, Tomikawa M, Sugimachi K: Laparoscopic gastric devascularization and splenectomy for sclerotherapy-resistant esophagogastric varices with hypersplenism. J Am Coll Surg 187:263-270, 1998
13. Watson DI, Coventry BJ, Chin T, Gill PG, Malycha P: Laparoscopic versus open splenectomy for immune thrombocytopenic purpura. Surgery 121:18-22, 1997
14. Tanoue K, Hashizume M, Morita M, Migoh S, Tsugawa K, Yagi S, Ohta M, Sugimachi K: Results of laparoscopic splenectomy for immune thrombocytopenic purpura. Am J Surg 177:222-226, 1999
15. Friedman RL, Fallas MJ, Carroll BJ, Hiatt JR, Phillips EH: Laparoscopic splenectomy for ITP. The gold standard. Surg Endosc 10:991-995, 1996
16. Tsiotos G, Schlinkert RT: Laparoscopic splenectomy for immune thrombocytopenic purpura. Arch Surg 132:642-646, 1997
17. Heniford BT, Park A, Walsh RM, Kercher KW, Matthews BD, Frenette G, Sing RF: Laparoscopic splenectomy in patients with normal-sized spleens versus splenomegaly: Does size matter? Am Surg 67:854-857, 2001
18. Nicholson IA, Falk GL, Mulligan SC: Laparoscopically assisted massive splenectomy: a preliminary report of the technique of early hilar devascularization. Surg Endosc 12:73-75, 1998
19. Mayo WJ: A consideration of some of the maladies in which splenectomy may be indicated. Lancet 2:889-892, 1916
20. Mayo WJ: The mortality and end results of splenectomy. Am J Med Sci 171:313-320, 1926
21. Schlinkert RT, Mann D, Weaver A: Laparoscopic splenectomy: reduction of hospital charges. J Gastrointest Surg 2:278-282, 1998

Chapter 24

MALIGNANT TUMORS OF THE SMALL INTESTINE

Hope J. Edmonds, M.D.
J. Kirk Martin, Jr., M.D.
Keith A. Kelly, M.D.

The small intestine is the largest segment of the gastrointestinal tract, making up 75% of its length and 90% of its surface area. Also, the small bowel is the major site for absorption of ingested materials and serves as a major endocrine and immunologic organ. Nonetheless, cancer of the small bowel is rare. Only about 1% of all detected neoplasms of the gastrointestinal tract are of small bowel origin.[1] Several histologic types of tumor are found in the small intestine: adenocarcinomas, carcinoids, lymphomas, leiomyosarcomas, and metastatic tumors. Appropriate diagnosis and treatment of each type depend on the histologic character and location. Diagnosis may be difficult because of the often vague and nonspecific presentation of these tumors and the lack of any highly specific diagnostic tests to confirm a suspected diagnosis. Furthermore, the relative rarity of the tumors may lead to a failure to consider them at all in a differential diagnosis.

ANATOMY

The small intestine, composed of the duodenum, jejunum, and ileum, extends from the pylorus to the ileocecal valve. It is about 3.5 m in length in situ at the operating table. The shortest and widest segment is the duodenum, whose length is approximately 30 cm. It is attached to the retroperitoneum and lies in proximity to the pancreas, making a C-shaped curve around the head of the pancreas. For the purpose of description, the duodenum is divided into four parts: superior, descending, horizontal, and ascending. The common bile duct and pancreatic ducts empty into the posteromedial portion of the descending duodenum at the ampulla of Vater. Blood supply to the duodenum comes through branches of the superior mesenteric and celiac arteries. The arterial supply is closely shared with the pancreas. This relationship necessitates pancreatoduodenectomy at the time of resection of many duodenal neoplasms. The duodenum terminates at the duodenojejunal flexure, where the suspensory muscle of the duodenum (ligament of Treitz) supports the organ as it bends abruptly anteriorly and becomes continuous with the jejunum.

The jejunum is composed of the first 40% of bowel distal to the ligament of Treitz. It is approximately 120 cm in length. Although there is no clear demarcation between the jejunum and the third segment of the small bowel (the ileum), anatomical localization is of surgical importance and thus gross characteristics are described. The jejunum is loosely tethered to the retroperitoneum by the mesentery with a blood supply derived from an extensive system of arterial branches of the superior mesenteric artery within the mesentery. This system also supplies most of the ileum. The jejunum occupies the periumbilical region of the abdomen. The internal wall of the jejunum is recognized by the plicae circulares, which are mucosal folds larger, taller, and more closely packed than in the ileum. The difference in these folds distinguishes ileum from jejunum. The folds may be visualized with radiologic contrast studies or palpated through the bowel wall at the time of operation.

The ileum is the most distal portion of the small bowel. It makes up 60% of the length of the small bowel distal to the ligament of Treitz, approximately 180 cm. It terminates at the ileocecal valve at the attachment site to the colon. The blood supply to the ileum is primarily through the branches of the superior mesenteric artery. The ileum typically inhabits the pelvic and hypogastric regions of the abdomen.

The plicae circulares in the ileum are low and sparse in the proximal ileum and absent in the terminal ileum.

Lymphatic drainage of the small bowel must be considered when addressing malignancy and metastasis. The duodenum contains lymph vessels within its anterior and posterior surfaces, and these inosculate freely with each other within the duodenal wall. The anterior lymph vessels follow the arterial supply and drain into the pancreatico-duodenal lymph nodes along the splenic artery and into the pyloric lymph nodes along the gastroduodenal artery. Efferent vessels then flow into the celiac nodes. The posterior lymph vessels drain into the superior mesenteric nodes located near the origin of the superior mesenteric artery. The villi of the jejunum and ileum contain lymphatics called lacteals, which empty their milky fluid into a plexus of lymph vessels within the walls of the bowel. The vessels then travel to the mesenteric lymph nodes, which lie close to the intestinal wall, along the superior mesenteric artery, and among the arcades. These nodes then drain into the superior mesenteric nodes.

INCIDENCE

Malignant tumors of the small bowel are rare, making up only 1.0% to 1.4% of all gastrointestinal tract tumors. In contrast, benign tumors of the small bowel are found in 0.2% to 0.3% of autopsy cases, which is a prevalence rate of more than 15 times that in surgical studies.[2,3] About 40% of small bowel malignant tumors are adenocarcinomas, 40% are carcinoids, 15% are sarcomas, and 5% are lymphomas.[4] Malignant small bowel tumors show an overall male predominance; in the United States, the incidence is 0.8 to 1.3/100,000 per year in men and 0.7 to 0.8/100,000 per year in women.[5,6] One of the largest series on small bowel adenocarcinoma is that of the Surveillance, Epidemiology, and End Results (SEER) program. That series included 1,832 small bowel tumors diagnosed between 1973 and 1982. According to the SEER program data,[7] small bowel adenocarcinomas and carcinoids are 40% and 70%, respectively, more common in black Americans than in white Americans, and small bowel lymphomas are twice as common in white Americans. Small bowel neoplasms are extremely rare during the first 3 decades of life. Mortality rates for small bowel cancer increase sharply at age 40 years and double every decade to the age of 75 years.[8]

PATHOPHYSIOLOGY

The mucosa of the small bowel rapidly regenerates. Dying cells are exfoliated, and new enterocytes migrate from the crypts, where they arise from less differentiated stem cells.

Replacement of cells occurs in a 5- to 7-day cycle. Although the turnover of cells in the small bowel is relatively quick, creating an increased potential for genetic errors or mutation during replication, the small bowel has a very low incidence of mucosal neoplasms. Transit time through the small bowel is short, about 2 hours. Ingested carcinogens likely are not in contact with bowel mucosa long enough to be a substantial cause of neoplastic transformation. Furthermore, the pH of the luminal contents is alkaline. This alkalinity and the activity of benzopyrene hydroxylase in the mucosa detoxify many carcinogens. The immune system of the small bowel provides another role in gut resistance to malignant transformation. IgA is secreted into the lumen. Immunocompetent lymphoid tissue also is found within the walls of the distal small bowel. These mechanisms seem to have a role in immunosurveillance against the development of malignancy.

DIAGNOSIS AND IMAGING

Diagnosis of small bowel tumors can be challenging because symptoms are often vague and nonspecific. It may be months or even years before a diagnosis is made. Pain is the most common presenting complaint; its frequency is 14% to 86% of subjects with small bowel cancers, depending on the series identified.[9] The pain is not predictable in character. It may be described as a crampy pain or a dull ache, accompanied by diffuse tenderness with or without peritoneal signs, depending on the presence of perforation. The pain may be misattributed to peptic ulcer or an inflammatory condition such as Crohn's disease or ulcerative colitis. Partial obstruction may occur with increasing size of tumor, causing characteristic symptoms of cramping pain, nausea, vomiting, and changes in bowel habits. Annular constriction, intussusception, or volvulus also may occur as tumor size increases. Complete obstruction occurs in only 5% to 38% of small intestinal cancers.[9] Adenocarcinomas are, by far, the most likely to obstruct the lumen of the bowel as they increase in size, whereas sarcomas or lymphomas are more likely to present as a palpable abdominal mass. Diarrhea, weight loss, gastrointestinal bleeding, anemia, and fever also are caused by small bowel tumors. Up to two-thirds of patients present with anorexia and weight loss.[9] Malabsorption also may contribute to weight loss in patients, especially in those with lymphoma. In carcinoid syndrome, flushing, diarrhea, wheezing, and palpitations also may be presenting complaints.

Physical examination may show no abnormality in a patient with small bowel neoplasm. Peritoneal signs may be present if acute perforation has occurred. In large sarcoma or lymphoma, an abdominal mass may be palpable. Occult bleeding likely will be found on examination of the stool. Jaundice may occur when a duodenal malignancy obstructs the bile duct. In most cases, results of physical examination are completely benign in the face of patient complaints of pain and any number of the symptoms described above.

Laboratory findings rarely show abnormalities other than microcytic, hypochromic anemia, signifying blood loss. If liver enzyme values are increased in the serum, liver metastasis or biliary obstruction due to a mass should be suspected. Carcinoid tumors can be diagnosed on the basis of an increased level of urinary 5-hydroxyindoleacetic acid (5-HIAA), but this is found in only 30% to 35% of patients with carcinoid tumor.[10] Levels of 5-HIAA usually increase when carcinoid tumors spread. Carcinoembryonic antigen is associated with tumors of the bowel, but it is not specific or sensitive enough for conclusive diagnosis of adenocarcinomas of the small bowel.

Other than laparotomy and direct visualization, radiologic imaging remains the best method to diagnose small intestinal malignancies. Radiologic abnormalities are present in 75% of cases of small bowel cancers at the time of diagnosis.[11] Supine and upright abdominal radiographs may show a mass. Free air may be found if perforation has occurred. With the use of barium contrast, the tumor can be localized. Good's review of small bowel tumors details the radiologic findings of several types of tumor.[12] Adenocarcinoma characteristically forms a napkin-ring stenosis of the bowel lumen (Fig. 1). Lymphomas also may constrict the lumen, but they also may form "aneurysmal" dilatation of the wall as a result of tumor necrosis. Sarcomas most often present as large extraluminal masses. Carcinoid tumors are usually small and rarely are detected on gastrointestinal contrast studies. Upper gastrointestinal series provide helpful diagnostic clues in 57% of primary malignancies, 43% of metastatic cases, and 25% of benign tumors.[13]

Computed tomography (CT) often is done in patients suspected of having a small bowel obstruction. CT is also a common, early diagnostic test done in cases of vague, unexplained abdominal pain. Because CT is a test that is likely to be available and often is ordered by evaluating clinicians, its appropriate use is necessary for detection of small bowel masses. Thickening of bowel wall, circumferential or focal discrete lesions, lymphadenopathy, and mesenteric fat involvement often can be readily seen with CT. In fact, it is highly sensitive (detection rate of 88%) for discovering mesenteric fat involvement. The sensitivity of CT for detection of regional lymphadenopathy is only 75%, and its specificity is only 20%.[14] It is limited in its ability to evaluate depth of tumor invasion. CT cannot distinguish submucosa, muscularis, and subserosal invasion. CT is adequate for detection of primary abnormalities of the bowel itself, but it has not been shown to be dependable for accurate staging of bowel lesions. Endoscopy is limited in its usefulness because of the inaccessibility of the small bowel. Only duodenal and terminal ileum lesions are within reach of a commonly used endoscope. Jejunal intubation can be used to perform small bowel endoscopy with biopsy. This technique is not commonly practiced.

SPECIFIC TUMOR TYPES

Adenocarcinoma
Adenocarcinoma is the most common of the small bowel malignancies, making up 40% of all cancers of the small bowel. In the SEER study,[7] the average incidence of small

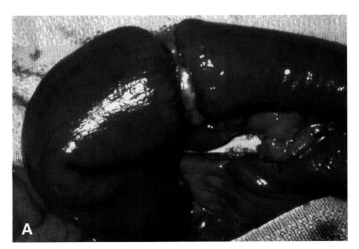
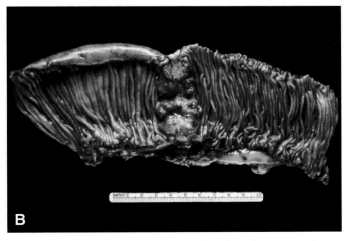

Fig. 1. (A), *A jejunal adenocarcinoma, showing the circumferential growth.* (B), *On exposure of the lumen of the bowel, tumor is shown to have infiltrated transmurally.*

bowel adenocarcinoma was 5.7 cases per million population per year in white Americans and 7.5 cases per million per year in black Americans. Patients are most often in their sixth or seventh decade of life, and there is a slight male predominance.[15] The average age of patients with small bowel adenocarcinoma is 65.4 years. More than two-thirds of patients are older than 60 years.[16] The location of the tumor appears to be more common proximally and to decrease in frequency distally, a finding suggesting that the mucosa of the duodenum is more sensitive to factors causing malignant transformation or, simply, that it is the first to be exposed to undiluted, ingested carcinogens. Substances inducing transformation may include ingested materials and those produced by the gastrointestinal tract, such as bile, pancreatic secretions, and gastric acid. Adenocarcinoma of the small bowel is found in the duodenum in 48.3% of cases, in the jejunum in 23.4%, in the ileum in 15.6%, and in other sites in 12.8%.[17] Within the duodenum, 65% of tumors are periampullary, 20% are proximal to the ampulla of Vater, and 15% are distal to the ampulla.[18]

Risk factors for the development of small bowel adenocarcinoma include, but are not limited to, familial adenomatous polyposis, presence of villous adenomas, and Crohn's disease.[19-21] The risk of duodenal carcinoma is increased 331 times in patients with familial adenomatous polyposis over that of the normal population.[18] Within the population of patients with villous adenomas, there is a high incidence of malignant transformation. Cancer occurs in 27% to 63% of patients with villous adenomas. Crohn's disease is associated with an 86-fold increase in the incidence of small bowel adenocarcinoma, and the majority of these tumors occur in the ileum.[22] The mechanism for development of small bowel adenocarcinoma in Crohn's disease is unclear. Most cases are in persons who have had Crohn's disease for more than 20 years.[23] Pathologically, multifocal mucosal dysplasia is often found with the adenocarcinoma, an association suggesting that the chronic inflammation of Crohn's disease results in progressive changes leading to the malignancy.[24]

Patients with small bowel adenocarcinoma may present with none or all of the following: pain, weight loss, occult bleeding or acute hemorrhage, small bowel obstruction (Fig. 2), palpable mass, perforation, or jaundice. Pain from partial luminal obstruction is common and often results in weight loss. Some patients may have a palpable mass or perforation, although these are both rare complications. If jaundice occurs, it is most likely due to adenocarcinoma of the duodenum rather than any other form of small bowel tumor.[15] Anemia is common as a result of occult bleeding. In fact, anemia is one of only two factors, the other being patient age, that are associated inversely

with survival in patients with small bowel adenocarcinoma.[22] Significant anemia or advanced age predicts relatively poor average survival. Upper gastrointestinal contrast radiographs are diagnostic in many cases of small bowel adenocarcinoma. CT may detect the primary tumor, distant metastases, and nodal involvement. Endoscopy can be done to obtain biopsy specimens of duodenal masses, but a high false-negative rate with biopsy of villous adenomas (25%-55%) makes dependence on such biopsy unwise.[25,26]

Staging of small bowel adenocarcinoma is done according to the TNM definitions of the American Joint Committee on Cancer (Table 1). Specimens taken at the time of operation provide the usual means of classifying an adenocarcinoma of the small bowel, and CT can provide limited information to classify tumors. CT is relatively effective for identifying distant metastases, but it is not useful for evaluation of the depth of tumor invasion. Metastatic disease can be suspected if the CT shows a small bowel wall thickness of more than 1.5 cm or if discrete mesenteric masses are more than 1.5 cm.[27] Because CT does not clearly distinguish among submucosal, muscularis, and subserosal layers, the depth of invasion cannot be derived from CT evaluation.

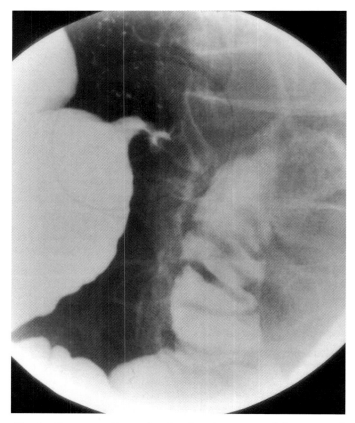

Fig. 2. Contrast radiography, showing obstruction of the intestinal lumen by an adenocarcinoma of the jejunum.

Table 1.—TNM Staging for Small Bowel Adenocarcinoma

Primary tumor (T)

TX	Primary tumor not evaluated
T0	No pathologic evidence of primary tumor
Tis	In situ carcinoma
T1	Tumor invades lamina propria or submucosa
T2	Tumor invades muscularis propria
T3	Tumor invades < 2 cm into the subserosa or into the nonperitonealized perimuscular tissue (mesentery or retroperitoneum)
T4	Tumor perforates the visceral peritoneum or invades the adjacent structures > 2 cm

Regional lymph nodes

NX	Regional lymph nodes not evaluated
N0	No regional lymph node involvement
N1	Regional lymph node metastasis

Distant metastases

MX	Distant sites not evaluated
M0	No distant metastasis
M1	Distant metastasis present

Stage grouping

Stage	T	N	M
0	Tis	N0	M0
I	T1 or T2	N0	M0
II	T3 or T4	N0	M0
III	Any T	N1	M0
IV	Any T	Any N	M1

Modified from American Joint Committee on Cancer. American Joint Committee on Cancer: Handbook for Staging of Cancer: From the Manual for Staging of Cancer, 4th edition. Edited by OH Beahrs, DE Henson, RVP Hutter, BJ Kennedy. Philadelphia, JB Lippincott Company, 1993, p 91. By permission of the American Joint Committee on Cancer.

Outcome for patients with small bowel adenocarcinoma is related to location of tumor, treatment rendered, age of patient, and stage of disease. Disease stage is the single most critical prognostic factor. If there is no nodal metastasis, the 5-year survival rate is 55%, decreasing to only 12% if local nodes are involved.[13] The 5-year survival rate is less with duodenal tumors (28.2%) than with ileal or jejunal tumors (37.8%).[16] This difference is likely due to the decreased frequency of cancer-directed surgical treatment for duodenal tumors (as a result of anatomical complexity) or to the disproportionately large number of patients older than 75 years who have duodenal adenocarcinomas and are not surgical candidates because of comorbidities. The decreased 5-year survival rate of patients with duodenal small bowel adenocarcinoma also may be due, in part, to the occasional need for pancreaticoduodenectomy if operation is attempted. Pancreaticoduodenectomy is associated with greater morbidity and mortality rates than segmental small bowel resection. Cancer-directed surgical treatment of adenocarcinomas of all sites is shown to increase the 5-year survival rate to 40.3%. Operation for limited disease is the only curative treatment. Of course, patients with unresectable tumors, those with distant metastases, and those with untreatable serious comorbidities do not usually undergo operative management. Metastatic disease and tumors of more poorly differentiated histologic type are associated with poorer 5-year survival rates, as with any other form of small bowel malignancy. Age also contributes to outcome; the relative risk of death increases by 1.8 times in patients older than 75 years. This is in part due to the greater proportion of duodenal tumors in persons 75 years or older and to the lesser frequency of surgical intervention. Adjuvant therapy, chemotherapy, and radiotherapy have been used infrequently in conjunction with operation, but their use has not shown any benefit in overall outcome.

Carcinoid Tumor

Carcinoid tumors, "karzinoids," were first described by Oberndorfer in 1907.[28] He described a tumor much like an adenocarcinoma, but its behavior was more benign. Later, less "benign" phenotypes were recognized. The term "carcinoid" is still used to describe a group of neoplasms arising from various neuroendocrine cells that perform various biological functions. The most frequent sites for carcinoids are the gastrointestinal tract (73.7%) and the bronchopulmonary system (25.1%).[29] Within the gastrointestinal tract, most tumors occur within the small bowel (28.7%), appendix (18.9%), and rectum (12.6%).[30] For all sites, the incidence is highest in black males (2.12 per 100,000 population per year). The incidence of carcinoids peaks in the sixth decade of life, but the age range is broad (20-80 years). For no known reason, these tumors are associated with noncarcinoid primary malignancies of the gastrointestinal tract and other nongastrointestinal tissues. Fifteen to thirty percent of patients have other neoplasms, most commonly of the breast, lung, colon, and stomach. The overall 5-year survival rate for all sites of small bowel carcinoid tumors is 50.4% ± 6.4% (mean ± SEM).

Carcinoid tumors arise from Kulchitsky cells, a type of enterochromaffin cell in the crypts of Lieberkühn. These cells belong to the amine precursor uptake decarboxylase system. Such cells are a group of pluripotent neuroendocrine cells, derived from the neural crest, that synthesize various vasoactive amines and regulatory peptides. Histologically, the tumors appear as a monotonous population of uniform cells with little cytoplasm and few mitotic figures. The term "carcinoid," meaning cancer-like, is indeed a misnomer, because these are true malignancies.

Like other small bowel malignancies, the presentation of carcinoids is nonspecific and the course is indolent. In fact, the median time from onset of symptoms to diagnosis is 2 years. A submucosal tumor may extend beyond the mesentery to shorten and thicken that mesentery, creating kinking of the bowel (Fig. 3). This leads to symptoms of partial small bowel obstruction. Some mucosal irritation may occur, but rarely is gross bleeding noted. Mesenteric ischemia or infarction is sometimes an acute complication occurring due to a form of mesenteric angiopathy. The cause of this angiopathy is poorly understood, but it consists of vascular thickening and sclerosis. The more common constitutional symptoms of carcinoid include weight loss, anorexia, and fatigue. These are usually attributed to metastatic disease, usually to the liver or adjacent nodes, which occurs in 90% of patients by the time of diagnosis. Despite the noted ability of carcinoid tumors to spread locally to adjacent lymph nodes or to adjacent organs, no TNM classification currently exists to portray the extent of spread of these tumors.

The carcinoid syndrome is a specific constellation of symptoms related to late-stage disease, most often with large metastatic lesions in the liver. The hallmarks of the syndrome are diarrhea and intermittent facial and upper body flushing. Symptoms are produced by certain foods, alcohol intake, or emotional stress. Less commonly, carcinoid syndrome presents with bronchospasm, venous telangiectasis of the face and neck, and pellegra (diarrhea, dementia, and dermatitis). Late in the clinical course, heart failure may develop as a result of endocarditis, and valvular fibrosis may occur as a result of increased levels of vasoactive amines circulating through the inferior vena cava to the heart. A potentially life-threatening complication of carcinoid syndrome is carcinoid crisis. This is manifested by intense flushing, diarrhea, and headache, sometimes followed by somnolence and coma. Cardiac manifestations are tachycardia, hypertension or hypotension, and arrhythmias. The diagnosis of carcinoid syndrome is most easily confirmed from evidence of serotonin overproduction, indicated by increased urinary excretion of 5-HIAA, a metabolite of serotonin. 5-HIAA levels are usually normal in patients with carcinoid tumors unless liver involvement is extensive or carcinoid syndrome is evident.

Detection of carcinoids, as with other indolent malignancies, is a challenge. Inflammatory causes of symptoms, such as Crohn's disease, must be ruled out. On small bowel radiography with contrast, tethering or pleating of the intestinal folds may be evident. Stenotic regions of bowel may be seen. More often, no primary lesion is noted, but CT may detect nodal metastases and stellate patterns of soft tissue stranding within adjacent mesentery. Hepatic nodules or metastases also may be evident on CT, ultrasonography, or magnetic resonance imaging. Endoscopy typically is of no use for detecting jejunal or ileal carcinoids, but it can detect duodenal or rectal tumors. Medical treatment and chemotherapy have been of some use in the management of small intestinal carcinoids.[30-33] The carcinoid crises, in particular, can be treated with octreotide. However, most patients will undergo operation, which is the only hope for a more permanent cure.[30]

Lymphoma

Lymphomas of the small bowel are relatively rare, making up only about 5% of all malignant tumors of the small bowel. They occur as primary lesions, without concurrent peripheral lymphadenopathy or splenomegaly, or as secondary sites of spread of a systemic disease. Five percent of all lymphomas are primary tumors of the gastrointestinal tract. Thus, they are the most common extranodal site of lymphoma primary tumors. In Western countries, small bowel lymphomas occur less often than gastric lymphomas, but they are more common than those in the large bowel. In contrast, in Mediterranean countries, and those of poor socioeconomic development, a form of lymphoma called immunoproliferative small intestinal disease predominates.[34,35] Chronic intestinal infection or parasitic infestation may contribute to the occurrence of this form. Small bowel lymphomas commonly occur during the fifth and sixth decades of life, and there is a slight male predominance. They also may occur in children 10 years or younger, usually as an advanced ileocecal Burkitt-type disease. Conditions such

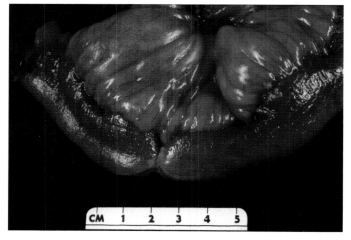

Fig. 3. Resected segment of jejunum shows a carcinoid tumor that has narrowed the bowel and shortened the adjacent mesentery.

as Crohn's disease, pharmacologic immunosuppression, and acquired immunodeficiency syndrome create an increased risk for the development of gastrointestinal lymphomas. Most small bowel lymphomas are of intermediate or high grade. They appear histologically with a nodular, diffuse growth pattern and are of B-cell origin. In contrast, lymphomas associated with celiac disease are often of T-cell type.

The initial presentation of small bowel lymphoma is often a surgical emergency. Symptoms of obstruction or perforation, and less likely massive hemorrhage, occur in 30% to 60% of patients. Unlike other small bowel malignancies that have an insidious onset of symptoms, lymphoma often presents with only 6 months of symptoms before diagnosis. Constitutional symptoms, occurring in two-thirds of patients, include fatigue, malaise, anorexia, and weight loss. Mechanical obstruction or functional impairment may produce cramping, diarrhea, constipation, or malabsorption. Anemia with heme-positive stool is common, although melena or hematochezia is rare. At presentation, 20% to 60% of patients have an abdominal mass.[35] In a patient with duodenal celiac disease who has increased malabsorption, lymphoma may be suspected. Patients with Mediterranean-type disease also may present with low-grade fever and vague abdominal pain. Those with the Western type of lymphoma may have the additional findings of clubbing and malabsorption.

Diagnosis is usually made from air-contrast gastrointestinal studies, which detect abnormalities in 90% of cases. Aneurysmal dilatation of a bowel loop is characteristic of lymphoma. Other radiologic findings may include submucosal masses, fistulas, obstructive masses, and ulcerations. CT may be helpful for detecting nodal involvement and the exact location of the tumor. The Ann Arbor system is commonly used for staging based on nodal involvement (Table 2). Jejunal aspirates may yield a diagnosis in the Mediterranean type, revealing many plasma cells. Although not diagnostic, an increased level of IgA heavy chains in the serum is also indicative of

Table 2.—Modified Ann Arbor Staging System of Primary Non-Hodgkin's Gastrointestinal Lymphomas

Stage	Description
IE	Tumor confined to small intestine
IIE	Spread to regional lymph nodes
IIIE	Spread to nonresectable lymph nodes beyond regional nodes
IVE	Spread to other organs within or beyond abdomen

Mediterranean type, also known as α chain disease or immunoproliferative small intestinal disease.[34,35] No specific diagnostic tests exist for Western lymphoma. Despite the aforementioned methods of diagnosis, many cases are diagnosed only at the time of celiotomy (Fig. 4).

Prognosis for patients with small bowel lymphoma, regardless of type, depends on the size of the primary tumor, stage of disease, the presence of multicentricity, and adjacent organ involvement.[31] Most tumors are stage III or IV. These are often fatal because of the extent of spread. Death usually ensues within 1 year. Patients with tumors of stage I or II are often able to undergo complete resection of the tumor. If so, they have a 5-year survival rate of 80%. Adjuvant chemotherapy or radiotherapy for stages IE or IIE is yet unproved. If disease has spread to stage III or IV and surgical, palliative debulking has occurred, a regimen of localized radiotherapy with systemic chemotherapy may provide some temporary relief.

Leiomyosarcoma

Leiomyosarcomas make up about 15% of all malignant neoplasms of the small bowel. They occur at all ages, but the peak incidence is in the sixth decade; there is a slight male predominance. There is no apparent association with race, occupational exposure, or hereditary factors. The tumors arise from mesodermal tissues. Other sarcomas (fibrosarcoma from connective tissue, neurofibrosarcoma from neural tissue, liposarcoma from adipose tissue, and angiosarcoma or Kaposi's sarcoma from vascular tissues) are extremely rare and are not addressed in this chapter. Kaposi's sarcoma in association with acquired immunodeficiency syndrome is actually a common malignancy,

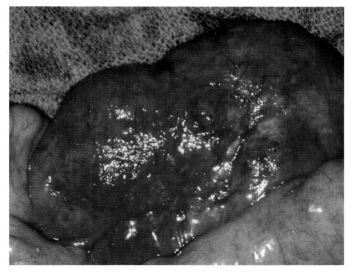

Fig. 4. Lymphosarcoma invading mesentery of the jejunum, discovered at celiotomy.

but it is a systemic disease with a gastrointestinal component, not a primary small bowel disease.

Leiomyosarcomas arise most commonly from the muscularis propria and less often from the muscularis mucosae and vascular musculature.[36] They occur most commonly in the jejunum, but also in the ileum and duodenum. Histologic distinction between leiomyosarcomas and benign leiomyomas is difficult. The distinction is based on number of mitotic figures per high-power microscopic field (more than two per high-power field signifies leiomyosarcoma), cellular atypia, presence of necrosis, and size of tumor. The distinction is made to aid in prognosis, because leiomyosarcoma is associated with a poorer prognosis than leiomyoma. Epithelioid leiomyosarcomas are characterized by irregular pleomorphic cells and have a better prognosis.

Symptoms of leiomyosarcoma are usually chronic, and the mean duration from symptoms to diagnosis is more than 1 year.[37] In fact, at diagnosis, most of the tumors have reached in excess of 5 cm in size. Patients may experience pain and weight loss. These tumors tend to grow extraluminally and rarely obstruct until late in their course. If obstruction occurs, it is usually due to external compression and, less commonly, intussusception or circumferential growth. Because of the large size and vascularity of the tumor, ischemia within the tumor leading to necrosis and hemorrhage (intra-abdominal, into the tumor, or intraluminal) is common, occurring in up to 66% of patients. Perforation occurs in 10% of patients. A palpable abdominal mass is found in 25% to 50% of cases. Jaundice may herald a duodenal mass or liver metastases. As with most of the other tumor types discussed, leiomyosarcoma is often seen on gastrointestinal barium radiographic studies. A barium-filled cavity may represent a space created by an area of central necrosis in the tumor. A mass effect with concomitant obstruction also may be seen. CT examination may show a large extraluminal mass, with or without central necrosis or calcification. Angiography should show a highly vascular mass, suggesting the diagnosis preoperatively.

Therapy for leiomyosarcoma is surgical. Sarcomas are relatively radioresistant. Doxorubicin-based chemotherapeutic agents may show some tumor response, but prognosis is poor without resection. Local lymph node resection is not indicated because leiomyosarcomas tend to spread hematogenously rather than through the lymphatic system. Metastasis occurs in 20% to 40% of cases, most often to the liver, lungs, and peritoneum (Fig. 5). Resectability is the key to prognosis. Five percent of tumors (those occurring in the duodenum) are often not resectable and are associated with a poor prognosis. For low-grade tumors that are resectable, 50% of operations are palliative and

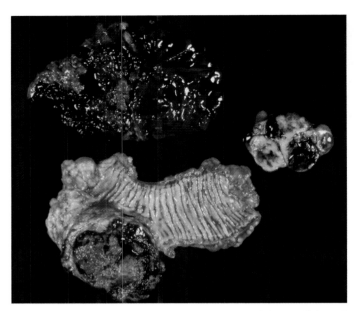

Fig. 5. Resected epithelioid leiomyosarcoma of the small bowel (bottom), *a metastatic lesion from elsewhere in the small bowel* (right), *and a metastatic lesion resected from the liver* (top).

50% are curative. At 5 years, 25% of patients with palliative resection are living and more than 50% with curative resection are living. If the tumor grade is high, 5-year survival, even with curative resection, is only 20%.

Metastatic Tumors

Metastasis to the small bowel may occur through direct spread, hematogenous spread, lymphatic dissemination, or peritoneal seeding from other intra-abdominal sources. Small bowel metastasis that does not develop by direct spread is rare. A 50-year review found only 76 cases of such metastasis; in these cases, the primary tumor was known and was biopsy proven.[38] The most common sites of tumor origin are the uterine cervix, large bowel, kidney, stomach, ovary, and melanoma (Fig. 6). The uterine body, esophagus, biliary tract, breast, head and neck, and thyroid are far less common primary sites. Symptoms of metastatic small bowel tumors are like those of any primary malignancy, including pain, obstructive symptoms, hemorrhage, and anemia. Surgical resection is the treatment of choice. The whole bowel must be examined for multiple metastases (Fig. 7). The prognosis is routinely poor; one series reported a 100% death rate 19 months after operation.

SURGICAL APPROACH

Two Mayo Clinic surgeons, Fred W. Rankin and Charles H. Mayo, initially stimulated interest in small bowel carcinoma when they published a review in 1930.[39] Some 70

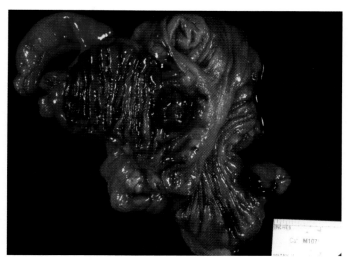

Fig. 6. Resected small bowel containing a metastasis from a renal cell carcinoma.

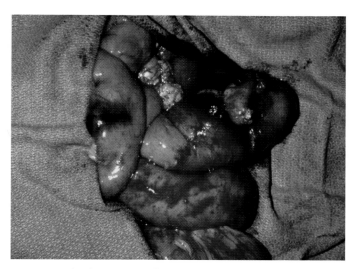

Fig. 7. Multiple metastatic lesions to the small bowel from a cutaneous melanoma.

years later, surgical resection remains the only potential curative treatment for small bowel cancer.

The resectability rate of small bowel carcinoma varies considerably by site: cancer-directed operation is used for 88.5% of jejunal and 92.9% of ileal cancers but for only 51.7% of duodenal carcinomas ($P < 0.0001$). During the most recent period examined in the National Cancer Database Report on Small Bowel Adenocarcinoma (1991-1995),[16] more than 91% of jejunal tumors and nearly 96% of ileal tumors were treated surgically, whereas only half of duodenal tumors (50.2%) were similarly managed.

The complexity of duodenal resections is undoubtedly an important factor in surgical management. Unfortunately, nearly half (48.3%) of small bowel carcinomas arise in the duodenum. Surgical management is guided by the location of the duodenal tumor and by the distance between the ampulla of Vater and the malignancy. Lesions arising in the first or second portions of the duodenum generally necessitate a pancreaticoduodenectomy, and reconstruction is made more difficult by the presence of a typically normal pancreas and a nondilated common duct. Carcinomas in the first portion of the duodenum usually are treated with a standard Whipple procedure, including resection of the gastric antrum. If the tumor is located in the second portion of the duodenum, then a pylorus-preserving Whipple procedure can be considered. It is important to bear in mind that regional lymphatics for the duodenum may drain to subpyloric, peripancreatic, portal, celiac, or even greater or lesser curve gastric lymph nodes. In a series of duodenal carcinomas treated at Memorial Sloan-Kettering Cancer Center between 1983 and 1994, only 53% of duodenal cancers were resected, and 90% of the resections required pancreaticoduodenectomy.

Similarly, M.D. Anderson Cancer Center found just 54% of duodenal tumors to be resectable, and pancreaticoduodenectomy was performed in 75% of these. The mortality rate after pancreaticoduodenectomy is inversely related to frequency of operation. The Veterans Administration Outcomes Group found that in-hospital mortality rates for pancreaticoduodenectomy were 3 to 4 times higher at hospitals performing one or two such operations or less per year than at hospitals performing five or more per year (12%-16% vs. 4%; $P < 0.001$). The 10 hospitals with the nation's highest volumes had the lowest mortality rates (2.1%).

Cancers in the third and fourth portions of the duodenum are technically more easily managed and may be treated with sleeve resection followed by duodenojejunostomy. Several options for the duodenojejunostomy have been described, including end-to-end anastomosis, or closure of the proximal transected duodenum and side-to-side anastomosis along the second portion of the duodenum. Care should be exercised during resections of the third portion of the duodenum. The superior mesenteric artery must be identified and preserved, and the midcolic vessels also should be saved, if possible. Duodenal diverticularization has been described, resecting the distal stomach and pylorus and then establishing a duodenojejunostomy Roux-en-Y and a gastrojejunostomy. The remaining second portion of the duodenum then receives only biliary and pancreatic secretions. This operation should be considered if intestinal continuity cannot be reestablished satisfactorily with the remaining duodenum. Simply stapling the pylorus closed has not been very successful in excluding the duodenum from gastric contents. Resections involving the first and second portions of the duodenum should probably be accompanied by cholecystectomy because bile stasis may occur after operation, and subsequent reoperation for symptomatic gallstones or cholecystitis may prove difficult. The inferior mesenteric vein should be preserved during mobilization of the ligament of Treitz.

Segmental resections for jejunal or ileal carcinomas should provide bowel margins that are grossly and microscopically free of involvement. This goal generally poses no special problem because of the length of the small bowel. Proximal and distal margins of 5 cm usually are preferred. In addition, en bloc resection of regional lymph nodes should be performed, carefully preserving superior mesenteric arterial branches to the remaining distal small intestine. Mesenteric vessels can be secured with transfixing sutures of 3-0 silk. The intestinal anastomoses should be watertight, have an adequate stoma, and be free of tension. In our practice, open, hand-sewn anastomosis and stapled anastomosis are performed with equal frequency. A hand-sewn anastomosis is generally fashioned with a mucosal (or through-and-through) running absorbable 3-0 suture and interrupted, inverting, seromuscular sutures of 3-0 silk or Dacron. The defect in the mesentery is carefully closed to prevent internal hernia. If the two ends of transected bowel are roughly equal in size, then an end-to-end anastomosis can be performed. If there is great disparity between the proximal and distal ends, the smaller, distal end can be "fish-mouthed" to enlarge its diameter for the anastomosis. Alternatively, the distal end can be closed (sutured in two layers, as described above, or stapled and the staple line inverted with interrupted 3-0 silk) and an end-to-side anastomosis performed. Side-to-side anastomosis generally is used for palliative bypass or to construct a functional end-to-end anastomosis with the stapler.

The National Cancer Database review found resection and regional lymphadenectomy to be the most common type of operation for small bowel carcinoma, accounting for 21.8% of 4,995 operations between 1985 and 1995.[16] During the first half (1985-1990) of the study period,

16.7% of patients were so treated, but this percentage increased to 25.7% during the second half (1991-1995) of the decade. Radical resections at the primary site accounted for 16.4% of the total, and excision without lymph node dissection was performed in 15.5% of the patients. Small bowel carcinoma is most often found in elderly patients; two-thirds of patients are 60 years or older at diagnosis. In the National Cancer Database review, older patients (> 75 years) were less likely to have curative resection (53.5%) than patients 60 to 75 years old (69%) or younger than 60 years (77.4%). The review also noted that patients who had operation without curative intent had 5-year disease-specific survival that was no different from that in patients who did not have operation (7.4% versus 11.7%, respectively; $P = 0.3260$). The 5-year disease-specific survival for patients who underwent cancer-directed operation (40.3%) was significantly better than that for patients who did not have cancer-directed operation (9.3%; $P < 0.0001$). Chemotherapy was given to 14.2% of patients with localized disease, 35.4% with metastatic regional lymph nodes, and 36.9% with distant metastases.

Survival varies by tumor location as well as histologic type. In the National Cancer Database,[16] the 5-year survival rate was 28.2% in patients with adenocarcinoma of the duodenum and 37.8% in those with jejunal or ileal adenocarcinoma ($P < 0.0001$). Median survival was 16.9 months vs. 29.6 months, respectively. Other significant factors in univariate analysis were age, curative intent, tumor stage, and tumor grade.

CONCLUSION

Although the small bowel is the largest segment of the gastrointestinal tract, small bowel tumors are relatively rare. They are difficult to diagnose because of the often vague presenting symptoms and indolent course of the disease. Treatment most often consists of surgical resection, which remains the only potentially curative therapy for most tumors. Depending on location, stage, and spread of malignancy, surgical intervention is of variable success.

REFERENCES

1. Cusack JC, Tyler DS: Small-bowel malignancies and carcinoid tumors. *In* The M.D. Anderson Surgical Oncology Handbook. Edited by DH Berger, BW Feig, GM Fuhrman. Boston, Little, Brown, 1995, p 142

2. Spiro HM: Clinical Gastroenterology. Third edition. New York, Macmillan, 1983

3. River L, Silverstein J, Tope JW: Benign neoplasms of the small intestine: a critical comprehensive review with reports of 20 new cases. Int Abst Surg 102:1-38, 1956

4. Martin RG: Malignant tumors of the small intestine. Surg Clin North Am 66:779-785, 1986

5. Heston JF, Kelly JB, Meigs JW, Flannery JT: Forty-five years of cancer incidence in Connecticut: 1935-79. Natl Cancer Inst Monogr 70:1-706, 1986

6. Cutler SJ, Young JL Jr (editors): Third National Cancer Survey: incidence data. Natl Cancer Inst Monogr 41:1-454, 1975

7. Weiss NS, Yang CP: Incidence of histologic types of cancer of the small intestine. J Natl Cancer Inst 78:653-656, 1987

8. Lilienfeld AM, Levin ML, Kessler II: Cancer in the United States. Cambridge, Massachusetts, Harvard University Press, 1972, pp 49-122

9. Wilson JM, Melvin DB, Gray GF, Thorbjarnarson B: Primary malignancies of the small bowel: a report of 96 cases and review of the literature. Ann Surg 180:175-179, 1974

10. Strodel WE, Talpos G, Eckhauser F, Thompson N: Surgical therapy for small-bowel carcinoid tumors. Arch Surg 118:391-397, 1983

11. Croom RD III, Newsome JF: Tumors of the small intestine. Am Surg 41:160-167, 1975

12. Good CA: Tumors of the small intestine. Am J Roentgenol 89:685-705, 1963

13. Bridge MF, Perzin KH: Primary adenocarcinoma of the jejunum and ileum: a clinicopathologic study. Cancer 36:1876-1887, 1975

14. Buckley JA, Siegelman SS, Jones B, Fishman EK: The accuracy of CT staging of small bowel adenocarcinoma: CT/pathologic correlation. J Comput Assist Tomogr 21:986-991, 1997

15. Adler SN, Lyon DT, Sullivan PD: Adenocarcinoma of the small bowel: clinical features, similarity of regional enteritis, and analysis of 338 documented cases. Am J Gastroenterol 77:326-330, 1982

16. Howe JR, Karnell LH, Menck HR, Scott-Conner C: the American College of Surgeons Commission on Cancer and the American Cancer Society: adenocarcinoma of the small bowel: review of the National Cancer Data Base, 1985-1995. Cancer 86:2693-2706, 1999

17. Severson RK, Schenk M, Gurney JG, Weiss LK, Demers RY: Increasing incidence of adenocarcinomas and carcinoid tumors of the small intestine in adults. Cancer Epidemiol Biomarkers Prev 5:81-84, 1996

18. Wood DA: Tumors of the intestines. *In* Atlas of Tumor Pathology, Section 6, Fascicle 22. Washington, DC, Armed Forces Institute of Pathology, 1967, pp 1-120

19. Offerhaus GJ, Giardiello FM, Krush AJ, Booker SV, Tersmette AC, Kelley NC, Hamilton SR: The risk of upper gastrointestinal cancer in familial adenomatous polyposis. Gastroenterology 102:1980-1982, 1992

20. Lightdale CJ, Sternberg SS, Posner G, Sherlock P: Carcinoma complicating Crohn's disease: report of seven cases and review of the literature. Am J Med 59:262-268, 1975

21. Hawker PC, Gyde SN, Thompson H, Allan RN: Adenocarcinoma of the small intestine complicating Crohn's disease. Gut 23:188-193, 1982

22. Veyrieres M, Baillet P, Hay JM, Fingerhut A, Bouillot JL, Julien M: Factors influencing long-term survival in 100 cases of small intestine primary adenocarcinoma. Am J Surg 173:237-239, 1997

23. Ribeiro MB, Greenstein AJ, Heimann TM, Yamazaki Y, Aufses AH Jr: Adenocarcinoma of the small intestine in Crohn's disease. Surg Gynecol Obstet 173:343-349, 1991

24. Collier PE, Turowski P, Diamond DL: Small intestinal adenocarcinoma complicating regional enteritis. Cancer 55:516-521, 1985

25. Galandiuk S, Hermann RE, Jagelman DG, Fazio VW, Sivak MV: Villous tumors of the duodenum. Ann Surg 207:234-239, 1988

26. Ryan DP, Schapiro RH, Warshaw AL: Villous tumors of the duodenum. Ann Surg 203:301-306, 1986

27. Minardi AJ Jr, Zibari GB, Aultman DF, McMillan RW, McDonald JC: Small-bowel tumors. J Am Coll Surg 186:664-668, 1998

28. Oberndorfer S: Karzinoide Tumoren des Dünndarms. Frankfurt Ztschr Path Wiesb 1:426-432, 1907

29. Modlin IM, Sandor A: An analysis of 8305 cases of carcinoid tumors. Cancer 79:813-829, 1997

30. Thompson GB, van Heerden JA, Martin JK Jr, Schutt AJ, Ilstrup DM, Carney JA: Carcinoid tumors of the gastrointestinal tract: presentation, management, and prognosis. Surgery 98:1054-1063, 1985

31. Kvols LK, Martin JK, Marsh HM, Moertel CG: Rapid reversal of carcinoid crisis with a somatostatin analogue. N Engl J Med 313:1229-1230, 1985

32. Marsh HM, Martin JK Jr, Kvols LK, Gracey DR, Warner MA, Warner ME, Moertel CG: Carcinoid crisis during anesthesia: successful treatment with a somatostatin analogue. Anesthesiology 66:89-91, 1987

33. Moertel CG, Johnson CM, McKusick MA, Martin JK Jr, Nagorney DM, Kvols LK, Rubin J, Kunselman S: The management of patients with advanced carcinoid tumors and islet cell carcinomas. Ann Intern Med 120:302-309, 1994

34. Rambaud JC: Small intestinal lymphomas and alpha-chain disease. Clin Gastroenterol 12:743-766, 1983

35. Al-Mondhiry H: Primary lymphomas of the small intestine: east-west contrast. Am J Hematol 22:89-105, 1986

36. Herbsman H, Wetstein L, Rosen Y, Orces H, Alfonso AE, Iyer SK, Gardner B: Tumors of the small intestine. Curr Probl Surg 17:121-182, 1980

37. Akwari OE, Dozois RR, Weiland LH, Beahrs OH: Leiomyosarcoma of the small and large bowel. Cancer 42:1375-1384, 1978

38. De Castro CA, Dockerty MB, Mayo CW: Metastatic tumors of the small intestines. Surg Gynecol Obstet 105:159-165, 1957

39. Rankin FW, Mayo C II: Carcinoma of the small bowel. Surg Gynecol Obstet 50:939-947, 1930

Chapter 25

VILLOUS TUMORS OF THE DUODENUM

Jeffrey M. Gauvin, M.D.
Michael B. Farnell, M.D.

Villous tumors of the duodenum (VTD) are premalignant neoplasms, first recognized more than 100 years ago by Perry[1] as broad-based, cauliflower-like masses and referred to as duodenal papillomas. In 1928, Golden[2] published the first definitive report of the treatment of a villous tumor of the duodenum. The term "villous" refers to the velvety texture and fingerlike projections of neoplastic mucosa that resemble villi. The diverse terminology applied to VTD in the past has been inconsistent and has led to confusion in the literature. The tumors have been called villous adenomas, villous papillomas, papillomas, papillomatous polyps, papillary tumors, papillary adenomas, tubulovillous adenomas, and villoglandular polyps.[3] Regardless of the different histologic elements that exist within any one tumor, the clinical presentation and optimal treatment of these variants are similar.

Although all the tumors are neoplasms, and a more correct term would be "villous neoplasms of the duodenum," most of the current literature refers to them as villous "tumors." Therefore, this is the term used in this chapter. The distinction is important because the premalignant nature of VTD was first suggested more than 40 years ago.[4,5] Their natural history is similar to that of villous tumors of the colon and rectum, having both a high rate of recurrence after local treatment and a high incidence of malignancy. About 25% of VTD harbor invasive malignancy at the time of surgical excision. Unlike colorectal lesions, however, the incidence of adenocarcinoma with VTD does not seem to increase as prominently with tumor size.[6,7] All evidence also suggests that the adenoma-carcinoma sequence (tubular adenoma, tubulovillous adenoma, villous adenoma, carcinoma in situ, invasive carcinoma) in colon cancer also occurs in the ampullary and periampullary regions. VTD should therefore be considered malignant (or at least premalignant) until proved otherwise.[3,8] In fact, up to 50% of VTD of the papilla of Vater contain foci of in situ adenocarcinoma at the time of diagnosis.[9,10]

Although VTD were thought to be rare, in that only 73 patients were described in a 1981 review article,[11] they are the most common benign periampullary neoplasm.[12,13] With the recent widespread use of upper endoscopy for evaluation of patients with gastrointestinal complaints, VTD are being recognized with increasing frequency. Moreover, recognition of the frequent association of VTD with colonic polyposis syndromes has heightened our awareness of these unusual neoplasms. Several institutions have published their experiences with VTD. Our recent review of 86 consecutive patients with histologically confirmed VTD treated surgically is the largest such series.[14]

Recurrence of VTD after endoscopic or surgical transduodenal, periampullary resection is common (in our experience, 43% at 10 years), and VTD may recur as an invasive cancer. These observations raise many questions about the appropriate treatment of VTD, especially in younger patients or those with polyposis syndromes.

SIZE AND HISTOLOGY

In our series, as in most others, the mean tumor size was 3 cm in greatest diameter, but the size ranged from 0.5 to 9 cm. Histologically, 75% of VTD were benign adenomas, of which 75% had several areas of atypia, 4% were adenomas containing areas of carcinoma in situ, and 22% contained foci of invasive carcinoma (Table 1). Interestingly, the mean size of each histologic type was 3.1, 1.5, and 3.3 cm, respectively, and did not correlate with the presence of cancer ($P = 0.53$). Because most tumors were in the periampullary region, some investigators have postulated an association between pancreaticobiliary secretions and mucosal transformation.[3] The continuous presence of these secretions bathing the VTD may help explain the differences between colorectal and duodenal villous tumors in terms of the relationship between size and the presence of malignant change.

DISTRIBUTION

About 90% of VTD are solitary and 10% multiple. Among solitary lesions, the vast majority (70%) are periampullary (within 1 cm of the ampulla), 10% occur in the non-periampullary second portion of the duodenum, 10% occur in the third portion of the duodenum, and only 5% are in the first portion. In our experience, only one patient had a lesion in the fourth portion of the duodenum. Interestingly, early in its development, adenomatous tissue involving the ampulla of patients with familial adenomatous polyposis, in particular, forms a goatee-shaped configuration distal to the ampulla, presumably in the area with the highest concentration of bile flow. This distribution also suggests that bile or pancreatic secretions may play a role in the development of duodenal adenomas and carcinomas.[3]

The recognition of a close association between polyposis syndromes of the colon and gastroduodenal villous tumors, and especially VTD, is a unique situation. When all patients with VTD are investigated, about 20% have an associated polyposis syndrome. Of patients with multiple VTD, 70% have an associated polyposis syndrome. Familial adenomatous polyposis was present in 7% of patients with VTD, Gardner variant in 11%, and Peutz-Jegher syndrome in 1%. Rarely, patients with Gardner's syndrome may have innumerable VTD involving all portions of the duodenum. In general, VTD occur equally in men and women and present at a mean age of 64 years. However, patients with an associated polyposis syndrome tend to be younger (mean age, 52 years) and more often have tumors at multiple sites of the duodenum than those with the sporadic form (44% vs. 6%, $P < 0.001$).

SYMPTOMS, SIGNS, AND DIAGNOSIS

VTD present with a wide spectrum of symptoms. Abdominal pain, nausea, weight loss, and symptoms of pancreatitis are the most common presenting complaints (Table 1). Anemia, obstructive jaundice, and weight loss are most prevalent in patients with VTD containing invasive carcinoma. Galandiuk et al.[7] found that jaundice was the most frequent presenting sign in 13 of 32 patients (41%). VTD are asymptomatic in about a third of patients, in which case the diagnosis is made at the time of upper endoscopy for an unrelated disorder or during screening for an associated polyposis syndrome.

Extended fiberoptic endoscopy with full visualization of the duodenum is the most useful and accurate tool for the diagnosis of VTD. Endoscopy allows both visualization and biopsy. All lesions at the ampulla of Vater should

Table 1.—The Relationship of Clinical Presentation to the Histologic Type of Villous Tumor of the Duodenum

Clinical presentation	Benign (n = 64) No.	Benign (n = 64) %	Carcinoma in situ (n = 3) No.	Carcinoma in situ (n = 3) %	Invasive carcinoma (n = 19) No.	Invasive carcinoma (n = 19) %	Overall (n = 86) No.	Overall (n = 86) %
Pain	29	45	1	33	5	26	35	41
Weight loss	8	12	-		7	37	15	17
Nausea, emesis	9	14	-		5	26	14	16
Pancreatitis	9	14	2	66	1	5	12	14
Anemia	5	8	-		4	21	9	11
Jaundice	4	6	-		4	21	8	9
Cholangitis	4	6	-		-		4	5
Melena	2	3	-		2	11	4	5
Asymptomatic; incidental finding	21	33	1	33	5	26	27	31

From Farnell et al.[14] By permission of The Society for Surgery of the Alimentary Tract.

be within reach of a side-viewing duodenoscope. In fact, a side-viewing scope is essential for a proper view of and access to the papilla. About half of VTD are missed with nonfocused, end-viewing endoscopic examinations.[15]

Although a side-viewing endoscopic examination is accurate for the diagnosis of VTD, histologic confirmation of malignancy by biopsy presents a very real risk of sampling error. When malignant change is absent on biopsy, the VTD cannot be considered benign with certainty. In all VTD, and especially in periampullary adenomas, geographic variability in the distribution of dysplasia is common. On endoscopic biopsy, the diagnosis of malignancy in VTD is missed in 40% to 60% of patients.[10,15] Indeed, in our experience, a false-negative diagnosis of malignancy was made preoperatively on the basis of direct endoscopic biopsy in 12 (55%) of 22 patients in whom malignancy was found after complete tumor excision.

Various other upper gastrointestinal imaging studies can be used to diagnose VTD, but they are much less reliable. We found that an upper gastrointestinal radiologic barium contrast study was positive in only 14 of 23 patients with VTD. Abdominal computed tomography showed the tumor in only 17 of 44 patients (Fig. 1). Percutaneous transhepatic cholangiography, performed in four patients with obstructive jaundice, was diagnostic of VTD in only one patient. In three patients, VTD were found incidentally with T-tube cholangiography during or after cholecystectomy and common bile duct exploration for presumed choledocholithiasis (Fig. 2). Subsequent upper gastrointestinal endoscopy confirmed the diagnosis of VTD in all of these patients.

Endoscopic retrograde cholangiopancreatography can be a valuable complementary method for evaluating the extension of villous changes into the common bile duct or pancreatic duct. Furthermore, endoscopic sphincterotomy at endoscopic retrograde cholangiopancreatography can be used for preoperative decompression of the biliary tree when indicated. Computed tomography and ultrasonography have little role in diagnosing VTD but are important for staging in patients with known or presumed malignant VTD. Endoscopic ultrasonography, however, is a promising new method for evaluating the malignant potential of periampullary VTD.[16] Unfortunately, it is not yet widely available, and its accuracy is highly operator-dependent.

CHOICE OF OPERATION

Although there is uniform agreement that most VTD should be resected, opinions differ widely regarding the optimal method. The difficulty in identifying underlying malignancy preoperatively, the potential morbidity and mortality associated with endoscopic resection, operative local resection, or pancreatoduodenectomy, imprecision

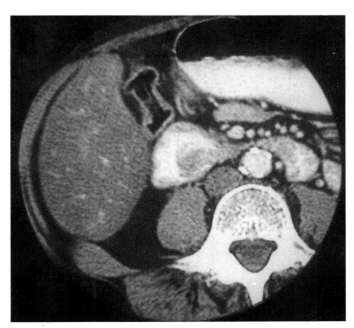

Fig. 1. Abdominal computed tomography with oral and intravenous contrast, demonstrating filling defect in medial wall of second portion of duodenum. (From Farnell et al.[14] By permission of The Society for Surgery of the Alimentary Tract.)

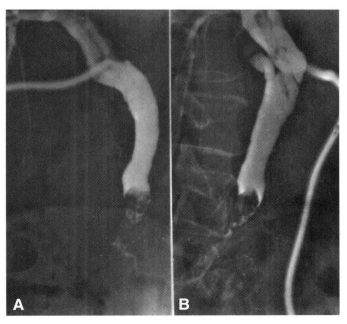

Fig. 2. Postoperative T-tube cholangiograms, showing luminal filling defect with characteristics of neoplasm. Subsequent upper esophagogastroduodenoscopy confirmed the presence of ampullary villous tumor. (A), Anteroposterior view. (B), Lateral view. These images demonstrate the propensity of ampullary villous tumors to extend proximally in the bile duct. (From Farnell et al.[14] By permission of The Society for Surgery of the Alimentary Tract.)

in confirming negative margins, and the high rate of recurrence after local excision combine to make management problematic in most patients. Pancreatoduodenectomy is considered the procedure of choice for VTD containing invasive carcinoma, but management of benign VTD with or without atypia or of VTD containing carcinoma in situ remains controversial.

For benign VTD less than 1 cm, endoscopic resection by an experienced interventional endoscopist is generally considered appropriate. However, for benign VTD more than 1 cm, the debate focuses on the role of transduodenal local excision versus pancreatoduodenectomy. Although transduodenal local excision is an organ-preserving operation with less morbidity and mortality than pancreatoduodenectomy, the complex anatomy of the ampullary region, the well-recognized coexistence of carcinoma within VTD, and the not infrequent recurrence of VTD after operation have led to the most controversy over this approach. In contrast, pancreatoduodenectomy virtually ensures the absence of recurrence and is the best "oncologic" procedure should the final pathologic analysis reveal the presence of an invasive adenocarcinoma. However, pancreatoduodenectomy is associated with greater perioperative morbidity and mortality and may have long-term complications affecting quality of life. Recent studies regarding perioperative and long-term outcome of pancreatoduodenectomy, however, have shown that in centers of excellence with defined experience with pancreatoduodenectomy, the operative mortality rate should be less than 4% and the quality of life after operation is often good.[17-19] An important study by McLeod et al.[20] showed that quality of life and gastrointestinal function after pancreatoduodenectomy, without recurrent tumor, were excellent and similar to these features after cholecystectomy. Accordingly, pancreatoduodenectomy should be considered an option for benign VTD in selected, fit patients, and especially for large or multicentric VTD.

On the basis of an earlier study from our institution,[21] our bias was to perform transduodenal excision for benign VTD, when feasible, because of a presumably low incidence (17%) of local recurrence. A meticulous technique, previously described,[21,22] was thought to be crucial for achieving good results. This study of short-term outcome suggested that pancreatoduodenectomy, as recommended by others,[12,23-25] was not essential for local control. However, our latest study of a much larger group of patients (86 vs. 36) with a much longer follow-up, demonstrated a recurrence rate of 32% at 5 years and of 43% at 10 years for histologically confirmed benign VTD after local excision. More importantly, 4 of the 17 benign tumors managed by local excision recurred as adenocarcinoma, and 3 of these 4 as invasive adenocarcinoma.

These new data call into question the role of local excision, even for benign VTD. This additional experience, coupled with the improved safety of pancreatoduodenectomy, prompted us to reassess the respective roles of local excision and pancreatoduodenectomy for this problematic neoplasm. Given this additional information, we now advocate pancreatoduodenectomy for many of the benign VTD in selected patients, especially in younger patients and those with very large VTD in which an adequate margin from the neoplasm would be problematic with local resection. When considering treatment options for VTD, two groups need to be considered: sporadic VTD and those associated with polyposis syndromes.

Sporadic VTD

When local excision for benign VTD is contemplated, factors affecting the propensity for recurrence must be considered. Hard areas on palpation, an ulcerated tumor, dilatation or obstruction of the common bile duct or the pancreatic duct on preoperative imaging, severe dysplasia on preoperative biopsies, or villous lesions extending into the bile or pancreatic ducts should be considered suspicious for underlying malignancy. In the presence of these factors, a pancreatoduodenectomy should be strongly entertained, especially in medically fit patients. When these factors are absent, local excision seems reasonable for compliant patients willing to undergo lifelong endoscopic surveillance at regular intervals or for patients unfit for a more radical operation. For benign VTD, without the above-mentioned factors, located on the lateral wall of the second portion of the duodenum and for those in the first, distal third, or fourth portions of the duodenum, full-thickness excision or even segmental resections are reasonable options. Whether preoperative endoscopic ultrasonography will allow better selection of candidates for local excision, as suggested by Rattner et al.,[16] is yet to be determined.

For VTD harboring invasive cancer that arises in the first, second, or proximal third portion, pancreatoduodenectomy is warranted. We prefer the pylorus-preserving technique for sporadic VTD, provided the tumor does not arise in the first portion of the duodenum and the patient does not have a polyposis syndrome. Among our 19 patients with VTD containing invasive cancer, the 5-year survival was 49%, which is similar to that in previous reports.[21,26] When VTD arise in the distal third or fourth portion of the duodenum, an extended segmental resection may be as effective as a pancreatoduodenectomy, because the classic pancreatoduodenectomy does not remove the primary lymph nodal basin of these distal duodenal cancers, namely, the nodes around the superior mesenteric artery.

Treatment for VTD containing only carcinoma in situ is much more controversial. In our series, only two such patients were treated with transduodenal local excision, and both remained recurrence-free 7 and 8 years postoperatively. Such a small experience prevents any firm recommendations. Nonetheless, given the expected high recurrence rate and the fact that VTD may recur as invasive cancer, we now believe that a medically fit person would benefit from a pancreatoduodenectomy for these lesions.

Recurrence after local excision can be treated either with local reexcision (open or endoscopic) or, as we prefer, with pancreatoduodenectomy. Unfortunately, recurrence may be in the form of invasive carcinoma, as occurred in 4 (23%) of our 17 patients. In such circumstances, pancreatoduodenectomy, when feasible, is the only reasonable option.

VTD Associated With Polyposis Syndromes

The duodenum and especially the periampullary region are second only to the colorectum as a site of polyp-associated malignancy in patients with familial adenomatous polyposis (FAP).[27-32] With the advent of prophylactic proctocolectomy, periampullary carcinoma is now the leading cause of mortality in FAP, affecting as many as 12% of patients.[29-32] In FAP, the relative risk of periampullary or duodenal cancer is 250 times that in the general population,[33,34] and mortality rates due to periampullary cancer are more than 300 times that in the general population.[27,35] For these reasons, patients with FAP should be enrolled in an established surveillance program of esophagogastroduodenoscopy once the diagnosis is established.

Our current recommendation for patients with FAP without a known VTD is an extended duodenoscopy with multiple ampullary biopsies once per year. Patients with positive ampullary biopsy specimens undergo snare ampullectomy, sphincterotomy, and thermal ablation of the periampullary adenomas with reexamination every 3 months until histologic resolution. Henceforth, patients are reexamined endoscopically and have biopsy annually. Recognition of high-grade dysplasia should prompt consideration of open surgical intervention. Because the entire duodenal mucosa is at risk, consideration should be given to pancreatoduodenectomy[36,37] or possibly the new operation of pancreas-sparing duodenectomy,[38,39] described below. Indeed, of the 11 patients with associated polyposis syndromes and benign VTD treated with local excision alone, 7 (64%) had recurrence.

Our experience with the theoretically attractive pancreas-sparing duodenectomy for the treatment of benign VTD in the series described above and since is limited to eight patients. Although technically demanding, the procedure eliminates the need for pancreatic resection and is associated with good intestinal absorption after operation, weight gain, and an excellent quality of life.[40] In our experience there were, however, five postoperative complications, including one reoperative intervention for hemorrhage, three temporary fistulas, and one wound infection. If pancreas-sparing duodenectomy is successful, long-term surveillance is still required. Moreover, it is clearly contraindicated in the setting of malignancy. Additional experience with the procedure will be needed before its role in the management of patients with FAP and VTD is established.

CONDUCT OF OPERATION

Pancreatoduodenectomy

We prefer the pylorus-preserving technique whenever possible. The length of the retained duodenal cuff is minimized with performance essentially of a pylorojejunostomy. If, however, tumor involves the first part of the duodenum, a standard pancreatoduodenectomy is performed. These procedures are described in Chapter 18.

Transduodenal Local Excision

Postoperative complications can be avoided and recurrence after local excision can be minimized if several key technical points and the complex periampullary anatomy are kept in mind (Fig. 3). After abdominal exploration, the head of the

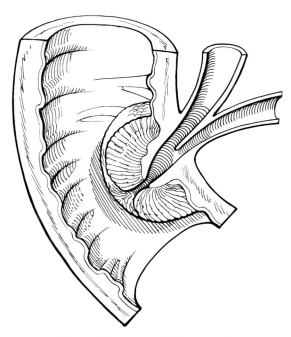

Fig. 3. Periampullary villous tumor. The regional anatomy complicates local excision. (From Sakorafas and Sarr.[22] By permission of Mayo Foundation.)

pancreas and the second and third portions of the duodenum are mobilized by an extended Kocher maneuver (Fig. 4). The appropriate site for the duodenotomy is chosen by transmural palpation. With a single finger, the adenoma and papilla are palpated through the lateral duodenal wall (Fig. 4). A longitudinal duodenotomy is then made laterally directly opposite the adenoma; adequate anterior mobilization of the duodenum is important. After the margin of the villous tumor is defined, the papilla is located. This can be done by identifying the site of egress of bile into the duodenum, by retrograde cannulation through the duodenotomy, or by inserting a Fogarty balloon catheter through the cystic duct remnant (after cholecystectomy) or, if necessary, through the common bile duct and advancing the catheter through the papilla (Fig. 5).

The submucosa surrounding the tumor is infiltrated with dilute adrenaline solution (1:100,000 solution) for a distance of 5 mm from the tumor's lateral border. This maneuver minimizes bleeding and facilitates submucosal excision by elevating the mucosa circumferentially around the tumor (Fig. 5). A distance of at least 5 mm is maintained from the lateral extent of the tumor, and the adenoma is circumscribed with electrocautery and dissected off the duodenal musculature. Finally, the papilla is transected, exposing the orifices of the pancreatic and common bile ducts (Fig. 6). These ducts maintain a direct connection with one another by way of the septal area.

Before reconstruction, the orifice of each duct is carefully inspected for residual adenomatous tissue that would necessitate excision. The pancreatico-biliary-duodenal junction is reconstructed by approximating the pancreaticobiliary mucosa to the duodenal mucosa with fine interrupted sutures (Fig. 6 A). An intraluminal probe, such as a Fogarty catheter, and optical magnification prevent inclusion of the opposite wall of the duct within the suture.

If the bile duct is not dilated, stricture of the reconstructed mucosal junction may be prevented by adding a sphincterotomy and, if necessary, a pancreatic ductal septectomy. In this event, the subsequent mucosal reapproximation results in a wider common pancreaticobiliary orifice

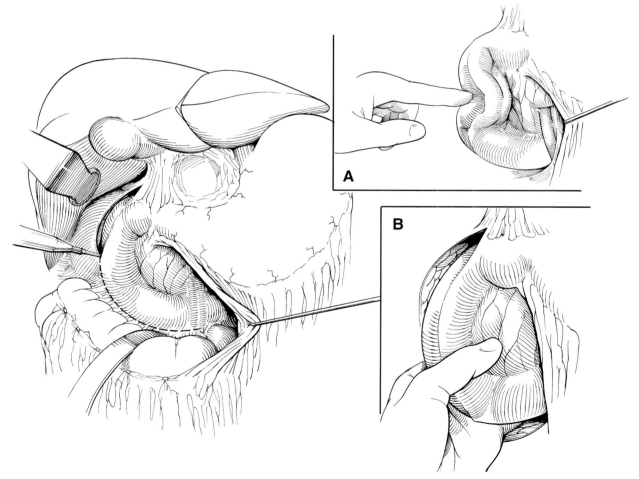

Fig. 4. Wide Kocher maneuver (left *and* B). *Transmural palpation to select the appropriate site for duodenotomy* (A). *(From Sakorafas and Sarr.[22] By permission of Mayo Foundation.)*

(Fig. 6 *B*). On completion, patency of both ducts should be assessed by cannulation with appropriately sized probes.

Intraductal extension of the tumor, which may not be evident on preoperative studies, requires excising a portion of one or both ducts. The ducts should be divided in a stepwise fashion, and the proximal end should be tagged with fine suture to prevent retraction into the pancreas (Fig. 7). Most importantly, the specimens must be carefully marked for anatomical orientation, such that any residual villous changes left at the margin of resection can be excised. Reconstruction involves precise approximation of the biliary and pancreatic ducts to the duodenal mucosa as two separate anastomoses (Fig. 7). Closure of the duodenotomy and drainage of the right subhepatic space complete the procedure.

MAYO CLINIC SURGICAL EXPERIENCE

Since 1980, we have operated on 86 patients with VTD, 64 with benign VTD, 3 with carcinoma in situ, and 19 with VTD containing invasive carcinoma.

Of the 64 patients with benign VTD, 50 with histologically confirmed benign VTD were treated by transduodenal local excision (combined with sphincteroplasty with or without pancreatic duct septotomy in 28 patients), 6 by pancreatoduodenectomy, 5 by pancreas-sparing duodenectomy, and 3 with VTD on the lateral wall of the duodenum by full-thickness excision.

Of the three patients with carcinoma in situ, two were treated by local excision. The presence of carcinoma in situ was recognized only on permanent histologic sections. These two patients received no further operation or other type of treatment. The other patient underwent a planned

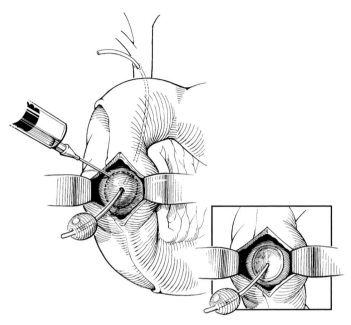

Fig. 5. Identification of the papilla by inserting a biliary Fogarty balloon catheter, and infiltration of the submucosa around the tumor with dilute adrenaline solution. Inset, Tumor has been excised and papilla transected, exposing the orifices of the pancreatic and common bile ducts. (From Sakorafas and Sarr.[22] By permission of Mayo Foundation.)

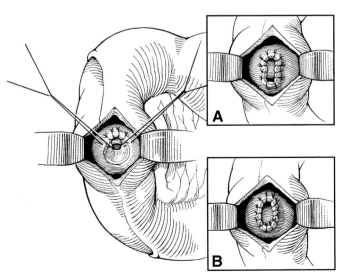

Fig. 6. Reconstruction of the pancreatico-biliary-duodenal junction, without (A) and with (B) sphincterotomy and pancreatic ductal septectomy. (From Sakorafas and Sarr.[22] By permission of Mayo Foundation.)

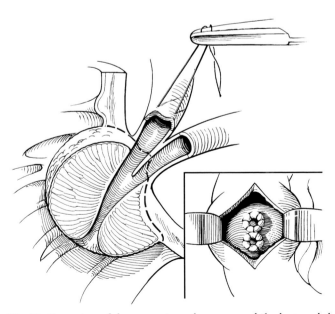

Fig. 7. Extension of the tumor into the common bile duct and the pancreatic duct. Inset, For reconstruction of the pancreatico-biliary-duodenal junction, biliary and pancreatic ducts are reapproximated with duodenal mucosa as two separate anastomoses. (From Sakorafas and Sarr.[22] By permission of Mayo Foundation.)

pancreatoduodenectomy because dilatation of the pancreatic duct was suspicious for underlying malignancy.

Of the 19 patients with VTD containing invasive carcinoma, 13 were managed with pancreatoduodenectomy. Of the 10 patients in whom invasive carcinoma within the VTD was known preoperatively, 8 were treated by pancreatoduodenectomy and 2 had unresectable lesions (liver metastasis; local extension) and underwent operative palliation. In the nine patients in whom cancer within the VTD was not known preoperatively, an initial attempt at local excision was converted to either pancreatoduodenectomy in five (because of suspicious findings or a frozen-section diagnosis of invasive carcinoma), to segmental resection in two, and to full-thickness excision in one with cirrhosis and portal hypertension and in one with extensive nodal metastases.

OPERATIVE MORBIDITY AND MORTALITY

Only one patient died after operation. This patient had sepsis after pancreatoduodenectomy from a leak at the hepaticojejunostomy. In total, 30 complications occurred in 23 (27%) of our 86 patients who had operation. Morbidity varied with the operative procedure and was 17% after local excision, 40% after pancreatoduodenectomy, 80% after pancreas-sparing duodenectomy (four of five patients), and 50% after full-thickness duodenal excision (two of four patients). The complications were typical of periampullary operation: postoperative pancreatitis, 3 patients; anastomotic leak, 13 patients; intra-abdominal abscess, 3 patients; and delayed gastric emptying, 7 patients. The mean duration of hospital stay was 15 days.

LONG-TERM FOLLOW-UP

For 82 of our 86 patients (95%), long-term follow-up data were available. The mean duration was 5.6 years (range, 0.3-16 years). Twenty-one patients (26%) died, 10 from recurrent metastatic adenocarcinoma and 11 from unrelated causes. No recurrences developed in patients with benign VTD managed by pancreatoduodenectomy, pancreas-sparing duodenectomy, or full-thickness excision. In contrast, benign VTD recurred in 17 of 52 patients who had undergone transduodenal local excision for benign tumors or for tumors containing carcinoma in situ. All recurrences were in the group with benign VTD, whereas none of the three VTD with carcinoma in situ recurred. Most recurrences were observed within 5 years, but late recurrences, even after 10 years, also were noted. The cumulative recurrence rate was 32% at 5 years and 43% at 10 years (Fig. 8). Of 19 patients with VTD containing invasive carcinoma (3 treated by local resection

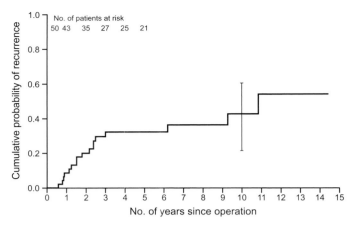

Fig. 8. Cumulative probability (Kaplan-Meier) of any recurrence in 50 patients with benign villous tumors of the duodenum (both sporadic and polyposis-associated) treated by local excision. The recurrence rate was 32% at 5 years and 43% at 10 years. The 95% confidence limits are shown. (From Farnell et al.[14] By permission of The Society for Surgery of the Alimentary Tract.)

and 16 by pancreatoduodenectomy), 11 died; the 5-year survival rate for this group was 49% (Fig. 9).

Most worrisome to us were the four patients with histologically confirmed benign VTD treated by local excision in whom the tumor recurred as adenocarcinoma 1.5, 2.5, 3, and 6 years later. These recurrences represent 23% (4 of 17) of recurrences, or about 8% of all patients undergoing local excision for benign VTD. Three of the four malignant recurrences had invasion; one of these proved to be unresectable. The fourth malignant recurrence was a carcinoma in situ. Although the numbers are small, there were no obvious differences in the size of the original tumor between patients with and those without recurrence as adenocarcinoma.

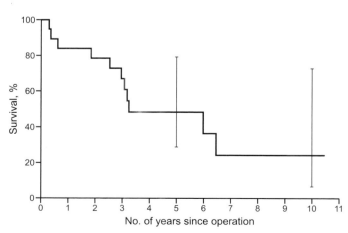

Fig. 9. Survival among 19 patients with villous tumors of the duodenum containing invasive cancer. Includes patients undergoing potentially curative and palliative procedures. The 95% confidence limits are shown. (From Farnell et al.[14] By permission of The Society for Surgery of the Alimentary Tract.)

The remaining 13 recurrences of VTD were treated by endoscopic resection in 10, local reexcision in 2, and pancreatoduodenectomy in 1. Four recurrences developed after endoscopic excision and were managed by transduodenal reexcision in three and pancreas-sparing duodenectomy in one. In patients with solitary sporadic, benign villous tumors managed by transduodenal local excision, recurrence was more likely to develop when the tumor was periampullary than when it was remote from the papilla (34% and 0%, respectively) ($P \leq 0.03$) (Fig. 10).

Of the 11 patients with an associated polyposis syndrome and a benign VTD treated by local excision, 7 had a recurrence. Recurrence rates were 60% at 5 years and 73% at 10 years. These rates are greater than those in patients without an associated polyposis syndrome (24% at 5 years and 30% at 10 years) ($P \leq 0.03$) (Fig. 11).

CONCLUSION

Surgical management of VTD is selective and based on clinical presentation, information from preoperative diagnostic evaluation, the presence of a polyposis syndrome, and intraoperative findings. Although local excision has a lower rate of operative complications, the high recurrence rate (32% at 5 years, 43% at 10 years) is disconcerting and especially so in patients younger than 60 years. If VTD are treated by local excision, a program of yearly endoscopic surveillance is mandatory.

Pancreatoduodenectomy prevents recurrence and is appropriate for selected patients at high risk with either benign VTD or VTD containing carcinoma. For patients with VTD associated with polyposis syndromes, the entire duodenal mucosa is at risk for malignancy. Dysplasia warrants complete removal of the duodenal mucosa by pancreatoduodenectomy or pancreas-sparing duodenectomy.

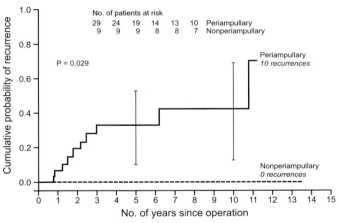

Fig. 10. Cumulative probability of recurrence (Kaplan-Meier) of solitary, sporadic benign villous tumors of the duodenum after local excision in 29 patients with periampullary location and in 9 patients with tumors remote from the papilla. The recurrence rates at 5 years were 34% and 0%, respectively (P = 0.029). The 95% confidence limits are shown. Patients with associated polyposis syndrome or with multiple tumors are excluded. (From Farnell et al.[14] By permission of The Society for Surgery of the Alimentary Tract.)

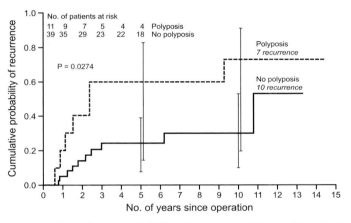

Fig. 11. Cumulative probability of recurrence (Kaplan-Meier) of benign villous tumors of the duodenum after local excision in 11 patients with associated polyposis syndrome and in 39 patients with sporadic tumors. The recurrence rates at 5 years were 60% and 24%, respectively (P = 0.0274). The 95% confidence limits are shown. (From Farnell et al.[14] By permission of The Society for Surgery of the Alimentary Tract.)

REFERENCES

1. Perry EC: Papilloma of the duodenum. Tr Pathol Soc Lond 44:84-88, 1892-1893
2. Golden R: Non-malignant tumors of the duodenum: report of 2 cases. Am J Roentgenol 20:405-413, 1928
3. Sakorafas GH, Friess H, Dervenis CG: Villous tumors of the duodenum: biologic characters and clinical implications. Scand J Gastroenterol 35:337-344, 2000
4. Baggenstoss AH: Major duodenal papilla: variations of pathologic interest and lesions of the mucosa. Arch Pathol 26:853-868, 1938
5. Cattell RB, Pyrtek LJ: Premalignant lesions of the ampulla of Vater. Surg Gynecol Obstet 90:21-30, 1950
6. Kutin ND, Ranson JH, Gouge TH, Localio SA: Villous tumors of the duodenum. Ann Surg 181:164-168, 1975
7. Galandiuk S, Hermann RE, Jagelman DG, Fazio VW, Sivak MV: Villous tumors of the duodenum. Ann Surg 207:234-239, 1988
8. Miller JH, Gisvold JJ, Weiland LH, McIlrath DC: Upper gastrointestinal tract: villous tumors. AJR Am J Roentgenol 134:933-936, 1980
9. Shabot MM, Asch MJ, Moore TC, State D: Benign obstructing papilloma of the ampulla of Vater in infancy. Surgery 78:560-563, 1975
10. Neumann RD, LiVolsi VA, Rosenthal NS, Burnell M, Ball TJ: Adenocarcinoma in biliary papillomatosis. Gastroenterology 70:779-782, 1976
11. Komorowski RA, Cohen EB: Villous tumors of the duodenum: a clinicopathologic study. Cancer 47:1377-1386, 1981
12. Asbun HJ, Rossi RL, Munson JL: Local resection for ampullary tumors. Is there a place for it? Arch Surg 128:515-520, 1993
13. Baczako K, Buchler M, Beger HG, Kirkpatrick CJ, Haferkamp O: Morphogenesis and possible precursor lesions of invasive carcinoma of the papilla of Vater: epithelial dysplasia and adenoma. Hum Pathol 16:305-310, 1985
14. Farnell MB, Sakorafas GH, Sarr MG, Rowland CM, Tsiotos GG, Farley DR, Nagorney DM: Villous tumors of the duodenum: reappraisal of local vs. extended resection. J Gastrointest Surg 4:13-21, 2000
15. Bleau BL, Gostout CJ: Endoscopic treatment of ampullary adenomas in familial adenomatous polyposis. J Clin Gastroenterol 22:237-241, 1996
16. Rattner DW, Fernandez-del Castillo C, Brugge WR, Warshaw AL: Defining the criteria for local resection of ampullary neoplasms. Arch Surg 131:366-371, 1996
17. Cameron JL, Pitt HA, Yeo CJ, Lillemoe KD, Kaufmann HS, Coleman J: One hundred and forty-five consecutive pancreaticoduodenectomies without mortality. Ann Surg 217:430-435, 1993
18. Fernandez-del Castillo C, Rattner DW, Warshaw AL: Standards for pancreatic resection in the 1990s. Arch Surg 130:295-299, 1995
19. Gordon TA, Burleyson GP, Tielsch JM, Cameron JL: The effects of regionalization on cost and outcome for one general high-risk surgical procedure. Ann Surg 221:43-49, 1995
20. McLeod RS, Taylor BR, O'Connor BI, Greenberg GR, Jeejeebhoy KN, Royall D, Langer B: Quality of life, nutritional status, and gastrointestinal hormone profile following the Whipple procedure. Am J Surg 169:179-185, 1995
21. Bjork KJ, Davis CJ, Nagorney DM, Mucha P Jr: Duodenal villous tumors. Arch Surg 125:961-965, 1990
22. Sakorafas GH, Sarr MG: Local excision of periampullary villous tumours of the duodenum. Eur J Surg Oncol 25:90-93, 1999
23. Chappuis CW, Divincenti FC, Cohn I Jr: Villous tumors of the duodenum. Ann Surg 209:593-598, 1989
24. Zinzindohoue F, Gallot D, Majery N, Malafosse M: A radical treatment of villous tumors of the duodenum [French]. Ann Chir 50:330-332, 1996
25. Ryan DP, Shapiro RH, Warshaw AL: Villous tumors of the duodenum. Ann Surg 203:301-306, 1986
26. Monson JR, Donohue JH, McEntee GP, McIlrath DC, van Heerden JA, Shorter RG, Nagorney DM, Ilstrup DM: Radical resection for carcinoma of the ampulla of Vater. Arch Surg 126:353-357, 1991
27. Offerhaus GJ, Giardiello FM, Krush AJ, Booker SV, Tersmette AC, Kelley NC, Hamilton SR: The risk of upper gastrointestinal cancer in familial adenomatous polyposis. Gastroenterology 102:1980-1982, 1992
28. Jagelman DG, DeCosse JJ, Bussey HJ: Upper gastrointestinal cancer in familial adenomatous polyposis. Lancet 1:1149-1151, 1988
29. Arvanitis ML, Jagelman DG, Fazio VW, Lavery IC, McGannon E: Mortality in patients with familial adenomatous polyposis. Dis Colon Rectum 33;639-642, 1990
30. Goedde TA, Rodriguez-Bigas MA, Herrera L, Petrelli NJ: Gastroduodenal polyps in familial adenomatous polyposis. Surg Oncol 1:357-361, 1992
31. Belchetz LA, Berk T, Bapat BV, Cohen Z, Gallinger S: Changing causes of mortality in patients with familial adenomatous polyposis. Dis Colon Rectum 39:384-387, 1996
32. Bertario L, Presciuttini S, Sala P, Rossetti C, Pietroiusti M: Causes of death and postsurgical survival in familial adenomatous polyposis: results from the Italian Registry. Italian Registry of Familial Polyposis Writing Committee. Semin Surg Oncol 10:225-234, 1994
33. Iwama T, Mishima Y, Utsunomiya J: The impact of familial adenomatous polyposis on the tumorigenesis and mortality at the several organs: its rational treatment. Ann Surg 217:101-108, 1993
34. Iwama T, Tomita H, Kawachi Y, Yoshinaga K, Kume S, Maruyama H, Mishima Y: Indications for local excision of ampullary lesions associated with familial adenomatous polyposis. J Am Coll Surg 179:462-464, 1994
35. Sanabria JR, Croxford R, Berk TC, Cohen Z, Bapat BV, Gallinger S: Familial segregation in the occurrence and severity of periampullary neoplasms in familial adenomatous polyposis. Am J Surg 171:136-140, 1996
36. Wallace MH, Phillips RK: Upper gastrointestinal disease in patients with familial adenomatous polyposis. Br J Surg 85:742-750, 1998
37. Penna C, Bataille N, Balladur P, Tiret E, Parc R: Surgical treatment of severe duodenal polyposis in familial adenomatous polyposis. Br J Surg 85:665-668, 1998
38. Chung RS, Church JM, vanStolk R: Pancreas-sparing duodenectomy: indications, surgical technique, and results. Surgery 117:254-259, 1995
39. Maher MM, Yeo CJ, Lillemoe KD, Roberts JR, Cameron JL: Pancreas-sparing duodenectomy for infra-ampullary duodenal pathology. Am J Surg 171:62-67, 1996
40. Sarmiento JM, Thompson GB, Nagorney DM, Donohue JH, Farnell MB: Pancreas-sparing duodenectomy for duodenal polyposis. Arch Surg 137:557-562, 2002

SMALL INTESTINAL DIVERTICULA

Daniel J. Ostlie, M.D.
Keith A. Kelly, M.D.

Diverticula are found throughout the small intestine. However, because of their relative rarity and the infrequency with which they cause complications, they have historically been viewed as anatomical curiosities rather than life-threatening disorders. Nonetheless, complications of small intestinal diverticula do occur, and when they do, serious morbidity and even mortality can result. The surgeon, thus, must be able to identify the diverticula and their complications and be prepared to intervene with appropriate surgical care to bring about an expeditious and successful outcome for the patient.

Meckel, in 1822, was the first to separate small intestinal diverticula into two categories: true and false. True diverticula contain all layers of the wall of the gastrointestinal tract, including a complete tunica muscularis. Conversely, false diverticula lack a tunica muscularis. They usually have only mucosal, submucosal, and serosal layers, the mucosa and submucosa having herniated through a defect in the tunica muscularis of the intestinal wall to form the diverticulum.

Krishnamurthy et al.[1] provided a more recent classification of the two diverticular types. The first, the acquired or pulsion diverticula, correspond to Meckel's false diverticula. They can be found in the duodenum, jejunum, and ileum. The second, the congenital, or true, diverticula, occur almost always in the ileum, where they are called Meckel's diverticula.

DUODENAL DIVERTICULA

Location, Incidence, and Cause

Chomel, in 1710, was the first to report a duodenal diverticulum, one that contained 22 calculi.[2] Since that time, multiple authors have documented the presence of these diverticula.[3-5] They are now recognized as the most common of all small intestinal diverticula. Approximately 75% are found near the ampulla of Vater on the pancreatic border of the second part of the duodenum. Rarely, they are found in the first, third, or fourth portions of the duodenum.[6]

Duodenal diverticula have been identified in up to 5% of persons undergoing radiographic studies[6] and nearly 25% of subjects having endoscopic or autopsy studies.[3] The incidence is the same among men and women, but it does increase with age. The diagnosis is usually made after the sixth decade of life and rarely before 40 years of age. In one series of 50 patients,[3] the mean age was 73 years, and only 2% of patients were younger than 40 years, findings similar to those of smaller series.[7,8] Because the vast majority of persons with duodenal diverticula are asymptomatic, the exact incidence is unknown.

The location of most duodenal diverticula along the pancreatic border lends support to the theory that the diverticula occur at points of vascular penetration into the bowel wall. Disordered duodenal motility and increased intraluminal duodenal pressure are other postulated causes.[9]

Symptoms and Signs

More than 90% of duodenal diverticula are asymptomatic.[10] When symptoms do occur, they are usually nonspecific and include nausea, vomiting, and postprandial epigastric pain. As noted above, most of these diverticula are adjacent to the papilla of Vater. Hence, it is not surprising that pancreatic or biliary symptoms are common.[3-5] Multiple authors have reported an increased incidence of pigmented biliary tract stones in persons with the diverticula.[11,12] The likely mechanism involves bacterial overgrowth in and around the diverticula with the bile duct being colonized with β-glucuronidase–producing bacteria. These bacteria deconjugate bilirubin to form free bilirubin, which binds to calcium, forming insoluble calcium bilirubinate.[9] Primary and recurrent common bile duct stones are much more common in persons with duodenal diverticula than in those without. In a study of 101 patients who had pancreatic or biliary symptoms after cholecystectomy, the probability of finding common bile duct stones was 88% when duodenal diverticula were present and 32% when they were not.[13] Interestingly, cholecystectomy does not prevent the development of common bile duct stones in persons with these diverticula.[14,15]

The relationship between acute and chronic pancreatitis and duodenal diverticula has been suggested in several series.[2,16] However, the diverticula cannot, at present, be considered a primary cause of pancreatitis, because biliary stones are often present in persons with pancreatitis; the stones could be causing the pancreatitis. Inspissated food causing distention of the diverticulum and compression of the pancreatic duct and ampullary dysfunction are other possible reasons for the development of pancreatitis in persons with the diverticula.[17,18]

Serious complications such as hemorrhage and perforation are, fortunately, rare. When present, they are associated with a mortality rate of up to 20%.[3] Bleeding can be massive and difficult to identify and control, especially if the diverticulum is found along the medial aspect of the duodenum. Only 102 patients in the world literature have been reported with duodenal perforation as a complication of duodenal diverticula.[10] The diagnosis is often difficult and made only at celiotomy. Complete kocherization of the duodenum at operation usually reveals the site of perforation.

Diagnosis

Diagnostic studies useful in identifying these diverticula include upper gastrointestinal radiologic examinations with contrast media and esophagogastroduodenoscopy. Diverticula originating along the lateral wall of the duodenum are readily identified during the radiologic examinations. Periampullary diverticula can be more difficult to diagnose radiographically. They often require endoscopy for accurate diagnosis.

The biliary tree must be evaluated with ultrasonography and cholangiography when symptoms consistent with biliary obstruction or infection are being considered in an individual with a duodenal diverticulum. Abnormalities of the biliary tree must be ruled out before assuming the symptoms are a result of the diverticula.

Treatment

Operation is usually necessary when duodenal diverticula become symptomatic. Treatment depends on the severity of the symptoms, the complication encountered, and the location of the diverticula. For periampullary diverticula, an endoscopic approach with a diathermy snare for excision has been described as a safe and effective technique.[19] More often, however, surgical excision is needed, especially for patients with emergency indications. Elective resection should be reserved for patients with intractable pain or obstructive symptoms caused by the diverticula.

For non-periampullary diverticula, we favor local excision with a two-layer closure using sutures or staples. A Kocher maneuver is performed, rolling the duodenum to the left to gain complete exposure. If this approach proves technically difficult or risks injury to the pancreatic or biliary tree because the diverticulum is deeply embedded within the head of the pancreas, invagination of the diverticulum with or without excision is an alternative.[3] A drain is placed near the site of operation for use postoperatively. When dealing with periampullary diverticula, excision also is preferred, but precise identification of the ampulla of Vater is required to avoid injury to it and subsequent stenosis. Identification is accomplished retrogradely with a probe through a duodenotomy or antegradely by way of a choledochotomy. When the common bile duct is opened, we leave a drain within it that is removed postoperatively. Diverticula within 1 cm of the papilla may necessitate a sphincteroplasty along with the diverticulectomy.

Emergency exploration for perforation, obstruction, or hemorrhage of duodenal diverticula should not be delayed.[10] Perforation with minimal or mild inflammation can be managed with diverticulectomy and closure of the duodenum, sometimes reinforced by an omental patch or serosal patch from a jejunal loop. For severe inflammation with obstruction, a duodenojejunostomy or gastrojejunostomy may be advisable to divert enteric flow away from the perforation site. If this is not possible, duodenal exclusion with bilioenteric anastomosis also can be considered.[20,21] The key to successful outcome is the maintenance of adequate drainage of the pancreatic and biliary ducts. Reimplantation of pancreatic or biliary ducts in cases of severe infection or inflammation should not be attempted because of the risk of poor healing and leak after operation.

Gastrointestinal hemorrhage due to a duodenal diverticulum is extremely rare. The specific bleeding vessel or ulcer can be difficult to localize. Precise localization with endoscopic or arteriographic techniques greatly facilitates operative intervention. Once identification is complete, diverticulectomy with ligation of the bleeding site is adequate. Acid suppression with medical therapy should be used in all cases.

JEJUNOILEAL DIVERTICULA

As with duodenal diverticula, jejunoileal diverticula have been medical curiosities for more than 200 years. Summerling and Baillie are credited as the first to describe false jejunoileal diverticula in 1794.[22] During the ensuing half century, sporadic cases of these diverticula were reported, including Sir Astley Cooper's case of jejunal diverticulosis described in his monograph on hernias in 1807.[23] Osler, in 1881, reported the first series of jejunoileal diverticula, consisting of 56 patients,[24] and in 1906 Gordinier and Sampson operated successfully on a patient with intestinal obstruction due to jejunal diverticula.[25] Radiologic diagnosis was first made by Case in 1920 with preoperative upper gastrointestinal contrast examination.[26]

Location, Incidence, and Cause

Jejunoileal diverticula are almost exclusively located on the mesenteric aspect of the intestine, at the entry or exit points of the vasa recta (Fig. 1). The larger vasa recta in the jenunum, as opposed to the ileum, are thought to account for the proclivity of diverticula to occur in the jejunum. Approximately 85% of the diverticula are jejunal, 10% are ileal, and 5% are in both locations. Multiplicity of diverticula is the general rule in the jejunum. However, multiplicity occurs less often distally; most diverticula are solitary in the ileum. The literature supports a slight male predilection, and the diverticula occur most often in the sixth and seventh decades of life. An association with diverticula in other parts of the gastrointestinal tract, most commonly duodenum and colon, is often present.[27,28]

When compared with the remainder of the intestinal tract (excluding stomach), jejunoileal false diverticula are the rarest forms of diverticular disease. Only 0.02% to 0.42% of patients examined with small intestinal radiologic contrast examinations have these lesions, whereas only 2.0% to 2.3% of patients who have enteroclysis studies have them. Autopsy series have revealed similar rates, ranging from 0.3% to 4%.[29,30]

The exact cause of jejunoileal diverticula remains elusive. That they may be pulsion diverticula has been commonly proposed. However, the pathogenesis has not been clearly delineated. The predisposition of diverticular formation on the mesenteric aspect of the intestine at "weak" points associated with the vasa recta has been suggested, as noted above. This concept is certainly an oversimplified explanation of a process that likely is multifactorial. Multiple authors have postulated theories that espouse dysmotility, abnormal innervation, or a combination of both as the cause. A functional deficit in the intrinsic innervation of the intestine distal to the diverticula with hypermotility and increased intraluminal pressure could lead to the formation of outpouchings. Altemeier et al.[31]

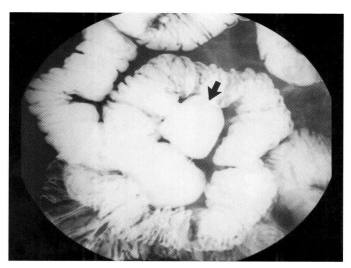

Fig. 1. Small intestinal radiograph obtained with barium sulfate contrast medium showing a jejunal diverticulum (arrow) arising from the mesenteric border of the mid jejunum.

suggested this as a mechanism based on the finding of uncoordinated hypermotility in a portion of thickened jejunum containing diverticula. Krishnamurthy et al.[1] reported abnormal smooth muscle and myenteric plexuses in intestine containing diverticula. They hypothesized that disordered contractions of the affected intestinal segment result in increased intraluminal pressures and subsequent prolapse of mucosa through vascular defects along the mesenteric border, leading to diverticular formation. These findings in combination with the high frequency of coexistent gastrointestinal diverticular disease suggest a more generalized motor disorder throughout the gastrointestinal tract. Attempts have been made to document abnormal motility throughout the gut. However, to date, they have yielded inconclusive results.[27]

Symptoms and Signs

The vast majority of patients with jejunoileal diverticula are asymptomatic, the diverticula being found incidentally at operation for other reasons or on routine radiologic examinations. Symptomatic diverticula can present variously, including malabsorption, inflammation, obstruction, or hemorrhage. A syndrome of chronic abdominal pain, flatulence, episodic diarrhea, and anemia has been identified as a distinct mode of presentation.[31,32]

Malabsorption due to jejunoileal diverticular disease is characterized by steatorrhea, megaloblastic anemia, nutritional depletion, and, in severe cases, neurologic complications caused by vitamin B_{12} deficiency.[33] Each of these conditions is the result of abnormal intestinal motility with stasis of luminal content within the diverticula. Stasis allows bacterial overgrowth of coliform organisms, which deconjugate bile acids. This process leads to decreased availability of conjugated bile salts and diminished solubilization of fats, resulting in impaired absorption and steatorrhea. Bacterial uptake of vitamin B_{12} competes with absorption of the vitamin by the mucosa and results in megaloblastic anemia. Prolonged and severe malabsorption of vitamin B_{12} can lead to subacute combined degeneration of the spinal cord and other neurologic complications.[34,35]

Inflammation of a diverticulum leading to diverticulitis and perforation is a rare but well-documented complication of jejunoileal diverticula, reported to occur in 2.3% of patients with jejunoileal diverticula (Fig. 2).[22] Perforation freely into the peritoneal cavity or into the adjacent mesentery usually results from obstruction of the diverticular orifice with poor drainage. In health, the proximal small intestine contains few bacteria. However, obstruction can lead to stasis with bacterial proliferation and mucosal damage. Moreover, increased intradiverticular pressure can occur and perforation result. Although much less common, jejunoileal diverticular perforation also has been reported after blunt abdominal trauma or after ingestion of a foreign body with impaction in the diverticulum.[35]

Diagnosis

The diagnosis is suggested by the presence of air-fluid levels within diverticula on upright abdominal radiographs. Small intestinal contrast studies can definitively provide the diagnosis when large diverticula retain contrast material after the remainder has passed distally into the colon. Prominent mucosal folds and dilated intestine around the diverticula are frequent.[36,37] Englund and Jensen[38] described a clinical triad of anemia, obscure abdominal

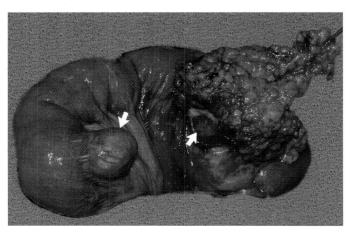

Fig. 2. *Surgical specimen of an inflamed, perforated jejunal diverticulum* (right arrow) *walled off by greater omentum, which has been lifted off the diverticulum. A second, uninflamed jejunal diverticulum* (left arrow) *is also present.*

pain, and dilated loops of bowel on barium study as suggestive of these diverticula.

Diagnosis of malabsorption can be difficult. Symptomatic patients more often harbor multiple rather than solitary diverticula.[27] The Schilling test and determination of serum concentrations of vitamin B_{12} and folate are helpful. However, recent evidence supports culture and identification of the bacterial overgrowth as the optimal diagnostic method.[39]

Clinically, diagnosis of jejunoileal diverticulitis or perforation is often difficult, leading to a delay in diagnosis and sometimes death. Presenting symptoms (fever, abdominal pain, and leukocytosis) mimic those of other abdominal disorders, such as perforated ulcer, cholecystitis, intussusception, appendicitis, and colonic diverticulitis. Frequently, the diagnosis is made only at laparotomy for what is believed to be one of these other conditions.[22,34,40] Previous documentation of the presence of jejunoileal diverticula can be helpful for establishing the diagnosis preoperatively. Computed tomography can be useful for identifying inflammation with or without air in the mesentery. Occasionally, intraluminal contrast material can be seen outlining a diverticulum adjacent to the inflammatory process.

The initial physical examination does not reveal the need for emergency surgical exploration in most patients. Because the diverticular location is within the mesentery, generalized peritonitis rarely results. Rather, the perforation occurs within the leaves of the mesentery, leading to localized peritonitis. Despite this seemingly autoprotective circumstance, the mortality rate associated with perforation is high when compared with that in the conditions mentioned above. Late presentation or delay in surgical intervention results in a higher mortality rate.[40,41] The longer the delay to diagnosis, the greater the intra-abdominal contamination. Koger et al.[40] described 13 patients with perforated jejunoileal diverticulitis. Five of these patients presented with severe soilage and prolonged time to operative intervention (74 hours), and eight patients had minimal soilage and more expeditious operative care (21 hours). Two patients, both with severe contamination, died of sepsis and multiorgan failure. Despite advances in preoperative and perioperative surgical care, the mortality rate in their series was 15%, a figure not substantially improved from earlier series, in which mortality rates varied from 21% to 40%.[42] The mortality rate remains high because of the age of the population at risk, the likelihood of comorbid diseases, and the delay in definitive care.

Intestinal obstruction is reported to be the most common complication of jejunoileal diverticula.[31] Mechanical obstruction results from volvulus, adhesions, enterolith formation, intussusception, or compression from a large diverticulum. Adhesions resulting from previous inflammation can lead to obstruction both extraluminally and intraluminally. Inflammation leads to serosal adhesion formation with classic extraluminal narrowing and obstruction of the intestinal lumen. Similarly, chronic intraluminal inflammation can lead to stricture formation with subsequent luminal narrowing and obstruction. An axial volvulus of a large diverticulum around its base can lead to obstruction of the main intestinal lumen.[43] Volvulus and adhesions usually require resection of the involved segments of small intestine.

More than 25 cases of an enterolith within a jejunoileal diverticulum causing ileus have been reported.[28] The cause of this rare event is believed to be a combination of events. Stasis, bile, and luminal debris within the diverticula predispose to anaerobic bacterial proliferation. The bacteria deconjugate taurine and glycine from bile salts. In addition, they also convert cholic acid to deoxycholic acid, which combines with palmitic and stearic fatty acids to form enteroliths. Obstruction results when these enteroliths are extruded from the diverticulum into the intestinal lumen, where they lodge usually at the level of the ileocecal valve. Resection of the diverticular-bearing intestine should not be undertaken unless there is a single diverticulum.[44]

Nonmechanical or pseudo-obstruction as a result of intestinal dyskinesia, as described previously, has been reported as a feature of jejunoileal diverticula in 10% to 25% of patients in published series.[22] Uncoordinated, abnormal, inefficient small intestinal motility can produce a bloated sensation, which in severe cases can present as mechanical obstruction. Histologic examination of intestinal specimens has revealed neural or smooth muscle abnormalities, the latter being similar to changes found in visceral myopathy or progressive systemic sclerosis.[1] Clinically, a thickened jejunum and dilated proximal small bowel have been identified. Patients with pseudo-obstruction have had effective relief of their symptoms after resection of the hypertrophied intestine and diverticula.[41]

First reported by Braithwaite in 1923,[45] intestinal *hemorrhage* occurs in up to 5% of patients with jejunoileal diverticula.[22,41] Usually the patient presents with hematochezia; however, melena and hematemesis can occur. Diagnostically, the difficulty is localization of the site of hemorrhage. The bleeding site usually is associated with ulceration within a specific diverticulum. Upper and lower endoscopy should be performed to rule out other sites of bleeding, such as colonic diverticulosis and peptic ulcer. Selective angiography should be used to identify precisely the site of bleeding. If angiography fails to localize the origin of blood loss, radionucleotide-tagged red blood cell scan should be obtained.[22] Occasionally, repeat esophagogastroduodenoscopy and colonoscopy are warranted.

Stable patients with recurrent blood loss should undergo enteroclysis. When the only disorder identified is jejunoileal diverticula, the involved segments should be resected.[27]

Treatment

Medical Therapy

Treatment of *malabsorption* due to jejunoileal diverticula is focused on eliminating bacterial overgrowth, restoring normal flora, and replacing deficient vitamins. A high-protein, low-residue diet with vitamin supplements is recommended.[28] Therapy with broad-spectrum antibiotics should be initiated; however, its success has been marginal. In the largest series to date, Tsiotos et al.[27] described 112 patients. Tetracycline, 250 mg three times daily for the first week of each month, followed by metronidazole, 250 mg twice daily the third week of each month, appeared to be a well-tolerated regimen. After a mean of 9 months of this regimen, the success rate for ameliorating symptoms in 45 patients with malabsorption was a disappointing 46%. The remaining 54% returned with recurrent complaints. Despite alteration of the antibiotic therapy, diet modification, and the administration of antidiarrheal agents, these patients continued to respond poorly to medical management.

Surgical Therapy

Patients with persistent or recurrent symptoms of malabsorption after prolonged medical therapy should be considered for segmental enteric resection. Although the literature lacks sufficient numbers of intestinal resections for malabsorption, the frequency of patients refractory to medical therapy and the lack of nutritional sequelae in surgically treated patients support segmental resection of the diverticula-bearing intestine when medical management has failed.[27]

An incorrect preoperative diagnosis of perforated jejunoileal diverticulum is not always easily corrected at operation. Because the diverticula develop within the mesentery and subsequent perforation is usually intramesenteric, identification of the offending diverticula can be difficult. In fact, the condition can be missed entirely, unless a meticulous exploration is undertaken. Suspicion of jejunoileal diverticular perforation should be raised when other small intestinal diverticula are present. Thorough examination of adherent bowel loops, especially the mesenteric aspect, is of absolute importance. Occasionally, noninflamed diverticula can be detected only with insufflation of the intestine.[40,41] This can be accomplished by occluding the proximal and distal segments of the length of intestine in question, followed by milking the intestinal contents and air toward each other, resulting in insufflation of the diverticula. Although rarely reported, asymptomatic pneumoperitoneum can be the initial clinical finding. It can be associated with pneumatosis cystoides intestinalis or subserosal air dissection around the bowel or surrounding structures. Mechanistic hypotheses include a leaking diverticulum with subsequent closure or equilibrium of gas across an attenuated intestinal wall. Because of its asymptomatic presentation, conservative management may be attempted; however, operation is usually required.[29]

Surgical therapy consists of segmental resection of the involved portion of intestine and primary anastomosis. Proximal diversion is not required.[27] If possible, other diverticula should be removed with the offending diverticulum. However, extensive resections should be avoided. Segmental resections of 75 cm of intestine have been tolerated in previous series. Distal ileal perforation may require resection of the ileocecal valve with ileocolic anastomosis. Local resection of the diverticulum (diverticulectomy) is not recommended because of the high complication rates resulting from breakdown at the site of closure.[40,46]

Patients presenting with obstruction from a diverticulum caused by an enterolith can have the enterolith milked proximally and removed through an enterotomy in nearly all cases. The diverticular-bearing intestine should not be resected unless there is a single diverticulum.[45]

At laparotomy, identifying the bleeding diverticulum among the many usually present can be difficult. Identification can be facilitated with preoperative instillation of methylene blue through an angiographic catheter directed at the bleeding site or by intraoperative endoscopy.[47,48] Regardless of location, treatment of hemorrhage due to jejunoileal diverticula is resection of the involved portion of small intestine with primary anastomosis. The operative mortality rate is 11%.[22,29]

MECKEL'S DIVERTICULUM

Meckel's diverticulum....Frequently suspected, often looked for, seldom found.[49]

Charles H. Mayo, 1933

Although the condition carries his name, Meckel was not the first to observe the presence of a congenital ileal diverticulum. Hildanus[50] reported one in 1598. A little more than a century later, in 1701, Ruysch[51] of Leyden published an illustration of this diverticulum in a copper engraving, and in 1700 Littre[52] reported the presence of the diverticulum in an inguinal hernia (Littre's hernia). It was not until 1809 that the anatomist Johann Friederich Meckel the Younger identified the origin of the diverticulum as a remnant of the omphalomesenteric duct[53] and

a potential cause of disease. His name subsequently was attached to this congenital anomaly. Shortly after these reports, Gramen described Meckel's diverticulitis,[54] and in 1898 Kettner reported small intestinal obstruction as a result of Meckel's diverticulum.[55] Salzer[56] first identified the presence of ectopic mucosa within the diverticulum in 1904.

Embryology and Anatomy

Meckel's diverticulum is often described by the "rule of twos": 2% incidence, found within 2 feet of the ileocecal valve, 2 inches long, and 2 types of heterotopic mucosa (pancreatic and gastric).

It is easiest to understand the congenital nature of a Meckel diverticulum if one views it as an abnormality arising during the embryologic development of the midgut. The primitive gut is attached to the yolk sac by the yolk stalk or omphalomesenteric (vitelline) duct at 3 weeks of gestation. Normally, elongation, narrowing, and eventually involution of the duct occur between the fifth and seventh week of fetal life, resulting in separation of the fetal intestine from the abdominal wall. Should this process be interrupted, various anomalies can result.

The usual Meckel diverticulum is found on the antimesenteric surface of the ileum within 100 cm of the ileocecal valve in the adult. It is a true diverticulum (containing mucosa, submucosa, tunica muscularis, and serosa) that is supported by its own arterial blood supply, a remnant of the paired vitelline arteries (Fig. 3). Failure of complete vitelline duct obliteration and separation from the abdominal wall or persistent vitelline artery remnants can result in a spectrum of vitelline (omphalomesenteric) duct anomalies (Fig. 4 and 5).

A Meckel diverticulum (distal obliteration and separation with the tip free in the abdominal cavity (Fig. 3) is the most common type of the anomaly, representing 74% of cases.[57] Other varieties include incomplete involution of the vitelline structures leading to fibrous bands fixing a Meckel diverticulum or the ileal serosa to the abdominal wall (Fig. 4 and 5). The pedicled intestine is able to rotate on or create a hernia around these bands, leading to obstruction. Patency of the omphalomesenteric duct results in a fistula between the intestine and umbilicus (an ileo-umbilical fistula). An umbilical sinus occurs when only the umbilical side of the duct fails to obliterate. Heterotopic gastric, duodenal, and colonic mucosa and pancreatic rests can be found in Meckel's diverticula. The embryologic origin of these tissues is not clearly understood. However, they likely develop from maturation of multipotential cells or mature cell rests that remain in the diverticulum during intestinal maturation.[58] The likelihood of finding heterotopic tissue and the type of

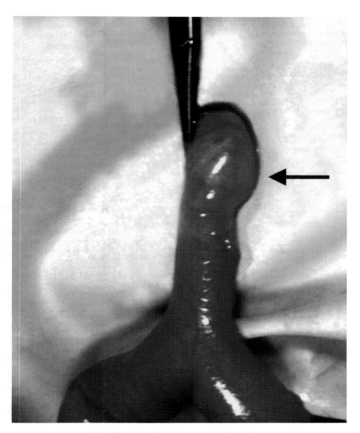

Fig. 3. A Meckel diverticulum (arrow) *found at operation.*

found with or without pancreatic tissue. The importance of aberrant gastric mucosa lies in its ability to secrete acid, leading to ulceration and hemorrhage. A "giant" Meckel diverticulum is an uncommon variant that can present with acute or chronic abdominal pain and obstruction.[59]

A Meckel diverticulum, the most common congenital anomaly of the gastrointestinal tract, has been reported to occur in 1.3% to 2.2% of the population.[60,61] When it is incidentally found, the distribution between men and women is equal, but in symptomatic cases males outnumber females 3-4:1.[62]

Symptoms and Signs

Most Meckel diverticula remain asymptomatic. When symptoms occur, they are related to the presence of heterotopic mucosa with hemorrhage or inflammation or to obstruction due to ductal remnants.

The most common clinical presentation of a Meckel diverticulum is lower gastrointestinal hemorrhage, which occurs in 40% to 50% of patients presenting with a complication.[63-65] The bleeding is usually painless, can present as melena or hematochezia, and can be massive or episodic. The source of the bleeding is an ulcer, usually located on the mesenteric aspect of the ileum. Ectopic gastric mucosa is found within the diverticulum.

The second most common complication of a Meckel diverticulum is intestinal obstruction reported in approximately 25% of patients with complications.[63] The obstruction can be the result of several mechanisms. Intussusception, with the Meckel diverticulum functioning as the lead point (Fig. 6), is responsible for nearly 45% of cases presenting as intestinal obstruction.[66] In a review of 160 patients, more than 50% of patients with intussusception were older than 10 years.[61] Intussusception

mucosa present depend on whether the diverticulum is symptomatic (more common) or incidental (uncommon). Heterotopic mucosa is found in approximately 55% of symptomatic patients but in only 15% of patients without symptoms. Gastric mucosa is the most commonly identified mucosa in symptomatic patients. It can be

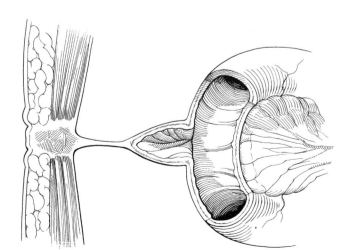

Fig. 4. A cordlike, nonpatent fibrous tract connecting a Meckel diverticulum to the posterior aspect of the anterior abdominal wall.

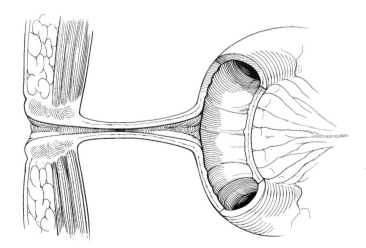

Fig. 5. A patent omphalomesenteric duct.

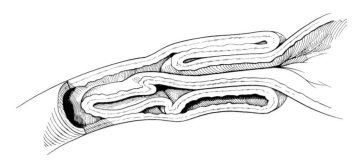

Fig. 6. An ileoileal intussusception with a Meckel diverticulum functioning as the lead point.

can present in multiple ways. In adults, mechanical obstruction, abdominal distention, and bloody stools predominate. Children may present with vomiting, intermittent abdominal pain, "currant jelly" stools, and palpable abdominal mass. With delay in diagnosis, dehydration and lethargy result.

Volvulus of the small bowel around persistent vascular or vitelline duct remnants is another mechanism by which obstruction can occur (Fig. 7) and is the cause in nearly 25% of cases with obstructive symptoms due to Meckel's diverticulum.[67] In these circumstances, patients present with evidence of intestinal ischemia necessitating emergency operation. Although rare, incarceration of a Meckel diverticulum within an inguinal hernia (Littre's hernia) can result in obstruction.

Inflammatory complications of Meckel's diverticula are the result of either local inflammation due to obstruction of the diverticular lumen with subsequent diverticulitis or peptic complications with perforation of an ulcer. Regardless, diverticulitis with or without perforation (Fig. 8) occurs in about 20% of patients with complications from a Meckel diverticulum.[58,67] The presenting symptoms of fever, leukocytosis, and abdominal pain, usually right lower quadrant pain, are often indistinguishable from those of acute appendicitis. The correct diagnosis of Meckel's diverticulitis is then made at operation. When a normal appendix is found at operation for suspected appendicitis, the terminal ileum must be examined for the presence of an inflamed Meckel diverticulum. Progression of the inflammation leads to perforation with peritonitis or abscess formation.

Finally, neoplasm, foreign bodies, and calculi have been found in Meckel's diverticula.[68] Carcinoids are the most common neoplasms found, but they occur in less than 2% of all Meckel's diverticula.[62,69,70] They resemble appendiceal carcinoids in that they are generally small, single, and asymptomatic. However, biologically and phenotypically, Meckel carcinoids resemble jejunoileal

carcinoids with greater metastatic potential than appendiceal carcinoids.[70] Less than 0.5% of patients presenting with complications of a Meckel diverticulum have a stone associated with the diverticulum.[67] These calculi can cause hemorrhage, obstruction, or perforation.

Diagnosis

Identifying a Meckel diverticulum as the source of enteric blood loss can be difficult. Often the patient will have undergone endoscopic examination with no definitive colonic source visualized. Occasionally blood can be seen coming through the ileocecal valve or within the ileum, raising the question of a possible bleeding Meckel diverticulum. Technetium Tc 99m scanning is a useful diagnostic tool in this setting. Jewett et al.[71] first described its use to identify ectopic gastric mucosa in 1970. Pertechnetate ions carrying technetium Tc 99m are stored in and secreted by the mucous cells of gastric-type mucosa. Increased uptake and excretion in intestinal areas away from the stomach suggest aberrant gastric tissue and the possibility of a Meckel diverticulum. The test can reliably detect 80% to 90% of Meckel diverticula in affected patients, and it excludes the condition in more than 90% of patients who do not have it.[72,73] Arteriography may be used to identify the site of bleeding when other measures fail.

The diagnosis of intussusception is most effectively made with ultrasonography, in which a doughnut (target or concentric ring) of intestinal segments is sought.[67] Contrast or pneumatic enema under fluoroscopic guidance is occasionally successful for identifying and reducing the intussusception. If this is the case, elective surgical diverticulectomy should be performed to obviate subsequent recurrence. When reduction is not successful through

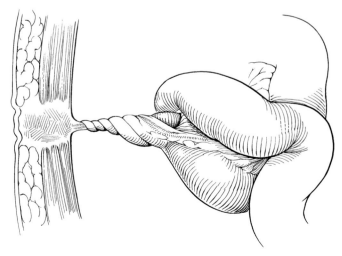

Fig. 7. A small intestinal volvulus around a vitelline ductal remnant resulting in intestinal obstruction.

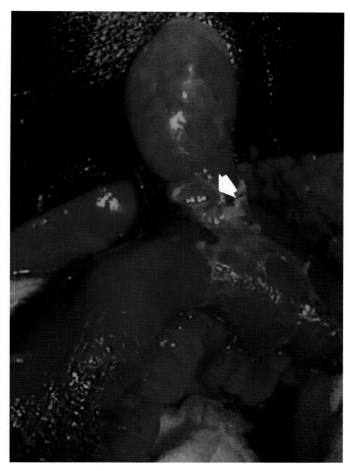

Fig. 8. An acutely inflamed Meckel diverticulum with perforation (arrow) *and acute peritonitis.*

radiologic methods, abdominal exploration is required. In most cases, it is only at operation that Meckel's diverticulum is identified as the inciting structure leading to the intussusception.

Surgical Therapy

Preoperatively, the patient is managed with nasogastric decompression for intestinal obstruction, intravenous resuscitation for correction of electrolyte abnormalities, blood transfusion for blood loss, antibiotics if strangulation is suspected, and minimal delay to operation.

Therapeutic Diverticulectomy

The surgical management of complications of Meckel's diverticula is centered on removal of the offending diverticulum. In each of the clinical scenarios presented, diverticulectomy is needed. The majority of patients can undergo removal of the diverticulum only, sparing the ileum to which it is attached. Occasionally inflammation, perforation, or ischemia mandates a more extensive removal. In these cases, either a wedge excision or

resection of the ileal segment containing the diverticulum with ileoileostomy may be required. Regardless, the operation can be performed with an open or laparoscopic approach.

Simple diverticulectomy is performed by dividing the diverticulum at its junction with the ileum. Stapled or two-layer suture closure is acceptable. A transverse closure decreases the possibility of narrowing the intestinal lumen. Wedge excision is generally done for hemorrhage. Removal of the Meckel diverticulim and a portion of the antimesenteric aspect of the congruent ileum allows for visualization of the bleeding ulcer bed. After oversewing the bleeding vessel, the ileum is closed in two layers. When a portion of ileum is resected, either a stapled or a two-layer suture anastomosis is appropriate.

Incidental Diverticulectomy

Although patients with the complications described should undergo surgical diverticulectomy, the decision to perform diverticulectomy for Meckel's diverticula found incidentally at operation is often debated. Johann Meckel reported that the risk of complications from resecting an asymptomatic diverticulum was about 25%, a figure repeated by Moses in 1947.[74] Although these outcomes generally have been accepted, few data were ever available to substantiate them. During the ensuing half decade, numerous reports quoted mortality rates of 0% to 20% in patients undergoing diverticulectomy for complications.[75-79] Reports on complication rates for patients undergoing incidental diverticulectomy during the same period cited complications in 1% to 9% after such operations.[64,80-82]

Opponents to incidental diverticulectomy cite Soltero and Bill,[75] who, in 1976, estimated that the lifetime risk of complications developing from an unoperated Meckel diverticulum was only 4.2%, and the risk decreases with age. They recommended that incidental diverticulectomy not be performed because of the potential postoperative complications resulting from an unnecessary procedure in an already low-risk population. Several other studies have supported this assumption.[64,83] Critics of these studies point out the retrospective nature of the data and the lack of evaluation of a defined population using epidemiologic tools.

We collected data on the question in a well-defined population in which age- and sex-specific incidence and complication rates were able to be determined. We reported a lifetime complication risk from an unresected Meckel diverticulum of 6.4%, with no appreciable change in risk with age. We also noted a postoperative complication rate of only 2% over 20 years for patients undergoing incidental diverticulectomy.[58] We advise incidental diverticulectomy in all patients regardless of age, unless the diverticulum is found during an emergency operation for another condition or the patient is not healthy enough to tolerate the additional operating time required.

Nonetheless, the decision to perform a Meckel diverticulectomy continues to be controversial. Morbidity and mortality from the procedure must be weighed against the possibility of Meckel's diverticula becoming symptomatic, multiplied by the risk of morbidity and mortality after operation for a symptomatic Meckel diverticulum. The risks are not constant and depend on multiple patient and diverticular variables, such as age, comorbid conditions, and size and type of diverticula. As noted above, the estimated lifetime risk of an asymptomatic Meckel diverticulum becoming symptomatic is 4.2% to 6.4%. The long-term risk of complications after incidental diverticulectomy is about 2%, whereas that after resection of a symptomatic diverticulum approaches 10%.[58]

If diverticulectomy is performed on every patient in the population at risk (which we do *not* advise), diverticulectomy has the following risk: 0.02 (population incidence) x 0.02 (long-term incidence) = 4/10,000. In contrast, the risk of morbidity associated with waiting to treat only patients who become symptomatic is as follows: 0.02 (population incidence) x 0.05 (chance of symptoms developing) x 0.1 (risk of operative complications) = 1/10,000.

It is obvious that not all asymptomatic diverticula will be removed. The risk of an incidental diverticulectomy versus that of no diverticulectomy may be similar. We have few data on patients in whom a Meckel diverticulum is discovered incidentally at operation but do not have resection and are subsequently followed over a long postoperative period. In the absence of such data, we advise diverticulectomy for the incidentally discovered diverticulum as being a reasonable choice during elective operations in healthy patients.

REFERENCES

1. Krishnamurthy S, Kelly MM, Rohrmann CA, Schuffler MD: Jejunal diverticulosis: a heterogenous disorder caused by a variety of abnormalities of smooth muscle or myenteric plexus. Gastroenterology 85:538-547, 1983

2. Neill SA, Thompson NW: The complications of duodenal diverticula and their management. Surg Gynecol Obstet 120:1251-1258, 1965

3. Psathakis D, Utschakowski A, Muller G, Broll R, Bruch HP: Clinical significance of duodenal diverticula. J Am Coll Surg 178:257-260, 1994

4. Skar V, Skar AG, Osnes M: The duodenal bacterial flora in the region of papilla of Vater in patients with and without duodenal diverticula. Scand J Gastroenterol 24:649-656, 1989

5. Scudamore CH, Harrison RC, White TT: Management of duodenal diverticula. Can J Surg 25:311-314, 1982

6. Donald JW: Major complications of small bowel diverticula. Ann Surg 190:183-188, 1979

7. Lotveit T, Skar V, Osnes M: Juxtapapillary duodenal diverticula. Endoscopy 20 Suppl 1:175-178, 1988

8. Shemesh E, Friedman E, Czerniak A, Bat L: The association of biliary and pancreatic anomalies with periampullary duodenal diverticula: correlation with clinical presentations. Arch Surg 122:1055-1057, 1987

9. Lobo DN, Balfour TW, Iftikhar SY, Rowlands BJ: Periampullary diverticula and pancreaticobiliary disease. Br J Surg 86:588-597, 1999

10. Akhrass R, Yaffe MB, Fischer C, Ponsky J, Shuck JM: Small-bowel diverticulosis: perceptions and reality. J Am Coll Surg 184:383-388, 1997

11. Eggert A, Teichmann W, Wittmann DH: The pathologic implication of duodenal diverticula. Surg Gynecol Obstet 154:62-64, 1982

12. Soreide JA, Seime S, Soreide O: Intraluminal duodenal diverticulum: case report and update of the literature 1975-1986. Am J Gastroenterol 83:988-991, 1988

13. Lotveit T, Osnes M, Larsen S: Recurrent biliary calculi: duodenal diverticula as a predisposing factor. Ann Surg 196:30-32, 1982

14. Kim MH, Myung SJ, Seo DW, Lee SK, Kim YS, Lee MH, Yoo BM, Min MI: Association of periampullary diverticula with primary choledocholithiasis but not with secondary choledocholithiasis. Endoscopy 30:601-604, 1998

15. Hall RI, Ingoldby CJ, Denyer ME: Periampullary diverticula predispose to primary rather than secondary stones in the common bile duct. Endoscopy 22:127-128, 1990

16. Leinkram C, Roberts-Thomson IC, Kune GA: Juxtapapillary duodenal diverticula: association with gallstones and pancreatitis. Med J Aust 1:209-210, 1980

17. Carey LC: Pathophysiologic factors in recurrent acute pancreatitis. Jpn J Surg 15:333-340, 1985

18. Afridi SA, Fichtenbaum CJ, Taubin H: Review of duodenal diverticula. Am J Gastroenterol 86:935-938, 1991

19. Hajiro K, Yamamoto H, Matsui H, Yamamoto T: Endoscopic diagnosis and excision of intraluminal duodenal diverticulum. Gastrointest Endosc 25:151-154, 1979

20. Trondsen E, Rosseland AR, Bakka AO: Surgical management of duodenal diverticula. Acta Chir Scand 156:383-386, 1990

21. Abdel-Hafiz AA, Birkett DH, Ahmed MS: Congenital duodenal diverticula: a report of three cases and a review of the literature. Surgery 104:74-78, 1988

22. Sibille A, Willocx R: Jejunal diverticulitis. Am J Gastroenterol 87:655-658, 1992

23. Cooper AP: On Hernia. Part II. The Anatomy and Surgical Treatment of Crural and Umbilical Hernia. London, Longman & Company, 1807, p 90

24. Osler W: Notes on intestinal diverticula. Ann Anat Surg 4:202-207, 1881

25. Gordinier HC, Sampson JA: Diverticulitis (not Meckel's) causing intestinal obstruction: multiple mesenteric (acquired) diverticula of the small intestine. JAMA 46:1585-1590, 1906

26. Case JT: Diverticulum of the small bowel other than Meckel's diverticulum. JAMA 75:1463-1470, 1920

27. Tsiotos GG, Farnell MB, Ilstrup DM: Nonmeckelian jejunal or ileal diverticulosis: an analysis of 112 cases. Surgery 116:726-731, 1994

28. Longo WE, Vernava AM III: Clinical implications of jejunoileal diverticular disease. Dis Colon Rectum 35:381-388, 1992

29. Palder SB, Frey CB: Jejunal diverticulosis. Arch Surg 123:889-894, 1988

30. Ross CB, Richards WO, Sharp KW, Bertram PD, Schaper PW: Diverticular disease of the jejunum and its complications. Am Surg 56:319-324, 1990

31. Altemeier WA, Bryant LR, Wulsin JH: The surgical significance of jejunal diverticulosis. Arch Surg 86:732-745, 1963

32. Lee RE, Finby N: Jejunal and ileal diverticulosis. Arch Intern Med 102:97-102, 1958

33. Knauer CM, Svoboda AC: Malabsorption and jejunal diverticulosis. Am J Med 44:606-610, 1968

34. Baskin RH Jr, Mayo CW: Jejunal diverticulosis: clinical study of 87 cases. Surg Clin North Am 32:1185-1196, 1952

35. Brown JE, Vallette R, Brown JE Jr: Recurrent jejunal diverticulosis. South Med J 78:352-353, 1985

36. Phillips JHC: Jejunal diverticulosis: some clinical aspects. Br J Surg 40:350-354, 1953

37. Salomonowitz E, Wittich G, Hajek P, Jantsch H, Czembirek H: Detection of intestinal diverticula by double-contrast small bowel enema: differentiation from other intestinal diverticula. Gastrointest Radiol 8:271-278, 1983

38. Englund R, Jensen M: Acquired diverticulosis of the small intestine: case reports and literature review. Aust N Z J Surg 56:51-54, 1986

39. Valdovinos MA, Camilleri M, Thomforde GM, Frie C: Reduced accuracy of ^{14}C-D-xylose breath test for detecting bacterial overgrowth in gastrointestinal motility disorders. Scand J Gastroenterol 28:963-968, 1993

40. Koger KE, Shatney CH, Dirbas FM, McClenathan JH: Perforated jejunal diverticula. Am Surg 62:26-29, 1996

41. Williams RA, Davidson DD, Serota AI, Wilson SE: Surgical problems of diverticula of the small intestine. Surg Gynecol Obstet 152:621-626, 1981

42. Roses DF, Gouge TH, Scher KS, Ranson JH: Perforated diverticula of the jejunum and ileum. Am J Surg 132:649-652, 1976

43. Munyaradzi OM, Wapnick S: Multiple jejunal diverticulosis and small bowel volvulus. Am J Surg 125:356-359, 1973

44. Beal SL, Walton CB, Bodai BI: Enterolith ileus resulting from small bowel diverticulosis. Am J Gastroenterol 82:162-164, 1987

45. Braithwaite LR: A case of jejunal diverticula. Br J Surg 11:184-188, 1923-1924

46. Wilcox RD, Shatney CH: Surgical implications of jejunal diverticula. South Med J 81:1386-1391, 1988

47. Rubio PA, Farrell EM: A new technique for identifying bleeding diverticula of the small bowel utilizing methylene blue infusion. Surgery 86:764, 1979

48. Flickinger EG, Stanforth AC, Sinar DR, MacDonald KG, Lannin DR, Gibson JH: Intraoperative video panendoscopy for diagnosing sites of chronic intestinal bleeding. Am J Surg 157:137-144, 1989

49. Mayo CW: Meckel's diverticulum. Proc Staff Meet Mayo Clin 8:230-232, 1933

50. Lichtenstein ME: Meckel's diverticulum: intestinal obstruction due to invagination and intussusception: peritonitis due to perforation by fish bone. Quart Bull Northwestern Univ M School 15:296-300, 1941

51. Ruysch F: Thesaurus Anatomicus I. Het eerste anatomisch cabinet. Amstelœdami, Wolters, 1701, p 7

52. Littre A: Observation sur une nouvelle espece de hernia. Hist Acad Roy Sc 2:300, 1700

53. Meckel J: Uber die divertikel am darmkanal. Arch Physiol 9:421-423, 1809

54. Amoury RA, Snyder CL: Meckel's diverticulum. In Pediatric Surgery. Fifth edition. Edited by JA O'Neill Jr, MI Rowe, JL Grosfeld, EW Fonkalsrud, AG Coran. St Louis, Mosby, 1998, pp 1173-1184

55. Amoury RA: Meckel's diverticulum. In Pediatric Surgery. Fourth edition. Edited by KJ Welch, JG Randolph, MM Ravitch, JA O'Neill Jr, MI Rowe. London, Year Book Medical Publishers, 1986, pp 859-867

56. Salzer H: Ueber das offene Meckel'sche Divertikel. Wien Klin Wchnschr 17:614-617, 1904

57. Soderlund S: Meckel's diverticulum; a clinical and histologic study. Acta Chir Scand Suppl 248:1-233, 1959

58. Cullen JJ, Kelly KA, Moir CR, Hodge DO, Zinsmeister AR, Melton LJ III: Surgical management of Meckel's diverticulum: an epidemiologic, population-based study. Ann Surg 220:564-568, 1994

59. Bell MJ, Ternberg JL, Bower RJ: Ileal dysgenesis in infants and children. J Pediatr Surg 17:395-399, 1982

60. Matsagas MI, Fatouros M, Koulouras B, Giannoukas AD: Incidence, complications, and management of Meckel's diverticulum. Arch Surg 130:143-146, 1995

61. Harkins HN: Intussusception due to invaginated Meckel's diverticulum: report of 2 cases with study of 160 cases collected from literature. Ann Surg 98:1070-1095, 1933

62. Androulakis JA, Gray SW, Lionakis B, Skandalakis JE: The sex ratio of Meckel's diverticulum. Am Surg 35:455-460, 1969

63. St-Vil D, Brandt ML, Panic S, Bensoussan AL, Blanchard H: Meckel's diverticulum in children: a 20-year review. J Pediatr Surg 26:1289-1292, 1991

64. Leijonmarck CE, Bonman-Sandelin K, Frisell J, Raf L: Meckel's diverticulum in the adult. Br J Surg 73:146-149, 1986

65. Vane DW, West KW, Grosfeld JL: Vitelline duct anomalies: experience with 217 childhood cases. Arch Surg 122:542-547, 1987

66. Kusumoto H, Yoshida M, Takahashi I, Anai H, Maehara Y, Sugimachi K: Complications and diagnosis of Meckel's diverticulum in 776 patients. Am J Surg 164:382-383, 1992

67. Holt S, Samuel E: Multiple concentric ring sign in the ultrasonographic diagnosis of intussusception. Gastrointest Radiol 3:307-309, 1978

68. Dovey P: Calculus in a Meckel's diverticulum: a preoperative radiological diagnosis. Br J Radiol 44:888-890, 1971

69. Weber JD, McFadden DW: Carcinoid tumors in Meckel's diverticula. J Clin Gastroenterol 11:682-686, 1989

70. Moyana TN: Carcinoid tumors arising from Meckel's diverticulum: a clinical, morphologic, and immunohistochemical study. Am J Clin Pathol 91:52-56, 1989

71. Jewett TC Jr, Duszynski DO, Allen JE: The visualization of Meckel's diverticulum with ^{99m}Tc-pertechnetate. Surgery 68:567-570, 1970

72. Bergstralh EJ, Offord K, Chu CP, O'Fallon WM, Melton LJ: Calculating incidence. Prevalence and mortality rates for Olmsted County, Minnesota: an update. Technical Report Series 49, 1992

73. Kurland LT, Molgaard CA: The patient record in epidemiology. Sci Am 245:54-63, 1981

74. Michas CA, Cohen SE, Wolfman EF Jr: Meckel's diverticulum: Should it be excised incidentally at operation? Am J Surg 129:682-685, 1975

75. Soltero MJ, Bill AH: The natural history of Meckel's diverticulum and its relation to incidental removal: a study of 202 cases of diseased Meckel's diverticulum found in King County, Washington, over a fifteen year period. Am J Surg 132:168-173, 1976

76. Simms MH, Corkery JJ: Meckel's diverticulum: its association with congenital malformation and the significance of atypical morphology. Br J Surg 67:216-219, 1980

77. von Hedenberg C: Surgical indications in Meckel's diverticulum. Acta Chir Scand 135:530-533, 1969

78. DeBartolo HM Jr, van Heerden JA: Meckel's diverticulum. Ann Surg 183:30-33, 1976

79. Weinstein EC: Meckel's diverticulum. J Am Geriatr Soc 13:903-907, 1965

80. Castleden WM: Meckel's diverticulum in an umbilical hernia. Br J Surg 57:932-934, 1970

81. Wansbrough RM, Thomson S, Leckey RG: Meckel's diverticulum: a 42-year review of 273 cases at the Hospital for Sick Children, Toronto. Can J Surg 1:15-21, 1957

82. Aubrey DA: Meckel's diverticulum: a review of the sixty-six emergency Meckel's diverticulectomies. Arch Surg 100:144-146, 1970

83. Snyder CL: Meckel's diverticulum. In Pediatric Surgery. Third edition. Edited by KW Ashcraft. Philadelphia, WB Saunders Company, 2000, pp 541-544

Chapter 27

CROHN'S DISEASE

Debora J. Fox, M.D.
Bruce G. Wolff, M.D.

First described in 1932 by Crohn et al.,[1] Crohn's disease is an inflammatory disorder of the gastrointestinal tract, involving most commonly the ileocolic region but manifesting in variations from the mouth to the anus. Crohn's disease continues to defy attempts at full characterization of its cause and development of effective treatments.

INCIDENCE

The incidence in the general population varies between 6 and 7 per 100,000 at risk.[2] It equally affects males and females. It has a bimodal distribution for age at onset: incidence is increased at about 20 years of age and again in the late 60s. Agrez et al.,[3] in a report on the Olmsted County, Minnesota, population between 1935 and 1975, found a peak incidence of surgical intervention in the third decade of life and cumulative risk of recurrence of 40% at 5 years and of 70% at 20 years. It is more prevalent in northern climates than southern climates and among white populations, and it may have a predisposition for certain ethnic groups, such as Scandinavians and Jews.[4]

ETIOLOGY

Immunologic, infectious, genetic, and environmental causes have been examined, but the actual cause has not been identified. Although the disease seems to have a familial predisposition, no clear pattern of inheritance has been found. Infectious and immunologic mechanisms continue to be investigated. *Mycobacterium paratuberculosis* has been isolated from segments of bowel involved with Crohn's disease, but no more definitive evidence has directly related the organism as causal. Environmental factors, such as dietary exposure to certain foods or chemicals, may result in a mucosal barrier immunologic reaction and subsequent disease. The disease is more common or more likely to occur in temperate environments, in heavy smokers,[5] and in spouses of patients with Crohn's disease. Several factors likely contribute to development of this disease.

NATURAL HISTORY

The initial lesion in Crohn's disease is the aphthous ulcer, which develops overlying a lymphoid follicle and is associated with active inflammation. Aphthous ulcers appear as small, flat ulcers with a whitish center and narrow rim of surrounding erythema. These are nonspecific and also may be present in infectious colitis. As Crohn's disease progresses, these ulcers enlarge and coalesce, forming deeper, erythematous, and friable ulcers consistent with inflammatory bowel disease. They may be linear and parallel other ulcers and have been described as "rake ulcers" or "bear claw ulcers." Normal intervening mucosa appears nodular and frequently is described as "cobblestoned" or is said to have pseudopolyps.

Although early disease may be difficult to distinguish from ulcerative colitis or infectious colitis, as the disease progresses the inflammation characteristically involves the full thickness of the bowel wall, including the serosal surface, which develops a serositis. The ulcers become deep fissures and may penetrate the full thickness of the bowel to perforate or become fistulous. The serositis results in fibrosis, abnormal serosal neovascularization, and "creeping" of the fat over the surface of the bowel beyond its normal mesenteric boundaries. Regional lymph nodes are often markedly enlarged, in contrast to the rarity of such enlargement in chronic ulcerative colitis.

As the inflammatory process continues, two main complications develop—strictures and fistulas. Acute inflammation may result in tissue edema and stricture formation, a process that is reversible with corticosteroid therapy. Chronic inflammation eventually results in fibrosis and stenosis, which at this point are no longer amenable to corticosteroid therapy. Full-thickness inflammation with fissure formation leads occasionally to perforation or fistula formation, heralded by abdominal pain, abdominal wall erythema, fever, or discharge. Fistula formation is an indication for operation.

The most frequent sites of disease are the terminal ileum and cecum; up to 90% of patients present with this pattern of distribution. Colon-only disease is the next most frequent pattern of involvement, followed by disease confined to the small bowel. In the report by Agrez et al.[3] on operation for Crohn's disease in the Olmsted County, Minnesota, population, Crohn's disease was found in both the large and the small bowel in 50% of patients, anal involvement was found more frequently in association with colon disease than with small bowel disease, and about 50% of patients had recurrence after operation. The risk of recurrence by site of disease was evaluated in a prospective randomized trial in which mesalamine was used to decrease postoperative recurrence (Table 1).[6]

Extraintestinal manifestations are frequent in Crohn's disease, occurring in more than 10% to 30% of patients. The disease may involve the skin (erythema nodosum, pyoderma gangrenosum), eyes (uveitis, conjunctivitis), joints (arthritis, ankylosing spondylitis), hematologic systems (anemia, hypercoagulability), liver (hepatitis, sclerosing cholangitis), kidney (nephrotic syndrome, amyloidosis), or pancreas (pancreatitis), or it may be multisystemic (amyloidosis).

DIAGNOSIS

Crampy abdominal pain associated with diarrhea is a common presentation of Crohn's disease. The diarrhea may be explosive and bloody. Obstructive-type symptoms are nonspecific and may accompany the disease as strictures develop. Eating induces symptoms, and thus patients often limit nutritional intake and lose weight.

Physical examination should begin with inspection of the oropharynx and includes a perianal examination looking for the characteristic lesions of Crohn's disease, such as thickened, bluish perianal skin, chronic ulcers or fissures, and fistulas.

Endoscopy is a useful diagnostic method for examining the upper and lower gastrointestinal tract. Esophagogastroduodenoscopy identifies aphthous ulcers or other lesions in these regions, estimated to be present in about half of patients with Crohn's disease.[4] Colonoscopy is useful for examining the pattern of colon involvement and for obtaining tissue for diagnosis; features such as segmental involvement and rake ulcers suggest Crohn's disease rather than ulcerative colitis.

The differential diagnosis includes ulcerative colitis, infectious colitis, and ischemic bowel.

Classic microscopic features help to distinguish Crohn's disease from other causes of bowel inflammation. Inflammation, characterized by a lymphocytic infiltrate, involves the full thickness of the wall, and lymphocytes are visible on the serosal surface. With chronic disease, the intestinal crypts exhibit distortion. Noncaseating granulomas, consisting of giant cells and inflammatory cells, are considered nearly pathognomonic for distinguishing Crohn's disease from other entities.

Small bowel follow-through radiography may provide further clues in the setting of indeterminate colitis. The presence of strictures in the small bowel suggests Crohn's disease rather than other causes.

A study by Orsoni et al.[7] examined the role of endosonography and magnetic resonance imaging as aids for characterizing complex perianal fistulas in Crohn's disease. This study found that the sensitivity for diagnosis of perianal fistula and abscess disease was 100% for ultrasonography and 55% for magnetic resonance imaging. The level of agreement with the surgical findings was 82% for ultrasonography and 50% for magnetic resonance imaging.

A similar study by Schwartz et al.[8] described results in 32 patients with perianal Crohn's disease who had magnetic resonance imaging, endoscopic ultrasonography, and examination under anesthesia by surgeons. The accuracy of all these examinations singly was more than 85%. The combination of endoscopic ultrasonography or magnetic resonance imaging with examination under anesthesia was 100% sensitive.

Although these tests are useful for defining the anatomy of complex perianal disease, it remains to be determined whether they will modify the intraoperative surgical plan.

Table 1.—Recurrence of Crohn's Disease, by Site of Disease

Site	Risk ratio	95% CI
Small bowel	1.00	
Small and large bowel	0.82	0.46-1.40
Large bowel*	0.41	0.18-0.94

*Small bowel compared with large bowel, $P = 0.0345$.

SURGICAL INDICATIONS

Patients with Crohn's disease characteristically have recurrent disease after operation and so often require multiple abdominal procedures. Each subsequent operation increases both the difficulty of the operation, because of adhesions, and the risk of malabsorption, because of short bowel. Thus, every attempt is made to treat patients conservatively by maximizing medical therapy.

Indications to proceed with an elective operation include the presence of chronic obstruction, fistula formation, abscess, chronic anemia due to bleeding, intractability despite medical management, and, in children, developmental delay (Table 2). Emergency surgical intervention is required for free perforation or acute gastrointestinal hemorrhage. Chronic obstruction is most likely due to stricture formation, but it may be due to adhesion or band formation. Crohn's disease is a transmural disease, and as such, perforation with abscess may occur. The presence of a fistula, with or without abscess, usually requires surgical intervention. Substantial chronic blood loss or frank gastrointestinal bleeding may develop as a sequela of Crohn's disease, and resection of gross disease may alleviate symptoms. Crohn's disease can have a considerable impact on the nutritional status and development of children. Active disease resulting in developmental delay necessitates surgical intervention.

PREOPERATIVE PREPARATION

Preoperative preparation is essentially identical to that for a patient undergoing intestinal surgery who does not have Crohn's disease. If the disease is primarily small bowel, no mechanical preparation is performed, with the exception that the patient may be asked to take a clear-liquid diet for several days before the procedure. If a colon resection or anastomosis is expected, then a bowel preparation consisting of a polyethylene glycol-balanced electrolyte solution or sodium phosphate in conjunction with oral antibiotics (neomycin and metronidazole) is

Table 2.—Indications for Operation in Crohn's Disease

Elective	Emergency
Intractability	Free perforation
Obstruction	Severe gastrointestinal hemorrhage
Fistula	
Abscess (contained)	
Bleeding (chronic)	
Growth retardation (children)	

administered over 4 to 5 hours on the day before operation to cleanse and disinfect the colon.

No studies have shown an advantage to the administration of intravenous antibiotics in addition to oral antibiotics preoperatively; however, we tend to administer a second-generation cephalosporin just before the skin incision. Patients undergoing a perianal examination and procedure are given metronidazole preoperatively and postoperatively. If the patient has been receiving systemic corticosteroids within the previous 12 months, we favor administration of a perioperative corticosteroid bolus and a slow postoperative taper.

Patients with Crohn's disease are subject to nutritional deficiencies. Some have anemia, either iron deficiency due to chronic blood loss from inflamed mucosa or anemia of chronic disease. Those with severe terminal ileitis or those who have previously undergone terminal ileal resection may have a deficiency in the fat-soluble vitamins and vitamin B_{12}. Generally poor nutrition may result in a vitamin K deficiency and subsequent coagulopathy. Severely malnourished patients may require preoperative hospitalization and parenteral nutrition support for several days before operation.

SURGICAL PRINCIPLES

Crohn's disease is a panenteric and multisystem disease that requires a conservative surgical approach. It may present in a single intestinal location, but it usually presents in a more widespread fashion, sometimes with skip lesions and normal intervening mucosa. Because it has a tendency to recur, more than 50% of patients will undergo subsequent bowel resections. The risk of becoming an enteric cripple is real; thus, every effort must be made through preoperative medical therapy and intraoperative strategy to conserve bowel. Operation involves techniques of resection and strictureplasty directed at symptomatic lesions.

The amount of margin to obtain during a bowel resection for Crohn's disease is controversial. The importance of a disease-free margin was examined by Wolff et al.,[9] who evaluated recurrence rates in 42 of 710 patients who had residual Crohn's disease at the anastomosis after surgical resection. Patients with microscopically positive margins had a recurrence rate of 89.4% at 8 years of follow-up. Several studies[10-12] have shown a lower recurrence rate with a more radical resection compared with resection leaving microscopically involved margins. Other studies have shown no benefit, including one prospective randomized trial by Fazio et al.[13] The need for a margin is at best controversial, and a more extensive resection of all involved bowel is often not optimal therapy, because the disease is widespread and resection leaves the patient with a short bowel. The advent of standard postoperative medical prophylaxis has further shifted the surgeon toward a more conservative resection. Whenever possible, we favor complete resection of disease with 2-cm negative margins, but we balance this goal with the extent of disease, resecting disease with lesser margins when more widespread disease is present.

ESOPHAGUS, DUODENUM, AND STOMACH

Often an unexpected diagnosis, classic signs of Crohn's disease in the esophagus, stomach, and duodenum are not readily discernible. Crohn's disease involving the third or fourth portion of the duodenum may mimic lymphoma, but it can be distinguished with a biopsy. The bowel wall is thickened and hyperemic, and stricture formation may result, especially in the distal stomach or duodenum. Peptic ulcer disease may coexist in up to 20% of patients with upper gastrointestinal involvement.[14]

Indications to operate include bleeding, perforation, or obstruction, duodenal obstruction being the most common reason to operate in this region.[4]

The treatment of choice in obstructing gastroduodenal Crohn's disease is a side-to-side gastrojejunostomy between a dependent portion of the stomach near the antrum and the proximal jejunum, usually without vagotomy (Fig. 1). Strictured areas are bypassed while maintaining intestinal continuity for biliopancreatic secretions. In short, limited strictures of the duodenum, strictureplasty (Fig. 2), as described under "Small Bowel" (see below), may be appropriate. Strictures of the third

and fourth portions of the duodenum may be amenable to a sleeve resection (Fig. 3) and an end-to-end duodenojejunostomy. Asymptomatic enteroenteric fistulas of this region are best treated conservatively. The duodenum may also be secondarily involved in fistula disease, the primary site being the distal ileum or colon. The site of the fistula origin on the small bowel or colon is resected and a primary anastomosis is created. The opening in the duodenum is examined and cleaned, and then either the opening is closed primarily or the site is excised with a wedge resection, including a few millimeters of surrounding "normal" wall. The defect is then closed primarily with sutures.[4]

SMALL BOWEL

The most common pattern of involvement is terminal ileitis, involving the distal-most small bowel for a 20- to 30-cm segment.

Keeping in mind that the recurrence rate approaches 90% at 7 years at an anastomosis where residual microscopic mucosal disease remains,[9] we resect limited segment disease with the goal of obtaining both microscopic and gross negative margins. In the presence of skip lesions or more extensive disease, we treat with a combination of resection and strictureplasty. Exclusion bypass of a strictured

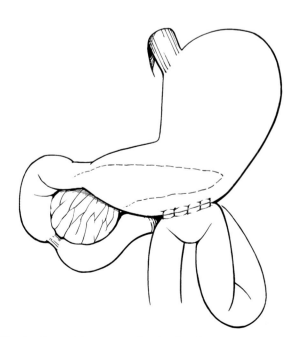

Fig. 1. Gastrojejunostomy for duodenal stricture.

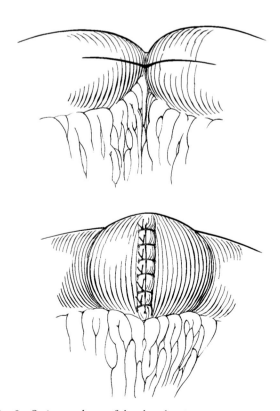

Fig. 2. Strictureplasty of duodenal stricture.

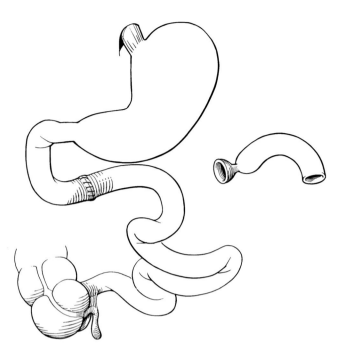

Fig. 3. Sleeve resection of a portion of the third and the fourth portions of duodenum.

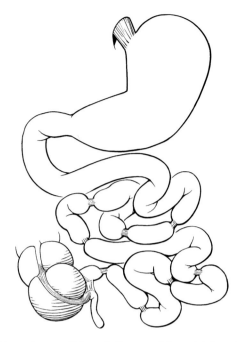

Fig. 4. Extensive small bowel disease with multiple strictures.

segment is contraindicated and should not be performed because of the risk of malignancy and bacterial overgrowth in the excluded segment. Nonetheless, we sometimes do bypass-in-continuity in patients with short bowel.

In extensive disease with multiple strictures (Fig. 4), strictureplasty is an effective therapy, allowing for relief of symptoms while conserving bowel length. For shorter strictures, a Heineke-Mikulicz–type strictureplasty is performed (Fig. 5). A longitudinal incision is made on the antimesenteric border of the small bowel, dividing the stricture and continuing onto nonstrictured bowel for 2 to 3 cm. The mucosa at the site of the stricture is inspected, and a mucosal specimen is sent for pathologic analysis to exclude malignancy. The stricture is closed transversely. The site of the stricture can be marked with a metal clip for future radiologic identification.

Longer strictures are not amenable to this type of strictureplasty, and consideration is given to either a Finney-type strictureplasty (Fig. 6) or resection of the grossly involved segment.

External inspection of the small bowel is an insensitive method for locating strictures. Intraoperative use of a long suction tube with a small inflatable balloon at the tip is useful for identifying all substantial strictures. During laparotomy for stricture disease, we begin by identifying a stricture near the terminal ileum. A longitudinal enterotomy is created across the stricture. The long tube is passed through this opening proximally through the small bowel lumen until the tip is at the ligament of Treitz (Fig. 7).

The balloon is inflated with 3 to 5 mL of saline, distending the small bowel but not overstretching the bowel. The tube is gently withdrawn, aspirating to decompress the bowel, toward the distal ileum. The balloon will "hang up" at the site of strictures or webs; we mark these sites with

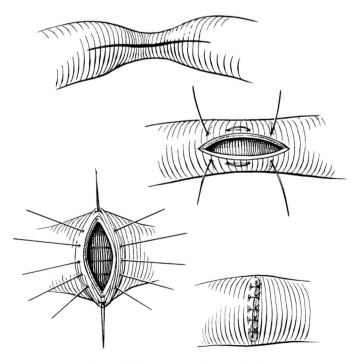

Fig. 5. Heineke-Mikulicz strictureplasty technique.

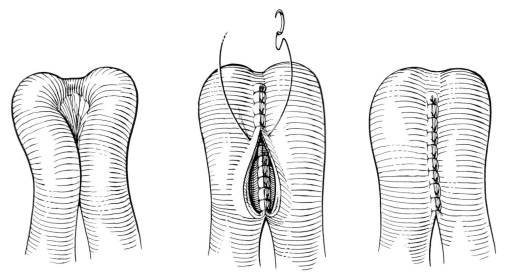

Fig. 6. Finney strictureplasty technique.

a suture. When the tube is completely withdrawn, all substantial stricture sites will have been marked and strictureplasty or resection can proceed. If the strictures are separated from each other by normal intervening bowel, then we liberally use strictureplasty. If the strictures are close together, either a Finney-type stapled anastomosis or a resection is appropriate.

Fistulous disease will develop in up to a third of patients with ileocolic Crohn's disease.[15] The fistula usually arises from the distal ileum and connects with another loop of bowel, to the skin, or to another hollow organ. About three-fourths of

fistulas are defined preoperatively on barium contrast studies.[16] If the fistula communicates with the colon, enteroscopy should be performed to examine the mucosa of the involved bowel for the presence of active Crohn's colitis. If active Crohn's disease is not found in the colon, correction requires resection of the involved loop of small bowel and simple oversewing of the tract in the target organ. In an ileosigmoid fistula, a segmental resection of the ileum is performed, a primary anastomosis is created, the tract is excised, and the sigmoid opening is oversewn. If the sigmoid also is involved by active Crohn's disease, then resection of

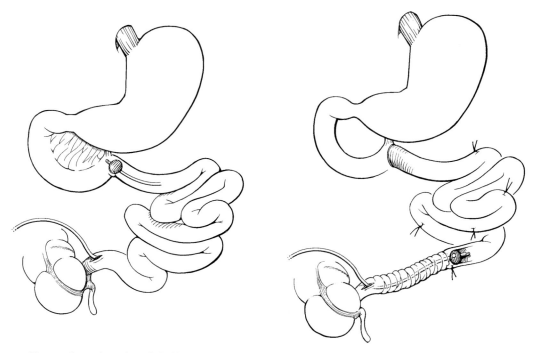

Fig. 7. Technique of long tube in bowel with balloon inflated and strictures identified with 3-0 silk suture.

it is reasonable (Fig. 8). Ileovesical fistulas due to Crohn's disease occurred in 7.7% of fistulas in our review,[16] and they are treated identically, oversewing the bladder opening with absorbable suture. We leave a urinary catheter in place for 7 days after repairing the bladder. Enterocutaneous fistulas are treated by resection of the ileum with primary anastomosis and curetting of the tract. The cutaneous opening is managed as is any open wound.

Laparoscopy is a useful adjunct in the surgical treatment of Crohn's disease of the small bowel. The "wet" edema frequently seen in association with the ileocolic disease enhances tissue planes and allows for a relatively easy laparoscopic dissection. Resection involves the general principles of laparoscopy.

COLON

Isolated Crohn's colitis is not an uncommon entity, but it may be difficult to distinguish from ulcerative colitis. Indications for operation include stricture, chronic obstruction, abscess, fistula, bleeding, extraintestinal complications, perforation, massive hemorrhage, and fulminant colitis. Surgical treatment of Crohn's colitis is identical to that of Crohn's disease involving the small bowel, with resection being the favored method of treatment for symptomatic stricturing. Surgical procedures for Crohn's colitis include segmental resection, colectomy with ileorectostomy, and proctocolectomy with end ileostomy.

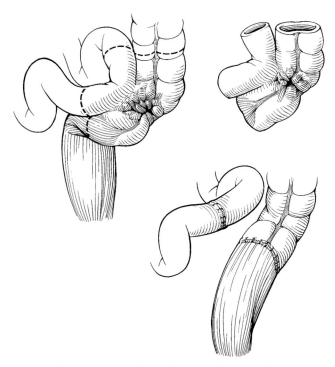

Fig. 8. Ileosigmoid fistula, before and after resection.

Strictures of the colon and the rectum are malignant until proved otherwise. Strictures of the large bowel in the setting of inflammatory bowel disease, in all circumstances, should be resected unless patient comorbidity prohibits an operative procedure. Malignancy in a colonic stricture is often a linitis plastica type and may be difficult to diagnose endoscopically or radiographically.

If the large bowel disease occurs in a segmental fashion and the anus is spared, limited resection is indicated (Fig. 9), followed by either a hand-sewn anastomosis (Fig. 10 A-D) or a stapled anastomosis (Fig. 10 E-G). We do not use strictureplasty for strictures in Crohn's colitis. In our series comparing segmental colectomy with abdominal colectomy and ileorectostomy, there was a higher risk for recurrent disease with segmental resection (59% vs. 40%), especially at the anastomosis, a higher need for subsequent medical or surgical therapy (44% vs. 20%), and a higher likelihood of eventually needing a permanent stoma (15% vs. 10%).[17] The sample size in that series was small and the difference in the likelihood of eventually needing a permanent stoma was not significant. The authors concluded that although the risk of recurrence was higher and subsequent surgical intervention was likely with a segmental resection, the risk of a permanent stoma was not lessened by doing a more extensive resection. Repeat operations for segmental colitis may delay permanent colostomy.

If the majority of the colon is involved by Crohn's disease and the rectum is spared, abdominal colectomy with ileorectostomy (Fig. 11) is appropriate. In our experience, 30% of patients have a satisfactory outcome; however, 30% eventually will require proctectomy.[18] Ileorectostomy is commonly known to be well tolerated in younger patients, but our series reported a good outcome in the elderly as well, with a low risk of incontinence and a minimal increase in stool frequency.[19] In the setting of disease in the colon and rectum, we perform either an anal-sparing proctocolectomy or an intersphincteric proctocolectomy with Brooke ileostomy (Fig. 12). The former can be considered if the anus is not involved by Crohn's disease, whereas the latter is preferred if anal disease is present. We do not use either a continent ileostomy or an ileal pouch-anal canal anastomosis for proven Crohn's disease because of the high rate of recurrence in the ileal pouch and the morbidity of subsequent operations to correct the complications. In the series by Sagar et al.,[20] inadvertent ileal pouch-anal canal anastomosis when Crohn's disease proved to be present was associated with a 45% pouch failure rate, a rate we consider unacceptable.

Appendiceal Crohn's disease is very rare, with fewer than 100 cases reported.[21] Treatment varies from simple appendectomy, if the appendiceal base is clear of involvement, to segmental ileocecal resection, if ileocecal involvement is present.

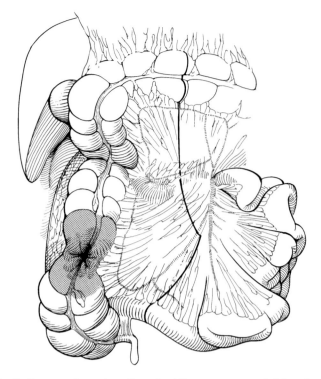

Fig. 9. Segmental resection of terminal ileum, cecum, and right colon.

ANUS AND RECTUM

Anorectal Crohn's disease can be severely disabling, presenting with a combination of anal tags, abscesses, and complex fistulas. A characteristic bluish perianal discoloration may be one of the first signs of perianal Crohn's disease. Anorectal Crohn's disease usually occurs in the setting of Crohn's colitis, but it may occur with isolated ileal disease. We support a conservative approach to the treatment of anorectal Crohn's disease.

We avoid proximal diversion because it does not result in satisfactory healing or abatement of symptoms. Removal of all diseased bowel proximal to the anus commonly results in healing of the anal lesions, although if any disease remains or recurs, the anal disease will recur.[22]

Proctectomy is reserved for strictures and severe non-healing perianal abscesses and fistulas that do not improve or progress with local care. An intersphincteric proctectomy is done in a standard fashion for benign disease but is technically more challenging in the region of inflammation near the anorectal ring. After resection of the specimen, hemostasis is achieved and the pelvis is irrigated thoroughly. The pelvic peritoneum is closed. Two large round silicone drains are placed into the pelvis

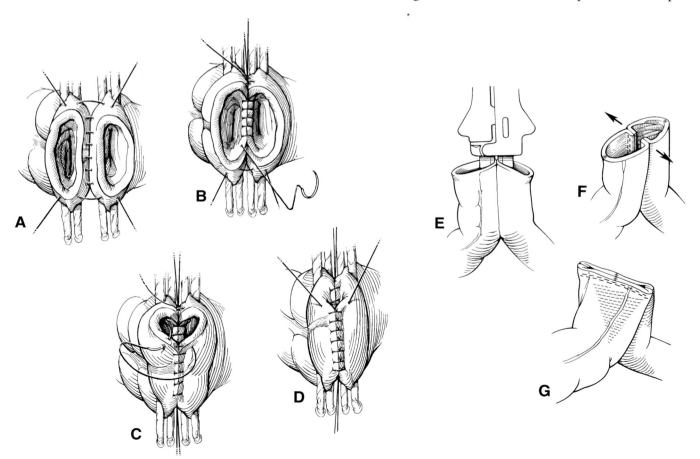

Fig. 10. Anastomosis after segmental resection. A-D, Hand-sewn anastomosis. E-G, Stapled anastomosis.

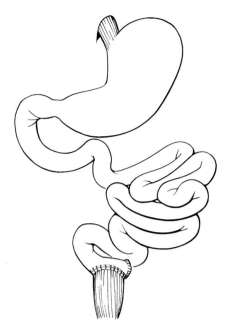

Fig. 11. Ileorectostomy.

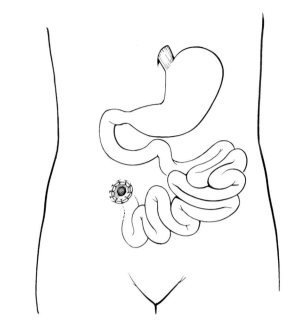

Fig. 12. Brooke ileostomy after proctocolectomy.

from the perineum, passing through the skin of the perineum bilaterally and traversing the ischiorectal fossa to enter the pelvic space through the levators (Fig. 13). The drains are placed somewhat anteriorly, so that they are not compressed when the patient sits. Alternatively, the drains may be brought out to the surface through the lower anterior abdominal wall rather than through the perineum. After drain placement, the perineum is closed with interrupted absorbable sutures. Postoperatively, drain irrigation is initiated with either 1 L of sterile normal saline or dilute povidone-iodine solution. The two drains are used in an alternating fashion every 4 hours for irrigation and drainage. At 48 to 72 hours, both drains are placed to wall suction and removed thereafter when drainage is minimal.

Anal strictures occur in severe Crohn's proctitis and generally are fibrotic and fixed. Distal rectal malignancy must be excluded. With the patient under anesthesia, the perianal region is examined, abscesses are drained, and the stricture is sequentially dilated. A lateral internal sphincterotomy may promote healing and decrease pain related to anal fissuring, but it has a risk of creating fecal incontinence. Deep, asymptomatic fissures should not be treated.

Perianal abscesses and fistulas in patients with active perianal Crohn's disease are treated more conservatively than those in patients without inflammatory bowel disease, but the basic principles of abscess and fistula operation are preserved, with adequate drainage of sepsis being the foremost goal. Surgical procedures in this area should be planned carefully and approached conservatively because

healing may be inadequate and there is a high risk of fecal incontinence. After any associated abscess is drained, a draining (noncutting) seton of a noninflammatory material (e.g., a 0.25-inch Penrose drain) is passed through the tract and left in place during the initiation of medical therapy, such as metronidazole or antitumor necrosis factor-α. The draining seton is placed through a fistula tract and tied loosely, its purpose being to maintain adequate drainage and avoid closed abscess formation rather than to erode through muscle in the manner of a cutting seton. The draining seton is removed at follow-up examination in the clinic when there is no evidence of ongoing infection and

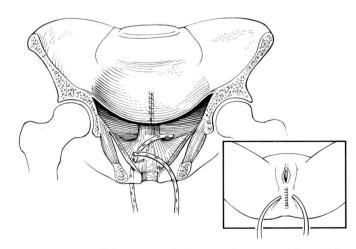

Fig. 13. Perineal drains placed into the pelvic space to be used for "circulation" of perfusate postoperatively.

the region of the seton appears relatively dry and noninflamed. Persistent fistulas may be treated with light debridement and application of fibrin glue.

More complex fistulas may be characterized with endoluminal ultrasonography or with the assistance of radiologic studies. Acute abscesses are drained. Again, we use draining setons, either a 0.25-inch Penrose drain or a polypropylene suture, which is left in place while medical therapy is optimized (Fig. 14).

Rectovaginal fistulas likewise are treated conservatively. We perform an examination with the patient under anesthesia to find and drain any abscesses. A draining seton is inserted with the expectation that it will remain in place long-term. We do not attempt a flap advancement-type procedure if active Crohn's proctitis is present. Fibrin glue is an option in the presence of a small, relatively quiescent fistula.

Hemorrhoidectomy is avoided in the presence of active disease.

Even in the setting of quiescent Crohn's disease, we approach "routine" perianal disease cautiously. Every attempt is made to treat fissures, abscesses, and fistulas conservatively. Active Crohn's disease must be excluded; if it is present, then medical therapy is optimized with the addition of anti-tumor necrosis factor-α agents.

If a fissure is present without active Crohn's disease, medical agents such as nitropaste and nifedipine are considered first-line therapy. Lateral internal sphincterotomy is performed if medical therapy fails, but it should be done in the operating room carefully and with excellent hemostasis.

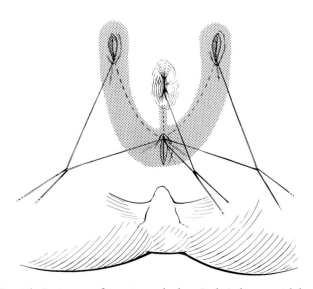

Fig. 14. Perineum of a patient who has Crohn's disease with horseshoe-type abscess and several polypropylene sutures looped, from right anterolateral to post midline, from left anterolateral to post midline.

Abscesses in a patient with quiescent Crohn's disease may be cryptogenic and are treated with incision and drainage. An examination with the patient under anesthesia can help distinguish simple fistulas from those related to recurrent Crohn's disease. Simple fistulas can be treated with fistulotomy, keeping in mind that healing may be impaired if the patient remains treated with corticosteroids or antimetabolites. Cutting setons are used in higher fistulas, again with caution and after ensuring that active Crohn's proctitis is absent.

Rectovaginal fistulas are often complex and difficult to manage. Again, we frequently use a draining seton to prevent a closed abscess, while simultaneously optimizing medical therapy. Fecal diversion rarely results in resolution of the problem. In quiescent Crohn's disease, there may be a role for advancement flap.

Severe perianal disease may require proctectomy for resolution. If the colon is mostly normal, then a colostomy is appropriate. If disease is more extensive, then a proctocolectomy and ileostomy are appropriate.

LAPAROSCOPY

We are using laparoscopy more frequently for the treatment of Crohn's disease, including obstructing and fistulizing disease. Intra-abdominal abscess is a contraindication to laparoscopic intervention. We apply the standard principles of laparoscopy to surgery for Crohn's disease. Often, the "wet" edema seen in the setting of acute inflammation facilitates the dissection, whereas fibrosis and fistula disease make the procedure more challenging. Using a low threshold for conversion to an open operation, we attempt to identify appropriate anatomical landmarks and proceed in a fashion similar to any other laparoscopic bowel resection. Although not yet studied in this setting, these minimal intervention procedures may be less traumatic for the patient and allow for quicker recovery postoperatively.

SURGICAL OUTCOMES

Early complications consist of those that occur with any abdominal operation and include intestinal obstruction due to adhesions, intra-abdominal abscess, wound infection, anastomotic leak, bleeding, deep venous thrombosis and pulmonary embolism, pulmonary infection, urinary retention, enterocutaneous fistula, and death.

Late complications are related to loss of small bowel absorptive area and include vitamin malabsorption, especially the fat-soluble vitamins and vitamin B_{12} absorbed in the distal ileum, bile salt malabsorption, and short bowel syndrome.

LONG-TERM OUTCOME

The cumulative risk of recurrence in young patients undergoing surgical resection is 70% at 20 years.[23] Risk factors for recurrence after operation for Crohn's disease have been examined by us.[24] We concluded that prophylactic treatment and proctocolectomy with Brooke ileostomy were the only two interventions that decreased disease recurrence. Several other factors were investigated but were not clinically significant, were statistically inconclusive, or were modifiable. Patients with an earlier age at onset of Crohn's disease have a higher risk of recurrence over time, which may be explained by a longer follow-up.[2,24] A patient's sex has not been consistently found to be a risk factor for increased postoperative recurrence rates.[24] The anatomical pattern of involvement of Crohn's disease predicts the risk of recurrent disease; patients with isolated Crohn's colitis who undergo proctocolectomy have the lowest risk of recurrent disease (Table 1). An ileocolic distribution is the most common anatomical pattern; more than 90% of patients have this presentation. It also has the highest risk for recurrence after resection. The risk of recurrence after resection for isolated small bowel disease is between that with Crohn's colitis and ileocolic Crohn's disease. Length of small bowel resected does not affect the recurrence rates. Obstructing disease has a tendency for a higher risk of recurrence than fistulizing disease. The risk of recurrence for patients who have more than one resection is slightly higher than that for patients who have only one resection, but this difference does not reach statistical significance.

Extended versus limited margins of gross disease have been examined at Mayo Clinic and at Cleveland Clinic,[13] as have histologic margins. Obtaining histologically negative margins does seem to lessen the chance of disease recurrence, but it is possible only in limited disease.

Our experience with strictureplasty for obstructive Crohn's disease was reported by Spencer et al.[25] Of 244 patients who underwent abdominal exploration for symptomatic Crohn's disease, 35 had a total of 71 strictureplasties. Strictureplasty was combined with resection in 67%. The perioperative complication rate was 14%, and there were no deaths, anastomotic leaks, fistulas, or abscesses during a 3-year follow-up.

Restarting medical therapy after surgical resection for symptomatic Crohn's disease seems to be beneficial for decreasing the risk of recurrent disease. In a study at Mayo Clinic,[6] prophylactic mesalamine in a dosage of 3.0 g/day was effective for preventing recurrence, reducing risk in the treated group versus the control group (treated, 31%; control, 53%).

After proctocolectomy for anorectal Crohn's disease, the disease recurrence rate is between 10% and 25%, wound healing difficulties occur in 50% to 60% of patients, and wound healing is delayed in up to 30% at 1 year.[21]

CONCLUSION

Crohn's disease is an inflammatory disease of the bowel with a tendency for progression and recurrence. Intestinal complications include obstruction and fistula formation. These are treated surgically if symptomatic and if refractory to medical therapy. Complete disease resection in the setting of isolated Crohn's colitis and postoperative prophylactic medical therapy with agents such as mesalamine and metronidazole decrease the likelihood of recurrence. Proper surgical principles and meticulous technique are necessary to minimize the risk of perioperative complications and ensure optimal patient outcome.

REFERENCES

1. Crohn BB, Ginzburg L, Oppenheimer GD: Regional ileitis: a pathologic and clinical entity. JAMA 99:1323-1329, 1932
2. Hellers G: Crohn's disease in Stockholm county 1955-1974: a study of epidemiology, results of surgical treatment and long-term prognosis. Acta Chir Scand Suppl 490:1-84, 1979
3. Agrez MV, Valente RM, Pierce W, Melton LJ III, van Heerden JA, Beart RW Jr: Surgical history of Crohn's disease in a well-defined population. Mayo Clin Proc 57:747-752, 1982
4. Harold KL, Kelly KA: Duodenal Crohn disease. Probl Gen Surg 16:50-57, 1999
5. Yamamoto T, Keighley MR: The association of cigarette smoking with a high risk of recurrence after ileocolonic resection for ileocecal Crohn's disease. Surg Today 29:579-580, 1999
6. McLeod RS, Wolff BG, Steinhart AH, Carryer PW, O'Rourke K, Andrews DF, Blair JE, Cangemi JR, Cohen Z, Cullen JB: Prophylactic mesalamine treatment decreases postoperative recurrence of Crohn's disease. Gastroenterology 109:404-413, 1995
7. Orsoni P, Barthet M, Portier F, Panuel M, Desjeux A, Grimaud JC: Prospective comparison of endosonography, magnetic resonance imaging and surgical findings in anorectal fistula and abscess complicating Crohn's disease. Br J Surg 86:360-364, 1999
8. Schwartz DA, Wiersema MJ, Dudiak KM, Fletcher JG, Clain JE, Tremaine WJ, Zinsmeister AR, Norton ID, Boardman LA, Devine RM, Wolff BG, Young-Fadok TM, Diehl NN, Pemberton JH, Sandborn WJ: A comparison of endoscopic ultrasound, magnetic resonance imaging, and exam under anesthesia for evaluation of Crohn's perianal fistulas. Gastroenterology 121:1064-1072, 2001
9. Wolff BG, Beart RW Jr, Frydenberg HB, Weiland LH, Agrez MV, Ilstrup DM: The importance of disease-free margins in resections for Crohn's disease. Dis Colon Rectum 26:239-243, 1983
10. Bergman L, Krause U: Crohn's disease: a long-term study of the clinical course in 186 patients. Scand J Gastroenterol 12:937-944, 1977
11. Krause U: Post-operative complication and early course of the surgical treatment of Crohn's disease. Acta Chir Scand 144:163-174, 1978
12. Nygaard K, Fausa O: Crohn's disease: recurrence after surgical treatment. Scand J Gastroenterol 12:577-584, 1977
13. Fazio VW, Marchetti F, Church M, Goldblum JR, Lavery C, Hull TL, Milsom JW, Strong SA, Oakley JR, Secic M: Effect of resection margins on the recurrence of Crohn's disease in the small bowel: a randomized controlled trial. Ann Surg 224:563-571, 1996
14. Nugent FW, Richmond M, Park SK: Crohn's disease of the duodenum. Gut 18:115-120, 1977
15. Farmer RG, Hawk WA, Turnbull RB Jr: Clinical patterns in Crohn's disease: a statistical study of 615 cases. Gastroenterology 68:627-634, 1975
16. Young-Fadok TM, Wolff BG, Meagher A, Benn PL, Dozois RR: Surgical management of ileosigmoid fistulas in Crohn's disease. Dis Colon Rectum 40:558-561, 1997
17. Prabhakar LP, Laramee C, Nelson H, Dozois RR: Avoiding a stoma: role for segmental or abdominal colectomy in Crohn's colitis. Dis Colon Rectum 40:71-78, 1997
18. Farnell MB, van Heerden JA, Beart RW Jr, Weiland LH: Rectal preservation in nonspecific inflammatory disease of the colon. Ann Surg 192:249-253, 1980
19. Beckwith PS, Wolff BG, Frazee RC: Ileorectostomy in the older patient. Dis Colon Rectum 35:301-304, 1992
20. Sagar PM, Dozois RR, Wolff BG: Long-term results of ileal pouch-anal anastomosis in patients with Crohn's disease. Dis Colon Rectum 39:893-898, 1996
21. Wolff BG: Crohn's colitis. In Current Therapy in Colon and Rectal Surgery. Edited by VW Fazio. Toronto, BC Decker, 1990, pp 195-198
22. Wolff BG, Culp CE, Beart RW Jr, Ilstrup DM, Ready RL: Anorectal Crohn's disease: a long-term perspective. Dis Colon Rectum 28:709-711, 1985
23. Wolff BG: Crohn's disease: the role of surgical treatment. Mayo Clin Proc 61:292-295, 1986
24. Wolff BG: Factors determining recurrence following surgery for Crohn's disease. World J Surg 22:364-369, 1998
25. Spencer MP, Nelson H, Wolff BG, Dozois RR: Strictureplasty for obstructive Crohn's disease: the Mayo experience. Mayo Clin Proc 69:33-36, 1994

Chapter 28

SMALL BOWEL OBSTRUCTION

Yvonne Baerga-Varela, M.D.

Small bowel obstruction (SBO) is one of the most common clinical problems faced by the general surgeon. SBO is unique in that multiple causes can result in the common physiologic end point of enteric obstruction. The specific cause usually is unknown at the time of initial diagnosis. The initial therapeutic approach is generic, based on the degree of obstruction and the clinical status of the patient.

Even though SBO was recognized in times before Christ, it was not until the 1900s that surgical therapy was accepted. The Mayo brothers published several reports regarding the surgical therapy of SBO. Despite more than a hundred years of surgical experience and several decades of advances in diagnostic techniques, many important challenges remain in the diagnosis and management of SBO. Ideally, timely surgical intervention should be offered to prevent lengthy hospitalization and to minimize morbidity. To accomplish this, we need to identify the cause of obstruction on presentation, the patients who will not improve with conservative management, and the patients with reversible intestinal ischemia.

HISTORY

Surgical treatment of SBO began centuries ago.[1] Praxagoras, in the 4th century B.C., cured a patient with SBO by creating an external intestinal fistula as he incised the inguinal swelling of the patient's incarcerated hernia. In 1561, Pierre Franco became known as the originator of the planned direct attack on a strangulated hernia, incising over the swelling and dividing the constricting band. In the 1700s, multiple surgeons in Paris had successfully operated for strangulated hernia with advanced intestinal gangrene.

Despite these reported successes, the surgical communities in Europe did not agree on surgical intervention for SBO. Multiple conservative measures were considered accepted methods of therapy for SBO through the 18th and 19th centuries. Dupuytren, of Paris, reported the use of phlebotomy by leeches before operation for strangulated hernias. In 1823, Astley Cooper, from England, reported the use of taxis, inverting the patient after the application of tobacco enemas. Duchenne used electric stimulation in 1855. Other reported methods for the therapy of SBO included oral metallic mercury, percutaneous intestinal puncture, and opium.

Overall, there was a reluctance to operate for intestinal obstruction during the 19th century. The British Medical Association (1878, 1883) and the First American Congress of Physicians & Surgeons (1888) agreed with the conservative management of SBO. In 1929, Miller reported a mortality rate of 65% with operative management for acute intestinal obstruction at Charity Hospital in New Orleans. These results emphasized the unacceptable operative mortality associated with this condition in the United States at that time, delaying the acceptance of operative intervention, probably related in large part to the inability to replace fluid and electrolytes adequately intraoperatively and postoperatively.

However, several reports of successful surgical intervention had been presented without acceptance. In 1871, Thomas Annandale read before the Medico-Chirurgical Society of Edinburgh his proposal for surgical intervention for the relief of intestinal obstruction. He concluded that operation is justifiable when the symptoms of sudden and complete intestinal obstruction are present and ordinary means have failed to give relief. He also recommended that operative intervention not be delayed for longer than 36 to 48 hours and that the operation be performed through a midline incision.[2] Lawson Tait, from Birmingham, protested in the British Medical Association in 1883, responding that the accurate diagnosis of SBO is obtained only on exploration—better before than after death. In 1885, Greves, from Liverpool, described a patient with acute intestinal obstruction, outlining the importance of surgical intervention and the specifics of preoperative and postoperative management.[3]

A better understanding of this condition and its therapy was being attained. In 1867, William Brinton described the different kinds of intestinal obstruction, presenting symptoms and stages, and he inclusively reported several clinical patient descriptions.[4] Brinton described the condition in the following manner: "The term 'intestinal obstruction' connotes with tolerable accuracy the class of cases to which it refers: a class made up of varieties very diverse in their origin and nature, but having this common feature—that, in all, the symptoms are caused mainly by an obstruction to the transit of contents through some part of the intestinal tube." In 1899, Frederick Treves, working in the London Hospital, also wrote a book on intestinal obstruction, describing its varieties, pathologic features, diagnosis, and treatment as a revised edition of his first book published in 1884.[5]

The concept of intestinal decompression for SBO had its origins in 1869, when Kussmaul reported the use of gastric lavage for the treatment of pyloric stenosis. It was not until the 1880s that proximal intestinal decompression was believed to provide relief of symptoms from mechanical obstruction or ileus.[1] Then, in the 1930s, Wangensteen began his seminal work on gastrointestinal intubation as effective treatment of postlaparotomy ileus.[6] Intravenous hydration was recognized as a crucial principle of care for SBO by the 1920s.

The Mayo brothers were proponents of surgical management. In 1897, William J. Mayo published his results of operative relief in five patients with pyloric obstruction due to cicatricial stenosis.[7] Again, in 1907, he described bowel resection for the relief of intestinal obstruction, in the Section of Surgery & Anatomy of the American Medical Association's 58th Annual Session, Atlantic City.[8] Charles H. Mayo read, before the Western Surgical Association on December 20th, 1910, his paper on SBO due to kinks and adhesions of the terminal ileum. He even presented his visions for prevention of postoperative adhesions.[9]

DEFINITIONS

The difference between a *mechanical* obstruction and a *functional*, or neurogenic, obstruction is important. A mechanical obstruction refers to a blockage of the bowel lumen, physically preventing luminal contents from passing through the gut. In a functional, or neurogenic obstruction, the luminal contents fail to pass because of disturbances in gut motility. A functional obstruction generally is referred to as an ileus when it occurs in the small and large bowel together and as colonic pseudo-obstruction when it affects the large bowel selectively.

Two other classifications of obstruction affect management and the urgency of surgical intervention. One distinction is between *simple* and *strangulated* obstruction, and the other is between *complete* and *incomplete* obstruction. Strangulation means that blood flow to the obstructed segment of bowel is compromised, necessitating immediate surgical intervention; the strangulation may be reversible or irreversible. As discussed later in this chapter, diagnosing impending strangulation can be very difficult and is commonly done too late. In contrast, simple obstruction refers to obstruction in which blood flow to the bowel is not compromised. Narrowing of the lumen that still allows passage of some fluid and air is known as a partial obstruction. A complete obstruction refers to totally occluded lumen. Along those lines, in a closed loop obstruction, both inflow and outflow of luminal contents to the involved segment of gut are blocked. In open loop obstruction, proximal decompression is possible.

SBO also has been classified according to anatomical location and on the basis of cause. When location is the means of classification, SBO can be divided into proximal (or high), intermediate, or distal. Proximal obstructions involve the pylorus, duodenum, or proximal jejunum, intermediate obstructions affect the mid jejunum or mid ileum, and distal obstructions involve the distal ileum. Depending on cause, SBO can be classified as intraluminal, intramural, or extrinsic (Table 1).

ETIOPATHOGENESIS

The most common cause of SBO in the Western Hemisphere is adhesions from prior abdominal operations. SBO due to neoplasm and hernias follows. The Mayo Clinic series reported by Mucha[10] in 1987 corroborated these three conditions as the most common causes of operative SBO in our practice. Several other reports have documented similar causes during the past 2 decades[11,12] (Table 2). Multiple miscellaneous causes occur to lesser extents (Fig. 1 and 2).

Despite its multiple causes, the local pathophysiologic effects of SBO are similar. Luminal obstruction causes proximal bowel distention due to accumulation of fluid and intestinal gas. Fluid accumulation in the lumen of the obstructed intestine results from decreased absorption and

Table 1.—Causes of Small Bowel Obstruction

Extrinsic
  Adhesions
  Hernias
    Internal
    External
  Volvulus
  External mass effect
    Neoplasm
    Benign tumor
    Inflammatory process
    Endometriosis
    Pregnancy
  Congenital bands
Intramural
  Neoplasms
    Primary
    Secondary
  Inflammatory process
    Crohn's disease
    Diverticulitis
    Appendicitis
  Chronic ischemia
    Radiation-induced
    Medication-induced
  Trauma
    Intramural hematoma
  Congenital
    Atresia, web, stenosis
Intraluminal
  Foreign bodies
  Intussusception
  Gallstone
  Parasites
  Exophytic lesions

Modified from Soybel.[6] By permission of Lippincott Williams & Wilkins.

increased secretion. Moderate increases of luminal pressure increase absorption, but as the mean intraluminal pressures increase to three or four times normal, absorption is impaired and a net secretion of fluid into the lumen occurs. Stasis of the intraluminal content increases bacterial proliferation.[6] With chronicity, the wall of the distended bowel becomes edematous; in addition, fluid loss into the peritoneum occurs from local serosal transudation. Motility with violent bursts of peristalsis occurs between quiescent intervals.[13]

The average intraluminal pressure in normal resting small bowel is 2 to 6 mm Hg. Resting pressures more than 30 mm Hg cause lymphatic and capillary stasis. Venous drainage is compromised at pressures more than 50 mm Hg, and arterial flow is impeded at pressures more than 90 mm Hg.[13] Sustained increases in intraluminal pressure can cause ischemia of the bowel, and the higher the pressure, the less time is needed to cause it.

In addition to the local effects of SBO, there are systemic manifestations. One of the most predominant systemic effects of SBO is hypovolemia. This is explained not only by the local fluid losses into the obstructed bowel lumen but also by substantial losses caused by vomiting. Other systemic effects include acid-base derangements based on the quantity and type of fluid lost. Decreased viability of the obstructed bowel with progression to necrosis is known to cause a systemic inflammatory response syndrome and sepsis with possible multiple organ failure and death.

DIAGNOSIS AND IMAGING

The most important clues to the diagnosis of SBO are the patient's history and results of physical examination. The first question that must be answered is whether the patient has SBO. The diagnosis of SBO is best ascertained on the basis of the clinical presentation, aided by laboratory studies and radiologic evaluations.

Two types of presentations are common. Some patients present with an acute episode of SBO, whereas

Table 2.—Common Causes of Small Bowel Obstruction

	Mucha, 1987[10]	Landercasper et al., 1993[11]	Fevang et al., 2000[12]
No. of patients	314	150	975
Cause, %			
Adhesion	49	52	54
Neoplasm	16	11	Excluded
Hernia	15	9	30
Other	20	29	16

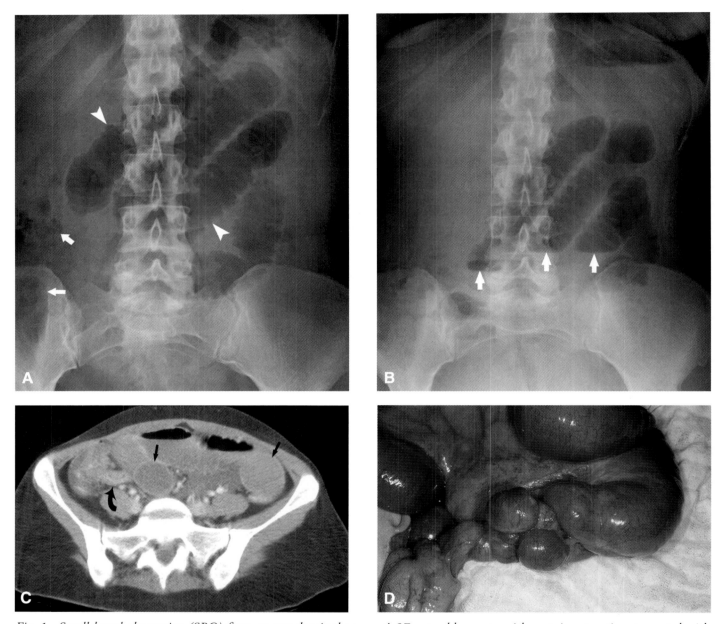

Fig. 1. Small bowel obstruction (SBO) from an extraluminal cause. A 37-year-old woman with no prior operations presented with abdominal distention, nausea, and vomiting. (A), Supine abdominal radiograph shows multiple dilated loops of small bowel (arrowheads) *with a small amount of air in the right colon* (arrows), *indicating SBO, either partial or early complete. (B), Upright radiograph shows multiple air-fluid levels* (arrows) *with dilated small bowel loops. (C), Computed tomogram shows marked dilatation of small bowel* (straight arrows) *to the level of the distal ileum, where there is a nondilated short segment of bowel* (curved arrow). *The colon is not distended. (D), Intraoperatively, the distal ileal obstruction was due to multiple serosal implants of endometriosis.*

others present with a history of chronic, recurrent symptoms. The diagnostic work-up and urgency of therapy differ between these two groups.

The clinical diagnosis of SBO is based on four key components: crampy abdominal pain, vomiting, obstipation, and abdominal distention. The clinical presentation varies depending on the level of obstruction, whether it is a closed or open loop obstruction, the duration from onset of symptoms, and the cause of the obstruction. Typically, the patient presents with a variable period of abdominal pain that tends to be colicky at first. This is followed by nausea, vomiting, passage of loose stools, and obstipation. On physical examination, varying degrees of abdominal distention are found, depending on the level of obstruction and the duration of symptoms. Peritoneal irritation suggests strangulation obstruction, which requires

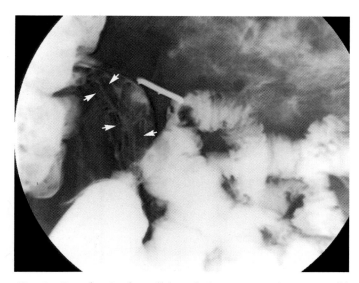

Fig. 2.   Intraluminal small bowel obstruction.   A 39-year-old woman with abdominal cramps.   Terminal ileum detail from a small bowel contrast examination shows multiple long, round filling defects (arrows) in the terminal ileum from Ascaris lumbricoides, causing partial obstruction.

emergency intervention.   During the physical examination, it is important to exclude external hernias as a possible cause of obstruction and blood or masses by rectal examination.

The stethoscope has been considered an important instrument in the clinical diagnosis of intestinal obstruction. Treves, in 1899, listened to the cecum during enema administration to decide whether a patient had a large bowel obstruction or SBO.[1] Charles H. Mayo preferred a gastric tube to a stethoscope for the evaluation of bowel obstruction. Presenting a paper on intestinal obstruction before the American Surgical Association, May 1922, he read: "I should prefer to see a stomach tube rather than a stethoscope hanging around the neck of my surgical intern."[14] Currently, both instruments are deemed important. Obstructive bowel sounds with rushes, tinkles, and borborygmi are unmistakable pathognomonic findings of obstruction, but they are not specific for mechanical versus functional obstruction. Another potentially important finding is the presence of a gastric succussion splash; in a patient who has not eaten during the previous 3 hours, a succussion splash is indicative of either gastric or intestinal obstruction (mechanical or functional).

In our practice, blood chemistry studies are of little or no value for determining the presence or absence of SBO or for clarifying the need for operative intervention.[10] However, they are of extreme value for determining serum electrolyte abnormalities and for allowing early recognition and resuscitation.

Radiologic investigations assist in evaluation and management of SBO. The most basic and frequently used is supine and upright plain abdominal radiography. Classic findings for SBO are distended loops of small bowel (>3 cm in diameter), air-fluid levels in the obstructed loops on upright views, and a paucity of colonic air (Fig. 3). Despite these typical characteristics, multiple studies have shown that plain radiography is diagnostic of SBO in only 50% to 80% of patients.[15-17] In the Mayo Clinic series,[10] flat and upright abdominal radiography also failed to demonstrate convincingly the presence of SBO in a large percentage of patients. Well-known pitfalls include the gasless abdomen caused by fluid-filled obstructed loops of small bowel (Fig. 4), the closed loop obstruction, and the high or proximal SBO.

If the diagnosis of SBO is not definitive, options for further radiologic evaluation include contrast studies of the gastrointestinal tract and abdominal computed tomography. These radiologic evaluations also can assist in management because they help in the differentiation of partial versus complete SBO and in identification of the particular cause.

Different types of contrast studies have been used in the diagnosis and management of SBO, and results have been mixed.[15] These studies include 1) upper gastrointestinal series (barium study of esophagus, stomach, and duodenum) (Fig. 5, 6, and 7), 2) small bowel follow-through (barium study of jejunum and ileum) (Fig. 8 and 9), 3) barium enema (colon study), 4) small bowel studies with meglumine diatrizoate, and 5) enteroclysis. The goals of these studies are to document the anatomical presence of obstruction, to localize the specific site, and, potentially, to identify the causative lesion. They are usually unnecessary when the diagnosis can be reached on the basis of the physical examination and history. Small bowel contrast studies are contraindicated when strangulation is suspected. Such contrast studies are used less frequently for evaluation of acute obstructive symptoms, and many times they are reserved for evaluation of chronic recurrent symptoms. Although enteroclysis is an excellent method to diagnose obstruction readily, even if multifocal, it is seldom used in our practice given its disadvantages. The barium used precludes other imaging methods such as computed tomography or angiography. Enteroclysis requires a large amount of radiation, is time-consuming, is operator-dependent, and is not well tolerated by patients with acute obstructive symptoms. In our practice, enteroclysis is reserved for selected patients with suspected partial mechanical obstruction or for those in whom a small bowel lesion is suspected. In contrast, a small bowel follow-through examination can be helpful when the SBO is not resolving, with the goal of documenting or excluding an anatomical finding that requires surgical intervention.

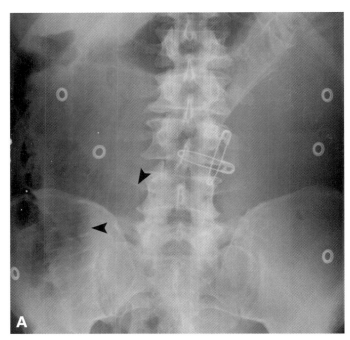

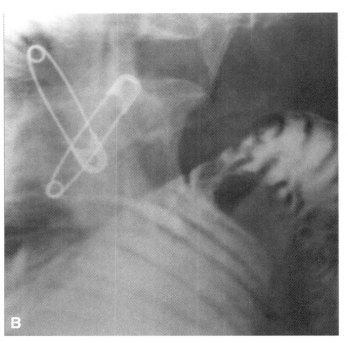

Fig. 3. Postoperative small bowel obstruction (SBO). A 57-year-old man who had been in a motor vehicle crash, which caused a ruptured spleen, necessitating splenectomy. Seven days later, signs and symptoms of bowel obstruction developed. (A), Abdominal radiograph shows dilated loops of small bowel (arrowheads) with paucity of gas in colon. (B), Contrast study shows typical appearance of SBO by an adhesive band, with tethering of the bowel toward one side of the bowel wall.

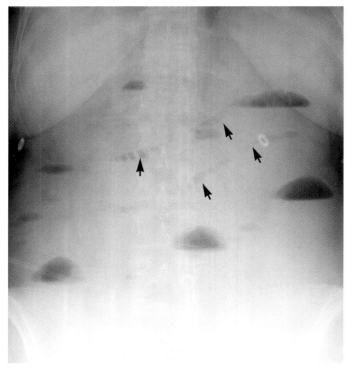

Fig. 4. Small bowel obstruction with fluid-filled obstructed bowel. Two weeks after cholecystectomy, an omental adhesion constricting a small bowel loop developed in a 56-year-old woman. Upright abdominal radiograph shows multiple air-fluid levels in the small bowel in a "string of beads" configuration (arrows). Dilated bowel loops are not seen because intraluminal air has been replaced by fluid.

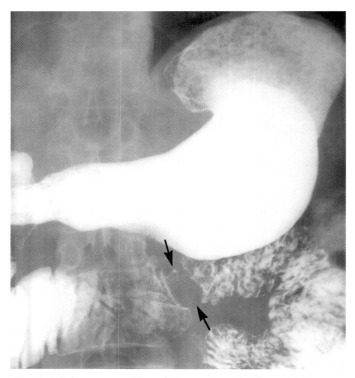

Fig. 5. Malignant small bowel obstruction. A 76-year-old woman with 2-month history of nausea and vomiting and 20-lb weight loss. Upper gastrointestinal study shows a dilated duodenum proximal to an annular constricting lesion (arrows) at the level of the ligament of Treitz. Pathologic analysis confirmed a primary grade 1 adenocarcinoma of jejunum.

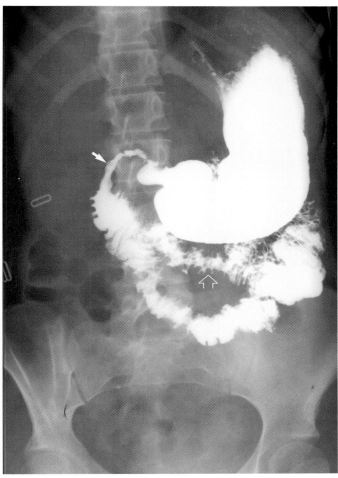

Fig. 6. *Crohn's disease of duodenum. A 15-year-old girl with a 10-lb weight loss and loose stools over 10 months. Upper gastrointestinal radiograph shows stricture of proximal duodenum with abnormal mucosa and marked deformity of pylorus and proximal duodenum (solid arrow). Superficial mucosal changes in proximal jejunum include ulceration and thickened folds (open arrow).*

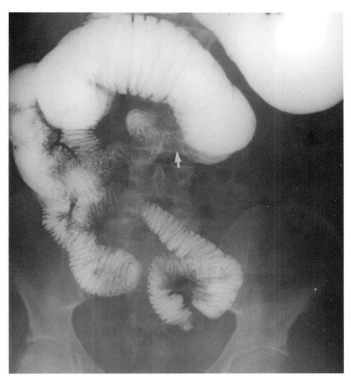

Fig. 7. *Chronic intermittent small bowel obstruction (SBO). A 27-year-old man with a 10-year history of intermittent nausea and vomiting. Upper gastrointestinal and small bowel radiograph shows distention of duodenum and proximal jejunum with a transition point (arrow). There is tapering and kinking of an abnormally rotated small bowel from Ladd bands of malrotation causing partial SBO. The small bowel distally is of normal caliber.*

In our practice, abdominal computed tomography with intravenous and oral contrast has become the radiographic study of choice in patients with suspected acute SBO not readily diagnosed from clinical presentation or plain film radiographic evaluations. Computed tomography has virtually revolutionized the evaluation of selected patients with SBO because it is simple, fast, and often diagnostic. Computed tomography is the preferred imaging method for the diagnosis of a malignant cause (primary or metastatic) and for associated inflammatory processes (i.e., appendicitis, diverticulitis, and Crohn's disease) causing SBO (Fig. 10). Computed tomography not only can help with the diagnosis of the condition (Fig. 11, 12, 13, and 14) but also can localize the obstructing segment and characterize it as complete or incomplete. In addition, it may establish the nature of

the obstructing lesion and can help detect strangulation.[6] The classic finding for the diagnosis of SBO on computed tomography is the presence of proximal dilated small bowel, collapsed distal bowel, and a focal transition zone. Passage of oral contrast into the colon or past the transition zone indicates partial or incomplete obstruction. Abdominal computed tomography with intravenous contrast can demonstrate a pattern of bowel wall enhancement useful for the diagnosis of intestinal ischemia and can on occasion reliably evaluate the patency of the mesenteric vessels.

Although there have been some reports of the use of ultrasonography and magnetic resonance imaging for evaluation of bowel obstruction,[18,19] we have not used these routinely in our practice. Although ultrasonography is readily available, gaseous distention of bowel loops confounds the interpretation and may prevent adequate visualization. Magnetic resonance imaging is similar to computed tomography, but because it is more expensive and much less readily available, it offers no notable advantages over computed tomography in most patients.

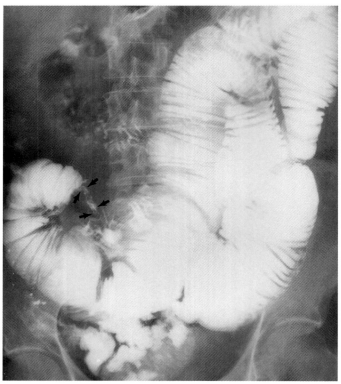

Fig. 8. Malignant small bowel obstruction from metastatic disease. A 68-year-old man, 5 years after resection for sigmoid colon carcinoma, had a 24-lb weight loss and several weeks of intermittent abdominal pain and distention. Small bowel follow-through radiograph shows dilated small bowel loops to level of distal ileum, where there is partial obstruction by an annular constricting lesion (arrows). The mucosa at the stricture site is abnormal, consistent with malignancy.

MANAGEMENT

Initial Therapeutic Steps

Once the diagnosis of SBO is established, several questions will influence management of the patient: 1) are there systemic manifestations of dehydration or electrolyte imbalances? 2) is the SBO partial or complete? 3) is the SBO simple or strangulated? and 4) what is the cause?

The two major options for initial management are operation and nonoperative (conservative) treatment. Nevertheless, before definitive therapy, some basic resuscitative maneuvers apply to all patients with suspected SBO. These patients have a large spectrum of clinical presentations. Some present early in the disease with only minimal dehydration. Others are dramatically dehydrated with electrolyte abnormalities and their sequelae. Some present with strangulated bowel with an unstable clinical condition, systemic inflammatory response, and even multiple organ dysfunction; these patients can present with

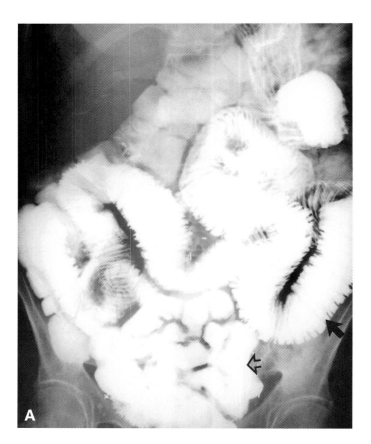

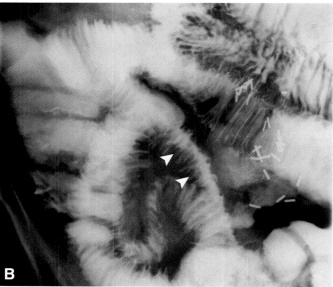

Fig. 9. Radiation enteropathy causing small bowel obstruction. A 60-year-old woman 14 months after external beam radiation therapy (1,200 rads) for endometrial adenocarcinoma with peritoneal spread. She presented with intermittent abdominal pain, diarrhea, nausea, and vomiting. (A), Small bowel examination shows caliber change from dilated jejunal loops (solid arrow) to normal-caliber loops of ileum (open arrow). (B), Close-up view of transition point shows considerable narrowing of distal jejunum with thickened folds, fixed loops, and poor peristalsis, consistent with radiation enteritis (arrowheads).

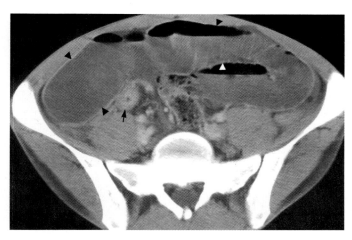

Fig. 10. Chronic small bowel obstruction. A 17-year-old boy with chronic obstructive symptoms. Computed tomogram shows diffuse small bowel dilatation and fluid-filled loops (arrowheads) *leading to a thick-walled, edematous terminal ileum* (arrow). *The differential diagnosis includes Crohn's disease, infection, or lymphoma.*

acute lung injury necessitating endotracheal intubation and mechanical ventilation. It is important that all patients presenting acutely have assessment and ensurance of proper airway, breathing, and circulation. Generic therapy includes intravenous hydration, gastric decompression, and bowel rest. After these basic therapeutic maneuvers, the surgeon must determine whether specific indications require surgical intervention, there is evidence of risk or signs of strangulation, and there is evidence of complete obstruction (Fig. 15).

The differentiation between partial and complete SBO is an important step in deciding the appropriate management. Partial obstruction is determined by the continued passage of flatus or stool after the onset of symptoms. In addition, persistence of colonic gas on radiographic evaluation for longer than 6 to 12 hours from the onset of symptoms is more consistent with a partial obstruction. Early in the course, an acute complete obstruction can present with loose stools. Nevertheless,

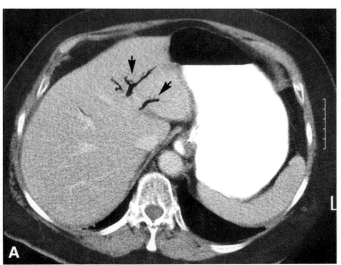

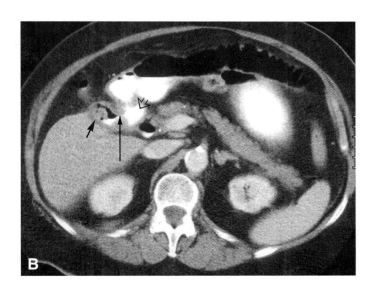

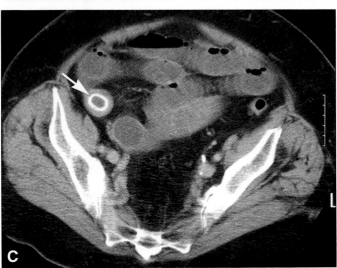

Fig. 11. Gallstone ileus. An 82-year-old woman with abdominal pain. (A), *Computed tomogram with oral and intravenous contrast shows pneumobilia* (arrows). (B), *A more inferior scan shows a contracted gallbladder with air* (short solid arrow) *and a communication* (long arrow) *with the duodenum* (open arrow). (C), *Dilated loops of distal small bowel lead to the level of the terminal ileum, where an obstructing, calcified ectopic gallstone is seen* (arrow).

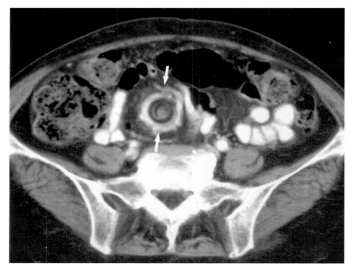

Fig. 12. Small bowel volvulus. A 74-year-old woman with intermittent abdominal pain. Contrast-enhanced computed tomogram shows swirling of the mesenteric structures, consistent with a volvulus (arrows).

it can be very difficult to differentiate between an early complete obstruction and a high-grade partial obstruction. Although in many patients it is safer to proceed with urgent operative intervention, in some patients the risk of an abdominal exploration is greater than the risk of watchful waiting.

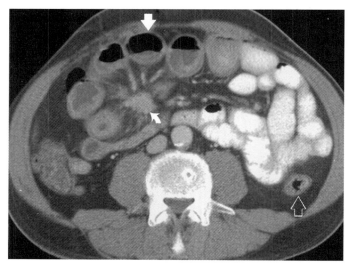

Fig. 13. Obstructing carcinoid tumor. A 54-year-old man with abdominal pain and cramping. Abdominal computed tomogram with oral and intravenous contrast demonstrates dilated loops of proximal small bowel (white arrow), normal-caliber distal small bowel and air in the colon (open arrow), consistent with partial small bowel obstruction. Spiculated mass in small bowel mesentery (curved white arrow) with thickened linear stranding of mesenteric tissues and tethering of small bowel. This appearance is typical of carcinoid metastasis to mesentery with a strong desmoplastic reaction.

The surgeon is forced to go the extra step to differentiate between a complete and a high-grade partial obstruction to determine whether conservative management is possible. Contrast studies can be very helpful in these situations. Our first option is abdominal computed tomography with oral and intravenous contrast. This allows visualization of the passage of contrast, or lack of passage, through the small bowel and into the cecum. Delayed films are obtained if necessary. Another alternative is the use of water-soluble contrast media—nonionic, low osmolar, or hyperosmolar. Disadvantages of water-soluble contrast include poor visualization of mucosal detail as it travels distally and is diluted with the intraluminal fluid and the risk of pulmonary injury if aspirated. Other investigators have suggested instillation of 50 mL of undiluted barium sulfate by nasogastric tube, clamping the nasogastric tube for 1 hour, and following the patient with serial abdominal plain radiography during the next 12 to 24 hours to determine whether the barium passes into the colon. The main question is how long to wait for the contrast to reach the colon. In an attempt to answer this question, Chen et al.[20] evaluated the use of a water-soluble contrast medium (Urografin) to differentiate partial and complete SBO. The presence of the contrast in the colon within 8 hours of ingestion as an indicator for nonoperative treatment had a sensitivity of 90%, a specificity of 100%, and an accuracy of 93%.

Although intestinal strangulation is a definite indication for immediate operative intervention, the surgeon is sometimes unable to make the diagnosis early and on clinical grounds (Fig. 16). Ideally, we should be able to

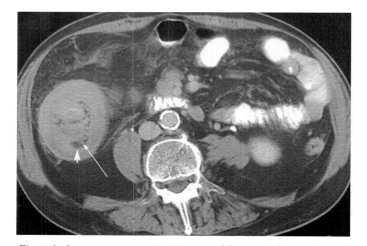

Fig. 14. Intussusception. An 83-year-old man with anemia and colicky abdominal pain from small bowel obstruction. Computed tomogram with oral and intravenous contrast shows dilated distal ileum loops leading to a low-density mass in right lower quadrant. This mass contains low-density fat (short arrow) and tiny vessels (long arrow) typical for an ileocolic intussusception.

Initial presentation

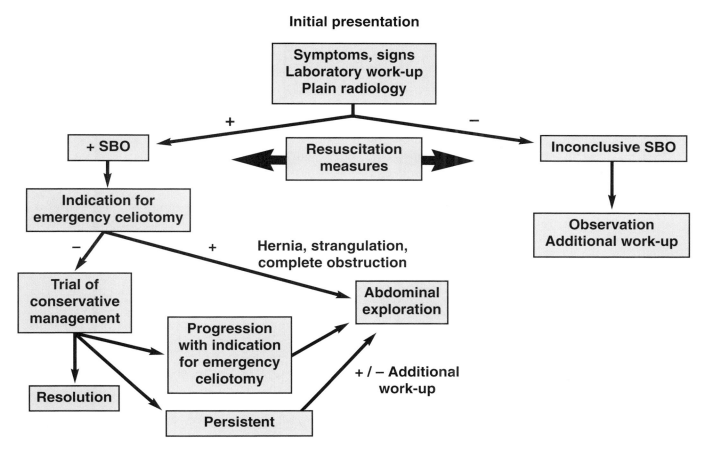

Fig. 15. *Management algorithm for small bowel obstruction (SBO).*

recognize when the obstructed bowel has early reversible ischemia. To date, there is no clinical marker or test that allows a confident diagnosis of the presence or absence of reversible vascular compromise. Continuous abdominal pain, fever, tachycardia, peritoneal signs, and leukocytosis are classic signs of strangulation obstruction. Other potential markers include metabolic acidosis, hyperkalemia, hyperphosphatemia, and increased values for serum amylase, alkaline phosphatase, lactate dehydrogenase, creatinine phosphokinase, D-lactate, intestinal fatty acid-binding protein, and aspartate and alanine aminotransferases. However, no particular marker or combination of these markers *accurately* and reliably predicts the presence of vascular compromise. In addition, multiple studies[6,21,22] have shown that the experienced clinical judgment of the surgeon is no better. Today, we agree with the results of the 1983 study by Sarr et al.,[23] which showed that the preoperative diagnosis of strangulation in patients with complete SBO cannot be made or excluded with any reliability on the basis of any known clinical variable, combination of variables, or the surgeon's clinical judgment.

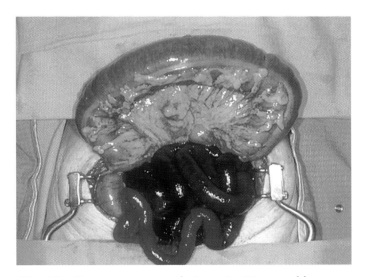

Fig. 16. *Gangrenous strangulation. An 82-year-old woman admitted for hydration who had vague abdominal pain, emesis, and a normal leukocyte count. Surgical consultation was obtained when her clinical condition deteriorated within a few hours of admission. She became hypotensive and evidence of acute lung injury developed. Abdominal exploration revealed necrosis of jejunum and ileum due to an adhesive volvulus.*

Several signs on well-performed, contrast-enhanced computed tomography have been reported to portend strangulation, such as bowel wall thickening, pneumatosis intestinalis, portal venous gas, increased bowel wall density without contrast, generalized ascites, and nonenhancement of bowel wall. The more signs present in a patient, the more likely vascular compromise exists. Despite advances in all the radiologic evaluations described, when encountered, these findings are usually related to late, irreversible intestinal ischemia. Alternatively, computed tomography can be overly sensitive because many of these signs are not specific and can be found in association with other inflammatory processes.[15] On evaluation of a patient, strangulation cannot be excluded. The risk of strangulation is negligible in a partial SBO (excluding a known incarcerated hernia, e.g., Richter type), but it increases to 20% to 40% with complete SBO.[23,24] Therefore, for a complete SBO, operation should be done as a semi-emergency after complete resuscitation with fluids and electrolyte correction. Nonoperative management of a complete SBO is a calculated risk.[23] This approach has led to the often quoted phrase, "The sun should never rise and set on a complete SBO."

The cause of SBO also plays a role in management. Patients with SBO caused by an incarcerated hernia need immediate operative repair. Other examples include obstruction due to tumor mass or an adjacent inflammatory process or abscess, in which the SBO will not resolve until the primary problem is addressed; emergency intervention is less crucial in this situation.

Conservative Therapy
Conservative, nonoperative management can be considered once the patient has been evaluated, resuscitative measures have been established, and indications for immediate operative intervention have been excluded. This is the approach for patients with partial SBO, possibly adhesive, or those in whom the diagnosis is not certain. The patient is committed to a period of observation and is monitored closely for clinical signs of compromised vital signs, breathing, circulation, urine output, abdominal examination, and gastrointestinal function. Most patients are hypovolemic because of decreased oral intake, vomiting, and fluid sequestration in both the bowel lumen and the peritoneal cavity. Aggressive fluid resuscitation must be continued with an isotonic saline solution such as lactated Ringer's solution. The use of central intravenous lines or even pulmonary artery catheters should be considered if indicated by the patient's condition or comorbid conditions. A urinary catheter should almost always be placed to monitor the urine output and the adequacy of rehydration.

Nasogastric suction must be established to provide symptomatic relief of nausea, vomiting, and pain and to facilitate administration of oral contrast if indicated; moreover, it helps prevent aspiration. There has been debate about the benefits of nasogastric versus long nasointestinal tube decompression in the treatment of SBO. Most retrospective and prospective reports have failed to show any differences between their use in regard to the decompression obtained and the success of nonoperative therapy.[24,25] Nasogastric decompression is preferred in our practice, given that the nasogastric tube is easy and quick to insert and does not have the risk of perforation or intussusception of the small bowel, as can occur, albeit rarely, with long intestinal tubes. Bowel rest with no oral intake is instituted. Parenteral nutrition should be considered if fasting is to exceed 7 days. Sixty to 85% of partial SBOs are reported to resolve with conservative management.[6,24] The patient may require abdominal exploration if the obstruction becomes complete, evidence of strangulation develops, or the obstruction fails to resolve after an appropriate interval (2-4 days) of nonoperative management.

The use of a water-soluble contrast agent (such as Gastrografin) has been proposed for the treatment of SBO. Many surgeons have had patients whose obstructive symptoms resolved after a water-soluble oral contrast agent was given. Because of these clinical experiences, Gastrografin has been studied as a therapeutic agent for bowel obstruction. Gastrografin, an ionic, monomeric, hyperosmolar, bitterly flavored mix of sodium diatrizoate, meglumine amidotrizoate, and polysorbate 80, is expected to reach the cecum in 30 to 90 minutes when taken orally by healthy subjects. It is proposed to assist in resolution of obstruction by drawing fluid into the lumen because of its hyperosmolar effects and thus increasing proximal bowel distention and presumably the pressure gradient across the obstruction. Other putative effects of the hyperosmolarity are dilution of the bowel contents and decreased bowel edema. In addition, Gastrografin allegedly increases peristalsis, and it has a "wetting agent" (polysorbate 80) that is considered to aid the slippery passage of bowel contents.

Assalia et al.[26] studied Gastrografin prospectively as a therapeutic agent for adhesive SBO. That study suggested a considerable decrease in time to resolution and mean hospital stay in patients who received the agent. In addition, no complications were associated with its use (e.g., aspiration pneumonia, exacerbation of obstructive symptoms, or fluid and electrolyte imbalances). The investigators concluded that Gastrografin promoted and hastened resolution of partial SBO. However, there was no difference in the need for operative intervention in patients who received Gastrografin. Feigin et al.[27] conducted a similar prospective randomized trial but were unable to prove any therapeutic benefit from the administration of water-soluble contrast for the treatment of postoperative SBO. In summary, although Gastrografin can be used safely in the evaluation of partial SBO, its therapeutic value remains controversial. In our practice, we are unconvinced of its putative therapeutic value, and we largely reserve its use as a diagnostic tool.

Operative Therapy

Operative intervention is always an option for bowel obstruction. It may be used on a relatively emergency basis after the initial work-up reveals the type and cause of the obstruction or after the failure of conservative management. The clinical scenario and surgeon's judgment are key factors in determining the timing of operation. Ideally, operation is performed in patients with impending or reversible strangulation obstruction who still have reversible ischemia, in those with an early complete SBO, and in those who will not respond to conservative therapy. In these patients, operative treatment decreases the overall length of hospital stay and the morbidity and mortality related to unsuccessful nonoperative treatment. The difficulty is the inability to make these determinations accurately and reliably on a patient's presentation.

Most commonly, operative intervention consists of an open abdominal exploration through a midline abdominal incision. The first step is identification of the obstructive cause. Multiple possible causes of obstruction exist, and a combination of these causes may coexist in the same patient. There are two points of caution in this step. The first is to use extreme care in handling the dilated, often very thin-walled, small bowel to prevent unnecessary bowel injury (especially at the site of obstruction) and abdominal contamination. The second caution is to perform a complete abdominal exploration to ensure that no incidental abnormality is missed. This can be done at the beginning of the procedure, or if the small bowel is massively distended it can be completed at the end of the procedure.

Once the cause of obstruction is identified, the second step of operation is to release it or repair it as indicated by the findings. The third step of operative therapy is to assess bowel viability. In many circumstances this determination is simple, and it is obvious to the surgeon that the loops of small bowel are either viable or not. Clinical criteria of bowel viability are the return of normal color, evidence of peristalsis, and the presence of arterial pulsations near or on the bowel wall. In some cases, the viability of the small bowel is questionable. The challenge in management then stems from the difficulty of accurately predicting intestinal recovery after an ischemic insult. Two adjuncts used in the intraoperative determination of small

bowel viability include intravenous fluorescein and Doppler evaluation of arterial signals in the antimesenteric surface of the bowel wall.

In 1942, Lange and Boyd[28] proposed intravenous sodium fluorescein as an accurate predictor of intestinal viability, given the assessment of tissue perfusion as indicated by the fluorescent pattern seen under an ultraviolet Wood light. Since then, this approach has been validated with definite viability end points.[29-32] The use of the Doppler ultrasonic flow probe to detect the presence of pulsatile blood flow within the wall of the bowel has been accurate in both experimental animals and humans.[33-35] However, most of the studies were not controlled and had equivocal viable and nonviable end points.

Bulkley et al.,[36] in a prospective controlled trial, compared the use of Doppler and fluorescein evaluations with standard clinical judgment for assessment of small intestinal viability intraoperatively. They established viability end points for patient follow-up according to definite histologic criteria. Overall clinical judgment was accurate (89%) but would have led to a relatively high rate of unnecessary bowel resections (i.e., false-positive rate of 46%). The Doppler method did not seem to improve the accuracy of any evaluation. The fluorescent pattern after intravenous administration of fluorescein was more sensitive, specific, and accurate than either clinical judgment or the Doppler method. A Mayo Clinic study[37] corroborated these findings in a small group of patients who underwent second-look abdominal explorations after revascularization for acute mesenteric ischemia. In 16 patients the overall accuracy of clinical judgment was 50%, fluorescein study 56%, and Doppler method 0%.

In our practice, clinical criteria are taken into consideration first. If these are not conclusive and intestinal viability is questionable, two ampules of sodium fluorescein (1,000 mg) are administered intravenously over 30 to 60 seconds. The room is darkened, and the operative field is illuminated with a handheld long-wave ultraviolet light. The bowel is deemed viable or not viable based on established criteria described by Bulkley et al.[32] for the fluorescent pattern observed. Bowel loops with normal, hyperemic, or fine granular patterns are considered viable, and those with patchy, perivascular, or nonfluorescent patterns are considered nonviable. Doppler is seldom used, but when it is used, it is mainly as a confirmatory adjunct. If these measures fail to ensure the surgeon of appropriate future intestinal viability, a second-look abdominal exploration is scheduled to occur in the next 12 to 24 hours regardless of a patient's improving clinical condition.

The fourth step of operative management is the definitive procedure. This depends on the cause, intestinal viability, local conditions of the tissue, the patient's clinical condition, and the surgeon's judgment. It can be as simple as release of an adhesive band with observation of the small bowel, a simple strictureplasty, or repair of abdominal wall or internal hernia, or it may require bypass of the obstructed segment. In more complex cases, it can involve segmental bowel resection due to tumor involvement, compromised viability, or injury to the bowel during adhesiolysis. The surgeon must decide whether to perform a primary anastomosis or to divert the enteral stream.

The last step of operation is abdominal wall closure. In most patients a primary closure is possible without difficulty. If intraoperative decompression of dilated small bowel is necessary to facilitate the abdominal wall closure, the retrograde manual decompression technique is preferred by our surgeons. In this technique, the intestinal contents are carefully milked retrograde (proximally) with compression by the index and middle fingers and concomitant gentle bowel traction. Noncrushing bowel clamps are positioned to hold back the intestinal contents, with care being taken to occlude only the lumen and not crush the bowel wall (a single click of the ratchets). It is important to palpate the duodenum intermittently to ensure proper drainage into the stomach and decompression by the nasogastric tube.[10] Temporary abdominal wall closure is seldom necessary.

Early Postoperative Small Bowel Obstruction
SBO occurs in the early postoperative period in 0.7% to 2% of all patients undergoing intraperitoneal operations.[38,39] Although encountered rarely, it is a diagnostic and therapeutic dilemma for the surgeon and has a definite mortality risk of 2% to 18%.[38,40-43]

The usual clinical features of SBO are clouded postoperatively by incisional pain, analgesics, abdominal distention, and the typical expectations of postoperative adynamic ileus. Abdominal radiography can be helpful but is not diagnostic. Computed tomography can assist in determination of complete versus partial obstruction and as an aid in recognition of the causes, such as abdominal sepsis or abscess. Contrast studies can be of great assistance for diagnosis. The same guidelines described for evaluation and management of an acute obstruction apply to postoperative SBO. Affected patients are unique given the increased difficulty of and morbidity associated with exploring the abdominal cavity 1 to 6 weeks after the initial operation.

A wide range of therapeutic options has been described, from early aggressive surgical intervention to compulsory conservative management. These confusing recommendations are due to the difficulty in diagnosis, the varying definitions of early SBO, and the weakness of retrospective reviews. Early SBO has been defined as obstruction occurring within 2 weeks, 30 days, 6 weeks, or the same hospitalization postoperatively. This entity occurs most often in patients with operations involving the abdominal cavity below the transverse mesocolon,[38] especially those relating to the left colon and rectum, pelvic procedures, and the appendix.[43] Studies have not found any clinical predictors of the need for operative intervention. In 20% to 60% of patients, the need for operative intervention is due to lack of symptom resolution.[40-42] The most common causes of early postoperative SBO found at reoperation are intra-abdominal adhesions, intra-abdominal sepsis or inflammatory processes, and preexisting abnormalities (intussusception, tumor, inflammatory bowel disease).[38,42,43]

Once early postoperative SBO is diagnosed, the need for and timing of operation necessitate evaluation of several criteria. First, the surgeon must determine whether emergency operative intervention is needed. The presence of an incarcerated hernia or signs or risk of intestinal strangulation necessitates emergency surgical intervention. In addition, the type of initial procedure, the status of the abdominal cavity at the time of the initial procedure, the patient's clinical condition, and the duration after the initial operation are key factors to be considered. The presence of an initial "unfriendly" abdomen (diffuse peritonitis, dense inflammatory adhesions, frozen abdomen with agglutinated bowel) should deter the wary surgeon from further exploration for fear of creating multiple enterotomies, which may mandate bowel resection or cause enterocutaneous fistulas. The clinical condition of the patient may be a contraindication for further surgical intervention, for example, after a definite postoperative myocardial infarction.

Patients can be divided into three groups based on the timing of presentation from the last abdominal procedure. Some patients present with definite obstruction early postoperatively, within 3 to 10 days from the last procedure. Conservative management can be considered as long as definite indications for emergency operative intervention are excluded and with the caution of not waiting so long that reoperation would be too risky given formation of dense adhesions. Other patients present late, more than 6 weeks from the last abdominal procedure. Surgical intervention in these patients can be considered without concern, unless the last operation on the abdominal cavity portends a high risk of dense adhesive reaction, for example, extensive adhesiolysis, multiple debridements for necrotizing pancreatitis, or prior closure of an open abdomen with a skin graft directly on the bowel. The most difficult group are patients who present between 10 days and 6 weeks postoperatively.

They present a technical challenge given the possibility of being unable to dissect the intestines safely. The risk of iatrogenic bowel injury with subsequent enterocutaneous fistulization is high. Charles H. Mayo recognized these risks as early as 1922 and published his concerns about reexploration.[14] Conservative management is the best choice for these patients. This approach may obligate a period of home total parenteral nutrition and bowel rest until the abdominal cavity is deemed operable again (3-12 months later). Patients who present with strangulated obstruction are the exception to this guideline. In these patients, even if there is a high risk of morbidity due to a poor clinical condition, a 10-day to 6-week interval since the initial operation, or even the presence of a previously unfriendly abdomen, surgical intervention may be required given the higher risk of progressive organ failure and death with attempted conservative management.

Prevention

The majority of SBOs in the Western Hemisphere are due to postoperative adhesions. An adhesion-related SBO is expected to develop in 4% to 15% of patients who undergo a celiotomy.[44] The highest general risk involves previous total colectomy. Although the cause of adhesions is not well understood, surgeons have striven to decrease the formation and morbidity of adhesions. Postoperative adhesions are a double-edged sword. Adhesions can form into dense permanent adhesions with the potential for SBO, but they also can protect by aiding in the healing of intra-abdominal injuries and sequestering sources of sepsis from the rest of the abdominal cavity.

The first step in prevention is to handle the tissues delicately, avoid tissue trauma and ischemia, and decrease the presence of intraperitoneal foreign material. In addition to these technical aids, multiple mechanical and chemical methods have been used for adhesion prevention throughout the past few decades. Chemical methods studied in the past have included the use of intraperitoneal heparin, streptokinase, dextran, prostaglandins, silicone, and corticosteroids. All have conflicting results of effectiveness and ineffectiveness.[45] Even in 1911, Charles H. Mayo presented a vision for prevention of postoperative adhesions. He wrote: "In some cases the application of sterile vaselin over the traumaticized peritoneal area seems to prevent the development of deleterious adhesions following the operation."[9] Several mechanical methods of orderly arrangement of loops of bowel have been reported and have had varying degrees of success. These methods include plication and internal stenting. Noble[46] introduced intestinal plication in 1937 with the idea of forming controlled adhesions. This concept was flawed because the placement of serosal sutures approximating adjacent loops of bowel was associated with an unacceptable rate of intestinal fistula formation. Childs and Phillips[47] proposed mesenteric plication, rather than plicating the bowel wall, to ensure a controlled gentle looping of the small bowel at risk for SBO. Although not complicated by fistulization, this technique was on occasion complicated by mesenteric hemorrhage and was contraindicated in patients with abdominal cavity contamination. In 1956, White[48] proposed internal splinting of the bowel with a long tube passed the whole length of the small bowel. Jones and Munro[44] reported the use of intraluminal small bowel splinting after extensive adhesiolysis in 140 patients without associated complications.

Recent techniques designed to separate tissue physically hold the greatest promise. Sheets of absorbable material used as separating "barriers" have been successful for decreasing adhesions between parietal and visceral peritoneum in the location where they have been placed.[49] Mayo Clinic participated in a prospective, randomized, double-blind multicenter study[50] of a bioabsorbable membrane composed of sodium hyaluronate and carboxymethylcellulose in patients undergoing colectomy with ileal pouch-anal anastomosis and diverting loop ileostomy. Adhesion formation was evaluated 8 to 12 weeks later with laparoscopy at the time of ileostomy closure. The study showed a statistically significant decrease of adhesion formation, without an increase in complications, in patients who received the membrane barrier compared with those who did not (15%-58% adhesion formation, respectively, $P < 0.0001$). Although promising, this substance would need to be applied throughout the abdominal cavity if adhesion formation were to be reduced overall. In addition, it is not yet clear whether these products will reduce the number of symptomatic adhesions or episodes of SBO. In our practice, few surgeons use these separating barriers routinely; rather, they use them on a selected basis.

Role of Laparoscopy

Until recently, acute SBO was a relative contraindication for laparoscopy not only because adhesions make visualization and dissection more difficult and risky but also because bowel distention decreases the visual field and increases the risk of iatrogenic bowel perforation. However, as our experience has increased, a laparoscopic operative approach has been applied to the management of acute SBO.

A minimally invasive approach has several potential benefits for the management of SBO. It decreases the duration of hospital stay and leads to a faster return of bowel function compared with conventional open abdominal exploration. It also lowers the risk of wound complications and incisional hernias and decreases the potential for postoperative adhesions and the risk of recurrent adhesive SBO. Disadvantages of a laparoscopic approach are the increased difficulty of the procedure in this setting, which may increase operative time. In addition, the dilated and fragile small bowel decreases the visual field and increases the risk of bowel injury.

Obviously, the benefits of laparoscopy become evident immediately when the cause of the obstruction is a single adhesive band that can be easily lysed. In 1991, Bastug et al.[51] published the first report of such a patient. Multiple reports have followed since, but all have a small number of patients. Laparoscopy is successful in evaluation and treatment of acute SBO in 50% to 70% of selected patients in several series.[52-56] Iatrogenic enterotomies have been reported in 6% to 10% of attempted laparoscopic operations for acute SBO (Table 3).

The role of laparoscopy in the treatment of acute SBO is yet to be defined. In a selected group of Mayo Clinic patients, the procedure was successful and had great benefit, but identifying these patients is difficult.[56] The incidence of unrecognized enterotomy leading to postoperative sepsis needs to be reduced. In addition, missed conditions requiring delayed reexploration need to be evaluated. In our practice, the standard remains open abdominal exploration; however, we have increased our use of laparoscopy as an initial approach in the treatment of presumed adhesive SBO in selected patients. This approach depends on the laparoscopic experience of the surgeon and on the exclusion of certain criteria in the patient's clinical condition. A laparoscopic approach is considered in the absence of the following criteria: peritoneal irritation, strong concerns of perforation or bowel necrosis, concern of dense and multiple adhesions due to multiple previous or recent major abdominal operations, and the presence of massively dilated bowel on preoperative imaging (small bowel more than 4 cm in diameter).

Certain technical aspects are key in performing laparoscopy for the management of SBO. The patient should be placed supine with the arms tucked on each side to allow for all extremes of positions that might be needed to aid exposure. The pneumoperitoneum is established with a Hasson catheter with a fully open technique rather than the Veress needle; all catheters are also placed under direct visualization to prevent inadvertent blind bowel injury of distended bowel. The trocars should be placed away from prior incisions and according to the position of the adhesions to be divided, but, in general, right upper quadrant and left lower quadrant cannulas allow maximal exposure for examining the entire jejunoileum. Distended fragile small intestine should be manipulated carefully and always completely under vision with large atraumatic forceps. At Mayo Clinic, we start at the ileocecal valve, grasping the distal nondilated small bowel until the area of obstruction is identified. When the bowel is very dilated, it is better to grasp its mesentery rather than the fragile bowel wall. Overall, it is important to have a liberal policy for conversion to open exploration.

OUTCOMES

An adhesion-related SBO will develop in 4% to 15% of all patients who undergo celiotomy.[44] The mortality rate associated with SBO has decreased dramatically during the past 100 years, from 60% in 1908[12] to 5% to 15% during the past 2 decades. Operative intervention is required in 40% to 70% of all hospitalized patients with SBO. In the series by Landercasper et al.[11] of 309 patients admitted for SBO, 150 (49%) required celiotomy.

Table 3.—Results of Laparoscopic Therapy for Small Bowel Obstruction

	Mayo Clinic series, 1998[56]		Strickland et al., 1999[53]		Agresta et al., 2000[55]		Suter et al., 2000[54]	
	No.	%	No.	%	No.	%	No.	%
No. of patients	40		40		63		83	
Successful laparoscopies*	26	65	24	60	52	83	47	57
Conversions to open exploration	14	35	16	40	11	18	36	43
Iatrogenic bowel injury during laparoscopy	3	8	4	10	1	2	13	16
Conversion for inadequate visualization	7	18	2	5	5	8	8	10

*Evaluation and therapy.

Once a patient has had SBO, the long-term risk of recurrence is high. As early as 1947, Krook[57] reported "every fresh intervention gives a result inferior to the preceding one." There is a paucity of studies evaluating outcome after hospital dismissal. In the retrospective review by Landercasper et al.,[11] the overall recurrence rate of SBO that necessitated hospitalization was 30% at 4 years and 42% at 10 years. The recurrence rates and need for celiotomy varied if the patients were stratified by conservative or operative therapy of the initial episode of SBO. According to this report, patients who require operation for SBO have an approximate 30% chance for development of recurrent SBO necessitating hospitalization and a 10% risk of needing a second celiotomy during the next 10 years. In contrast, patients initially treated conservatively have a 53% risk of recurrence and a 17% risk of requiring operative therapy during the following 10 years.

The mortality rate associated with the surgical therapy of SBO is reported to be between 5% and 10%.[10-12] In the Mayo Clinic series, Mucha[10] found a hospital mortality rate of 10% in patients requiring operation for SBO. He noted, similar to other investigators,[12] that the mortality increased with a patient's age. In addition, the variation in mortality depended on the cause of obstruction: 5% for adhesive obstruction, 4% for obstructions caused by hernia, and 21% for those caused by neoplasm. The prognosis was dismal for patients with obstruction caused by neoplastic disease, with a mortality rate of 50% at 6 months, 71% at 1 year, and 95% at 4 years. Similar findings were reported by Landercasper et al.[11]; no patient was alive 5 years after operation for malignant SBO. In contrast, 21% of the adhesive SBOs in the Mayo Clinic series occurred in patients with prior malignancy. Accordingly, patients should not be denied operative intervention because of a prior history of malignancy.

The postoperative complication rate for patients treated surgically for SBO has varied between 20% and 50%.[10-12,58] These complications can involve all organ systems and include gastrointestinal, respiratory, renal, cardiac, neurologic, hematologic bleeding or thrombosis, abdominal sepsis, or wound problems. The Mayo Clinic series[10] found an overall morbidity rate of 30%; the wound infection rate was 4% and the wound dehiscence rate was 1%. The presence of strangulated bowel at abdominal exploration increases the complication and mortality rates.[12,59] Strangulated bowel was found in a greater proportion (28%) of patients in whom hernia was the cause of obstruction.

CONCLUSION

SBO remains a common problem faced by the abdominal surgeon. The key to management of this condition is appropriate diagnosis and timely surgical intervention. Causes are varied despite similar local physiologic conditions and clinical presentation. Postoperative adhesions, neoplasm, and hernias remain the most common causes of SBO through the past several decades. The diagnosis is established on the basis of clinical presentation with the aid of radiologic studies. Abdominal computed tomography has become the study of choice for patients with acute presentation and an uncertain diagnosis of SBO. Abdominal computed tomography documents the anatomical presence of obstruction, defines whether it is partial or complete, may aid in determination of the cause, and can suggest strangulation. Initial conservative therapy is appropriate in patients with early postoperative obstruction, presumed malignant neoplasm, comorbidities, and evidence of partial or incomplete obstruction, provided the patient has no signs of strangulation. Immediate surgical intervention is indicated in all patients with a high risk of bowel necrosis, including those with incarcerated hernias, complete SBO, and concern for intestinal strangulation. Early postoperative SBO still poses a challenge for management. A laparoscopic approach has been increasingly used in the surgical management of SBO. Careful technique has made it possible in selected patients, but its role has yet to be defined. Intraoperative prevention of adhesion formation has been the focus of many years of research. The newer barrier membranes show some promise for decreasing adhesion formation between the parietal peritoneum and the visceral peritoneal surfaces, but prevention of adhesions between visceral peritoneal surfaces (e.g., loops of bowel) remains unsolved. Although the overall mortality rate associated with SBO has decreased dramatically throughout the past century, the risk of recurrence remains high. Several challenges in the diagnosis and management of SBO persist, including reliable preoperative recognition of reversible bowel ischemia, preoperative identification of the cause of obstruction, intraoperative determination of intestinal viability after ischemic insult, prevention of adhesion formation, and determination of the role for a minimally invasive approach to therapy. Solving these challenges could have a great impact on the care and outcome of patients.

REFERENCES

1. Wangensteen OH: Understanding the bowel obstruction problem. Am J Surg 135:131-149, 1978
2. Annandale T: Case in Which an Internal Intestinal Obstruction was Removed by the Operation of Gastrotomy. Edinburgh, Oliver and Boyd, 1871
3. Greves EH: On a case of acute intestinal obstruction in a boy, with remarks upon the treatment of acute obstruction. Liverpool M Chir J 5:118-153, 1885
4. Brinton W: Intestinal Obstruction. Edited by T Buzzard. London, John Churchill and Sons, 1867
5. Treves F: Intestinal Obstruction: Its Varieties with their Pathology, Diagnosis, and Treatment. Second edition, revised. New York, William Wood and Company, 1899
6. Soybel DI: Ileus and bowel obstruction. In Surgery: Scientific Principles and Practice. Second edition. Edited by LJ Greenfield. Philadelphia, Lippincott-Raven Publishers, 1997, pp 817-831
7. Mayo WJ: Cicatricial stenosis and valve formation as a cause of pyloric obstruction: a report of five cases relieved by operation. JAMA 29:778-782, 1897
8. Mayo WJ: Resection for the relief of intestinal obstruction. JAMA 49:903-905, 1907
9. Mayo CH: Intestinal obstruction due to kinks and adhesions of the terminal ileum. Surg Gynecol Obstet 12:227-230, 1911
10. Mucha P Jr: Small intestinal obstruction. Surg Clin North Am 67:597-620, 1987
11. Landercasper J, Cogbill TH, Merry WH, Stolee RT, Strutt PJ: Long-term outcome after hospitalization for small-bowel obstruction. Arch Surg 128:765-770, 1993
12. Fevang BT, Fevang J, Stangeland L, Soreide O, Svanes K, Viste A: Complications and death after surgical treatment of small bowel obstruction: a 35-year institutional experience. Ann Surg 231:529-537, 2000
13. Nadrowski LF: Pathophysiology and current treatment of intestinal obstruction. Rev Surg 31:381-407, 1974
14. Mayo CH: The cause and relief of acute intestinal obstruction. JAMA 79:194-197, 1922
15. Frager DH, Baer JW: Role of CT in evaluating patients with small-bowel obstruction. Semin Ultrasound CT MR 16:127-140, 1995
16. Baker S: The Abdominal Plain Film. Norwalk, Connecticut, Appleton & Lange, 1990, pp 155-242
17. Markus JB, Somers S, Franic SE, Moola C, Stevenson GW: Interobserver variation in the interpretation of abdominal radiographs. Radiology 171:69-71, 1989
18. Suri S, Gupta S, Sudhakar PJ, Venkataramu NK, Sood B, Wig JD: Comparative evaluation of plain films, ultrasound and CT in the diagnosis of intestinal obstruction. Acta Radiol 40:422-428, 1999
19. Regan F, Beall DP, Bohlman ME, Khazan R, Sufi A, Schaefer DC: Fast MR imaging and the detection of small-bowel obstruction. AJR Am J Roentgenol 170:1465-1469, 1998
20. Chen SC, Chang KJ, Lee PH, Wang SM, Chen KM, Lin FY: Oral urografin in postoperative small bowel obstruction. World J Surg 23:1051-1054, 1999
21. Stewardson RH, Bombeck CT, Nyhus LM: Critical operative management of small bowel obstruction. Ann Surg 187:189-193, 1978
22. Pain JA, Collier DS, Hanka R: Small bowel obstruction: computer-assisted prediction of strangulation at presentation. Br J Surg 74:981-983, 1987
23. Sarr MG, Bulkley GB, Zuidema GD: Preoperative recognition of intestinal strangulation obstruction: prospective evaluation of diagnostic capability. Am J Surg 145:176-182, 1983
24. Bass KN, Bulkley GB: Small bowel obstruction. In Current Surgical Therapy. Sixth edition. Edited by JL Cameron. St Louis, Mosby, 1998, pp 122-131
25. Meissner K: Intestinal splinting for uncomplicated early postoperative small bowel obstruction: Is it worthwhile? Hepatogastroenterology 43:813-818, 1996
26. Assalia A, Schein M, Kopelman D, Hirshberg A, Hashmonai M: Therapeutic effect of oral Gastrografin in adhesive, partial small-bowel obstruction: a prospective randomized trial. Surgery 115:433-437, 1994
27. Feigin E, Seror D, Szold A, Carmon M, Allweis TM, Nissan A, Gross E, Vromen A, Freund HR: Water-soluble contrast material has no therapeutic effect on postoperative small-bowel obstruction: results of a prospective, randomized clinical trial. Am J Surg 171:227-229, 1996
28. Lange K, Boyd LJ: The use of fluorescein to determine the adequacy of the circulation. Med Clin North Am 26:943-952, 1942
29. Papachristou D, Fortner JG: Prediction of intestinal viability by intra-arterial dye injection: a simple test. Am J Surg 132:572-574, 1976
30. Marfuggi RA, Greenspan M: Reliable intraoperative prediction of intestinal viability using a fluorescent indicator. Surg Gynecol Obstet 152:33-35, 1981
31. Stolar CJ, Randolph JG: Evaluation of ischemic bowel viability with a fluorescent technique. J Pediatr Surg 13:221-225, 1978
32. Bulkley GB, Wheaton LG, Strandberg JD, Zuidema GD: Assessment of small intestinal recovery from ischemic injury after segmental, arterial, venous, and arteriovenous occlusion. Surg Forum 30:210-213, 1979
33. Cooperman M, Pace WG, Martin EW Jr, Pflug B, Keith LM Jr, Evans WE, Carey LC: Determination of viability of ischemic intestine by Doppler ultrasound. Surgery 83:705-710, 1978
34. O'Donnell JA, Hobson RW II: Operative confirmation of Doppler ultrasound in evaluation of intestinal ischemia. Surgery 87:109-112, 1980
35. Cooperman M, Martin EW Jr, Carey LC: Evaluation of ischemic intestine by Doppler ultrasound. Am J Surg 139:73-77, 1980
36. Bulkley GB, Zuidema GD, Hamilton SR, O'Mara CS, Klacsmann PG, Horn SD: Intraoperative determination of small intestinal viability following ischemic injury: a prospective, controlled trial of two adjuvant methods (Doppler and fluorescein) compared with standard clinical judgment. Ann Surg 193:628-637, 1981
37. Ballard JL, Stone WM, Hallett JW, Pairolero PC, Cherry KJ: A critical analysis of adjuvant techniques used to assess bowel viability in acute mesenteric ischemia. Am Surg 59:309-311, 1993
38. Stewart RM, Page CP, Brender J, Schwesinger W, Eisenhut D: The incidence and risk of early postoperative small bowel obstruction: a cohort study. Am J Surg 154:643-647, 1987
39. Sarr MG, Nagorney DM, McIlrath DC: Postoperative intussusception in the adult: A previously unrecognized entity? Arch Surg 116:144-148, 1981
40. Quatromoni JC, Rosoff L Sr, Halls JM, Yellin AE: Early postoperative small bowel obstruction. Ann Surg 191:72-74, 1980
41. Frykberg ER, Phillips JW: Obstruction of the small bowel in the early postoperative period. South Med J 82:169-173, 1989
42. Pickleman J, Lee RM: The management of patients with suspected early postoperative small bowel obstruction. Ann Surg 210:216-219, 1989

43. Sykes PA, Schofield PF: Early postoperative small bowel obstruction. Br J Surg 61:594-600, 1974

44. Jones PF, Munro A: Recurrent adhesive small bowel obstruction. World J Surg 9:868-875, 1985

45. Fabri PJ, Rosemurgy A: Reoperation for small intestinal obstruction. Surg Clin North Am 71:131-146, 1991

46. Noble TB Jr: Plication of the small intestine as prophylaxis against adhesions. Am J Surg 35:41-44, 1937

47. Childs WA, Phillips RB: Experience with intestinal plication and a proposed modification. Ann Surg 152:258-265, 1960

48. White RR: Prevention of recurrent small bowel obstruction due to adhesions. Ann Surg 143:714, 1956

49. Wilson MS, Ellis H, Menzies D, Moran BJ, Parker MC, Thompson JN: A review of the management of small bowel obstruction. Ann R Coll Surg Engl 81:320-328, 1999

50. Becker JM, Dayton MT, Fazio VW, Beck DE, Stryker SJ, Wexner SD, Wolff BG, Roberts PL, Smith LE, Sweeney SA, Moore M: Prevention of postoperative abdominal adhesions by a sodium hyaluronate-based bioresorbable membrane: a prospective, randomized, double-blind multicenter study. J Am Coll Surg 183:297-306, 1996

51. Bastug DF, Trammell SW, Boland JP, Mantz EP, Tiley EH III: Laparoscopic adhesiolysis for small bowel obstruction. Surg Laparosc Endosc 1:259-262, 1991

52. Chevre F, Renggli JC, Groebli Y, Tschantz P: Laparoscopic treatment of small bowel obstruction arising on adhesions [French]. Ann Chir 51:1092-1098, 1997

53. Strickland P, Lourie DJ, Suddleson EA, Blitz JB, Stain SC: Is laparoscopy safe and effective for treatment of acute small-bowel obstruction? Surg Endosc 13:695-698, 1999

54. Suter M, Zermatten P, Halkic N, Martinet O, Bettschart V: Laparoscopic management of mechanical small bowel obstruction: Are there predictors of success or failure? Surg Endosc 14:478-483, 2000

55. Agresta F, Piazza A, Michelet I, Bedin N, Sartori CA: Small bowel obstruction: laparoscopic approach. Surg Endosc 14:154-156, 2000

56. Leon EL, Metzger A, Tsiotos GG, Schlinkert RT, Sarr MG: Laparoscopic management of small bowel obstruction: indications and outcome. J Gastrointest Surg 2:132-140, 1998

57. Krook S: Obstruction of the small intestine due to adhesions and bands: an investigation of the early and late results after operative treatment and an aetiological study of recurrences. Acta Chir Scand 95 Suppl 125:1-200, 1947

58. Larsen E, Pories WJ: Frequency of wound complications after surgery for small bowel obstruction. Am J Surg 122:384-386, 1971

59. Deutsch AA, Eviatar E, Gutman H, Reiss R: Small bowel obstruction: a review of 264 cases and suggestions for management. Postgrad Med J 65:463-467, 1989

Chapter 29

ACUTE MESENTERIC ISCHEMIA

Richard J. Fowl, M.D.

Acute mesenteric ischemia (AMI) is a formidable clinical problem. Despite considerable advances in the care of patients with vascular disease, the mortality rate from AMI has not improved much during the past 30 years. Most studies report a mortality rate of 70% to 90% (Table 1).[1-12] The main reason for the high mortality rate is delay in diagnosis.

PATHOPHYSIOLOGY AND ETIOLOGY

Three main arteries supply blood to the intestine: 1) the celiac artery, which is the origin of the hepatic, splenic, and left gastric arteries, 2) the superior mesenteric artery (SMA), and 3) the inferior mesenteric artery. These arteries have abundant interconnecting collaterals, and if one becomes occluded, the collaterals from the other arteries usually can compensate. However, acute occlusion, especially of the SMA, may result in ischemic bowel injury if collateral pathways are inadequate to compensate for the sudden change in hemodynamics.

Three mechanisms cause AMI: 1) emboli that originate from another site, most commonly the heart, 2) thrombosis of an artery with preexisting atherosclerotic stenosis, or 3) nonocclusive mesenteric ischemia caused by severe visceral vasoconstriction in the peripheral arteries of the intestine without occlusion of the proximal arteries. Acute occlusive intestinal ischemia is usually caused by an arterial embolus. The SMA is the most common site, but emboli to the celiac artery have been reported.[13] In addition to the heart, the thoracic aorta also may be a source of emboli.[14] Cholesterol emboli lodging in the distal mesenteric arterial tree may be produced after the thoracic aorta is clamped during a cardiac or thoracic aortic

operation or after a diagnostic or therapeutic cardiac catheterization. An embolus in the SMA usually lodges distal to the origin of the middle colic artery (Fig. 1). This blockage permits some limited perfusion of the proximal small intestine through the middle colic arterial collaterals that often can maintain some bowel viability and reduce the extent of infarction. Therefore, the prognosis for embolic occlusion is better than that for ischemia due to acute thrombosis or nonocclusive ischemia. Acute thrombosis of the SMA occurs with sudden occlusion of a severely stenotic atherosclerotic lesion. In contrast to an embolism, thrombosis typically occurs at the origin of the artery,

Table 1.—Mortality Rates From Acute Mesenteric Ischemia in Published Reports

Reference	Year	Patients, no.	Mortality rate, %
Ottinger and Austen[1]	1967	51	84
Singh et al.[2]	1975	30	81
Smith and Patterson[3]	1976	23	91
Kairaluoma et al.[4]	1977	44	70
Ottinger[5]	1978	136	85
Boley et al.[6]	1977	35	45
Krausz and Manny[7]	1978	40	78
Sachs et al.[8]	1982	37	76
Finucane et al.[9]	1989	32	78
Levy et al.[10]	1990	62	40
Batellier and Kieny[11]	1990	65	52
Klempnauer et al.[12]	1997	60	80

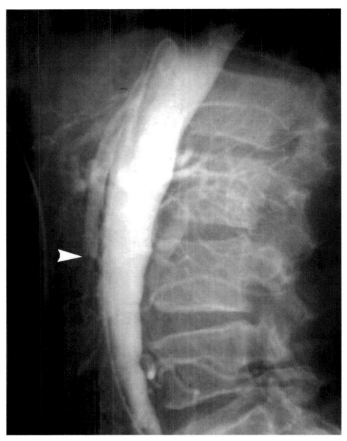

Fig. 1. Mesenteric angiogram shows a normal proximal superior mesenteric artery with a meniscus sign (arrowhead), a sharp cutoff that is diagnostic of an embolism.

patients with AMI are women. Risk factors include known cardiac disorders that cause thrombus formation in a heart chamber (e.g., atrial fibrillation, valvular disease, ventricular aneurysm, prosthetic heart valves with subtherapeutic anticoagulation, dilated cardiomyopathy). The presence of a supraceliac thoracic aortic aneurysm could be a rare source of emboli. Patients with a chronic history of weight loss and postprandial abdominal pain, which are symptoms of intestinal angina, may have atherosclerotic mesenteric occlusive disease.

These patients typically present with acute onset of severe abdominal pain often not localized to one area. The duration of pain may be a few hours to 14 days.[5] Other symptoms include nausea, vomiting, and diarrhea. The absence of abdominal pain in patients who are mentally intact usually excludes a diagnosis of AMI. However, we have seen one coherent elderly patient who denied any abdominal pain. His clinical deterioration led to an abdominal exploration that showed diffuse intestinal gangrene. He eventually died.

The hallmark early physical finding is minimal abdominal tenderness despite complaints of severe abdominal pain. This feature is well known as "pain out of proportion to the physical findings." Abdominal distention may be absent, and bowel sounds may be present. Occult blood in the rectum is found in only 25% of these patients.[5] Frequently, diarrhea (with or without blood in the stool) and vomiting also are present. Marked

usually resulting in severe ischemia to the entire small intestine. Thus, survival is rare after an acute thrombosis of the SMA. Thrombosis of the SMA that results in extensive bowel ischemia usually is accompanied by severe atherosclerotic disease of the celiac artery, which eliminates a major source of collateral blood supply (Fig. 2).

Nonocclusive mesenteric ischemia results from severe, prolonged arterial spasm in the peripheral arterial branches. The most common cause is cardiac failure.[15-17] Other causes include cocaine or ergot ingestion,[18,19] gastroenteritis, appendicitis, spinal shock, obstetrical complications, or any condition causing a state of shock.[16,20,21] Digitalis preparations commonly used in patients with congestive heart failure may cause visceral arterial vasospasm and aggravate conditions that produce intestinal ischemia.

DIAGNOSIS

Clinical Presentation
In contrast to the male predominance in vascular disease that occurs elsewhere in the body, about two-thirds of

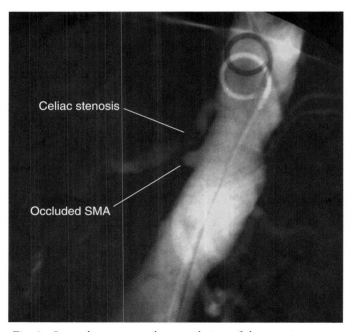

Fig. 2. Lateral aortogram shows occlusion of the superior mesenteric artery (SMA) and a high-grade stenosis of the celiac trunk due to atherosclerotic disease.

peritoneal tenderness after bowel infarction is a late and usually ominous finding.

Laboratory Examination

Routine laboratory tests are not helpful in making an early diagnosis of AMI. Leukocytosis is present in 90% of patients. About half of them will have a leukocyte count of 10 to 20 x 10^9/L; the other half will have a count of more than 20 x 10^9/L.[5] A leukocyte count of more than 25 x 10^9/L may indicate bowel infarction. Other laboratory markers (e.g., serum amylase, phosphate, lactate dehydrogenase, and creatine phosphokinase) are potential diagnostic markers for AMI but are not consistently reliable.[22,23]

Radiologic Examination

Plain abdominal radiographs are also nonspecific for the diagnosis of AMI, but radiography should be performed to evaluate for other possible causes of abdominal pain, such as bowel obstruction. In AMI, abdominal radiographs usually demonstrate only an ileus, or they may reveal nothing atypical.

Computed tomography is especially helpful in diagnosing other causes of abdominal pain. It also may be useful in diagnosing AMI, but it does not always provide the definitive information required to proceed with urgent surgical treatment. Findings on computed tomograms that are consistent with AMI include a dilated, thickened bowel wall, engorgement of the mesenteric veins, gas in the bowel wall or portal vein, nonfilling of the mesenteric arteries by contrast media given intravenously, and heavy calcification at the origins of the SMA or the celiac artery.[24,25] None of these findings are specific for AMI, and supplemental information provided by angiography is required to confirm the diagnosis and plan appropriate therapy. Valuable time may be lost while waiting for a computed tomogram, especially during late evening or weekend hours when technicians have to be called in to conduct these tests. Such delays can adversely affect patient outcome.

The most valuable diagnostic examination for AMI is mesenteric angiography. The study must be biplanar to image the origins of the SMA and the celiac artery (lateral view) as well as the distal branch vessels (anterior-posterior view). The angiogram defines the anatomical lesions and usually can distinguish acute thrombosis, embolism, or nonocclusive mesenteric ischemia. In arterial thrombosis, the mesenteric arteries often are occluded at their origin from the aorta. An arterial embolus usually lodges at or beyond the origin of the middle colic artery, with the proximal 2 cm to 3 cm of the SMA being entirely healthy. A sharp cutoff (meniscus sign) is observed with embolism (Fig. 1). A more tapered occlusion often occurs with thrombotic disease, but these two entities may have similar angiographic findings. In nonocclusive disease, the proximal vessels are healthy but the branch vessels show severe narrowing or multiple irregularities. In extreme cases, the distal branch vessels are barely visible or even absent.

Because angiography may result in excessive delay to treatment, making a decision to obtain this study is not easy. When the patient has had symptoms for several hours and classic findings of AMI are present, prompt surgical intervention may be the best approach, because irreversible bowel ischemia will occur 6 to 8 hours after mesenteric arterial occlusion. A surgeon experienced with mesenteric arterial disorders usually can determine whether to do an embolectomy or an arterial bypass without a preoperative angiogram. Without an angiogram to provide anatomical information, however, it may be more difficult to determine the most appropriate type of operation. Moreover, when nonocclusive ischemia is suspected, an angiogram can be both diagnostic and therapeutic. Vasodilatation can occur after angiography.

INDICATIONS FOR OPERATION

The diagnosis of acute occlusive mesenteric ischemia is an indication to operate for either an embolus or a thrombus. For nonocclusive mesenteric ischemia, laparotomy is called for when peritoneal signs indicate bowel infarction or perforation. In the nonresponsive patient, another indication is clinical deterioration during administration of intra-arterial vasodilator therapy. Delay to diagnosis is the major reason for the excessive mortality rate in persons with this disorder. Therefore, prompt surgical intervention is the most important life-saving measure to avert irreversible bowel infarction.

CONDUCT OF OPERATION

Preoperative Preparation

While tests are being performed to ascertain the diagnosis of AMI, the patient also should receive proper preoperative therapy. Fluid resuscitation should be started, and urine output should be monitored closely with a Foley catheter. These patients may be dehydrated enough to require a considerable amount of intravenous fluid. Hemodynamic monitoring is ideal, but trying to insert a central venous catheter can delay treatment and increase the likelihood of extensive, irreversible bowel infarction. These patients usually arrive in the operating room in suboptimal condition, but delaying an operation to try to improve the patient's condition is not indicated.

Embolic Occlusive Disease

The preferred treatment for an embolus in the mesenteric arteries is surgical embolectomy. It permits revascularization of the intestine and examination of the bowel to assess its viability.

The most common site for clinically significant mesenteric emboli is the SMA. Consequently, most of the reported surgical experience is with this vessel rather than with the celiac artery. In case a saphenous vein is needed for a bypass graft, the patient is prepared for the surgical procedure bilaterally from the nipples to the knees. The SMA is exposed by retracting the transverse colon superiorly and the small-bowel mesentery inferiorly and to the patient's right. Exposure of the SMA is obtained at the junction of the transverse colon and the small-bowel mesentery. After proximal and distal control of this artery is obtained, a transverse or longitudinal incision is made (Fig. 3). A no. 2 or no. 3 Fogarty balloon catheter is passed distally until no more thrombus can be removed, then it is passed proximally into the aorta. Removal of the proximal thrombus should allow pulsatile blood flow. After inflow is obtained, the transverse incision is closed primarily with several interrupted 6-0 polypropylene sutures. A longitudinal arteriotomy should be closed with a vein patch.

Thrombotic Occlusive Disease

The surgical management of acute thrombosis due to atherosclerotic disease of the SMA or celiac artery is much more complicated technically, because it requires bypass grafts of the occluded vessels. Both the celiac artery and the SMA should be revascularized. For patients undergoing a mesenteric bypass graft for chronic intestinal ischemia, Hollier and colleagues[26] at our institution found a much better survival rate and fewer complications with the revascularization of multiple mesenteric vessels rather than with the reconstruction of the SMA alone.

Various techniques for mesenteric reconstruction have been described. At Mayo Clinic, we prefer to use the antegrade bypass, with a graft that originates from the supraceliac aorta. The distal anastomosis is performed just beyond the atherosclerotic plaque that usually occurs at the origin of the SMA. In AMI, when there is infarcted or marginally viable bowel and bowel resection is required, a prosthetic graft is contraindicated because of the risk of graft infection in the postoperative period. Instead, we use a saphenous vein graft. After the abdomen is opened, the lesser curvature of the stomach is retracted to the patient's left to expose the diaphragmatic crura overlying the supraceliac aorta. The crura are divided with both sharp and blunt dissection to expose the aorta, of which 4 cm to 5 cm is dissected. The celiac trunk is dissected or, when there is extensive inflammation, the common hepatic artery may be exposed just

superior and proximal to the pylorus. The distal anastomosis should be performed to the distal celiac artery or to one of its major branches if the proximal celiac artery is diseased. As previously described, the SMA is exposed, and the site for the distal anastomosis is usually 3 cm to 5 cm beyond its origin. After the SMA is fully exposed, the saphenous vein is removed from the thigh and reversed. The proximal anastomosis is performed to the supraceliac aorta using a side-biting clamp (e.g., a Satinsky clamp) to occlude it. The vein graft is placed anterior to the pancreas, and the distal anastomosis is performed to the SMA. Another segment of vein can be sutured to the vein graft (piggybacked) or sutured separately to the aorta if there is enough room, then anastomosed to the celiac artery or the common hepatic artery. When the intestine is viable, a bifurcated polyethylene terephthalate or polytetrafluoroethylene prosthetic graft may be used instead. When the suprarenal aorta is calcified,

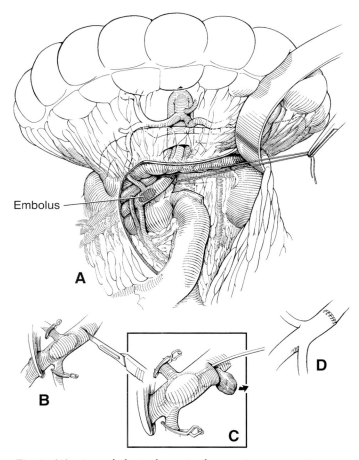

Fig. 3. (A), *An embolus is shown in the superior mesenteric artery after this artery has been exposed.* (B), *A transverse arteriotomy is made in the superior mesenteric artery proximal to the embolism, because the artery is larger at that point.* (C), *The embolus is removed using a balloon catheter.* (D), *The arteriotomy is closed with polypropylene sutures. (Modified from Kazmers.[27] By permission of Springer-Verlag New York.)*

the infrarenal aorta or iliac artery also may be used as an inflow source for a retrograde bypass graft.[27]

Nonocclusive Disease

Because most patients who develop nonocclusive AMI are often critically ill, methods to optimize supportive care must be initiated. For example, fluid and pharmacologic therapy may maximize cardiac output, and removal of vasopressor agents and treatment of an underlying condition such as an abscess may help prevent septic shock.

The mainstay of therapy is direct infusion of papaverine into the SMA. After a mesenteric angiogram confirms the diagnosis of nonocclusive intestinal ischemia, an intra-arterial catheter in the SMA provides a constant infusion of papaverine (30-60 mg/h).[6] The infusion is continued for at least 24 hours, and angiography is repeated to evaluate the patient's response. A longer interval may be required, depending on the patient's clinical response. The clinical examination also must be followed carefully to identify peritoneal signs or hemodynamic instability, which could signify bowel infarction. When clinical deterioration occurs, the patient should be transferred promptly to the operating room to undergo an exploratory laparotomy to check for bowel infarction. If the bowel is marginally viable, papaverine infusion should be continued for another 24 hours, and a repeat laparotomy should be done to determine whether bowel viability has improved with additional vasodilator therapy. However, when extensive bowel infarction is found, which is common, a decision must be made either to perform a major bowel resection that could leave the patient with a crippling short-bowel syndrome or to allow the patient to expire.

ASSESSMENT OF INTESTINAL VIABILITY

An important aspect in surgical management of patients with intestinal ischemia is assessment of bowel viability to determine how much bowel, if any, requires resection. Several techniques can be used to evaluate the extent of bowel infarction. Clinical assessment includes examining the color of the bowel, observing the bowel for contractions, and palpating pulsations in the mesenteric arteries. Doppler flow assessment consists of listening for arterial signals on the antimesenteric surface of the intestine with a continuous-wave Doppler probe. In the fluorescein method, 100 mg of fluorescein is administered intravenously, then the intestine is examined under a Wood lamp. Viable bowel appears bright yellow under the lamp, and nonviable bowel appears dark. One study comparing these three techniques found that clinical judgment was 89% accurate, Doppler assessment was 84% accurate, and fluorescein was 100% accurate.[28] We have found, as others have,[29] that clinical judgment and Doppler assessment are a useful, readily available, and accurate combination for determining bowel viability in most patients. We also have found fluorescein helpful in some patients who have equivocal findings on clinical assessment of Doppler tests.

Despite multiple methods to assess intestinal viability, assessing whether a segment of intestine is viable may not be possible during the initial operation. In such cases, marginally viable bowel should be left alone, and the patient should be returned to the operating room 24 hours later for a "second-look" laparotomy. Often, marginal bowel will appear normal during the second procedure, and the patient can be spared an excessive and unnecessary bowel resection that results in short-bowel syndrome. However, it also allows marginal bowel that is necrotic after 24 hours to be resected before perforation that causes further deterioration in the patient's overall condition. Rather than continuing to observe the patient who is doing well clinically the day after the initial operation, the surgeon should perform a second laparotomy if that was the original plan. Patients with evolving bowel ischemia or infarction often appear clinically well for a few days before they suddenly and rapidly deteriorate and die.[29]

SURGICAL OUTCOMES

Table 1 summarizes the mortality rates from AMI in 12 reports spanning 30 years. Although there have been at least three reports with mortality rates of less than 70%,[6,10,11] most series report higher mortality rates, despite major advances in patient care. The main reason for the continued high mortality rate is the delay in diagnosis and treatment. The prognosis for embolic disease is better than that for nonocclusive or thrombotic disease. Studies from the 1990s report mortality rates for mesenteric emboli of 50% to 76%.[11,12,30] For mesenteric arterial thrombosis, the mortality rate is nearly 100%.[12,30] For nonocclusive disease, the mortality rate is 67% to 83%,[12,30] although one report found that aggressive treatment using early angiography and intra-arterial vasodilator therapy resulted in a lower mortality rate.[6]

Few data exist on the long-term outcome of patients after surgical treatment of AMI. However, one German study reported survival in only 12 of 60 patients who presented with AMI (80% early mortality).[12] At 3-year follow-up, only 5 of those 12 patients were still alive. None of the five patients treated for mesenteric arterial thrombosis were still alive. Causes of death were mainly cardiovascular in nature. Only one patient died from recurrent intestinal ischemia. This study demonstrated both excessive early and late mortality rates in these patients.[12]

CONCLUSION

The mortality rate for AMI remains high because of the difficulty in making an early diagnosis and initiating prompt treatment. The main step toward reducing mortality is for physicians to be aware that patients with acute abdominal pain who have risk factors for AMI may have this disorder. When blood flow can be restored to the intestine in less than 6 hours after the initial ischemic event, the patient's prognosis, especially for ischemia due to embolism, is greatly improved. Despite improved care of patients during the past three decades, AMI is likely to remain a major clinical challenge.

REFERENCES

1. Ottinger LW, Austen WG: A study of 136 patients with mesenteric infarction. Surg Gynecol Obstet 124:251-261, 1967
2. Singh RP, Shah RC, Lee ST: Acute mesenteric vascular occlusion: a review of thirty-two patients. Surgery 78:613-617, 1975
3. Smith JS Jr, Patterson LT: Acute mesenteric infarction. Am Surg 42:562-567, 1976
4. Kairaluoma MI, Karkola P, Heikkinen D, Huttunen R, Mokka RE, Larmi TK: Mesenteric infarction. Am J Surg 133:188-193, 1977
5. Ottinger LW: The surgical management of acute occlusion of the superior mesenteric artery. Ann Surg 188:721-731, 1978
6. Boley SJ, Sprayregan S, Siegelman SS, Veith FJ: Initial results from an aggressive roentgenological and surgical approach to acute mesenteric ischemia. Surgery 82:848-855, 1977
7. Krausz MM, Manny J: Acute superior mesenteric arterial occlusion: a plea for early diagnosis. Surgery 83:482-485, 1978
8. Sachs SM, Morton JH, Schwartz SI: Acute mesenteric ischemia. Surgery 92:646-653, 1982
9. Finucane PM, Arunachalam T, O'Dowd J, Pathy MS: Acute mesenteric infarction in elderly patients. J Am Geriatr Soc 37:355-358, 1989
10. Levy PJ, Krausz MM, Manny J: Acute mesenteric ischemia: improved results: a retrospective analysis of ninety-two patients. Surgery 107:372-380, 1990
11. Batellier J, Kieny R: Superior mesenteric artery embolism: eighty-two cases. Ann Vasc Surg 4:112-116, 1990
12. Klempnauer J, Grothues F, Bektas H, Pichlmayr R: Long-term results after surgery for acute mesenteric ischemia. Surgery 121:239-243, 1997
13. Fratesi SJ, Barber GG: Celiac artery embolism: case report. Can J Surg 24:512-513, 1981
14. Porembka DT, Johnson DJ, Fowl RJ, Reising J, Dick BL: Descending thoracic aortic thrombus as a cause of multiple system organ failure: diagnosis by transesophageal echocardiography. Crit Care Med 20:1184-1187, 1992
15. Aldrete JS, Han SY, Laws HL, Kirklin JW: Intestinal infarction complicating low cardiac output states. Surg Gynecol Obstet 144:371-375, 1977
16. Williams LF Jr, Anastasia LF, Hasiotis CA, Bosniak MA, Byrne JJ: Nonocclusive mesenteric infarction. Am J Surg 114:376-381, 1967
17. Britt LG, Cheek RC: Nonocclusive mesenteric vascular disease: clinical and experimental observations. Ann Surg 169:704-711, 1969
18. Greene FL, Ariyan S, Stansel HC Jr: Mesenteric and peripheral vascular ischemia secondary to ergotism. Surgery 81:176-179, 1977
19. Myers SI, Clagett GP, Valentine RJ, Hansen ME, Anand A, Chervu A: Chronic intestinal ischemia caused by intravenous cocaine use: report of two cases and review of the literature. J Vasc Surg 23:724-729, 1996
20. Landreneau RJ, Fry WJ: The right colon as a target organ of nonocclusive mesenteric ischemia: case report and review of the literature. Arch Surg 125:591-594, 1990
21. Howard TJ, Plaskon LA, Wiebke EA, Wilcox MG, Madura JA: Nonocclusive mesenteric ischemia remains a diagnostic dilemma. Am J Surg 171:405-408, 1996
22. Moneta GL: Diagnosis of intestinal ischemia. In Vascular Surgery. Vol 2. Fifth edition. Edited by RB Rutherford. Philadelphia, WB Saunders Company, 2000, pp 1501-1511
23. Jamieson WG, Marchuk S, Rowsom J, Durand D: The early diagnosis of massive acute intestinal ischaemia. Br J Surg 69 Suppl:S52-S53, 1982
24. Bartnicke BJ, Balfe DM: CT appearance of intestinal ischemia and intramural hemorrhage. Radiol Clin North Am 32:845-860, 1994
25. Taourel PG, Deneuville M, Pradel JA, Regent D, Bruel JM: Acute mesenteric ischemia: diagnosis with contrast-enhanced CT. Radiology 199:632-636, 1996
26. Hollier LH, Bernatz PE, Pairolero PC, Payne WS, Osmundson PJ: Surgical management of chronic intestinal ischemia: a reappraisal. Surgery 90:940-946, 1981
27. Kazmers A: Operative management of acute mesenteric ischemia. Part 1. Ann Vasc Surg 12:187-197, 1998
28. Bulkley GB, Zuidema GD, Hamilton SR, O'Mara CS, Klacsmann PG, Horn SD: Intraoperative determination of small intestinal viability following ischemic injury: a prospective, controlled trial of two adjuvant methods (Doppler and fluorescein) compared with standard clinical judgment. Ann Surg 193:628-637, 1981
29. Taylor LM Jr, Moneta GL, Porter JM: Treatment of acute intestinal ischemia caused by arterial occlusions. In Vascular Surgery. Vol 2. Fifth edition. Edited by RB Rutherford. Philadelphia, WB Saunders Company, 2000, pp 1512-1519
30. Inderbitzi R, Wagner HE, Seiler C, Stirnemann P, Gertsch P: Acute mesenteric ischaemia. Eur J Surg 158:123-126, 1992

ACUTE MESENTERIC VENOUS THROMBOSIS

Peter Gloviczki, M.D.
Kenneth J. Cherry, Jr., M.D.
Thomas C. Bower, M.D.
Corey J. Jost, M.D.

Mesenteric venous thrombosis is a rare severe form of acute mesenteric ischemia. Its clinical presentation is frequently insidious; signs and symptoms of the disease may be nonspecific, and delay in diagnosis is frequent. Mortality due to mesenteric venous thrombosis is substantial. The main causes of death are bowel infarction with peritonitis leading to septic shock and short-bowel syndrome after extensive resection.

In recent decades, there has been considerable progress in the diagnosis and treatment of mesenteric venous thrombosis. Risk factors for venous thrombosis have been defined better, previously unknown abnormalities of coagulation have been discovered, and physicians are increasingly aware of this abdominal emergency. The availability and more frequent use of abdominal imaging techniques (e.g., ultrasonography, computed tomography [CT], magnetic resonance imaging [MRI]) have helped detect acute mesenteric venous thrombosis at earlier stages.

In this chapter, we review the incidence, pathogenesis, and clinical presentation of acute mesenteric venous thrombosis. We discuss the difficulty in reaching an early diagnosis, review the accuracy of available imaging studies, and discuss nonsurgical and surgical treatment options and results. Finally, we recommend an algorithm for optimal management of patients who have this potentially lethal condition.

INCIDENCE

The true incidence of mesenteric venous thrombosis is not known. In one large autopsy series, thrombus was found in the mesenteric veins of 1.5% of the cases.[1]

Clinically significant mesenteric venous thrombosis is diagnosed less frequently, and a review of the literature to 1984 revealed only 372 published cases.[2] Ottinger and Austen[3] found that mesenteric venous thrombosis led to 0.006% of hospital admissions and less than 2% of autopsy cases. Kazmers[4] estimated that intestinal infarction due to mesenteric venous thrombosis is encountered in fewer than 1 in 1,000 laparotomies for acute abdomen. Rhee et al.[5] at Mayo Clinic identified 72 patients (6.2%) with mesenteric venous thrombosis among 1,167 patients treated for mesenteric ischemia.

Mesenteric venous thrombosis represents 5% to 15% of all cases of acute mesenteric ischemia.[5,6] Earlier reports noted a greater incidence, probably because venous thrombosis could not be distinguished from nonocclusive mesenteric ischemia.[7]

ETIOLOGY

The term "primary" or "idiopathic" mesenteric venous thrombosis is reserved for cases of mesenteric venous thrombosis that have no known cause. The number of patients in this group has decreased because of improved diagnosis and recognition of additional causes of thrombotic disorders. Therefore, the number of patients with secondary mesenteric venous thrombosis is increasing.

Various genetic disorders (e.g., protein C and S deficiencies, antithrombin-III deficiency, factor V Leiden mutation, dysfibrinogenemia, abnormal plasminogen) have been diagnosed in patients with mesenteric venous thrombosis.[8-12] Antiphospholipid antibodies (e.g., lupus anticoagulant, anticardiolipin antibody), plasminogen-activator deficiency, and hyperhomocystinemia have been noted also.[13-15] Factor V Leiden mutation has emerged as the most common genetic cause of deep venous thrombosis. Deficiency in protein S, a cofactor of protein C, is associated with 5% of all cases of venous thrombosis. However, about one-third of the patients who have protein S deficiency and an associated thrombotic event have an associated factor V Leiden mutation.

Secondary mesenteric venous thrombosis also can be caused by inflammation, abdominal infection, pancreatitis, pregnancy, use of oral contraceptives, myeloproliferative disease, polycythemia, thrombocytosis, malignant tumors, portal hypertension, or open abdominal or laparoscopic surgical interventions.[16-25] Mesenteric venous thrombosis occurs more frequently after splenectomy, when a long remnant of the splenic vein forms a cul-de-sac prone to thrombosis or to becoming a nidus for thrombus propagation.[26,27]

Penetrating or blunt abdominal trauma, iatrogenic injury to the mesenteric vessels, and endoscopic sclerotherapy are additional causes of mesenteric venous thrombosis.[28] Congestive heart failure also may be a cause, but nonocclusive mesenteric ischemia due to a low flow state must be excluded in patients with left heart failure. Localized mesenteric venous thrombosis caused by volvulus, intussusception, or strangulation of the bowel has a different pathogenesis and will not be discussed in this chapter.

In the Mayo Clinic series, the most frequent etiologic factors were previous abdominal surgical procedures, hematologic abnormalities, and previous mesenteric venous thrombosis (Table 1).

CLINICAL CLASSIFICATION

Patients with symptoms lasting less than 4 weeks are classified as having acute mesenteric venous thrombosis. Those with symptoms lasting longer than 4 weeks but with no evidence of bowel infarction or those who were asymptomatic but found to have mesenteric venous thrombosis during evaluation for other pathologic conditions of the abdomen are classified as having chronic mesenteric venous thrombosis. Patients who have symptoms of portal hypertension (e.g., gastrointestinal bleeding) and documented mesenteric venous thrombosis also belong to the chronic group. Our discussion focuses on the management of patients who have acute mesenteric venous thrombosis.

ACUTE MESENTERIC VENOUS THROMBOSIS

Intestinal infarction due to acute thrombosis of the mesenteric and portal veins was first described by Fagge in

Table 1.—Conditions Associated With Mesenteric Venous Thrombosis in 72 Patients

Condition	Patients	
	No.	%
Previous abdominal surgical procedure	37	51
Hypercoagulable state	30	42
Previous mesenteric venous thrombosis	25	35
Smoking	23	32
Previous deep venous thrombosis	20	28
Alcohol abuse	15	21
Malignant tumor	13	18
Cirrhosis	13	18
Oral contraceptive use	4	6

Modified from Rhee et al.[5] By permission of Mosby.

1876.[29] In 1895, Elliot[30] performed the first resection of an infarcted bowel due to venous thrombosis. In 1935, Warren and Eberhard[31] provided the first detailed description and review of acute mesenteric venous thrombosis.

Clinical Presentation

Demographic Data
In the Mayo Clinic series, 53 patients (30 men, 23 women) with a mean age of 56.6 years (range, 23-81 years) were treated for acute mesenteric venous thrombosis.[5] In a collected series of 116 patients, mean age was 64 years (range, 17-88 years).[5,32-35] The male-to-female ratio was 1.5:1 (69:47) with men having a greater risk for mesenteric venous thrombosis.

Symptoms and Signs
The spectrum of presentation ranges from mild abdominal pain and distention of several days' duration to full-blown peritonitis with sepsis. The patient may present with typical symptoms and signs of acute bowel ischemia characterized by pain out of proportion to physical findings, nausea, vomiting, and constipation with or without bloody diarrhea. Such acute presentation, however, is rare. More frequent is a constant or sometimes intermittent diffuse abdominal pain and bloating of several days' or even weeks' duration. Four (8%) of the 53 Mayo Clinic patients presented with symptoms lasting less than 24 hours, and 75% had symptoms lasting longer than 48 hours. Abdominal pain was the most frequent symptom, followed by anorexia and diarrhea (Table 2). One-fourth of the patients had gastrointestinal tract bleeding, and 13% had constipation. The abdominal pain was diffuse

Table 2.—Symptoms of Acute Mesenteric Venous Thrombosis in 53 Patients

Symptom	Patients No.	%
Abdominal pain	44	83
Anorexia	28	53
Diarrhea	23	43
Nausea and vomiting	22	41
Upper gastrointestinal bleeding	15	28
Lower gastrointestinal bleeding	12	23
Constipation	7	13

Modified from Rhee et al.[5] By permission of Mosby.

and nonspecific in 57% of patients. When the pain was localized, it occurred in the right lower quadrant in three of every four patients. Abdominal distention was the most frequent sign, and only one of every three patients presented with clinical signs of peritonitis (Table 3).

Diagnostic Tests

Findings of laboratory tests provide supportive information that is nondiagnostic. However, leukocytosis, increased concentrations of serum lactates, and electrolyte abnormalities may indicate bowel ischemia. Elevated serum D-lactate is the finding most predictive of mesenteric ischemia.[36,37] We found leukocytosis in 51% of the 53 patients, and lactates were above 1.65 mmol/L in 28% of patients (Table 3).[5]

Table 3.—Signs of Acute Mesenteric Venous Thrombosis in 53 Patients

Sign	Patients No.	%
Abdominal distention	27	51
Leukocytosis (> 10 x 10^9/L)	27	51
Peritonitis	19	36
Blood on rectal examination	17	32
Elevated lactates (> 1.65 mmol/L)	15	28
Fever (> 38°C)	13	24
Tachycardia (> 110/min)	11	21
Elevated amylase (> 115 U/L)	10	19
Ascites	5	9
Elevated creatine kinase (> 350 U/L)	4	8
Hypotension (< 90 mm Hg)	3	6

Modified from Rhee et al.[5] By permission of Mosby.

When appropriate, patients with mesenteric venous thrombosis should undergo screening for hypercoagulable states. It is important to determine factor V Leiden, lupus anticoagulant, hyperhomocystinemia, prothrombin mutation, plasminogen-activator deficiency, antithrombin-III deficiency, and deficiencies in proteins C and S. These tests, however, play a minimal role in the early management of acute mesenteric ischemia.

Abdominal radiographs without contrast show a pattern of ileus in only two-thirds of cases. Marked abdominal wall thickening is observed most frequently. Air in the portal system or in the abdominal cavity is a rare finding of advanced disease.

When mesenteric venous thrombosis is suspected, CT is the preferred test. Rosen et al.[38] described the typical CT findings of a dense venous wall and central lucency in 15 patients with mesenteric venous thrombosis whose diagnosis was confirmed with mesenteric venography or exploration. Of 20 patients in our series who were studied with CT, thrombus in the superior mesenteric vein was found in 11 (55%), as exemplified by Figure 1. Portal vein thrombosis and splenic vein thrombosis were documented in 35%. CT also is helpful for imaging other signs of bowel ischemia (e.g., thickened bowel wall, pneumatosis, "streaky" mesentery), and it aids in the diagnosis of secondary pathologic conditions. CT was 100% sensitive in showing abdominal findings suggestive of mesenteric venous thrombosis or ischemic bowel. Other authors report similar diagnostic accuracy. Mesenteric venous thrombosis was diagnosed correctly with CT in 14 patients studied by Vogelzang et al.[39] and in nine of 10 patients studied by Harward et al.[32]

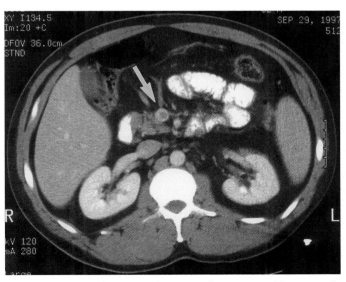

Fig. 1. Computed tomographic scan of a 35-year-old man with acute mesenteric venous thrombosis due to thrombus in superior mesenteric vein (arrow).

If findings of CT are not diagnostic or unequivocal, or if they do not allow the exclusion of mesenteric arterial occlusion, mesenteric arteriography with radiographs of the venous phase should be performed. With CT, we identified thrombus or nonvisualization of the mesenteric vein in five (71%) of seven patients.

Abdominal ultrasonography also was sensitive in our experience. Ultrasound findings confirmed thrombus in the superior mesenteric vein in 8 (80%) of 10 patients, as exemplified by Figure 2. Miller and Berland[40] found that duplex ultrasonography of the abdomen was as useful as CT in diagnosing mesenteric venous thrombosis.

MRI is used with increasing frequency to diagnose pathologic conditions of the abdomen. With MRI, Gehl et al.[41] diagnosed abdominal venous thrombosis in 15 consecutive patients. The results of MRI are similar to those obtained with CT.

The diagnosis of acute mesenteric venous thrombosis also can be established using upper gastrointestinal tract endoscopy.[42,43] A potential future diagnostic technique is the superconducting quantum interference device magnetometer. Experiments with this noninvasive device show promise for early and rapid diagnosis of mesenteric venous thrombosis before it results in bowel necrosis.[44]

Despite advanced imaging techniques, mesenteric venous thrombosis is frequently diagnosed only during an operation.[5] In our series, 16 (30%) of 53 patients had a diagnosis of acute mesenteric venous thrombosis that was established only on abdominal exploration. Median delay to diagnosis was 48 hours (mean, 83 ± 17 hours).

Treatment

Patients who have acute mesenteric venous thrombosis require early diagnosis, immediate anticoagulation with heparin, and rapid fluid resuscitation to increase their intravascular volume. Patients who have peritoneal signs of acute mesenteric venous thrombosis should be treated with broad-spectrum antibiotics directed at both aerobic and anaerobic organisms. Those patients who have bowel infarction and peritonitis require early exploration and resection of the nonviable portion of the bowel.

Nonsurgical Management

Patients who do not have peritonitis but who do have documented acute mesenteric venous thrombosis can be observed and managed nonsurgically with fluid resuscitation and heparin for anticoagulation. Most patients require long-term anticoagulation with warfarin, unless it is contraindicated by bleeding complications caused by portal venous hypertension or other pathologic conditions.

Transcatheter Thrombolysis

Patients who have increasing symptoms indicative of mesenteric venous thrombosis but no evidence of peritonitis or bowel infarction may require thrombolytic therapy. A few reports have noted successful thrombolytic therapy with the use of a catheter placed either in the superior mesenteric artery or in the portal or mesenteric veins through the liver.[45-47] Thrombolytic therapy is contraindicated in patients with peritonitis or gastrointestinal tract bleeding. Because urokinase is unavailable, further studies with tissue plasminogen activators and other new thrombolytic

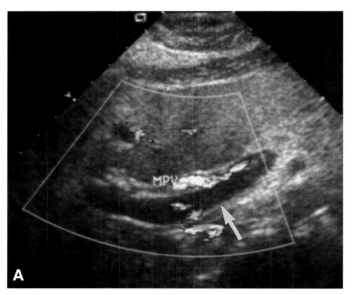
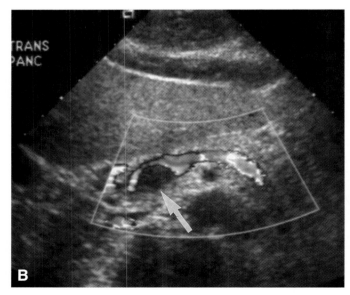

Fig. 2. Duplex ultrasonogram of an 82-year-old woman with acute mesenteric venous thrombosis. (A), Thrombus in the superior mesenteric vein at its confluence with the portal vein (arrow). *(B), Nonocclusive thrombus projecting into the portal vein* (arrow).

medications are needed to define the correct indications for this promising, minimally invasive treatment.

Surgical Treatment

Open or laparoscopic abdominal exploration is necessary in patients who show signs of peritonitis. In the Mayo Clinic series, 34 (64%) of 53 patients with acute mesenteric venous thrombosis underwent abdominal exploration.[5] Edema of the mesentery and cyanotic discoloration of the involved bowel are characteristic of mesenteric venous thrombosis. Thrombus is found most often in the superior mesenteric vein (Fig. 3), then in the splenic vein or portal vein (Fig. 4). Frequently, thrombosed veins in the cut edge of the mesentery are noted. Intestinal infarction caused by mesenteric venous thrombosis usually affects the jejunum or the distal ileum. In our experience, the ascending colon was involved in only 13% of patients and the duodenum in only 8%. Transmural bowel necrosis was present in 85% of the patients, of whom 21% had bowel perforation.

Before a bowel resection, intraoperative assessment should be made of the perfusion of the bowel and mesentery. To confirm adequate perfusion, we inject two ampules of fluorescein intravenously and observe the bowel under a Wood lamp. Absent, perivascular, or patchy patterns indicate poor perfusion. The arterial supply is frequently intact, with pulsatile flow palpable in the superior mesenteric artery and pulsatile flow demonstrated with Doppler in the small-bowel mesentery. In the Mayo Clinic series, bowel resection was necessary in 88% of patients during the first operation.

If the diagnosis of mesenteric ischemia has not been confirmed before the operation and if anticoagulant

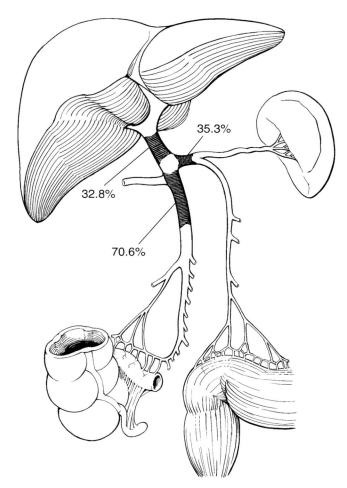

Fig. 4. Frequency of thrombosis in the superior mesenteric (71%), splenic (35%), and portal (33%) veins in patients with acute mesenteric venous thrombosis. (Modified from Rhee RY, Gloviczki P: Mesenteric venous thrombosis. Surg Clin North Am 77:327-338, 1997. By permission of WB Saunders Company.)

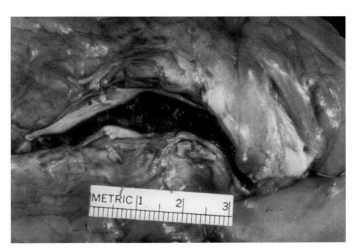

Fig. 3. Disease specimen of small-bowel mesentery shows thrombus in superior mesenteric vein. (From Rhee et al.[5] By permission of Mosby.)

therapy has not been initiated, 5,000 units of heparin are given, and nonfractionated heparin infusion is started intraoperatively at a rate of 1,000 units per hour. The activated partial thromboplastin time is monitored continuously to keep it at more than 80 seconds. This type of acute mesenteric ischemia is the only one for which we fully heparinize the patient intraoperatively and maintain continuous heparin perfusion even in the early perioperative period. Despite the increased risk of bleeding complications, perioperative anticoagulation decreases the risk of rethrombosis and improves the rate of survival.

Single case reports have noted successful thrombectomy of the superior mesenteric vein using a Fogarty balloon catheter and manual expression of the thrombus from the mesenteric vein.[4,33,48-50] Frequently, thrombosis is extensive and involves the small distal veins as well as the intrahepatic portal outflow. Adjuncts to thrombectomy, such as local thrombolytic therapy,[50] also have been successful. In one patient who underwent thrombectomy, early rethrombosis required resection of additional bowel during a second-look procedure. Although an occasional case of early thrombosis can be treated with thrombectomy, most patients present with diffuse venous thrombosis, frequently after a previous thrombotic episode, and with extension of the thrombus into the distal mesenteric veins. It is unlikely that these patients can be treated successfully with venous thrombectomy.

To preserve bowel length and avoid short-bowel syndrome, we recommend resection of only the obviously nonviable portion of the bowel. Primary anastomosis can be performed in most patients. As in the management of acute mesenteric arterial occlusion, the decision to do a second-look operation is made during the first operation. Bowel of questionable viability is assessed again within 24 hours. During 14 second-look operations, we resected additional bowel in all 14 patients.[5] The benefit of the second-look laparotomy also has been noted by Levy et al.[35] and Khodadadi et al.[51] Other authors have used second-look laparoscopy.[52]

Clinical Outcome

Most patients who present with peritonitis and an infarcted bowel that requires resection have multiple complications and must undergo a prolonged hospitalization. In our experience, the mean hospital stay for patients with acute venous thrombosis was 22 days (range, 1-98 days).[5] Complications, most frequently short-bowel syndrome, wound infection, and sepsis, occurred in 55% of patients (Table 4). Five patients, only one of whom was taking anticoagulant therapy at the time, had a pulmonary embolism.

The 30-day rate of mortality for patients with acute mesenteric venous thrombosis is clinically significant; in our 53 patients, it was 27%. The 30-day rate of mortality decreased between the first and last decades of the study from 32% in the early period to 24% in the last, but this difference was not statistically significant due to the small sample size (Fig. 5). Early mortality in other published series was similar (range, 13%-50%).[11,12,15-18] Death is often caused by a concurrent severe medical condition, which confounds the mortality rate from this disease.[32,34] Patients who present with necrotic bowel have a worse prognosis and higher complication rates.[5] The use of anticoagulant medication, however, greatly increases early survival (Fig. 6).

Long-term survival of patients with acute mesenteric venous thrombosis is poor. In the Mayo Clinic series, it was 36% at 3 years. The cause of death in 38% of the patients was mesenteric venous thrombosis.

Table 4.—Complications of Acute Mesenteric Venous Thrombosis in 53 Patients

Complication	Patients No.	Patients %
Short-bowel syndrome	12	23
Wound infection	11	21
Sepsis	9	17
Pneumonia	7	13
Pulmonary embolus	5	9
Renal failure	5	9
Gastrointestinal bleeding	3	6

From Rhee et al.[5] By permission of Mosby.

Summary of Current Management

Abdominal pain of several days' duration and peritonitis in a patient who has had previous lower extremity or mesenteric venous thrombosis are suggestive of a diagnosis of mesenteric venous thrombosis. Leukocytosis and elevated lactates in a middle-aged patient who has known coagulation abnormalities but no risk factors for atherosclerosis should increase suspicion of the diagnosis. If the diagnosis is correct, CT scans will confirm mesenteric ischemia and likely show thrombus in the mesenteric vein. Absence of peritonitis permits nonsurgical management with anticoagulant therapy and fluid resuscitation. For patients who have progressive symptoms but no peritonitis and no contraindication to thrombolysis, transcatheter thrombolytic treatment can be considered. Patients who have localized or diffuse peritonitis, however, require abdominal exploration (Fig. 7). During the operation, resection of the nonviable portion of the bowel

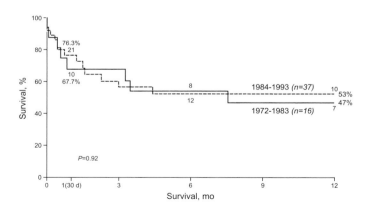

Fig. 5. Survival of patients with acute mesenteric venous thrombosis during the early (1972–1983) and late (1984–1993) periods of the Mayo Clinic study. (From Rhee et al.[5] By permission of Mosby.)

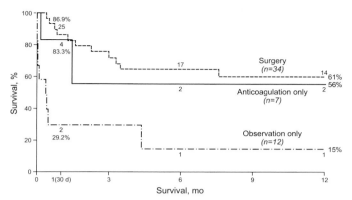

Fig. 6. Survival of patients with acute mesenteric venous thrombosis treated with surgery and anticoagulation medication, anticoagulation medication alone, or observation alone. (From Rhee et al.[5] By permission of Mosby.)

can be performed, and a venous thrombectomy can be considered. If the viability of the remaining bowel is questionable, a decision to do a second-look laparotomy 24 hours later should be made during the first operation.

Patients receive heparin for anticoagulation and can be given oral anticoagulants after surgical exploration is no longer planned.

CONCLUSION

Acute mesenteric venous thrombosis is a lethal disease, with a 30-day mortality of 27% in our experience. Although CT is a sensitive diagnostic test, clinical presentation and findings of laboratory tests are frequently nonspecific and result in a delay in diagnosis. Patients who have documented or suspected mesenteric venous thrombosis but no peritonitis can be managed nonsurgically with anticoagulant therapy and fluid resuscitation. Those patients who have peritonitis should undergo early exploration and resection of the infarcted bowel. Immediate use of anticoagulants provides the best prognosis, but long-term survival remains dismal, mostly because of underlying severe comorbidity and because recurrent mesenteric thrombosis is likely. Patients who have mesenteric venous thrombosis will require life-long treatment with anticoagulants.

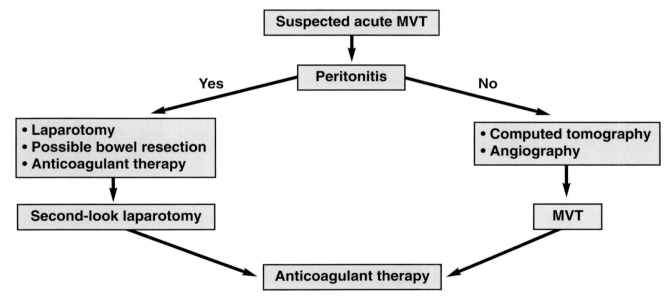

Fig. 7. Management algorithm for patients with acute mesenteric venous thrombosis (MVT). (From Rhee et al.[5] By permission of Mosby.)

REFERENCES

1. Grendell JH, Ockner RK: Mesenteric venous thrombosis. Gastroenterology 82:358-372, 1982

2. Abdu RA, Zakhour BJ, Dallis DJ: Mesenteric venous thrombosis—1911 to 1984. Surgery 101:383-388, 1987

3. Ottinger LW, Austen WG: A study of 136 patients with mesenteric infarction. Surg Gynecol Obstet 124:251-261, 1967

4. Kazmers A: Intestinal ischemia caused by venous thrombosis. *In* Vascular Surgery. Vol 2. Fourth edition. Edited by RB Rutherford. Philadelphia, WB Saunders Company, 1995, pp 1288-1300

5. Rhee RY, Gloviczki P, Mendonca CT, Petterson TM, Serry RD, Sarr MG, Johnson CM, Bower TC, Hallett JW Jr, Cherry KJ Jr: Mesenteric venous thrombosis: still a lethal disease in the 1990s. J Vasc Surg 20:688-697, 1994

6. Howard TJ, Plaskon LA, Wiebke EA, Wilcox MG, Madura JA: Nonocclusive mesenteric ischemia remains a diagnostic dilemma. Am J Surg 171:405-408, 1996

7. Boley SJ, Kaleya RN, Brandt LJ: Mesenteric venous thrombosis. Surg Clin North Am 72:183-201, 1992

8. Green D, Ganger DR, Blei AT: Protein C deficiency in splanchnic venous thrombosis. Am J Med 82:1171-1174, 1987

9. Broekmans AW, van Rooyen W, Westerveld BD, Briet E, Bertina RM: Mesenteric vein thrombosis as presenting manifestation of hereditary protein S deficiency. Gastroenterology 92:240-242, 1987

10. Leebeek FW, Lameris JS, van Buuren HR, Gomez E, Madretsma S, Sonneveld P: Budd-Chiari syndrome, portal vein and mesenteric vein thrombosis in a patient homozygous for factor V Leiden mutation treated by TIPS and thrombolysis. Br J Haematol 102:929-931, 1998

11. Boyko OB, Pizzo SV: Mesenteric vein thrombosis and vascular plasminogen activator. Arch Pathol Lab Med 107:541-542, 1983

12. Gruenberg JC, Smallridge RC, Rosenberg RD: Inherited antithrombin-III deficiency causing mesenteric venous infarction: a new clinical entity. Ann Surg 181:791-794, 1975

13. Lee HJ, Park JW, Chang JC: Mesenteric and portal venous obstruction associated with primary antiphospholipid antibody syndrome. J Gastroenterol Hepatol 12:822-826, 1997

14. Blanc P, Barki J, Fabre JM, Larrey D, Domergue J, Michel H, Lavabre-Bertrand T: Superior mesenteric vein thrombosis associated with anticardiolipin antibody without autoimmune disease (letter). Am J Hematol 48:137, 1995

15. Marie I, Levesque H, Lecam-Duchez V, Borg JY, Ducrotte P, Philippe C: Mesenteric venous thrombosis revealing both factor II G20212A mutation and hyperhomocysteinemia related to pernicious anemia (letter). Gastroenterology 118:237-238, 2000

16. Graubard ZG, Friedman M: Mesenteric venous thrombosis associated with pregnancy and oral contraception: a case report. S Afr Med J 71:453, 1987

17. De Luca M, Dugo M, Arduini R, Liessi G: Acute venous thrombosis of spleno-mesenteric portal axis: an unusual localization of thromboembolism in the nephrotic syndrome. Am J Nephrol 11:260-263, 1991

18. Tossou H, Iglicki F, Casadevall N, Delamarre J, Dupas JL, Capron JP: Superior mesenteric vein thrombosis as a manifestation of a latent myeloproliferative disorder (letter). J Clin Gastroenterol 13:597-598, 1991

19. Whelan MA, Kaim P: Mesenteric complications in a patient with polycythemia vera. Am J Gastroenterol 77:526-528, 1982

20. Venturini I, Cioni G, Turrini F, Gandolfo M, Modonesi G, Cosenza R, Miglioli L, Cristani A, D'Alimonte P, De Santis M, Zeneroli ML: Mesenteric vein thrombosis: a rare cause of abdominal pain in cirrhotic patients—two case reports. Hepatogastroenterology 45:44-47, 1998

21. Sanabria JR, Hiruki T, Szalay DA, Tandan V, Gallinger S: Superior mesenteric vein thrombosis after the Whipple procedure: an aggressive, combined treatment approach. Can J Surg 40:467-470, 1997

22. Millikan KW, Szczerba SM, Dominguez JM, McKenna R, Rorig JC: Superior mesenteric and portal vein thrombosis following laparoscopic-assisted right hemicolectomy: report of a case. Dis Colon Rectum 39:1171-1175, 1996

23. Krummen DM, Cannova J, Schreiber H: Conservative management strategy for pancreatitis-associated mesenteric venous thrombosis. Am Surg 62:432-434, 1996

24. Cornu-Labat G, Kasirajan K, Simon R, Smith DJ, Herman ML, Rubin JR: Acute mesenteric vein thrombosis and pancreatitis: a rare association. Int J Pancreatol 21:249-251, 1997

25. Farin P, Paajanen H, Miettinen P: Intraoperative US diagnosis of pylephlebitis (portal vein thrombosis) as a complication of appendicitis: a case report. Abdom Imaging 22:401-403, 1997

26. Kowal-Vern A, Radhakrishnan J, Goldman J, Hutchins W, Blank J: Mesenteric and portal vein thrombosis after splenectomy for autoimmune hemolytic anemia. J Clin Gastroenterol 10:108-110, 1988

27. Rattner DW, Ellman L, Warshaw AL: Portal vein thrombosis after elective splenectomy: an underappreciated, potentially lethal syndrome. Arch Surg 128:565-569, 1993

28. Goldberg H, Fabry TL: Mesenteric thrombosis following sclerotherapy during vasopressin infusion: mechanism and therapeutic implications. J Clin Gastroenterol 11:56-57, 1989

29. Fagge CH: A case of acute thrombosis of the superior mesenteric and portal veins, attended with rapidly fatal collapse. Trans Pathol Soc London 27:124-128, 1875-1876

30. Elliot JW: The operative relief of gangrene of intestine due to occlusion of the mesenteric vessels. Ann Surg 21:9-23, 1895

31. Warren S, Eberhard TP: Mesenteric venous thrombosis. Surg Gynecol Obstet 61:102-121, 1935

32. Harward TR, Green D, Bergan JJ, Rizzo RJ, Yao JS: Mesenteric venous thrombosis. J Vasc Surg 9:328-333, 1989

33. Gertsch P, Matthews J, Lerut J, Luder P, Blumgart LH: Acute thrombosis of the splanchnic veins. Arch Surg 128:341-345, 1993

34. Grieshop RJ, Dalsing MC, Cikrit DF, Lalka SG, Sawchuk AP: Acute mesenteric venous thrombosis: revisited in a time of diagnostic clarity. Am Surg 57:573-577, 1991

35. Levy PJ, Krausz MM, Manny J: The role of second-look procedure in improving survival time for patients with mesenteric venous thrombosis. Surg Gynecol Obstet 170:287-291, 1990

36. Murray MJ, Gonze MD, Nowak LR, Cobb CF: Serum D(-)-lactate levels as an aid to diagnosing acute intestinal ischemia. Am J Surg 167:575-578, 1994

37. Gunel E, Caglayan O, Caglayan F: Serum D-lactate levels as a predictor of intestinal ischemia-reperfusion injury. Pediatr Surg Int 14:59-61, 1998

38. Rosen A, Korobkin M, Silverman PM, Dunnick NR, Kelvin FM: Mesenteric vein thrombosis: CT identification. AJR Am J Roentgenol 143:83-86, 1984

39. Vogelzang RL, Gore RM, Anschuetz SL, Blei AT: Thrombosis of the splanchnic veins: CT diagnosis. AJR Am J Roentgenol 150:93-96, 1988

40. Miller VE, Berland LL: Pulsed Doppler duplex sonography and CT of portal vein thrombosis. AJR Am J Roentgenol 145:73-76, 1985

41. Gehl HB, Bohndorf K, Klose KC, Gunther RW: Two-dimensional MR angiography in the evaluation of abdominal veins with gradient refocused sequences. J Comput Assist Tomogr 14:619-624, 1990

42. Leiser A, Wysjenbeek A, Kadish U: Mesenteric venous infarction presenting as an upper GI bleeding and diagnosed by upper GI endoscopy. Endoscopy 17:119-120, 1985

43. Wade TP, Jewell WR, Andrus CH: Mesenteric venous thrombosis: modern management and endoscopic diagnosis. Surg Endosc 6:283-284, 1992

44. Allos SH, Staton DJ, Bradshaw LA, Halter S, Wikswo JP Jr, Richards WO: Superconducting quantum interference device magnetometer for diagnosis of ischemia caused by mesenteric venous thrombosis. World J Surg 21:173-177, 1997

45. Rivitz SM, Geller SC, Hahn C, Waltman AC: Treatment of acute mesenteric venous thrombosis with transjugular intramesenteric urokinase infusion. J Vasc Interv Radiol 6:219-223, 1995

46. Poplausky MR, Kaufman JA, Geller SC, Waltman AC: Mesenteric venous thrombosis treated with urokinase via the superior mesenteric artery. Gastroenterology 110:1633-1635, 1996

47. Ludwig DJ, Hauptmann E, Rosoff L Jr, Neuzil D: Mesenteric and portal vein thrombosis in a young patient with protein S deficiency treated with urokinase via the superior mesenteric artery. J Vasc Surg 30:551-554, 1999

48. Inahara T: Acute superior mesenteric venous thrombosis: treatment by thrombectomy. Ann Surg 174:956-961, 1971

49. Bergentz SE, Ericsson B, Hedner U, Leandoer L, Nilsson IM: Thrombosis in the superior mesenteric and portal veins: report of a case treated with thrombectomy. Surgery 76:286-290, 1974

50. Klempnauer J, Grothues F, Bektas H, Pichlmayr R: Results of portal thrombectomy and splanchnic thrombolysis for the surgical management of acute mesentericoportal thrombosis. Br J Surg 84:129-132, 1997

51. Khodadadi J, Rozencwajg J, Nacasch N, Schmidt B, Feuchtwanger MM: Mesenteric vein thrombosis: the importance of a second-look operation. Arch Surg 115:315-317, 1980

52. Spittler C, Chari V, Husni E, Patzakis J, Li P, Zelis J, Chung R: Second-look laparoscopy for visceral ischemia facilitated by preinstalled ports. Am Surg 63:732-734, 1997

Chapter 31

Chronic Mesenteric Ischemia

W. Andrew Oldenburg, M.D.

Chronic mesenteric ischemia occurs when the blood flow to the intestine has been reduced to an amount that is inadequate to support the bowel's metabolic demands for secretion, absorption, and motility. Although it typically is caused by progressive atherosclerotic occlusive disease affecting the proximal portion of the mesenteric vessels, rarely, mechanical causes (e.g., dissection, median arcuate ligament compression), collagen vascular disorders, and other vasculopathies are the cause.[1] Effective treatment of chronic mesenteric ischemia is confounded by difficulties in making the diagnosis, the presence of coexisting diseases, and the technically difficult procedures needed in patients who are usually emaciated and malnourished. Although treatment of the disease is challenging, management is rewarding for clinicians able to correct the underlying mesenteric arterial stenoses or occlusions and restore the patient to a well-nourished person who is able to eat without fear of abdominal pain.

PREVALENCE

Chronic mesenteric ischemia is a rare disease. In fact, only 332 affected patients were described in the literature between 1977 and 1996.[2] Of all peripheral vascular procedures performed, only 0.5% are mesenteric reconstructive procedures.[3,4] Only a few series have described more than 50 patients who have had mesenteric revascularization for chronic mesenteric ischemia. Because of the tertiary referral practice at Mayo Clinic in Rochester, Jacksonville, and Scottsdale, we have treated more than 125 patients with chronic mesenteric ischemia since 1960.

CLINICAL PRESENTATION

Typically, chronic mesenteric ischemia occurs in older persons. The mean age at diagnosis has been in the mid 60s. Females are affected more frequently than males (4:1 ratio), probably because they have smaller arteries requiring less plaque "burden" before extensive stenosis occurs. Unknown is whether females have a greater predilection to form plaque at the origins of visceral vessels than males. The classic symptom of chronic mesenteric ischemia is postprandial diffuse abdominal pain that progresses to the point that patients have a "fear of foods." They stop eating and experience substantial weight loss. Interestingly, J. E. Dunphy, while a surgical resident at the Peter Bent Brigham Hospital in 1936, reported that 7 of 12 patients who died of acute mesenteric ischemia had prodromal symptoms of abdominal pain associated with meals.[5] In our experience, essentially 100% of patients present with abdominal pain. Weight loss occurs in 60% to 70% and is less of a predictor. Not infrequently, patients have learned that nutritional needs can be maintained and abdominal pain avoided by eating small amounts more frequently. As a result, their presentation to a surgeon is delayed. Other associated symptoms may include diarrhea due to malabsorption, constipation, nausea, vomiting, and bloating.

Because of the indolent nature of chronic mesenteric ischemia, the average patient has had symptoms for at least a year before diagnosis.[6,7] As a result, malnutrition occurs in a high proportion of patients. One in six patients evaluated recently at Mayo Clinic with the condition had lost more than 30% of ideal body weight by the time they came to diagnosis and treatment (Table 1). In addition, 60%

Table 1.—Weight Loss in Patients Presenting With Chronic Mesenteric Ischemia

Weight at presentation, % of ideal body weight	Patients (n = 103)	
	No.	%
< 90	51	50
< 80	31	30
< 70	17	16
< 60	4	4

of patients have concomitant vascular disease affecting other arteries (i.e., cerebral, coronary, or peripheral arteries). These factors contribute to the increased morbidity and mortality associated with treatment.

DIAGNOSIS

Any attempt to diagnose chronic mesenteric ischemia must first start with a high suspicion based on the above-mentioned clinical clues. Frequently, the patient has undergone a multitude of noncontributory tests by the time the diagnosis of chronic mesenteric ischemia is entertained. Testing the blood usually reveals no specific abnormalities, although an occasional patient has anemia, hypoalbuminemia, or abnormal results of liver function tests. Radiographs of the abdomen typically show a nonspecific gas pattern. Ultrasonography of the gallbladder may show stones or, rarely, a thickened gallbladder wall suggesting acalculous cholecystitis. These findings frequently divert the clinician away from the diagnosis of chronic mesenteric ischemia and lead to cholecystectomy with little subsequent improvement in symptoms. Occasionally, a patient has evidence of gastric erosions on upper endoscopy as a result of concomitant chronic gastric ischemia.

Although noninvasive diagnosis of mesenteric artery stenosis was first described in 1984,[8] criteria for diagnosis with duplex ultrasonography were not established until the report of Moneta et al. in 1991.[9] The criteria were based on the principle that peak systolic velocity and end-diastolic velocity of blood flow through the artery increase in extensive mesenteric artery stenosis. In the superior mesenteric artery (SMA), a peak systolic velocity more than 275 cm/s or no flow accurately predicts a 70% to 100% stenosis with a sensitivity of 89%, a specificity of 92%, and an accuracy of 96%.[9,10] An end-diastolic velocity in the SMA of 45 cm/s or more is predictive of a 50% or more stenosis with a sensitivity of 90%, a specificity of 91%, and an accuracy of 91%.[11,12] Criteria for establishing a substantial celiac artery stenosis are not as accurate. Celiac peak systolic velocity 200 cm/s or more

has a sensitivity of 87%, specificity of 82%, and accuracy of 100%, and celiac end-diastolic velocity of 35 cm/s or more has a sensitivity of 80%, specificity of 93%, and accuracy of 95%.[9-12] Other supportive information suggestive of celiac stenosis or occlusion includes documentation of retrograde flow in the hepatic artery. Although combining fasting and postprandial duplex ultrasonography may improve specificity and positive predictive value, it has not been shown to improve overall accuracy.[13] For this reason, we have stopped performing postprandial duplex studies. The results of duplex ultrasonography of the mesenteric vessels may be technician- and patient-dependent. In 10% of patients, the results of duplex ultrasonography are nondiagnostic. In addition, duplex ultrasonography examines only the proximal portions of the SMA and celiac artery. Therefore, when the diagnosis of stenosis is highly suspected, a negative result should not deter the clinician from performing a more definitive test, such as magnetic resonance angiography of the abdomen or visceral arteriography.

Computed tomography, although frequently negative, is usually performed to rule out other potential conditions, such as pancreatitis or malignancy. Calcific plaques at the origins of the celiac artery and SMA are suggestive of chronic mesenteric ischemia but are not diagnostic. Computed tomography is helpful for planning the appropriate mesenteric reconstructive procedure by demonstrating the extent of calcific atherosclerotic plaques involving the supraceliac, paravisceral, and infrarenal aorta. If the visceral arteries are heavily involved with long atherosclerotic plaques and yet the aorta is relatively spared, mesenteric bypass is preferred over transaortic visceral endarterectomy. However, if the aorta is diffusely involved and yet the plaque in the visceral arteries extends only 1 to 2 cm from the origin, then transaortic visceral endarterectomy may be an excellent option.

Visceral arteriography has been the standard test for demonstrating the anatomy of the mesenteric circulation ever since being introduced in 1929 by dos Santos et al.[14] It must be performed in the anterior-posterior and lateral projections not only to demonstrate the branches of the celiac artery, the SMA, and the inferior mesenteric artery but also to visualize the origins of these arteries, because they arise off the anterior aspect of the aorta. The arteriography must be sequenced so that delayed films are obtained to identify the collateral mesenteric circulation and the direction of flow through these collateral vessels. Determining directional flow through these collateral vessels provides a functional importance to stenoses and occlusions. Unfortunately, the finding of extensive mesenteric occlusive disease is not uncommon and does not necessarily correlate with the presence of symptoms typical of chronic mesenteric ischemia. In fact, the frequency of asymptomatic extensive (defined as >50% stenosis) visceral artery disease increases with age and approaches 6% to 8% of patients studied.[15,16] Thus, the decision to operate on patients with visceral artery stenosis or occlusion must be placed into context with the presenting symptoms.

Debatable is the management of asymptomatic patients with substantial visceral artery stenosis or occlusion (i.e., >50% stenosis of at least two of the three major visceral vessels). The potential risk for development of subsequent acute or chronic mesenteric ischemic symptoms must be weighed against the risk of a major operation.[16,17] We have tended to be on the conservative side because of the extensive nature of the operation and the usual presence of substantial comorbidity in this group of patients. We advocate close observation unless the patient becomes symptomatic. Prophylactic mesenteric revascularization may be indicated in the rare patient who is undergoing an infrarenal aortic operation, who has extensive obstructive disease of the SMA and celiac arteries, and in whom the inferior mesenteric artery provides most of the collateral circulation to the intestine. Similarly, in the patient with renovascular disease undergoing transaortic renal endarterectomy, the endarterectomy may be extended to include the origins of the SMA and celiac artery if substantial disease is present in those vessels.

Most recently, interest has been increasing in magnetic resonance angiography of the visceral vessels, especially contrast-enhanced magnetic resonance angiography. Because of spatial limitations, only the main portions of the visceral vessels may be demonstrated. Typically, this includes the major divisions of the celiac artery, the proximal 5 to 8 cm of the SMA, and the main portion of the inferior mesenteric artery, but not its branches. Magnetic resonance angiography of the visceral vessels has the same limitations as conventional angiography in that the anatomy of the circulation is identified but not the functional importance of the identified lesions. Its advantages over conventional arteriography are that it is less costly and less invasive and does not require the use of potentially nephrotoxic contrast media. When magnetic resonance angiography was compared with conventional visceral arteriography, both tests found a substantial stenosis in 92% of arteries studied[18] (Fig. 1). This mirrors our experience with contrast-enhanced magnetic resonance angiography. As we have gained experience and confidence with this technique, we are increasingly using it without conventional angiography. Preliminary work with two-dimensional phase contrast magnetic resonance angiography and magnetic resonance oximetry has been done to measure oxygen extraction by the bowel and blood flow to assess the consequences of an extensive visceral artery

stenosis.[19-24] Because of the complexity and the time involved to generate this information, this has remained mainly a research tool to date.

TREATMENT

Choice of Operation

Appropriate treatment for chronic mesenteric ischemia has centered around reestablishing normal mesenteric blood flow by surgical revascularization, by percutaneous transluminal angioplasty, or by stenting. Despite recognition of this disease early in the 20th century, the first successful mesenteric revascularization for chronic mesenteric ischemia was not reported until 1958.[25] Since that time, controversy mainly has centered around the best revascularization technique and the number of visceral vessels to be reconstructed. Surgical revascularization techniques have been based either on visceral bypass with an antegrade or a retrograde approach or on transaortic visceral endarterectomy. Rarely, reimplantation or patch angioplasty of the origin of the visceral vessels may be an option. In our experience, nearly 80% of visceral reconstructions have been done with antegrade bypass grafts, 14% with retrograde bypass grafts, and 8% with visceral endarterectomy.

We have favored antegrade bypass grafts because the supraceliac aorta is relatively spared of atherosclerotic plaque. We are able to sew a bifurcated graft to the supraceliac aorta, providing a wide proximal anastomosis and allowing multiple bypasses distally to the celiac artery and the SMA. We have preferred this approach over the lower thoracic aorta because of the increased morbidity associated with a combined transthoracic and transperitoneal approach. Theoretically, an antegrade graft causes less turbulence in the bloodstream because blood is flowing in a prograde fashion. Therefore, the long-term patency may be better with antegrade than with retrograde grafts.

In the literature, there are proponents for both antegrade[3,7,26-31] and retrograde[32-36] grafts. Statistically, there is no clear advantage of one type of graft over the other. We also have favored multiple visceral artery revascularizations, when indicated, to lessen the risk of recurrent symptoms and to improve long-term survival. Symptomatic recurrence has been reported to be as high as 50% when only one visceral artery is bypassed. In our experience with multiple visceral artery revascularizations, the recurrence rate was only 11%.[6,7] The surgeon treating patients with chronic mesenteric ischemia should be well versed in all three surgical approaches, because any particular patient may require one type of reconstruction and not another, depending on the anatomical or clinical constraints.

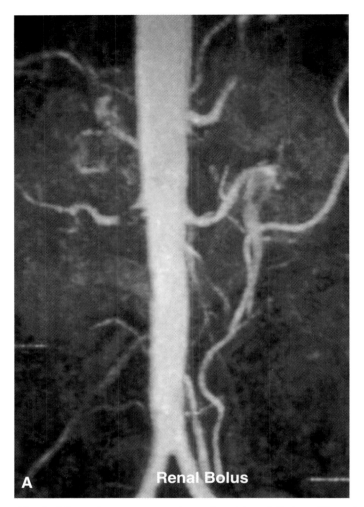 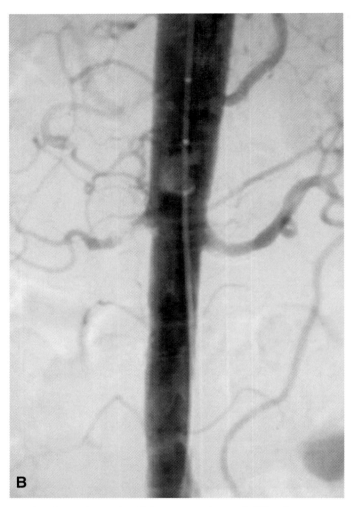

Fig. 1. Magnetic resonance angiography with gadolinium (A) *and conventional arteriography of the mesenteric vessels* (B). *Anteroposterior views.*

Operative Technique

An upper midline abdominal incision is performed from the xiphoid to just below the umbilicus. After a thorough abdominal exploration to exclude an undetected malignancy and to document the presence or absence of visceral artery pulsations, the triangular ligament of the left lobe of the liver is divided. The left lobe of the liver is then retracted to the patient's right. The gastrohepatic ligament is divided and the lesser sac is entered. The stomach is retracted inferiorly by the first assistant's left hand, and the distal intra-abdominal esophagus is retracted to the patient's left. The anterior aspect of the supraceliac aorta is palpated, and the crura of the diaphragm are divided over the aorta. Dissection is carried superiorly and inferiorly to expose the aorta from the upper aspect of the diaphragm down to the celiac artery. Care is taken to expose the anterior and lateral aspects of the aorta but not the posterior aspect for fear of causing injury and bleeding from the intercostal or lumbar arteries. Once this has

been accomplished, the distal target arteries are exposed. Because the patient is usually cachectic, the common hepatic artery is easily identified just superior to the distal stomach in the lesser sac. The common hepatic artery is exposed distally until it bifurcates into the proper hepatic and gastroduodenal branches. This allows an adequate length of hepatic artery for a spatulated distal anastomosis.

Exposure of the SMA is achieved by reflecting the transverse colon and its mesocolon superiorly. The ligament of Treitz is taken down to allow passage of the operator's right hand around the base of the small bowel mesentery. The SMA is identified by rolling one's thumb over the anterior aspect of the base of the small bowel mesentery, feeling for a tubular structure. This part of the operation may be difficult because of the lack of pulsations in the SMA. Dissection is done through a longitudinal incision in the base of the small bowel mesentery to expose the anterior aspect of the SMA. If the superior mesenteric vein is encountered first, dissection must be done to the patient's left to identify the

SMA. The SMA is exposed for a distance of 3 to 4 cm, and its branches are carefully controlled with small vessel loops. We occasionally have used a self-retaining retractor to spread the mesentery and help expose the SMA. A tunnel is created from the SMA back up to the supraceliac aorta. This may be done either anterior or posterior to the pancreas. We have preferred the posterior route because the graft is protected from the stomach and bowel in this position. The tunnel is created by making a hole through the base of the transverse mesocolon on the left side of the middle colic artery. With finger dissection, one finger is passed superiorly to inferiorly from the supraceliac aorta, behind the celiac artery, and to the left of the aorta. The other finger is passed inferiorly to superiorly through the hole in the transverse mesocolon, behind the pancreas until the two fingers meet. Frequently, a Kelly clamp must be passed to make an opening through the crura of the diaphragm.

The patient is then systemically heparinized. Frequently, mannitol and furosemide also are administered before suprarenal aortic clamping to promote a vigorous diuresis. A bifurcated graft (12 x 7 mm) is chosen. Five minutes after the heparin and other drugs are given, the supraceliac aorta is clamped. This can be done with a partial occlusion clamp, but our preference has been to occlude the proximal and distal aspects of the supraceliac aorta with individual clamps. A longitudinal aortotomy is made as high up on the supraceliac aorta as is comfortable. The body of the bifurcated graft is cut not only on the bevel but also slightly on the oblique so the left limb of the graft once sewn in will lie slightly posterior to the right limb. This directs the left limb toward the tunnel behind the pancreas. On completion of the proximal anastomosis (Fig. 2), the supraceliac aortic clamps are removed—first the proximal one to allow flushing of the proximal aorta out the limbs of the graft, followed by the distal aortic clamp. This allows any clot or atheromatous debris to be removed before reestablishing distal flow down the aorta. With the common hepatic artery controlled proximally and distally, a longitudinal incision is made on the anterosuperior aspect of the common hepatic artery. The right limb is brought to the common hepatic artery, cut to fit in a beveled fashion, and sewn in with a 5-0 or 6-0 polypropylene suture (Fig. 3). Once this anastomosis is complete, flow is restored through the right limb into the common hepatic artery. Next, the left limb is passed through the previously created retropancreatic tunnel down to the SMA. With control of the SMA and its branches, a longitudinal arteriotomy of about 2 cm in length is made on the anterior aspect of the SMA. The left limb of the graft is cut to fit and sewn in with a 6-0 polypropylene suture. Flow is restored through the left limb into the SMA.

Retrograde bypass grafts originate from the infrarenal aorta or iliac arteries depending on the location of substantial aortic plaque. Traditionally, these grafts have originated from the proximal infrarenal aorta. Unfortunately, because of the short distance between the proximal infrarenal aorta and the SMA, the grafts are frequently made too long. This leads to kinking of the graft when the small bowel is returned to its anatomical position. Foley et al.[36] recommend making a reverse C-loop configuration of the graft, with the origin of the graft arising from the distal infrarenal aorta or the iliac arteries and curving around to end on the anterior aspect of the SMA at the base of the small bowel mesentery (Fig. 4). We have used this technique on several occasions.

Interest in transaortic endarterectomy dates back to Stoney and Wylie's report in 1973,[37] in which they describe approaching the paravisceral aorta through a thoraco-abdominal approach. Unfortunately, this approach was associated with increased morbidity and mortality because two body cavities are entered. In 1994, Reilly et al.,[38] from the same institution, reported on the use of the transperitoneal left medial visceral rotation for exposure of the paravisceral aorta for elective visceral artery reconstruction. Compared with the thoracoabdominal approach, this operation was

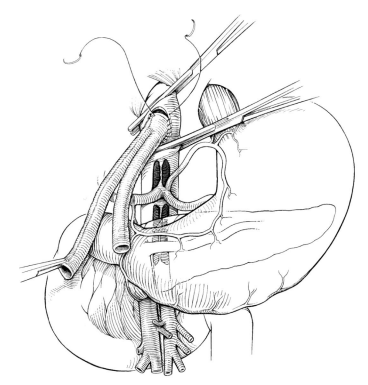

Fig. 2. Supraceliac antegrade aortic bifurcated graft anastomosis. (Modified from Kazmers A: Operative management of chronic mesenteric ischemia. Ann Vasc Surg 12:299-308, 1998. By permission of the journal.)

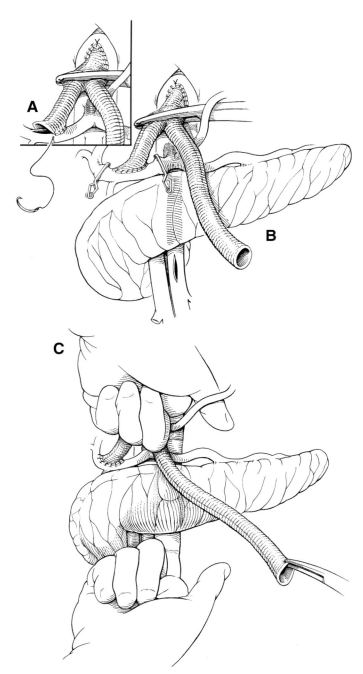

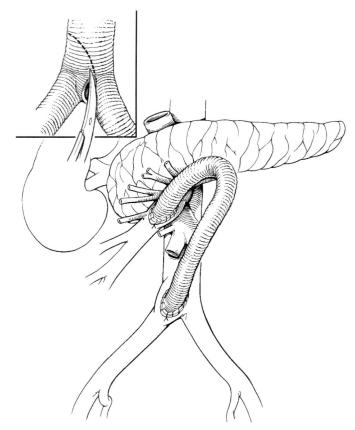

Fig. 4. *C-shaped retrograde graft from the distal abdominal aorta to the superior mesenteric artery. This is used to avoid kinking. (Modified from Foley et al.[36] By permission of Mosby.)*

Fig. 3. *Supraceliac aortic bifurcated graft to the hepatic artery (A and B) and to the superior mesenteric artery (not illustrated). Note the retropancreatic tunnel created for the limb going to the superior mesenteric artery (C). (Modified from Kazmers A: Operative management of chronic mesenteric ischemia. Ann Vasc Surg 12:299-308, 1998. By permission of the journal.)*

associated with reduced mortality. In properly selected patients, this approach provides excellent exposure for transaortic visceral endarterectomy by way of a "trapdoor" aortotomy. Visceral revascularization with this approach is best suited for patients with proximal occlusive disease

(involving the first 1-2 cm of the visceral vessels) and those with concomitant renal artery occlusive disease.

After a midline transperitoneal incision from xiphoid to pubis, the lateral peritoneal attachments to the left colon and splenic flexure of the colon are divided. A retroperitoneal plane behind the colon is created and is extended superiorly behind the spleen and pancreas through the splenophrenic ligament. The spleen, pancreas, and colon are retracted medially, and the plane is extended anterior to the fascia of Gerota, leaving the left kidney posterior. The left crus of the diaphragm is divided longitudinally along the left lateral wall of the aorta. The supraceliac aorta is exposed and mobilized to allow proximal aortic control. Dissection is extended inferiorly, exposing the origins of the celiac and SMA arteries. The left renal vein is identified, and the left adrenal and gonadal veins are ligated and divided. This provides extensive mobilization of the left renal vein to allow better exposure of the renal arteries and the pararenal aorta.

Once all the visceral arteries have been exposed and adequately mobilized, the patient is heparinized. Each of the visceral arteries is controlled distally with either vessel loops or clamps. The infrarenal aorta is controlled, followed by the supraceliac aorta. A longitudinal aortotomy is made in a "trapdoor" fashion extending between the renal arteries, running on the left lateral wall of the aorta around the origins of the superior mesenteric and celiac arteries and curving to the right side of the supraceliac aorta. The endarterectomy plane is begun in the aortic wall and extended around the origins of the visceral vessels. Only after this has been done can the eversion endarterectomy of the visceral arteries begin (Fig. 5 and 6). The key to adequate transaortic endarterectomy is to expose and mobilize each of the arteries for 3 to 4 cm distally. This facilitates delivery of the arterial branch into the lumen of the aorta, helping with the eversion endarterectomy. On completion of the transaortic endarterectomy, the aortotomy is closed with 3-0 or 4-0 polypropylene. Before completion of the closure, the proximal aorta is flushed out by way of the aortotomy, and heparin is instilled into the aorta. Once the aortotomy is completed, the aortic clamps are removed, followed by the renal artery clamps and then by the SMA and celiac artery clamps. About 5 minutes before release of the aortic clamps, the anesthesiologist needs to be alerted, so that time is allowed to increase the patient's intravascular volume and blood pressure so as to avoid severe hypotension after the unclamping.

We have used intraoperative flow probes to measure flow through the limbs of the grafts. Typically, the flow is more than 1,000 mL/min. Flows less than 400 mL/min are suggestive of eventual graft failure.[7] We also have used intraoperative duplex ultrasonography to document patency of our grafts and to document prograde flow through the common hepatic and superior mesenteric arteries. Intraoperative duplex ultrasonography is especially useful when performing a transaortic endarterectomy, because this test can demonstrate clearly the distal end point of the endarterectomy to ensure that there is not a residual obstructing plaque or an intimal flap. Because of the loss of arteriolar tone and the subsequent development of the capillary leak syndrome, patients frequently require 10 to 20 L of crystalloid to maintain their intravascular filling pressures for the first 24 to 48 hours postoperatively. This tremendous shift in fluids must be anticipated so the patient does not become hypotensive and hypercoagulable. This capillary leak syndrome typically corrects itself in 48 to 72 hours with a swing of extravascular fluids into the intravascular compartment. This fluid shift also should be anticipated and diuretic therapy begun on the second or third day to avoid pulmonary edema.

Results of Operation

Results from visceral artery revascularization are durable and effective for relieving symptoms of mesenteric ischemia. Objective long-term graft patency has been found in 71% to 95% of patients.[30,36,39,40] Long-term relief from symptoms of chronic mesenteric ischemia is achieved in about 90% of patients (Table 2).[7] Operative mortality and long-term survival are adversely affected when concomitant vascular procedures are performed (i.e., renal or

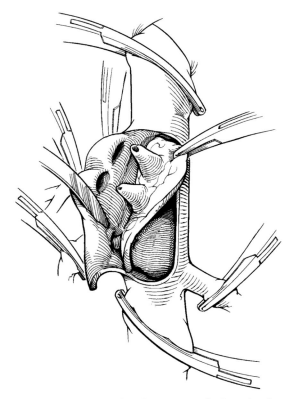

Fig. 5. Transaortic visceral endarterectomy by "trapdoor" approach by way of the left side of the proximal abdominal aorta.

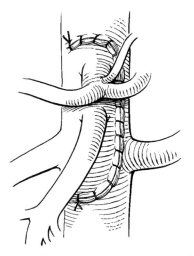

Fig. 6. Closure of the "trapdoor" aortotomy after transaortic endarterectomy.

aortic revascularizations).[7] For this reason, we try to focus the operation toward only revascularization of the mesenteric vessels. We do not add concomitant procedures unless circumstances dictate otherwise.

Angioplasty and Stenting of Visceral Arteries

Because of the high incidence of extensive comorbidity in patients with chronic mesenteric ischemia, percutaneous transluminal angioplasty with stenting of the visceral arteries has seemed to be a logical approach. In 1980, Furrer et al.[45] reported the first case of percutaneous transluminal angioplasty of the SMA. Since then, several case reports and a few small series have been reported. Results of series containing five or more patients are reviewed in Table 3. According to these studies, angioplasty with stenting has a high initial technical success

Table 2.—Results of Operative Management of Chronic Mesenteric Ischemia

Reference	Year	No. of patients	No. of vessels revascularized	Follow-up, mo	Technical success	Immediate pain relief	Long-term pain relief	Complications	Mortality rate	Patency
Kieny et al.[41]	1990	60	69	102	100	NA	NA	NA	3.5	75
Cormier et al.[42]	1991	32	90	69	100	NA	NA	NA	9	91
Cunningham et al.[26]	1991	74	194	71	100	100	86	17	12	NA
McAfee et al.[7]	1992	58	119	60	100	NA	90	41	10	90
Calderon et al.[32]	1992	20	36	36	100	100	100	20	0	100
Christensen et al.[43]	1994	90	109	55	100	NA	63	NA	13	NA
Gentile et al.[13]	1995	26	29	48	100	100	89	NA	10	89
Johnston et al.[3]	1995	21	43	120	100	NA	NA	19	0	86
Moawad and Gewertz[2]	1997	24	38	60	100	100	78	45	4	78
Kasirajan et al.[44]	2001	85	130	36	100	100	87	33	8	76
Mean		49	86	66	100	100	85	29	7	86
SD		28	53	27			12	12		9

NA, not available.
From Kasirajan et al.[44] By permission of Mosby.

Table 3.—Results of Percutaneous Management of Chronic Mesenteric Ischemia

Reference	Year	No. of patients	No. of vessels revascularized	Follow-up, mo	Technical success	Immediate pain relief	Long-term pain relief	Complications	Mortality rate	Patency
Matsumoto et al.[46]	1995	19	20	25	79	63	52	32	0	NA
Hallisey et al.[47]	1995	16	25	28	84	81	75	6	6	75
Allen et al.[48]	1996	19	24	39	95	79	79	5	5	NA
Maspes et al.[49]	1998	23	41	27	90	77	75	9	0	88
Nyman et al.[50]	1998	5	6	21	100	80	80	40	0	40
Sheeran et al.[51]	1999	12	13	16	92	92	75	NA	8	74
Kasirajan et al.[44]	2001	28	32	36	100	NA	66	18	11	73
Mean		17	23	27	91	79	72	18	4	70
SD		7	12	8	8	9	10	15		18

NA, not available.
From Kasirajan et al.[44] By permission of Mosby.

rate (79%-100%), restenosis occurs in 10% to 25% of patients, and results from stenting appear to be better than results from angioplasty and are slightly inferior to those from surgical revascularization.

Despite these encouraging results with percutaneous transluminal angioplasty and stenting, we continue to advocate surgical visceral artery revascularization in patients who are of acceptable risk. We believe that this provides the most successful and durable results. Among patients who are not surgical candidates and who have symptomatic visceral artery stenosis or short segment occlusions, angioplasty with stenting is a reasonable alternative.

CONCLUSION

Patients with chronic mesenteric ischemia present late. Usually, they are malnourished and dehydrated at presentation. This condition creates distinct challenges for effective diagnosis and treatment of this disorder. Successful and prompt diagnosis is centered on a high suspicion. Duplex ultrasonography and magnetic resonance arteriography are excellent tests for identifying extensive visceral artery stenosis or occlusions, although conventional angiography remains the standard. In carefully selected patients, surgical revascularization provides long-lasting relief. In those unsuitable for operation, percutaneous transluminal angioplasty with stenting offers a reasonable alternative.

REFERENCES

1. Shanley CJ, Ozaki CK, Zelenock GB: Bypass grafting for chronic mesenteric ischemia. Surg Clin North Am 77:381-395, 1997
2. Moawad J, Gewertz BL: Chronic mesenteric ischemia: clinical presentation and diagnosis. Surg Clin North Am 77:357-369, 1997
3. Johnston KW, Lindsay TF, Walker PM, Kalman PG: Mesenteric arterial bypass grafts: early and late results and suggested surgical approach for chronic and acute mesenteric ischemia. Surgery 118:1-7, 1995
4. Rheudasil JM, Stewart MT, Schellack JV, Smith RB III, Salam AA, Perdue GD: Surgical treatment of chronic mesenteric arterial insufficiency. J Vasc Surg 8:495-500, 1988
5. Dunphy JE: Abdominal pain of vascular origin. Am J Med Sci 192:109-113, 1936
6. Hollier LH, Bernatz PE, Pairolero PC, Payne WS, Osmundson PJ: Surgical management of chronic intestinal ischemia: a reappraisal. Surgery 90:940-946, 1981
7. McAfee MK, Cherry KJ Jr, Naessens JM, Pairolero PC, Hallett JW Jr, Gloviczki P, Bower TC: Influence of complete revascularization on chronic mesenteric ischemia. Am J Surg 164:220-224, 1992
8. Jager KA, Fortner GS, Thiele BL, Strandness DE: Noninvasive diagnosis of intestinal angina. J Clin Ultrasound 12:588-591, 1984
9. Moneta GL, Yeager RA, Dalman R, Antonovic R, Hall LD, Porter JM: Duplex ultrasound criteria for diagnosis of splanchnic artery stenosis or occlusion. J Vasc Surg 14:511-518, 1991
10. Moneta GL, Lee RW, Yeager RA, Taylor LM Jr, Porter JM: Mesenteric duplex scanning: a blinded prospective study. J Vasc Surg 17:79-84, 1993
11. Bowersox JC, Zwolak RM, Walsh DB, Schneider JR, Musson A, LaBombard FE, Cronenwett JL: Duplex ultrasonography in the diagnosis of celiac and mesenteric artery occlusive disease. J Vasc Surg 14:780-786, 1991
12. Zwolak RM, Fillinger MF, Walsh DB, LaBombard FE, Musson A, Darling CE, Cronenwett JL: Mesenteric and celiac duplex scanning: a validation study. J Vasc Surg 27:1078-1087, 1998
13. Gentile AT, Moneta GL, Lee RW, Masser PA, Taylor LM Jr, Porter JM: Usefulness of fasting and postprandial duplex ultrasound examinations for predicting high-grade superior mesenteric artery stenosis. Am J Surg 169:476-479, 1995
14. dos Santos R, Lamas A, Pereira Caldas J: L'artéropgraphie des membres de l'aorte et de ses branches abdominales. Bull Mem Soc Natl Chir 55:587-601, 1929
15. Croft RJ, Menon GP, Marston A: Does 'intestinal angina' exist? A critical study of obstructed visceral arteries. Br J Surg 68:316-318, 1981
16. Thomas JH, Blake K, Pierce GE, Hermreck AS, Seigel E: The clinical course of asymptomatic mesenteric arterial stenosis. J Vasc Surg 27:840-844, 1998
17. Kaleya RN, Sammartano RJ, Boley SJ: Aggressive approach to acute mesenteric ischemia. Surg Clin North Am 72:157-182, 1992
18. Meaney JF, Prince MR, Nostrant TT, Stanley JC: Gadolinium-enhanced MR angiography of visceral arteries in patients with suspected chronic mesenteric ischemia. J Magn Reson Imaging 7:171-176, 1997
19. Li KC, Whitney WS, McDonnell CH, Fredrickson JO, Pelc NJ, Dalman RL, Jeffrey RB Jr: Chronic mesenteric ischemia: evaluation with phase-contrast cine MR imaging. Radiology 190:175-179, 1994

20. Naganawa S, Cooper TG, Jenner G, Potchen EJ, Ishigaki T: Flow velocity and volume measurement of superior and inferior mesenteric artery with cine phase contrast magnetic resonance imaging. Radiat Med 12:213-220, 1994

21. Li KC, Hopkins KL, Dalman RL, Song CK: Simultaneous measurement of flow in the superior mesenteric vein and artery with cine phase-contrast MR imaging: value in diagnosis of chronic mesenteric ischemia. Radiology 194:327-330, 1995

22. Burkart DJ, Johnson CD, Reading CC, Ehman RL: MR measurements of mesenteric venous flow: prospective evaluation in healthy volunteers and patients with suspected chronic mesenteric ischemia. Radiology 194:801-806, 1995

23. Li KC, Wright GA, Pelc LR, Dalman RL, Brittain JH, Wegmueller H, Lin DT, Song CK: Oxygen saturation of blood in the superior mesenteric vein: in vivo verification of MR imaging measurements in a canine model. Radiology 194:321-325, 1995

24. Li KC, Dalman RL, Ch'en IY, Pelc LR, Song CK, Moon WK, Kang MI, Wright GA: Chronic mesenteric ischemia: use of in vivo MR imaging measurements of blood oxygen saturation in the superior mesenteric vein for diagnosis. Radiology 204:71-77, 1997

25. Shaw RS, Maynard EP III: Acute and chronic thrombosis of the mesenteric arteries associated with malabsorption: report of two cases successfully treated by thromboendarterectomy. N Engl J Med 258:874-878, 1958

26. Cunningham CG, Reilly LM, Rapp JH, Schneider PA, Stoney RJ: Chronic visceral ischemia: three decades of progress. Ann Surg 214:276-287, 1991

27. MacFarlane SD, Beebe HG: Progress in chronic mesenteric arterial ischemia. J Cardiovasc Surg (Torino) 30:178-184, 1989

28. Moawad J, McKinsey JF, Wyble CW, Bassiouny HS, Schwartz LB, Gewertz BL: Current results of surgical therapy for chronic mesenteric ischemia. Arch Surg 132:613-618, 1997

29. Stoney RJ, Ehrenfeld WK, Wylie EJ: Revascularization methods in chronic visceral ischemia caused by atherosclerosis. Ann Surg 186:468-476, 1977

30. Beebe HG, MacFarlane S, Raker EJ: Supraceliac aortomesenteric bypass for intestinal ischemia. J Vasc Surg 5:749-754, 1987

31. Rapp JH, Reilly LM, Qvarfordt PG, Goldstone J, Ehrenfeld WK, Stoney RJ: Durability of endarterectomy and antegrade grafts in the treatment of chronic visceral ischemia. J Vasc Surg 3:799-806, 1986

32. Calderon M, Reul GJ, Gregoric ID, Jacobs MJ, Duncan JM, Ott DA, Livesay JJ, Cooley DA: Long-term results of the surgical management of symptomatic chronic intestinal ischemia. J Cardiovasc Surg (Torino) 33:723-728, 1992

33. Taylor LM Jr, Porter JM: Colonic ischemia following aortic reconstruction. Semin Vasc Surg 3:200-205, 1990

34. McCollum CH, Graham JM, DeBakey ME: Chronic mesenteric arterial insufficiency: results of revascularization in 33 cases. South Med J 69:1266-1268, 1976

35. Baur GM, Millay DJ, Taylor LM Jr, Porter JM: Treatment of chronic visceral ischemia. Am J Surg 148:138-144, 1984

36. Foley MI, Moneta GL, Abou-Zamzam AM Jr, Edwards JM, Taylor LM Jr, Yeager RA, Porter JM: Revascularization of the superior mesenteric artery alone for treatment of intestinal ischemia. J Vasc Surg 32:37-47, 2000

37. Stoney RJ, Wylie EJ: Surgical management of arterial lesions of the thoracoabdominal aorta. Am J Surg 126:157-164, 1973

38. Reilly LM, Ramos TK, Murray SP, Cheng SW, Stoney RJ: Optimal exposure of the proximal abdominal aorta: a critical appraisal of transabdominal medial visceral rotation. J Vasc Surg 19:375-389, 1994

39. McMillan WD, McCarthy WJ, Bresticker MR, Pearce WH, Schneider JR, Golan JF, Yao JS: Mesenteric artery bypass: objective patency determination. J Vasc Surg 21:729-740, 1995

40. Mateo RB, O'Hara PJ, Hertzer NR, Mascha EJ, Beven EG, Krajewski LP: Elective surgical treatment of symptomatic chronic mesenteric occlusive disease: early results and late outcomes. J Vasc Surg 29:821-831, 1999

41. Kieny R, Batellier J, Kretz JG: Aortic reimplantation of the superior mesenteric artery for atherosclerotic lesions of the visceral arteries: sixty cases. Ann Vasc Surg 4:122-125, 1990

42. Cormier JM, Fichelle JM, Vennin J, Laurian C, Gigou F: Atherosclerotic occlusive disease of the superior mesenteric artery: late results of reconstructive surgery. Ann Vasc Surg 5:510-518, 1991

43. Christensen MG, Lorentzen JE, Schroeder TV: Revascularisation of atherosclerotic mesenteric arteries: experience in 90 consecutive patients. Eur J Vasc Surg 8:297-302, 1994

44. Kasirajan K, O'Hara PJ, Gray BH, Hertzer NR, Clair DG, Greenberg RK, Krajewski LP, Beven EG, Ouriel K: Chronic mesenteric ischemia: open surgery versus percutaneous angioplasty and stenting. J Vasc Surg 33:63-71, 2001

45. Furrer J, Gruntzig A, Kugelmeier J, Goebel N: Treatment of abdominal angina with percutaneous dilatation of an arteria mesenterica superior stenosis: preliminary communication. Cardiovasc Intervent Radiol 3:43-44, 1980

46. Matsumoto AH, Tegtmeyer CJ, Fitzcharles EK, Selby JB Jr, Tribble CG, Angle JF, Kron IL: Percutaneous transluminal angioplasty of visceral arterial stenoses: results and long-term clinical follow-up. J Vasc Interv Radiol 6:165-174, 1995

47. Hallisey MJ, Deschaine J, Illescas FF, Sussman SK, Vine HS, Ohki SK, Straub JJ: Angioplasty for the treatment of visceral ischemia. J Vasc Interv Radiol 6:785-791, 1995

48. Allen RC, Martin GH, Rees CR, Rivera FJ, Talkington CM, Garrett WV, Smith BL, Pearl GJ, Diamond NG, Lee SP, Thompson JE: Mesenteric angioplasty in the treatment of chronic intestinal ischemia. J Vasc Surg 24:415-421, 1996

49. Maspes F, Mazzetti di Pietralata G, Gandini R, Innocenzi L, Lupattelli L, Barzi F, Simonetti G: Percutaneous transluminal angioplasty in the treatment of chronic mesenteric ischemia: results and 3 years of follow-up in 23 patients. Abdom Imaging 23:358-363, 1998

50. Nyman U, Ivancev K, Lindh M, Uher P: Endovascular treatment of chronic mesenteric ischemia: report of five cases. Cardiovasc Intervent Radiol 21:305-313, 1998

51. Sheeran SR, Murphy TP, Khwaja A, Sussman SK, Hallisey MJ: Stent placement for treatment of mesenteric artery stenoses or occlusions. J Vasc Interv Radiol 10:861-867, 1999

Chapter 32

VISCERAL ARTERY ANEURYSMS

William M. Stone, M.D.
Maher A. Abbas, M.D.

Aneurysmal degeneration of the arteries that supply the abdominal viscera is an uncommon but potentially lethal condition. Only about 3,500 patients with visceral artery aneurysm have been reported in the English biomedical literature, most within the past 30 years. The most frequently affected vessel is the splenic artery, which accounts for almost 65% of all cases. Hepatic artery aneurysm is the next most common type, accounting for 20% of the total, whereas superior mesenteric artery (SMA) aneurysm accounts for 5%, celiac 4%, gastric and gastroepiploic 4%, jejunal, ileal, and colic 3%, and pancreatic, pancreaticoduodenal, and gastroduodenal 2% (Table 1). The frequency distribution of the various aneurysms has varied little over time.

In contrast, the etiologic and pathologic findings of visceral artery aneurysms do vary from one type of aneurysm to another. For example, splenic artery aneurysms are more common in women than in men and are more likely to be associated with cirrhosis and portal hypertension than are other types of visceral artery aneurysms. The natural history and risk of rupture also may vary from one type of aneurysm to another, but this difference is less clear-cut. Data on natural history and risk of rupture are scarce because of the lack of careful natural history studies, including population-controlled studies. Obtaining this information is difficult because these lesions are so rare.

Historically, visceral artery aneurysms were discovered only after they ruptured. However, with the increasing use of diagnostic imaging for nonspecific abdominal complaints, visceral aneurysms are being recognized more frequently at earlier stages. Computed tomography (CT), in particular, has facilitated the identification of unsuspected visceral artery aneurysms. After these lesions have been diagnosed, their management requires careful consideration.

Certainly, there is no question that operating is the best course of action to take when an aneurysm becomes symptomatic, enlarges rapidly, or ruptures. However, management of the asymptomatic aneurysm, which is based primarily on the limited data available about the risk of rupture, requires a different approach. Although any aneurysm can rupture, a complication that carries significant morbidity and mortality, the risk of rupture seems minimal for most lesions. Nonetheless, newly evolving endovascular and laparoscopic techniques have increased the tendency to intervene electively for pathologic conditions of the arteries. As these techniques become more advanced, elective operations for asymptomatic visceral artery aneurysms may be used more frequently.

Table 1.—Distribution of Visceral Artery Aneurysms

Artery site*	Percent of all visceral aneurysms
Splenic	65
Hepatic	20
Superior mesenteric	5
Celiac	4
Gastric, gastroepiploic	4
Jejunal, ileal, colic	3
Pancreatic, pancreaticoduodenal, gastroduodenal	2

*Some patients may have an aneurysm in two or more locations.

Because the etiologic and pathologic characteristics, and probably the natural history, of visceral artery aneurysms apparently vary from one type of aneurysm to another, we discuss each type separately.

SPLENIC ARTERY ANEURYSM

The splenic artery is the most common and most investigated visceral vessel with aneurysmal degeneration. Splenic artery aneurysms represent 60% to 70% of all aneurysms of the visceral vessels (Table 1). They have been described in more than 1,900 patients.[1] However, their true incidence and rate of rupture are not known. The reported incidence has been 0.098% to 10.4% of patients examined, depending on how rigorous a search for the entity is conducted.[2] True incidence remains elusive. Splenic artery aneurysms were identified in only 217 of 2,091,965 patients registered at Mayo Clinic (Rochester, Minnesota; Scottsdale, Arizona; and Jacksonville, Florida) between January 1980 and December 1998.[3] This figure represents an incidence of 0.01%, which is not a true incidence but one that underscores the rarity of the lesion. Stanley and Fry[4] reported an incidental finding of splenic artery aneurysm of 0.78% in more than 3,000 patients undergoing angiography. This figure most likely is representative of the actual incidence.

Most patients with splenic artery aneurysms are women, with a female-to-male ratio of about 4:1. This sex predilection probably is related to hormonal fluctuations, which have been implicated in the pathogenesis of these aneurysms. Although the precise cause of splenic artery aneurysms remains unclear, several possible causes have been suggested. These include atherosclerosis, arterial fibroplasia (with concomitant renal disease), arteritis, collagen vascular disease, α_1-antitrypsin deficiency, inflammatory and infectious disorders, hemodynamic and endocrine changes of pregnancy, pancreatitis, cirrhosis, and portal hypertension with splenomegaly.[5]

Multiple pregnancies are the most recognized factor; about 40% of all women with splenic artery aneurysms have had six or more pregnancies.[4] The hemodynamic changes of pregnancy include excessive blood flow through the splanchnic bed, which may contribute to the formation of aneurysmal degeneration. Hormonal changes may contribute to a loss of arterial wall integrity, perhaps because of the presence of estrogen and progesterone receptors in the arterial wall.[1] Human and animal studies have found degenerative changes in the splenic artery, including disruption of the internal elastic lamina, fragmentation of the elastic fibers, and fibroplasia of the media. Furthermore, relaxin, a gestational hormone secreted late in pregnancy that enhances the elasticity of the pubic symphysis, may act similarly on the arterial wall.[1]

Patients with portal hypertension also seem to have a predilection for splenic artery aneurysms. The hyperdynamic circulation that occurs with portal hypertension has been postulated as a key factor in the development of this aneurysmal degeneration. Patients with cirrhosis and portal hypertension also are known to have increased estrogen production.[6] These changes may be similar to those in patients who have had multiple pregnancies, thus accounting for the increased incidence of this type of aneurysm in patients with portal hypertension.

Atherosclerotic changes that occur in patients with splenic artery aneurysms are believed by many authors to be due to the aneurysms. Calcification of the aneurysm is a common finding; it has been noted in 90% of the patients with aneurysms who were examined at Mayo Clinic.[3] Unfortunately, calcification has no protective effect against rupture, as documented by several series.[6] Splenic artery aneurysms are generally solitary and saccular. They usually develop at branch points along the distal vessel or infrequently at proximal locations.[7]

Because of frequent calcification of these aneurysms, the first diagnosis is often made by radiography (Table 2). Plain radiography may show the first evidence of an aneurysm and usually is the only test required. Often, a calcified "ring" is observed in the left upper quadrant (Fig. 1). CT is used increasingly and can help to establish the diagnosis (Fig. 2). CT may show noncalcified aneurysms and evidence of a ruptured aneurysm, but it is probably used more typically for patients who present with symptoms. Ultrasonography also may be used diagnostically (Fig. 3). Angiography may show the aneurysm as an incidental finding (Fig. 4), which can be most useful in patients with portal hypertension who are undergoing angiography before a liver transplantation. Occasionally, magnetic resonance imaging may facilitate diagnosis, but this test plays a small role in the evaluation of these patients.

In most patients, the aneurysm is small (< 1.0 cm in diameter) and is an incidental finding. At Mayo Clinic, more than 90% of patients with an aneurysm presented without symptoms from it.[3] However, in another large series, 15% to 20% of patients presented with symptoms.[4] The most common symptom is vague abdominal pain often associated with rupture. The pain usually is located

Table 2.—Radiologic Tests Useful in the Diagnosis of Visceral Artery Aneurysms

Plain radiography of the abdomen
Computed tomography
Ultrasonography
Angiography

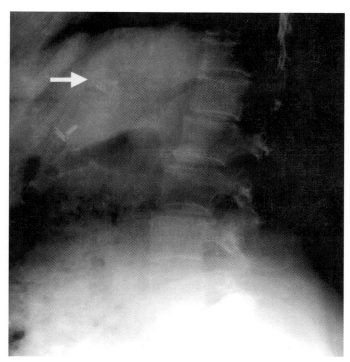

Fig. 1. Plain radiograph shows calcification (arrow) *in a splenic artery aneurysm.*

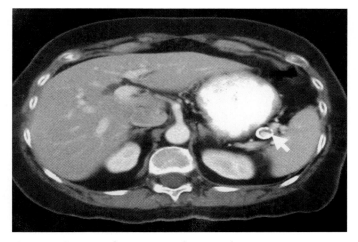

Fig. 2. Computed tomogram depicts splenic artery aneurysm (arrow).

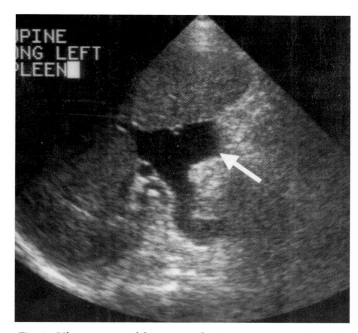

Fig. 3. Ultrasonogram delineates a splenic artery aneurysm (arrow).

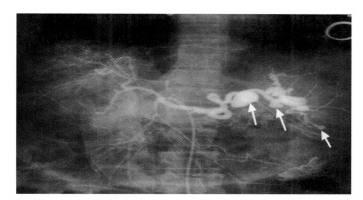

Fig. 4. Angiogram shows multiple splenic artery aneurysms (arrows).

in the epigastrium or left upper quadrant of the abdomen and may result in rapid aneurysmal expansion. The sudden onset of pain should alert the clinician to the possibility of a rupture. With the rupture of an aneurysm, bleeding generally fills the lesser sac and causes local symptoms. The lesser sac initially contains the hemorrhage, but then blood passes through the foramen of Winslow into the abdominal cavity. This "double rupture" phenomenon occurs in about 25% of patients.[8] Rupture during pregnancy may be confused with other obstetrical emergencies, which can cause inordinate delay to appropriate treatment.

The risk of rupture of a splenic artery aneurysm appears minimal. Most reports indicate about 2% of female patients who are not pregnant are at risk.[8] However, some authors report rupture rates during pregnancy as high as 95%.[9] Although most authors agree that the risk of rupture increases during pregnancy, aneurysms in pregnant women have a low risk of rupture. Aneurysmal calcification does not appear to have a protective effect. Several reports have linked the risk of rupture to the size of the aneurysm, cirrhosis, liver transplantation, and α_1-antitrypsin deficiency. As first noted by Trastek et al.[10] in 1982, the risk of rupture appears to be greater in patients with aneurysms that are more than 2 cm in diameter. The later Mayo data support this earlier finding.[3] The risk of rupture has been well documented in cirrhotic patients undergoing liver transplantation, because it often occurs within days of the transplantation. In a survey of 126 transplantation centers, Gaglio and colleagues[11] reported on 21 patients with ruptured splenic artery aneurysms who were awaiting transplantation or who had become transplant recipients. Of note is that 47% of these patients had α_1-antitrypsin deficiency. In most series, rupture mortality is 20% to 25%. However, if rupture occurs during pregnancy, maternal mortality is 70% and fetal mortality is 90% to 95%.[1] These high mortality rates have caused most authors to advocate intervention in pregnant patients.

Appropriate indications for intervention for patients with a splenic artery aneurysm are elusive. No treatment controversy exists for patients who present with a ruptured aneurysm, because this condition usually requires surgical exploration with ligation of the aneurysm and splenectomy. Endovascular embolization of ruptured aneurysms has been reported but is not the standard treatment. Splenectomy is required more often after a rupture and, in the Mayo Clinic series,[3] was required for all patients who had a ruptured aneurysm. Patients who present with symptoms or with an expanding aneurysm should undergo urgent intervention. When elective intervention is indicated, the potential rupture risk should be weighed against the risk of intervention. Intervention is warranted in pregnant women or in women of childbearing age, in patients with portal hypertension (particularly with α_1-antitrypsin deficiency), or in patients who have an aneurysm with a diameter of more than 2 cm. Ligation, using either an open procedure or a laparoscopic technique, is the primary elective intervention. Traditionally, splenectomy has been an elective intervention. However, recent experiences have led to simple ligation in most patients. Percutaneous embolization also should be considered, particularly for patients at increased risk during surgical intervention. Nonetheless, embolization is a less attractive option because of complications, such as splenic infarction and dissection of the celiac artery, and because of the possibility of inadequate embolization.

HEPATIC ARTERY ANEURYSM

The hepatic artery aneurysm makes up about 20% of all visceral artery aneurysms and is the second most common type of aneurysm.[12] Historically, this type of aneurysm has been found to be related to infectious causes. More contemporary reports suggest that infection is an atypical finding and that infectious agents cause less than 10% of all such aneurysms.[13] Atherosclerotic changes are the most common pathologic finding, but much debate has focused on whether these changes are primary or secondary. Most authors believe that atherosclerotic changes are due to hepatic artery aneurysms. Medial degeneration

of the hepatic artery is a frequent pathologic finding and may resemble the changes in other visceral artery aneurysms. In the Mayo Clinic series, atherosclerosis was the most typical pathologic finding, but medial degeneration was found in about 20% of patients.[14] Traumatic hepatic artery pseudoaneurysms also may be increasing, as intrahepatic and extrahepatic interventional techniques become more routine. Less frequently, connective tissue disorders may cause these lesions.

Most hepatic aneurysms are solitary and have a sex predilection for men, with a ratio as high as 2:1.[15] This male predominance may correlate with the increased frequency of atherosclerotic changes in these aneurysms identified by pathologic examination. The mean age at presentation is sometime in the 50s or 60s, with traumatic aneurysms occurring at a slightly younger age.[13] About 80% of all hepatic aneurysms are extrahepatic; the remainder are within the hepatic parenchyma.[13] Of the Mayo Clinic patients, 38% had an associated nonvisceral arterial aneurysm and 30% had associated malignancies.[14]

Symptoms of hepatic artery aneurysms may be related to rupture, rapid expansion, or erosion into surrounding structures. However, most aneurysms are discovered incidentally and rarely cause symptoms. Epigastric and right upper quadrant discomfort are the most common symptoms. With erosion into surrounding structures, biliary colic may occur and can lead to an erroneous diagnosis of acute cholecystitis. Diagnosis usually is made by CT or ultrasonography. Historically, these aneurysms were found on radiographs of the gastrointestinal tract using contrast media that revealed an extraluminal mass causing an indentation of the upper gastrointestinal tract. Most of these aneurysms are not calcified. Therefore, plain radiography is not sensitive in establishing the diagnosis. When symptoms do occur, CT is the preferred diagnostic test. Rupture of this type of aneurysm generally produces abdominal pain. Frequently, the aneurysm also has eroded into surrounding structures. Erosion is reported to accompany as many as 50% of all ruptures.[16] Erosion into the biliary tree may cause biliary colic or gastrointestinal bleeding. Symptoms may mimic those of pancreatitis. Intraperitoneal hemorrhage may result in hemodynamic instability. Intrahepatic aneurysms have a greater risk of rupture, but extrahepatic aneurysms occur more often.[17] The size of the aneurysm does not correlate with the risk of rupture.

We consider the presence of hepatic artery aneurysms to be an indication for operation. In most series, the risk of rupture was high (40%).[7] In the Mayo Clinic patients, 22% presented with rupture, mostly at intrahepatic locations.[14] Although surgical intervention is warranted when rupture occurs or symptoms develop because of the aneurysm, it also is justified for patients whose lesions are found incidentally. The smallest aneurysm that ruptured in our series was 1.8 cm in diameter.[14] The reported mortality from rupture is about 35%.[13]

Operative intervention should be planned preoperatively with as much anatomical information as possible. Preoperative angiography can be used to assess the exact location of the aneurysm and the status of any collateral blood flow. Aneurysms of the common hepatic artery that have excellent collateral blood flow may be ligated without concomitant revascularization,[13] which seems to be well tolerated. However, proper hepatic artery aneurysms frequently require concomitant revascularization. In the Mayo Clinic series, only 40% of hepatic aneurysms required revascularization.[14] The preferred conduit for reconstruction was usually the saphenous vein. However, prosthetic grafts were equally effective. Hepatic resection may be necessary occasionally but is unusual with extrahepatic aneurysms. Intervention with percutaneous embolization for intrahepatic artery aneurysms is used increasingly and appears justifiable in this group of patients.[18] Some hepatic necrosis may result from embolization, but it may be tolerated better in a given patient than would a major hepatic resection. Complications from embolization always should be considered both before and after embolization. An evaluation of the success of the procedure requires additional follow-up diagnostic studies.

SUPERIOR MESENTERIC ARTERY ANEURYSM

The SMA is the third most commonly affected visceral vessel with aneurysmal degeneration, accounting for 5% to 6% of all visceral artery aneurysms.[8] Historically, SMA aneurysms often seem to be infectious. Syphilitic aneurysms were the most frequent type of SMA aneurysm in the past, but they are now quite rare. Bacterial endocarditis also has been implicated in the development of SMA aneurysms, and it may be the most common cause.[13] However, in the Mayo Clinic series, only 5% of all SMA aneurysms had an infectious component.[19] Atherosclerotic changes in the SMA predominate in pathologic findings. However, as with hepatic aneurysms, these may be secondary rather than primary. Medial degeneration of the vessel wall also is prevalent.

Historically, women have been affected more than men. However, some authors have found no sex predilection.[13] Nevertheless, in the Mayo Clinic series, there was a male preponderance, with a ratio of 2:1.[19] Most patients who present with infection are younger than 50 years of age. However, recent findings suggest that SMA aneurysms occur more commonly in older patients in their 50s or 60s.[13] Most SMA aneurysms are located in the first 5 cm

of the artery and tend to be solitary. Calcification occurs less often than with other visceral aneurysms, affecting only 62% of all SMA aneurysms.

Symptoms were noted frequently in earlier reports,[20] but in recent series, patients have presented without symptoms.[13] Again, the infectious nature of the SMA aneurysm may explain the higher percentage of symptomatic patients in past reports. Epigastric or midabdominal pain tends to be the most typical symptom. Intestinal angina is unusual but may occur. When intestinal angina is present, it is most likely caused by a secondary complication of the aneurysm that results in thrombosis. A pulsatile, usually tender mass has been found in many patients. When rupture occurs, it generally produces pain, especially when there is extensive intra-abdominal hemorrhage.

Reports vary on the risk of rupture from an SMA aneurysm. The risk has been stated to be quite low.[20] However, in the Mayo Clinic patients, there was almost a 40% risk of rupture, even though few (5%) aneurysms were mycotic.[19] Also of note is that men and patients with noncalcified aneurysms were at higher risk. When rupture occurred in the Mayo Clinic patients, mortality was 38%.[19]

Surgical management of these lesions primarily has involved ligation with or without revascularization. With emergency rupture or ischemia or both, ligation alone may be reasonable. Collateral perfusion to the viscera may be adequate at exploration, but careful assessment with intraoperative Doppler ultrasonography and intravenous fluorescein testing is warranted. Bowel resection may be necessary but was not required in any of the recent Mayo Clinic patients.[19] Percutaneous embolization also may be used in emergency conditions. However, it does not offer the advantage of being able to assess the extent of bowel ischemia. Elective intervention for SMA lesions has been advocated for most patients who are at reasonable operative risk. When surgical intervention is elective, revascularization is more likely to be done. The preferred conduit for revascularization depends on bowel viability; venous conduits usually are selected when the bowel is acutely ischemic. When intervention is elective, long-term results may be excellent.

CELIAC ARTERY ANEURYSM

Aneurysms of the celiac artery represent 4% to 5% of all visceral artery aneurysms.[8] These aneurysms, similar to those of the SMA, historically have been viewed as infectious. Recent reports, however, do not suggest an infectious pathogenesis as the main cause.[13] At Mayo Clinic, only 11% of patients were mycotic, and the remaining patients showed pathologic changes consistent with atherosclerosis.[21] As with other visceral artery aneurysms, these atherosclerotic changes were likely due to the aneurysm rather than being the cause of the aneurysm. However, in the Mayo Clinic series, 67% of patients had associated nonvisceral artery aneurysms, including aortic, femoral, and popliteal artery aneurysms.[21] This finding suggests that atherosclerosis may play an extensive role in the pathogenesis of these lesions. Most reports have noted that men and women are equally affected.[13] However, among the Mayo Clinic patients, there was a preponderance of men, with a ratio of 2:1.[21] This finding also may explain the increased incidence of atherosclerotic changes and concomitant nonvisceral aneurysms.

Most authors report vague abdominal discomfort in patients. However, these symptoms also have been identified as incidental, nonspecific findings. CT and ultrasonography are the most common diagnostic tests used to identify these lesions. Angiography is a critical diagnostic test before consideration of surgical intervention (Fig. 5). Angiography also may uncover the diagnosis coincidentally in patients who are undergoing the test for other reasons.

The reported risk of rupture for these aneurysms has been as low as 13% and as high as 80%.[22] The risk may be related to the etiology of the aneurysm and is increased by the presence of infection (Fig. 6). The Mayo Clinic series identified a 7% risk of rupture, but only 11% of patients had an infectious cause of the aneurysm.[21] When rupture occurs, epigastric pain develops in most patients, who subsequently have severe intra-abdominal hemorrhage. Initially, the hemorrhage may be contained briefly within the lesser sac.

When these lesions are an emergency, intervention carries greater risk. Exposure of the most proximal celiac trunk may require a thoracoabdominal incision. Ligation of the celiac artery is an option but has significant risk of hepatic infarction. Adequate assessment of hepatic perfusion must be undertaken before ligation. Most authors recommend revascularization, even in emergency conditions. Authors also agree that most patients should undergo elective intervention whenever feasible.[22] The elective approach should include revascularization. Autologous vein or prosthetic grafts are the most frequently used conduits. However, long-term follow-up at Mayo Clinic[21] has identified an increased rate of thrombosis with venous conduits. Therefore, prosthetic grafts may be a better alternative. The risks of an elective operation appear minimal, with the interventions well tolerated.

GASTRIC AND GASTROEPIPLOIC ARTERY ANEURYSMS

Gastric artery aneurysms are much more common than gastroepiploic artery aneurysms. Together, they make up

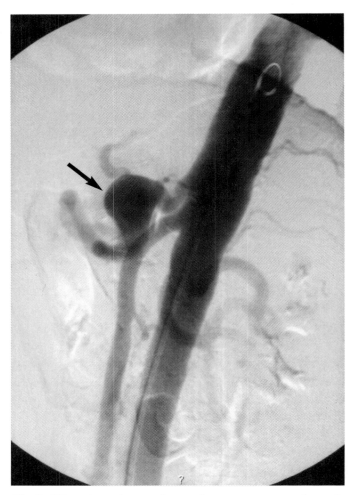

Fig. 5. Visceral arteriogram shows celiac artery aneurysm (arrow).

about 4% of all visceral artery aneurysms.[8] There is a male predominance, with a ratio of 3:1. Gastric and gastroepiploic artery aneurysms typically occur in the sixth decade of life. Their pathogenesis is varied, but most are due to medial degeneration. Less commonly, atherosclerosis may be the cause and is thought to be a secondary process.

Most patients present with symptoms, although many also present with rupture. Few of these lesions are found incidentally. Rupture has been reported in as many as 90% of cases, resulting in mortality as high as 70%.[7] Gastrointestinal hemorrhage is as common as intra-abdominal hemorrhage. Diagnostic imaging includes CT and ultrasonography. CT has shown intra-abdominal hemorrhage in patients with rupture, but it may not detect small lesions. For patients undergoing an elective procedure, preoperative angiography is reasonable but not mandatory. No data exist on the size or natural history of the aneurysm to assist with management decisions.

Operative intervention is recommended for any patient who is a reasonable candidate. Ligation with or without

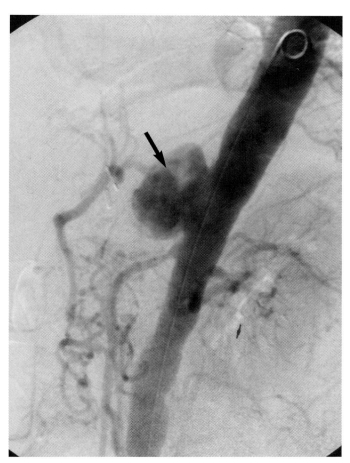

Fig. 6. Angiogram depicts an infected celiac artery aneurysm (arrow).

resection of the aneurysm is adequate, and revascularization is not warranted. Occasionally, wedge resection of the adjacent gastric wall may be necessary, generally for aneurysms within the gastric wall. Elective operations have a high rate of success, with minimal perioperative morbidity and mortality and a small incidence of recurrent gastric bleeding.

JEJUNAL, ILEAL, AND COLIC ARTERY ANEURYSMS

Arterial aneurysms of branches of the SMA, including the jejunal, the ileal, and the colic arteries, account for about 3% of all visceral artery aneurysms. There appears to be no sex predilection, and patients are usually in their 50s or 60s. Multiple aneurysms are found in about 10% of patients.[8] Atherosclerosis is an unusual finding, but medial degeneration is found in most patients. Septic emboli to multiple branch visceral vessels may occur, resulting in multiple aneurysms.[23]

Most patients present with symptoms, and rupture is not unusual. Because diagnostic imaging studies are becoming more routine, more patients without symptoms are being identified. However, most of these aneurysms are not identified in the asymptomatic state, so most reports are of ruptured aneurysms. The true incidence of rupture may be about 30%.[8] In our series, a 25% incidence of rupture was found.[24] In our experience, all ruptures were in colic arteries. In the past, ileal aneurysms were usually found to be ruptured, and rupture of jejunal aneurysms was relatively unusual.[25] When rupture occurs, there also may be free intraperitoneal hemorrhage or gastrointestinal hemorrhage. The mortality as a result of rupture has been reported by others to be about 20%.[25]

Most authors recommend intervention for branch arterial aneurysms, and ligation with or without aneurysmal resection is the most common procedure.[25,26] Bowel resection may be necessary if viability is compromised by ligation. In the Mayo Clinic series, 50% of patients underwent surgical intervention, including ligation with or without bowel resection, with no operative mortality.[24] Percutaneous embolization has been reported but carries some risk of bowel ischemia or infarction. In light of this risk, we do not advocate embolization.

PANCREATIC, PANCREATICODUODENAL, AND GASTRODUODENAL ARTERY ANEURYSMS

The least common of all visceral artery aneurysms are those that affect the pancreatic, pancreaticoduodenal, or gastroduodenal arteries. These vessels tend to develop aneurysmal degeneration as a consequence of pancreatic or peripancreatic inflammatory processes. These aneurysms represent 1% to 2% of all visceral artery aneurysms and occur more often in men, with a reported ratio of 4:1.[8] Most patients who have these lesions are in their 40s, a decade younger than patients with other types of visceral artery aneurysms. Atherosclerosis is a rare finding. Usually, the aneurysms are pseudoaneurysms related to an adjacent inflammatory process or trauma.

Most patients who present with these lesions are symptomatic and have vague epigastric discomfort. Pain from pancreatitis also may be an important finding. Chronic relapsing pancreatitis is the most common type of pancreatitis in patients in whom these aneurysms develop. As many as 50% of patients with gastroduodenal artery aneurysms have chronic pancreatitis, whereas 30% of patients with pancreatic artery aneurysms have chronic pancreatitis.[26]

The exact rupture rate for these aneurysms is not known. However, when inflammation is the cause, rupture occurs in more than 50% of patients at risk.[26] Hemorrhage generally causes abdominal pain; however, this pain may be confused with pain from pancreatic inflammation. Rupture is best diagnosed with CT, which can be used to identify blood in the retroperitoneum. Rupture into the gastrointestinal or biliary tract also may occur. Angiography may be of diagnostic benefit, and it also may have some therapeutic benefit when embolization is used.

The mortality rate from rupture of these arteries is 25% to 50%. Operative intervention is particularly hazardous, because of adjacent severe pancreatic inflammation.

Be that as it may, ligation of the aneurysm is the preferred intervention. Ligation from within the aneurysm sac has been advocated by some authors, who argue that it allows for a more secure closure.[26] Pancreatic resection may be necessary occasionally. However, this operation should be used only for selected lesions and patients. Percutaneous embolization remains an alternative treatment that has been used with some success.[27] Unfortunately, recurrent hemorrhage, which limits the usefulness of this technique, has been associated with it.

REFERENCES

1. Hallett JW Jr: Splenic artery aneurysms. Semin Vasc Surg 8:321-326, 1995
2. Bedford PD, Lodge B: Aneurysm of the splenic artery. Gut 1:312-320, 1960
3. Abbas MA, Stone WM, Fowl RJ, Gloviczki P, Oldenburg WA, Pairolero PC, Hallett JW, Bower TC, Panneton JM, Cherry KJ: Splenic artery aneurysms: two decades experience at Mayo Clinic. Ann Vasc Surg 16:442-449, 2002
4. Stanley JC, Fry WJ: Pathogenesis and clinical significance of splenic artery aneurysms. Surgery 76:898-909, 1974
5. Carr SC, Pearce WH, Vogelzang RL, McCarthy WJ, Nemcek AA Jr, Yao JS: Current management of visceral artery aneurysms. Surgery 120:627-633, 1996
6. Ohta M, Hashizume M, Ueno K, Tanoue K, Sugimachi K, Hasuo K: Hemodynamic study of splenic artery aneurysm in portal hypertension. Hepatogastroenterology 41:181-184, 1994
7. Stanley JC, Thompson NW, Fry WJ: Splanchnic artery aneurysms. Arch Surg 101:689-697, 1970
8. Stanley JC, Zelenock GB: Splanchnic artery aneurysms. In Vascular Surgery. Vol 2. Fourth edition. Edited by RB Rutherford. Philadelphia, WB Saunders Company, 1995, pp 1124-1139
9. Angelakis EJ, Bair WE, Barone JE, Lincer RM: Splenic artery aneurysm rupture during pregnancy. Obstet Gynecol Surv 48:145-148, 1993
10. Trastek VF, Pairolero PC, Joyce JW, Hollier LH, Bernatz PE: Splenic artery aneurysms. Surgery 91:694-699, 1982
11. Gaglio PJ, Regenstein F, Slakey D, Cheng S, Takiff H, Rinker R, Dick D, Thung SN: α-1 antitrypsin deficiency and splenic artery aneurysm rupture: An association? Am J Gastroenterol 95:1531-1534, 2000
12. Iseki J, Tada Y, Wada T, Nobori M: Hepatic artery aneurysm. Report of a case and review of the literature. Gastroenterol Jpn 18:84-92, 1983
13. Shanley CJ, Shah NL, Messina LM: Common splanchnic artery aneurysms: splenic, hepatic, and celiac. Ann Vasc Surg 10:315-322, 1996
14. Abbas MA, Fowl RJ, Stone WM, Panneton JM, Oldenburg WA, Bower TC, Cherry KJ, Gloviczki P: Hepatic artery aneurysms: factors predicting complications. J Vasc Surg (in press)
15. Lumsden AB, Mattar SG, Allen RC, Bacha EA: Hepatic artery aneurysms: the management of 22 patients. J Surg Res 60:345-350, 1996
16. Harlaftis NN, Akin JT: Hemobilia from ruptured hepatic artery aneurysm: report of a case and review of the literature. Am J Surg 133:229-232, 1977
17. Erskine JM: Hepatic artery aneurysm. Vasc Surg 7:106-125, 1973
18. Kadir S, Athanasoulis CA, Ring EJ, Greenfield A: Transcatheter embolization of intrahepatic arterial aneurysms. Radiology 134:335-339, 1980
19. Stone WM, Abbas M, Cherry KJ, Fowl RJ, Gloviczki P: Superior mesenteric artery aneurysms: Is presence an indication for intervention? J Vasc Surg 36:234-237, 2002
20. Blumenberg RM, David D, Slovak J: Abdominal apoplexy due to rupture of a superior mesenteric artery aneurysm: clip aneurysmorrhaphy with survival. Arch Surg 108:223-226, 1974
21. Stone WM, Abbas MA, Gloviczki P, Fowl RJ, Cherry KJ: Celiac arterial aneurysms: a critical reappraisal of a rare entity. Arch Surg 137:670-674, 2002
22. Graham LM, Stanley JC, Whitehouse WM Jr, Zelenock GB, Wakefield TW, Cronenwett JL, Lindenauer SM: Celiac artery aneurysms: historic (1745-1949) versus contemporary (1950-1984) differences in etiology and clinical importance. J Vasc Surg 2:757-764, 1985
23. Trevisani MF, Ricci MA, Michaels RM, Meyer KK: Multiple mesenteric aneurysms complicating subacute bacterial endocarditis. Arch Surg 122:823-824, 1987
24. Tessier DJ, Abbas MA, Fowl RJ, Stone WM, Bower TC, McKusick MA, Gloviczki P: Management of rare mesenteric arterial branch aneurysms. Ann Vasc Surg 16:586-590, 2002
25. Diettrich NA, Cacioppo JC, Ying DP: Massive gastrointestinal hemorrhage caused by rupture of a jejunal branch artery aneurysm. J Vasc Surg 8:187-189, 1988
26. Shanley CJ, Shah NL, Messina LM: Uncommon splanchnic artery aneurysms: pancreaticoduodenal, gastroduodenal, superior mesenteric, inferior mesenteric, and colic. Ann Vasc Surg 10:506-515, 1996
27. Mandel SR, Jaques PF, Sanofsky S, Mauro MA: Nonoperative management of peripancreatic arterial aneurysms: a 10-year experience. Ann Surg 205:126-128, 1987

COLONIC MOTOR DISORDERS: CONSTIPATION

Luca Stocchi, M.D.
John H. Pemberton, M.D.

Constipation is a very common complaint. Despite the common use of the word, various symptoms are attributed to constipation, and thus its definition is complex. The American Gastroenterological Association has recommended that a patient has *functional* constipation if at least two of the following symptoms are present for 3 or more months: straining at defecation at least a fourth of the time, lumpy or hard stools at least a fourth of the time, sensation of incomplete evacuation at least a fourth of the time, and two or fewer bowel movements per week.[1] A recent survey of 10,018 individuals which examined the epidemiology of constipation in the United States found an overall prevalence of 14.7%. In particular, the subset of patients with functional constipation, as defined above, had a relative prevalence of 4.6%.[2]

There are two fundamental causes of functional constipation: anorectal dysfunction and slow colonic transit. In most patients only one factor predominates, but the two conditions can present together. Anorectal dysfunction also has been referred to as outlet obstruction, anismus, pelvic floor dyssynergia, and paradoxic contraction of the pelvic musculature. Several synonyms also have been used to describe functional constipation of colonic origin, including slow-transit constipation, slow colonic transit, colonic inertia, or Arbuthnot Lane's disease. The myriad complexities of "definable" constipation are not discussed here. This chapter examines the cause and pathogenesis of functional constipation, the methods currently used for its diagnosis, the options available for surgical treatment, and the immediate and long-term surgical results.

ETIOLOGY AND PATHOGENESIS

The cause of constipation is unclear but is probably multifactorial. It is reasonable to presume that different factors might explain different subtypes of slow colonic transit. For example, some patients relate the onset of their symptoms to a specific event, such as childbirth[3] or hysterectomy.[4-6] In addition, several neurologic conditions are associated with slow colonic transit, including Parkinson's disease, multiple sclerosis, cerebrovascular accidents, spinal trauma, and spinal tumor. In other cases, more direct damage to the myenteric autonomic plexuses of the colon is postulated, such as in diabetes, Chagas' disease, or laxative abuse. However, because most patients do not have associated diseases or potentially inciting events in their past medical histories, the term "idiopathic constipation" is used.

Regardless of possible causes, most patients with slow-transit constipation have reduced contractile colonic activity compared with normal subjects. In particular, the number, intensity, and duration of high-amplitude propagated contractions, which are responsible for advancement of colonic content, are decreased.[7] In addition, patients with slow colonic transit do not respond to feeding with increased colonic motor activity, which is a physiologic response in normal individuals.[8] In this regard, when anorectal dysfunction coexists, it has been postulated that, at least in some patients, decreased colonic contractility might result from a viscero-visceral inhibitory reflex originating from the distended rectum.

Several histopathologic findings have been noted in the colon of patients with slow-transit constipation.

"Neuronal dysplasia"[9] with submucosal hypergangliono-sis and reduced mucosal innervation has been observed.[10] Other investigators have emphasized the correlation of slow colonic transit with a functional deficit of cholinergic fibers,[11,12] decreased concentration of vasoactive inhibitory peptide,[13] excessive production of nitric oxide,[14] and increased serotonin concentration.[15] However, such findings are not consistently observed by different investigators, and no unifying pathogenetic theory has been formulated. In particular, whether the alterations in the myenteric plexuses are a consequence or a cause of the slow transit is still being discussed.

DIAGNOSIS AND IMAGING

Despite the frequency of functional constipation, only a few patients are actually candidates for operation. An accurate diagnostic work-up is essential to plan the most appropriate management of patients with refractory constipation. The work-up becomes a crucial element in achieving favorable postoperative outcomes.

Besides the numerous conditions causing constipation which are amenable to medical treatment, it is of foremost importance to rule out any organic colonic sources of constipation, especially colorectal cancer. In this regard, colonoscopy or barium enema and flexible sigmoidoscopy is recommended. Other structural colorectal abnormalities causing functional disorders should be ruled out, such as rectocele, sigmoidocele, megarectum, or megacolon.

The cost-effectiveness of the often extensive diagnostic work-up necessary for patients with functional constipation has been questioned. In particular, it has been argued that such evaluations change the management of relatively few patients.[16] However, only about 1% or less of all patients with constipation present for further evaluation when medical treatment has failed. Within this subpopulation, quantifying anorectal and colonic function is the only possible way to select surgical candidates. A careful history and physical examination remain essential, but further evaluations are therefore necessary and should focus on evaluation of colonic transit and anorectal function.

History and Physical Examination

A careful history often effectively addresses the need for further testing, and symptoms have been shown to be good predictors of colonic transit time.[17] In this regard, it is particularly valuable to have the patient with constipation keep a symptom diary. This practice also should be encouraged because it is a reliable and inexpensive method to monitor patient compliance and the efficacy of treatment.

Physical examination rules out systemic or neurologic disorders that cause constipation and reveals anorectal abnormalities, such as rectal prolapse. Some clues suggest the diagnosis of anorectal dysfunction. For example, a patient reporting frequent or prolonged straining at defecation is typical. During physical examination, patients should be asked to strain while in the left decubitus position. Posterior motion of the puborectalis muscle usually indicates preservation of pelvic floor function. In addition, the presence of pelvic floor descent usually can be assessed. In regard to pelvic descent, both an excessive and an insufficient degree of descent indicate a pelvic floor anomaly. Digital examination should provide basic information on the adequacy of sphincter tone at rest and during squeezing. Straining during digital rectal examination provides further information regarding the adequacy of pelvic floor and sphincter relaxation.

Psychologic Evaluation

Mental status evaluation is important because many patients with constipation also harbor psychologic and psychiatric conditions. Moreover, patients with psychologic problems are more likely to seek medical attention for constipation at a lower threshold than normal subjects. Importantly, there is evidence that patients with psychologic or psychiatric conditions are less likely to benefit from operation,[18] a factor that, of course, becomes important when counseling a patient on the outcomes of operation.

Evaluation of Colonic Transit

Colonic transit is evaluated with radiopaque markers or scintigraphy. The most common technique uses radiopaque markers and a series of plain abdominal radiographs. The technique originally described uses 20 inert, nonabsorbable markers ingested simultaneously. In normal subjects, 80% of the ingested markers should be eliminated per rectum by the end of the fifth day.[19] In addition, a visual subdivision into colorectal segments is obtained by drawing an inverted Y-shaped line on the plain abdominal radiograph which connects the fifth lumbar vertebral body with the posterior superior iliac spines bilaterally. This method facilitates better estimation of transit in specific colonic segments.[20] A variant of this technique has been advocated as being more effective for obtaining information on transit times in specific segments of the colon. This procedure entails ingestion of the 20 markers followed by daily abdominal radiography until the markers completely disappear from the colon. Segmental transit times are then calculated by applying a mathematic formula.[21] A second variant is based on the ingestion of 10 markers per day for 10 days followed by abdominal radiography on the 11th day.[22] These modifications of the original Hinton technique never gained widespread popularity. A more recent modification has been proposed to reduce the radiation exposure while maintaining the capability to collect data on segmental colonic transit. In this variant, described by Metcalf et al.,[23] patients ingest 20 markers each day for 3 consecutive days (a different type of marker is used each day); a single plain abdominal radiograph is obtained on the fourth day. An additional radiograph can be obtained on the seventh day when the transit is prolonged (Fig. 1).

The radiopaque marker technique is simple and inexpensive and uses conventional technology that is readily available in any radiologic suite. However, it requires multiple radiologic examinations or at least follow-up of a few days after the markers have been ingested. In addition, the patient needs to avoid use of laxatives and enemas during the examination period.

Scintigraphy solves the problems of the radiopaque procedure.[24,25] In this technique, pellets containing indium In 111 are coated with a pH-sensitive polymer that releases the isotope only when the colon has been reached. The distribution of the isotope throughout the various colonic segments can be recorded by averaging the radioactive counts. During the same examination, it is possible to add a technetium Tc 99m pellet-egg meal for the measurement of gastric emptying and small bowel transit time (Fig. 2).

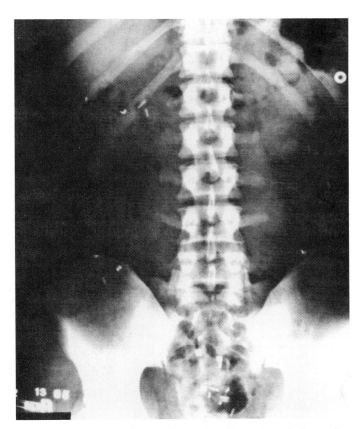

Fig. 1. Low-kilovolt plain abdominal radiograph depicting radiographic markers still present in the colon 7 days after ingestion.

Results from scintigraphic evaluation of colonic transit are comparable to those obtained with conventional methods.[24] The advantages of scintigraphy are decreased radiation exposure, increased accuracy in the assessment of transit in each colonic segment, and, of course, additional information regarding stomach emptying and small bowel transit. In addition, all of the data are available within 24 hours. This is an attractive diagnostic tool in tertiary referral centers. However, the scintigraphic method costs approximately 5 times more than a conventional radiopaque marker transit test, and a specific expertise in nuclear medicine is required for preparation of the isotopic reagents. Both factors limit its broad applicability.

Moreover, the upper gastrointestinal tract can, in any case, be examined separately to assess the motility of the small bowel. In fact, the presence of concurrent dysmotility disorders in other segments of the gastrointestinal tract generally portends a worse prognosis (see below).

Evaluation of Anorectal Function

The various colonic transit studies are generally accurate for establishing the diagnosis of slow-transit constipation, but there is no single standard for assessment of anorectal function. Rather, the combination of several tests offers complementary pieces of information useful to establish the diagnosis of anorectal dysfunction. Although this workup is sometimes tedious, it is critical for the decision to operate or to delay or avoid operation altogether. Several tests are available, including anorectal manometry, evacuation proctography (defecography), balloon expulsion, and electromyography. Some tests such as intraluminal measurement of colonic myoelectrical and motor function are useful in the research setting but have no role in the clinical management of patients. The American Gastroenterological Association currently recommends confirming of the diagnosis of constipation or impaired defecation by at least two different tests.[2]

Anorectal Manometry

Measurement of anal canal pressures is useful as a complementary test to confirm the diagnosis of anorectal dysfunction (Fig. 3). Similar to defecography, anorectal manometry lacks accuracy when used alone. In fact, the same manometric pattern suggestive of paradoxic contraction of the puborectalis muscle also can be found in normal subjects and only partially reflects the respective findings from defecography.[26] Anorectal manometry does rule out the diagnosis of Hirschsprung's disease in patients with constipation; the presence of a rectoanal inhibitory reflex rules out the disease. An additional application of anorectal manometry is for monitoring a patient's response to pelvic floor retraining. Other than

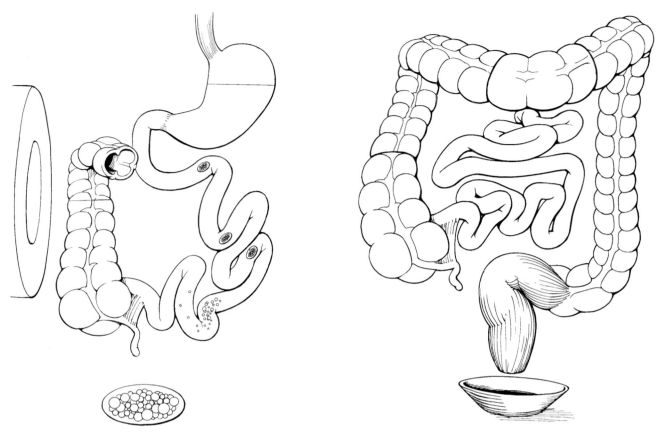

Fig. 2. Scintigraphic transit method. Dual-labeled markers and gamma camera facilitate concurrent determination of colonic transit, gastric emptying, and small bowel transit. The geometric center of the radiolabeled markers is calculated. At 4 hours, the center should be at the hepatic flexure, and at 24 hours, it should be in the distal descending or proximal sigmoid colon.

these specific indications, its routine use is not recommended in patients with constipation.

Evacuation Proctography (Defecography)

In this test, the patient evacuates contrast medium, previously injected into the rectum, under radiologic visualization.[27,28] Defecography is particularly useful for detecting anatomical abnormalities such as rectocele and enterocele and specific functional disorders such as paradoxic contraction of the puborectalis muscle. Unfortunately, these abnormalities are not pathognomonic of any one disorder. In fact, pathologic findings frequently overlap between symptomatic patients and normal subjects.[29-31] A variant of conventional evacuation proctography is measurement of the rate of evacuated contrast medium.[32] In addition, isotope-labeled artificial stools also have been used.[33,34] However, neither of these adds substantial accuracy. For defecography to be helpful, there must be dedicated radiologic expertise and the ability to correlate the defecography with the clinical history. Although it can confirm the diagnosis of anorectal dysfunction obtained by other tests, it is not sufficiently

accurate as a single test. The American Gastroenterological Association does not recommend its routine use except for the specific indications mentioned here.[2]

Balloon Expulsion Test

This test usually is conducted in association with anorectal manometry to determine the presence of anorectal dysfunction. It consists of defecating a balloon inflated with 50 mL of water with the patient placed in the left lateral decubitus position. If the balloon is not subsequently expelled promptly, weights up to 500 g can be attached. Inability to expel the balloon at any weight above 200 g is diagnostic of anorectal dysfunction.[35,36] Although some authors estimate that this test in combination with a careful history and physical examination has a diagnostic accuracy of 90%,[37] it is generally agreed that it is of unproven value when used as the sole test to assess anorectal function.[2] However, it is simple, inexpensive, and easily tolerated. In addition, there is evidence that inability to expel the balloon is associated with an increased likelihood of functional failure after colectomy.[38]

be evaluated initially with a colonic transit test. If results are normal, a further therapeutic trial should be attempted and the tests repeated. If all the testing then is normal for the second time, the patient is not a candidate for operation and empiric treatment is recommended. Whenever abnormalities in defecation or straining are clinically evident or suspected, the patient should be referred for tests of pelvic floor function. Patients with slow colonic transit also should undergo pelvic floor function tests to rule out a concomitant pelvic floor disorder. In patients with both slow colonic transit and pelvic floor disorders, pelvic floor retraining is performed first (Fig. 5). At completion of the biofeedback course, the patient should be reevaluated. If symptoms persist and slow colonic transit is confirmed, colectomy becomes the treatment of choice.

INDICATIONS FOR OPERATION

Operation should be considered for patients with a diagnosis of slow colonic transit not amenable to any further medical management. In the presence of normal anorectal function, colectomy is recommended. However, when anorectal dysfunction coexists, it should be addressed first by pelvic floor retraining (biofeedback). This technique, initially described in patients hospitalized for prolonged periods,[40] is currently offered on an outpatient basis in most centers. The success rate for anorectal dysfunction should approximate 80%, although variations are possible depending on the specific causes of anorectal dysfunction and the method used to evaluate the efficacy of the procedure (Table 1). At completion of the pelvic floor retraining sessions, the patient should be reevaluated. Some authors have reported correction of both slow colonic transit and anorectal dysfunction with a liberal initial use of biofeedback in an unselected population with refractory constipation.[56] However, if symptoms persist and slow transit constipation is confirmed, the patient should then undergo colectomy.

It is very important to exclude from operation patients with anorectal dysfunction alone and those with symptoms but no functional abnormalities identified during evaluation. Patients with anorectal dysfunction should be treated with pelvic floor retraining, and those with symptoms but no functional problem likely belong to the nonsurgical group of patients with irritable bowel syndrome and need appropriate medical treatment. Pelvic floor retraining is currently the standard of care for patients with anorectal dysfunction because the results of operations designed primarily to "relax" the pelvic floor surgically have been disappointing. For example, Pinho et al.[58] reported an overall improvement rate of only 31% after

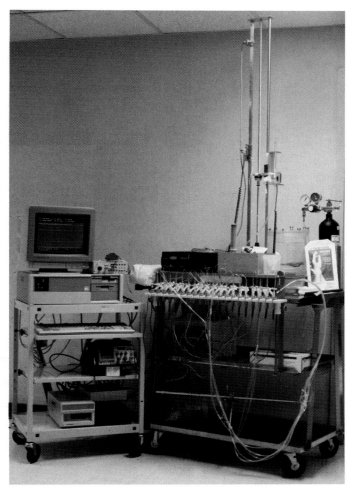

Fig. 3. Anorectal manometry is performed with multiple recording channels and computerized analysis.

Electromyography

Needle electromyography provides an accurate mapping of the functional activity of the striated muscles of the pelvic floor by placement of electrodes into the muscle layer. As might be expected, this procedure is painful, not well tolerated by patients, and subject to sampling errors. Surface electromyography is less invasive and might have more merit in the evaluation of sphincter function, especially to monitor sphincter performance during biofeedback training. There is evidence suggesting that this technique is more effective than balloon biofeedback.[39] However, as a diagnostic test, electromyography should not be considered among the primary options for the evaluation of anorectal function.

Approach to Constipation in a Tertiary Referral Practice

The algorithm for the evaluation of patients with intractable constipation is shown in Figure 4. Patients with intractable constipation without organic cause should

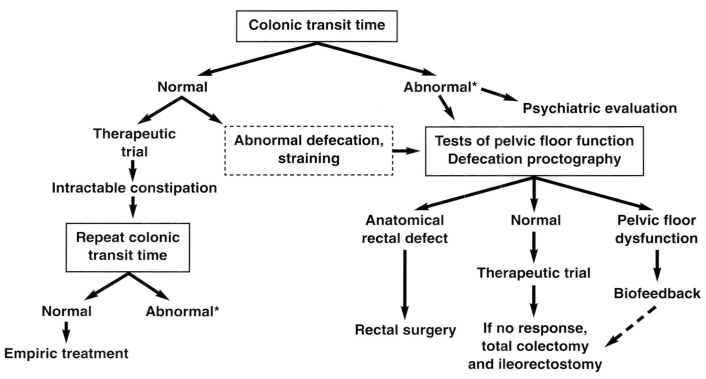

Fig. 4. *Algorithm for intractable complex constipation. All other anatomical, pathologic, drug- or disease-related causes have been eliminated. Colonic transit and tests of pelvic floor function categorize patients into those with slow transit, those with pelvic floor dysfunction, or those with both. Patients with normal test results are treated empirically and not subjected to unnecessary pelvic floor retraining or ileorectostomy. *If colonic transit is abnormal, follow pathway on right.*

anorectal myectomy in patients with outlet obstruction, including a subpopulation of patients with megarectum. Contemporary series examining more selected patient populations have not offered better outcomes. In 15 patients with idiopathic constipation, Kamm et al.[59] reported a 20% success rate after lateral division of the puborectalis muscle.

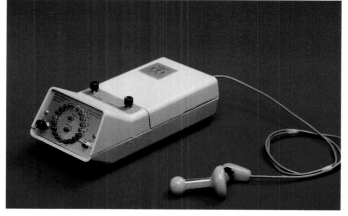

Fig. 5. *A portable device (and, if necessary, used at home) that provides visual reinforcement during pelvic floor retraining.*

It is now well accepted that the indiscriminate consideration of patients who indeed harbor anorectal dysfunction as surgical candidates results inevitably in an increased risk of surgical failure and persistent constipation. For patients in whom conservative treatments fail to correct anorectal dysfunction, the construction of a continent colonic conduit to allow irrigation and evacuation of the distal colon and rectum has been described as a possible salvage treatment.[60] Although successful in the hands of proponents, experience with this procedure is still limited.

CONDUCT OF OPERATION

Colectomy and Ileorectostomy

The procedure of choice for the treatment of slow colonic transit is abdominal colectomy with ileorectal anastomosis (Fig. 6). The intraperitoneal cecum and colon should be mobilized with a limited, non-oncologic mesenteric excision. Therefore, the lymphovascular ligation does not need to be done at the origin of the vessels with wide mesenteric excision, such as is often done for colon cancer. The dissection of the rectum should be very limited, and care should be exerted to avoid damage to the pelvic nerves

Table 1.—Functional Outcomes After Pelvic Retraining Techniques (Biofeedback)

Reference	Year	No. of patients treated	Follow-up, mo	Successes No.	%
Bleijenberg and Kuijpers[40]	1987	10	1-14	7	70
Dahl et al.[41]	1991	14	> 6	13	93
Kawimbe et al.[42]	1991	15	6 (mean)	13	87
Lestar et al.[43]	1991	16	> 12	11	69
Fleshman et al.[44]	1992	9	> 6	9	100
Wexner et al.[45]	1992	18	9 (mean)	16	89
Juhasz et al.[46]	1993	69	22	61	88
Papachrysostomou and Smith[47]	1994	22	After therapy	19	86
Ho et al.[48]	1996	62	15 (mean)	56	90
Gilliland et al.[49]	1997	194	After therapy	87*	49
Glia et al.[50]	1997	20	6	15	75
Karlbom et al.[51]	1997	19	14 (median)	12	43†
Ko et al.[52]	1997	17	7 (mean)	13	76
Patankar et al.[53]	1997	30	After therapy	25	83
Rieger et al.[54]	1997	19	> 6	2	11
Rao et al.[55]	1997	25	After therapy	23	92‡
Chiotakakou-Faliakou et al.[56]	1998	100	23 (median)	57	57
McKee et al.[57]	1999	30	> 12	9	30

*Only 178 patients were available for follow-up.
†A total of 28 patients had treatment (9 had no improvement at 3 months).
‡Subjective improvement. Objective improvement by anorectal testing was 76%.

when the presacral space is entered. The anastomosis should be done between the terminal ileum and the upper rectum. Construction of an ileosigmoid anastomosis must be avoided. In the absence of well-controlled comparative studies, there is evidence from retrospective studies that preservation of an excessively long rectosigmoid predisposes to recurrent constipation postoperatively.[61,62] Conversely, when the anastomosis is fashioned deep in the pelvis, the volume of the rectal reservoir may be reduced, which might lead to diarrhea. The anastomosis can be done with a hand-sewn or a stapled technique and can be end-to-end or side-to-end, according to the preference of the operating surgeon.

The same operation also can be completed successfully with a laparoscopy-assisted technique.[63] Further experience is needed to confirm the applicability of this approach.

Other Operations
Other procedures have been proposed as alternatives to colectomy. Some authors have advocated segmental colonic resection as a less "aggressive" operation that also might prevent postoperative diarrhea. Segmental resections have been done based on the results of colonic transit tests that demonstrate a specific area of slow colonic transit within the colon. The outcome of these procedures has been unpredictable.[64] In general, a limited resection predisposes the patient to recurrent constipation, which then requires a subsequent subtotal colectomy.

In work examining the outcome of segmental colectomy for slow colonic transit, You et al.[65] reported that 3 of 28 patients treated with segmental colectomy had recurrent constipation, all followed up for at least 2 years, corresponding to a failure rate of almost 11%. The patients with failed segmental resections were then treated with completion colectomy. In addition, although limited colonic resections have been advocated as the solution to postoperative diarrhea after ileorectal anastomosis, there is evidence that diarrhea also can occur after segmental colectomy.[66] Importantly, these findings and those of other authors remain difficult to interpret because patients did not undergo complete evaluations of intestinal transit.

Another alternative that is claimed to solve the problem of diarrhea is cecorectal anastomosis.[67] Despite its theoretical advantages over ileorectal anastomosis, the operative results of this procedure have not been convincing. No substantial improvement has been found in bowel transit and incidence of postoperative abdominal distention.[68] In some cases, the functional results have been decidedly poor,[69] and resection of the cecorectal anastomosis with conversion to ileorectal anastomosis has been necessary in up to 30% of patients.[70] Therefore, there is no evidence that cecorectal anastomosis offers any advantages over ileorectal anastomosis.

Although success is expected when patients are properly selected, in several cases constipation may persist even after colectomy with ileorectal anastomosis in the presence of normal anorectal function. A permanent ileostomy is the most straightforward option when this occurs, but patients are sometimes reluctant to accept the idea of a permanent stoma. In these cases, completion proctectomy and ileal pouch-anal anastomosis is an option. The functional results of this procedure for such an unusual indication also have been generally satisfactory.[71-73]

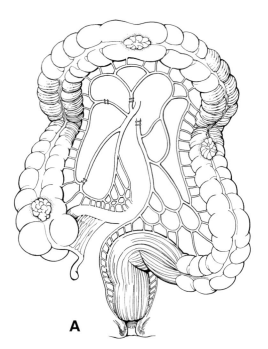
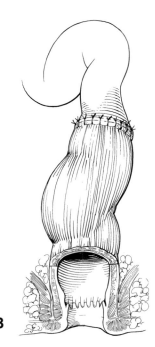

Fig. 6. Colectomy and ileorectostomy (at 8-12 cm above the dentate line) is the operation of choice for patients with slow-transit constipation. (A), Before operation. (B), After operation. (A modified from Keighley MRB: Colorectal cancer. In Atlas of Colorectal Surgery. Edited by MRB Keighley, JH Pemberton, VW Fazio, R Parc. New York, Churchill Livingstone, 1996, pp 189-241. By permission of the publisher.)

SURGICAL OUTCOMES

Mortality should be zero when the indication for operation is a benign colonic functional disorder. Occasional anastomotic leaks occur and generally are managed conservatively. Small bowel obstruction is the most frequent complication after ileorectal anastomosis for slow colonic transit. The frequency ranges between 0% and 71%, depending on the number of patients analyzed, the duration of follow-up, and the presence of concurrent dysmotility disorders. However, larger series generally report a rate of 10% to 20% (Table 2). Interestingly, it appears that small bowel obstruction is more common after ileorectal anastomosis performed for slow colonic transit than for other indications. Small bowel obstructions may resolve with conservative treatment, but nonoperative management fails in 0% to 48% of patients and they require a subsequent re-celiotomy for lysis of adhesions.

There is evidence that patients with coexistent pan-gastrointestinal motility disorders are at increased risk of postoperative complications after colectomy with ileorectal anastomosis. In a group of 20 patients followed up for a median of 96 months, preoperative testing revealed that overall 86% of the patients had at least one abnormality in gastrointestinal motility, bladder function, or autonomic function. In this very selected population, 71% of patients had to be readmitted for intestinal obstruction, and 48% needed celiotomy for lysis of adhesions.[79]

LONG-TERM FOLLOW-UP

Functional outcome after ileorectal anastomosis for slow colonic transit frequently has been based on the evaluations of postoperative diarrhea with possible incontinence and recurrent constipation. The definitions of these conditions have been variable among different authors, who have variably emphasized the number of bowel movements using different cutoff values, the consistency of the stools, or the need for antidiarrheal medications. Incontinence has been rarely scored, and the definition of "disabling" has been empirically used to delineate the group of patients with the most serious forms of such complications. Similarly, the definition of constipation has included the inability to increase the number of bowel movements postoperatively and also the persistence of nonspecific "difficulties" at defecation or the continued need for laxatives.

Unfortunately, there is a lack of uniform definitions that can be used to evaluate functional outcomes after ileorectal anastomosis for slow colonic transit, and this in turn corresponds with the difficulty of evaluating the quality of life of patients who undergo this procedure. For example, several patients who experience diarrhea after ileorectal anastomosis consider this a remarkable improvement compared with their preoperative constipation.[81] In view of these discrepancies, functional benefits derived from operation most commonly have been evaluated by

Table 2.—Results After Colectomy and Ileorectostomy for Slow Colonic Transit*

Reference	Year	No. of patients evaluated	No. of patients operated	Follow-up, mo	No. of deaths	SBO No.	SBO %	Operation for SBO No.	Operation for SBO %	Satisfaction rate, %
Pemberton et al.[62]	1991	277	38[†]	20	0	4	11	3	8	NA
Rex et al.[74]	1992	224	14	12 (minimum)	0	4	29	3	21	86
Sunderland et al.[72]	1992	288	18	24 (median)	0	2	11	2	11	89
Mahendrarajah et al.[75]	1994	19	9	16 (median)	0	1	11		0	89
Piccirillo et al.[76]	1995	416	54	27 (mean)	0	5	9	2	4	94
Redmond et al.[77]	1995	NA	21	90 (mean)	0	NA	18	1	5	90
Christiansen and Rasmussen[78]	1996	138	11	12-60	0	0		0		91
de Graaf et al.[66]	1996	346	20	12 (minimum)	0	NA		1	2	63[‡]
Ghosh et al.[79]	1996	NA	21	96 (median)	0	15	71	10	48	NA
Lubowski et al.[80]	1996	NA	52	42 (median)	0	9	17	7	14	90
Platell et al.[70]	1996	NA	86[§]	60 (mean)	2	10	12	31	36	81
Pluta et al.[81]	1996	188	24	65 (NA)	0	5	21	2	8	92
Ho et al.[63]	1997	411	24	24/12 (mean)[∥]	0	4	17	2	8	96
Nyam et al.[82]	1997	1,009	74	56 (mean)	0	7	9[¶]	5	7	97
You et al.[65]	1998	NA	12[#]	24	0	2	5	1	3	100
Bernini et al.[83]	1998	NA	106	78 (mean)	0	31	29	19	18	78
Lahr et al.[84]	1999	2,042	52	20 (mean)	0	6	12	NA		91

NA, not available; SBO, small bowel obstruction.

*These patients did not have physiologic evaluation of colonic transit and pelvic floor function.

†Includes two patients who underwent ileosigmoidostomy.

‡Includes four patients who underwent subtotal colectomy with ileostomy. Incidence of small bowel obstruction in a total of 42 different procedures.

§Ten additional patients underwent cecorectal anastomosis. Follow-up based on a total of 87 patients.

∥Follow-up for 17 open ileorectal anastomoses/7 laparoscopic-assisted ileorectal anastomoses.

¶Nine (12%) additional patients had prolonged postoperative ileus (same institution as Pemberton et al.[62]).

#Ileosigmoidostomy. Twenty-eight additional patients underwent partial colectomy.

reporting the percentage of patients who were satisfied with the results of their procedures.

In contemporary series, the overall satisfaction rate after ileorectal anastomosis should be about 90%. The main reason for such a high success rate is appropriate patient selection. In fact, earlier series, which reported operations in patients treated for functional constipation with more limited (or no) evaluation, generally reported less satisfactory outcomes (Table 3). It is important to note that such a high success rate depends on proper patient selection and on enhanced patient expectations. Patients with constipation often present with an array of accompanying symptoms, especially abdominal pain and bloating. Although operation is effective for increasing the number of bowel movements, it generally does not correct concurrent symptoms. Therefore, it is important to warn patients that operation has the potential to address only a specific aspect of their bowel function. In fact, patients who

have idiopathic constipation present with disturbed gastric and small bowel transit.[91] Therefore, not surprisingly, patients with generalized gastrointestinal motility disorders have a higher chance of recurrent symptoms or other abdominal complaints after colectomy. In a long-term study with a mean follow-up of 7.5 years, 90% of patients with pure colonic inertia had a successful long-term outcome postoperatively, but only 13% of patients with generalized intestinal dysmotility had prolonged relief. In particular, within 5 years after colectomy, 80% had recurrent constipation.[77] However, 88% of this same subgroup had an initial improvement. Therefore, operation should be offered with caution to these patients and only after ensuring that they are willing to accept an increased risk of long-term failure.

We recently reported the long-term results of operation for chronic constipation at Mayo Clinic.[82] Among patients referred for severe constipation refractory to aggressive

Table 3.—Results After Total or Subtotal Colectomy for Constipation*

Reference	Year	No. of patients evaluated	No. of patients operated	Follow-up, mo	No. of deaths	SBO No.	%	Satisfaction rate, %
Preston et al.[85]	1984	NA	16	42 (mean)	0	7	44	81
Roe et al.[86]	1986	74	9[†]	8 (mean)	0	0		71
Leon et al.[87]	1987	45	13	31	0	13	100	77
Akervall et al.[88]	1988	NA	12	41 (mean)	0	4	33	67
Kamm et al.[89]	1988	NA	44	48	0	8	18	69
Vasilevsky et al.[90‡]	1988	NA	52	46	2 (3.8%)	18	35	79
Yoshioka and Keighley[68]	1989	135	40	36 (median)	0	4	14[§]	58

NA, not available; SBO, small bowel obstruction.

*These patients did not have physiologic evaluation of colonic transit and pelvic floor function.

†Follow-up on seven patients.

‡Same institution as Bernini et al.[83] (partial overlap of patients who had operation between 1982 and 1985).

§Follow-up on 28 patients who did not have further operation.

medical management, 1,009 were evaluated with colonic transit studies and functional assessment of the pelvic floor. Among these, 52 showed evidence of slow colonic transit alone and underwent colectomy with ileorectal anastomosis. In addition, 22 patients had both slow colonic transit and anorectal dysfunction. These patients initially had pelvic floor retraining, followed by colectomy once the anorectal dysfunction was corrected. The mean follow-up of all 74 patients was 56 months. There was no operative mortality, and seven patients (9%) had a small bowel obstruction. An additional nine patients (12%) had prolonged postoperative ileus. Despite these complications, 90% of the patients had a good or improved quality of life. No cases of disabling diarrhea or recurrent constipation were reported. Interestingly, there was no difference in outcome between patients with slow colonic transit alone or slow colonic transit and pelvic floor dysfunction, because patients with a combined disorder underwent

pelvic floor retraining and then ileorectal anastomosis. These satisfactory results replicate the outcomes from other series (Tables 2 and 3).

CONCLUSION

Few patients presenting with constipation are surgical candidates. The outcome of operation is difficult to predict unless patients are carefully selected. Selection of operative candidates is based on evaluation of colonic transit with either radiopaque markers or scintigraphy. Moreover, pelvic floor function should be assessed with several different tests, which provide complementary information. Among these, no single test is currently accepted as the standard. Patients with anorectal dysfunction should be treated with pelvic floor retraining. Only patients with persistent slow colonic transit are candidates for operation. If selection is done correctly, satisfaction rates of about 90% are achieved.

REFERENCES

1. Barnett JL, Hasler WL, Camilleri M: American Gastroenterological Association medical position statement on anorectal testing techniques. American Gastroenterological Association. Gastroenterology 116:732-760, 1999
2. Stewart WF, Liberman JN, Sandler RS, Woods MS, Stemhagen A, Chee E, Lipton RB, Farup CE: Epidemiology of constipation (EPOC) study in the United States: relation of clinical subtypes to sociodemographic features. Am J Gastroenterol 94:3530-3540, 1999
3. MacDonald A, Baxter JN, Bessent RG, Gray HW, Finlay IG: Gastric emptying in patients with constipation following childbirth and due to idiopathic slow transit. Br J Surg 84:1141-1143, 1997
4. Roe AM, Bartolo DC, Mortensen NJ: Slow transit constipation: comparison between patients with or without previous hysterectomy. Dig Dis Sci 33:1159-1163, 1988
5. Smith AN, Varma JS, Binnie NR, Papachrysostomou M: Disordered colorectal motility in intractable constipation following hysterectomy. Br J Surg 77:1361-1365, 1990
6. Vierhout ME, Schreuder HW, Veen HF: Severe slow-transit constipation following radical hysterectomy. Gynecol Oncol 51:401-403, 1993
7. Bassotti G, Chiarioni G, Vantini I, Betti C, Fusaro C, Pelli MA, Morelli A: Anorectal manometric abnormalities and colonic propulsive impairment in patients with severe chronic idiopathic constipation. Dig Dis Sci 39:1558-1564, 1994
8. Ferrara A, Pemberton JH, Grotz RL, Hanson RB: Prolonged ambulatory recording of anorectal motility in patients with slow-transit constipation. Am J Surg 167:73-79, 1994
9. Stoss F, Meier-Ruge W: Diagnosis of neuronal colonic dysplasia in primary chronic constipation and sigmoid diverticulosis endoscopic biopsy and enzyme-histochemical examination. Surg Endosc 5:146-149, 1991
10. Krishnamurthy S, Schuffler MD, Rohrmann CA, Pope CE II: Severe idiopathic constipation is associated with a distinctive abnormality of the colonic myenteric plexus. Gastroenterology 88:26-34, 1985
11. Burleigh DE: Evidence for a functional cholinergic deficit in human colonic tissue resected for constipation. J Pharm Pharmacol 40:55-57, 1988
12. Bassotti G, Chiarioni G, Imbimbo BP, Betti C, Bonfante F, Vantini I, Morelli A, Whitehead WE: Impaired colonic motor response to cholinergic stimulation in patients with severe chronic idiopathic (slow transit type) constipation. Dig Dis Sci 38:1040-1045, 1993
13. Koch TR, Carney JA, Go L, Go VL: Idiopathic chronic constipation is associated with decreased colonic vasoactive intestinal peptide. Gastroenterology 94:300-310, 1988
14. Cortesini C, Cianchi F, Infantino A, Lise M: Nitric oxide synthase and VIP distribution in enteric nervous system in idiopathic chronic constipation. Dig Dis Sci 40:2450-2455, 1995
15. Lincoln J, Crowe R, Kamm MA, Burnstock G, Lennard-Jones JE: Serotonin and 5-hydroxyindoleacetic acid are increased in the sigmoid colon in severe idiopathic constipation. Gastroenterology 98:1219-1225, 1990
16. Rantis PC Jr, Vernava AM III, Daniel GL, Longo WE: Chronic constipation—is the work-up worth the cost? Dis Colon Rectum 40:280-286, 1997
17. Glia A, Lindberg G, Nilsson LH, Mihocsa L, Akerlund JE: Clinical value of symptom assessment in patients with constipation. Dis Colon Rectum 42:1401-1408, 1999
18. Kamm MA: Role of surgical treatment in patients with severe constipation. Ann Med 22:435-442, 1990
19. Hinton JM, Lennard-Jones JE, Young AC: A new method for studying gut transit times using radioopaque markers. Gut 10:842-847, 1969
20. von der Ohe MR, Camilleri M: Measurement of small bowel and colonic transit: indications and methods. Mayo Clin Proc 67:1169-1179, 1992
21. Arhan P, Devroede G, Jehannin B, Lanza M, Faverdin C, Dornic C, Persoz B, Tetreault L, Perey B, Pellerin D: Segmental colonic transit time. Dis Colon Rectum 24:625-629, 1981
22. Mollen RM, Claassen AT, Kuijpers JH: The evaluation and treatment of functional constipation. Scand J Gastroenterol Suppl 223:8-17, 1997
23. Metcalf AM, Phillips SF, Zinsmeister AR, MacCarty RL, Beart RW, Wolff BG: Simplified assessment of segmental colonic transit. Gastroenterology 92:40-47, 1987
24. Stivland T, Camilleri M, Vassallo M, Proano M, Rath D, Brown M, Thomforde G, Pemberton J, Phillips S: Scintigraphic measurement of regional gut transit in idiopathic constipation. Gastroenterology 101:107-115, 1991
25. Camilleri M, Zinsmeister AR: Towards a relatively inexpensive, noninvasive, accurate test for colonic motility disorders. Gastroenterology 103:36-42, 1992
26. Wald A, Caruana BJ, Freimanis MG, Bauman DH, Hinds JP: Contributions of evacuation proctography and anorectal manometry to evaluation of adults with constipation and defecatory difficulty. Dig Dis Sci 35:481-487, 1990
27. Mahieu P, Pringot J, Bodart P: Defecography: I. Description of a new procedure and results in normal patients. Gastrointest Radiol 9:247-251, 1984
28. Mahieu P, Pringot J, Bodart P: Defecography: II. Contribution to the diagnosis of defecation disorders. Gastrointest Radiol 9:253-261, 1984
29. Bartram CI, Turnbull GK, Lennard-Jones JE: Evacuation proctography: an investigation of rectal expulsion in 20 subjects without defecatory disturbance. Gastrointest Radiol 13:72-80, 1988
30. Turnbull GK, Bartram CI, Lennard-Jones JE: Radiologic studies of rectal evacuation in adults with idiopathic constipation. Dis Colon Rectum 31:190-197, 1988
31. Shorvon PJ, McHugh S, Diamant NE, Somers S, Stevenson GW: Defecography in normal volunteers: results and implications. Gut 30:1737-1749, 1989
32. Kamm MA, Bartram CI, Lennard-Jones JE: Rectodynamics—quantifying rectal evacuation. Int J Colorectal Dis 4:161-163, 1989
33. Wald A, Jafri F, Rehder J, Holeva K: Scintigraphic studies of rectal emptying in patients with constipation and defecatory difficulty. Dig Dis Sci 38:353-358, 1993
34. Hutchinson R, Mostafa AB, Grant EA, Smith NB, Deen KI, Harding LK, Kumar D: Scintigraphic defecography: quantitative and dynamic assessment of anorectal function. Dis Colon Rectum 36:1132-1138, 1993
35. Fleshman JW, Dreznik Z, Cohen E, Fry RD, Kodner IJ: Balloon expulsion test facilitates diagnosis of pelvic floor outlet obstruction due to nonrelaxing puborectalis muscle. Dis Colon Rectum 35:1019-1025, 1992
36. Pezim ME, Pemberton JH, Levin KE, Litchy WJ, Phillips SF: Parameters of anorectal and colonic motility in health and in severe constipation. Dis Colon Rectum 36:484-491, 1993

37. Camilleri M, Thompson WG, Fleshman JW, Pemberton JH: Clinical management of intractable constipation. Ann Intern Med 121:520-528, 1994

38. van der Sijp JR, Kamm MA, Bartram CI, Lennard-Jones JE: The value of age of onset and rectal emptying in predicting the outcome of colectomy for severe idiopathic constipation. Int J Colorectal Dis 7:35-37, 1992

39. Bleijenberg G, Kuijpers HC: Biofeedback treatment of constipation: a comparison of two methods. Am J Gastroenterol 89:1021-1026, 1994

40. Bleijenberg G, Kuijpers HC: Treatment of the spastic pelvic floor syndrome with biofeedback. Dis Colon Rectum 30:108-111, 1987

41. Dahl J, Lindquist BL, Tysk C, Leissner P, Philipson L, Jarnerot G: Behavioral medicine treatment in chronic constipation with paradoxical anal sphincter contraction. Dis Colon Rectum 34:769-776, 1991

42. Kawimbe BM, Papachrysostomou M, Binnie NR, Clare N, Smith AN: Outlet obstruction constipation (anismus) managed by biofeedback. Gut 32:1175-1179, 1991

43. Lestar B, Penninckx F, Kerremans R: Biofeedback defaecation training for anismus. Int J Colorectal Dis 6:202-207, 1991

44. Fleshman JW, Dreznik Z, Meyer K, Fry RD, Carney R, Kodner IJ: Outpatient protocol for biofeedback therapy of pelvic floor outlet obstruction. Dis Colon Rectum 35:1-7, 1992

45. Wexner SD, Cheape JD, Jorge JM, Heymen S, Jagelman DG: Prospective assessment of biofeedback for the treatment of paradoxical puborectalis contraction. Dis Colon Rectum 35:145-150, 1992

46. Juhasz ES, Pemberton JH, Rath DM: Early and late results of pelvic floor retraining for pelvic floor discoordination (abstract). Gastroenterology 104:A530, 1993

47. Papachrysostomou M, Smith AN: Effects of biofeedback on obstructive defecation—reconditioning of the defecation reflex? Gut 35:252-256, 1994

48. Ho YH, Tan M, Goh HS: Clinical and physiologic effects of biofeedback in outlet obstruction constipation. Dis Colon Rectum 39:520-524, 1996

49. Gilliland R, Heymen S, Altomare DF, Park UC, Vickers D, Wexner SD: Outcome and predictors of success of biofeedback for constipation. Br J Surg 84:1123-1126, 1997

50. Glia A, Gylin M, Gullberg K, Lindberg G: Biofeedback retraining in patients with functional constipation and paradoxical puborectalis contraction: comparison of anal manometry and sphincter electromyography for feedback. Dis Colon Rectum 40:889-895, 1997

51. Karlbom U, Hallden M, Eeg-Olofsson KE, Pahlman L, Graf W: Results of biofeedback in constipated patients: a prospective study. Dis Colon Rectum 40:1149-1155, 1997

52. Ko CY, Tong J, Lehman RE, Shelton AA, Schrock TR, Welton ML: Biofeedback is effective therapy for fecal incontinence and constipation. Arch Surg 132:829-833, 1997

53. Patankar SK, Ferrara A, Levy JR, Larach SW, Williamson PR, Perozo SE: Biofeedback in colorectal practice: a multicenter, statewide, three-year experience. Dis Colon Rectum 40:827-831, 1997

54. Rieger NA, Wattchow DA, Sarre RG, Saccone GT, Rich CA, Cooper SJ, Marshall VR, McCall JL: Prospective study of biofeedback for treatment of constipation. Dis Colon Rectum 40:1143-1148, 1997

55. Rao SS, Welcher KD, Pelsang RE: Effects of biofeedback therapy on anorectal function in obstructive defecation. Dig Dis Sci 42:2197-2205, 1997

56. Chiotakakou-Faliakou E, Kamm MA, Roy AJ, Storrie JB, Turner IC: Biofeedback provides long-term benefit for patients with intractable, slow and normal transit constipation. Gut 42:517-521, 1998

57. McKee RF, McEnroe L, Anderson JH, Finlay IG: Identification of patients likely to benefit from biofeedback for outlet obstruction constipation. Br J Surg 86:355-359, 1999

58. Pinho M, Yoshioka K, Keighley MR: Long-term results of anorectal myectomy for chronic constipation. Dis Colon Rectum 33:795-797, 1990

59. Kamm MA, Hawley PR, Lennard-Jones JE: Lateral division of the puborectalis muscle in the management of severe constipation. Br J Surg 75:661-663, 1988

60. Williams NS, Hughes SF, Stuchfield B: Continent colonic conduit for rectal evacuation in severe constipation. Lancet 343:1321-1324, 1994

61. Kuijpers HC: Application of the colorectal laboratory in diagnosis and treatment of functional constipation. Dis Colon Rectum 33:35-39, 1990

62. Pemberton JH, Rath DM, Ilstrup DM: Evaluation and surgical treatment of severe chronic constipation. Ann Surg 214:403-411, 1991

63. Ho YH, Tan M, Eu KW, Leong A, Choen FS: Laparoscopic-assisted compared with open total colectomy in treating slow transit constipation. Aust N Z J Surg 67:562-565, 1997

64. Kamm MA, van der Sijp JR, Hawley PR, Phillips RK, Lennard-Jones JE: Left hemicolectomy with rectal excision for severe idiopathic constipation. Int J Colorectal Dis 6:49-51, 1991

65. You YT, Wang JY, Changchien CR, Chen JS, Hsu KC, Tang R, Chiang JM, Chen HH: Segmental colectomy in the management of colonic inertia. Am Surg 64:775-777, 1998

66. de Graaf EJ, Gilberts EC, Schouten WR: Role of segmental colonic transit time studies to select patients with slow transit constipation for partial left-sided or subtotal colectomy. Br J Surg 83:648-651, 1996

67. Costalat G, Garrigues JM, Didelot JM, Yousfi A, Boccasanta P: Subtotal colectomy with ceco-rectal anastomosis (Deloyers) for severe idiopathic constipation: an alternative to total colectomy reducing risks of digestive sequelae [French]. Ann Chir 51:248-255, 1997

68. Yoshioka K, Keighley MR: Clinical results of colectomy for severe constipation. Br J Surg 76:600-604, 1989

69. Fasth S, Hedlund H, Svaninger G, Oresland T, Hulten L: Functional results after subtotal colectomy and caecorectal anastomosis. Acta Chir Scand 149:623-627, 1983

70. Platell C, Scache D, Mumme G, Stitz R: A long-term follow-up of patients undergoing colectomy for chronic idiopathic constipation. Aust N Z J Surg 66:525-529, 1996

71. Nicholls RJ, Kamm MA: Proctocolectomy with restorative ileoanal reservoir for severe idiopathic constipation: report of two cases. Dis Colon Rectum 31:968-969, 1988

72. Sunderland GT, Poon FW, Lauder J, Finlay IG: Videoproctography in selecting patients with constipation for colectomy. Dis Colon Rectum 35:235-237, 1992

73. Hosie KB, Kmiot WA, Keighley MR: Constipation: another indication for restorative proctocolectomy. Br J Surg 77:801-802, 1990

74. Rex DK, Lappas JC, Goulet RC, Madura JA: Selection of constipated patients as subtotal colectomy candidates. J Clin Gastroenterol 15:212-217, 1992

75. Mahendrarajah K, Van der Schaaf AA, Lovegrove FT, Mendelson R, Levitt MD: Surgery for severe constipation: the use of

radioisotope transit scan and barium evacuation proctography in patient selection. Aust N Z J Surg 64:183-186, 1994

76. Piccirillo MF, Reissman P, Wexner SD: Colectomy as treatment for constipation in selected patients. Br J Surg 82:898-901, 1995

77. Redmond JM, Smith GW, Barofsky I, Ratych RE, Goldsborough DC, Schuster MM: Physiological tests to predict long-term outcome of total abdominal colectomy for intractable constipation. Am J Gastroenterol 90:748-753, 1995

78. Christiansen J, Rasmussen OO: Colectomy for severe slow-transit constipation in strictly selected patients. Scand J Gastroenterol 31:770-773, 1996

79. Ghosh S, Papachrysostomou M, Batool M, Eastwood MA: Long-term results of subtotal colectomy and evidence of noncolonic involvement in patients with idiopathic slow-transit constipation. Scand J Gastroenterol 31:1083-1091, 1996

80. Lubowski DZ, Chen FC, Kennedy ML, King DW: Results of colectomy for severe slow transit constipation. Dis Colon Rectum 39:23-29, 1996

81. Pluta H, Bowes KL, Jewell LD: Long-term results of total abdominal colectomy for chronic idiopathic constipation: value of preoperative assessment. Dis Colon Rectum 39:160-166, 1996

82. Nyam DC, Pemberton JH, Ilstrup DM, Rath DM: Long-term results of surgery for chronic constipation. Dis Colon Rectum 40:273-279, 1997

83. Bernini A, Madoff RD, Lowry AC, Spencer MP, Gemlo BT, Jensen LL, Wong WD: Should patients with combined colonic inertia and nonrelaxing pelvic floor undergo subtotal colectomy? Dis Colon Rectum 41:1363-1366, 1998

84. Lahr SJ, Lahr CJ, Srinivasan A, Clerico ET, Limehouse VM, Serbezov IK: Operative management of severe constipation. Am Surg 65:1117-1121, 1999

85. Preston DM, Hawley PR, Lennard-Jones JE, Todd IP: Results of colectomy for severe idiopathic constipation in women (Arbuthnot Lane's disease). Br J Surg 71:547-552, 1984

86. Roe AM, Bartolo DC, Mortensen NJ: Diagnosis and surgical management of intractable constipation. Br J Surg 73:854-861, 1986

87. Leon SH, Krishnamurthy S, Schuffler MD: Subtotal colectomy for severe idiopathic constipation: a follow-up study of 13 patients. Dig Dis Sci 32:1249-1254, 1987

88. Akervall S, Fasth S, Nordgren S, Oresland T, Hulten L: The functional results after colectomy and ileorectal anastomosis for severe constipation (Arbuthnot Lane's disease) as related to rectal sensory function. Int J Colorectal Dis 3:96-101, 1988

89. Kamm MA, Hawley PR, Lennard-Jones JE: Outcome of colectomy for severe idiopathic constipation. Gut 29:969-973, 1988

90. Vasilevsky CA, Nemer FD, Balcos EG, Christenson CE, Goldberg SM: Is subtotal colectomy a viable option in the management of chronic constipation? Dis Colon Rectum 31:679-681, 1988

91. Nightingale JM, Kamm MA, van der Sijp JR, Morris GP, Walker ER, Mather SJ, Britton KE, Lennard-Jones JE: Disturbed gastric emptying in the short bowel syndrome: evidence for a 'colonic brake.' Gut 34:1171-1176, 1993

DIVERTICULAR DISEASE OF THE COLON

Tonia M. Young-Fadok, M.D.

At the beginning of the 20th century, diverticular disease was uncommon. Since then, however, it has become perhaps the most common affliction of the colon, although many patients remain completely asymptomatic. Despite the fact that Rochester, Minnesota, is a small community and common diseases have a tendency to be overshadowed in tertiary care centers, Mayo Clinic surgeons have made important contributions to the safety of operative intervention for diverticulitis. In fact, William J. Mayo, M.D., and colleagues, in 1907, were the first to report surgical resection for a small series of nine patients with complicated diverticulitis.[1] All patients presented with what would now be considered florid symptoms and signs, one with a mass "as large as a child's head...in the region of the sigmoid," a description indicating the unusual nature of the diagnosis at that time. All nine patients underwent resection; two patients died and two had persistent fistulas. The authors had reason for pride in their presentation, however, because these patients were the first in whom the pathologic diagnosis of diverticulitis was established during life. Dr. Mayo later described a series of 42 patients,[2] 13 of whom had coexistent carcinoma of the sigmoid; even today, differentiation preoperatively may be impossible, and the inability to exclude carcinoma remains an indication for surgical intervention. More recently, Mayo Clinic surgeons have contributed to improved safety of surgical resection.

TERMINOLOGY

The underlying entity of diverticulitis is a *diverticulum* (plural, diverticula), which is a saccular protrusion of mucosa through the muscle wall of the colon. The mere presence of diverticula is indicated by the term *diverticulosis*, which usually denotes the absence of symptoms. Inflammation in association with diverticula is *diverticulitis*. Finally, the term *diverticular disease* includes all manifestations of diverticula, i.e., their existence, inflammation, or bleeding. Diverticulitis may be complicated or simple. *Complicated* diverticulitis refers to the development of abscess, fistula, obstruction (from edema in the acute setting or fibrosis and stricturing as a chronic sequela), bleeding, and perforation. *Simple* diverticulitis describes the presence of diverticulitis in the absence of these complications.

PATHOLOGY AND PATHOPHYSIOLOGY

A colonic diverticulum is a false or pulsion diverticulum because it does not contain all layers of the wall. Mucosa herniates through the muscle layer and is covered only by the serosa. Diverticula develop in four "rows" at points in the colonic circumference where the vasa recta penetrate the circular muscle layer,[3] on each side of the mesenteric taenia and on the mesenteric border of the two antimesenteric taeniae (Fig. 1). Diverticula do not develop in the rectum, possibly because of the coalescence of taeniae into a longitudinal muscle layer.

Diverticula are distributed unevenly throughout the colon. In Western cultures, 95% of patients with diverticula have sigmoid involvement. Diverticula are limited to the sigmoid colon in 65% of patients, and diverticula involve the sigmoid predominantly but other segments of the colon also are involved to a lesser degree in 24%.[4]

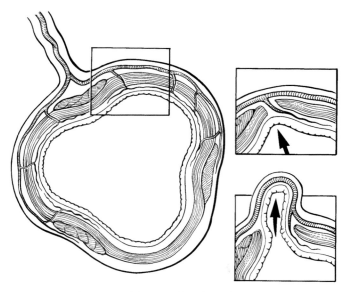

Fig. 1. Development of diverticula where the vasa recta penetrate the muscularis (arrows).

which states that pressure (P) is proportional to wall tension (T) and inversely proportional to radius (R) of the colon (P = kT/R), where "k" is a constant.

Diverticulitis, or inflammation associated with diverticula, is thought to involve a microscopic or macroscopic perforation of a thin-walled diverticulum. An early belief was that obstruction of the ostia of the diverticula, for example, by fecoliths or seeds, led to increased intradiverticular pressure and perforation, but this is now thought to be rare.[11] Increased intraluminal pressure or local trauma of inspissated food particles may erode the wall of the diverticulum. Inflammation and focal necrosis result in perforation. A small perforation often becomes walled off by pericolic fat and mesentery, resolving without further consequence or forming a localized abscess. In contrast, with more extensive inflammatory reaction, surrounding hollow organs adhere to the inflamed segment of colon, and intestinal obstruction or an internal fistula may develop. Poor containment, as may occur in antimesenteric diverticula, results in peritonitis.

Similarly, 95% of all operations for diverticular disease involve resection of the sigmoid colon.[5] This frequency contrasts with that in Asian countries, where right-sided involvement is more common.[6]

The points at which diverticula develop,[7] where the vasa recta penetrate the colon wall, are areas of potential weakness. Many patients have myochosis, i.e., thickening of the circular muscle layer, shortening of the taeniae, and luminal narrowing. There is no hypertrophy or hyperplasia of the muscular layer of the colonic wall, but deposition of elastin in the taeniae is increased.[8] Structural changes in collagen content of the wall of the sigmoid are similar to those resulting from aging but are greater in magnitude[9] and may decrease resistance of susceptible segments of the wall to abnormal increases in intraluminal pressure. Similar changes in patients with connective tissue disorders may explain the appearance of diverticula at an early age.

Abnormal motility has been implicated in the development of diverticula. Normally, intraluminal pressure is the same throughout the colon. However, segmentation of the colon (a motility process in which proximal and distal segmental muscular contractions separate the lumen into isolated chambers) is exaggerated in diverticulosis. Painter et al.[10] postulated that strong occlusive contractions at both ends of the chamber lead to marked segmental increases in intraluminal pressures (Fig. 2), which may predispose to herniation of mucosal diverticula. Because the sigmoid colon is the colon segment with the smallest diameter, it also may be the site of the greatest intraluminal pressure, according to the law of Laplace,

CLINICAL PRESENTATION

The presentation of colonic diverticular disease depends on the presence and degree of underlying inflammation. *Diverticulosis* may exist in the absence of symptoms and be diagnosed when noted as an incidental finding on a test performed for other indications. Some patients with diverticulosis complain of cramping, bloating, flatulence, and irregular defecation. Because these symptoms also may

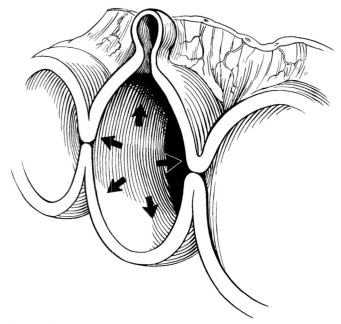

Fig. 2. Segmentation of the colon.

be present with irritable bowel syndrome, which frequently coexists with diverticulosis, it can be unclear which diagnosis is responsible for the symptoms. Fortunately, the treatment for both conditions is often similar and simple: increased dietary fiber.

Diverticulitis results from microscopic or macroscopic perforation of a diverticulum. Hence, the clinical presentation is determined by the degree of perforation and the patient's ability to contain it. The inflammation is frequently mild, and a small perforation may be walled off by pericolic fat or contained within the mesentery. This may result in a localized abscess, in a fistula if adjacent organs are involved, or obstruction. Conversely, poor containment, more likely in elderly and immunoincompetent patients, results in peritonitis. Thus, patients may present with manifestations ranging from abdominal discomfort to perforated diverticulitis with fecal peritonitis, sepsis, and death.

Left lower quadrant pain is the most common complaint in Western countries, occurring in 70% of patients.[12] Pain frequently is present for several days before presentation, and this time course aids in the differentiation of diverticulitis from other causes of acute abdominal pain. In one series, only 17% of patients had symptoms for less than 24 hours.[5] A helpful pointer in the history is that up to half of patients have had one or more previous episodes of similar pain. Other symptoms include nausea and vomiting in 20% to 62%, constipation in 50%, diarrhea in 25% to 35%, and urinary symptoms (dysuria, urgency, frequency, pneumaturia) in 10% to 15%.[12]

On physical examination, left lower quadrant tenderness is characteristic.[13] The tenderness may extend across the suprapubic region and even into the right lower quadrant if the sigmoid is redundant. Pure right lower quadrant tenderness is uncommon with sigmoid diverticulitis, but it also may result from right-sided diverticulitis, which is rare in Western countries but common in Asia.[13-15] Generalized tenderness is ominous, suggesting free perforation and peritonitis. A tender mass is present on abdominal or rectal examination in 20% of patients.[16]

Low-grade fever and mild leukocytosis are common. However, a normal temperature and leukocyte count do not exclude the diagnosis. In one series, 45% of patients had a normal leukocyte count.[17] Urinalysis may show sterile pyuria, which is a result of the adjacent inflammation in the sigmoid. Colonic flora or mixed bacteria on urine culture suggest the development of a colovesical fistula.

DIAGNOSIS AND IMAGING

Acute diverticulitis frequently can be diagnosed on the basis of the history and physical examination alone. When the clinical picture is clear, additional tests are unnecessary for a diagnosis.[18,19] We find, however, that the lack of additional testing may do the patient a disservice. A clinical diagnosis alone may be incorrect in up to a third of patients.[20,21] In addition, if additional unconfirmed attacks occur, the patient may be at risk when surgical management is refused, whereas had there been evidence, a surgical approach might have been prudent and the decision to proceed with resection would have been possible. Thus, in the patient who has symptoms of sufficient severity to merit hospitalization, our preference is to obtain radiographic confirmation.

Traditionally, abdominal and chest radiographs are obtained in the setting of acute abdominal pain. They are useful for excluding free air and other causes of abdominal pain, such as obstruction, rather than for helping make the diagnosis of diverticulitis. Contrast enema, ultrasonography, and computed tomography have a role in establishing the diagnosis of diverticulitis. Computed tomography has become our preferred method, because it is both diagnostic and potentially therapeutic and allows evaluation of the extramural inflammatory process. Features of diverticulitis on computed tomography include increased soft tissue density within pericolic fat in 98%, colonic diverticula in 84%, bowel wall thickening in 70%, and soft tissue masses representing phlegmon, or pericolic fluid collections representing abscesses, in 35%.[22,23]

In 10% of patients, diverticulitis cannot be distinguished from carcinoma because both can have bowel wall thickening. Features more suggestive of diverticulitis are fluid at the base of the mesentery and mesenteric vascular engorgement.[24] Helical computed tomography with colonic contrast alone is up to 99% accurate for diagnosing diverticulitis and avoids the risks, costs, and delays associated with oral and intravenous contrast studies, in addition to suggesting an alternative diagnosis in 58% of patients who do not have diverticulitis.[25]

With computed tomography, the extent of pericolic inflammation can be staged, a feature that is underestimated by contrast enema examination in 41% of patients.[23] Inflammation can be classified as mild (localized colonic wall thickening and inflammation of pericolic fat) or severe (extensive pericolic thickening and stranding, extraluminal gas, and pericolic abscess). For patients with severe inflammation, elective resection can be offered to those who respond to medical therapy. Finally, computed tomography also may be therapeutic. Computed tomography-guided percutaneous drainage of localized abscesses may avoid emergency operation and allow a later single-stage procedure.

High-resolution compression ultrasonography may reveal a thickened colonic wall or cystic masses with echogenic densities suggestive of abscess.[26] In 85% of patients, an abnormal colonic segment, thicker than 4 mm over a segment of 5 cm or longer, is found at the point of maximal tenderness.[27] The colon has a target-like appearance in cross-section. Reported sensitivities range from 85% to 98% and specificities from 80% to 98%.[27,28] The technique is limited by being operator-dependent and is hampered by the presence of abdominal distention.

Contrast enema examination is safe in the acute setting if single-contrast technique is used. In the presence of free air, barium is absolutely contraindicated,[29] but water-soluble contrast is safe and may indicate the site of perforation. Even in the absence of peritoneal signs, water-soluble contrast is most often preferred in any patient with suspected diverticulitis. With the ready availability of computed tomography, contrast enema testing is used rarely, but it does have a role if the diagnosis is equivocal on computed tomography.

Endoscopic evaluation (rigid proctoscopy or flexible sigmoidoscopy) is relatively contraindicated in acute diverticulitis. Air insufflation may convert a sealed perforation to a free leak. Limited sigmoidoscopy occasionally is necessary to rule out, for example, inflammatory bowel disease, and in experienced hands a gentle examination with minimal air insufflation is considered safe.[30]

MEDICAL THERAPY AND INDICATIONS FOR OPERATION

The presentation of sigmoid diverticulitis and its medical and surgical management are the subject of practice guidelines published by the American Society of Colon and Rectal Surgeons (ASCRS)[19] and the Society for Surgery of the Alimentary Tract (SSAT).[31] This outline of our approach conforms to these standards.

From a clinical and therapeutic viewpoint, diverticulitis is divided into simple and complicated presentations. Simple diverticulitis, which affects 75% of patients, is not associated with complications, and most of these patients respond to medical therapy. Complicated diverticulitis refers to the presence of perforation, obstruction, abscess, or fistula, which arises in 25% of patients in the first episode. Nearly all of these patients require operation, but in some an emergency procedure can be converted to an elective procedure.

Medical Therapy

In the absence of systemic symptoms and signs, patients with mild abdominal tenderness can be treated as outpatients. Treatment includes a low-residue diet and oral antibiotics such as metronidazole (500 mg three times a day) or ciprofloxacin (500 mg twice a day). Oral ciprofloxacin reaches blood levels similar to those with intravenous administration and requires only twice-daily dosing, thus improving compliance. Hospitalization is recommended for increasing abdominal tenderness, fever, or inability to tolerate oral intake. Patients who have comorbid conditions that may mask reliable symptoms and signs, such as patients with immunosuppression or diabetes, should not be treated as outpatients.

Hospitalization is indicated for patients with more severe disease, substantial pain, or localized peritonitis. Initial therapy is conservative, aiming to obtain a response and avoid operation or to convert an urgent situation to an elective one. Therapy includes bowel rest (a nasogastric tube is usually required only if there is an obstructive picture with an incompetent ileocecal valve and small bowel distention) and intravenous fluids. Intravenous broad-spectrum antibiotics should cover anaerobic and gram-negative flora. Recommended regimens, based on consensus rather than randomized trials, include antianaerobic coverage with metronidazole or clindamycin and gram-negative coverage with an aminoglycoside (e.g., gentamicin), monobactam (e.g., aztreonam), or a third-generation cephalosporin (e.g., ceftazidime, ceftriaxone).[32] Single-agent coverage with second-degree cephalosporins (e.g., cefotetan) or β-lactamase inhibitor combinations (e.g., ampicillin-sulbactam, ticarcillin-clavulanate) are also reasonable.[33] Intravenous analgesia is important for patient comfort, but titration is needed so as not to preclude accurate assessment of abdominal signs. Some clinicians prefer meperidine rather than morphine,[34] but the evidence for morphine causing increased intracolic pressure is old and possibly unreliable. Abscesses found on computed tomography should be drained. An abscess less than 4 cm in diameter is often not amenable to catheter drainage and often can be treated successfully with antibiotics. In this situation, we collaborate closely with a radiologist.

The three possible outcomes are improvement, failure to improve, and deterioration. Improvement should be apparent within 48 hours, with decreased tenderness, fever, and leukocytosis. Persistent signs suggest an incorrect diagnosis or a nonresolving phlegmon or abscess, and computed tomography may identify those in whom an abscess has developed which may respond to percutaneous drainage. Patients who improve are dismissed with instructions for a low-residue diet. Six weeks later they are evaluated with colonoscopy or with flexible sigmoidoscopy and barium enema examination. After resolution of symptoms, a high-fiber diet is recommended because long-term use of fiber may prevent recurrences.[35,36]

Indications for Operation

Emergency Indications

Diffuse peritonitis mandates resuscitation, broad-spectrum antibiotics, and emergency exploration. Extensive diagnostic testing is rarely necessary. Examples of antibiotic regimens are ampicillin (1 to 2 g intravenously every 4-6 h) and gentamicin (1.5 to 2 mg/kg intravenously every 8 h) and metronidazole (500 mg intravenously every 8 h), imipenem-cilastatin (500 mg intravenously every 6 h), and piperacillin-tazobactam (3.375 to 4.5 g intravenously every 6 h).

Certain patients who initially fulfill criteria for conservative management will require emergency surgical intervention. If a patient's condition deteriorates (increasing pain, more localized peritonitis or diffuse tenderness, increasing leukocyte count), a search should be made for a reversible condition (i.e., computed tomography to rule out drainable abscess). Operation is necessary if there is no reversible condition, if an abscess cannot be drained, or if drainage does not result in improvement. Sometimes the most difficult patients to treat are those who do not respond to medical therapy but whose condition does not deteriorate. Failure to improve is also an indication for operation.

Elective Indications

Elective resection is advocated for patients who have had one episode of complicated diverticulitis (e.g., abscess, obstruction, or fistula) that responded to initial conservative management. Elective resection is usually performed 6 to 8 weeks after the acute episode to allow inflammation to subside. Elective operation is also offered to those who have had two confirmed episodes of acute diverticulitis. Generally, the episodes should have been severe enough to require hospitalization, but a careful history will sometimes reveal patients (often physicians) with symptoms of sufficient severity to have merited admission but who treated themselves at home with antibiotics. Conversely, it is often wiser not to offer resection to the patient who has had multiple "episodes" treated by their primary physician with antibiotics on an outpatient basis and has no documented abnormality in leukocyte count, barium enema, or computed tomography during an episode. It is prudent to recommend documentation with the next attack.

Special Cases

In certain circumstances, surgical resection is offered after only one attack, even in the absence of complicated diverticulitis. These include immunocompromised patients and those with connective tissue disorders. The immunocompromised patient is predisposed to infection and exhibits delayed wound healing. Such patients often fail to demonstrate typical symptoms and signs of acute inflammatory processes of the abdomen. It is unclear whether patients receiving exogenous steroid therapy or chemotherapy or those with chronic renal failure have a greater incidence of diverticulosis. Diverticulosis is reported in 45% to 50% of patients with renal failure and in 13% of those who have had transplantation.[37] A particularly high incidence of diverticulosis is associated with polycystic kidney disease.[38] It is clear, however, that there is an increased incidence of complicated diverticulitis in immunocompromised patients. In one series of 209 patients,[39] free perforation occurred in 43% of immunocompromised patients and in only 14% of immunocompetent patients. Postoperative morbidity rates were 65% and 24%, and mortality rates were 39% and 2%, respectively. Patients with polycystic kidney disease constituted only 9% of one transplant series but 46% of cases of diverticulitis. Hence, immunocompromised patients having one episode of documented diverticulitis should undergo elective resection.

The approach is similar in patients with connective tissue disorders. Many are already immunocompromised from treatment with corticosteroids, but they seem to have an additional risk of complicated diverticulitis related to the underlying disorder. In one study, 27 patients with lupus who underwent colectomy were compared with patients who had inflammatory bowel disease in an attempt to match for steroid use. Diverticulitis was the most common indication for colectomy in the patients with lupus— 13 of the 27, and 6 of those presented with perforation. Postoperative morbidity was also substantially increased in the lupus group, resulting in the recommendation that patients with lupus should be offered resection after a single attack of diverticulitis.[40]

Young patients are traditionally offered surgical intervention after recovery from a single episode. The recommendation is based on two premises. The first is that young patients manifest a more virulent form of the disease (i.e., are more likely to have complications and more often require operation for the first episode). The second premise is that young patients who respond to medical management are more likely to have recurrent episodes.

Closer evaluation of available data suggests that the approach in young patients is less straightforward. Because diverticulitis is relatively unusual in young patients, the natural history is unclear. Patients younger than 40 years constitute only 12% to 29% of larger series.[12,17,41-43] Certain features are common to most series. There is a consistent male dominance in young patients, the ratio ranging from 2:1 to 4:1.[12,17,41,42] Comorbid conditions are unusual with the exception of obesity in 84% to 96% of these patients.[12,41] The percentage who undergo resection, however, varies widely, as does the rate of pre-operative misdiagnosis.

Concern that the disease is more virulent in young patients arises from series showing that a high percentage of these patients undergo operative intervention. The frequency of operation, however, varies markedly. For comparison, studies of all patients with diverticulitis report operation rates of 27% to 33%.[4,5] Support for the more virulent theory comes from series of young patients in whom operation rates range from 48% to 88%.[12,42,43] In disagreement are other series of young patients with operation rates at first admission of 15% to 41%.[17,41]

This situation is partly explained by consideration of misdiagnosis rates. Many young patients undergo urgent operation after incorrect preoperative diagnosis.[44] Series with high rates of misdiagnosis, of 41% to 50%, have higher operation rates.[12,42] In one series of 63 patients younger than 45 years, conservative treatment was successful in 65%.[45] Of the 22 patients (35%) who underwent exploration, 12 had a misdiagnosis. Thus, only 10 of the 63 patients (16%) actually required emergency intervention. In another study, preoperative computed tomographic and contrast studies were extensively used; the operative rate was only 15% in patients younger than 40 years but was 33% in older patients.[17] That study, however, also found that younger patients had more severe diverticulitis by computed tomographic criteria and an increased risk of poor outcomes (persistent inflammation, residual abscess, fistula, stenosis) that ultimately necessitated operation.

Young patients may have a predisposition to recurrence of symptoms. In 77 patients younger than 50 years, 23% required operation at presentation for peritonitis, abscess, obstruction, and fistula.[46] A fourth of the whole group, and two-thirds of those requiring resection, had a prior hospitalization for complicated diverticulitis. Other investigators have reported that young patients initially treated medically had more emergency room visits and complications than those who underwent resection.[47] Some studies have confirmed this finding, reporting readmission rates of up to 55%[48] and subsequent operative rates of 20% to 41%.[44,48,49] However, other series have reported no subsequent operation after 4 years of follow-up.[50]

One way to make sense of these conflicting data is to consider the *overall* operative rate for the first admission and subsequently.[51] This overall rate is more consistent, in the range of 50%. Thus, some series suggest a high operative rate at first presentation,[12,42,43] and others show a lower rate at first admission of 15% to 25% but with a poor outcome at first admission in up to 29% of patients[17] and subsequent operation in 32% of patients.[49] The data are relatively consistent when examined in this way, but, again, discrepancies develop when different authors have

different interpretations. Some state that after medical therapy a risk of subsequent operation of 32% to 41% in patients followed for 5 to 9 years does not justify elective resection.[49] Others disagree and recommend elective operation on the basis of the same data.[48]

Thus, evidence suggests an ultimate operative rate of 50%. High rates at first presentation occur in the presence of misdiagnosis (the diagnosis is often not considered in a young patient with peritoneal signs). Although the operative rate at first admission may decrease with wider use of computed tomography, a larger proportion of those responding to medical therapy ultimately may require resection. Our approach is to advise younger patients whose first episode has responded to medical therapy of the risks and benefits of operation versus observation. This issue thus rests on the patient's own evaluation of risks and lifestyle concerns.[51] In a patient with no comorbid conditions, elective operation after a single episode remains a reasonable option, whereas another patient with the same risks may be equally justified in choosing observation.

CONDUCT OF OPERATION

The conduct of the operation is governed by the setting: emergency or elective. These circumstances essentially describe the stability of the patient, the degree of contamination or inflammation present, and the ability to perform a bowel preparation, and these factors, in turn, dictate the procedure selected.

Laparotomy: Emergency

An emergency exists in the presence of free perforation with purulent or fecal peritonitis (Hinchey stages III and IV)[52] and an acute abdomen. Sepsis from an undrainable abscess and unrelieved large bowel obstruction are also in this category. Bowel preparation is not indicated, and attention is focused on rapid resuscitation, correction of fluid and electrolyte abnormalities, and administration of broad-spectrum antibiotics. The patient should be informed of the need for stoma; if time permits, the right and left lower quadrants are marked for ileostomy or colostomy by an enterostomal therapist.

The basic tenets include control of sepsis, resection of diseased tissue, and restoration of intestinal continuity, if possible, with or without a protective stoma. The four basic surgical options are 1) the outdated three-stage approach with only colostomy and drainage at a first operation, followed by colonic resection at a second operation and closure of the colostomy at a third operation; 2) two-stage approach with colonic resection, closure of proximal rectum, and colostomy at the first operation (Hartmann's procedure), followed by takedown of the colostomy and anastomosis at a second operation; 3) two-stage approach with colonic resection, anastomosis, and proximal colostomy or ileostomy at the first operation, followed by closure of the stoma at the second operation; and 4) primary resection with anastomosis in one operation (Table 1).

Three-Stage Procedure: Transverse Colostomy and Drainage

The three-stage procedure is rarely indicated, and in most settings it is condemned. Nagorney et al.[53] from Mayo Clinic and Finlay and Carter[54] reported more morbidity in patients treated with colostomy and drainage alone as the first of three operations. The Mayo Clinic series also noted a higher mortality rate for the three-stage procedure: 26% vs. 7% with resection. Only rarely are the inflammatory changes so extensive as to preclude mobilization and resection because of concerns regarding the safety of the ureter and iliac vessels. The procedure may have merit when advanced surgical care is not immediately available, as a temporizing procedure before the patient is transferred to a tertiary center.

Two-Stage Procedure Versus Primary Anastomosis

The patient is placed in synchronous lithotomy position to permit access to the perineum. An adequate incision is made. A dense inflammatory reaction around the focal point in the sigmoid often precludes initiation of dissection in this area. It is helpful to begin dissection peripherally, both proximally along the lateral peritoneal reflection of the descending colon and distally in the rectum. This approach allows a "proximal-to-distal" resection, in which the colon is divided proximal to the phlegmon with a linear stapler and the colon is dissected proximal to distal rather than the usual lateral-to-medial dissection.[51] Ureteral stents may help in identifying the ureters in softer tissues distant from the inflammatory process, allowing them to be followed more easily. Once the diseased segment has been mobilized, a decision must be made to perform an anastomosis or a colostomy.

Two-Stage: Hartmann's Procedure

Contraindications to primary anastomosis include both intraoperative findings and comorbid conditions. A primary anastomosis should not be performed in the presence of feculent peritonitis, malnutrition, immunosuppression, severe anemia, and uncertain viability of the bowel. In these cases, Hartmann's procedure should be performed. The rectal stump can be stapled or sutured. I prefer to leave drains in the pelvis or use a rectal tube to control or prevent disruption of the rectal stump. Use of long, nonabsorbable, monofilament sutures to mark the top of the rectal stump assists in identification when the colostomy is closed at a second operation.

Two-Stage: Resection, Primary Anastomosis, and Proximal Stoma

Hartmann's procedure removes the source of sepsis, but reversal of the colostomy is often difficult because of adhesions and difficulty identifying the rectal stump. Up to a third of patients are left with a permanent stoma.[55] Relative contraindications to an unprotected anastomosis include presence of a chronic abscess cavity and mild systemic illness, in which case the patient may be served better by creation of a primary anastomosis that is protected by a proximal diverting colostomy or ileostomy. Our practice is for a loop ileostomy (in the absence of substantial fecal loading of the colon) because it is easy to close, less bulky, and easier to manage than a loop colostomy.

Table 1.—Choice of Operation for Colonic Diverticulitis

Hinchey stage	Description	Recommended procedure	Alternative procedures
I	Simple diverticulitis	Elective sigmoid resection, primary anastomosis Emergency sigmoid resection, primary anastomosis, ± proximal diverting stoma	Sigmoid resection, end colostomy, and rectal stump in lupus or collagen vascular disorders
II	Contained abscess	Percutaneous drainage, then elective sigmoid resection, primary anastomosis Emergency sigmoid resection, primary anastomosis, ± proximal diverting stoma	Consider Hartmann's procedure in immunocompromised patient
III	Purulent peritonitis	Hartmann's procedure Emergency sigmoid resection, primary anastomosis, proximal diverting stoma	Three-stage procedure in rare cases
IV	Fecal peritonitis	Hartmann's procedure	Three-stage procedure in rare cases

Single-Stage Procedure With On-table Lavage

In the emergency setting, preoperative bowel preparation is not possible, and a large fecal load precludes a primary anastomosis. Consideration may be given to intraoperative colonic lavage in selected patients to permit primary resection and anastomosis. In addition to mobilization of the affected sigmoid, mobilization of the splenic and sometimes the hepatic flexure may help.[51] Bowel proximal to the sigmoid is occluded with tape, and immediately above this the lumen is cannulated with large-bore, corrugated plastic tubing (anesthesia ventilator tubing). The end of the tube is passed off the field. The cecum or appendix base is cannulated with a Foley catheter, through which warm saline is infused until the efflux is clear. Lavage was performed in 33 of 62 patients undergoing nonelective operation for diverticulitis: 18 Hinchey stage I, 10 stage II, and 5 stage III disease.[56] Only one anastomotic complication occurred.

Laparotomy: Elective

Elective resection is usually performed 6 to 8 weeks after the most recent episode. This interval allows the inflammatory process to subside. A longer wait may increase the risk of another attack, but there are no clear data for this commonly held belief. Usual bowel preparation is used. At Mayo Clinic, either two 45-mL bottles of sodium phosphate (at 5 PM and 10 PM) or 2 to 4 liters of polyethylene glycol solution (at 5 PM) is used, in addition to 2 g each of metronidazole and neomycin at 7 PM and 11 PM. The patient is placed in synchronous position. Ureteral catheters are used rarely and selectively in patients with considerable prior phlegmon, prior abscess drainage, or persistent discomfort in the left lower quadrant suggestive of continued inflammation.

In quiescent disease, the standard lateral-to-medial approach is possible. In the presence of inflammation or heavy scarring and obliteration of the normal plane, the previously described method of commencing peripherally in normal planes and "moving in" on the difficult area is successful. The proximal resection margin should be in soft, pliable bowel, usually the distal descending colon. This area does not have to be free of diverticula but must be free of bowel wall thickening. The distal resection margin must be in the proximal rectum. Below this, diverticula rarely, if ever, occur. Benn et al.[57] described 501 patients who had sigmoid resection for diverticular disease at Mayo Clinic. Recurrent diverticulitis occurred in 12.5% of patients when the distal sigmoid was retained and in 6.7% of patients in whom the rectum formed the distal margin (P = 0.03).[57] The splenic flexure should be mobilized if necessary to achieve a tension-free anastomosis, but it is not necessary in all cases. Dissection of the upper presacral space and mobilization of the proximal rectum also may assist with creation of the anastomosis.

Laparoscopic Resection

Laparoscopic techniques have a role in several facets of diverticular disease.[58] These include diagnosis, diversion, resection of the affected segment of colon, and restoration of colonic continuity (either as a staged procedure or primarily). Free perforation and fecal peritonitis or extensive purulent peritonitis are absolute contraindications to the laparoscopic approach because of the limitations on complete exploration and clearance of contaminated material. Both single-institution[59,60] and multicenter studies[61] have shown benefits of the approach in terms of reduced ileus and hospital stay and complication rates comparable to those of laparotomy. Randomized trials confirming superiority of the approach, however, have not been performed.

The inflammation that may accompany diverticulitis is often challenging, even in open procedures. Resolution of the inflammatory component allows for a successful laparoscopic approach in most cases.[58] The presence of a colovesical, colovaginal, or coloenteric fistula reduces the chances of completing the procedure laparoscopically, as does prior use of a drain, but it is not an absolute contraindication to this approach. Even in open cases, the bladder side of a colovesical fistula frequently requires nothing more than pinching off the fibrous fistula tract and leaving the bladder decompressed with catheter drainage. The same principles apply to the laparoscopic approach. Ureteral stents may be helpful. Lighted stents are not necessary because the firm tubular structure of the stent in the retroperitoneum usually can be detected with the laparoscopic instruments. As with open procedures, it is helpful to approach the mass in the sigmoid from both cephalad and caudad directions, normal tissue planes away from the phlegmon having been identified. A low threshold for conversion to laparotomy should be maintained to avoid damage to vessels and ureter. The same extent of resection should be accomplished laparoscopically, namely, proximal resection of the sigmoid back to soft, pliable tissue and distal resection to a point where the taeniae have coalesced, necessitating resection to a point below the sacral promontory. This approach thus precludes an extracorporeal anastomosis.

Patient Preparation

A routine bowel preparation is used. It is helpful to add 2 tablets of bisacodyl toward the end of the preparation (at 10 PM) because it reduces residual liquid in the small bowel, avoids handling of heavy fluid-filled bowel loops, and improves visualization.

Equipment and Instruments

Certain basic laparoscopic equipment is required. The surgeon's familiarity and comfort with the equipment are more important than the specific details. A 30° laparoscope is most helpful, particularly for mobilization of the flexures and when working in the pelvis. Basic instruments include graspers and some means of dividing tissue. Bowel-handling instruments should be atraumatic and used with care to prevent serosal injury or even enterotomy. The Mayo Clinic approach is to attempt, when possible, grasping the peritoneal edge adjacent to the bowel rather than the bowel wall itself. Instruments should be of sufficient length to reach up to the flexures and down into the pelvis. For minimizing the risk of complications, whether electrocautery (monopolar or bipolar) or ultrasonic cutting devices are used is less important than awareness of potential limitations of the energy source used. A suction or irrigation device is helpful, as is a smoke filter.

At Mayo Clinic, the procedure has been simplified by using a standardized approach that minimizes disposable equipment. Two 10- to 12-mm trocars and two 5-mm trocars are used in a diamond-shaped pattern. Most of the mobilization is done with electrocautery scissors and two bowel-handling instruments (e.g., 5-mm Babcock). A 5-mm grasper with cautery attachment is useful to control small bleeding vessels. Because the anastomosis needs to be at the confluence of the taeniae in the proximal rectum, this position is too low to permit simple mobilization of a loop of sigmoid, followed by exteriorization and extracorporeal anastomosis, which does not achieve the extent of resection that is usually advocated. The laparoscopic approach should not be an excuse for performing a less than adequate resection. Hence, intracorporeal bowel division and anastomosis are necessary. Intracorporeal division of the proximal rectum requires a linear stapler. An ultrasonic dissector is useful for division of the mesorectum, but this also can be achieved with electrocautery and clips.

Patient Position and Room Setup
The patient is placed in the combined synchronous or modified lithotomy (Lloyd-Davies) position with Allen stirrups, and the arms are padded and tucked at the sides. The thighs are level with the abdominal wall to avoid interference with laparoscopic instruments used in the lower ports. The surgeon stands on the right facing the lesion; the first assistant is on the left to assist in placing traction on the sigmoid and rectum as dissection proceeds. This position also allows the surgeon to stand between the patient's legs if the splenic flexure needs to be mobilized. The nurse stands on the patient's right, above the surgeon. The camera holder stands next to the surgeon to avoid reverse images. Two monitors are used, one on each side of the patient.

Procedure
Cut-down technique is used to place a blunt trocar in the supraumbilical position. The 30° laparoscope is used

through this, a 10/12-mm trocar is placed in the right lower quadrant, and two 5-mm trocars are inserted in the left lower quadrant and the suprapubic midline. It is important to insert the lower quadrant trocars lateral to the epigastric vessels.

The operating table is positioned in the Trendelenburg position with the left side inclined up to expose the pelvis and the lateral attachments of the sigmoid colon (Fig. 3). The peritoneum lateral to the sigmoid colon is grasped and pulled medially to expose the left lateral peritoneal reflection (Fig. 4). The reflection is opened along the white line of Toldt, and the sigmoid and descending colon are mobilized medially as far as the splenic flexure. By remaining precisely on the medial aspect of the peritoneal reflection, the ureter is identified at the base of the sigmoid fossa. Remaining in the correct retroperitoneal plane exposes the ureter and Gerota's fascia and avoids dissection behind the left kidney.

The splenic flexure can be mobilized at this point in the procedure if needed, otherwise later. The splenocolic attachments are divided with cautery or ultrasonic scissors, a step allowing the whole flexure to be mobilized. The omentum is dissected off the distal transverse colon. This combination of dissection off the retroperitoneum and off the omentum usually results in the splenic flexure reaching to just below the umbilicus, which is sufficient for subsequent exteriorization.

With the left side still banked up, the rectum is retracted anteriorly and to the right, a maneuver that allows the peritoneum of the left lateral aspect of the rectum to be scored as a continuation of the previous dissection of the left lateral peritoneal reflection. This exposes the connective tissue of the proximal aspect of the presacral space, which can be entered and developed from the left side. With the proximal rectum elevated toward the anterior abdominal wall, the right pararectal peritoneum is scored. Traction on the peritoneum allows gas to enter the presacral space through the peritoneal scoring and helps to identify the correct presacral plane. The right side of the presacral space is developed to meet the previous dissection started from the left (Fig. 5).

The rectum is elevated anteriorly to maintain sufficient traction (Fig. 6). As the posterior dissection proceeds, this puts tension on the lateral pararectal peritoneum, which is divided. The presacral space is developed to a point in the proximal third of the rectum, where one can be sure that the taeniae have completely coalesced. Leaving too long a rectal stump not only predisposes to recurrent diverticulitis but also can cause difficulty maneuvering the handle of the circular stapler to the end of the stump. The mesorectum is divided at the chosen resection margin with ultrasonic scissors, and the rectum can be divided at this point with a linear stapler (Fig. 7).

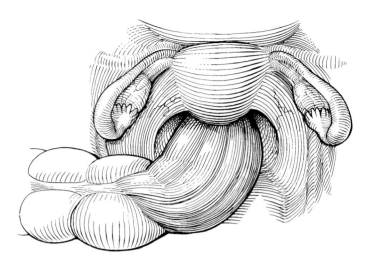

Fig. 3. Laparoscopic view of sigmoid colon and pelvis.

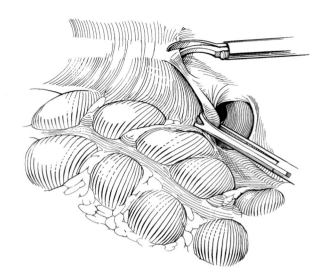

Fig. 4. Opening left lateral peritoneal reflection along white line of Toldt.

By continuing scoring of the right pararectal peritoneum in a cephalad direction, the origin of the superior hemorrhoidal artery or the inferior mesenteric artery can be exposed. This vascular pedicle can be divided if necessary to achieve sufficient mobilization for exteriorization; often, it is not necessary. Anterior traction of the rectosigmoid junction facilitates this identification. The windows in the mesentery on either side of the vessels are identified and developed. It is important to inspect the left lateral side of the mesentery to ensure that the ureter is not incorporated before dividing the vessels at their base

with a laparoscopic linear stapler with a vascular cartridge (Fig. 8). The chosen proximal resection margin (removing the entire sigmoid and choosing bowel that is soft) is brought down to the level of the transected rectum to ensure sufficient length of the proximal limb. If necessary, the splenic flexure is mobilized at this point.

Exteriorization is performed by enlargement of the supraumbilical port site incision around the umbilicus. The distal transected rectal margin is pulled up, and the whole specimen can be exteriorized (Fig. 9). The remaining mesentery and the proximal margin of the specimen are

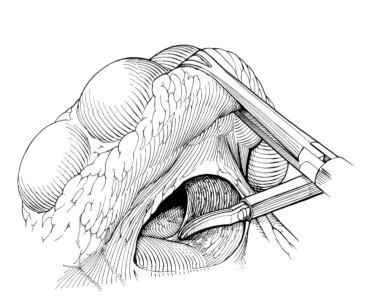

Fig. 5. Entry into superior portion of presacral space from the right side of the rectum, joining prior dissection from left side.

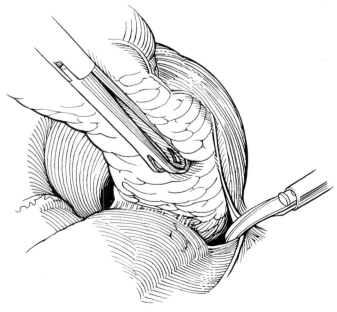

Fig. 6. Dissection in presacral plane with retraction of rectum anterosuperiorly.

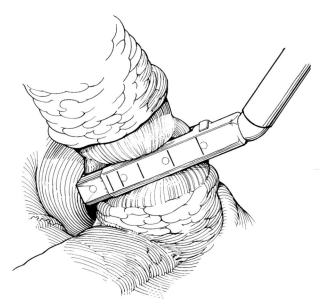

Fig. 7. Transection of rectum with laparoscopic linear stapler.

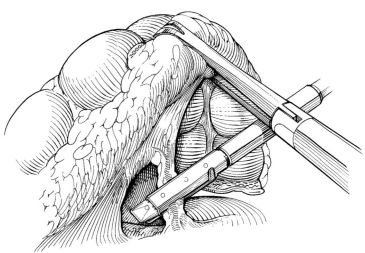

Fig. 8. Division of superior rectal vessels (if necessary to achieve adequate mobility for exteriorization).

resected extracorporeally. A purse-string suture is placed in the proximal resection margin and the head of an end-to-end anastomosis stapler is secured before retaining this to the abdominal cavity and closing the extraction incision. The pneumoperitoneum is reestablished. The anvil is grasped, and the ability of the proximal margin to reach the distal resection level is rechecked.

Before the end-to-end anastomosis stapler is inserted by way of the anus, a suture is tied through the hole in the spike to allow it to be removed more easily. The stapler

is inserted and advanced to the distal staple line, where the spike is brought out adjacent to the staple line. The suture in the spike is grasped (Fig. 10) and the spike is removed. The anvil is docked onto the handle (Fig. 11) and the stapler is reapproximated while correct orientation of the proximal limb is confirmed. The stapler is fired and removed, and the tissue donuts are checked for integrity. The anastomosis is checked by filling the pelvis with saline, compressing the bowel proximal to the anastomosis, and performing rigid sigmoidoscopy with air insufflation. Absence of air bubbles indicates an intact anastomosis. After irrigation of the abdomen, the pneumoperitoneum is evacuated and the port sites are closed.

OUTCOMES AND LONG-TERM FOLLOW-UP

The overall need for operation with the first attack of diverticulitis is 20% to 29%; most patients have complicated diverticulitis.[17] The mortality rate is 1.3% to 5%.[62] Almost all patients with simple diverticulitis initially are treated conservatively. Approximately 85% respond and 15% require operation.[62] Following successful conservative therapy for a first attack, 30% to 40% of patients remain asymptomatic, 30% to 40% have episodic abdominal cramps without confirmed diverticulitis, and 33% have a second attack.[16] Long-term follow-up shows a readmission rate for diverticulitis of 2% per patient year for patients in whom conservative therapy was successful.[62] Thus, elective resection is not necessary for all patients who respond to medical therapy. There is an increased risk of complications, however, after a second attack; the rate of complicated diverticulitis approaches 60% and the mortality

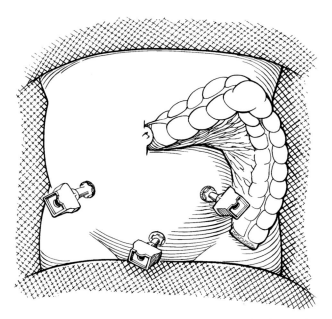

Fig. 9. Exteriorization of the mobilized sigmoid colon and transected proximal rectum.

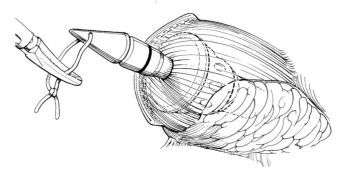

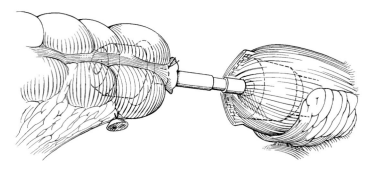

Fig. 10. Spike of endoanal circular stapler brought out adjacent to staple line in rectum with suture placed through spike to allow its removal.

Fig. 11. Docking of anvil of stapler onto handle.

rate is doubled.[4,63] Only 10% of patients subsequently remain asymptomatic. These values form the basis for recommending elective resection after two confirmed attacks. These figures are from older literature. It is unclear whether earlier diagnosis with more widespread use of computed tomography will result in more patients presenting with simple diverticulitis and whether earlier institution of therapy improves outcomes and avoids operation.

Patients treated operatively are generally considered cured. Progression of diverticulosis in the remaining colon occurs in 15%,[64] and further operation is needed in only 2% to 11%.[57,64] There is a mortality rate of 6% for purulent peritonitis and 35% for fecal peritonitis.[53]

DIVERTICULAR BLEEDING

Diverticula and vascular ectasias account for the majority of episodes of lower gastrointestinal bleeding. Three recent large series, comprising more than 500 patients in total, indicated that diverticular bleeding was the most common cause, occurring in 24% to 42% of episodes.[65-67] Bleeding occurs in 15% of patients with extensive diverticulosis; in a third of these patients (5%), it is massive.[63]

Pathophysiology

Diverticular bleeding is arterial, from the vasa recta. As a diverticulum herniates, the vessel responsible for the weakness in the wall of the colon becomes draped over the dome of the diverticulum, separated from the lumen only by mucosa. Eccentric intimal thickening and thinning of the media occur in the vasa recta along the side adjacent to the lumen.[7] These changes may result in segmental weakness of the artery and predispose to rupture into the lumen, but precipitating factors have not been clearly elucidated. Inflammation does not seem to be a predisposing factor. The wider ostia and domes of right-sided diverticula compared with those in the left colon, possibly exposing vasa recta to injury over a greater length of

the vessel wall, may explain the higher incidence of hemorrhage from right-sided diverticula.[7]

Natural History

Comorbid conditions in elderly patients (mean age, 68-77 years)[68,69] contribute to morbidity and mortality rates of 10% to 20%.[69,70] Bleeding stops spontaneously in 70% to 80% of episodes. Blood transfusion of less than 4 units in 24 hours is associated with spontaneous cessation of bleeding in 99% of patients.[71] The risk of rebleeding, however, ranges from 14% to 38%;[68,71] with a second episode, the risk of further hemorrhage approaches 50%,[71] leading to the recommendation that surgical resection be performed after a second bleeding episode. The right colon is the source of diverticular bleeding in 48% to 90% of these patients.[7,68,72]

Clinical Presentation

Diverticular bleeding is characterized by painless, bright-red rectal bleeding. Most episodes are minor (<1 unit of blood), and up to 50% of patients[72] have a prior history of passage of maroon or bright-red blood. Abdominal pain is usually absent, and bleeding with acute diverticulitis is extremely rare.[7] Physical examination is unremarkable, without abdominal tenderness or mass. Less than 5% of patients have massive hemorrhage requiring transfusion.

Management

Diagnosis and treatment of diverticular bleeding require a coordinated approach by gastroenterologists, radiologists, and surgeons.[33] At Mayo Clinic, skilled gastroenterologists spearhead a specialized bleeding team; this approach has been shown to reduce mortality.[68] Management of massive colonic bleeding has three components: resuscitation, diagnosis and localization of the site of bleeding, and subsequent management. The American College of Gastroenterology has published practice guidelines addressing lower gastrointestinal bleeding.[73]

Resuscitation and Initial Assessment

Initial assessment comprises aggressive fluid resuscitation and cross-matching of blood. An upper gastrointestinal source must be excluded by nasogastric lavage (bile-stained aspirate must be obtained) or by upper endoscopy, if indicated, because 10% to 15% of patients with hematochezia have an upper tract cause.[33] Rectal examination, anoscopy, or proctoscopy should be part of the initial assessment; massive hemorrhoidal bleeding, although rare, can be excluded easily. Further evaluation is then performed to localize or treat the source. Colonoscopy, radionuclide bleeding scanning, and mesenteric angiography have all been used, depending on the rate of bleeding and on available expertise.[33] A combination of diagnostic methods can identify the source preoperatively in 90% of patients with massive bleeding.[74]

Diagnosis

Colonoscopy

The role of colonoscopy in acute diverticular bleeding is evolving. Endoscopic management of a bleeding diverticulum, with irrigation of 1:1,000 epinephrine, was first reported in 1985.[75] Success has since been reported with the heater probe,[76] bipolar cautery probe,[77] injection therapies,[78,79] and fibrin sealant.[80] Endoscopic "stigmata" with prognostic value have been reported.[81] Cumulative results of small studies suggest a hemostasis rate of 75%.[82] Some authors have reported use of emergency colonoscopy in unprepared bowel because blood is cathartic.[83] Others use enemas or rapid preparation with balanced electrolyte solutions given orally or by nasogastric tube.[84,85] When performed successfully (i.e., satisfactory visualization of the mucosal surface), colonoscopy has a diagnostic accuracy of 72% to 86%.[83-85] Advantages include precise localization and the potential for therapeutic intervention. Only a selected few patients, however, are realistically amenable to colonoscopy, those with low-volume, intermittent colonic bleeding.

Radionuclide Imaging

Tagged red cell scanning uses technetium Tc 99m pertechnetate to label or tag autologous red blood cells from the patient before reinjection. Abdominal images are obtained frequently during the first 30 minutes and then every few hours for up to 24 hours. Advantages are its noninvasiveness and sensitivity. One series demonstrated a sensitivity of 97%, specificity of 83%, and positive predictive value of 94%.[86] The disadvantages are that bleeding is localized to a general area of the abdomen without necessarily localizing the bleeding source to a specific organ, and thus accuracy rates range from 24% to 91%.[63] Poor

organ localization occurs because extravasated blood may move within the colon in a peristaltic or antiperistaltic direction; in addition, localization to an area of the *abdomen* cannot define a site in the *colon*. For example, bleeding from a redundant sigmoid colon may appear as extravasation in the right lower quadrant, suggesting bleeding from the right colon or the distal small bowel.

Angiography

The first mesenteric vessel examined is the superior mesenteric artery because 50% to 80% of diverticular bleeding and virtually all bleeding from angiodysplasia occur in the territory of this artery.[87] If no source is found, the inferior mesenteric and celiac vessels are studied. Successful localization of the site of bleeding varies from 14% to 72%[69,70,84,88] and depends on the rate of bleeding (sensitivities are as low as 0.5 mL/minute), timing (the patient must be actively bleeding at the time of the intravenous administration of contrast), and expertise. Angiographic localization is 100% specific, but sensitivity varies with the pattern of bleeding. With acute bleeding, sensitivity approaches 50% but decreases to 30% with a pattern of recurrent hemorrhage.[89] A positive angiogram is associated with an 86% likelihood of operative treatment.[89] The use of radionuclide imaging to screen for active bleeding before angiography may reduce the frequency of negative arteriograms,[90] but some groups maintain that the incidence of negative arteriograms is increased by the delay inherent in performing radionuclide scanning.[69] Complications, which occur in 9% of patients, include arterial thrombosis, mesenteric or peripheral embolization of atherosclerotic debris from the aorta, and renal failure.[84]

Advantages of angiography are that there is no requirement for bowel preparation and anatomical localization is organ-accurate. Also, angiographic techniques allow therapeutic infusion of vasoconstrictor agents or vascular embolization. With a subselectively positioned intra-arterial catheter, vasopressin can be infused directly into the artery supplying the segment of bleeding colon. Infusion begins at 0.2 U/minute, with repeat angiography after 20 minutes; if bleeding persists, the rate is increased to 0.4 to 0.6 U/minute.[91] If the bleeding is controlled, the infusion is continued in an intensive-care setting for 24 to 36 hours and then tapered over 24 hours.[91] In up to 91% of patients receiving intra-arterial vasopressin, bleeding stops; however, up to 50% have rebleeding on cessation of vasopressin infusion.[69] In the latter patients, however, vasopressin may permit resuscitation, stabilization, and bowel preparation with the goal of resection and primary reanastomosis.[69] Transcatheter embolization is a more definitive means of controlling hemorrhage, but it is associated with colonic infarction in up to 20% of patients. Attempts to reduce the risk have included use of temporary occluding agents or a "superselective" catheterization technique.[92]

Surgical Intervention

Surgical resection for *acute* lower gastrointestinal bleeding is reserved until medical, endoscopic, or angiographic methods have failed. Persistent instability despite aggressive resuscitation requires emergency operative intervention in 18% to 25% of patients with diverticular bleeding who require blood transfusion.[71,93] The surgical approach is highly dependent on whether a bleeding source has been identified. Every attempt should be made to exclude an upper gastrointestinal source of bleeding (e.g., nasogastric intubation or emergency gastroscopy). Segmental resection is possible if the bleeding site has been identified. The most difficult clinical situation is the hemodynamically unstable patient with no identified source of bleeding.

At operation, careful exploration searches for an obvious source or a mass. Because diverticular bleeding is not associated with acute diverticulitis, the involved diverticulum is not immediately evident externally. Most patients are elderly and thus many have colonic diverticula. Without preoperative localization, the decision of what to resect becomes problematic. Various techniques have been described, including dividing the colon into sections by applying occlusive clamps and determining which section fills with blood. This technique, which requires ongoing massive bleeding, is generally unsatisfactory. A better approach involves intraoperative colonoscopy[74] after a rapid on-the-table intraoperative bowel preparation; an infusion catheter is placed into the cecum, through which a warmed electrolyte solution is rapidly infused, and a transanal catheter (or anesthesia tubing) controls the efflux of fluid from below. This approach allows the possibility of a localized segmental colectomy involving only the site of bleeding.

If no obvious colonic site can be identified and the bleeding is massive and life-threatening, an abdominal colectomy is performed involving the entire colon susceptible to diverticula and angiodysplasia (i.e., from the terminal ileum to the proximal rectum). The decision to perform ileorectal anastomosis (with or without diverting loop ileostomy) versus a Brooke ileostomy with rectal stump depends on standard surgical factors, including ability to irrigate the rectal stump clean, hemodynamic stability, age of the patient, comorbid conditions, and preoperative fecal continence. Thus, all possible attempts at specific localization preoperatively and intraoperatively are important to limit the extent of colectomy required. A source of bleeding is ultimately identified in 78% of patients undergoing emergency operation for lower gut bleeding.[74]

Surgical intervention in the patient who has an identified bleeding source is guided by the presence of hemodynamic stability, which in turn determines the ability to undergo bowel preparation. A segmental resection is made possible by preoperative localization. The advisability of anastomosis, with or without protective stoma, depends on standard surgical principles: hemodynamic stability, comorbid conditions, and bowel preparation (at Mayo Clinic, a right-sided anastomosis is performed in an "unprepped" but hemodynamically stable patient).

In the hemodynamically stable patient, a laparoscopic approach can be used. The treatment of diverticular bleeding by resection of an identified source is relatively straightforward. The difficulty arises from identifying the segment containing the bleeding. If this is initially identified with colonoscopy, the site of bleeding can be tattooed by colonoscopic injection of 0.1 mL of India ink into the submucosa. This should be injected in at least three positions around the circumference to avoid mesenteric fat from obscuring the site of the tattoo on the serosal surface.

Outcomes of Operative Treatment

The need for operative intervention varies with the degree of bleeding. With severe or massive bleeding, 24% to 78% of patients require operative intervention.[69,71,74,84] Preoperative localization of the site of bleeding and the use of vasopressin as a temporizing measure have reduced operative morbidity from 37% after emergency resection to 9% after segmental colectomy. The operative mortality rate of 9% to 11% reflects generally comorbid conditions.[69,74,93]

When the source of bleeding is localized, a segmental colectomy is performed, and the rate of rebleeding is 0% to 14%.[69,71,94] The rebleeding rate was 6% in one series of segmental resection performed after angiographic identification of a bleeding site.[69] Blind segmental resection of the most involved diverticula-bearing segment carries a rebleeding rate as high as 42%,[94] a morbidity rate of 83%, and a mortality rate of 57% and so is contraindicated.[94] If the site of bleeding has been objectively localized, even in patients with extensive diverticular disease, a segmental resection eradicating the bleeding site is adequate.[69] Total colectomy is reserved for patients who continue to bleed without a documented site of bleeding, but it is associated with a high morbidity rate (37%) and a high mortality rate (11%-33%).[69,71,95] Although the rebleeding rate after abdominal colectomy approaches 0%,[94] in the elderly the procedure is associated with relatively disabling diarrhea in about 15% and socially unsatisfactory diarrhea in a larger percentage. Thus, this extent of operation should not be undertaken lightly.

REFERENCES

1. Mayo WJ, Wilson LB, Giffin HZ: Acquired diverticulitis of the large intestine. Surg Gynecol Obstet 6:8-15, 1907
2. Mayo WJ: Diverticulitis of the large intestine. JAMA 69:781-785, 1917
3. Meyers MA, Volberg F, Katzen B, Alonso D, Abbott G: The angioarchitecture of colonic diverticula: significance in bleeding diverticulosis. Radiology 108:249-261, 1973
4. Parks TG: Natural history of diverticular disease of the colon: a review of 521 cases. Br Med J 4:639-642, 1969
5. Rodkey GV, Welch CE: Changing patterns in the surgical treatment of diverticular disease. Ann Surg 200:466-478, 1984
6. Lee YS: Diverticular disease of the large bowel in Singapore: an autopsy survey. Dis Colon Rectum 29:330-335, 1986
7. Meyers MA, Alonso DR, Gray GF, Baer JW: Pathogenesis of bleeding colonic diverticulosis. Gastroenterology 71:577-583, 1976
8. Whiteway J, Morson BC: Elastosis in diverticular disease of the sigmoid colon. Gut 26:258-266, 1985
9. Wess L, Eastwood MA, Wess TJ, Busuttil A, Miller A: Cross linking of collagen is increased in colonic diverticulosis. Gut 37:91-94, 1995
10. Painter NS, Truelove SC, Ardran GM, Tuckey M: Segmentation and the localization of intraluminal pressures in the human colon, with special reference to the pathogenesis of colonic diverticula. Gastroenterology 49:169-177, 1965
11. Rege RV, Nahrwold DL: Diverticular disease. Curr Probl Surg 26:133-189, 1989
12. Konvolinka CW: Acute diverticulitis under age forty. Am J Surg 167:562-565, 1994
13. Fischer MG, Farkas AM: Diverticulitis of the cecum and ascending colon. Dis Colon Rectum 27:454-458, 1984
14. Sugihara K, Muto T, Morioka Y, Asano A, Yamamoto T: Diverticular disease of the colon in Japan: a review of 615 cases. Dis Colon Rectum 27:531-537, 1984
15. Ngoi SS, Chia J, Goh MY, Sim E, Rauff A: Surgical management of right colon diverticulitis. Dis Colon Rectum 35:799-802, 1992
16. Parks TG: Natural history of diverticular disease of the colon. Clin Gastroenterol 4:53-69, 1975
17. Ambrosetti P, Robert JH, Witzig JA, Mirescu D, Mathey P, Borst F, Rohner A: Acute left colonic diverticulitis in young patients. J Am Coll Surg 179:156-160, 1994
18. Roberts P, Abel M, Rosen L, Cirocco W, Fleshman J, Leff E, Levien D, Pritchard T, Wexner S, Hicks T: Practice parameters for sigmoid diverticulitis. The Standards Task Force American Society of Colon and Rectal Surgeons. Dis Colon Rectum 38:125-132, 1995
19. Wong WD, Wexner SD, Lowry A, Vernava A III, Burnstein M, Denstman F, Fazio V, Kerner B, Moore R, Oliver G, Peters W, Ross T, Senatore P, Simmang C: Practice parameters for the treatment of sigmoid diverticulitis—supporting documentation: the Standards Task Force. The American Society of Colon and Rectal Surgeons. Dis Colon Rectum 43:290-297, 2000
20. Ming S-C, Fleischner FG: Diverticulitis of the sigmoid colon: reappraisal of the pathology and pathogenesis. Surgery 58:627-633, 1965
21. Morson BC: The muscle abnormality in diverticular disease of the sigmoid colon. Br J Radiol 36:385-392, 1963
22. Birnbaum BA, Balthazar EJ: CT of appendicitis and diverticulitis. Radiol Clin North Am 32:885-898, 1994
23. Hulnick DH, Megibow AJ, Balthazar EJ, Naidich DP, Bosniak MA: Computed tomography in the evaluation of diverticulitis. Radiology 152:491-495, 1984
24. Padidar AM, Jeffrey RB Jr, Mindelzun RE, Dolph JF: Differentiating sigmoid diverticulitis from carcinoma on CT scans: mesenteric inflammation suggests diverticulitis. AJR Am J Roentgenol 163:81-83, 1994
25. Rao PM, Rhea JT, Novelline RA, Dobbins JM, Lawrason JN, Sacknoff R, Stuk JL: Helical CT with only colonic contrast material for diagnosing diverticulitis: prospective evaluation of 150 patients. AJR Am J Roentgenol 170:1445-1449, 1998
26. Parulekar SG: Sonography of colonic diverticulitis. J Ultrasound Med 4:659-666, 1985
27. Yacoe ME, Jeffrey RB Jr: Sonography of appendicitis and diverticulitis. Radiol Clin North Am 32:899-912, 1994
28. Schwerk WB, Schwarz S, Rothmund M: Sonography in acute colonic diverticulitis: a prospective study. Dis Colon Rectum 35:1077-1084, 1992
29. Trenkner SW, Thompson WM: Since the advent of CT scanning, what role does the contrast enema examination play in the diagnosis of acute diverticulitis? AJR Am J Roentgenol 162:1493-1494, 1994
30. Young-Fadok TM, Roberts PL, Spencer MP, Wolff BG: Colonic diverticular disease. Curr Probl Surg 37:457-514, 2000
31. Stabile BE: Surgical treatment of diverticulitis. The Society for Surgery of the Alimentary Tract. Patient Care Guidelines 2000. Manchester, MA, SSAT, 2000, pp 22-25
32. Chow AW: Appendicitis and diverticulitis. In Infectious Diseases: a Treatise of Infectious Processes. Edited by PD Hoeprich, MC Jordan, AR Ronald. Philadelphia, JB Lippincott Company, 1994, pp 878-881
33. Stollman NH, Raskin JB: Diagnosis and management of diverticular disease of the colon in adults. Ad Hoc Practice Parameters Committee of the American College of Gastroenterology. Am J Gastroenterol 94:3110-3121, 1999
34. Ferzoco LB, Raptopoulos V, Silen W: Acute diverticulitis. N Engl J Med 338:1521-1526, 1998
35. Larson DM, Masters SS, Spiro HM: Medical and surgical therapy in diverticular disease: a comparative study. Gastroenterology 71:734-737, 1976
36. Painter NS: Diverticular disease of the colon: the first of the Western diseases shown to be due to a deficiency of dietary fibre. S Afr Med J 61:1016-1020, 1982
37. Starnes HF Jr, Lazarus JM, Vineyard G: Surgery for diverticulitis in renal failure. Dis Colon Rectum 28:827-831, 1985
38. Scheff RT, Zuckerman G, Harter H, Delmez J, Koehler R: Diverticular disease in patients with chronic renal failure due to polycystic kidney disease. Ann Intern Med 92:202-204, 1980
39. Tyau ES, Prystowsky JB, Joehl RJ, Nahrwold DL: Acute diverticulitis: a complicated problem in the immunocompromised patient. Arch Surg 126:855-858, 1991
40. Young-Fadok T, Sgambati S, Wolff B: Increased morbidity and mortality after colectomy in patients with lupus: a case-matched series (abstract). Dis Colon Rectum 43:A57, 2000
41. Acosta JA, Grebenc ML, Doberneck RC, McCarthy JD, Fry DE: Colonic diverticular disease in patients 40 years old or younger. Am Surg 58:605-607, 1992
42. Schauer PR, Ramos R, Ghiatas AA, Sirinek KR: Virulent diverticular disease in young obese men. Am J Surg 164:443-446, 1992

43. Freischlag J, Bennion RS, Thompson JE Jr: Complications of diverticular disease of the colon in young people. Dis Colon Rectum 29:639-643, 1986

44. Chodak GW, Rangel DM, Passaro E Jr: Colonic diverticulitis in patients under age 40: need for earlier diagnosis. Am J Surg 141:699-702, 1981

45. Spivak H, Weinrauch S, Harvey JC, Surick B, Ferstenberg H, Friedman I: Acute colonic diverticulitis in the young. Dis Colon Rectum 40:570-574, 1997

46. Anderson DN, Driver CP, Davidson AI, Keenan RA: Diverticular disease in patients under 50 years of age. J R Coll Surg Edinb 42:102-104, 1997

47. Cunningham MA, Davis JW, Kaups KL: Medical versus surgical management of diverticulitis in patients under age 40. Am J Surg 174:733-735, 1997

48. Ouriel K, Schwartz SI: Diverticular disease in the young patient. Surg Gynecol Obstet 156:1-5, 1983

49. Vignati PV, Welch JP, Cohen JL: Long-term management of diverticulitis in young patients. Dis Colon Rectum 38:627-629, 1995

50. Simonowitz D, Paloyan D: Diverticular disease of the colon in patients under 40 years of age. Am J Gastroenterol 67:69-72, 1977

51. Young-Fadok TM, Sarr MG: Diverticular disease of the colon. In Textbook of Gastroenterology. Vol 2. Third edition. Edited by T Yamada. Philadelphia, Lippincott Williams & Wilkins, 1999, pp 1926-1945

52. Hinchey EJ, Schaal PG, Richards GK: Treatment of perforated diverticular disease of the colon. Adv Surg 12:85-109, 1978

53. Nagorney DM, Adson MA, Pemberton JH: Sigmoid diverticulitis with perforation and generalized peritonitis. Dis Colon Rectum 28:71-75, 1985

54. Finlay IG, Carter DC: A comparison of emergency resection and staged management in perforated diverticular disease. Dis Colon Rectum 30:929-933, 1987

55. Belmonte C, Klas JV, Perez JJ, Wong WD, Rothenberger DA, Goldberg SM, Madoff RD: The Hartmann procedure: first choice or last resort in diverticular disease? Arch Surg 131:612-615, 1996

56. Lee EC, Murray JJ, Coller JA, Roberts PL, Schoetz DJ Jr: Intraoperative colonic lavage in nonelective surgery for diverticular disease. Dis Colon Rectum 40:669-674, 1997

57. Benn PL, Wolff BG, Ilstrup DM: Level of anastomosis and recurrent colonic diverticulitis. Am J Surg 151:269-271, 1986

58. Morales Conde S, Fleshman JW: Laparoscopic colon resection. In Current Surgical Therapy. Sixth edition. Edited by JL Cameron. St Louis, Mosby, 1998, pp 1195-1201

59. Franklin ME Jr, Dorman JP, Jacobs M, Plasencia G: Is laparoscopic surgery applicable to complicated colonic diverticular disease? Surg Endosc 11:1021-1025, 1997

60. Schlachta CM, Mamazza J, Poulin EC: Laparoscopic sigmoid resection for acute and chronic diverticulitis: an outcomes comparison with laparoscopic resection for nondiverticular disease. Surg Endosc 13:649-653, 1999

61. Kockerling F, Schneider C, Reymond MA, Scheidbach H, Scheuerlein H, Konradt J, Bruch HP, Zornig C, Kohler L, Barlehner E, Kuthe A, Szinicz G, Richter HA, Hohenberger W: Laparoscopic resection of sigmoid diverticulitis: results of a multicenter study. Laparoscopic Colorectal Surgery Study Group. Surg Endosc 13:567-571, 1999

62. Sarin S, Boulos PB: Long-term outcome of patients presenting with acute complications of diverticular disease. Ann R Coll Surg Engl 76:117-120, 1994

63. Imbembo AL, Bailey RW: Diverticular disease of the colon. In Textbook of Surgery: the Biological Basis of Modern Surgical Practice. Fourteenth edition. Edited by DC Sabiston Jr. Philadelphia, WB Saunders Company, 1991, pp 910-920

64. Wolff BG, Ready RL, MacCarty RL, Dozois RR, Beart RW Jr: Influence of sigmoid resection on progression of diverticular disease of the colon. Dis Colon Rectum 27:645-647, 1984

65. Peura DA, Lanza FL, Gostout CJ, Foutch PG: The American College of Gastroenterology Bleeding Registry: preliminary findings. Am J Gastroenterol 92:924-928, 1997

66. Bramley PN, Masson JW, McKnight G, Herd K, Fraser A, Park K, Brunt PW, McKinlay A, Sinclair TS, Mowat NA: The role of an open-access bleeding unit in the management of colonic haemorrhage: a 2-year prospective study. Scand J Gastroenterol 31:764-769, 1996

67. Longstreth GF: Epidemiology and outcome of patients hospitalized with acute lower gastrointestinal hemorrhage: a population-based study. Am J Gastroenterol 92:419-424, 1997

68. Gostout CJ, Wang KK, Ahlquist DA, Clain JE, Hughes RW, Larson MV, Petersen BT, Schroeder KW, Tremaine WJ, Viggiano TR, Balm RK: Acute gastrointestinal bleeding: experience of a specialized management team. J Clin Gastroenterol 14:260-267, 1992

69. Browder W, Cerise EJ, Litwin MS: Impact of emergency angiography in massive lower gastrointestinal bleeding. Ann Surg 204:530-536, 1986

70. Uden P, Jiborn H, Jonsson K: Influence of selective mesenteric arteriography on the outcome of emergency surgery for massive, lower gastrointestinal hemorrhage: a 15-year experience. Dis Colon Rectum 29:561-566, 1986

71. McGuire HH Jr: Bleeding colonic diverticula: a reappraisal of natural history and management. Ann Surg 220:653-656, 1994

72. Casarella WJ, Kanter IE, Seaman WB: Right-sided colonic diverticula as a cause of acute rectal hemorrhage. N Engl J Med 286:450-453, 1972

73. Zuccaro G Jr: Management of the adult patient with acute lower gastrointestinal bleeding. American College of Gastroenterology. Practice Parameters Committee. Am J Gastroenterol 93:1202-1208, 1998

74. Wagner HE, Stain SC, Gilg M, Gertsch P: Systematic assessment of massive bleeding of the lower part of the gastrointestinal tract. Surg Gynecol Obstet 175:445-449, 1992

75. Mauldin JL: Therapeutic use of colonoscopy in active diverticular bleeding (letter). Gastrointest Endosc 31:290-291, 1985

76. Johnston J, Sonnes J: Endoscopic heater probe coagulation of the bleeding colonic diverticulum (abstract). Gastrointest Endosc 32:160, 1986

77. Savides TJ, Jensen DM: Colonoscopic hemostasis for recurrent diverticular hemorrhage associated with a visible vessel: a report of three cases. Gastrointest Endosc 40:70-73, 1994

78. Bertoni G, Conigliaro R, Ricci E, Mortilla MG, Bedogni G, Fornaciari G: Endoscopic injection hemostasis of colonic diverticular bleeding: a case report. Endoscopy 22:154-155, 1990

79. Kim YI, Marcon NE: Injection therapy for colonic diverticular bleeding: a case study. J Clin Gastroenterol 17:46-48, 1993

80. Andress HJ, Mewes A, Lange V: Endoscopic hemostasis of a bleeding diverticulum of the sigma with fibrin sealant (letter). Endoscopy 25:193, 1993

81. Foutch PG: Diverticular bleeding: Are nonsteroidal anti-inflammatory drugs risk factors for hemorrhage and can colonoscopy predict outcome for patients? Am J Gastroenterol 90:1779-1784, 1995

82. Foutch PG, Zimmerman K: Diverticular bleeding and the pigmented protuberance (sentinel clot): clinical implications, histopathological correlation, and results of endoscopic intervention. Am J Gastroenterol 91:2589-2593, 1996

83. Rossini FP, Ferrari A, Spandre M, Cavallero M, Gemme C, Loverci C, Bertone A, Pinna Pintor M: Emergency colonoscopy. World J Surg 13:190-192, 1989

84. Jensen DM, Machicado GA: Diagnosis and treatment of severe hematochezia: the role of urgent colonoscopy after purge. Gastroenterology 95:1569-1574, 1988

85. Van Gossum A, Bourgeois F, Gay F, Lievens P, Adler M, Cremer M: Operative colonoscopic endoscopy. Acta Gastroenterol Belg 55:314-326, 1992

86. Nicholson ML, Neoptolemos JP, Sharp JF, Watkin EM, Fossard DP: Localization of lower gastrointestinal bleeding using in vivo technetium-99m-labelled red blood cell scintigraphy. Br J Surg 76:358-361, 1989

87. Reinus JF, Brandt LJ: Vascular ectasias and diverticulosis: common causes of lower intestinal bleeding. Gastroenterol Clin North Am 23:1-20, 1994

88. DeMarkles MP, Murphy JR: Acute lower gastrointestinal bleeding. Med Clin North Am 77:1085-1100, 1993

89. Fiorito JJ, Brandt LJ, Kozicky O, Grosman IM, Sprayragen S: The diagnostic yield of superior mesenteric angiography: correlation with the pattern of gastrointestinal bleeding. Am J Gastroenterol 84:878-881, 1989

90. Steer ML, Silen W: Diagnostic procedures in gastrointestinal hemorrhage. N Engl J Med 309:646-650, 1983

91. Rosen RJ, Sanchez G: Angiographic diagnosis and management of gastrointestinal hemorrhage: current concepts. Radiol Clin North Am 32:951-967, 1994

92. Guy GE, Shetty PC, Sharma RP, Burke MW, Burke TH: Acute lower gastrointestinal hemorrhage: treatment by superselective embolization with polyvinyl alcohol particles. AJR Am J Roentgenol 159:521-526, 1992

93. Bokhari M, Vernava AM, Ure T, Longo WE: Diverticular hemorrhage in the elderly: Is it well tolerated? Dis Colon Rectum 39:191-195, 1996

94. Parkes BM, Obeid FN, Sorensen VJ, Horst HM, Fath JJ: The management of massive lower gastrointestinal bleeding. Am Surg 59:676-678, 1993

95. Setya V, Singer JA, Minken SL: Subtotal colectomy as a last resort for unrelenting, unlocalized, lower gastrointestinal hemorrhage: experience with 12 cases. Am Surg 58:295-299, 1992

Chapter 35

COLON CANCER

Debora J. Fox, M.D.
Heidi Nelson, M.D.

Colon cancer will affect 6% of the population in the United States and is the second leading cause of death due to cancer. It is diagnosed in 130,000 patients per year; about 50,000 of them will die of the disease. Because most cancers are thought to arise from polyps, many are preventable with proper screening and evaluation. Certain families and persons at increased risk have been identified as knowledge of the genetic basis of colon cancer has developed. Proper decision making and appropriate surgical technique are critical to optimal patient outcome.

The exact cause and mechanism of colon cancer are unknown. Environmental and dietary practices contribute, as evidenced by the widely varying incidence and mortality rates worldwide.[1] Various dietary and medical modifications have been examined as agents related to the risk of colon cancer, including vitamins and folate,[2] calcium carbonate, red meat,[3] medications such as nonsteroidal anti-inflammatory agents,[4] bile salt-binding agents, and fiber.[5]

Screening programs for colon cancer facilitate early identification of polyps and cancer and can decrease mortality from cancer. Despite the availability of these programs, only 17% to 32% of adults receive fecal occult blood testing and only 9% to 11% undergo flexible sigmoidoscopy according to recommended guidelines.[6,7] National attention to this problem and education of both patients and health care providers are necessary to establish appropriate screening and lessen further the impact of this disease.

PHYSIOLOGY, BIOCHEMISTRY, MOLECULAR BIOLOGY, AND PATHOLOGY

Although the majority of cases of colon cancer are spontaneous, risk increases if a first-degree relative is affected, suggesting an underlying genetic basis. Studies of families with a cancer predisposition, such as found in hereditary nonpolyposis colon cancer and familial adenomatous polyposis, have improved our understanding of the genetic basis of colon cancer.[8,9]

The adenoma-carcinoma sequence, recognized in the 1970s, refers to the concept that colon cancer arises in adenomatous polyps. This was supported by certain registries showing an increase in the frequency of adenomatous polyps around age 45 years, preceding an increase in the frequency of colon cancers by 5 to 10 years. In the early 1970s, colonoscopic polypectomy became more prevalent, and the risk of dysplasia in adenomatous polyps was noted to increase with increasing polyp size. Polyps more than 1 cm in size had a rate of high-grade dysplasia of more than 10%, whereas polyps more than 2 cm in size had a rate of dysplasia and neoplasia exceeding 46%.[10] Sessile polyps were more likely to contain malignancy.[11] In the mid-1980s, several reports of flat adenomas, tubular adenomas that flattened with air insufflation, led to new diagnostic endoscopic challenges. These lesions were much more prone to malignant degeneration with increased size. Subsequent molecular analysis has shown that they have a higher rate of aneuploidy than typical polypoid adenomas.[12]

Improvements in DNA analysis have led to further elucidation of the adenoma-carcinoma sequence at a genetic level for polypoid lesions. Genes, including *APC*, K-*ras*, *p53*, and *DCC*, have been isolated and characterized, and patterns of sequential disruption have been correlated to polyp growth and eventual malignant change.[13] The sequence of change in nonpolypoid lesions differs from that in polypoid lesions, and yet a final presentation, the de novo lesion, must be further investigated.[11]

DIAGNOSIS AND IMAGING

Colon cancer is most often asymptomatic until it reaches advanced stages. Early symptoms, including rectal bleeding and change in bowel habits, are often attributed to other causes and ignored until the cancer is advanced. In a study of a primary care population presenting with visible rectal bleeding, the overall rate of serious abnormality was 24%, polyps were present in 13%, and cancer was present in 6.5%. In the same study, 6 (16%) of a subgroup of 37 patients with identifiable anal abnormalities (fissures, hemorrhoids) also had polyps or cancer.[14]

Colon screening is reserved for the asymptomatic population and may be achieved with a combination of fecal occult blood testing and radiologic and endoscopic techniques. In the presence of symptoms such as rectal bleeding, the colon evaluation is no longer considered a screening test but is rather a *diagnostic examination*. *Colon surveillance* is done for patients with a propensity for polyp formation, in the setting of a strong family history, or as part of the postoperative follow-up regimen.

Fecal occult blood testing is used routinely as a screening tool, administered on an annual basis, as supported by recommendations of the American Cancer Society and the American Society of Colon and Rectal Surgeons. It is a cost-effective tool that lowers mortality from colorectal cancer, but is imperfect in that it is not specific and thus provides many false-positive results that lead to unnecessary colonoscopy.

Flexible sigmoidoscopy is recommended about once every 5 years in the asymptomatic population and more frequently in the presence of lower gastrointestinal symptoms. Because it visualizes only the rectum and lowest portion of the colon, its ability to detect colon cancer is limited. Ideally, the finding of neoplasia would prompt an examiner to refer the patient for colonoscopy. Read et al.,[15] from Lahey-Hitchcock, studied the prevalence of higher lesions found on colonoscopy in a group of patients referred with the finding of polyps on flexible sigmoidoscopy. The rate of proximal neoplasm was 29% with distal polyps less than 5 mm in size, 29% with polyps 6 to 10 mm in size, and 57% with polyps larger than 1 cm. Advanced proximal neoplasms (defined as polyps more than 1 cm in size with a villous

component, advanced dysplasia, or carcinoma) were present in 6%, 10%, and 29% of these groups, respectively. Netzer et al.,[16] in a study of the prevalence and distribution of neoplasms in relation to the rectosigmoid in 11,760 patients undergoing colonoscopy, found neoplasia in 19.3% of patients. Of the patients with proximal lesions, 79% had an index polyp in the rectosigmoid and 78% of the cancers coexisted with a distal index polyp. Age older than 65 years, multiple polyps, and a positive family history increase the likelihood of proximal neoplasm in the presence of a lesion found on sigmoidoscopy.[17]

Colonoscopy is the standard for examination of the colon; it provides superior visualization of the entire colonic mucosa and a greater sensitivity for detection of small polyps than radiologic studies.[18] Colonoscopy allows snare excision of most lesions, providing both a diagnostic and a therapeutic role in the treatment of polypoid lesions. Its role for reducing mortality from colon cancer has been investigated.[18] The use of colonoscopy is limited because it is more expensive than a barium enema, physician reimbursement is limited (although expanding rapidly), and most institutions do not have sufficient endoscopists and resources to offer the procedure to all patients. Furthermore, and probably more relevant, is the fact that colonoscopy is not complication-free—our institution has a perforation rate of 0.075%[19]—and the frequency of postpolypectomy bleeding is between 0.5% and 2.0%.[20]

Barium enema is an alternative method for evaluation of the colon. It has a sensitivity of 50% to 75% for polyps more than 1 cm in size.[21] Identification of a lesion requires subsequent endoscopic examination.

Computed tomographic colography and magnetic resonance colography are currently being evaluated as alternatives to conventional methods of colon evaluation. Diagnostic tests only, these methods require an excellent bowel preparation on the part of the patient and implementation of specific regimens and techniques by the radiologist. Their sensitivity and specificity exceed those of the barium enema.[21] In our review[22] of computed tomographic colography for polyps more than 1 cm, sensitivity was 75% and specificity was 90%. The sensitivity for smaller polyps decreased to less than 45%. Currently, computed tomographic colography cannot be recommended as a routine diagnostic test, but it shows promise as a noninvasive screening technique.

INDICATIONS FOR OPERATION

The presence of cancer in the colon is an absolute indication for operation unless comorbid conditions or the presence of metastatic disease favors a nonoperative approach or the cancer is superficial in an endoscopically resected polyp.

All patients having polyps with a Haggitt level 4 cancer require a subsequent colon resection with associated resection of the vascular pedicle and regional nodal tissue. A Haggitt level 2 or 3 cancer necessitates further colon resection if the cancer is higher grade (grade 3 or 4), there is angiolymphatic invasion, the stalk margin is grossly or microscopically positive, or there is uncertainty as to whether the margin was truly negative or the polyp was pedunculated.

Before operation, a thorough history and physical examination should be performed, and careful attention is given to family history and to general health as it relates to the ability to tolerate an operation. As part of the general physical examination, special attention is directed to the supraclavicular lymph nodes and the liver to detect metastases. Staging is completed with chest radiography to exclude pulmonary metastases and with liver function tests to exclude liver metastases. Any suspicion of metastases should prompt further work-up with thoracic, abdominal, or pelvic computed tomography.

Despite recently published studies exploring colon operation without a bowel preparation, we prefer a preoperative bowel preparation with a balanced electrolyte solution, such as polyethylene glycol 3350 or a sodium phosphate solution. When polyethylene glycol 3350 is used, we administer 2 liters of the solution, 1 glass every 15 minutes beginning at 5 pm until gone. Patient compliance may be enhanced by the addition of flavored unsweetened soft drink mix to the solution. Oral neomycin and metronidazole are administered, 1 g of each at 6 PM and at 11 PM. Sodium phosphate is administered similarly, with one bottle taken at 5 PM and 1 bottle at 9 PM.

Any patient who may require a stoma meets preoperatively with an enterostomal nurse for education and literature. The site of the potential stoma is marked preoperatively and is located in an optimal position to ensure excellent appliance adherence, ease of care, and minimal interference with clothing.

CONDUCT OF OPERATION

General Oncologic Principles
Pertinent to all colon resections for cancer, we agree with and adhere to the recently published guidelines for colon and rectal cancer surgery (Table 1). The extent of the surgical resection is determined by tumor location relative to the lymphovascular supply of the bowel.

Right Hemicolectomy
The distal 10 cm of ileum and right colon supplied by the ileocolic, right colic, and right branch of the middle colic arteries is resected en bloc with the arterial supply and

Table 1.—Summary of Surgical Guidelines for Colon Cancer

Lymphadenectomy should extend to the level of the origin of the primary feeding vessel; suspected positive lymph nodes outside the standard resection should be removed when feasible

Bowel margins ≥ 5 cm proximally and distally should be used

Laparoscopic colectomy for cancer should be confined to clinical trials

En bloc resection should be performed for tumors adherent to local structures

Inadvertent bowel perforation increases the risk of recurrence and should be avoided

Thorough abdominal exploration for metastatic, locally advanced primary and lymph node disease should be performed

The no-touch technique is debated, but little evidence supports it

Bowel washout may have theoretical benefits in rectal cancer, but such benefits have not been proved

Ovaries grossly involved with tumor should be removed; prophylactic oophorectomy cannot be supported

Modified from Nelson H, Petrelli N, Carlin A, Couture J, Fleshman J, Guillem J, Miedema B, Ota D, Sargent D: Guidelines 2000 for colon and rectal cancer surgery. J Natl Cancer Inst 93:583-596, 2001. By permission of Oxford University Press.

accompanying lymphatic tissue. Evidence supports only a limited resection of small bowel in association with a right colon cancer, because lymphatic spread toward the small bowel rarely occurs.

After the right colon is exposed, a peritoneal incision is made with cautery, freeing the retroperitoneal attachments of the ileum and cecum (Fig. 1 A). The lateral peritoneal attachments of the ascending colon are taken down, elevating the colon off the duodenum but leaving the duodenum retroperitoneal (Fig. 1 B). The dissection is carried around the hepatic flexure to the region of the middle colic artery. The ileocolic artery is ligated (Fig. 1 C).

The specimen is removed, preserving blood flow to the remaining distal ileum through a preserved ileal vascular arcade from the superior mesenteric artery and preserving the right branch of the middle colic artery. In a modification of this procedure, the entire middle colic artery can be resected and an extended right hemicolectomy done, but adequate blood supply must be preserved to the distal transverse colon to ensure healing at the subsequent anastomosis.

We reconstruct the anastomosis with either a hand-sewn or a stapled technique. Our hand-sewn technique is performed in a double-layer fashion, with an inner layer of absorbable running suture and an outer layer of interrupted suture, either absorbable or permanent (Fig. 2). The stapled anastomosis is done with two firings of a linear 90-mm stapler.

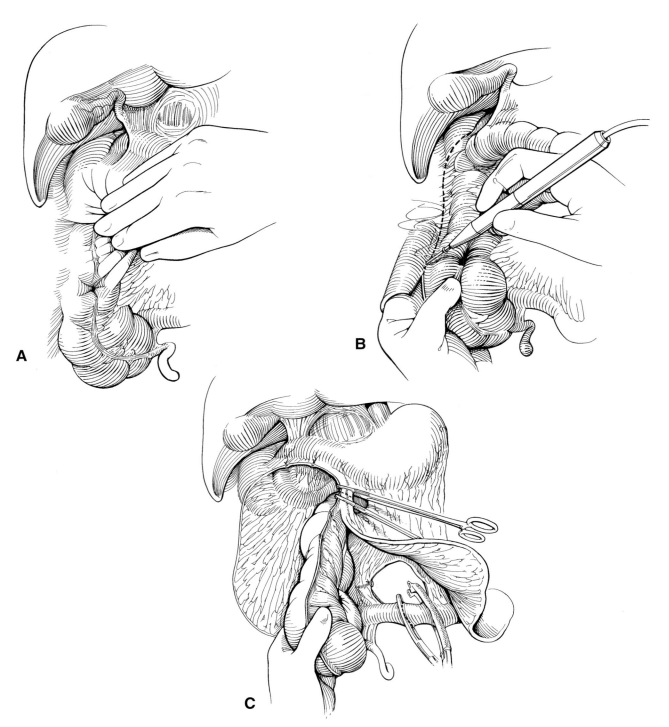

Fig. 1. Right hemicolectomy, open technique. (A and B), Mobilization of the ascending colon. (C), The ileocolic vessels have been ligated, noncrushing clamps placed on the distal ileum, and hemostats placed on the middle colic vessels before their division. The ileum will be transected at the dotted line.

Transverse Colon Resection

The specimen is inspected, and the relationship of the tumor to the middle colic vessels is noted. If the specimen directly overlies the middle colic vessels, we perform a resection incorporating this vascular pedicle and associated lymphatic drainage. If the tumor lies partway between the middle colic vessels and the left colic branches, we resect the bowel en bloc with both of these vascular pedicles. If the tumor lies between the middle colic and right colic vessels, an extended right hemicolectomy is our procedure of choice. For most tumors of the left side of the colon from the transverse to the sigmoid, the splenic flexure often must be mobilized.

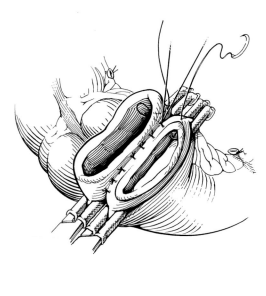

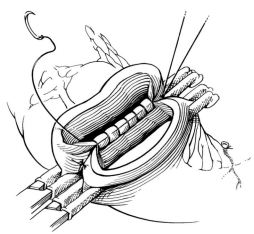

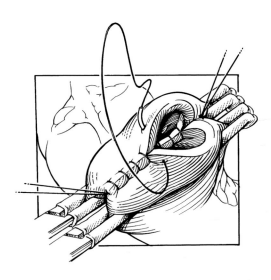

Fig. 2. Suture anastomosis. An end-to-end enteric anastomosis is constructed with a seromuscular layer of interrupted silk sutures and a running mucosal layer of polyglycolic acid suture.

Left Hemicolectomy

A specimen based on the left colic artery or ascending branch of the sigmoid artery is removed en bloc with the arterial supply and associated mesenteric lymph nodes. Adequate blood supply must be preserved to the proximal and distal cut ends of bowel to allow anastomosis of viable tissue. The anastomosis is constructed either in a double-layer hand-sewn fashion or with a double firing of the linear 90-mm stapler.

Sigmoid Colonic Anterior Resection and Low Anterior Resection

The patient is placed in a synchronous, or legs-up position, and a self-retaining ring retractor is used to facilitate exposure for a sigmoid colonic or a low anterior resection. The sigmoid colon is resected with sigmoid arterial branches, associated mesentery, and lymph drainage; the arterial supply is ligated at the origin of the sigmoid arteries and the superior hemorrhoidal branch is preserved. Ligating the vessels at this level does not adversely affect outcome and preserves blood supply to the upper rectum for the anastomosis. Mobilization of the rectum allows the proximal mesorectum to be removed with the specimen.

If the anastomosis is at or above the sacral promontory, we create it in a double-layer, hand-sewn fashion. If the distal extent of the resection is below the promontory, we perform either a hand-sewn, double-layer anastomosis or an end-to-end anastomosis with a circular stapling device.

Laparoscopic Right Hemicolectomy

After presurgical preparation and institution of general anesthesia, the patient is placed in the supine position. Both a urinary catheter and a nasogastric tube are inserted. Ankle straps are applied in anticipation of steep table rotation to facilitate exposure. A sterile skin preparation and draping are performed. The following is adapted from our previously described five-step method.[23]

A 10-mm port is placed in an open fashion, either supraumbilically (if no prior abdominal operation has been done) or in the left upper quadrant (if a previous abdominal scar is present). After port placement, air insufflation is commenced with a flow rate of 6 L/min and a maximal pressure of 14 to 15 mm Hg. A 30° angled laparoscope is advanced through this port, and an abdominal survey is completed.

Two additional 10-mm ports are placed under direct vision, one suprapubic in the midline, avoiding the bladder dome, and one in the left upper quadrant of the abdomen. The bowel is manipulated along its peritoneal edge with graspers to determine mobility and adhesions. We practice early conversion to an open operation for massive adhesions, inability to mobilize the distal ileum, bulky or large lesions, atypical anatomy, or other unexpected findings.

The patient is positioned in steep Trendelenburg position, with the right side up to allow the abdominal contents to fall to a dependent position away from the surgical site. The small bowel is flipped up out of the pelvis, exposing the retroperitoneal attachments of the distal small bowel and cecum. The peritoneum in this region is opened horizontally, and the ureter is identified and left in the retroperitoneum. The line of dissection is carried around to the lateral attachments of the cecum and ascending colon, which are taken down sharply; tension is maintained by grasping the peritoneum near the bowel wall with either a Babcock or an alligator clamp and pulling the cecum toward the left upper quadrant.

Before mobilization of the hepatic flexure, the patient is repositioned to reverse Trendelenburg position with the right side up to allow the abdominal contents to fall away from the right upper quadrant. The peritoneum is grasped near the colon at the hepatic flexure, and the colon is elevated ventrally and caudally. The peritoneum overlying the gastrocolic ligament is divided sharply, and dissection is carried down, separating the underlying tissues from the mesocolon. The duodenum is encountered and is avoided, leaving it retroperitoneal. The dissection is continued until the entire right colon is mobilized to the midline. The vascular pedicle can be ligated intracorporeally or the specimen delivered, and the vascular pedicle ligated extracorporeally.

A Babcock clamp is placed through the inferior midline port, and the peritoneum near the region of the cecum is grasped. The supraumbilical port is removed, and the incision is extended around the umbilicus for a total length of 4 to 6 cm. The Babcock clamp is used to bring the desired bowel up and out of the open abdominal incision, after which it is removed. The entire terminal ileum, cecum, ascending colon, and hepatic flexure are mobilized out of the abdomen. Under direct vision, the mesentery is taken down, extracorporeal ligation being performed in the thin patient and intracorporeal ligation in the obese patient. The specimen is resected, and an anastomosis is created according to the surgeon's preference. The bowel is placed back into the abdomen, and the abdomen is thoroughly irrigated with saline. The irrigant is thoroughly aspirated from the abdomen. Laparoscopic reexploration is warranted if the irrigant returns bloody or does not readily clear of blood on further irrigation.

The two remaining ports are removed, and the fasciae of port sites and midline are closed with interrupted absorbable suture. The skin is closed with a running absorbable suture.

Laparoscopic Left Hemicolectomy, Sigmoid Colonic Resection, and Low Anterior Resection

The laparoscopic left hemicolectomy is performed in the same manner as the laparoscopic right hemicolectomy, reversing the left upper quadrant to the mirror image of the right upper quadrant. The abdominal cavity is explored and conversion to an open procedure is given consideration. The camera is moved between the supraumbilical position and the other port sites as needed for optimal visualization and instrument maneuverability.

For sigmoid colon resection, the patient is placed in the left side-up, steep Trendelenburg position, and sigmoid mobilization is begun (Fig. 3 A and B). Peritoneum near the sigmoid colon is grasped, and the sigmoid is retracted toward the right upper quadrant. The lateral peritoneal attachments are incised, and the retroperitoneal attachments are teased away from the bowel (Fig. 3 B). The ureter is identified and protected throughout the dissection. The lateral attachments of the descending colon are taken down with a combination of sharp dissection and electrocautery until the splenic flexure is reached.

The patient is repositioned in left side-up, steep reverse Trendelenburg position to allow the abdominal contents to fall away from the left upper quadrant. Peritoneum near the colon is grasped, and the splenic flexure of the colon is retracted anterocaudally, toward the midline. The peritoneal surface is opened with cautery, and the colon is dissected free from its retroperitoneal attachments. The dissection is continued until the midline is reached.

Although we prefer extracorporeal ligation of vessels for ease and safety, if the patient is obese or the mesentery is short, then we ligate the sigmoid artery at its origin from the inferior mesenteric artery, thus facilitating mobilization of the specimen out of the abdomen (Fig. 3 C). The sigmoid is elevated anteriorly and the vasculature is identified. The peritoneum overlying the origin of the vessel is opened, and the bare space on either side of the vessel is developed. A linear stapler with a vascular staple cartridge is used to ligate and transect the vessels. The midline port is removed, and a 4- to 6-cm periumbilical midline incision is created. The specimen is exteriorized through this wound, and extracorporeal ligation of the vessels is continued and completed.

The specimen is resected, and an anastomosis is constructed extracorporeally with either sutures or stapler. Alternatively, the anastomosis can be completed intracorporeally below the sacral promontory with a circular stapling device. Preoperatively, if the surgeon anticipates performing an intracorporeal, stapled anastomosis, the patient is positioned with the legs in stirrups, and the legs are appropriately padded. The colon is mobilized, and the vasculature is identified and ligated. A site distal to the tumor is chosen, and the mesentery is cleaned in this area to allow application of a laparoscopic linear stapling device (Fig. 3 *D*). The proximal transected end of bowel is brought out through the wound, and vessel ligation is completed extracorporeally. A site proximal to the tumor is chosen, and the bowel is transected, removing the specimen for pathologic analysis. A purse-string suture is run around the proximal cut end of bowel, and the anvil por-

tion of the circular stapler is placed into the bowel (Fig. 3 *E*). The purse-string suture is tightened down around the center pin. The bowel is placed back into the abdomen. The circular stapling device is placed into the anus, and under direct vision with the laparoscope, the central pin is advanced through the stapled stump of distal bowel (Fig. 3 *F*). The trocar is removed, and the anvil and arm are connected. The stapler is fired and removed.

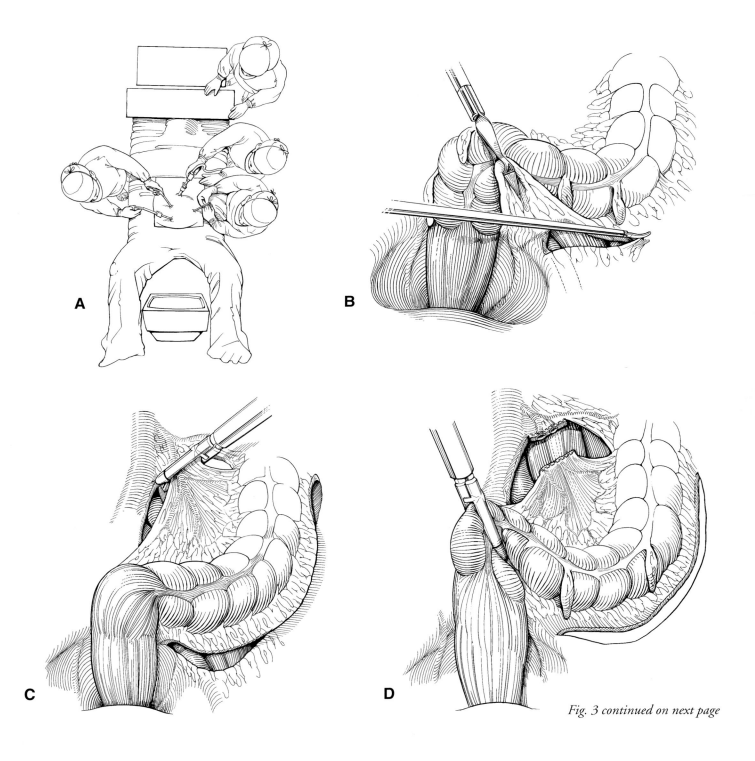

Fig. 3 continued on next page

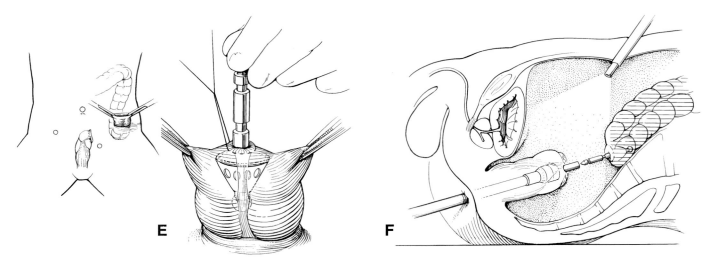

Fig. 3. Sigmoid resection, laparoscopic technique. (A), Patient is positioned with legs up (synchronous) with a monitor between the legs. Three or four cannulas are placed; the camera is best positioned in the left upper quadrant. (B), The peritoneal reflection is grasped, elevated, and incised and left ureter is identified early. (C), The vascular pedicle is ligated intracorporeally with a linear vascular stapler. (D), The distal bowel is transected with one or more applications of the endoscopic linear stapler. The proximal end then can be exteriorized. (E), The bowel is divided proximal to the tumor to complete the resection, a purse-string suture is placed, and the anvil of a circular stapler is secured in the distal end of the proximal limb of bowel. (F), The central pin of the circular stapler is advanced across the rectal staple line. The anvil and stapler shaft are attached to each other and closed, and the stapler is fired.

The ports are removed and the abdomen is irrigated. The fasciae of the periumbilical wound and the two port sites are closed with interrupted absorbable suture. The skin is closed with running absorbable suture.

Special Circumstances

An operation to excise the site of a prior polypectomy offers a special challenge to the surgeon. For the open procedure, we prefer to position all patients with prior polypectomy who are undergoing colectomy in the combined, or legs-up, position in anticipation of intraoperative colonoscopy. We first enter the abdomen and expose the colon with minimal dissection, then we subsequently perform colonoscopy. After locating the site of the lesion, we mark the site with a seromuscular suture. For laparoscopic colon resection, the polyp site can be marked with India ink during colonoscopy a day or two before the laparoscopic procedure, or a plain radiograph of the abdomen can be obtained during colonoscopy to identify the exact location of the tip of the scope with the polypectomy site in direct view. For some cases in which a polyp is still present but in a hard-to-discern location, it may be necessary to rely on a barium enema for precisely locating the site of abnormality before resection. Marking the site with India ink at the time of colonoscopy allows intraoperative localization of the disease site, whereas a delay from colonoscopy to the laparoscopy allows clearance of the intracolonic air and provides for an easier operation.

SURGICAL OUTCOMES

Perioperative risks can be minimized with adequate preoperative preparation and attention to detail during patient positioning. Laparoscopic colectomy has an expected conversion rate of 20%, a morbidity rate of 14%, and a mortality of about 1%.[24,25] Wound infection occurs in approximately 4% of patients who have colon resection.

Bleeding occurs perioperatively, either due to a technical error intraoperatively or in a delayed fashion from the anastomotic site. The presence of ongoing bleeding perioperatively in an amount exceeding that expected from the surgical dissection and intraoperative blood loss prompts a return to the operating room and exploration. Colonic bleeding postoperatively is presumed to be from the anastomotic line and generally is self-limited. Blood transfusion is performed if there are hemodynamic changes, and all efforts are made to find and correct any coagulopathy. Gentle endoscopy and directed therapy occasionally have a role but must be undertaken conservatively with minimal insufflation. Direct operative intervention with ligation in the operating room is therapeutic in ongoing bleeding.

Neuropathy is a dreaded but infrequent complication that generally resolves spontaneously but can persist with drastic results. Prevention depends on careful attention to positioning of the patient and retractors in the operating room. We position the patient's upper extremities to pad and protect the ulnar nerve at the elbow and minimize traction on the median nerve. The combined, or legs-up, position is used whenever access is needed to the anus, either for intraoperative colonoscopy or if use of the circular stapler is anticipated for a low anastomosis. For these cases, there must be no sustained pressure on the calves in order to avoid pressure necrosis and a compartment syndrome. Likewise, sustained pressure on the peroneal nerves must be avoided. Femoral nerve injury can occur from abdominal retractors pressing too deeply into the retroperitoneum.

We routinely use elastic stockings and sequential compression devices on the legs of our patients to minimize the development of deep venous thrombosis. In high-risk patients, we administer subcutaneous heparin or other anticoagulants as an additional safety measure.[26,27]

Perioperative events, such as cardiac and respiratory events, are minimized by performing complete preoperative histories and physical examinations. If problems are identified, the advice of appropriate specialists is obtained. For the higher-risk patient, a team approach involving the medical specialist, surgeon, and anesthesiologist is important for determining the most appropriate preoperative, intraoperative, and postoperative care, identifying issues such as a need for invasive monitoring, admission to the intensive care unit, cardioprotective medications, and pulmonary hygiene maneuvers.

In general, we favor early removal of the nasogastric tube, reserving longer periods of nasogastric decompression for patients with chronic or severe bowel and gastric obstruction or in any situation in which bowel rest is desired. Ambulation is encouraged either the night of operation or the following morning. The Foley catheter is removed as soon as the patient is comfortable in all abdominal cases or on the fourth morning after dissection in the pelvis. In the latter situation, we check post-void residual volumes with ultrasonography or "in-and-out" catheterization after the first urine void to exclude bladder stasis. We resume feeding as early as possible, gauging resumption of oral intake either on patient desire to eat or passage of flatus. In general, patients who have had laparoscopy eat earlier, mobilize surgical fluids sooner, and experience a speedier recovery.

At Mayo Clinic, adjuvant chemotherapy is administered by medical oncologists. Standard 5-fluorouracil–based chemotherapy regimens are clearly indicated for patients with stage III disease.[28] The precise regimens are constantly evolving. Current regimens include 5-fluorouracil and leucovorin, and future regimens likely will include camptothecin-11. Chemotherapy is considered in patients with stage II disease who have worrisome prognostic features such as aneuploidy, a high proportion of S-phase tumor cells, or cancer that was obstructing or perforated. Patients with stage IV disease may be eligible for standard or experimental chemotherapy regimens at the discretion of the medical oncologist. Radiation generally does not have a role in the therapy of colon cancer, but occasionally it is used in an attempt to improve outcome in patients with cancer locally invading contiguous organs or a considerable portion of the abdominal wall.

LONG-TERM FOLLOW-UP

Patients are seen on an annual basis for 5 years after their operation for follow-up history, physical examination, and laboratory tests. Colonoscopy is performed at the first annual visit and 4 to 5 years afterward. The frequency of interval endoscopy is intensified if the patient has hereditary nonpolyposis colon cancer or other genetic risk factors or if the patient has recurrent polyps or symptoms warranting evaluation. Liver function tests, a complete blood count, and a chest radiograph are obtained annually for 5 years to exclude metastasis of disease to the lungs or liver. Disease recurrence at either of these sites results in referral to a thoracic or hepatic surgeon for consideration of resection.

The likelihood of recurrence of disease is based on stage of the tumor; recurrence exceeds 50% in transmural tumors with lymph node metastases. Clear margins are important for maximal survival. Colonic perforation increases the likelihood of recurrence (Table 2).

CONTROVERSIES

Laparoscopy in Colon Cancer Surgery

In the mid 1990s, as interest in the application of laparoscopic techniques to colon cancer surgery gained momentum, a randomized, prospective trial to examine the feasibility and safety of laparoscopic colon cancer surgery was instituted.[25] Reported benefits of laparoscopic surgery included decreased hospital stay, decreased postoperative pain, shorter length of postoperative ileus, fewer adhesions, and faster return to work, but it was not clear that laparoscopy could provide an oncologic procedure equivalent to the traditional open method of colon resection. Opponents raised concerns that margins would be inadequate, fewer lymph nodes would be obtained and staging ability would be limited, pneumoperitoneum might disperse tumor intra-abdominally, and, therefore, port site recurrence rates would be prohibitively high. Cost was a further issue.

The trial closed to accrual: results from this controlled trial are not yet available. Progress reports are promising,

Table 2.—Five-Year Survival Rates by Stage of Colon Cancer

Stage	5-year survival, % of patients
I	82-97
II	63-80
III	30-74
IV	< 20

Data from Cohen et al.[28]

demonstrating that, in experienced hands, laparoscopic surgery for colon cancer provides an equivalent operation from the standpoint of cancer-free specimen margins, ability to stage, and risk of cancer recurrence in the surgical wounds (open incision or port site). Concerns of spread due to pneumoperitoneum are still under investigation, but several current series show the ability to perform the laparoscopic procedure with recurrence rates at the trocar or wound site comparable to those with open surgery.

Several studies have examined specific indications for laparoscopic operation and the different populations who might benefit from it. One study showed that elderly populations may especially benefit from laparoscopic operation. Stocchi and Nelson[25] showed that patients older than 75 years undergoing laparoscopic operations had improved postoperative outcome compared with those having open colectomy for cancer. Benefits included less postoperative morbidity and narcotic use, faster recovery of bowel function (bowel movements), and reduced duration of hospital stay. More patients who underwent laparoscopic colectomy were able to remain independent at dismissal compared with those who had the open procedure; this result must be considered a substantial social and economic benefit.

Prophylactic Oophorectomy

Between 1% and 11% of women will have metastases from their colon cancer to their ovaries; thus, preoperative discussion of the need for oophorectomy is needed when counseling female patients. A controversial topic, some physicians argue that the ovaries should be removed prophylactically in all postmenopausal women and selectively in premenopausal women with colon cancer. The vast majority of women will have normal, disease-free ovaries, and for psychosocial reasons many women are not willing to undergo prophylactic resection. In our series of 155 patients, oophorectomy in 77 patients who had operation for colon cancer did not yield a single positive specimen, yet Kaplan-Meier curves of recurrence-free survival suggested a survival advantage.[29] In general,

we remove grossly abnormal ovaries in all patients, but with greater reservation in females of childbearing age. In our experience, preoperative discussion with the patient greatly facilitates acceptance and understanding if oophorectomy is necessary intraoperatively. About 2% of women undergoing large bowel resection for cancer who do not have their ovaries removed will require a second operation at a future date for an abnormal ovarian mass.

Obstructing Colon Cancer

Obstructing tumors of the large bowel may be associated with a poor prognosis. A retrospective review by Carraro et al.[30] examined the characteristics of 107 patients receiving a one-stage curative operation for obstructing colon cancer over a 10-year period comparing the results with those in 256 patients with nonobstructing tumors who had curative operations during the same period. Obstruction occurred most frequently in the left colon and at the splenic flexure. Univariate analysis showed that significant prognostic factors for poor outcome included obstruction, age older than 70 years, advanced stage of carcinoma, high histologic grade, and disease recurrence. Obstruction, however, was excluded as a risk factor in multivariate analysis. Other studies have shown similar results. Thus, further work is needed.

Complete resection of the tumor with either primary or delayed anastomosis is preferable. The tumor should be excised en bloc with any attached structures. Locally unresectable tumors most often will necessitate a proximal diverting colostomy or an ileostomy, with consideration of a mucous fistula to avoid a blind loop. Alternatively, an expanding wire stent may be placed across the lesion by the interventional endoscopist, allowing temporary relief of the obstruction. Thereafter, the bowel will clear of fecal matter, decompressing the bowel proximal to the lesion and allowing for bowel preparation, preoperative staging studies, and elective operation.

Perforated Colon Cancer

Perforated viscus frequently presents as an acute surgical abdomen, leading to urgent stabilization and surgical exploration. Free or mesenteric air in association with the colon inevitably raises the question of perforated diverticular disease; however, colon carcinoma must be considered in the differential diagnosis. Colon cancer must be considered in surgical planning because induration in the region of a colon perforation along with a lack of appropriate preoperative colon evaluation will make intraoperative diagnosis difficult.

During resection, oncologic surgical principles should be followed, preferably with complete tumor resection and negative margins. If, preoperatively, the colon was not evaluated radiologically with water-soluble contrast, the rectum should be examined with rigid proctoscopy. Whenever possible, resection of the perforated segment of colon is desirable to limit sepsis. Caution must be used during dissection to avoid injuring retroperitoneal and adhesed structures. Cutting across tumor should be avoided. Further spillage of bowel contents during resection should be prevented, both to avoid abdominal sepsis and to limit theoretic tumor spillage. Leaving the perforated segment in place with proximal diversion will delay final diagnosis and should be avoided. Options after resection include colostomy with delayed anastomosis or primary anastomosis with protective proximal loop ileostomy or loop colostomy. The abdomen should be thoroughly irrigated before closure, including the subdiaphragmatic regions and the pelvis.

Bleeding Colon Cancer

Bleeding is a common symptom of colorectal cancer and, when present, should prompt a full colon evaluation, even in the presence of anal conditions such as hemorrhoids. Frequently, bleeding is occult, allowing for a full evaluation before any surgical planning. Iron deficiency anemia discovered on routine laboratory tests or a positive fecal occult blood test performed as part of the annual examination should prompt further evaluation, including a complete endoscopic colon evaluation.

Bleeding may be overt and, on occasion, life-threatening. Colonoscopy during overt lower gastrointestinal bleeding is challenging but may provide invaluable diagnostic information and therapeutic opportunities. Tagged red cell scanning and angiography may provide further diagnostic information and may help to localize the site of bleeding.

Once a bleeding tumor is localized, appropriate judgment is needed to determine the urgency of operative intervention. Preoperative resuscitation of the patient with fluids and blood products is critical. Anticoagulation should be reversed. This step alone may result in rapid cessation of bleeding. Whenever possible, a bowel preparation should be performed, allowing for optimal resection and primary anastomosis, according to oncologic principles.

CONCLUSION

Colon cancer is a common malignancy; its rate in the general population is about 6%. Between a third and half of patients with colon cancer will die of it. Cure rates more than 90% are achievable in patients who undergo operation for early-stage cancer.

Controversy exists regarding the best screening strategy. For patients at average risk, annual fecal occult blood testing with interval endoscopy is considered adequate screening. Patients at moderate or high risk, that is, those with a family history of colon cancer, prior polyps, or inflammatory bowel disease, should undergo colonoscopic surveillance at least every 5 years or more frequently, as determined by the clinician.

The outcome of operation for colon cancer depends on early diagnosis, proper staging, and appropriate surgical intervention. Open colectomy is the standard for oncologic operation. In selected circumstances, resection of hepatic metastases and pulmonary metastases provides the possibility of a cure.

Laparoscopic colectomy is still under investigation for its adequacy as a cancer operation, but early results of ongoing trials are favorable. Certain subgroups, such as the elderly, benefit greatly from this approach in terms of a more rapid return to independent living after operation.

REFERENCES

1. Lang NP: Thomas G. Orr Memorial Lectureship. Colon cancer from etiology to prevention. Am J Surg 174:578-582, 1997

2. Giovannucci E, Stampfer MJ, Colditz GA, Hunter DJ, Fuchs C, Rosner BA, Speizer FE, Willett WC: Multivitamin use, folate, and colon cancer in women in the Nurses' Health Study. Ann Intern Med 129:517-524, 1998

3. Truswell AS: Diet and prevention of cancer: whether meat is a risk factor for cancer remains uncertain (letter). BMJ 319:187, 1999

4. Sturmer T, Glynn RJ, Lee IM, Manson JE, Buring JE, Hennekens CH: Aspirin use and colorectal cancer: post-trial follow-up data from the Physicians' Health Study. Ann Intern Med 128:713-720, 1998

5. Fuchs CS, Giovannucci EL, Colditz GA, Hunter DJ, Stampfer MJ, Rosner B, Speizer FE, Willett WC: Dietary fiber and the risk of colorectal cancer and adenoma in women. N Engl J Med 340:169-176, 1999

6. Screening for colorectal cancer—United States, 1992-1993, and new guidelines. MMWR Morb Mortal Wkly Rep 45:107-110, 1996

7. Pignone MP, Harris R, Kinsinger L: Changing cancer screening practice: physician or patient activation? (Abstract.) J Gen Intern Med 12 Suppl 1:110, 1997

8. Pignatelli M: The adenomatous polyposis coli tumour suppressor gene regulates c-MYC transcription in colon cancer cells. Gut 44:596, 1999

9. Lerman C, Hughes C, Trock BJ, Myers RE, Main D, Bonney A, Abbaszadegan MR, Harty AE, Franklin BA, Lynch JF, Lynch HT: Genetic testing in families with hereditary nonpolyposis colon cancer. JAMA 281:1618-1622, 1999

10. Muto T, Bussey HJ, Morson BC: The evolution of cancer of the colon and rectum. Cancer 36:2251-2270, 1975

11. Muto T, Nagawa H, Watanabe T, Masaki T, Sawada T: Colorectal carcinogenesis: historical review. Dis Colon Rectum 40 Suppl:S80-S85, 1997

12. Muto T, Masaki T, Suzuki K: DNA ploidy pattern of flat adenomas of the large bowel. Dis Colon Rectum 34:696-698, 1991

13. Vogelstein B, Fearon ER, Hamilton SR, Kern SE, Preisinger AC, Leppert M, Nakamura Y, White R, Smits AM, Bos JL: Genetic alterations during colorectal-tumor development. N Engl J Med 319:525-532, 1988

14. Helfand M, Marton KI, Zimmer-Gembeck MJ, Sox HC Jr: History of visible rectal bleeding in a primary care population: initial assessment and 10-year follow-up. JAMA 277:44-48, 1997

15. Read TE, Read JD, Butterly LF: Importance of adenomas 5 mm or less in diameter that are detected by sigmoidoscopy. N Engl J Med 336:8-12, 1997

16. Netzer P, Buttiker U, Pfister M, Halter F, Schmassmann A: Frequency of advanced neoplasia in the proximal colon without an index polyp in the rectosigmoid. Dis Colon Rectum 42:661-667, 1999

17. Levin TR, Palitz A, Grossman S, Conell C, Finkler L, Ackerson L, Rumore G, Selby JV: Predicting advanced proximal colonic neoplasia with screening sigmoidoscopy. JAMA 281:1611-1617, 1999

18. Winawer SJ, Zauber AG, Ho MN, O'Brien MJ, Gottlieb LS, Sternberg SS, Waye JD, Schapiro M, Bond JH, Panish JF, Ackroyd F, Shike M, Kurtz RC, Hornsby-Lewis L, Gerdes H, Stewart ET: Prevention of colorectal cancer by colonoscopic polypectomy. The National Polyp Study Workgroup. N Engl J Med 329:1977-1981, 1993

19. Farley DR, Bannon MP, Zietlow SP, Pemberton JH, Ilstrup DM, Larson DR: Management of colonoscopic perforations. Mayo Clin Proc 72:729-733, 1997

20. Hernandez EJ, Ellington RT, Harford WV: Isolated transverse mesocolon laceration during routine colonoscopy. J Clin Gastroenterol 28:46-48, 1999

21. Rex DK: CT and MR colography (virtual colonoscopy): status report. J Clin Gastroenterol 27:199-203, 1998

22. Hara AK, Johnson CD, Reed JE, Ahlquist DA, Nelson H, MacCarty RL, Harmsen WS, Ilstrup DM: Detection of colorectal polyps with CT colography: initial assessment of sensitivity and specificity. Radiology 205:59-65, 1997

23. Young-Fadok TM, Nelson H: Laparoscopic right colectomy: five-step procedure. Dis Colon Rectum 43:267-271, 2000

24. Nelson H: Laparoscopic surgery. In Surgery of the Colon & Rectum. Edited by RJ Nicholls, RR Dozois. New York, Churchill Livingstone, 1997, pp 865-878

25. Stocchi L, Nelson H: Laparoscopic colectomy for colon cancer: trial update. J Surg Oncol 68:255-267, 1998

26. Cook DJ, Guyatt GH, Laupacis A, Sackett DL: Rules of evidence and clinical recommendations on the use of antithrombotic agents. Chest 102 Suppl 4:305S-311S, 1992

27. Sackett DL: Rules of evidence and clinical recommendations on the use of antithrombotic agents. Chest 95 Suppl 2:2S-4S, 1989

28. Cohen AM, Kelsen D, Saltz L, Minsky BD, Nelson H, Farouk R, Gunderson LL, Michelassi F, Arenas RB, Schilsky RL, Willet CG: Adjuvant therapy for colorectal cancer. Curr Probl Surg 34:601-676, 1997

29. Young-Fadok TM, Wolff BG, Nivatvongs S, Metzger PP, Ilstrup DM: Prophylactic oophorectomy in colorectal carcinoma: preliminary results of a randomized, prospective trial. Dis Colon Rectum 41:277-283, 1998

30. Carraro PG, Segala M, Cesana BM, Tiberio G: Obstructing colonic cancer: failure and survival patterns over a ten-year follow-up after one-stage curative surgery. Dis Colon Rectum 44:243-250, 2001

Chapter 36

ISCHEMIC COLITIS

Mark D. Sawyer, M.D.

Ischemic colitis, first described by Boley et al.[1] in 1963 and given its current appellation by Marston et al.[2] in 1966, is the most common form of intestinal ischemia. It may be described most simply as the end pathophysiologic result of an interruption or diminution of blood flow to the colon. A definitive, pragmatic classification of this disease is problematic, because a broad array of underlying causes impede the precise identification of the elements that precipitate a particular clinical episode. At Mayo Clinic, we prefer a treatment-based, patient-oriented classification; namely, patients are categorized as those who will or will not respond to nonoperative therapy, as delineated by Robert et al.[3] Although most patients will not require surgery, early involvement of the surgeon is crucial to identifying those patients for whom early operative intervention may be lifesaving.

COLONIC VASCULAR ANATOMY AND VARIATIONS

In the healthy state, the colon derives its blood supply from the superior mesenteric artery and the inferior mesenteric artery (Fig. 1). The superior mesenteric artery gives off the right colic artery and terminates as the ileocolic artery, together supplying the right colon, the hepatic flexure, and the proximal transverse colon. The middle colic artery arises more proximally from the superior mesenteric artery and provides the blood supply to the transverse colon. The right and middle colic arteries may each be absent in as many as 20% of patients.[4] The inferior mesenteric artery supplies the splenic flexure and the descending and sigmoid colon. Its most distal inferior

branch becomes the superior rectal artery, which supplies the proximal rectum. Collateral flow between the systemic and visceral circulation takes place through small

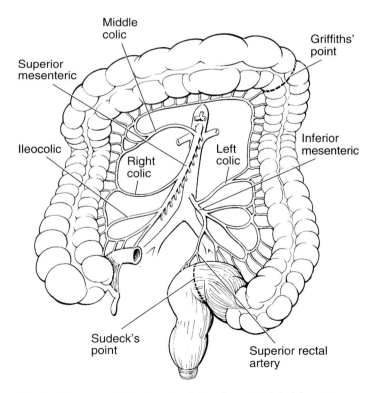

Fig. 1. The arterial blood supply of the colon. (Modified from Mayo CW: Surgery of the Small & Large Intestine: a Handbook of Operative Surgery. 2nd ed. Chicago, Year Book Medical Publishers, 1962, p 99. By permission of Mayo Foundation.)

vessels that join the superior to the middle rectal arteries, an area known as Sudeck's point.[5] Although some authors debate the clinical importance of these vessels, ischemia has been found in this area.[6]

Branches of the visceral vessels near the border of the colon inosculate with each other to form the so-called marginal artery of Drummond. The continuity of this vessel may be interrupted near the splenic flexure, at a potential watershed area known as Griffiths' point.[7] This area may be partially or completely bridged by the "meandering mesenteric artery," a more centrally located analogy to the marginal artery of Drummond that runs between the middle and left colic arteries. Historically, it has been called the "Arch of Riolan," but the former term is preferred because of the vagaries of translating Riolan's original manuscript from the French.[8,9] When present, this vessel connects the circulations of the superior mesenteric artery and the inferior mesenteric artery. However, it should not be depended on to provide circulation after a resection, because it is not always present. At Mayo Clinic, preoperative angiography is rarely used in patients who have ischemic colitis, because the angiogram may be normal, but ischemic colitis may still be present. Nonetheless, knowledge of the colonic vascular anatomy and its variations is crucial to appropriate resection, particularly when a patient has had previous aortic or colonic surgery.[10]

PATHOLOGIC CONDITIONS

The natural course of ischemic colitis with hematochezia as an early symptom presents an interesting conundrum: why is bleeding a manifestation of the disease? In actuality, many patients may seek treatment sometime after an ischemic episode. Some patients recover spontaneously, many without a distinct cause being identified. Others recover with treatment by intravenous fluids and antibiotic therapy. Those patients who are treated as inpatients may have a passage of bloody diarrhea (i.e., hematochezia) a few days after they are adequately rehydrated. Usually self-limited, this passage of blood presumably occurs as the infarcted mucosa sloughs off the underlying reperfused tissue. Thus, hematochezia may more accurately represent a reperfusion injury rather than ischemia per se.

ETIOLOGIC FACTORS AND PATIENT GROUPS

The etiology of ischemic colitis is often idiopathic; Table 1 lists some of the more common causes. Simple dehydration in a patient who has predisposing factors may be enough to induce clinically significant ischemia.

Table 1.—Causes of Ischemic Colitis

Nonocclusive	Occlusive
Idiopathic	Large vessel
Shock	Thrombus
Colonic dilatation or distention	Embolus
Ogilvie's syndrome	Surgical ligation[11]
Colonic obstruction	Small vessel
Medications[12]	Diabetes mellitus[13]
Oral contraceptives	Radiotherapy
NSAIDs[14]*	Atherosclerosis
Catecholamines	
Vasopressin	
Ergot alkaloids	
Pseudoephedrine[15]	
Cocaine[16]	

*NSAIDs, nonsteroidal anti-inflammatory drugs.

Nonocclusive Ischemic Colitis in Elderly Patients
Most ischemic colitis is secondary to nonocclusive vascular disease. No distinct causative factor can be implicated positively in as many as 50% of these patients. This common form of the disease occurs more often in men than in women, usually in the left colon near the watershed area of the splenic flexure. The ravages of age, atherosclerosis (especially of the inferior mesenteric artery), decreasing cardiac output, microvascular disease (e.g., diabetes mellitus, vasculitis), and the accruing effects of various medications all may contribute to a diminished blood flow. Thus, a subsequent event such as hypovolemia or vasospasm may decrease blood flow to the colon below a critical point and result in ischemia. In these cases, ischemic colitis may respond to the optimization of hemodynamics, intravenous antibiotics, and bowel rest, but surgical intervention may be required in 50% to 75% of elderly patients.

Ischemic Colitis in Young Adults
Ischemic colitis in young adults (< 50 years of age) has pathologic similarities to the nonocclusive disease that occurs in elderly patients, but it differs in patient demographics, severity, necessity for surgical intervention, and mortality.[17-21] Most patients in this age group are women, and as many as 50% of the cases are associated with oral contraceptive use.[18,22-24] In our 8-year review of 38 Mayo Clinic patients under age 50 who had ischemic colitis,[24] 75% of them were successfully managed nonoperatively. In those patients who needed an operation, the most common indication was perforation of the colon.

Acute Occlusive Ischemic Colitis

Acute types of ischemic colitis that are secondary to occlusive vascular disease nearly always require surgical intervention. The area of midgut that is rendered ischemic because of thromboemboli of the superior mesenteric artery will depend on how far the embolus is from the ostium of the artery's origin. The most distal branches of the artery are the right colic and ileocolic arteries. Occlusion at this level affects only the right colon. The more proximal the embolus, the more extensive is the attendant ischemia of the small intestine, and the more likely it is to affect the middle colic artery. Thrombi that lodge in the proximal superior mesenteric artery are particularly harmful. The attendant necrosis of the small intestine which they produce portends a poor prognosis.

Ischemic Colitis After Abdominal Aortic Reconstruction

Patients with ischemic colitis that occurs after an operation for an abdominal aortic aneurysm are at risk for overwhelming sepsis, which has an attendant mortality of 57%.[11] In addition, the as-yet-unendothelialized prosthetic graft is particularly vulnerable to infection. If the graft has been contaminated, it may be necessary to resect it and do an extra-anatomical bypass, although a prolonged course of antibiotic treatment may be satisfactory. In these circumstances, ischemia is more akin to acute occlusive disease precipitated by the acute loss of the blood supply from the inferior mesenteric artery during aortic reconstruction. The remaining blood supply to the sigmoid colon comes from systemic collateral flow through the middle rectal arteries below the sigmoid and from visceral collateral flow through the middle colic artery above it. Patients with mild ischemia may recover with hemodynamic optimization, intravenous antibiotics, and bowel rest. When surgical resection is required, surgeons at Mayo Clinic prefer to use a colostomy to divert the fecal stream and avoid possible intra-abdominal contamination in already compromised patients. To prevent contamination of the aortic prosthesis, the surgeon should avoid primary anastomosis of the bowel.

CLINICAL PRESENTATION AND DIAGNOSIS

Physical Examination

As a rule, patients who present with ischemic colitis have tenderness over the affected area of the colon. Peritoneal signs, however, are often absent, particularly in elderly patients. Thus, the conclusions reached from the physical examination must take into consideration the patient's age. Most patients with ischemic colitis are elderly, and they may not manifest as much abdominal tenderness as would truly reflect the extent of their pathologic condition. When peritoneal signs are elicited during a physical examination, they most likely indicate transmural necrosis, which requires urgent surgical intervention. Other factors that suggest the need for surgery are those associated with the systemic inflammatory response syndrome (e.g., hypotension, fever, oliguria, altered mental status). Of course, the presence of diffuse peritonitis indicates extensive necrosis or perforation and mandates urgent exploration of the abdomen.

Abdominal pain and bloody diarrhea are the most prevalent symptoms in patients with ischemic colitis. The typical chronology is crampy abdominal pain first, followed by a strong urge to defecate, and then diarrhea and hematochezia. These symptoms may be accompanied by anorexia, nausea, and emesis caused by ischemia and the resulting functional obstruction. These symptoms may worsen for several days before the patient seeks treatment. In patients with low-flow ischemia, the resulting dehydration will worsen the ischemia and any clinical symptoms.

Colonoscopy

In patients whose symptoms do not indicate the need for immediate surgical treatment, colonoscopy is the preferred diagnostic test.[25,26] At Mayo Clinic, colonoscopy is used instead of a less complete examination of the colon such as sigmoidoscopy. Because areas of ischemia may not be contiguous, the absence of direct, localizing peritoneal signs makes it difficult to exclude involvement of particular areas of the colon without direct visualization. Flexible sigmoidoscopy may be used in patients whose ischemia is secondary to aortic reconstruction, but care must be taken not to overlook the possibility of proximal ischemia due to atherosclerosis in the superior mesenteric artery. In addition to direct visualization of the colonic mucosa, biopsy specimens may aid in distinguishing ischemic colitis from other forms of colitis. Colonoscopic findings depend on the severity of the ischemic insult and the stage in the course of the disease at which the colonoscopy is performed. Transmural necrosis, the most serious manifestation, is suggested by blackened epithelium shaggy from furfuraceous desquamation. These areas of frank necrosis may be bordered by areas of the colon that are receiving increased perfusion. Superficial ischemia causes patchy mucosal necrosis surrounded by viable epithelium. Other colonoscopic signs of ischemic colitis (e.g., edema, erythema, submucosal hemorrhage) suggest a reperfusion phase of the injury. Repeat endoscopy at 24-hour to 72-hour intervals can document regression or progression of the disease and may be helpful in its management.[26]

Radiographic Diagnosis

Computed tomography is frequently and increasingly used to assess patients who have abdominal pain. Although findings for colitis tend to be nonspecific,[27] computed tomography may be helpful in conjunction with a review of the patient's clinical presentation. On computed tomograms, ischemic colitis shows as a thickened colonic wall, analogous to the thumbprinting observed on a barium enema radiograph, which used to be the chief diagnostic test for the disease.[28] More serious signs are pneumatosis coli or the more deadly portent of gas within the portal venous system. Although not pathognomonic, the presence of air within the colonic wall or the portal vein of patients with ischemic colitis usually indicates transmural necrosis that mandates urgent surgical exploration.

INDICATIONS FOR OPERATION

Most cases of ischemic colitis occur in elderly patients, although younger adults also may be affected. The disease is often caused or influenced by underlying systemic disease such as a low-flow state resulting from congestive heart failure. Furthermore, these same conditions lessen the patient's ability to withstand sepsis, the resultant systemic inflammatory response syndrome, and operative therapy. The substantial morbidity and mortality associated with surgery in these patients make an accurate assessment of those who require such treatment of paramount importance. Certainly, patients with peritoneal signs or systemic sepsis and the attendant symptoms thereof require surgical exploration. Lesser manifestations in elderly patients require expert clinical judgment as to whether the risks of operating are greater or lesser than the risks of not operating.

CONDUCT OF OPERATION

Surgical treatment involves anatomical resection of all nonviable areas of the colon, with care taken to resect back to vascularized margins that have viable mucosa (Fig. 2). As a general rule, we ligate the mesenteric vessels close to the colon to preserve maximal collateral circulation. This approach may be an appropriate antithesis to an operation for malignancy (i.e., conserving vasculature rather than sacrificing it). Mesenteric fat may preclude easy palpation or visualization of the colonic vasculature. Tools such as a Doppler probe or intravenous fluorescein may help determine areas of vascular perfusion, the presence of blood flow in a particular vessel, or the viability of questionable areas of the colon. A reassessment of the surgical margins after the resection should check for poor collateral blood supply that would mandate a proximal diversion of the colon or ileum with a distal mucous fistula or a Hartmann pouch. A primary anastomosis may be feasible after a right hemicolectomy for limited disease without clinically significant contamination or sepsis but should be considered with care. Unfortunately, ischemia increases the risk of anastomotic failure, and its underlying cause is often not alleviated by an operation.

SURGICAL OUTCOMES

The most influential variables affecting outcome in patients with ischemic colitis are age and whether the ischemia is segmental or involves the whole colon.[29] Three-fourths of patients with total colonic ischemia die. About 3% of the deaths in patients who are younger than 50 years of age are directly attributable to the ischemic colitis, and 5% more die of related causes. Patients older than age 50 have a mortality rate of about 50% and an operative mortality of as much as 65%. As might be expected, postoperative

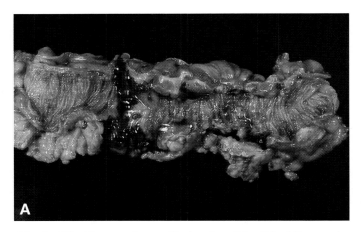
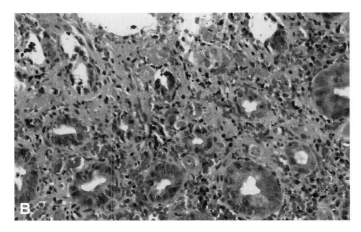

Fig. 2. (A), *Gross specimen of ischemic colitis.* (B), *Microscopic specimen of ischemic colitis.* (Hematoxylin-eosin; x400.)

mortality is rare in young patients, in whom there are differing causes and fewer of the general health detriments that are present with advanced age. In elderly patients, the pathophysiology generally has an adverse effect on overall health, predisposing them to have colonic ischemia. Younger patients with ischemic colitis do not have the extensive atherosclerosis that accompanies old age; thus, the disease is usually treatable nonsurgically. Conditions in the younger population that lead to ischemic colitis (e.g., vasculitis, thromboembolism, dehydration, oral contraceptive use) are usually more reversible with treatment than the common causes present in elderly patients (e.g., atherosclerosis, congestive heart failure, diabetes mellitus).

Complications after nonsurgical treatment have been reported but are not common. If the underlying pathophysiologic conditions are chronic and recalcitrant to treatment, ischemia may recur or affect a new area of the colon. After single or multiple ischemic episodes, strictures may develop as late complications of the disease.[30] As previously mentioned, hematochezia, although often a presenting symptom, is probably more accurately conceptualized as a complication of reperfusion.

LONG-TERM FOLLOW-UP

Long-term outcome in ischemic colitis depends on the etiology, the treatment, and the age of the patient. Younger patients in whom the underlying cause is treated successfully can be expected to do well and to have little chance of recurrence. Elderly patients who have an underlying chronic condition as the cause (e.g., atherosclerosis, congestive heart failure) are at greater risk for recurrent episodes of ischemic colitis.

Any patient, especially an elderly one who has had an episode of ischemic colitis treated nonsurgically, may be faced with strictures that develop during the healing process. These strictures may eventually require operative correction.

CONCLUSION

Ischemic colitis is the end pathologic condition observed when any of several factors diminish blood flow to the colon. The typical patient, whose diagnosis is confirmed with colonoscopy, usually responds well to treatment with intravenous fluids, antibiotics, and bowel rest. Transmural necrosis, which requires urgent surgical intervention, should be suspected in patients who have signs of peritonitis or sepsis. A surgical approach also may be indicated for complications of ischemic colitis such as perforation, recurrence, or strictures. When resecting the ischemic colon, the surgeon should be cognizant of the patient's vascular anatomy, particularly in patients who have had a colectomy that has changed the usual pattern of collateral blood supply to the colon.

REFERENCES

1. Boley SJ, Schwartz S, Lash J, Sternhill V: Reversible vascular occlusion of the colon. Surg Gynecol Obstet 116:53-60, 1963
2. Marston A, Pheils MT, Thomas ML, Morson BC: Ischaemic colitis. Gut 7:1-15, 1966
3. Robert JH, Mentha G, Rohner A: Ischaemic colitis: two distinct patterns of severity. Gut 34:4-6, 1993
4. Marston A: Vascular Disease of the Gastrointestinal Tract: Pathophysiology, Recognition and Management. Second edition. Baltimore, Williams & Wilkins, 1986, pp 1-15
5. Sudeck P: Ueber die Gefässversorgung des Mastdarmes in Hinsicht auf die operative Gangrän. München Med Wchnschr 54:1314-1317, 1907
6. Yamazaki T, Shirai Y, Tada T, Sasaki M, Sakai Y, Hatakeyama K: Ischemic colitis arising in watershed areas of the colonic blood supply: a report of two cases. Surg Today 27:460-462, 1997
7. Meyers MA: Griffiths' point: critical anastomosis at the splenic flexure. Significance in ischemia of the colon. Am J Roentgenol 126:77-94, 1976
8. Steward JA, Rankin FW: Blood supply of the large intestine: its surgical considerations. Arch Surg 26:843-891, 1933
9. Fisher DF Jr, Fry WJ: Collateral mesenteric circulation. Surg Gynecol Obstet 164:487-492, 1987
10. Bower TC: Ischemic colitis. Surg Clin North Am 73:1037-1053, 1993
11. Van Damme H, Creemers E, Limet R: Ischaemic colitis following aortoiliac surgery. Acta Chir Belg 100:21-27, 2000
12. Neitlich JD, Burrell MI: Drug-induced disorders of the colon. Abdom Imaging 24:23-28, 1999
13. Nagai T, Tomizawa T, Monden T, Mori M: Diabetes mellitus accompanied by nonocclusive colonic ischemia. Intern Med 37:454-456, 1998
14. Carratu R, Parisi P, Agozzino A: Segmental ischemic colitis associated with nonsteroidal antiinflammatory drugs. J Clin Gastroenterol 16:31-34, 1993
15. Dowd J, Bailey D, Moussa K, Nair S, Doyle R, Culpepper-Morgan JA: Ischemic colitis associated with pseudoephedrine: four cases. Am J Gastroenterol 94:2430-2434, 1999
16. Linder JD, Monkemuller KE, Raijman I, Johnson L, Lazenby AJ, Wilcox CM: Cocaine-associated ischemic colitis. South Med J 93:909-913, 2000
17. Newell AM, Deckert JJ: Transient ischemic colitis in young adults. Am Fam Physician 56:1103-1108, 1997
18. Deana DG, Dean PJ: Reversible ischemic colitis in young women: association with oral contraceptive use. Am J Surg Pathol 19:454-462, 1995
19. Judge JS, Hoffman NE, Levitt MD: Transient ischaemic colitis in young adults. Aust N Z J Surg 64:721-722, 1994
20. Matsumoto T, Iida M, Kimura Y, Nanbu T, Fujishima M: Clinical features in young adult patients with ischaemic colitis. J Gastroenterol Hepatol 9:572-575, 1994
21. Barcewicz PA, Welch JP: Ischemic colitis in young adult patients. Dis Colon Rectum 23:109-114, 1980
22. Gurbuz AK, Burbuz B, Salas L, Rosenshein NB, Donowitz M, Giardiello FM: Premarin-induced ischemic colitis. J Clin Gastroenterol 19:108-111, 1994
23. Mann DE Jr, Kessel ER, Mullins DL, Lottenberg R: Ischemic colitis and acquired resistance to activated protein C in a woman using oral contraceptives. Am J Gastroenterol 93:1960-1962, 1998
24. Preventza OA, Lazarides K, Sawyer MD: Ischemic colitis in young adults: a single-institution experience. J Gastrointest Surg 5:388-392, 2001
25. Habu Y, Tahashi Y, Kiyota K, Matsumura K, Hirota M, Inokuchi H, Kawai K: Reevaluation of clinical features of ischemic colitis: analysis of 68 consecutive cases diagnosed by early colonoscopy. Scand J Gastroenterol 31:881-886, 1996
26. Longo WE, Ballantyne GH, Gusberg RJ: Ischemic colitis: patterns and prognosis. Dis Colon Rectum 35:726-730, 1992
27. Philpotts LE, Heiken JP, Westcott MA, Gore RM: Colitis: use of CT findings in differential diagnosis. Radiology 190:445-449, 1994
28. Balthazar EJ, Yen BC, Gordon RB: Ischemic colitis: CT evaluation of 54 cases. Radiology 211:381-388, 1999
29. Longo WE, Ward D, Vernava AM III, Kaminski DL: Outcome of patients with total colonic ischemia. Dis Colon Rectum 40:1448-1454, 1997
30. Simi M, Pietroletti R, Navarra L, Leardi S: Bowel stricture due to ischemic colitis: report of three cases requiring surgery. Hepatogastroenterology 42:279-281, 1995

Chapter 37

APPENDICITIS

Michael P. Bannon, M.D.

In the centuries after the appendix was first drawn by Leonardo da Vinci, it and the nature of its associated abnormality, appendicitis, generated much controversy. This controversy seemingly had resolved by the time Reginald Fitz urged prompt appendectomy for acute appendicitis in 1886.[1] Now, more than a century later, appendicitis is considered an elementary surgical problem often managed by junior members of the operative team. Yet, this disease can be extremely difficult to diagnose and even more difficult to exclude. Seemingly, the 21st century should have brought certainty to the diagnosis of appendicitis, but it has not. The definitive diagnostic aid for appendicitis remains to be found. This diagnostic uncertainty has generated recent controversy about the appropriate applications of computed tomography for the diagnosis of appendicitis. Controversy also continues about the treatment of appendicitis. The simple resection of a cecal appendage should be straightforward. However, the advent of laparoscopy has introduced a new option, and the appropriate application of and relative indications for open and laparoscopic resection continue to evolve.

DIAGNOSIS

Despite current trends emphasizing imaging studies, history and physical examination remain the diagnostic mainstays for appendicitis.[2] The clinician begins by asking the patient to recall when he or she last felt well and the symptom that first prompted recognition of illness. With appendicitis, this symptom will be vague abdominal pain. In most patients, the initial pain is periumbilical in location. The periumbilical region is the expected location of visceral pain emanating from a midgut structure such as the appendix; however, some patients with appendicitis describe an initial low epigastric pain. Anorexia and nausea usually follow the onset of pain but are not universally present. One or two episodes of emesis occur commonly. The bowel habit is generally unaffected, although the patient may pass loose stool. Appendiceal perforation with abscess adjacent to the rectum may cause diarrhea as a result of perirectal inflammation and irritability.

Within 6 to 24 hours, the pain localizes in the right lower quadrant, and the patient describes signs of peritoneal irritation. This is the parietal pain emanating from irritation of the anterior abdominal wall in contact with the inflamed appendix, and it primarily manifests as considerable to severe exacerbation of pain with movement.

A differential diagnosis of appendicitis is outlined in Table 1. Although emesis is common with appendicitis, it is not usually a dominant complaint. Repeated episodes of emesis as the dominant symptom suggest gastroenteritis. Symptoms of dysuria and urinary frequency and urgency should be sought as clues to urinary tract infection. Vaginal discharge suggests pelvic inflammatory disease. A menstrual history should be obtained, with particular attention given to the duration and amount of flow of recent menses. A missed prior menses or spotting in place of menses may indicate pregnancy and raise the possibility of an ectopic gestation. Symptomatic anemia or shock in a young woman with abdominal pain must lead to immediate presumption of ruptured ectopic pregnancy. Diarrhea as a prominent complaint suggests the presence of a colon disorder.

While obtaining the history, the clinician should note the patient's demeanor and physical attitude. Patients

Table 1.—Diseases in the Differential Diagnosis of Right Lower Quadrant Pain

Sigmoid diverticulitis
Meckel's diverticulitis
Perforated cecal neoplasm
Crohn's ileitis
Gastroenteritis
Ruptured ovarian cyst
Ectopic pregnancy
Pelvic inflammatory disease
Omental infarction
Acute cholecystitis
Urinary tract infection
Renal calculus

experiencing parietal appendiceal pain typically lie perfectly still. If the appendix lies posteriorly, the patient may flex the right hip because of irritation of the psoas muscle. The abdominal examination is greatly facilitated by the patient's trust. This should be gained through the rapport the examiner establishes while taking the history. The examination must be gentle and begin with soft percussion far removed from the quadrant of maximal pain and tenderness. If prior harsh examiners have left the patient wary, soft percussion taps to the patient's shoulder can be used to demonstrate the gentle nature of the current examination. The examiner should slowly move the point of percussion toward the point of maximal tenderness while watching the patient's face. Peritoneal irritation will be apparent as an objective change in the patient's facial expression with soft percussion. Peritoneal irritation can be recognized definitively in this way. There is no need to attempt to elicit rebound tenderness; indeed, harsh depression and then quick release of the abdominal wall cause the patient with peritonitis severe, unnecessary pain.

Patients with appendicitis have peritoneal irritation in a localized area of the right lower quadrant. Usually this is near the classic McBurney point, lying one-third the distance along a line from the anterior superior iliac spine to the umbilicus. Patients with retrocecal appendicitis have a classic history and tenderness in the classic location, but the tenderness is not dramatic and peritoneal irritation is not present. This blunted response results from the protection that cecal interposition provides the peritoneum of the anterior abdominal wall from the inflammatory process. The psoas sign is likely to be positive in these patients.

Rectal and vaginal examinations must be performed. The intraperitoneal but pelvic appendix will present only modest abdominal tenderness, much like the retrocecal

appendix. However, pelvic appendicitis may be associated with considerable tenderness on rectal or vaginal examinations. A speculum examination must be performed in search of cervical exudate indicative of pelvic inflammatory disease; if present, this exudate should be examined for *Chlamydia* and cultured for bacteria.

Fever is usually present but is modest. Leukocytosis is present; the leukocyte count is between 10×10^9/L and 15×10^9/L and the number of polymorphonuclear leukocytes is increased. Temperature more than 39°C or a leukocyte count more than 15×10^9/L raises concern for perforation. Only a small percentage of patients with appendicitis are afebrile and have a normal leukocyte count and a normal differential at presentation.

Other laboratory studies are useful primarily for differential diagnosis. Anemia may corroborate suspicion of a perforated cecal carcinoma in an elderly patient. Urinalysis may reveal bacteria and leukocytes indicative of urinary tract infection or microscopic hematuria indicative of a renal calculus. A pregnancy test excludes ectopic gestation and the possibility of other early obstetric complications in women of childbearing years. Serum amylase and liver function tests may be useful in the few patients atypically describing right upper quadrant or true epigastric pain.

IMAGING STUDIES

Plain abdominal radiography is not useful for evaluation of suspected appendicitis. Most patients with appendicitis do not have an opaque appendicolith (or renal stone) (Fig. 1); an appendicolith is found in, at most, 10% to 20% of patients with appendicitis.[3-5] Other signs of appendicitis such as loss of the psoas shadow or localized right lower quadrant ileus are nonspecific.[6] Plain abdominal radiography is useful only if bowel obstruction is a serious differential consideration. In all other circumstances, this study can be omitted.

The diagnosis of appendicitis based on the history, physical examination, temperature, and leukocyte count may be inaccurate in up to 30% of cases. Some investigators have found an increase in the C-reactive protein level helpful for establishing a clinical diagnosis of appendicitis.[7] However, most recent efforts to improve diagnostic accuracy have focused on ultrasonography and computed tomography (CT). In several studies, CT has proved superior to ultrasonography;[8-10] in another study, ultrasonography did not add to CT and physical examination.[11] Because ultrasonography eliminates radiation exposure, it is most applicable in pediatric populations.[12]

CT for suspected appendicitis should be performed using cuts at 5- to 7-mm intervals and with colon contrast.[13,14] The contrast agent is most expeditiously administered rectally. CT signs of appendicitis include

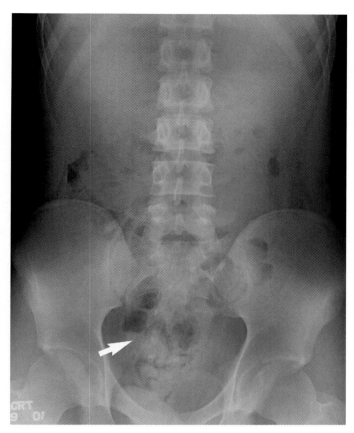

Fig. 1. Abdominal radiograph, showing appendicolith (arrow).

During the past several years, CT has increased in popularity for preoperative diagnosis or exclusion of appendicitis and has been championed as the standard of care by some investigators. The study by Rao et al.[16] of routine CT for patients with an emergency room diagnosis of appendicitis or a suspicion warranting hospital observation showed clinical and cost-savings benefits attributable to CT. In 100 patients, appendicitis was correctly diagnosed with CT in 52, and there were no false-negative results and one false-positive result. Overall, in 81 patients, CT led to a correct specific diagnosis. CT changed treatment plans in 59 of 100 patients and thus, for example, prevented unnecessary appendectomy and diminished the need for hospital observation. Nonetheless, the indiscriminate or routine application of CT to the evaluation of all patients with right lower quadrant pain seems to devalue dramatically clinical assessment and is likely inappropriate. The current dilemma is to define the circumstances under which CT can provide the greatest benefit.

The classic negative appendectomy rate of 15% is actually comprised of negative appendectomy rates of approximately 10% for men and up to 50% for women. Hospital resources are used for observation in 25% to 50% of patients with suspected appendicitis before operation or before hospital dismissal without operation. CT, then, may have the greatest potential benefit in the evaluation of women with right lower quadrant pain and men with equivocal presentations otherwise warranting in-hospital observation.

A recent study suggests that this benefit is indeed the case.[11] A clinical pathway using CT followed by a second physical examination changed the initial disposition in 34 of 99 patients with suspected appendicitis. CT added nothing to the management of male patients in whom

appendiceal distention and wall thickening, periappendiceal fat stranding, and the presence of an appendicolith[13,15] (Fig. 2, 3, and 4). Signs of advanced appendicitis include free fluid, extraluminal air, and abscess or phlegmon. The enlarged, distended appendix is very specific for appendicitis, whereas fat stranding is very sensitive.

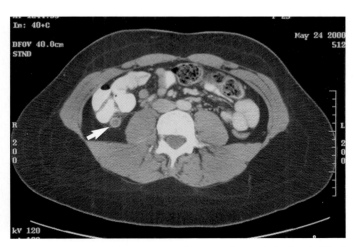

Fig. 2. Computed tomogram, showing dilated, fluid-filled appendix with a thickened wall (arrow) *and periappendiceal fat stranding.*

Fig. 3. Computed tomogram, showing distended, fluid-filled appendix (arrow).

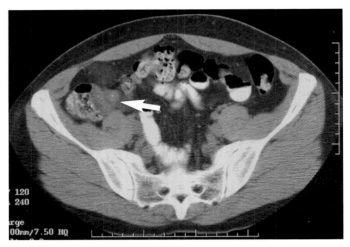

Fig. 4. Computed tomogram, showing thickened appendix containing tiny calcifications (arrow). *Stranding in periappendiceal fat.*

appendicitis was diagnosed by a surgeon; the negative appendectomy rate was 8%. However, CT in combination with reexamination reduced the negative appendectomy rate from 50% to 17% in women. Of patients initially designated for hospital observation, nearly 50% were managed more expeditiously when the CT pathway was used; 20% underwent immediate operation and 26% were dismissed without a specific observation period.

Our current practice, considering recently available information, is to perform appendectomy without preoperative imaging for male patients with a diagnosis of appendicitis and to perform CT for male patients with equivocal presentations and for all female patients. Further data will be necessary to refine the application of CT for women with right lower quadrant pain.

TREATMENT

General Supportive Care

Patients admitted to the hospital for suspected appendicitis should be hydrated with intravenous fluid and should undergo repeated physical examinations and monitoring of temperature and leukocyte count. Analgesics are generally withheld until a definitive diagnosis is made so that potential progression of abdominal pain and tenderness is not blunted. However, once a decision to perform appendectomy has been made, narcotic analgesics should be administered promptly and in doses that ameliorate the pain. For the rare patients who present in septic shock from perforated appendicitis with generalized peritonitis, aggressive restitution of blood volume and possibly respiratory support are necessary before induction of anesthesia.

Antibiotics

All patients who have appendectomy should receive antibiotics preoperatively.[17] Antibiotics should be chosen to provide broad coverage of gram-negative organisms and anaerobic organisms.[14,18] In general, a second-generation cephalosporin or an extended-spectrum penicillin is appropriate. Patients with penicillin allergy are treated with a quinolone in combination with metronidazole. Patients found to have a normal appendix or simple appendicitis do not receive antibiotics postoperatively. Patients with perforated or gangrenous appendicitis receive intravenous antibiotics for 5 days followed by oral quinolone with metronidazole for 1 week.

Open Appendectomy

Open appendectomy is routinely performed through a muscle-splitting right lower quadrant incision. The skin incision follows the skin lines and is centered over the point of maximal tenderness. Most often this approach centers the incision over the classic McBurney point. The goal of exposure is to bring the cecum and appendix onto the anterior abdominal wall. The incision should be placed with care. If an incision is placed too high, the cecum and appendix can be brought to the anterior abdominal wall but only by dividing lateral peritoneal attachments and mobilizing the cecum and distal ascending colon. An incision placed too low requires that the operation be performed in the peritoneal cavity with compromised exposure through a "tunnel" created by retracting the superior portion of the incision. The appendiceal-cecal junction lies in the lateral iliac fossa and should be exposed by an incision lateral to the rectus abdominus muscle; entry into the rectus sheath and division of the rectus abdominus muscle are both unnecessary.

After division of the subcutaneous tissue and Scarpa's fascia, the external oblique aponeurosis is divided in line with its fibers. Internal oblique and transversus abdominus muscles are in turn separated in line with their fibers, but not divided. The peritoneum then is opened transversely and entered. If the incision is placed correctly, the peritoneum will be opened directly over the anterior taenia of the cecum. Cloudy fluid often is encountered. Frank pus is present in cases of perforation and abscess. There is no need for bacterial cultures.[19,20] The cecum is grasped with a gauze square, retracted inferiorly, and then rotated anteriorly. If the appendix lies free in an intraperitoneal location, the cecum and appendix will rotate onto the anterior abdominal wall. In more advanced inflammation, adhesions between the appendix and intraperitoneal structures need to be divided (often blindly and bluntly) before this maneuver will be successful. If the appendix lies in a retroperitoneal location, the cecum and distal ascending colon need to be mobilized to achieve adequate exposure.

Once the appendix and cecum are mobilized to the anterior abdominal wall, appendiceal resection proceeds rapidly. The mesoappendix is clamped, divided, and ligated. The base of the appendix is ligated, divided, and invaginated. The cecum is returned to the abdominal cavity, and the right lower quadrant is irrigated and suctioned dry. The abdominal wound is closed in layers. If a proper muscle-splitting incision has been made, the opening in each muscle layer is buttressed by intact portions of the other two muscles. The risk of postoperative hernia is minimal, and patients are advised to return to full activity immediately unless limited by pain.

LAPAROSCOPIC APPENDECTOMY

Laparoscopic appendectomy is performed with the patient supine. Nasogastric and urinary catheters are placed to avoid injury to the stomach and urinary bladder during initial cannulation of the peritoneal cavity. The surgeon and camera operator stand on the patient's left; the first assistant is on the patient's right. Because the camera is facing the first assistant, this surgeon may experience directional (left-right) confusion, which can be overcome by looking at the patient's abdomen to orient the initiation of movements and looking at the video monitor to fine-tune the motion; once experience is gained, appropriate movements become second nature.

Pneumoperitoneum is established with the Veress needle inserted in the periumbilical position. Insufflation pressures are kept to less than 15 mm Hg. A 10-mm cannula is placed in the umbilical position, and the laparoscope is introduced into the abdomen for an initial visual inspection. This allows examination of the gallbladder, anterior proximal duodenum, and colon for signs of inflammation. The pelvis is examined for serous or purulent fluid. Exposure of the appendix may require retraction of the terminal ileum or cecum.

Once the initial inspection is completed, three additional cannulas are placed under direct laparoscopic vision (Fig. 5). The 12-mm cannula placed in the left lower quadrant serves as the working port. A grasper inserted through the 5-mm cannula in the right anterior axillary line at the level of the umbilicus is used to retract the anterior taenia of the cecum cephalad to facilitate exposure of the appendiceal-cecal junction. A second 5-mm cannula is placed in the inferolateral right lower quadrant; through this, the distal appendix is snared with an endoscopic loop ligature to allow safe caudad retraction (Fig. 6). Direct traction with a grasper risks rupturing a friable, inflamed appendix.

The inflamed appendix may be adherent to one or more of the following structures: cecum, terminal ileum, and posterolateral peritoneum of the right "gutter." Gentle blunt dissection with a closed grasper breaks these fibrinous, inflammatory adhesions and mobilizes the appendix for caudad retraction. Some patients have a lateral peritoneal attachment of the appendix, which can be divided with electrocautery.

Cephalad traction applied to the cecum and caudad traction applied to the appendix expose the mesoappendix (Fig. 6). Placing the patient in the Trendelenburg position with the left side down often enhances this exposure by dropping the small intestine out of the laparoscopic field. Through the lower midline 12-mm cannula, the peritoneum overlying the mesoappendix is opened with a hook cautery. Depending on exposure, either the appendiceal artery or its primary branches are dissected from mesoappendiceal fat. Each isolated vessel is occluded with hemostatic clips and divided with endoscopic scissors (Fig. 7). Mesoappendiceal fat is divided with electrocautery. The base of the appendix is closed and divided with a linear stapling device. A small appendix can be removed directly through the 12-mm cannula; a turgid, edematous appendix too large to fit through the cannula is placed in a specimen bag before withdrawal through the left lower quadrant cannula incision. The appendiceal stump, anterior taenia coli of the cecum, and mesoappendix are checked for mechanical integrity and hemostasis. The operative field and pelvis are irrigated with saline and suctioned dry. The fascial defects of the 10-mm and 12-mm incisions are closed with interrupted 2-0 polyglycolic acid suture, and the skin incisions are closed with a subcuticular 4-0 polyglycolic acid suture.

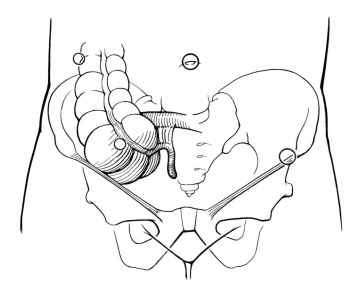

Fig. 5. Position of cannulas (circles) *for laparoscopic appendectomy.*

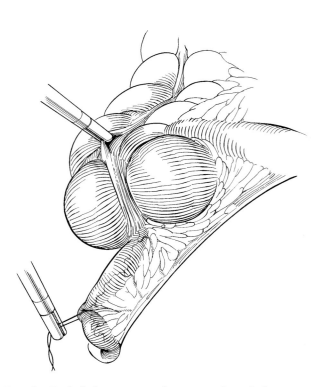

Fig. 6. Cephalad retraction of cecum and caudad retraction of appendix during laparoscopic appendectomy.

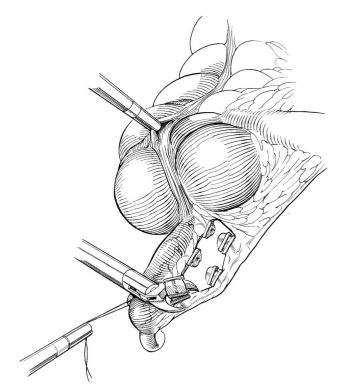

Fig. 7. Isolation, clip ligation, and division of mesoappendiceal vessels during laparoscopic appendectomy.

Variations of the technique may be appropriate. The superior right cannula can be eliminated if cecal retraction is not necessary to splay out the mesoappendix; this is often the case if the appendix is minimally inflamed or normal. Ligation and division of the mesoappendix with a linear stapling device can be substituted for specific dissection of appendiceal vessels. Also, the appendiceal stump can be closed with endoscopic loop ligatures rather than with a linear stapling device.

COMPLICATED APPENDICITIS

Gangrene and perforation are two complications of appendicitis identified in the operating room which greatly increase the risk of postoperative infection. In most instances, a standard appendectomy can be performed for a gangrenous or perforated appendix. However, if the appendiceal base is necrotic or extremely friable, closure of the appendiceal stump is unsafe because of the risk of dehiscence of the closure. In these circumstances, a cuff of noninflamed cecum about the appendiceal base can be resected with the appendix by application of a linear stapler. In rare cases, cecectomy or ileocecectomy is necessary. These advanced forms of appendicitis necessitate full therapeutic courses of antibiotics postoperatively. Intravenous administration of antibiotics is continued until fever and

leukocytosis resolve, usually a period of at least 5 days. Therapy can be completed out of hospital with additional antibiotics administered orally—usually a quinolone in combination with metronidazole.

Appendiceal abscess results from neglected appendicitis with perforation. This can present as a palpable mass, but more commonly it is identified as a periappendiceal fluid collection with CT. Appendiceal abscess is best treated with percutaneous drainage[21-23] and intravenous antibiotics. The rare abscess that cannot be drained percutaneously can be drained operatively through an extraperitoneal incision. Eight to 12 weeks after resolution of the abscess, a colon radiograph is obtained. If a residual appendix is identified, interval appendectomy is performed. If no residual appendix is identified, patients are offered a choice of expectant management or interval appendectomy. Interval appendectomy is not performed routinely.[24,25]

Occasionally, appendiceal perforation is not contained and leads to diffuse peritonitis. Patients with this complication undergo exploration through a midline celiotomy.

POSTOPERATIVE COMPLICATIONS

The most common early complication after appendectomy is wound infection, and the most concerning is intraperitoneal abscess. The frequency of wound infection may be as low as 2% to 3%[26] but is likely as high as 10%. Abscess occurs in less than 0.01% of cases.[26] Wound infection should be treated by opening the cutaneous and subcutaneous wound closures; if associated cellulitis is present, this should be treated with intravenous antibiotics. Postoperative intraperitoneal abscess should be treated with percutaneous drainage.

The main long-term complication is intestinal obstruction caused by adhesions in the right lower quadrant. The frequency of obstruction caused by appendectomy as a sole prior operation, however, is rare (less than 2%).[27] However, it often requires reoperation.[26,28]

LAPAROSCOPIC VERSUS OPEN APPENDECTOMY

A prospective randomized Mayo Clinic study of laparoscopic versus open appendectomy found advantages of the laparoscopic approach which were highly statistically significant.[29] These advantages were earlier resumption of general diet, shorter duration of parenteral analgesia, fewer milligrams of parenteral narcotic used, shorter postoperative hospital stay, and an earlier return to full activity. Despite statistical significance, the clinical magnitude of these differences was underwhelming. The difference in postoperative stay was less than 1 full day. Although return to full activity was 2 weeks for patients undergoing the laparoscopic approach and 3 weeks for those undergoing the open approach, the laparoscopic approach was not associated with an earlier return to work. The inability of the laparoscopic approach to confer an earlier return to work diminishes the impact of the otherwise impressive finding of an earlier return to full activity. In subgroup analyses, all the benefits of laparoscopic appendectomy were conferred to patients who had either uncomplicated appendicitis or active lifestyles. The laparoscopic approach conferred a modest cost savings compared with the open approach. Although laparoscopic appendectomy was associated with greater in-hospital costs, overall cost for this procedure (including indirect societal costs) was on average $2,400 less. The Mayo Clinic findings are consistent with those of other studies.[30,31] Laparoscopic appendectomy confers slight advantages over open appendectomy. The slight advantages identified may be due to the bias inherent in non-blinded studies.

Laparoscopic appendectomy is very clearly a safe procedure. The Mayo Clinic study and others have shown that the laparoscopic approach does not lead to more technical or general postoperative complications. Although laparoscopic appendectomy is a safe and effective operation, its merits relative to open appendectomy are questionable. The simple truth is that laparoscopic appendectomy is better than open appendectomy—but only very slightly better.

The advantages of laparoscopic appendectomy are not great enough to suggest that the open approach be abandoned. The modest clinical and economic advantages of laparoscopic appendectomy must be balanced against the pure simplicity of open appendectomy. On balance, the magnitudes of the laparoscopic advantages are not enough to outweigh the technical simplicity of open appendectomy. Simply stated, laparoscopic appendectomy is a long run for a short slide. Thus, open appendectomy still has a prominent role in the management of appendicitis.

Laparoscopy clearly provides for more complete inspection of the peritoneal cavity than a right lower quadrant celiotomy. This difference has led to the advocacy of laparoscopic appendectomy for women and obese patients. The further development of preoperative CT likely will negate this potential advantage of laparoscopy. Obese patients may benefit from laparoscopy because of smaller wound(s) and fewer wound infections, but this has not been documented.

In the Mayo Clinic emergency surgical practice, laparoscopic appendectomy is selectively offered to patients who are most likely to benefit from this approach. According to the Mayo Clinic study, these are patients with uncomplicated appendicitis who have a very active lifestyle. Such patients are, for example, the high school athletes with appendicitis during the sports season, the farmer during planting or harvest season, and the laborer with limited disability coverage. The vast majority of patients continue to undergo open appendectomy.

REFERENCES

1. Fitz RH: Perforating inflammation of the vermiform appendix: with special reference to its early diagnosis and treatment. Am J Med Sci 92:321-346, 1886
2. Bergeron E, Richer B, Gharib R, Giard A: Appendicitis is a place for clinical judgement. Am J Surg 177:460-462, 1999
3. Graham AD, Johnson HF: The incidence of radiographic findings in acute appendicitis compared to 200 normal abdomens. Mil Med 131:272-276, 1966
4. Beneventano TC, Schein CJ, Jacobson HG: The roentgen aspects of some appendiceal abnormalities. Am J Roentgenol Radium Ther Nucl Med 96:344-360, 1966
5. Hatten LE, Miller RC, Hester CL Jr, Moynihan PC: Appendicitis and the abdominal roentgenogram in children. South Med J 66:803-806, 1973
6. Fee HJ Jr, Jones PC, Kadell B, O'Connell TX: Radiologic diagnosis of appendicitis. Arch Surg 112:742-744, 1977
7. Andersson RE, Hugander AP, Ghazi SH, Ravn H, Offenbartl SK, Nystrom PO, Olaison GP: Diagnostic value of disease history, clinical presentation, and inflammatory parameters of appendicitis. World J Surg 23:133-140, 1999
8. Balthazar EJ, Birnbaum BA, Yee J, Megibow AJ, Roshkow J, Gray C: Acute appendicitis: CT and US correlation in 100 patients. Radiology 190:31-35, 1994
9. Stroman DL, Bayouth CV, Kuhn JA, Westmoreland M, Jones RC, Fisher TL, McCarty TM: The role of computed tomography in the diagnosis of acute appendicitis. Am J Surg 178:485-489, 1999
10. Wise SW, Labuski MR, Kasales CJ, Blebea JS, Meilstrup JW, Holley GP, LaRusso SA, Holliman J, Ruggiero FM, Mauger D: Comparative assessment of CT and sonographic techniques for appendiceal imaging. AJR Am J Roentgenol 176:933-941, 2001
11. Wilson EB, Cole JC, Nipper ML, Cooney DR, Smith RW: Computed tomography and ultrasonography in the diagnosis of appendicitis: When are they indicated? Arch Surg 136:670-675, 2001
12. Garcia Pena BM, Mandl KD, Kraus SJ, Fischer AC, Fleisher GR, Lund DP, Taylor GA: Ultrasonography and limited computed tomography in the diagnosis and management of appendicitis in children. JAMA 282:1041-1046, 1999
13. Curtin KR, Fitzgerald SW, Nemcek AA Jr, Hoff FL, Vogelzang RL: CT diagnosis of acute appendicitis: imaging findings. AJR Am J Roentgenol 164:905-909, 1995
14. Barie PS: Management of complicated intra-abdominal infections. J Chemother 11:464-477, 1999
15. Rao PM, Rhea JT, Novelline RA: Sensitivity and specificity of the individual CT signs of appendicitis: experience with 200 helical appendiceal CT examinations. J Comput Assist Tomogr 21:686-692, 1997
16. Rao PM, Rhea JT, Novelline RA, Mostafavi AA, McCabe CJ: Effect of computed tomography of the appendix on treatment of patients and use of hospital resources. N Engl J Med 338:141-146, 1998
17. Bauer T, Vennits B, Holm B, Hahn-Pedersen J, Lysen D, Galatius H, Kristensen ES, Graversen P, Wilhelmsen F, Skjoldborg H: Antibiotic prophylaxis in acute nonperforated appendicitis. The Danish Multicenter Study Group III. Ann Surg 209:307-311, 1989
18. Cinat ME, Wilson SE: New advances in the use of antimicrobial agents in surgery: intra-abdominal infections. J Chemother 11:453-463, 1999
19. McNamara MJ, Pasquale MD, Evans SR: Acute appendicitis and the use of intraperitoneal cultures. Surg Gynecol Obstet 177:393-397, 1993
20. Bilik R, Burnweit C, Shandling B: Is abdominal cavity culture of any value in appendicitis? Am J Surg 175:267-270, 1998
21. vanSonnenberg E, Wittich GR, Casola G, Neff CC, Hoyt DB, Polansky AD, Keightley A: Periappendiceal abscesses: percutaneous drainage. Radiology 163:23-26, 1987
22. Jeffrey RB Jr, Federle MP, Tolentino CS: Periappendiceal inflammatory masses: CT-directed management and clinical outcome in 70 patients. Radiology 167:13-16, 1988
23. Jeffrey RB Jr: Management of the periappendiceal inflammatory mass. Semin Ultrasound CT MR 10:341-347, 1989
24. Hoffmann J, Lindhard A, Jensen HE: Appendix mass: conservative management without interval appendectomy. Am J Surg 148:379-382, 1984
25. Eriksson S, Styrud J: Interval appendicectomy: a retrospective study. Eur J Surg 164:771-774, 1998
26. Hale DA, Molloy M, Pearl RH, Schutt DC, Jaques DP: Appendectomy: a contemporary appraisal. Ann Surg 225:252-261, 1997
27. Riber C, Soe K, Jorgensen T, Tonnesen H: Intestinal obstruction after appendectomy. Scand J Gastroenterol 32:1125-1128, 1997
28. Meagher AP, Moller C, Hoffmann DC: Non-operative treatment of small bowel obstruction following appendicectomy or operation on the ovary or tube. Br J Surg 80:1310-1311, 1993
29. Long KH, Bannon MP, Zietlow SP, Helgeson ER, Harmsen WS, Smith CD, Ilstrup DM, Baerga-Varela Y, Sarr MG: A prospective randomized comparison of laparoscopic appendectomy with open appendectomy: clinical and economic analyses. Surgery 129:390-400, 2001
30. McCall JL, Sharples K, Jadallah F: Systematic review of randomized controlled trials comparing laparoscopic with open appendicectomy. Br J Surg 84:1045-1050, 1997
31. Slim K, Pezet D, Chipponi J: Laparoscopic or open appendectomy? Critical review of randomized, controlled trials. Dis Colon Rectum 41:398-403, 1998

Chapter 38

CHRONIC ULCERATIVE COLITIS

Keith A. Kelly, M.D.
Roger R. Dozois, M.D.

Ulcerative colitis, an inflammatory, ulcerating disease of the mucosa of the large intestine of unknown cause, varies in severity from a chronic, low-grade process requiring little treatment to an acute, fulminating process requiring intensive therapy. Although there is no curative medical treatment, management of the disease remains primarily medical. Therapy varies with the severity and extent of the illness and with patient factors, such as age, tolerance and response to medication, associated systemic problems, and preference or reluctance for operation. Operation continues to have a major role in the management of ulcerative colitis because it may save the patient's life, eliminate cancer or the long-term risk of it, and, most important, abolish the large intestinal disease. Also, advances in recent years have increased understanding of the role and timing of operation. Finally, the development and establishment of novel, sphincter-saving procedures that improve the quality of life of patients after proctocolectomy, superior stomal care, and improved stomal appliances are important considerations that currently influence decisions regarding surgical treatment.

This chapter presents the approach and experience with this disease at Mayo Clinic, although the work of others also is cited. Another review of our work has been published elsewhere.[1]

SYMPTOMS AND SIGNS

The classic intestinal symptoms and signs of ulcerative colitis are abdominal pain, cramps, tenesmus, fecal urgency, bloody diarrhea, and fecal incontinence. Patients have a mean of about 12 watery bowel movements a day. Extreme urgency often accompanies the movements. Failure to reach a toilet quickly enough commonly results in fecal incontinence. Systemic symptoms, such as fever, malaise, anorexia, and weight loss, may accompany the intestinal symptoms. On examination, some patients appear surprisingly healthy, whereas others appear chronically or acutely ill. The abdomen may be distended, tympanitic, and tender. When colon cancer accompanies the colitis, a mass may be felt.

Extraintestinal manifestations of ulcerative colitis are present in about 30% of patients (Table 1). These usually produce associated symptoms and signs, although they may not. For example, sclerosing cholangitis may cause no symptoms, signs, or biochemical changes in the blood, but it can be found on cholangiography.

DIAGNOSIS

The diagnosis is most commonly made with endoscopic or radiographic examinations of the large intestine and by

Table 1.—Common Extraintestinal Manifestations of Ulcerative Colitis

Skin	Eyes
Pyoderma gangrenosum	Uveitis
Erythema nodosum	Iritis
Liver	Blood
Hepatic "triaditis"	Hypercoagulability
Sclerosing cholangitis	Vascular thrombosis
Joints	Anemia
Peripheral arthritis	Hyperproteinemia
Rheumatoid spondylitis	Thrombocytosis

biopsy. The columnar mucosa of the large intestine appears reddened, edematous, and hemorrhagic on endoscopy. Tiny ulcerations can be seen. The mucosa is friable on rubbing. The mucosal changes are most severe in the rectum and sigmoid colon. The severity of inflammation often gradually decreases as the transverse colon, ascending colon, and cecum are approached. The appendix can be involved. The distal ileum shows "backwash" ileitis in about 15% of patients. More proximal parts of the small intestine are not involved. Moreover, the distal two-thirds of the anal canal, which is lined by squamous mucosa, also is not inflamed. The radiologist may note a "shortened" colon that has lost its haustra and is not distensible. Segmental strictures and cancers can be found.

Biopsy of the inflamed mucosa reveals the microscopic changes of mucosal inflammation and often the characteristic abscess at the base of the intestinal mucosal crypts. The inflammation and ulceration are mucosal, not transmural.

Enteric infection should be excluded by stool culture and examination for ova and parasites. The two main confounding diseases are Crohn's disease and indeterminate colitis. Crohn's disease usually can be diagnosed from the segmental and transmural nature of the disease and its propensity to involve all parts of the alimentary canal from the mouth to the anus. For example, "right-sided colitis" with an anal fistula suggests Crohn's disease rather than ulcerative colitis. Indeterminate colitis is diagnosed when clinical, endoscopic, radiographic, and pathologic features of both ulcerative colitis and Crohn's disease are present. We have found that about 15% of patients with indeterminate colitis eventually are proved to have Crohn's disease after proctocolectomy and ileal pouch-anal canal anastomosis, whereas only about 2% of patients with ulcerative colitis subsequently will be shown to have Crohn's disease after operation.[2]

MEDICAL TREATMENT

Medical treatment of ulcerative colitis commonly includes corticosteroids and other anti-inflammatory agents, immunosuppressive agents, antibiotics, and monoclonal antibodies directed toward cytokines active in the inflammatory cascade (Table 2). Most patients (80%) will respond and not require operation. The remaining 20% of patients will have operation.

INDICATIONS FOR OPERATION

Operation is indicated in ulcerative colitis either because of failure of medical treatment or because of acute or chronic complications of the disease (Table 3).

Table 2.—Medications Commonly Used to Treat Ulcerative Colitis

Corticosteroids: prednisone, hydrocortisone, budesonide
Aminosalicylic acids (ASA): 5-ASA and its derivatives
Immunosuppressives: 6-mercaptopurine, cyclosporine
Antibiotics: ciprofloxacin, amoxicillin/clavulanate potassium

Failure of Medical Treatment

In general, the response to medical treatment is good, the success rate ranging from 87% to 92% for moderate-to-mild disease. In severe disease, the remission rates are less favorable. Although some patients will experience a partial response and continue to live with mild-to-moderate symptoms, in others treatment fails altogether. Attacks of colitis can be so severe that medical treatment has no or minimal effect. Responses to medical treatment may be achieved only with large doses of medications. Consequently, patients experience unacceptable and intolerable side effects from the medications. Some patients may not tolerate medical treatment and opt for surgical excision of their disease. Unfortunately, this type of patient tends to be least able to cope with complications of operation or with the subsequent need for a permanent stoma. Poor nutrition and failure to grow in children with colitis, despite medical therapy, may also necessitate operation.

Fulminant Colitis

Fulminant disease occurs in approximately 10% of patients with ulcerative colitis, and such severe attacks may be the first manifestation of the disease. These patients have severe abdominal pain associated with fever, tachycardia, bloody diarrhea, dehydration, and weight loss. A leukocytosis usually is present. The patients should be managed aggressively with medication, but failure to improve within 48 hours or continued deterioration necessitates prompt surgical intervention. Indeed, although historically

Table 3.—Indications for Operation

Intractable to medical therapy
Severe side effects of medical therapy
Weight loss, failure to thrive or grow
Fulminant colitis
Toxic megacolon
Bleeding, obstruction, and perforation of colon
Colonic mucosal dysplasia
Cancer of large intestine
Severe extraintestinal manifestations of colitis

fulminant colitis has been associated with a high mortality rate, that rate now has decreased to less than 3% when aggressive medical treatment is used in combination with early operation.

Toxic Megacolon

Toxic megacolon may be the initial manifestation of ulcerative colitis. In the past, toxic megacolon occurred in 6% of hospitalized patients with ulcerative colitis, but its current frequency is less. Factors contributing to toxic megacolon include hypokalemia, anticholinergics, and administration of a barium sulfate enema during a radiologic examination of the colon. Patients with toxic megacolon are seriously ill with abdominal pain, tenderness, increased stool frequency, fever, tachycardia, leukocytosis, and malnutrition. Corticosteroids may mask symptoms and make the clinical diagnosis less obvious. Most often, segmental dilatation of the colon is present on abdominal radiography. Perforation of a toxic megacolon is not infrequent and is associated with a high mortality rate (20% to 40% with perforation, 4% without perforation).

Patients should have operation early. Urgent colectomy with rectal preservation and end ileostomy is indicated if no clinical improvement is noted within 24 hours after initiation of appropriate medical treatment or if the clinical situation continues to deteriorate as evidenced by persistent tachycardia, low blood pressure, and increasing abdominal pain and tenderness. Even patients who respond to medical treatment initially have a high probability of a second attack of fulminant colitis or toxic megacolon (30%) or subsequent colonic resection (50%), often as an emergency.[3] Thus, medical management in this subset of patients is increasingly regarded as preparatory to early operation.

Perforation

Perforation is rare in the absence of toxic megacolon complicating ulcerative colitis, and its occurrence should raise questions about the possibility of Crohn's disease. The risk of perforation is greatest at the time of the first attack and correlates with the extent and severity of the disease. Large doses of corticosteroids may mask symptoms. Therefore, a strong suspicion must be maintained in patients with severe colitis who are receiving corticosteroids, especially if the clinical status changes. The mortality rate associated with perforation can be decreased only with early operation.

Hemorrhage

Massive bleeding occurs infrequently in patients with ulcerative colitis (less than 4%) but causes 10% of emergency colectomies and often is associated with toxic megacolon.

If transfusion requirements remain excessive, operation is indicated. The choice between an abdominal colectomy and a proctocolectomy should be made at the time of operation. If there is continued massive rectal bleeding from the rectal stump at the time of operation and the patient is of advanced age or not suitable for a later restorative procedure, immediate proctocolectomy should be performed. In younger patients, near-total proctocolectomy with ileal pouch-anal canal anastomosis sometimes can be done.

Obstruction

Obstruction in a patient with long-standing ulcerative colitis almost always results from malignancy. Thus, even if barium enema, colonoscopy, and histologic findings seem to favor a benign stricture, one must remain suspicious of malignancy, and colectomy should be recommended.

Cancer

The association between ulcerative colitis and cancer is well recognized. The incidence of cancer is increased in patients with extensive and long-standing colitis. Although controlled studies suggest that the true risk of carcinoma is much less than that previously reported from referral centers, the risk remains great in patients who have had the disease 10 years or longer, when the disease involves the entire colon, and especially when the colitis had its onset in childhood. Such patients should undergo either prophylactic proctocolectomy or, at least, enter a rigorous surveillance program.

Surveillance, however, has many limitations. When a patient has quiescent or mild disease, it may be difficult to persuade the patient to undergo biannual colonoscopy and biopsy. Dysplasia does not always precede carcinoma, and a carcinoma may be flat or mainly submucosal and escape detection. Finally, all too often carcinoma already is present in patients when dysplasia is first detected. Unfortunately, carcinomas continue to develop while patients are in surveillance programs, and these carcinomas often may be advanced. If dysplasia or a dysplasia-associated lesion or mass develops in a patient under surveillance, operation is indicated because such a development is associated with a greater than 50% chance of invasive cancer being present.

Extraintestinal Manifestations

Approximately 30% of patients with ulcerative colitis will have at least one extraintestinal manifestation of the colonic disease. Cutaneous, joint, and vascular manifestations usually regress and do not recur after resection of the entire colonic and rectal mucosa.[4] Others, such as ankylosing spondylitis and rheumatoid arthritis, which are separate disease processes that have genetic predisposition in common with ulcerative colitis, do not. Primary sclerosing cholangitis may progress to cirrhosis or cholangiocarcinoma after operation.[5] Many of these extracolonic manifestations improve as the severity of disease decreases, but if they continue to cause considerable symptoms, proctocolectomy should be considered.

SURGICAL TREATMENT

The rationale behind operation is that removal of the colon and rectum cures patients of their large intestinal disease and improves their health. In the past, operations for ulcerative colitis often were delayed or postponed indefinitely despite strong indications for surgical intervention. Reluctance to consider operation by patients and their treating physicians was based, in part, on the fear of ileostomy and its physical, social, and psychologic consequences. Indeed, a conventional ileostomy leaves a patient with complete fecal incontinence. An appliance must be worn day and night to collect the stomal output. Unwelcome noises may issue from the stoma from time to time, embarrassing some patients. The appliances themselves are somewhat unsightly, uncomfortable, and odoriferous, and there is the ever-present threat of leakage of stool or gas at the site of attachment of the appliance to the skin. Peristomal skin irritation and ulceration may occur. Moreover, appliances are expensive. Thus, alternatives to the incontinent Brooke ileostomy were needed.

Today, alternative operations, used primarily in patients having elective operation for their disease, are available that allow the diseased intestine to be removed and yet fecal continence to be preserved (Table 4). These newer operations include proctocolectomy with ileal pouch-anal canal anastomosis and proctocolectomy with ileal pouch-distal rectal anastomosis. Proctocolectomy and Brooke ileostomy and proctocolectomy with continent ileostomy (Kock pouch) remain options for some patients. Colectomy and ileorectal anastomosis have a limited role today.

PROCTOCOLECTOMY AND ILEAL POUCH-ANAL CANAL ANASTOMOSIS

Proctocolectomy and ileal pouch-anal canal anastomosis (IPAA) has become the operation of choice for many patients with ulcerative colitis. The operation is attractive because it avoids a permanent ileostomy and cures the patient of the disease while preserving anorectal function.[6,7] Referral for operation is occurring sooner after the onset of ulcerative colitis, perhaps in part because of the newer operative approach.[8]

Table 4.—Operations Currently in Use for Ulcerative Colitis

Proctocolectomy, ileal pouch-anal canal anastomosis
Proctocolectomy, ileal pouch-distal rectal anastomosis
Proctocolectomy, end ileostomy (Brooke)
Proctocolectomy, continent ileostomy (Kock pouch)
Colectomy, ileorectostomy
Colectomy, end ileostomy, closure of rectum

Rationale

The rationale for the IPAA is that excision of the cecum, colon, and proximal rectum and stripping of the mucosa from the distal rectum and proximal anal canal remove all the large intestinal disease in patients with ulcerative colitis, and yet the operation preserves the anal sphincters. Construction of the ileal pouch maintains an adequate fecal reservoir. Anastomosis of the pouch to the anal canal allows voluntary transanal defecation and reasonable fecal continence and avoids ileostomy. In addition, because the distal rectal and proximal anal mucosa are removed endorectally, the chance of damage to the innervation of the bladder and genitalia during the operation is minimized. Finally, because a complete proctectomy is not performed, there is no perineal wound, a wound that sometimes is difficult to heal.

Preparation for Operation

The nutritional status of the patient should be stabilized before operation. This may require the use of parenteral nutritional supplementation. Severe anemia should be treated with blood transfusions. For patients currently receiving or recently (within a year) having received corticosteroid therapy, additional therapy, usually 100 mg of hydrocortisone intravenously every 8 hours, is given to ensure adequate hormonal support during the operative period. The colon is cleansed with 2 L of an electrolyte solution given by mouth the night before the operation. Diet is restricted to clear liquids the day before the operation. Additionally, neomycin (1.0 g) and metronidazole (0.5 g) are given orally the night before the procedure at 5 PM and 11 PM.

The Procedure

The technique currently used in most patients at Mayo Clinic consists of excision of the cecum, colon, and proximal rectum, stripping of the distal rectal and proximal anal mucosa, construction of a J-shaped ileal pouch, and ileal pouch-anal canal anastomosis. We use the two-stage operative approach most of the time, protecting the pouch-anal anastomosis with a diverting loop ileostomy at the first operation and closing the loop ileostomy at a second operation about 2 months later. However, we have completed the operation in one stage without a loop ileostomy in some patients. We believe, though, that this approach increases the risk of anastomotic leaks, pelvic sepsis, and anastomotic stricture.

The anesthetized patient is positioned on the operating table in the modified lithotomy-Trendelenburg position to provide access to both abdomen and perineum. A vertical midline incision is made. The abdomen is explored and the presence of ulcerative colitis established. The cecum and colon are mobilized, preserving the greater omentum.[9] The rectum is freed down to the pelvic floor, keeping close to the rectal wall, thereby avoiding damage to the pelvic autonomic nerves. The mobilized rectum then is divided near the pelvic floor. A stapling device can be used to facilitate the division. The cecum, colon, and proximal rectum are removed and sent for pathologic examination to confirm the diagnosis.

The ileal pouch is next constructed from the distal 30 to 35 cm of ileum. Several types of ileal reservoirs have been used by other surgeons, including the J-shaped, S-shaped, W-shaped, and the lateral-lateral pouch. We prefer the J-shaped reservoir. The J-shaped reservoir is simpler to construct, requires less intestine, and can be done more rapidly than the other, more complex types of reservoir, thus decreasing the chance of contamination and infection. Moreover, the J pouch gives clinical results comparable to those obtained with the other reservoirs. Also, physiologically, the J pouch ultimately accommodates nearly 400 mL of fecal content and gas, preserves the anorectal angle by fitting into the concavity of the sacrum, generates low but coordinated propulsive contractions, and, most important, can be emptied spontaneously under voluntary control.

Pouch construction is begun by mobilizing the small intestinal mesentery from the retroperitoneum to allow the distal ileum to reach the level of the dentate line. Dividing the visceral peritoneum along the right side of the superior mesenteric artery allows the mesentery to stretch and increases its length. If additional length is required, the ileocolic vessels or branches of the superior mesenteric vessels or both can be transected. When it is clear that the ileum will reach the dentate line, construction of the J pouch is begun with the terminal 30 to 35 cm of the ileum. The ileum is folded into the shape of the J and its 15-cm limbs are approximated with continuous 2-0 chromic catgut or 2-0 polyglycolic acid sutures in the seromuscular layer (Fig. 1). The antimesenteric border of the limbs is incised and the mucosal surface of the newly formed pouch is exposed. A second row of sutures is used on the mucosal layer of the posterior wall. The anterior wall then is completed in the same two-layer fashion. Alternatively, the pouch can be constructed with several applications of a stapling device.

The surgeon then moves to the perineum to excise the distal rectal and proximal anal mucosa. The anus is effaced and dilated slightly either by placing and opening two Gelpi self-retaining retractors at the anal verge or by using a circular retractor. A dilute (1:100,000) solution of epinephrine is injected into the submucosa at the dentate line to aid in separation of the mucosa from the underlying muscularis and to reduce bleeding. Dissection of the diseased proximal anal and distal rectal columnar mucosa with cautery or scissors in the submucosal plane begins at the dentate line and extends proximally and circumferentially for a distance of 3 to 4 cm. After the first 2 cm of mucosa is mobilized, the dissection can be completed either endoanally or extra-anally after the distal rectum is everted onto the perineum. The mucosal dissection is extended to a point 4 to 5 cm above the dentate line beyond which all layers of the remaining rectum are removed. Leaving only a short, 3- to 4-cm distal rectal tunica muscularis cuff reduces operating time, bleeding, and contamination (and thus the risk of pelvic sepsis), allows for better subsequent expansion of the ileal pouch, and decreases the chance of leaving behind potentially premalignant mucosal cells.

The previously constructed ileal J pouch then is pulled endorectally through the muscular cuff. Its most distal portion is anastomosed to the anoderm at the dentate line, working intraluminally and with 2-0 and 3-0 absorbable sutures (Fig. 1). A soft plastic suction catheter is placed in

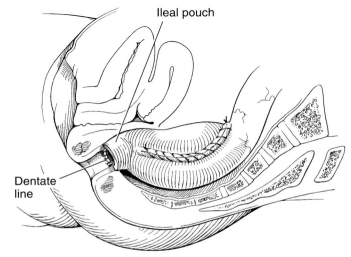

Fig. 1. After near-total proctocolectomy, a J-shaped ileal pouch is constructed from the terminal ileum. The pouch is then sewn to the dentate line of the anal canal to restore enteric continuity.

the presacral space behind the pouch and brought to the surface through the left anterior abdominal wall to drain the space postoperatively. A loop ileostomy then is established through an opening made in the right anterior abdominal wall.

The patient is allowed a minimum of 2 months to recover from this first procedure, after which complete healing of the pouch and the anastomosis is confirmed radiographically with a barium sulfate enema. The loop ileostomy is mobilized at a second operation through a small transverse, biconvex incision that encompasses the stoma. The defect in the bowel is closed with sutures or staples. The repair can be done with or without performing bowel resection, including the stoma.

Proctocolectomy and ileal pouch-anal canal anastomosis can be done laparoscopically, but it is not yet clear that the laparoscopic approach is faster, cheaper, safer, or followed by a speedier recovery and fewer complications than the open technique. Thus, we continue to perform the operation with the open technique in most patients. In almost all patients, the operation can be completed successfully.[10]

Clinical Results

More than 2,000 patients underwent the operation at Mayo Clinic–affiliated hospitals between January 1981 and January 2001, and approximately equal numbers of men and women received the procedure. The mean age of the patients was 32 years; the ages ranged from 14 to 64 years.

Early Results

A detailed analysis of an initial group of 1,310 patients who underwent J pouch IPAA showed that the mean hospital stay was 10 days after the first stage of the operation and 7 days after the second.[11] These lengths of postoperative stay have decreased in recent years. Three patients died in the immediate postoperative period (0.2%): one of massive pulmonary embolism 3 weeks after dismissal to home, 1 of complications of a perforated, corticosteroid-induced gastric ulcer that led to fatal sepsis, and one of a subarachnoid hemorrhage. This experience, as well as that of others, indicates that the operation can be done safely. Indeed, mortality rates in other reported series have ranged from 0% to 1.5%.

Morbidity, however, remains an important concern; the overall complication rate ranges between 13% and 58%, depending on the report. Patients should be informed of the morbidity preoperatively. Most complications occur early after the operation, with a frequency similar to that after other abdominal procedures for ulcerative colitis. Moreover, the complications do not often result in long-term disability, such as would occur with loss of the pouch and the need to convert to a permanent ileostomy.

Early Complications

The most frequent complication after the IPAA, both at Mayo Clinic and elsewhere, is small bowel obstruction, which occurred in 13% of our patients. About half of the patients with obstruction required reoperation; in the other half, the symptoms resolved with nonoperative measures.[12,13] This rate of small bowel obstruction is similar to that reported in the literature for IPAA and for other types of operations for ulcerative colitis.

Once the most feared complication after ileoanal anastomosis, pelvic sepsis manifesting as either a pelvic phlegmon or frank abscess has occurred in only 6% of Mayo Clinic patients.[14] Since 1991, postoperative sepsis rates have decreased to 3%, although the frequency remains greater in patients with indeterminate colitis (17%). The symptoms and signs have included fever, pelvic or perineal pain, and leukocytosis. Computed tomography has helped to confirm the presence of abscess. Patients with phlegmons were treated successfully with antibiotics alone, whereas those with abscesses required computed tomography-guided transperineal or transabdominal drainage or surgical drainage. The rate of pelvic sepsis has diminished substantially, possibly because the long rectal muscular cuff previously left in place is no longer used, and possibly because the operation is more carefully and rapidly performed now that the learning curve has been negotiated. Of the patients who required laparotomy for control of sepsis, however, 41% lost their pouch and only 29% ever had a functioning operation. Pelvic sepsis, if it occurs, is a primary cause of pouch failure. However, if no reoperation was required, 92% of patients with sepsis had a functional ileoanal anastomosis. Wound infections, both deep and superficial, were rare, occurring in only 3% of all patients. Urinary dysfunction also was uncommon, occurring transiently in only 5% of patients, with 2% requiring intermittent catheterization on dismissal from the hospital. None of the patients has required a permanent catheter, and all patients were able to void spontaneously at the time of follow-up.

After ileostomy closure, small bowel obstruction again was the most common complication, occurring in 9% of patients, about half of them requiring reoperation. When the frequencies after the first and second operations were combined, 22% of patients had small bowel obstruction develop after ileoanal anastomosis. Leakage at or near the site of closure of the loop ileostomy occurred in 2% of patients after closure of the ileostomy. The leak often occurred in that segment of bowel dissected free of the abdominal wall and unfolded in an attempt to avoid bowel resection.[15] Bowel resection, including the stoma itself, and performance of an end-to-end anastomosis may reduce the likelihood of this complication.

Late Results

Stool frequency, pattern of continence, ability to discriminate gas from stool, and the use of medication after ileoanal anastomosis were reviewed after the procedure was done in 1,130 patients with ulcerative colitis at Mayo Clinic hospitals. The daytime and nocturnal stool frequency remained stable at five or six stools per day and one or two stools per night and did not change significantly over a mean of 5 years after operation.[16,17] Similar results have been reported by other investigators.

Fecal incontinence occurs after ileoanal anastomosis but with variable manifestations. Daytime incontinence is uncommon, whereas occasional (twice per week or less) nighttime spotting occurs in 20% to 30% of patients more than 12 months after operation. An attempt to determine the correct percentage of nocturnal incontinence by reporting the frequency of pad use is misleading, because 60% of all female patients use a pad sometimes at night mostly as a precautionary measure. Also, the frequency of nocturnal incontinence and dependence on medication declined considerably with time after the operation. After IPAA, stool frequency is greater in older patients (8 ± 4 stools per day in those older than 50 years, 6 ± 3 stools per day in those 50 years or younger; $P = 0.05$), and older patients have more fecal incontinence.[8] Women and men have the same number of stools each day and the same pattern of fecal spotting.[18] Of interest is the finding that the frequency of fecal spotting after IPAA seems to be affected by the preoperative stool frequency; the greater the number of stools before the operation, the more likely patients are to be incontinent after the operation ($P < 0.03$).[19] Among patients who have the operation for indeterminate colitis, about 15% eventually are shown to have Crohn's disease and not ulcerative colitis. These patients have more pelvic sepsis on long-term follow-up than patients with ulcerative colitis (17% vs. 7%, $P < 0.001$), more pouch fistulas (31% vs. 9%), and more pouch failures (27% vs. 11%, $P < 0.001$). Patients with indeterminate colitis in whom Crohn's disease does not develop have complication rates similar to those of patients with straightforward ulcerative colitis, except for pouch fistula.[2]

Quality of Life

The clinical results support the observation that the ileoanal operation is safe and effective for restoring anorectal function and eradicating the disease. Because IPAA functions as an alternative to the once widely performed Brooke ileostomy, it is reasonable to anticipate that it should provide an improved quality of life over that of the ileostomy if it is to be widely acceptable to both patients and their treating physicians. In a study comparing the performance of seven daily activities among patients with Brooke ileostomy ($n = 406$) and patients with an ileal pouch ($n = 298$), patients with an ileal pouch outperformed those with Brooke ileostomy in every activity, including sexual activity, sports, social functions, recreation, family relationships, work around the house, and travel.[20] Patients with an ileoanal operation also had a better quality of life than patients with a continent ileostomy (Kock pouch).[21] These results largely agree with those of other investigators who studied the functional outcome of the operation and clearly indicate that patients not only regain their health but also are satisfied with the operation and perform daily activities in a normal or near-normal fashion.[22]

Sexual Function, Pregnancy, and Delivery

In most patients, ulcerative colitis develops during their reproductive years; therefore, the impact of proctocolectomy on all aspects of sexual function is an important consideration. Men are concerned with potency and sterility, and women are concerned about their future ability to conceive and carry a pregnancy to term. Moreover, the pelvic location of the ileal reservoir raises anxieties in patients and obstetricians alike regarding the effect of pregnancy and delivery on the function of the ileal pouch and the potential interference with the pelvic reservoir and anal sphincter during the delivery process.

In general, sexual activity increased dramatically after operation compared with preoperative levels, most likely due to an improvement in general health.[23] Postoperatively, sexual dysfunction occurred in 11% of men and 12% of women overall. Impotence occurred in 1.5% of men and retrograde or lack of ejaculation in 4%. The remainder reported that "lack of motivation" or fatigue was the principal cause of sexual dysfunction. In women, dyspareunia was the primary complaint in 7%, and 3% feared leakage of stool during intercourse. It is important to remember that 49% of patients stated that they were sexually dysfunctional before the operation. Also, complaints of sexual dysfunction have been fewer in women with pelvic reservoirs than in those with an end ileostomy, even if continent, or after ileorectostomy.

The ability to conceive appears to be decreased somewhat after the ileoanal operation. This may be due to postoperative adhesions decreasing the patency of the fallopian tubes or their fimbriated ends. Pregnancy and delivery are safe after IPAA, even vaginal delivery. Among women who had at least one successful pregnancy, no maternal deaths occurred, and pouch function was only minimally altered during and after pregnancy. Moreover, the type of delivery, whether vaginal or cesarean section, did not alter postpartum pouch function substantially. On the basis of this information, patients can be reassured that pregnancy and delivery are safe and should have no prolonged adverse effect on the function of their pelvic reservoir. Use of cesarean section should be dictated primarily by obstetric reasons, although some patients prefer a cesarean section to protect their pouch and anal sphincter. If a vaginal delivery and episiotomy are contemplated, a mediolateral episiotomy is preferred to avoid possible damage to the ileal pouch and anal sphincter. In addition, if the pelvic floor is scarred and not supple, vaginal delivery may pose a greater risk of perineal tear and postpartum incontinence. In such patients, a cesarean section is preferred. The long-term effects of pregnancy and delivery, especially if multiple, on pelvic ileal reservoir function are unknown and may prompt greater use of cesarean section.

Late Complications

Pouchitis

Pouchitis is suspected when patients have abdominal cramps, frequent stools, watery and sometimes bloody diarrhea, urgency, incontinence, malaise, and fever.[24] The incidence of pouchitis has increased steadily as the length of follow-up has increased. The cumulative probability of having at least one episode of "clinical" pouchitis increased from 18% at 1 year postoperatively to 48% at 10 years after operation. Pouchitis recurred after treatment in two-thirds of patients and was thought to be a chronic problem in about half of those with recurrence.

Pouchitis can be defined with clinical, endoscopic, and histologic criteria. The major problem with histologic criteria alone is that biopsy specimens from the pouch are heterogeneous. For example, a biopsy specimen from one part of the pouch may be interpreted as normal "colon," from another part as normal ileum, from another as chronic inflammation, and, finally, from another as chronic and acute inflammation. Although histologic criteria may be theoretically helpful, the authors' experience has been that patients with classic signs and symptoms of pouchitis do not always have such histologic changes, and vice versa. A combination of clinical, endoscopic, and histologic findings is required to establish the diagnosis.

The cause of pouchitis remains unknown.[24] It may be caused by abnormal pouch motility leading to poor emptying, by bacterial overgrowth or an immunologic reaction to bacterial products, or by ischemia and reperfusion injury or chemical injury. Pouchitis also may be a novel manifestation of inflammatory bowel disease.

Patients with ulcerative colitis who have primary sclerosing cholangitis are at increased risk of pouchitis[25] (63% in those who have cholangitis and 32% in those who do not), and the pouchitis may be chronic in nearly all.[15,25]

On the contrary, the incidence of pouchitis is not influenced by the type of pouch constructed, by the presence or absence of pelvic sepsis, or by the age and sex of the patient. Patients with extraintestinal manifestations of colitis, however, may be at greater risk for pouchitis.[26] Indeed, when extraintestinal manifestations were present preoperatively, pouchitis occurred in 39% of patients, but it occurred in only 26% when no extraintestinal manifestations were present ($P < 0.001$).[26] Anecdotally, in seven patients the extraintestinal manifestations recurred when pouchitis occurred and abated when the pouchitis was treated. These findings suggest that there is an association between pouchitis and the extraintestinal manifestations. The pathophysiologic mechanisms underlying pouchitis appear to provoke a systemic response similar to that which occurs in response to chronic ulcerative colitis itself.

In a great majority of patients with pouchitis in Mayo Clinic studies and in other studies, treatment with metronidazole or ciprofloxacin has been successful. The same medications have been successful for recurrent episodes. Of interest, pouchitis is rare in patients with polyposis,[27,28] in whom the rates of stagnation of enteric content, overgrowth of bacteria, and ischemia should not differ from those present after operation in patients with colitis. The rarity of pouchitis in patients with polyposis suggests that whatever causes colitis predisposes to pouchitis.

Strictures

Strictures of the anastomosis may be caused by one or more of the following problems: sepsis, excess tension at the anastomosis, and ischemia. Undue tension may lead to ischemia and poor healing of the anastomosis with subsequent excessive scarring, or the pouch may pull away from its anastomosis at the dentate line, leaving the underlying internal sphincter denuded and exposed. Heavy scarring may ensue, leading to the formation of a dense stricture of variable length. Local sepsis may produce similar results and, if severe, may be associated with scarring of the pelvic floor itself. Long, dense strictures are difficult to treat successfully by conservative means, although in some patients repeated dilations may offer considerable relief of obstructive symptoms, at least temporarily. Most often, however, such long strictures need to be treated operatively, either through the perineal approach, excising the stricture and advancing the pouch distally, or through an abdominal approach that includes freeing and elevating the pouch out of the pelvis, repairing it or constructing a new one, incising the pelvic floor scarring carefully, and reanastomosing the apex of the pouch to the mid anal canal.[29]

Fistulas

Pouch-perineal fistulas usually are associated with pelvic sepsis, which must be treated, often with fecal diversion, before the fistulas will heal. Late fistulas, especially if originating from the dentate line, may be the result of crypto-glandular infection. They can be treated like any similar fistula, although conservatism and the wide use of a seton drain are highly recommended to avoid damage to the anal sphincter. In most patients with pouch-vaginal fistulas, especially when they occur before closure of the temporary ileostomy, the fistula resolves spontaneously if closure of the ileostomy is deferred for several months. If the fistula does not heal, local repair, preferably under the cover of the ileostomy, may be necessary. The development of peri-anal fistulas, especially if complex and not originating from the dentate line area, should raise the suspicion that the patient may have Crohn's disease.

Mid pouch or proximal pouch leaks are now less common because of improved technique. However, they are more common in patients with indeterminate colitis (31%) than in patients with classic ulcerative colitis (9%). Conservative treatment entails prolonged diversion. Aggressive treatment, with mobilization of the pouch, repair of the defect, and reanastomosis of the pouch to the anal canal, may be used if conservatism fails.

Cancer

The possibility that a cancer might occur in the pouch itself is remote. Indeed, to the authors' knowledge, cancer has developed in only one of our patients with Kock pouches (continent ileostomies) during extended periods of follow-up. Cancer after ileoanal anastomosis, however, has been reported by at least three separate groups. In two instances, the patient had a long rectal muscular cuff left in place, as practiced several years ago, and in one of these two patients severe dysplasia was present at the time of the original operation. Quite possibly, premalignant or even malignant cells might have been left behind at the time of the anal mucosal stripping, later leading to the development of a frank carcinoma. These disturbing observations help to substantiate our recommendation that the rectal muscular cuff should be short and circumferential, thus reducing the risk of performing an incomplete rectal mucosal excision. Also, we believe that the distal rectal and proximal anal columnar mucosa should be completely removed. In at least two patients, cancer has developed in the distal rectum or proximal anal canal after a stapled ileal pouch–distal rectal anastomosis. These reports should serve as a warning to surgeons who do not do a "mucosectomy," and thus leave behind variable amounts of residual disease. These reports also emphasize the need to perform endoscopic surveillance of ileal pouches with biopsy, regardless of whether the pouches remain in intestinal continuity.

Reoperation for Late Complications

In some cases, late complications after IPAA can be corrected by reoperation.[30] Because these complications often are complex and difficult to manage, they may necessitate more than one procedure, and the procedures are not always successful for salvaging the reservoir. Various operations have been used to correct pouch problems and their postoperative complications.[31] Patients with ileoanal anastomotic stricture initially are treated with dilation while under anesthesia, but the presence of recurrent strictures, especially if associated with other complications, may require operative division of the stricture, partial or even complete reconstruction of the ileal reservoir, or even excision of the reservoir with establishment of a permanent ileostomy. Patients with perianal abscesses, fistulas, and sinuses also can be treated, at least initially, with local perianal operations. The risk of postoperative complications, however, is substantial, and further operations, such as fistulotomy, primary fistula closure, diverting ileostomy, and even pouch reconstruction, are sometimes required. In the authors' experience, nearly 20% of such patients may need to have their pouch excised.

Intra-abdominal abscess, with or without fistula, is the most serious complication of ileoanal anastomosis. In all instances, drainage of the abscess is needed, and the diverting ileostomy needs to be reestablished if it already has been closed. In some patients, especially those with a low-lying retropouch abscess, percutaneous computed tomographic–guided drainage may be feasible and successful.

Patients with unsatisfactory function also may require reoperation. These patients may have poor pouch emptying due to a long efferent intestinal limb interposed between the pouch and the anal canal, incontinence related to too small or too large a reservoir, obstruction due to a J-pouch septum, and outlet obstruction due to mucosal prolapse. Some patients will require shortening or elimination of the pouch's efferent limb, or even excision of the existing reservoir with reconstruction of a new reservoir. Although a transperineal approach can be used, the transabdominal approach often is needed to accomplish the reconstructive operation.

These rather difficult salvage procedures for pouch-related complications have resulted in a loss of the ileal reservoir in 20% of patients, especially if the indication for operation was a poor functional result. In our experience, none of the patients who had reoperation died. These reoperations restored pouch function in two-thirds of patients, 70% of whom had an excellent clinical outcome, with stool frequency and incontinence comparable to those in patients who did not have postoperative complications after their original pouch construction. Although salvage procedures for pouch complications can be done safely and can restore function in a large proportion of patients, the risk of further complications and reoperation, including pouch excision, is considerable. These observations should be shared with patients and their families before such procedures are undertaken.

Failure

After 10 years of follow-up, IPAA ultimately failed in 9% of our patients.[10,14,30,32] In these patients, excision of the pouch or construction of a permanent abdominal ileostomy was necessary. The most frequent causes of failure, occurring alone or in combination, were pelvic sepsis, gross fecal incontinence at night, frequent stools, and Crohn's disease. Patients with indeterminate colitis who eventually were recognized as having clear-cut Crohn's disease during follow-up had a failure rate of 27%. Only rarely did pouchitis alone lead to failure of the operation (2% of all patients for whom the procedure failed). Of the failures, 75% occurred within 1 year, 12% within 2 years, and 12% after 3 or more years.

Physiologic Results

Detailed physiologic studies have been performed postoperatively to define the physiologic alterations that occur as a result of the IPAA operation.[5] Several physiologic factors important for achieving fecal continence are addressed here. These factors include the anal sphincters, anorectal sensation, the puborectal and the anorectal angles, the rectoanal inhibitory reflex, the distensibility and capacity of the pouch, pouch motility, the ability to defecate, the rapidity of transit through more proximal bowel, and the quality and quantity of the enteric content.

Resting pressure of the anal sphincter is decreased about 15% after operation, a value not great enough to result in incontinence in most patients. In contrast, the squeeze pressure of the anal sphincter is unchanged or increased after operation in most patients. In a few patients, however, squeeze pressures are less than in healthy subjects. In these patients, the likelihood of incontinence is increased.

Anal-rectal sensation is usually intact after operation because the squamous lining of the distal anal canal and its innervation are preserved. The patient can detect the difference between flatus and feces presenting at the anal canal. Also, the anorectal angle is maintained at about 100° after operation, which helps to preserve continence. In contrast, the rectal-anal inhibitory reflex is almost always abolished postoperatively. Loss of the reflex, however, does not mean that incontinence will ensue. Patients in whom the reflex is lost may still have perfect continence, and vice versa.

The distensibility and capacity of the ileal pouch are nearly identical to those of a healthy, disease-free rectum, but the contractility of the pouch is increased. When the pouch is distended to only 100 mL, large-amplitude pressure waves appear in the pouch; the healthy rectum can be distended to more than 350 mL before such waves appear. These waves signal the call to stool for the patient with a pouch, and defecation must proceed. Interestingly, about 100 mg of stool is passed with each bowel movement in patients with a pouch. Emptying of the pouch by the patient is facilitated by the Valsalva maneuver and occurs rapidly and almost as completely as in health. Patients with a pouch empty about 55% of an artificial stool instilled into the pouch, whereas patients with a healthy rectum empty about 75% of the instillate.

The fecal output and body content of water and extracellular fluid in patients with IPAA are similar to those in patients with ileostomy. About 650 mL of semisolid stool is passed per day in five to seven 100-mL bowel movements. Dietary restriction and the use of bulk-forming agents have little effect on the volume excreted, but they reduce urgency and perineal irritation by making the stool less liquid and possibly by binding the enteric bile salts. The use of agents such as loperamide hydrochloride to slow transit, improve absorption, and strengthen the anal sphincter also is helpful in the initial weeks after ileostomy closure. The persistent passage of a large volume of semiformed stool in the early postoperative period, however, is a major factor in the frequent stooling, mild incontinence, and perineal irritation experienced by some patients soon after IPAA. The less the volume of stool passed, the fewer the number of bowel movements and the better the result.

Of interest, the transit of chyme through the small intestine of patients with IPAA actually is slower than that of healthy control subjects, and the ileal mechanisms that exert hormonal and neural braking effects on the transit remain intact.[33] These factors ensure that sufficient time is present for small bowel digestion and absorption and that ileal output is not excessive. Nonetheless, measures that would slow small bowel transit and enhance intestinal absorption would be welcome.

PROCTOCOLECTOMY AND ILEAL POUCH-DISTAL RECTAL ANASTOMOSIS

The lack of complete continence at night in some patients after IPAA has caused some surgeons to explore another operation for ulcerative colitis—proctocolectomy and ileal pouch-distal rectal anastomosis (Fig. 2).[34] In this procedure, 1 to 3 cm of bowel above the dentate line, including the transitional mucosa, is left intact. The ileal pouch is either sewn or, more often, stapled to the distal rectum or proximal anal canal at the pelvic floor. The rationale is that the operation is easier to perform than the conventional IPAA; preservation of the transitional mucosa maintains anal sensation, anal sphincter function, and postoperative continence, especially at night; and the transitional mucosa is not involved or is only minimally involved with colitis and can safely be left behind. Some authors also have postulated that inflammation in the transitional mucosa, even if present, subsides after operation.

Early results of pilot studies suggest that this operation is faster than the IPAA procedure and that anal sensation and anal sphincter strength may be better preserved. Whether this operation is safer is uncertain. Fecal continence, which also has been reported as improved, especially at night, has been attributed to these findings. These favorable results, however, have been reported by investigators who base their conclusions on retrospective studies. In contrast, randomized trials conducted prospectively in small numbers of patients have shown no difference in function between conventional IPAA and ileal pouch-distal rectal anastomosis.[35]

A concern with the ileal pouch-distal rectal anastomosis is that the operation leaves diseased mucosa behind.[36] Histologic examination of 50 colitis specimens removed at conventional proctocolectomy at Mayo Clinic showed that ulcerative colitis was present in the transitional zone within 1 cm of the dentate line in 90% of specimens.[37] Preserving anal canal mucosa proximal to the dentate line therefore leaves residual disease in 90% of patients. Moreover, other authors have noted that 19 of 20 distal "donuts" of the rectum removed at the time of the stapled anastomosis without mucosectomy for ulcerative colitis harbored inflammatory mucosa. Finally, others also have shown

that dysplasia or neoplasia can be present or may develop in this mucosa in patients with ulcerative colitis. Long-term prospective, randomized clinical trials comparing these two operations in a larger number of patients therefore are needed. Unless a dramatic improvement in nighttime continence is subsequently noted, our preference will continue to be the conventional IPAA operation.

PROCTOCOLECTOMY AND BROOKE ILEOSTOMY

The advent of improved appliances and better surgical technique made proctocolectomy and Brooke ileostomy the standard operation for ulcerative colitis for many years. The ileostomy is constructed from the terminal ileum and is positioned in the right lower quadrant of the abdomen. The patient's fecal effluent discharges through the stoma and is collected by an appliance that the patient wears continuously day and night. Although the role of this operation now is more limited, it retains a place in certain patients.

Advantages and Disadvantages

The advantages of the operation are that it is simple, it is associated with few postoperative complications, and it removes all the diseased large intestine. The major disadvantage is that the patient is left with a permanent, incontinent stoma requiring the wearing of an appliance at all times. Also, the perineal wound created by removing the rectum and anal canal may be slow to heal in some cases, causing discomfort and inconvenience. Finally, any operation involving removal of the entire rectum may result in urinary or sexual dysfunction.

Indications

This operation may be preferable to IPAA in patients who are not suitable candidates for a sphincter-saving procedure because of either their age or the incompetency of their anal sphincter. It also may be indicated when malignancy has supervened in the rectum and requires removal of the rectum or when other medical problems are of such severity that a more complex, complication-prone, longer operation may be considered too risky. The operation also may be more suitable for patients whose work makes it easier for them to handle an appliance as opposed to a pelvic ileal reservoir or Kock pouch.

Preoperative Preparation

At a preoperative interview among the treating surgeon, the stoma therapist, and the patient, the exact description of the procedure and the new anatomy produced by the operation should be thoroughly discussed. The patient must

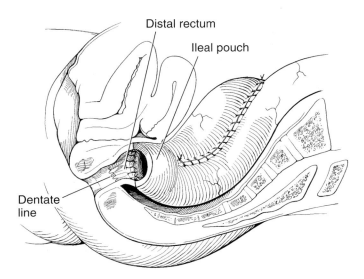

Fig. 2. Ileal pouch-distal rectal anastomosis.

Distal rectum

Ileal pouch

Dentate line

understand that the ileostomy provides a permanent abdominal stoma and that an appliance must be worn continuously to collect the fecal effluent. At times, a visit with a person who already has made a successful adjustment to an ileostomy is warranted and may be most useful in dispelling the patient's fears and misconceptions. In addition, before operation, an appropriate abdominal site is selected by the surgeon and the stoma therapist. The site usually is just lateral and inferior to the umbilicus midway between the midline and the right anterior superior iliac spine, avoiding abdominal skin folds, creases, and scars that may hinder effective sealing of the appliance to the skin.

Operative Technique

The patient is placed in the modified lithotomy position to allow the surgeon access to both the abdomen and the perineum. A catheter is inserted in the urinary bladder, and the skin of the abdomen and perineum are prepared with a dilute solution of povidone-iodine.

Through a vertical midline abdominal incision, abdominal contents are inspected thoroughly to confirm the presence of the disease. The diseased large intestine then is excised, and every effort is made to preserve as much of the small intestine as possible. Usually, all but a centimeter of terminal ileum can be saved. The greater omentum and the mesentery of the small intestine also are preserved.

The terminal ileum is next prepared for use as a stoma by dividing its secondary and tertiary vascular arcades while preserving its marginal artery and vein. The abdominal skin at the exact center of the site preselected for the ileostomy is grasped with a Kocher clamp and elevated so that a circular defect 3 cm in diameter can be created in it. The anterior and posterior laminas of the rectus abdominis sheath are then incised and the peritoneal cavity is entered. The final defect created should be approximately 4 cm in diameter and allow admittance of the index and middle fingers simultaneously. The distal ileum then is grasped with a noncrushing clamp and brought out to the skin surface through the defect. The ileum should project above the skin surface for a distance of approximately 5 cm. The ileum then is anchored to the endoabdominal fascia and posterior sheath of the rectus abdominis with interrupted 4-0 nonabsorbable sutures. Next, the space lateral to the terminal ileum should be closed, approximating the ileal mesentery to the retroperitoneum and the right lateral parietal peritoneum with a continuous 2-0 absorbable suture.

The ileal stoma is constructed by turning the terminal ileum inside out so its mucosal surface is exposed and its serosal surface is covered by the eversion (Fig. 3). The distal cut edge of the everted ileum is sewn to the dermis at the site of the stoma with interrupted 3-0 absorbable sutures. Some of these sutures also include the seromuscular layer of the inner wall of the ileum at the skin level to ensure that the stoma does not retract.

After the rectum has been mobilized to the pelvic floor anteriorly, posteriorly, and laterally, with care taken to stay close to the rectal wall, the rectum and anus are excised in the intersphincteric plane. The perineal wound is closed primarily, and a soft plastic catheter is left in the deep pelvis. The catheter is brought out to the skin surface through a stab wound in the left flank or in the perineum. The pelvic floor is reconstructed with absorbable sutures and the abdominal incision is closed with absorbable sutures.

Postoperative Care

The ileostomy usually begins discharging its contents on the second or third postoperative day, at which time the patient is ready to begin oral feedings. The diet is increased gradually, starting with clear liquids and gradually increasing the solid content so that by the fifth day the patient can consume a general diet. Before dismissal from the hospital, the patient should be taught self-care of the ileostomy by the stoma therapist. Patients generally do not require long-term medications. Also, patients are encouraged to eat all types of food but are cautioned not to consume

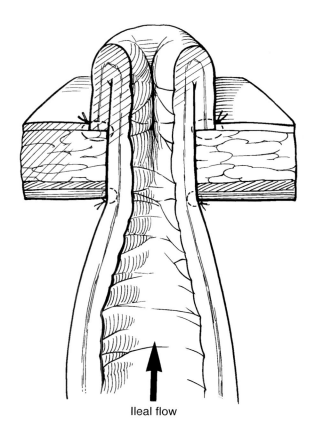

Ileal flow

Fig. 3. End (Brooke) ileostomy.

undispersed vegetable fiber that may obstruct the stoma. Mushrooms, raw vegetables, and nuts are of particular concern. Finally, patients are advised to care properly for the skin surrounding the stoma.

Results

Complications from this operation are infrequent but not negligible. With the use of meticulous surgical technique, infection and bleeding usually are avoided. After proctectomy for inflammatory bowel disease, delayed perineal wound healing can be observed. Complete failure to heal is most unusual. When it does occur, patients usually require some type of reconstructive operation. Stomal complications occur in 5% to 25% of patients, although most authors report a complication rate less than 15%. Complications such as retraction, prolapse, hernia, bleeding, varices, stenosis, and obstruction usually require surgical revision.[38]

In the long term, patients may be prone to chronic dehydration, urinary stone formation, and gallstone formation. Depending on the amount of distal ileum resected, the loss of water, sodium, chloride, potassium, and bicarbonate through the stoma may be greater than in health and lead to mild chronic dehydration and slight acidosis. The low output of acidic urine may lead to precipitation of uric acid stones in the urinary tract. Adequate fluid intake, including alkali, should help prevent these complications. Resection of the terminal ileum also predisposes to bile acid malabsorption and gallstones.

Urinary and sexual dysfunction may result from damage to innervation during removal of the rectum and from psychologic factors. Impotence occurs in 3% to 12% of male patients, but it is more likely in older patients. Women may be troubled by dyspareunia and episodic vaginal discharge as a result of pelvic floor disruption. These complications can be minimized by careful dissection in proximity to the rectum and by excising the rectum and anus in the intersphincteric plane.

The quality of life of patients undergoing proctocolectomy and Brooke ileostomy is greatly improved, primarily because of eradication of the disease and restoration of the general health of the patient. Presence of the stoma, however, may limit social, sexual, and sporting activities. However, more than 90% of patients adapt to these limitations, have a nearly normal lifestyle, and are satisfied with the results.

PROCTOCOLECTOMY AND CONTINENT ILEOSTOMY (KOCK POUCH)

The continent reservoir ileostomy (Kock pouch) also offers an alternative to a Brooke ileostomy for certain patients with ulcerative colitis requiring a proctocolectomy. The continent ileal reservoir is constructed entirely from the distal ileum. It consists of a pouch that collects and stores the ileal effluent, a valve that makes the pouch continent for both gas and feces, and a conduit leading to the stoma. Because the pouch is continent, no external appliance need be worn.

Background and Rationale

In 1967, in Sweden, Kock reasoned that if an internal reservoir were constructed of terminal ileum, it would store fecal matter internally until emptied voluntarily with catheterization, obviating an external appliance.[18] The pouch would need to hold about 400 mL, so frequent emptying would be unnecessary. Kock further suggested that incising the ileum along the antimesenteric border when making the pouch would help prevent ileal contractions, thereby keeping pressure low in the pouch as it filled.

Kock further recognized that an internal valve, also constructed from the terminal ileum, would be needed to separate the pouch from the stoma if continence were to be achieved. A catheter then could be passed through the stoma, through the valve, and into the pouch to drain the feces at appropriate intervals convenient to the patient. Between intubations, no stool should leak from the reservoir and, therefore, an external collecting device or bag would be unnecessary.

Kock devised a "nipple" valve made by intussuscepting the efferent ileal limb into the pouch for a distance of 5 cm. The intussusceptum was anchored in place with nonabsorbable sutures or staples. This valve proved successful and provided continence in Kock's patients and in our patients.[19,39,40] The method of anchoring the intussusceptum has continued to evolve, but, to date, the nipple valve remains the valve of choice.

Indications and Contraindications

Although the IPAA now is preferred by most patients requiring proctocolectomy, the continent ileostomy remains a viable alternative to the Brooke ileostomy for certain patients. Candidates are those who have a conventional Brooke ileostomy after proctocolectomy and want to improve their quality of life, those who need a proctocolectomy and want to preserve fecal continence but are not candidates for an ileoanal anastomosis (usually because of poor anal sphincter function), those who prefer a continent ileostomy to an ileoanal anastomosis because daily work takes them away from toilet facilities for prolonged periods, and those with a failed ileoanal anastomosis who want to preserve fecal continence and avoid an external appliance. The operation should be discouraged in older patients, who may be more prone to postoperative complications, including valve dysfunction, and may not tolerate a reoperation; patients with Crohn's disease; obese patients; patients who have had a large portion of small intestine resected; critically ill patients, such as those with toxic megacolon in whom a staged procedure may be safer; and psychologically unfit patients because of the inability to intubate properly and to tolerate reoperation should it be required.

The Operation

The terminal 45 cm of ileum is used to form the pouch. At 15 cm from the distal cut end of the ileum, a 30-cm segment of ileum is measured and fashioned into a U shape (Fig. 4). The antimesenteric borders of the two 15-cm limbs of the U are then approximated with continuous 2-0 absorbable suture. The antimesenteric borders of the limbs are then incised, exposing the mucosa. The incision is made 4 to 5 cm longer on the afferent limb than on the efferent limb of the ileum so that the afferent and efferent limbs of the pouch separate as the pouch is constructed. A second row of absorbable sutures is used to control oozing from the cut edges of the bowel on what will become the posterior wall of the pouch.

The valve is fashioned from the terminal ileum. The serosal surface of the efferent limb of the ileum is scarified with electrocautery beginning at the pouch and extending for a distance of 10 cm toward the distal cut end. The peritoneum is stripped off the mesentery adjacent to the 10-cm segment and the mesentery is "defatted." These maneuvers are designed to promote adherence of the ileum and its mesentery when the efferent limb is intussuscepted into the pouch to form the valve.

The efferent limb is intussuscepted into the pouch, forming a "nipple valve" about 5 cm in length. The

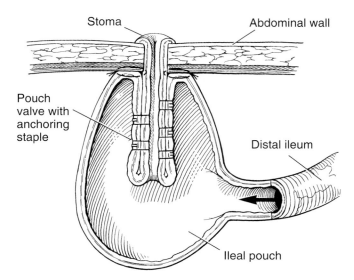

Fig. 4. Continent ileostomy (Kock pouch). Arrow *shows direction of ileal flow.*

intussusceptum is anchored in place with four cartridges of stainless steel staples placed along the long axis of the intussusceptum at 90° intervals. An autosuture apparatus is used to place the staples. Care is taken to avoid placing the staples through the vascular supply of the intussuscepted bowel. Placement of the staples is facilitated by using a catheter (28F) as a stent in the lumen of the intussusceptum.

The bottom of the U then is folded over to form the anterior wall of the pouch. Closure is completed with two layers of continuous 2-0 chromic catgut. The efferent limb of the ileum, which will lead from the pouch to the skin, is sutured to the pouch with interrupted 3-0 nonabsorbable sutures just at the exit of the limb from the pouch to further anchor the intussusceptum in place.

The site of the ileal stoma is located just above the pubic hairline in the right lower quadrant of the abdomen. After an elliptical defect has been created in the skin and another just below in the fascia, the terminal ileum leading from the pouch to the exterior is brought through the defects and cut off flush with the skin. The length of ileum between the pouch and the stoma is made as short as possible to prevent tortuosity and to facilitate later catheterization of the pouch. The pouch is sutured to the undersurface of the anterior abdominal wall just at the exit of the terminal ileum from the abdomen to prevent the pouch from retracting into the abdominal cavity postoperatively. These stitches also ensure that the nipple valve is directly posterior to the stoma. The distal cut end of the ileum then is sewn to the edges of the surrounding skin with interrupted 3-0 chromic catgut.

A catheter (28F) is passed through the stoma and valve, and its tip is positioned within the lumen of the pouch just before the abdominal incision is closed. A suture is tied around the catheter at the level of the stoma so that the exact position of the catheter can be easily ascertained postoperatively. The catheter is left in place for 1 month after operation.

Posthospitalization Care

On leaving the hospital, patients are given a catheter designed specifically for use in draining the pouch, an ileal pouch catheter. The catheter has a diameter of 1 cm (30F) and a length of 64 cm. It has a thick wall and large holes at the insertion end just proximal to its blunt tip. The patient keeps the catheter in a small plastic case, which is carried at all times.

Patients report a sensation of fullness when the pouch needs to be emptied. To empty the pouch, the patient passes the catheter through the stoma into the pouch, usually while in the sitting position. The ileal contents are allowed to drain spontaneously (by gravity) through the catheter directly into the toilet or another suitable receptacle. The Valsalva maneuver and direct manual compression of the abdomen over the pouch are sometimes used to facilitate drainage, but irrigations are not required. Once the pouch is empty, the catheter is removed, rinsed clean, and placed in its case for later use. A soft gauze pad with a waterproof external surface is taped over the stoma to absorb any mucus secreted by the stoma. Patients rapidly become expert at this procedure, which requires about 5 to 10 minutes to complete. None of our patients have ever perforated the pouch with the catheter.

Some patients have found that partially digestible substances, such as seeds, apple skins, celery, and mushrooms, plug the catheter and so have avoided these foods. However, others have found that all foods can be eaten, provided they are thoroughly chewed before being swallowed. Bezoars have not developed in the pouches.

No restrictions are placed on physical activities when the patient has fully recovered, about 4 to 6 weeks after the operation. Pregnancy is not contraindicated; many of our patients have become pregnant. Some have had cesarean section, and others have had normal vaginal delivery.

Results

Mayo Clinic Patient Population

Continent ileal reservoirs were constructed in 460 patients at two Mayo Clinic–affiliated hospitals from November 1, 1971, to January 1, 1982.[39] There were nearly equal numbers of men and women in the series; their ages ranged from 16 to 67 years (mean, 32 years). These operations are still being done, but in much smaller numbers. Today, most patients choose the IPAA rather than the Kock pouch.

Most of the patients (92%) with Kock pouches had chronic ulcerative colitis. About two-thirds of patients had the pouch constructed in conjunction with proctocolectomy and chose a continent ileostomy to avoid a conventional ileostomy. Three-tenths of patients were dissatisfied with the incontinent Brooke ileostomy and sought change to a continent ileostomy. Sixteen patients had a continent ileostomy constructed elsewhere and came to Mayo Clinic for revision of a poorly functioning pouch.

Safety

No pouch-related deaths occurred intraoperatively or postoperatively, and most patients generally convalesced satisfactorily. The mean postoperative stay in the hospital was 10 days. Compared with patients who had a conventional Brooke ileostomy, the patients with ileal reservoirs experienced more abdominal cramps and distention postoperatively and returned to a general diet more slowly, a reflection of the intestinal obstruction produced by the pouch and its valve. The symptoms gradually disappeared as the pouch dilated postoperatively.

With increasing experience, we have been able to reduce the need for excision of the reservoir from about 10% in the first 10 years to about 3%. This was accomplished by avoiding its use in patients with Crohn's colitis and by favoring revision over excision when serious complications took place.

Effectiveness

Long-term follow-up (up to 6 years) has shown excellent results in the series. Most of the pouches have remained continent, with almost no peristomal irritation of the skin or unpleasant odors from the stoma. Moreover, social, sexual, and psychologic disability are absent or minimal. In general, the patients have gained weight, returned to good health, and taken up their previous employment or occupation.

Malfunction of the Nipple Valve

Incontinence and difficult intubation of the pouch due to malfunction of the nipple valve have been the major difficulties in our overall series, necessitating reoperation in about 20% of patients. The malfunction has developed between 1 month and 20 years after construction of the pouch. However, most instances occur within the first year. The risk of malfunction necessitating revision or excision of the pouch decreases with time.

The reason for malfunction of the nipple valve appears to be as follows. The intestine, in an effort to relieve the complete intestinal obstruction created by the valve, spontaneously extrudes the valve out along its mesenteric attachment, rendering the pouch partially incontinent. The efferent ileal limb leading from the pouch to the exterior becomes longer and more tortuous with the valve extruded. The pouch leaks and yet is difficult to intubate because the catheter used for draining the pouch becomes entrapped in the folds of the efferent limb and cannot be advanced into the lumen of the pouch. Persistent efforts at intubation usually are successful. However, occasionally it has been necessary to intubate the pouch with an endoscope first and then to pass the catheter through the instrument into the pouch.

Reoperation is required when the valve malfunctions.[19,40] The pouch and ileostomy are taken down from the anterior abdominal wall. An incision is made through the anterior wall of the pouch. The nipple valve is pulled back into the pouch and reanchored with stainless steel staples. The incision in the anterior wall of the pouch is closed, and the pouch and stoma are fixed again in the right lower quadrant of the abdomen, as described earlier. Revision of the nipple valve has been successful in that ultimately 95% of patients intubate successfully and do not have to wear an appliance. Several factors seem to influence the risk of valve revision. Younger patients (less than 40 years) require fewer revisions than older patients (40 years or older); the older the patient, the greater the probability of revision. Fewer revisions are required in women, in patients who have their continent reservoir constructed at the same time as the procto-colectomy, and in nonobese patients than in men, those who had a previously constructed Brooke ileostomy con-verted to a continent ileostomy, and in obese patients. With the technical modifications described, we have con-siderably reduced this nagging problem; currently, only about 10% of patients need revision of the valve at some point postoperatively.

Diarrhea and Pouchitis

About a third of our patients have had episodes of watery diarrhea late postoperatively. *Staphylococcus aureus*, *Campylobacter*, or other pathogens have been cultured from the ileal content in some of the patients, and the diarrhea subsided when appropriate antibiotic therapy was given. Other patients have had diarrhea because of a mechanical obstruction of the small intestine. Lysis of adhesions resolved the diarrhea. Still other patients had reddened, friable, edematous mucosa in the pouch with-out evidence of abnormal fecal flora or mechanical obstruc-tion of the small intestine proximal to the nipple valve. They seem to have the same type of cryptogenic pouchi-tis as that occurring in patients after IPAA. Moreover, the frequency of pouchitis in the two groups of patients is nearly identical. Patients with the Kock pouch who have pouchitis usually respond to oral metronidazole, as do the patients with the ileoanal anastomosis.

Quality of Life

The crucial consideration in assessing the value of the con-tinent ileostomy is whether it is continent enough so that patients need not wear an external appliance. At the time of follow-up, 75% of patients stated they had always been continent for gas and stool, and ultimately 95% of the entire group never wore an appliance. Others who work in large referral centers have reported similar results. When quality of life after continent ileostomy was compared with that after Brooke ileostomy, we found that satisfaction was greater and the desire for change was less in Kock pouch patients than in Brooke ileostomy patients. Also, in each performance category, more patients with continent ileostomy improved in their daily activities than patients with Brooke ileostomy.

ABDOMINAL COLECTOMY AND ILEORECTAL ANASTOMOSIS

Colectomy with ileorectostomy is used rarely today in Mayo Clinic hospitals as an elective operative treatment of ulcerative colitis. The operation does not excise the diseased rectum, which may continue to cause symptoms, such as bleeding, pain, and diarrhea, does not ameliorate the extraintestinal manifestations of colitis, and does not decrease the risk of rectal carcinoma. Nonetheless, some patients, especially those with minimal rectal involvement by the disease, may be candidates for this procedure.[41]

The operation may be indicated in patients who are not suitable candidates for an IPAA or a continent ileosto-my but who want to maintain the anal route of defecation. It also may serve a useful role in young male patients who are anxious to avoid any type of ileostomy and its disabili-ties or any risk of sexual or urinary dysfunction occasioned by proctectomy. The colitis should be of short duration because of the increased risk of rectal carcinoma with long-standing disease. Patients with relative sparing of the rectum and maintenance of rectal capacity and distensibility achieve the best postoperative results. It also may be a useful alter-native in patients in whom Crohn's disease cannot be excluded and occasionally in patients with ulcerative colitis complicated by advanced metastatic malignancy of the colon, especially if the rectum is relatively spared.

The operation should be avoided in patients with severe rectal disease, especially those with a rigid, noncompliant rectum. It also should be avoided when precancerous dys-plastic changes are present in the rectum. Finally, the oper-ation should not be performed in emergency situations because of the increased risk of anastomotic breakdown. In this circumstance, the cut end of the proximal rectum should be sutured or stapled closed and a temporary Brooke ileostomy constructed. These patients then may be can-didates later for the IPAA.

Advantages and Disadvantages

The obvious advantage of ileorectostomy is maintenance of the anal route of defecation. It also is a relatively safe operation associated with minimal immediate complica-tions. However, its significant disadvantages, including persistent diarrhea, continuing active rectal disease, the necessity for close endoscopic follow-up, and the cumulative risk of cancer, make the operation less attractive, especially now that IPAA can be offered.

The Operation

Colectomy and ileorectal anastomosis may be performed as a one-stage procedure in the elective setting (Fig. 5) or as a two-stage procedure in patients requiring emergency operation. In the two-stage procedure, the first stage comprises colectomy with ileostomy and either mucous fistula or oversewing of the rectal stump, and the second stage consists of restoring bowel continuity with an ileorectal anastomosis.

Results

In the Mayo Clinic experience, the procedure was performed in less than 10% of patients requiring operation for ulcerative colitis in the 1960s and 1970s, when IPAA was not available. Of 63 patients, 2 (3.2%) died postoperatively and 1 (1.6%) had anastomotic leaks. In the long term, only 55% of patients had satisfactory functional results.[41] The less-than-desirable results were due to excessive frequency of stooling (more than eight per day), the continued need for corticosteroids, incontinence, and poor health. Eventually, 30% of the patients required proctectomy within a few years. Other studies have shown a spectrum of results, with a perioperative mortality rate ranging from 0% to 7%, a leak rate ranging from 0% to 11%, and eventual proctectomy in 4% to 37% of patients. Satisfactory rectal function also has varied, being reported in from 32% to 96% of patients. These varied results reflect the selection of patients for the procedure, the varying duration of follow-up, and the degree of an individual surgeon's enthusiasm for the operation.

The risk of cancer in the residual rectum has been reported to be 6% after 20 years of disease and 15% after 30 years. The risk is high, considering that most patients who have the operation are young and will need continued surveillance. By contrast, impotence and urinary dysfunction are uncommon sequelae, although retrograde ejaculation and impotence have been reported.

The operation has a very limited role in our current surgical management of ulcerative colitis, especially since the advent of IPAA. Indeed, comparative studies have shown no major benefit of colectomy and ileorectal anastomosis over IPAA in terms of morbidity, mortality, stool frequency, continence, and sexual dysfunction.

PROCTOCOLECTOMY AND JEJUNAL POUCH-ANAL CANAL ANASTOMOSIS

We have been studying a newer approach to rectal reconstruction in the Mayo Clinic surgical research laboratories: proctocolectomy and jejunal pouch-anal canal anastomosis.

Advantages

A jejunal pouch used as a rectal substitute after proctocolectomy might have advantages over an ileal pouch so used. The jejunum is larger than the ileum and would form a more capacious pouch. This could mean fewer bowel movements per day and less fecal leakage. The jejunum is seldom inflamed in ulcerative colitis, whereas the ileum is inflamed more commonly. Thus, a jejunal pouch might intrinsically be more resistant to postoperative pouchitis than an ileal pouch. Moreover, interposing a jejunal pouch between the distal ileum and the anal canal might preserve ileal mucosal functions better than when the ileum itself is used to form a pouch. Bile salts and vitamin B_{12} might be absorbed better by the ileum if it were not used to form a pouch. Bacterial overgrowth occurs in ileal pouches, and the toxic products of the bacteria or the bile salts they deconjugate and dehydroxylate might damage ileal mucosa and impair its absorptive functions. Moreover, the ileal mucosa also secretes peptide YY, a hormone that exerts a brake on transit of chyme through more proximal small intestine. Slower transit usually means better absorption, less ileal effluent, and, hence, fewer bowel movements in the postprandial period.

Another point follows from the fact that the bacterial overgrowth in ileal pouches deconjugates and dehydroxylates luminal bile salts, possibly rendering them more toxic to ileal mucosa. Interposing a jejunal pouch between the terminal ileum and the pouch might preserve ileal bile salt absorption, with perhaps fewer bile salts passing into the jejunal pouch, less fecal bile salt loss, and less pouch inflammation.

The Operation

A 30-cm segment of jejunum is isolated from the mid small bowel and fashioned into a J-shaped jejunal pouch with 15-cm limbs (Fig. 6). Jejunoileal continuity is restored with an end-to-end jejunoileostomy. The afferent limb of the jejunal pouch is anastomosed to the distal cut end of ileum. The pouch is then brought down endorectally and sewn to the dentate line in the anal canal, just as with an IPAA.

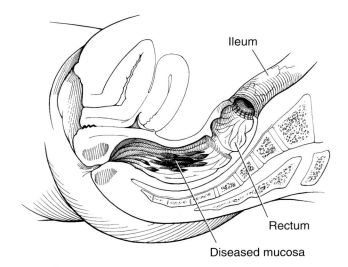

Ileum

Rectum

Diseased mucosa

Fig. 5. Ileorectostomy.

Results

Experiments in our surgical research laboratory have provided evidence to support some of these hypotheses.[31,42,43] Dogs with jejunal pouch-distal rectal anastomosis have slower transit of chyme through the small intestine than dogs with ileal pouches, perhaps in part due to the greater serum PYY levels in the blood postprandially. Jejunal pouches are larger and more distensible than ileal pouches. Dogs with the jejunal pouch had slower transit through their small intestine, fewer bowel movements, and larger bowel movements than dogs with the ileal pouch. The jejunal pouch dogs remained healthy and gained weight during a 6-month interval after operation, as did ileal pouch dogs. Bacterial overgrowth occurred in the lumens of both types of pouches, but neither type of canine pouch developed "pouchitis." Moreover, 7-dehydroxylation and passive absorption of bile salts still occurred in dogs after jejunal pouch-anal canal anastomosis, as they did after IPAA, thus bile acid malabsorption was prevented.

This operation has not yet been used in patients at Mayo Clinic.

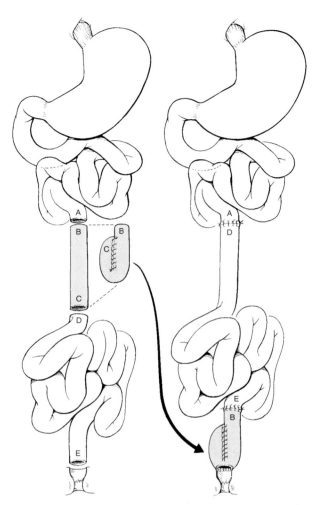

Fig. 6. Jejunal pouch-anal canal anastomosis after near-total proctocolectomy. A segment of distal jejunum (B-C) is used to form the pouch (left panel), which is interposed between the terminal ileum (E) and the anal canal (right panel). Jejunoileal continuity is restored with a jejunoileostomy (A-D, right panel).

REFERENCES

1. Dozois RR, Kelly KA: The surgical management of ulcerative colitis. *In* Inflammatory Bowel Disease. Fifth edition. Edited by JB Kirsner. Philadelphia, WB Saunders Company, 2000, pp 626-657

2. Yu CS, Pemberton JH, Larson D: Ileal pouch-anal anastomosis in patients with indeterminate colitis: long-term results. Dis Colon Rectum 43:1487-1496, 2000

3. Grant CS, Dozois RR: Toxic megacolon: ultimate fate of patients after successful medical management. Am J Surg 147:106-110, 1984

4. Goudet P, Dozois RR, Kelly KA, Ilstrup DM, Phillips SF: Characteristics and evolution of extraintestinal manifestations associated with ulcerative colitis after proctocolectomy. Dig Surg 18:51-55, 2001

5. Cangemi JR, Wiesner RH, Beaver SJ, Ludwig J, MacCarty RL, Dozois RR, Zinsmeister AR, LaRusso NF: Effect of proctocolectomy for chronic ulcerative colitis on the natural history of primary sclerosing cholangitis. Gastroenterology 96:790-794, 1989

6. Pemberton JH, Kelly KA, Beart RW Jr, Dozois RR, Wolff BG, Ilstrup DM: Ileal pouch-anal anastomosis for chronic ulcerative colitis: long-term results. Ann Surg 206:504-513, 1987

7. Kelly KA, Pemberton JH, Wolff BG, Dozois RR: Ileal pouch-anal anastomosis. Curr Probl Surg 29:57-131, 1992

8. Goudet P, Dozois RR, Kelly KA, Melton LJ III, Ilstrup DM, Phillips SF: Changing referral patterns for surgical treatment of ulcerative colitis. Mayo Clin Proc 71:743-747, 1996

9. Ambroze WL Jr, Wolff BG, Kelly KA, Beart RW Jr, Dozois RR, Ilstrup DM: Let sleeping dogs lie: role of the omentum in the ileal pouch-anal anastomosis procedure. Dis Colon Rectum 34:563-565, 1991

10. Browning SM, Nivatvongs S: Intraoperative abandonment of ileal pouch to anal anastomosis: the Mayo Clinic experience. J Am Coll Surg 186:441-445, 1998

11. Meagher AP, Farouk R, Dozois RR, Kelly KA, Pemberton JH: J ileal pouch-anal anastomosis for chronic ulcerative colitis: complications and long-term outcome in 1,310 patients. Br J Surg 85:800-803, 1998

12. Priedhomme M, Farouk R, Dozois RR: Complications after ileal pouch-anal canal anastomosis. Perspect Colon Rectal Surg 11:57, 2000

13. Francois Y, Dozois RR, Kelly KA, Beart RW Jr, Wolff BG, Pemberton JH, Ilstrup DM: Small intestinal obstruction complicating ileal pouch-anal anastomosis. Ann Surg 209:46-50, 1989

14. Farouk R, Dozois RR, Pemberton JH, Larson D: Incidence and subsequent impact of pelvic abscess after ileal pouch-anal anastomosis for chronic ulcerative colitis. Dis Colon Rectum 41:1239-1243, 1998

15. Kartheuser AH, Dozois RR, Wiesner RH, LaRusso NF, Ilstrup DM, Schleck CD: Complications and risk factors after ileal pouch-anal anastomosis for ulcerative colitis associated with primary sclerosing cholangitis. Ann Surg 217:314-320, 1993

16. Farouk R, Pemberton JH, Wolff BG, Dozois RR, Browning S, Larson D: Functional outcomes after ileal pouch-anal anastomosis for chronic ulcerative colitis. Ann Surg 231:919-926, 2000

17. Horgan AF, Pemberton JH: Long-term follow-up after surgery for chronic ulcerative colitis. Probl Gen Surg 16:151-157, 1999

18. Kock NG: Intra-abdominal "reservoir" in patients with permanent ileostomy: preliminary observations on a procedure resulting in fecal "continence" in five ileostomy patients. Arch Surg 99:223-231, 1969

19. Dozois RR, Dozois EJ: Continent ileostomy. *In* Mastery of Surgery. Fourth edition. Edited by RJ Baker, JE Fischer. Philadelphia, Lippincott Williams & Wilkins, 2001, pp 1425-1434

20. Pemberton JH, Phillips SF, Ready RR, Zinsmeister AR, Beahrs OH: Quality of life after Brooke ileostomy and ileal pouch-anal anastomosis: comparison of performance status. Ann Surg 209:620-626, 1989

21. Kohler LW, Pemberton JH, Zinsmeister AR, Kelly KA: Quality of life after proctocolectomy: a comparison of Brooke ileostomy, Kock pouch, and ileal pouch-anal anastomosis. Gastroenterology 101:679-684, 1991

22. Kohler LW, Pemberton JH, Hodge DO, Zinsmeister AR, Kelly KA: Long-term functional results and quality of life after ileal pouch-anal anastomosis and cholecystectomy. World J Surg 16:1126-1131, 1992

23. Metcalf AM, Dozois RR, Kelly KA: Sexual function in women after proctocolectomy. Ann Surg 204:624-627, 1986

24. Heppell J, Kelly K: Pouchitis. Current Opin Gastroenterol 14:322-326, 1998

25. Penna C, Dozois R, Tremaine W, Sandborn W, LaRusso N, Schleck C, Ilstrup D: Pouchitis after ileal pouch-anal anastomosis for ulcerative colitis occurs with increased frequency in patients with associated primary sclerosing cholangitis. Gut 38:234-239, 1996

26. Lohmuller JL, Pemberton JH, Dozois RR, Ilstrup D, van Heerden J: Pouchitis and extraintestinal manifestations of inflammatory bowel disease after ileal pouch-anal anastomosis. Ann Surg 211:622-627, 1990

27. Kartheuser AH, Parc R, Penna CP, Tiret E, Frileux P, Hannoun L, Nordlinger B, Loygue J: Ileal pouch-anal anastomosis as the first choice operation in patients with familial adenomatous polyposis: a ten-year experience. Surgery 119:615-623, 1996

28. Nyam DC, Brillant PT, Dozois RR, Kelly KA, Pemberton JH, Wolff BG: Ileal pouch-anal canal anastomosis for familial adenomatous polyposis: early and late results. Ann Surg 226:514-519, 1997

29. Galandiuk S, Scott NA, Dozois RR, Kelly KA, Ilstrup DM, Beart RW Jr, Wolff BG, Pemberton JH, Nivatvongs S, Devine RM: Ileal pouch-anal anastomosis: reoperation for pouch-related complications. Ann Surg 212:446-452, 1990

30. Sagar PM, Dozois RR, Wolff BG, Kelly KA: Disconnection, pouch revision and reconnection of the ileal pouch-anal anastomosis. Br J Surg 83:1401-1405, 1996

31. Teixeira FV, Hofmann AF, Hagey LR, Pera M, Kelly KA: Bile acid absorption after near-total proctocolectomy in dogs: ileal pouch vs. jejunal pouch-distal rectal anastomosis. J Gastrointest Surg 5:540-545, 2001

32. Farouk R, Dozois RR, Pemberton JH: Aetiology of pouch failure after restorative proctocolectomy for ulcerative colitis: an analysis based on patient age (abstract). Gut 44 Suppl 1:103A, 1999

33. Soper NJ, Chapman NJ, Kelly KA, Brown ML, Phillips SF, Go VL: The "ileal brake" after ileal pouch-anal anastomosis. Gastroenterology 98:111-116, 1990

34. Kelly KA: Anal sphincter-saving operations for chronic ulcerative colitis. Am J Surg 163:5-11, 1992

35. Reilly WT, Pemberton JH, Wolff BG, Nivatvongs S, Devine RM, Litchy WJ, McIntyre PB: Randomized prospective trial comparing ileao pouch-anal anastomosis performed by excising the anal mucosa to ileal pouch-anal anastomosis performed by preserving the anal mucosa. Ann Surg 225:666-676, 1997

36. Dozois RR, Juhasz E: Ileoanal pouches—Is mucosectomy essential? Can J Gastroenterol 7:258-265, 1993
37. Ambroze WL, Pemberton JH, Dozois RR, Carpenter HA: Does retaining the anal transition zone (ATZ) fail to extirpate chronic ulcerative colitis (CUC) after ileal pouch-anal anastomosis (IPAA)? (Abstract.) Dis Colon Rectum 34:P20, 1991
38. Roy PH, Sauer WG, Beahrs OH, Farrow GM: Experience with ileostomies: evaluation of long-term rehabilitation in 497 patients. Am J Surg 119:77-86, 1970
39. Dozois RR, Kelly KA, Beart RW Jr, Beahrs OH: Improved results with continent ileostomy. Ann Surg 192:319-324, 1980
40. Dozois RR, Kelly KA, Ilstrup D, Beart RW Jr, Beahrs OH: Factors affecting revision rate after continent ileostomy. Arch Surg 116:610-613, 1981
41. Farnell MB, Adson MA: Current results: the Mayo Clinic experience. In Alternatives to Conventional Ileostomy. Edited by RR Dozois. Chicago, Year Book Medical Publishers, 1985, pp 100-121
42. Teixeira FV, Hinojosa-Kurtzberg M, Pera M, Hanson RB, Williams JW, Kelly KA: The jejunal pouch as a rectal substitute after proctocolectomy. J Gastrointest Surg 4:207-216, 2000
43. Teixeira FV, Pera M, Kelly KA: Enhancing release of peptide YY after near-total proctocolectomy: jejunal pouch vs. ileal pouch-anal rectal anastomosis. J Gastrointest Surg 5:108-112, 2001

Chapter 39

COLONIC VOLVULUS

Richard M. Devine, M.D.

Colonic volvulus occurs when a portion of the colon twists around its mesentery, resulting in a closed-loop obstruction. Volvulus of the sigmoid colon and cecum are the most common types. Volvulus also occurs in the transverse colon and at the splenic flexure, but these locations account for only 2% to 3% of all cases.

INCIDENCE AND AGE OF PATIENTS

The incidence of colonic volvulus varies by the area of the world. In the United States and Great Britain, volvulus accounts for about 1% to 7% of all cases of large-bowel obstruction.[1] In some areas of Africa, the incidence is much higher, with one West Africa series reporting colonic volvulus in 20% to 50% of patients with intestinal obstructions.[2] In a population-based study in Olmsted County, Minnesota, the incidence of colonic volvulus was about 3 cases per 100,000 persons per year. The incidence was much greater in patients older than 60 years. The incidence in the population younger than 60 years was only 1 per 100,000 persons per year, whereas it was 14 per 100,000 persons per year in the population older than 60 years.[3]

In the Olmsted County study, 56% of cases involved the sigmoid colon, 41% the cecum, and 3% the splenic flexure. This distribution is similar to the reported incidence from other U.S. series of about 60% involving the sigmoid colon and 40% involving the cecum.[4] Elsewhere around the world, the distribution is more heavily weighted toward sigmoid volvulus. In a collected series of cases outside the United States, 82% involved the sigmoid colon.[4]

Patients presenting with colonic volvulus are, on average, 60 to 70 years of age. In a series of 137 patients at Mayo Clinic, the mean age of patients was 61 years for those with sigmoid volvulus and 59 years for those with cecal volvulus.[3] In a series of 37 patients at the Cleveland Clinic, the mean age was 63 years (range, 11-85).[1] In a series of 58 patients at the Hennepin County Medical Center in Minneapolis, Minnesota, the average age was 66 years (70.9 years in sigmoid volvulus, 61.5 years in cecal volvulus).[5] Colonic volvulus also occurs in the pediatric age group. Fifty-six cases of sigmoid volvulus in patients under age 20 have been reported, with the youngest patient being only 2 days old.[6,7] In published series on cecal volvulus, the age range often extends into the pediatric age group.[6,8] One patient in the Mayo Clinic series who had cecal volvulus was less than 1 year old. There are 11 reports of transverse colonic volvulus in children, the youngest of whom was 2 years old.[9]

ETIOLOGY

Many factors are associated with the development of colonic volvulus, but the single unifying element is a freely mobile segment of colon.

Cecal volvulus occurs when the terminal ileum, cecum, and proximal ascending colon twist around the axis of the ileocolic artery. In most adults, the cecum is fused to the retroperitoneum well enough to prevent a cecal volvulus. Postmortem studies, however, show that 10% to 20% of adults have a cecum mobile enough to allow a volvulus to develop.[10,11] Associated factors that may influence the development of cecal volvulus include adhesions from previous operations, congenital adhesive bands, incomplete rotation of the colon during fetal development, pregnancy, and distal colonic strictures.

Occasionally, acute distention of the cecum occurs because of a folding of the mobile cecum anteriorly and superiorly over the ascending colon. This condition is not a true volvulus, because there is no axial rotation. Instead, it is referred to as a "cecal bascule." A bascule is a device similar to a seesaw in that it is balanced so that when one end is lowered, the other is raised. In patients with cecal bascule, the cecum is raised but the ascending colon stays in place.

The unifying element in patients with sigmoid volvulus is a long, redundant sigmoid colon with a narrow mesocolon (Fig. 1). The narrow base of the sigmoid mesocolon is probably congenital, but the long redundant sigmoid colon can be an acquired condition caused by various factors. In Brazil, megacolon as a result of Chagas' disease is a major cause of volvulus. A redundant colon also may develop in patients who have chronic constipation, which may explain why persons in long-term inpatient treatment for medical or psychiatric reasons tend to be overrepresented in reported series.[12]

Intestinal obstruction due to volvulus during pregnancy occurs once in every 1,500 to 66,000 deliveries.[13,14] After adhesions, volvulus is the second most common cause of intestinal obstruction during pregnancy. Volvulus of the cecum and of the sigmoid colon can both occur during pregnancy. Cecal volvulus represents 25% to 44% of these cases.[15] About 75% occur during the third trimester near the time of delivery.[16]

CECAL VOLVULUS

Diagnosis
Patients with an acute volvulus of the right colon present with abdominal pain and distention. An analysis of 50 patients in Baltimore, Maryland, found that the duration of symptoms before presentation was 12 hours to 10 days (average, 2 days). Nine (18%) of these 50 patients had chronic intermittent symptoms and underwent elective operations, and seven more patients (14%) had a history of previous episodes that resolved spontaneously.[8] Anderson and Welch[17] reported similar data from a series of 64 patients in Glasgow, Scotland. The duration of symptoms in their series ranged from 8 hours to 11 days (average, 2 days). Nineteen (30%) of their patients had a history of previous episodes.

Supine and upright radiographs of the abdomen will show a dilated cecum. Classically, the dilated cecum is found in the epigastric area or left upper quadrant, and it will have the shape of a kidney bean or comma with the

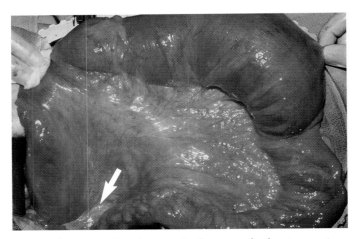

Fig. 1. Intraoperative photograph of a sigmoid colon in a patient who presented with sigmoid volvulus shows a dilated redundant sigmoid on a narrow mesenteric pedicle (arrow).

hilus of the bean facing toward the right side of the abdomen (Fig. 2). On upright radiographs, the distended cecum may contain a large air-fluid level. Distended loops of small bowel are often present and air-filled loops of the terminal ileum can be observed in an abnormal position to the right of the distended cecum. If plain radiographs alone are equivocal, a contrast enema may be used. A water-soluble contrast medium should be used if there is any suspicion of a bowel perforation. The area of obstruction on the contrast examination will appear in the proximal right colon as a tapered configuration shaped like a beak. Dye may pass through the narrowed area and outline the distended cecum.[18]

With the increasing availability and use of computed tomography to evaluate patients with signs and symptoms of acute abdominal pain, many patients will have this test. It will show the dilated small bowel proximal to the obstruction and the large air- and fluid-filled cecum. In addition, it may show a "whirl sign" in the area of obstruction that is caused by loops of bowel twisting around an axis of the ileocolic artery (Fig. 3).[19]

Diagnosing cecal volvulus on the basis of only plain radiographs is more difficult. Rabinovici et al.[20] reviewed 561 cases of cecal volvulus reported between 1959 and 1989. They found that the diagnosis was suspected 46% of the time on plain films of the abdomen but that a definitive diagnosis relying on plain films alone was made in only 7% of cases.[20] A barium enema was used in 50% of the patients with an accuracy of 88%. In a review by O'Mara et al.,[8] 38 patients had plain abdominal radiographs, and the preoperative diagnosis was made with these alone in only 2 patients. Of 29 patients who had plain abdominal radiographs, 20 (69%) were diagnosed preoperatively with colonic radiography using a barium contrast enema.

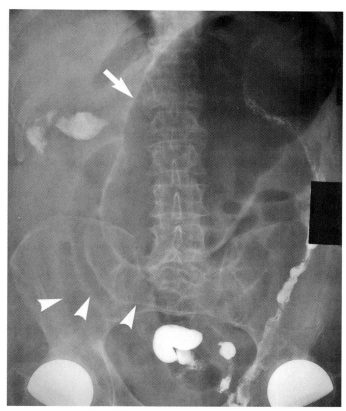

Fig. 2. Radiograph of a cecal volvulus shows a large dilated cecum in the left upper quadrant (arrow) *and mildly dilated loops of small bowel* (arrowheads). *Barium sulfate remains in the colon from a previous barium enema.*

Although it is satisfying to make the correct diagnosis before operating, the most critical decision is whether the patient requires an operation. Patients who present with signs and symptoms of an acute abdomen may require no further work-up beyond radiographs of the abdomen taken with the patient in supine and upright positions. If a decision can be made to explore the patient surgically on the basis of the patient's presentation and radiographs, then further testing may be superfluous.

Treatment

As a diagnostic procedure, a barium enema may reduce the obstruction.[3,8] However, this result should be regarded as fortuitous; no authors recommend barium enema as a therapeutic maneuver because of its low success rate and potential danger. Successful and unsuccessful attempts at colonoscopic decompression have been reported,[21,22] but most authors do not recommend it. Physical examinations and leukocyte counts are unreliable predictors of the presence or absence of gangrenous bowel, and colonoscopy is potentially dangerous because the colonoscope may perforate gangrenous areas that may be present in the volvulus.

Percutaneous decompression has been described by Patel et al.[23] They decompressed a gas-filled cecum with a 16-gauge catheter inserted using a catheter-over-needle technique. The catheter was removed after a few minutes when it became clogged with feces. The patient was discharged 4 days later.

Absent unusual circumstances, a patient with suspected cecal volvulus should be taken immediately to the operating room. We prefer to explore such patients through a generous midline incision. When the abdomen is opened, the surgeon may encounter a tense, massively dilated cecum that could burst with the slightest manipulation. Thus, the bowel should be decompressed with a large-gauge needle. Just aspirating the air should decrease the tension enough to allow the cecum to be manipulated with less risk of rupture and gross contamination of the abdominal cavity. When the cecal wall contains patches of frank necrosis or areas of questionable viability, resection is necessary. The surgeon then has the option of doing either an ileostomy or a primary anastomosis. The surgeon should base this decision on the patient's overall condition, the presence or absence of fecal contamination, and the condition of the bowel at the site of the anastomosis. Although published reports neither support nor contraindicate primary anastomosis, we at Mayo Clinic believe that it adds little to the morbidity and mortality of most patients.

When the bowel is viable, the alternatives are to resect with or without anastomosis or to conduct cecopexy, cecostomy, cecopexy with cecostomy, or detorsion alone. Tejler and Jiborn[24] compiled the results of operations from 15

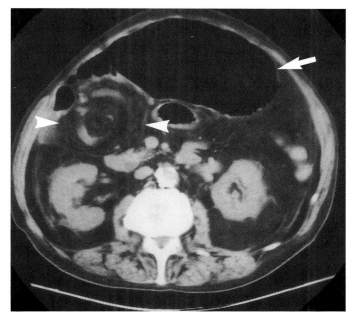

Fig. 3. A computed tomogram of a large, air-filled cecal volvulus (arrow) *and a whirl sign* (arrowheads) *caused by twisted mesentery.*

reports published from 1972 to 1986. They examined only the results for patients who had cecal volvulus without gangrene. The recurrence rates were 13% for detorsion alone, 13% for cecopexy, and 1% for cecostomy. Mortality was not significantly different for the procedures, ranging from 5% with cecopexy to 13% for detorsion alone. Patients with resection had an 8% mortality rate.

In the absence of a prospective randomized study, no firm recommendations can be made about which procedure is best. Any of these options is a viable alternative. In the Mayo Clinic series reported by Ballantyne et al.,[3] the most common procedure was resection with primary anastomosis. Thirty-five of 66 patients who had surgery for cecal volvulus had this procedure. Twelve patients had cecopexy, 11 had detorsion alone, and 4 had cecostomy. The mortality was 8.3% to 14% and did not differ significantly among the groups. The only recurrence was in the patients with detorsion alone. A more recent report from Mayo Clinic by Benacci and Wolff[25] updated their experience with tube cecostomy for treatment of cecal volvulus. They reported three postoperative deaths in nine cases. No death was related to placement of the cecostomy tube but instead resulted from severe preexisting medical conditions.

I have found that the large dilated cecum will not lay satisfactorily in the right lower quadrant. Thus, it is technically difficult to do either a cecopexy or a cecostomy. In most cases, I favor resection with primary anastomosis.

VOLVULUS OF THE SIGMOID COLON

Diagnosis

The most prominent features in patients who present with sigmoid colonic volvulus are abdominal pain and distention, which are also most prominent in cecal volvulus. The mean duration of symptoms before presentation is 3 to 4 days.[12,26] Plain radiographs can be diagnostic, but in many cases a barium enema is necessary to establish the diagnosis. In the study by Ballantyne,[4] plain abdominal radiographs were diagnostic in 37% of patients. A barium enema established the diagnosis in 20% more, for an overall diagnosis with preoperative radiographs of 57%. Hiltunen et al.[12] reported that plain radiographs were suggestive of the diagnosis in 62% of patients.

Plain abdominal radiographs will show a dilated sigmoid loop that extends upward from the pelvis into the upper abdomen. The dilated loop will lack haustra and will have a paucity of fecal material; a white line is observable where the two loops of sigmoid colon are juxtaposed (Fig. 4). When the colon is dilated proximal to the obstruction, plain radiographs are more difficult to interpret.[27] A colonic radiograph using contrast media given by enema will demonstrate a tapering obstruction called a "bird's beak" deformity at the site of the torsion. As in cecal volvulus, computed tomography may demonstrate the whirl sign, a round soft-tissue mass in a whirled configuration[28] that is created by the torsed limbs of the colon.

Treatment

The initial treatment of sigmoid colonic volvulus is endoscopic decompression, which can be done with a rigid or flexible sigmoidoscope with an expected success rate of about 80%. At Mayo Clinic, 25 of 31 attempts (81%) at sigmoidoscopic decompression were successful.[3] Usually, the point of torsion can be reached with a rigid proctoscope, but a flexible sigmoidoscope should be tried if torsion cannot be reduced with a proctoscope. Friedman et al.[5] reduced sigmoid volvulus with a flexible sigmoidoscope in three patients who had a volvulus beyond the reach of the rigid endoscope.

When endoscopic decompression cannot be accomplished or there are signs of ischemic bowel, an immediate operation is indicated. Ischemic, ulcerated mucosa on endoscopy also is an indication for an operation. Any patient

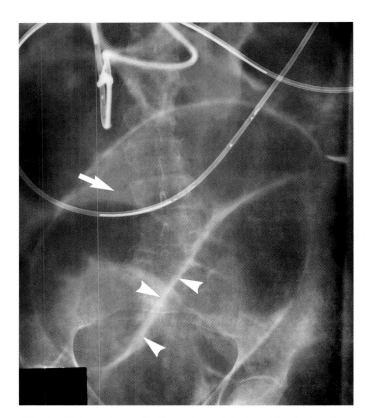

Fig. 4. Plain radiograph of a patient with sigmoid colonic volvulus shows the lack of haustra, a dilated viscus folded back on itself (arrow), and a white line where the two loops of dilated bowel are juxtaposed (arrowheads). A tube has been placed by mouth for decompression of the small bowel.

whose volvulus is successfully decompressed should nevertheless continue to be observed. In the series by Hiltunen et al.,[12] necrosis could not be predicted by preoperative symptoms, signs, or laboratory tests, and the sigmoid colon was later found to be necrotic in 12% of patients.

A successful endoscopic decompression should be regarded only as a temporary measure because of the high incidence of recurrent volvulus. In a series by Chung et al.,[29] 12 of 14 patients (86%) who refused surgery after successful endoscopic decompression had recurrent volvulus a median of 2.8 months later. Other reported rates of recurrence vary from 29% to 90%.[12,22,30,31] Arnold and Nance[31] and Peoples et al.[32] recommended that patients older than 70 years with a first episode of volvulus that is decompressed successfully should be managed by observation alone. They based this recommendation on the high operative mortality in patients older than 70 years. However, they also recommended surgical intervention in all patients younger than 70 years. Bak and Boley[33] recommended surgery in all appropriate candidates, regardless of age. Their recommendation was based on the low mortality rate for elective procedures (5.6% in patients 65 years old or older) and the high mortality rate for recurrent volvulus (22%). The experience at Mayo Clinic is similar. Forty-two patients had operations for volvulus with no mortality: 7 had detorsion alone, 25 had resection with primary anastomosis, and 10 had resection with end-sigmoid colostomy. Regardless of age, patients who can tolerate an operation should have the procedure.

Conventional surgical procedures in either emergency or elective surgery for sigmoid volvulus include detorsion alone, detorsion with sigmoidopexy, resection with stoma, or resection with primary anastomosis. More novel treatments are mesosigmoidoplasty,[34] extraperitonealization,[35,36] or endoscopic sigmoidopexy.[37,38]

When there is gangrene or necrosis of the sigmoid colon, resection is necessary. In this situation, the safest procedure is probably resection and an end colostomy with either a mucous fistula or oversewing of the distal end. In low-risk patients, a primary anastomosis may be considered with or without proximal intraoperative colon lavage.

When the sigmoid colon is viable, nonresective alternatives such as sigmoidopexy or detorsion alone are alternatives, but they both have a high risk of recurrence. In a series of 84 patients, Bhatnagar and Sharma[35] had 36 who had previous operations for volvulus. Fifteen patients had had a laparotomy with detorsion alone, and 21 had had a sigmoidopexy.

If possible, patients who undergo successful decompression with an endoscope should have a bowel preparation and elective surgery during the same hospitalization. In most cases, resection with primary anastomosis can be done with low morbidity. Reports have indicated a high incidence of recurrence in patients who have a sigmoid resection and an associated megacolon. Chung et al.[29] found that 6 (22%) of 27 patients who had a sigmoid resection had recurrence and that 4 of these 6 patients had megacolon. Morrissey and Deitch[39] reported recurrent volvulus in 7 (37%) of 19 patients who had a sigmoid resection and anastomosis. The recurrence rate was 82% in patients with megacolon and only 6% in patients without it. Harbrecht and Fry[40] also reported three cases of recurrent volvulus despite sigmoid resection in patients who had associated megacolon. Thus, a subtotal colectomy should be considered in patients who have sigmoid volvulus and associated megacolon.

Endoscopic sigmoidopexy was reported in two patients deemed too ill to undergo a surgical procedure.[37,38] The same equipment and procedure were used to place percutaneous endoscopic gastrostomy tubes. One patient had two tubes placed to fix the colon, and the other had one tube placed. Both patients did well and eventually died of heart disease without recurrent volvulus.

Elective extraperitonealization was recommended by Bhatnagar and Sharma[35] and Avisar et al.[36] This procedure involves creating a space between the peritoneum and the left lateral endoabdominal fascia and the posterior rectus fascia, then placing the redundant sigmoid colon in this space through an opening made in the peritoneum of the left lower pericolic gutter. Avisar et al. treated 11 patients this way without mortality or recurrence. All 11 patients had previous nonoperative endoscopic reduction. Bhatnagar and Sharma treated 84 patients similarly with a 9% operative mortality.

At Mayo Clinic, elective resection of sigmoid colonic volvulus with primary anastomosis of the sigmoid colon to the rectum has been done with a low mortality rate (0%). This operation is our preferred procedure in patients who are surgical candidates.

VOLVULUS OF THE TRANSVERSE COLON

The diagnosis of volvulus of the transverse colon and its splenic flexure usually can be made from plain abdominal radiographs, computed tomograms, or contrast radiographs using barium sulfate or meglumine diatrizoate. Treatment almost always involves resection with primary anastomosis or colostomy. The latter is used when patients present with shock, peritonitis, or severe comorbid conditions.

REFERENCES

1. Jones IT, Fazio VW: Colonic volvulus: etiology and management. Dig Dis 7:203-209, 1989
2. Bagarani M, Conde AS, Longo R, Italiano A, Terenzi A, Venuto G: Sigmoid volvulus in west Africa: a prospective study on surgical treatments. Dis Colon Rectum 36:186-190, 1993
3. Ballantyne GH, Brandner MD, Beart RW Jr, Ilstrup DM: Volvulus of the colon: incidence and mortality. Ann Surg 202:83-92, 1985
4. Ballantyne GH: Review of sigmoid volvulus: clinical patterns and pathogenesis. Dis Colon Rectum 25:823-830, 1982
5. Friedman JD, Odland MD, Bubrick MP: Experience with colonic volvulus. Dis Colon Rectum 32:409-416, 1989
6. Khanna PR, Gangopadhyay AN, Shahoo SP, Khanna AK: Sigmoid volvulus in childhood: report of six cases. Pediatr Surg Int 16:132-133, 2000
7. Smith SD, Golladay ES, Wagner C, Seibert JJ: Sigmoid volvulus in childhood. South Med J 83:778-781, 1990
8. O'Mara CS, Wilson TH Jr, Stonesifer GL, Cameron JL: Cecal volvulus: analysis of 50 patients with long-term follow-up. Ann Surg 189:724-731, 1979
9. Houshian S, Sorensen JS, Jensen KE: Volvulus of the transverse colon in children. J Pediatr Surg 33:1399-1401, 1998
10. Wolfer JA, Beaton LE, Anson BJ: Volvulus of the cecum: anatomical factors in its etiology; report of a case. Surg Gynecol Obstet 74:882-894, 1942
11. Donhauser JL, Atwell S: Volvulus of the cecum, with review of 100 cases in literature and report of 6 new cases. Arch Surg 58:129-148, 1949
12. Hiltunen KM, Syrja H, Matikainen M: Colonic volvulus: diagnosis and results of treatment in 82 patients. Eur J Surg 158:607-611, 1992
13. Montes H, Wolf J: Cecal volvulus in pregnancy. Am J Gastroenterol 94:2554-2556, 1999
14. Lopez Carral JM, Esen UI, Chandrashekar MV, Rogers IM, Olajide F: Volvulus of the right colon in pregnancy. Int J Clin Pract 52:270-271, 1998
15. Connolly MM, Unti JA, Nora PF: Bowel obstruction in pregnancy. Surg Clin North Am 75:101-113, 1995
16. Goldthorp WO: Intestinal obstruction during pregnancy and the puerperium. Br J Clin Pract 20:367-376, 1966
17. Anderson JR, Welch GH: Acute volvulus of the right colon: an analysis of 69 patients. World J Surg 10:336-342, 1986
18. Haskin PH, Teplick SK, Teplick JG, Haskin ME: Volvulus of the cecum and right colon. JAMA 245:2433-2435, 1981
19. Frank AJ, Goffner LB, Fruauff AA, Losada RA: Cecal volvulus: the CT whirl sign. Abdom Imaging 18:288-289, 1993
20. Rabinovici R, Simansky DA, Kaplan O, Mavor E, Manny J: Cecal volvulus. Dis Colon Rectum 33:765-769, 1990
21. Anderson MJ Sr, Okike N, Spencer RJ: The colonoscope in cecal volvulus: report of three cases. Dis Colon Rectum 21:71-74, 1978
22. Brothers TE, Strodel WE, Eckhauser FE: Endoscopy in colonic volvulus. Ann Surg 206:1-4, 1987
23. Patel D, Ansari E, Berman MD: Percutaneous decompression of cecal volvulus. AJR Am J Roentgenol 148:747-748, 1987
24. Tejler G, Jiborn H: Volvulus of the cecum: report of 26 cases and review of the literature. Dis Colon Rectum 31:445-449, 1988
25. Benacci JC, Wolff BG: Cecostomy: therapeutic indications and results. Dis Colon Rectum 38:530-534, 1995
26. Khanna AK, Kumar P, Khanna R: Sigmoid volvulus: study from a north Indian hospital. Dis Colon Rectum 42:1081-1084, 1999
27. Javors BR, Baker SR, Miller JA: The northern exposure sign: a newly described finding in sigmoid volvulus. AJR Am J Roentgenol 173:571-574, 1999
28. Shaff MI, Himmelfarb E, Sacks GA, Burks DD, Kulkarni MV: The whirl sign: a CT finding in volvulus of the large bowel. J Comput Assist Tomogr 9:410, 1985
29. Chung YF, Eu KW, Nyam DC, Leong AF, Ho YH, Seow-Choen F: Minimizing recurrence after sigmoid volvulus. Br J Surg 86:231-233, 1999
30. Hines JR, Geurkink RE, Bass RT: Recurrence and mortality rates in sigmoid volvulus. Surg Gynecol Obstet 124:567-570, 1967
31. Arnold GJ, Nance FC: Volvulus of the sigmoid colon. Ann Surg 177:527-537, 1973
32. Peoples JB, McCafferty JC, Scher KS: Operative therapy for sigmoid volvulus: identification of risk factors affecting outcome. Dis Colon Rectum 33:643-646, 1990
33. Bak MP, Boley SJ: Sigmoid volvulus in elderly patients. Am J Surg 151:71-75, 1986
34. Subrahmanyam M: Mesosigmoplasty as a definitive operation for sigmoid volvulus. Br J Surg 79:683-684, 1992
35. Bhatnagar BN, Sharma CL: Nonresective alternative for the cure of nongangrenous sigmoid volvulus. Dis Colon Rectum 41:381-388, 1998
36. Avisar E, Abramowitz HB, Lernau OZ: Elective extraperitonealization for sigmoid volvulus: an effective and safe alternative. J Am Coll Surg 185:580-583, 1997
37. Chiulli RA, Swantkowski TM: Sigmoid volvulus treated with endoscopic sigmoidopexy. Gastrointest Endosc 39:194-196, 1993
38. Choi D, Carter R: Endoscopic sigmoidopexy: a safer way to treat sigmoid volvulus? J R Coll Surg Edinb 43:64, 1998
39. Morrissey TB, Deitch EA: Recurrence of sigmoid volvulus after surgical intervention. Am Surg 60:329-331, 1994
40. Harbrecht PJ, Fry DE: Recurrence of volvulus after sigmoidectomy. Dis Colon Rectum 22:420-424, 1979

Chapter 40

Familial Adenomatous Polyposis

Eric J. Dozois, M.D.
Roger R. Dozois, M.D.

Familial adenomatous polyposis (FAP) is a dominantly inherited, tumor-predisposing disease typically characterized by a myriad of adenomas distributed throughout the gastrointestinal tract, but predominantly in the colon and rectum, where the risk of early cancer is nearly certain. The number of polyps can range from a few to hundreds and even thousands. The polyps are often associated with extracolonic manifestations involving the ectodermal, endodermal, and mesodermal tissues. The oft-cited number of 100 polyps varies predominantly with age in a disease that usually manifests during adolescence. The genetic disorder transmitted autosomally is caused by a mutation of the *APC* gene located on chromosome 5q21-22; the estimated gene frequency is 1 in 13,000 to 1 in 24,000 people.[1] Because of the autosomal dominant pattern of inheritance, first-degree relatives have a 50% chance of carrying the gene responsible for the genesis of FAP.

A better understanding of the natural history of the disease and of its molecular genetics is increasingly important for establishing an accurate diagnosis, providing appropriate treatment, and planning surveillance.

COLORECTAL DISEASE

Natural History and Clinical Course

Adenomatous polyps, especially those of the colon and rectum, begin to appear at puberty or even earlier in life. Symptoms such as bleeding, change in bowel habit, and abdominal pain are unusual before the age of 20 years and may herald large or very dense polyps, desmoid tumors, or even carcinomas. Most patients are 20 to 35 years old before symptoms appear. They may have iron deficiency anemia, weight loss, and a palpable abdominal or rectal mass. Symptomatic FAP is rare in children younger than 10 years. By age 40 years, cancer almost always complicates the polypoid disease and may be unresectable in patients with symptoms. The diagnosis of FAP should be strongly suspected in younger patients with a family history of colorectal cancer, duodenal cancer, or desmoid tumors; colorectal symptoms; a palpable soft tissue mass; and the finding of congenital hypertrophy of the retinal pigment epithelium on retinoscopy.

An attenuated phenotype of FAP may be suspected when polyps are few, the disease expresses itself later in life (third or fourth decade), and when the polyps are located more proximally in the right colon.[1] The attenuated form may be the result of mutations in the region of the *APC* gene 5q21 and may be particularly difficult to recognize, especially if the germline mutation is spontaneous and not associated with a family history suggestive of the disease.

Colorectal Cancer, Extracolonic Manifestations and Genetics

Somatic mutation of the normal APC allele coupled with prior inherited or spontaneous germline mutation of the other allele may lead to development of dysplastic colorectal epithelium and microscopic adenomas early in life.[1]

Also, phenotypic variants of FAP with mutations of the same *APC* gene 5q21 exist but are of a different type or site.[2] Such mutations lead to various extracolonic manifestations, including osteomas, epidermoid cysts, dental abnormalities, desmoid tumors (particularly in the mesentery), and tumors of the central nervous system, thyroid, liver, adrenal cortex, biliary tract, and pancreas. The term "familial adenomatous polyposis" is preferred to eponyms such as Gardner's syndrome (referring to the association of osteomas, epidermoid cysts, dental abnormalities, and desmoid tumors) or Turcot's syndrome (the association of certain tumors of the central nervous system and FAP). Retinoscopy to detect congenital hypertrophy of the retinal pigment epithelium, once used as a marker of FAP, has been largely replaced by genetic testing.

Evaluation

In addition to a careful history and physical examination, evaluation should include endoscopy of the upper and lower gastrointestinal tract, imaging, and genetic testing.

The finding of numerous adenomatous polyps on screening sigmoidoscopy or colonoscopy is diagnostic of FAP. Even the presence of a single adenoma in a patient younger than 40 years should raise suspicion of an inherited predisposition to colorectal cancer. Family members at risk and those with positive results of genetic testing should undergo annual flexible sigmoidoscopy beginning at puberty.

Colonoscopy is helpful for determining the extent of the disease and timing of operation and is useful in patients suspected of having the attenuated form of FAP.

Genetic Testing

Indirect testing by linkage analysis was the first genetic test to identify the mutation site of FAP in a small region of chromosome 5q21.[3] Because several family members are needed for this type of analysis, the benefits of linkage analysis are limited to only patients with FAP who have a known family history of the disease.

Direct genetic testing became feasible when the *APC* gene on chromosome 5q21 was observed to be mutated in the germline in FAP, such mutations resulting in a truncated protein.[4] Because of the detection of this abnormal protein, a clinical test became available which is useful for determining whether other family members are affected. In about 30% of patients, FAP can develop as a result of the new germline mutation that occurred at the time of their conception.[4]

The APC mutation detected by protein truncation testing has a sensitivity of 80% and a specificity of 100%; the mutation detected by linkage analysis has a sensitivity of 95% and a specificity of 98% to 99%.[1] Uncovering the mutation by protein truncation testing or the gene predicting carrier status by linkage analysis is useful to make appropriate surveillance recommendations to patients with FAP.

Recent and future studies of genotype-phenotype correlations may help predict the risk of cancer in the duodenum or rectum or elsewhere in the gastrointestinal tract.

Surgical Treatment

Indications and Timing for Operation

The principal indication for operation in FAP is the need to excise adenomatous-bearing mucosa to prevent the development of large bowel cancer. Even though patients may be asymptomatic and at low risk for cancer when the polyps first appear in adolescence, cancer may appear at any age and occasionally has been reported in patients younger than 10 years. Thus, operation is usually advised when the polyps are first discovered, in most instances when patients are in their mid-teenage years. Waiting until a patient is in the late teens or 20s before operating may be risky. Operation should be performed earlier if malignant transformation of the polyps is identified or if patients have complications, such as bleeding.

Choice of Operation

Because adenocarcinoma of the colon or rectum or both will develop in virtually all patients with untreated FAP, prophylactic proctocolectomy is indicated. The two principal surgical options are 1) colectomy with initial ileorectal anastomosis (IRA), often followed at a later age by proctectomy with ileal pouch-anal anastomosis (IPAA) (secondary IPAA), and 2) immediate restorative proctocolectomy with IPAA (primary IPAA). Proctocolectomy with ileostomy, either continent (Kock pouch) or incontinent (Brooke ileostomy), is seldom used and only under unusual circumstances. Each of these operations has its advantages and disadvantages.

Colectomy With Ileorectal Anastomosis

The rationale for IRA is that it removes most of the cancer-prone, large-intestinal mucosa in a straightforward, one-stage operation while preserving anorectal function. The advantages are numerous. It is a safe operation associated with minimal complications (Table 1), and it can be performed by well-trained surgical generalists. Also, because little, if any, perirectal dissection is done, the risk of damage to the sympathetic and parasympathetic pelvic nerves with consequent urinary and sexual dysfunction is minimal.

Some authors further argue that because the risk of rectal cancer is greatest after patients are older (50 to 55 years old), IRA is preferable initially in most young patients.[5] A secondary IPAA may be indicated later in life. The reasoning behind this proposal is further sustained by the observations that patients with IRA have fewer complications, lesser stool frequency, and better continence than their IPAA counterparts.[6]

The major disadvantage of IRA is that the rectum, with its propensity to form polyps and cancer, is left in place.[5,7] Thus, patients need close and frequent surveillance

Table 1.—Outcome of Ileorectal Anastomosis in Patients With Familial Adenomatous Polyposis

| Institution | No. of patients | Mean no. of stools per 24 hours | % of patients | | | | | |
| | | | Complications | Fecally continent | | Seepage of stool | | Quality of life (good or excellent) |
				Day	Night	Day	Night	
Mayo Clinic	21	4	17	83	89	11	11	NR
Cleveland Clinic	51	4	17	82	NR	8		93
St. Mark's Hospital	62	3	21	72	NR	NR		NR
St.-Antoine Hospital	23	3	NR	98	96	NR		NR
University of Toronto	60	< 6 (75%)	23	90	87	10	13	80

NR, not reported.
Modified from Soravia et al.[15] By permission of the American Society of Colon and Rectal Surgeons.

of the rectal remnant with the necessity of endoscopically destroying polyps, which in itself is not always problem-free and relies heavily on the assiduity of the patient to have the frequent examinations. Also, despite rigorous endoscopic surveillance, invasive cancer not only may appear but also may be difficult to detect.

Finally, and most importantly, the risk of rectal cancer remains, and the cancer is potentially lethal. In the Mayo Clinic series, the rectal cancer risk was 32% 20 years after IRA.[7] More recently, almost identical data have been reported by the St. Mark's Hospital in London, England.[5] Of even greater concern, the cancers may be advanced and incurable. In the St. Mark's series, 5 of 11 cancers were Dukes' class C.[8] In many such patients, the entire rectum needs to be resected to maximize the possibility of cure. Thus, the opportunity to perform an IPAA may be lost. In the Leeds Castle Polyposis Group data, the 5-year survival rate after proctectomy for rectal cancer after previous IRA was 71%.[9] Another serious concern derives from the findings of Penna et al.[10] in France and of Heiskanen and Jarvinen[11] in Finland. The French group reported that in a series of 29 patients with IRA, cancer developed in 7; 3 had the diagnosis preoperatively, and 4 had cancer discovered only intraoperatively. The Finnish group reported that despite rigorous surveillance, rectal cancer was diagnosed in 9 of 100 patients with FAP treated by IRA. We found that the two rectal cancers in 49 teenagers with FAP were found only intraoperatively, one being a stage III cancer.[12] In the St. Mark's experience, as well as ours at Mayo Clinic, rectal cancers may be recognized as soon as 6 months after a previous endoscopy.[5]

Proctocolectomy With Primary IPAA

The rationale for this operation is that it removes all of the cancer-prone colorectal mucosa while preserving rectal functions by constructing a neorectum. The major advantage is that it theoretically eliminates the risk of rectal cancer. Also, the operation avoids a permanent stoma and a potentially troublesome perineal wound. Finally, surveillance of the neorectum need not be so rigorous.

The disadvantages of the operation are that it is more complex to perform and the risk of complications may be greater, at least in theory, especially in less experienced hands. Dissection and removal of the rectum may affect continence and cause sexual and bladder dysfunction. Finally, the development of ileal reservoir adenomas may predispose to carcinoma, and thus postoperative surveillance of the neorectum is necessary.

Mayo Clinic Experience

Between 1981 and 1994, 187 patients with FAP had proctocolectomy and IPAA at Mayo Clinic in Rochester, Minnesota.[13] Their ages ranged from 11 to 59 years, and they were followed for an average of 60 months. All patients had a transanal "mucosectomy" and a hand-sewn anastomosis of the ileal reservoir to the anal canal at the dentate line. A temporary ileostomy was established in 85% of patients.

No patient died in the early postoperative period, although two patients died later of metastatic colorectal carcinoma. The overall postoperative morbidity rate was 24%, small bowel obstruction being the most common complication (13%). It necessitated reoperation in 3.2% of patients. Pelvic sepsis and pouchitis were rare (1.6% and 3%, respectively). Patients had four bowel movements per 24 hours and good but not perfect fecal control (Table 2). No patient had a new cancer develop after IPAA.

Results were nearly identical in a more recent series of 48 teenagers who had operation at Mayo Clinic.[12] Of interest, one patient with a colonic carcinoma diagnosed preoperatively died of metastatic disease. Also, in two

Table 2.—Outcome of Ileal Pouch-Anal Anastomosis in Patients With Familial Adenomatous Polyposis

Institution	No. of patients	Mean no. of stools per 24 hours	% of patients					
			Complications	Continence		Seepage		Quality of life (good or excellent)
				Day	Night	Day	Night	
Mayo Clinic	187	4	24	84	80	12	22	98
Cleveland Clinic	62	5	NR	75	74	25	20	95
St. Mark's Hospital	37	5	60	60	NR	NR		NR
St.-Antoine Hospital	171	4	27	98	96	3.2	6.4	NR
University of Toronto	50	< 6 (70%)	26	75	51	25	49	93

NR, not reported.
Modified from Soravia et al.[15] By permission of the American Society of Colon and Rectal Surgeons.

other patients, rectal cancer, previously unsuspected, was found intraoperatively, and the stage of the disease was stage III in one. Importantly, none had sexual dysfunction, and the following activities were either improved or unchanged: social (83% of patients), sexual (87%), sport (80%), housework (90%), recreation (80%), family (93%), travel (78%), and work (89%).

IRA Versus IPAA
More and more groups favor IPAA, but the debate persists as to which operation is best. Surgeons need to be mindful of several issues. Neither operation is a perfect solution for all situations, and the choice of operation must be individualized. IRA can be reasonably contemplated in the rare patients who have few or no rectal polyps, because the likelihood for development of rectal cancer may be diminished.[14] IRA also may be considered in patients with advanced colon cancer that is unlikely to be cured and will necessitate adjuvant therapy, especially if the rectum is minimally involved. Finally, IRA may be preferable if desmoid disease involves the distal small bowel mesentery, making IPAA difficult or even impossible technically. In most patients, our preference is primary IPAA.

Comparison of results of IRA and IPAA in many large referral centers with extensive experience with both operations shows minimal differences in the postoperative morbidity and mortality rates. Indeed, when Soravia et al.[15] from the University of Toronto compared results from Cleveland Clinic, Mayo Clinic, St.-Antoine Hospital in Paris, St. Mark's Hospital in London, and the University of Toronto, the complication rates and functional results were remarkably similar among the five institutions, and no institution reported perfect continence with either operation. Each center witnessed some degree of daytime and nighttime seepage after both operations. Seepage was

present in 8% to 49% of patients at risk (Tables 1 and 2). Furthermore, when quality of life after operation was assessed, no major difference between the two operations was discerned (Tables 1 and 2).

Secondary IPAA, namely, the conversion from IRA to IPAA at a later age, may not always be technically feasible and is associated with a greater risk of complications than is primary IPAA. Penna et al.[10] showed that such a conversion may not be feasible technically or may be ill advised for oncologic reasons. In another study, the risk of postoperative complications was nearly doubled when a secondary IPAA was performed (60%)[6] as opposed to a primary IPAA (30%). In our hands, the risk of sexual dysfunction after secondary IPAA was also greater.[13] In yet another study, the overall risk of complications was 40% after primary IPAA and 56% after secondary IPAA.[16] Admittedly, in some patients who have IPAA, the operation may fail and necessitate a permanent abdominal stoma. This is a tragic outcome, considering the patients' young age. But even more tragic is the development of rectal cancer, which not only may result in the need for permanent stoma but also, more importantly, may jeopardize the patient's life. For all of these reasons, most authors now favor IPAA as the initial operation for the majority of patients with FAP.

Surgical Decision Making Based on Genetic Testing
Molecular genetic testing has been proposed as a guide to decision making in the surgical management of patients with FAP. Some authors have suggested that patients with an APC mutation before codon 1250 may have a lower risk for development of rectal carcinoma and should, therefore, be reasonable candidates for colectomy and IRA.[17] In another study, among 31 patients with a mutation on APC outside codon 1309 and 1328 sites who had IRA,

only 1 patient required secondary proctectomy because of florid proliferation of rectal polyps.[18]

However, in both of these reports, the decision to perform IRA instead of IPAA was not made according to the actual mutation location but rather was based on the degree of rectal involvement by polyps, and this clinical criterion alone could explain the findings. In the future, these observations will need to be supported by longer follow-up and further genotype-phenotype correlation before the value of molecular genetic testing in surgical decision making can be clearly established in FAP carriers. Also, even though the risk of rectal cancer in such a subset of IRA patients might be less, it would not be eliminated.

Proctocolectomy With Ileostomy

Proctocolectomy with an incontinent Brooke end ileostomy or a Kock continent ileostomy, the so-called Kock pouch, is rarely performed because patients generally prefer other options that allow preservation of anorectal function and the avoidance of a permanent stoma.

These operations may, however, be the best and indeed the only options in patients with invasive cancers of the lower rectum, in whom oncologic results would be compromised by an IPAA, and in patients with incompetent anal sphincters.

The operations also may be feasible in patients with a failed IRA or a failed IPAA when a secondary IPAA is not possible. In these circumstances, and if the patient wants to preserve continence and avoid an appliance, the existing ileal reservoir may be used to create a Kock pouch.[19] A Brooke ileostomy is preferable in older, obese patients, in whom a Kock pouch is fraught with a high complication rate, especially relating to use of the nipple valve that provides continence to the pouch, or in patients who want to have a simple, single-stage operation.

Surveillance After Operation

Because the rate of cancer has been reported to be as high as 32% in a retained rectum of FAP patients at risk 20 years after colectomy[7] and 29% at 60 years of age in patients who have had ileostomy,[5] proctoscopy and biopsies of the residual rectum are necessary every 6 months. The development of clusters of polyps or a carpeting of polyps in the rectum, the need for more and more frequent endoscopic ablations, the appearance of malignant changes, or the impossibility to control adequately the rectal polyposis are all indications for proctectomy.

Adenomas can develop in the ileal reservoir after IPAA or after the Kock pouch operation.[20-23] Although the natural history of ileal pouch polyps is unknown, polyps have been reported as early as 3 to 4 years after establishment of an ileostomy or ileal reservoir, but most

carcinomas have been reported after 20 years.[21] Surveillance of the ileal pouch is needed (Fig. 1). Because there appears to be a close correlation between the frequency of duodenal adenomas and neorectal adenomas, it has been proposed that "pouchoscopy" be performed as frequently as upper gastrointestinal endoscopy, namely, every 2 to 3 years.[23] This approach will need to be further defined. In patients who had a stapled IPAA without mucosectomy and in whom some residual anal canal mucosa remains distal to the stapled anastomosis, endoscopy possibly should be as frequent as that recommended after IRA.

DESMOID DISEASE

Desmoid tumors are rare, benign fibromatous lesions forming a heterogeneous group of pathologic entities resulting from the proliferation of well-differentiated fibroblasts.[24,25] Desmoid tumors may be well encapsulated and have the appearance of a well-defined mass in the mesentery (Fig. 2), most often at the site of a previous operation (Fig. 3), or within the abdominal wall itself or both. Sometimes, desmoid tumors lack encapsulation and have a whitish, infiltrative plaquelike appearance, often referred to as mesenteric fibromatosis (Fig. 4). Other important observations now documented by several authors include familial clustering of the disease among certain kindreds, preponderance of women, and variable growth patterns.[24] In some patients the disease progresses rapidly and aggressively, whereas in others it is more indolent.

The cause of the disease and what regulates its rate of growth are unknown. Operation seems to have a definite triggering effect on desmoid growth. Some observations

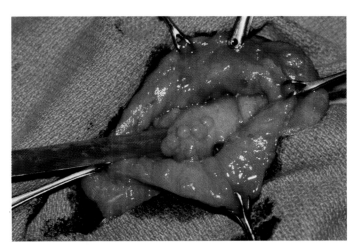

Fig. 1. Multiple adenomas of Kock pouch reservoir in a patient with familial adenomatous polyposis. The ileum immediately proximal to the pouch was free of polyps.

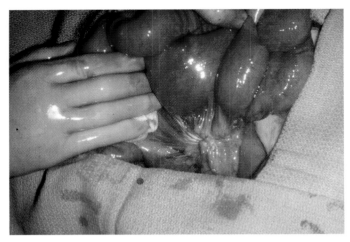

Fig. 2. Infiltrative, whitish desmoid mass located at root of mesentery, causing retraction, kinking, and shortening of the small intestinal mesentery.

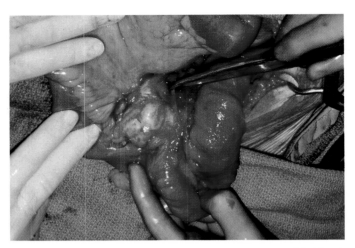

Fig. 3. Desmoid tumor forming a mass at the junction of the distal ileum and cecum, at the site of a previous appendectomy.

also suggest, although do not clearly prove, that hormones, especially estrogen, play some sort of regulatory role.[26] These include the higher incidence of desmoid tumors in women during their reproductive years, the apparent tendency of these tumors to develop during pregnancy or soon after, their occasional disappearance after menopause, the production of similar lesions in laboratory animals by estrogen administration, and the potential benefit of anti-estrogen drugs.[26]

The association of FAP with desmoid tumors was first described by Nichols at Mayo Clinic in 1923[27] and is now well recognized to be present in at least 10% of patients with FAP and to be hereditary.

More recently, genetic studies have suggested a close genotypic-phenotypic correlation between the *APC* gene mutation, the number of colonic polyps, and the presence of desmoid tumors.[25] *APC* germline mutations between codons 1445 to 1578 seem to be associated with extensive polyposis and severe desmoid disease, whereas mutations in codons 1924, 1962, and 1987 correlate with less severe desmoid disease and fewer polyps.[25]

Treatment

Despite the benign histologic appearance of desmoid tumors, their biologic behavior can be rather "malignant" and even cause death. Their high propensity to recurrence and to engulfing surrounding viscera and vessels complicates their management.

Management of desmoid tumors is difficult and controversial with regard to early detection, the role of operation, type of operation, and the value of nonoperative therapies.

Prospective imaging may be of value in planning operation, especially when there is a family history of desmoid

disease. The unexpected finding of a sizable yet asymptomatic desmoid tumor might alter surgical decision making with regard to the type of operation needed. In such instances, an IPAA or an IRA may not be feasible and a conventional ileostomy may prove necessary because of technical reasons. Such a possibility needs to be discussed with the patient and patient's family preoperatively.

Because surgical trauma may predispose to the development of desmoid tumors, it becomes readily apparent that operative management should be reserved for lesions causing major complications and that operation should be minimized as much as feasible.

Excision with minimal sacrifice of intestine is desirable but seldom possible unless the lesions are small, do not involve major portions of the mesenteric blood supply, or are not located at the root of the mesentery. In our experience, two-thirds of patients have unresectable lesions.[26] Even when feasible, total resection is not only often

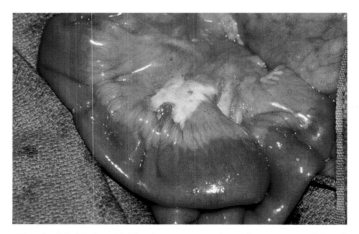

Fig. 4. Multiple whitish plaques on surface of mesentery of distal ileum, often referred to as mesenteric fibromatosis.

ineffective but also may actually promote recurrence and catastrophic complications. For all these reasons, conservatism is favored. Biopsy is preferred to excision. If clinical obstruction warrants operative therapy, bypass, as opposed to major resection, is indicated, followed by a trial of medical therapy. In our experience, small bowel obstruction occurred in nearly half of patients, and in 70% of them diffuse, dense fibrotic adhesions were responsible.[26] Debulking has no place. It almost invariably leads to more aggressive and infiltrative desmoid growth.[25]

When desmoid tumors are located within the abdominal wall and if, after a reasonable period of observation, the lesion is enlarging, operative excision with clear margins should be considered. Incomplete excision is associated with a high likelihood of recurrence.[28] Also, it is important to excise desmoid tumors before they become large. Otherwise, reconstruction of the abdominal wall with synthetic materials or myocutaneous flaps may be necessary.[24] Alternatively, abdominal wall desmoid tumors may be treated with chemotherapeutic agents, especially if there is a mesenteric component or if the abdominal lesion is a recurrence after previous excision.[29]

The unexpected finding of a mesenteric desmoid tumor at the time of a planned IPAA may alter the choice of operation. If the lesion is large and shortens the mesentery, an IRA may be considered, depending on the status of the rectal polyposis. In rare situations, a proctocolectomy and ileostomy may be the only option. If the lesion is small, plaquelike, and away from the distal ileum, an IPAA may still be feasible technically, and there is no clear-cut evidence that it will favor further desmoid disease more than other types of operations.

It has been suggested, however, that the added manipulations associated with IPAA, especially manipulations of the mesentery, might increase the risk of future desmoid disease. In our own experience, among 196 patients who had IPAA, desmoid tumors developed in 11: 4 in the abdominal wall and 7 in the mesentery.[24] Three of the four abdominal wall desmoid tumors were excised locally without recurrence or loss of the ileal pouch, but four of the seven mesenteric desmoid tumors led to a permanent ileostomy.[24] The risk of desmoid tumors has been estimated to be 17% after IRA and 12% after IPAA.[30] Most patients should be treated conservatively at first. Treatments include noncytotoxic pharmacologic agents, chemotherapy, and radiotherapy.

Pharmacologic agents such as antiestrogens, tamoxifen, and nonsteroidal anti-inflammatory drugs, such as sulindac, although they can inhibit in vitro desmoid cell proliferation,[31] have had limited value, especially in the long term.[26,30,32,33] There have been no prospective, randomized trials reporting success.

In the presence of large, unresectable desmoid tumors, especially if they are rapidly growing, a chemotherapeutic regimen, including doxorubicin and dacarbazine, has been successful in our experience and in that of others.[29] The regimen may be used to decrease the size of the lesions preoperatively or as a palliative measure.

Radiotherapy is used as a last resort because it may cause small intestinal injury and is associated with a high rate of failure or recurrence.[25,34] Combination chemotherapy, radiation, and operation has been successful in a few patients, including some of ours, in whom the large mass underwent total necrosis and liquefaction and was amenable to surgical extension.[25,34]

Surveillance Guidelines

Routine computed tomography of the abdomen is not recommended, except in patients with known desmoid tumors. Magnetic resonance imaging may be preferable to computed tomography to assess vascular involvement and predict rate of growth.[33]

UPPER GASTROINTESTINAL DISEASE

Adenomas of the stomach, duodenum, and small intestine occur in nearly all patients with FAP. The second portion of the duodenum, particularly the periampullary region, is most prone to adenomatous transformation. The risk of cancer in this area hovers around 5% or more if there is a family history of such occurrence.[1] Gastric fundic polyps are common (up to 60%), small (1-5 mm), and often diffuse and hyperplastic. If they are an isolated finding, repeat gastroduodenoscopy at 5-year intervals is sufficient.[1] In contrast, gastric antral polyps are less common, are most often adenomatous, and can be found in conjunction with cancer. Gastric adenocarcinomas have been found in our FAP registry patients, but they are uncommon.

The reported risk of duodenal cancer in patients with FAP has varied between 0.5% and 5%. Most authors report a range of 0.3% to 2%.[34] This rate, however, far exceeds that in the general population. The lesions are often located in the periampullary region, where they are surrounded by polyps, a finding that supports the adenoma-carcinoma sequence.[34] Incriminating risk factors include a family history of duodenal neoplasia, the bilious milieu, and possibly the severity of rectal polyposis.[35]

Small intestinal adenomas are rare and carcinomas even more so. Jejunal cancers developed in 5 (0.4%) of 1,255 patients with FAP, as documented by the Leeds Castle Polyposis Group survey of 10 registries.[34]

Treatment

Preoperative staging of neoplasms with computed tomography and endoscopic ultrasonography, including the intraductal approach, may be useful, especially for lesions in the vicinity of the papilla of Vater.[1] When polyps increase in size or number or both or show premalignant features such as villous transformation or severe dysplasia during surveillance, treatment is advisable. Endoscopic ablation of benign ampullary and duodenal lesions by various electrothermal methods or laser is appropriate as initial therapy for smaller benign lesions.[1] When lesions become larger (> 2-3 cm) or are malignant, operation is preferable. This may include "ampullectomy" alone, pancreas-sparing duodenectomy, or even pylorus-preserving pancreaticoduodenectomy.[36,37] Duodenal polyps 2 mm or smaller may regress with sulindac. Larger polyps, especially if more than 10 mm, do not seem to respond.[34] Nugent[38] suggested that sulindac may be useful for lesions smaller than 5 mm with early APC mutations. In the Toronto series, a periampullary cancer developed in one patient receiving the chemopreventive medication.[34] More data from randomized trials are needed to establish the effectiveness of chemoprevention.

Surveillance Guidelines

Esophagogastroduodenoscopy should be done whenever colorectal polyps are discovered. Frequent repeat examinations are advisable when the patient reaches age 20 years to assess rapidity of change and to determine the rate of future endoscopic follow-up. The upper gut examination is recommended every 3 years if polyps are small (< 5 mm) and few (< 20) and if the papilla appears normal.[1] Otherwise, more frequent examinations, perhaps every 1 to 2 years, are advised if polyps are more than 5 mm in size, more than 20 in number, or have worrisome histologic features, especially if the polyps are near the papilla. If no polyps are noted in the presence of a normal papilla, a repeat upper gastrointestinal endoscopy is necessary only every 3 to 5 years.

REFERENCES

1. King JE, Dozois RR, Lindor NM, Ahlquist DA: Care of patients and their families with familial adenomatous polyposis. Mayo Clin Proc 75:57-67, 2000
2. Fodde R, Khan PM: Genotype-phenotype correlations at the adenomatous polyposis coli (APC) gene. Crit Rev Oncog 6:291-303, 1995
3. Leppert M, Dobbs M, Scambler P, O'Connell P, Nakamura Y, Stauffer D, Woodward S, Burt R, Hughes J, Gardner E, Lathrop M, Wasmuth J, Lalouel J-M, White R: The gene for familial polyposis coli maps to the long arm of chromosome 5. Science 238:1411-1413, 1987
4. Petersen GM: Genetic testing and counseling in familial adenomatous polyposis. Oncology (Huntingt) 10:89-94, 1996
5. Nugent KP, Phillips RK: Rectal cancer risk in older patients with familial adenomatous polyposis and an ileorectal anastomosis: a cause for concern. Br J Surg 79:1204-1206, 1992
6. Madden MV, Neale KF, Nicholls RJ, Landgrebe JC, Chapman PD, Bussey HJ, Thomson JP: Comparison of morbidity and function after colectomy with ileorectal anastomosis or restorative proctocolectomy for familial adenomatous polyposis. Br J Surg 78:789-792, 1991
7. Bess MA, Adson MA, Elveback LR, Moertel CG: Rectal cancer following colectomy for polyposis. Arch Surg 115:460-467, 1980
8. Bussey HJ, Eyers AA, Ritchie SM, Thomson JP: The rectum in adenomatous polyposis: the St. Mark's policy. Br J Surg 72 Suppl:S29-S31, 1985
9. De Cosse JJ, Bulow S, Neale K, Jarvinen H, Alm T, Hultcrantz R, Moesgaard F, Costello C: Rectal cancer risk in patients treated for familial adenomatous polyposis. The Leeds Castle Polyposis Group. Br J Surg 79:1372-1375, 1992
10. Penna C, Kartheuser A, Parc R, Tiret E, Frileux P, Hannouon L, Nordlinger B: Secondary proctectomy and ileal pouch-anal anastomosis after ileorectal anastomosis for familial adenomatous polyposis. Br J Surg 80:1621-1623, 1993
11. Heiskanen I, Jarvinen HJ: Fate of the rectal stump after colectomy and ileorectal anastomosis for familial adenomatous polyposis. Int J Colorectal Dis 12:9-13, 1997
12. Parc YR, Moslein G, Dozois RR, Pemberton JH, Wolff BG, King JE: Familial adenomatous polyposis: results after ileal pouch-anal anastomosis in teenagers. Dis Colon Rectum 43:893-898, 2000
13. Nyam DC, Brillant PT, Dozois RR, Kelly KA, Pemberton JH, Wolff BG: Ileal pouch-anal canal anastomosis for familial adenomatous polyposis: early and late results. Ann Surg 226:514-519, 1997
14. Kelly KA, Heppell JP, Dozois RR: Familial adenomatous polyposis. In Current Surgical Therapy. Sixth edition. Edited by JL Cameron. St Louis, Mosby, 1998, pp 214-217
15. Soravia C, Klein L, Berk T, O'Connor BI, Cohen Z, McLeod RS: Comparison of ileal pouch-anal anastomosis and ileorectal anastomosis in patients with familial adenomatous polyposis. Dis Colon Rectum 42:1028-1033, 1999
16. Bjork JA, Akerbrant HI, Iselius LE, Hultcrantz RW: Risk factors for rectal cancer morbidity and mortality in patients with familial

adenomatous polyposis after colectomy and ileorectal anastomosis. Dis Colon Rectum 43:1719-1725, 2000

17. Vasen HF, van der Luijt RB, Slors JF, Buskens E, de Ruiter P, Baeten CG, Schouten WR, Oostvogel HJ, Kuijpers JH, Tops CM, Meera Khan P: Molecular genetic tests as a guide to surgical management of familial adenomatous polyposis. Lancet 348:433-435, 1996

18. Wu JS, Paul P, McGannon EA, Church JM: APC genotype, polyp number, and surgical options in familial adenomatous polyposis. Ann Surg 227:57-62, 1998

19. Dozois RR, Dozois EJ: Continent ileostomy. In Mastery of Surgery. Fourth edition. Edited by RJ Baker, JE Fischer. Philadelphia, Lippincott Williams & Wilkins, 2001, pp 1425-1434

20. Wu JS, McGannon EA, Church JM: Incidence of neoplastic polyps in the ileal pouch of patients with familial adenomatous polyposis after restorative proctocolectomy. Dis Colon Rectum 41:552-556, 1998

21. Geller A, Wang KK, Dozois RR, Batts KP: Laser photoablation of ileal reservoir adenomas. Gastrointest Endosc 44:473-477, 1996

22. Stryker SJ, Carney JA, Dozois RR: Multiple adenomatous polyps arising in a continent reservoir ileostomy. Int J Colorectal Dis 2:43-45, 1987

23. Parc YR, Olschwang S, Desaint B, Schmitt G, Parc RG, Tiret E: Familial adenomatous polyposis: prevalence of adenomas in the ileal pouch after restorative proctocolectomy. Ann Surg 233:360-364, 2001

24. Sagar PM, Moslein G, Dozois RR: Management of desmoid tumors in patients after ileal pouch-anal anastomosis for familial adenomatous polyposis. Dis Colon Rectum 41:1350-1355, 1998

25. Moslein G, Dozois RR: Desmoid tumors associated with familial adenomatous polyposis. Perspect Colon Rectal Surg 10:109-126, 1998

26. Lotfi AM, Dozois RR, Gordon H, Hruska LS, Weiland LH, Carryer PW, Hurt RD: Mesenteric fibromatosis complicating familial adenomatous polyposis: predisposing factors and results of treatment. Int J Colorectal Dis 4:30-36, 1989

27. Nichols RW: Desmoid tumors: a report of 31 cases. Arch Surg 7:227-236, 1923

28. Posner MC, Shiu MH, Newsome JL, Hajdu SI, Gaynor JJ, Brennan MF: The desmoid tumor: not a benign disease. Arch Surg 124:191-196, 1989

29. Schnitzler M, Cohen Z, Blackstein M, Berk T, Gallinger S, Madlensky L, McLeod R: Chemotherapy for desmoid tumors in association with familial adenomatous polyposis. Dis Colon Rectum 40:798-801, 1997

30. Heiskanen I, Jarvinen HJ: Occurrence of desmoid tumours in familial adenomatous polyposis and results of treatment. Int J Colorectal Dis 11:157-162, 1996

31. Tonelli F, Valanzano R, Brandi ML: Pharmacologic treatment of desmoid tumors in familial adenomatous polyposis: results of an in vitro study. Surgery 115:473-479, 1994

32. Penna C, Tiret E, Parc R, Sfairi A, Kartheuser A, Hannoun L, Nordlinger B: Operation and abdominal desmoid tumors in familial adenomatous polyposis. Surg Gynecol Obstet 177:263-268, 1993

33. Clark SK, Phillips RK: Desmoids in familial adenomatous polyposis. Br J Surg 83:1494-1504, 1996

34. Berk T, Cohen Z: Hereditary gastrointestinal polyposis syndromes. In Surgery of the Colon and Rectum. Edited by RJ Nicholls, RR Dozois. New York, Churchill Livingstone, 1997, pp 390-410

35. Spigelman AD, Williams CB, Phillips RK: Rectal polyposis as a guide to duodenal polyposis in familial adenomatous polyposis. J R Soc Med 85:77-79, 1992

36. Kadmon M, Tandara A, Herfarth C: Duodenal adenomatosis in familial adenomatous polyposis coli: a review of the literature and results from the Heidelberg Polyposis Register. Int J Colorectal Dis 16:63-75, 2001

37. Penna C, Bataille N, Balladur P, Tiret E, Parc R: Surgical treatment of severe duodenal polyposis in familial adenomatous polyposis. Br J Surg 85:665-668, 1998

38. Nugent KP: Colorectal cancer: surgical prophylaxis and chemoprevention. Ann R Coll Surg Engl 77:372-376, 1995

Chapter 41

CANCER OF THE RECTUM

Jacques P. Heppell, M.D.
Elizabeth J. McConnell, M.D.
Steven E. Schild, M.D.

Mayo Clinic surgeons of the past were pioneers in the operative treatment of rectal cancer. They provided a large clinical experience in the evaluation of prognostic factors and operative strategies. Mayo Clinic surgeons of today have improved preoperative staging and operative care and determined effective adjuvant therapy. A multidisciplinary approach to the treatment of locally advanced and recurrent disease has been adopted.

Despite the high prevalence of rectal cancer, optimal surgical, medical, and radio-oncologic care remains controversial. The purpose of this chapter is to challenge the surgeon to select the most appropriate approach to cure the patient yet minimize morbidity, recurrence, and mortality. Surgical treatment of rectal cancer should not be viewed as a tumor-specific operation but rather as a patient-specific operation, providing not only improved survival but also an excellent quality of life.[1]

LANDMARKS IN TREATMENT AT MAYO CLINIC

A century ago, Charles H. Mayo, M.D., described his technique of combined abdominal-perineal resection for cancer of the rectum. On August 30, 1904, at the Oregon State Medical Society meeting, he presented a report entitled "Carcinoma of the Large Bowel." It was later published in the Oregon *Medical Sentinel*.[2] Dr. Mayo demonstrated that the combined operation could be performed with less bleeding by defining the avascular plane and leaving intact the short mesentery of the rectum within the fascia.

The following is an excerpt from Dr. Mayo's report:

Our usual method of performing the combined operation is with the patient in Trendelenburg position. Through a median abdominal incision the bowels are pushed into the upper abdomen, where they are retained by a gauze pack. A careful examination of the upper rectum, sigmoid, and lymph-glands is now made, and at times the liver region is also explored, to determine the question whether the operation is to be palliative or an attempt is to be made to secure a permanent cure.

If total extirpation is decided upon, a horseshoe incision of the peritoneum is made, cutting on each side of the rectum and across it below. With dry gauze the fatty tissue of the short mesentery is separated, and the lower sigmoid loosened by blunt dissection. The bowel is now clamped as low as possible, but at least two inches above the cancer, by two pairs of heavy forceps placed close together. The bowel is severed between them: one cut end of the bowel and forceps is protected by gauze; the other end of the bowel is turned in and closed with a purse-string suture, done with the other end, which has been covered by gauze. With both ends closed there is no danger of soiling the peritoneum in the further steps of the operation.

The superior hemorrhoidal artery is ligated, and the proximal sigmoid segment is separated sufficiently to be brought through a McBurney gridiron incision in the iliac fossa. This incision is peculiar in the skin incision, being at a distance of one and one-half inches to one side of the muscle separation. The end of the bowel is brought out and sutured to the skin incision; also a few sutures unite the bowel to the peritoneum at the point of exit....

The distal bowel is now separated and pushed below the uterus and bladder or the bladder and prostate. A gauze pack is placed over this, and the peritoneum nearly closed, forming a pelvic floor, and the abdominal wound is closed, the remainder of the operation being completed from below. A gauze pack is placed in the rectum, to render it palpable, and the anus closed by a purse-string suture. An incision is made around the anus, and separation of the rectum is made until the point is reached where it was loosened from above. All the glands and fascia in front of the coccyx and sacrum are removed at the same time. A portion of the pack previously placed in the pelvis is now withdrawn through the perineal wound for drainage, the remainder of the incision being closed. If the surgeon has a good assistant, the perineal operation, with the removal of the rectum, can be performed by him during the time the abdominal work is advancing above....

C. H. Mayo, M.D.
Rochester, Minn.
Surgeon at St. Mary's Hospital of Rochester, Minn.

As early as 1910, D.C. Balfour, M.D.,[3] described a method of anastomosis between the sigmoid colon and rectum with a rubber tube support. C.F. Dixon, M.D.,[4] further refined the colorectal anastomosis and reemphasized the approach of sharp dissection around the lamina propria, following the guidelines of meticulously cleaning the hollow of the sacrum: "The entire pelvic portion of the colon is now mobilized by manual elevation of the gland-bearing tissues from the hollow of the sacrum...an end-to-end anastomosis is made between the first portion of the sigmoid or the lower end of the descending colon and the upper end of the rectum...." Dixon recognized that the lymphatic spread of rectal cancer typically followed a proximal route, and his technique of anterior resection allowed extirpation of the lymphatics and preservation of the anal sphincter. The anterior resection described by Dixon became known worldwide as the "Mayo Clinic operation." Gradually, this operation gained in popularity and today remains the operation of choice for carcinomas of the rectosigmoid region and upper third of the rectum. Waugh et al.[5] reviewed 444 consecutive patients who had operation during the 10 years from 1941 through 1950 for carcinoma located up to 15 cm from the anal margin. They reported an operative mortality rate of 3.8% and an overall 5-year survival rate of 65.6% with anterior resection, 53% with the sphincter-saving procedure, and 51.6% with the combined abdominoperineal resection. They stated that "technically, the sphincter-preserving procedure should be just as extensive an operation above the levator muscle as the combined abdominoperineal operation of Miles when used for lesions of the mid portion or upper portion

of the rectum." Important contributions to the management of rectal cancer have continued to be made by Mayo Clinic physicians, residents, and alumni (Table 1).[2-20]

SCREENING

Colorectal cancer is the second most common visceral malignancy in the United States. In approximately 40% of cases, the cancer originates from the rectum. In 1999,

Table 1.—Contributions to the Evaluation and Treatment of Rectal Cancer by Mayo Clinic Consultants, Residents, and Alumni

Year	Reference	Contribution
1904	Mayo[2]	Combined abdominoperineal resection
1910	Balfour[3]	Colorectal anastomosis
1939	Dixon[4]	First anterior resection
1952	Black[6]	Abdomino-endorectal resection
1953	Quer, Dahlin, Mayo[7]	Distal margin of resection
1955	Waugh et al.[5]	Comparison of abdominoperineal resection and sphincter-saving operations
1961	Jackman[8]	Local therapy in selected cases
1963	Hallenbeck et al.[9]	An instrument for colorectal anastomosis without sutures
1980	Knight, Griffen[10,11]	Double-stapled anastomosis for rectal reconstruction
1980	Adson et al.[12]	Rectal cancer in familial polyposis
1981	Beart, Kelly[13]	Comparison of hand-sewn and stapled rectal anastomosis. First prospective randomized clinical trial in surgery at Mayo Clinic
1983	Beart, O'Connell[14]	Postoperative follow-up
1985	Ahlquist et al.[15]	Screening of colorectal cancer
1985	GITSG (Moertel)[16]	Prolonged disease-free survival with adjuvant chemoradiation
1989	Dozois et al.[17]	Extended resection for locally advanced disease
1994	Wolff, Pemberton, et al.[18]	Long-term effect of adjuvant chemoradiation therapy on bowel function
1996	Gunderson, Nelson, et al.[19]	Multidisciplinary team approach for local recurrence (IOERT)
1998	Thibodeau et al.[20]	Microsatellite instability as prognostic factor

IOERT, intraoperative electron radiotherapy.

there were 36,400 cases of rectal cancer and about 8,600 patients died of this disease.[21] The majority of patients die with distant metastasis, others with uncontrolled local disease, the symptoms of which are often difficult to palliate.

Colorectal cancer is highly curable when detected early, but almost half of Americans older than 50 years have never been screened for the disease.[22] Because of its high prevalence, its long asymptomatic phase, and the presence of a treatable precancerous lesion, colorectal cancer ideally meets the criteria for screening. In theory, improved detection and removal of premalignant rectal lesions should lead to complete eradication of rectal cancer. Digital rectal examination, flexible sigmoidoscopy, and the fecal occult blood test have been accepted as the screening method for a normal-risk, asymptomatic population, performed every 5 years starting at age 50 years.[23] Despite these recommendations, patients still present with advanced rectal cancer. Ahlquist et al.,[24] at Mayo Clinic, reported that detection of altered human DNA in stool with a multitarget assay panel is a feasible method to screen for both cancers and premalignant adenomas of the colorectum. They are now conducting a large clinical study to determine the usefulness of this noninvasive, sensitive, and specific fecal screening tool. The hope is that the widespread availability of cost-effective, mass population screening programs will allow earlier detection at a better prognostic stage that may be treatable with less invasive procedures.

FACTORS INFLUENCING THE TREATMENT OF RECTAL CANCER

In the evaluation of a patient with rectal cancer, the surgeon must consider many factors that can influence the outcome of treatment. Recommendations then are based on what is the appropriate procedure for each person. Factors related to the patient, the tumor, and the experience of the surgeon must be considered.

Patient-Related Factors

Age

In Mayo Clinic's recent experience, the mean age at diagnosis of rectal cancer was 67 years (range, 23-99).[25] The diagnosis is made before age 40 years in less than 4% of cases.[26] Younger patients have a prognosis similar to that of any age group compared stage for stage.[27] Elderly patients have a slower progression of the disease. Also, they may have weak anal sphincters and poor tolerance to staged operations and adjuvant treatment.[28]

Sex and Physique

Male sex may be a factor in poorer prognosis.[29,30] A sphincter-saving procedure can be technically easier in

women than in men because they have a broader pelvis, which facilitates rectal dissection and lower anastomosis.

The operation is often more difficult in obese or mesomorphic patients. The body mass index may help to determine the likelihood of a successful low colorectal anastomosis.

Symptoms

Patients who present with symptoms from rectal cancer have prognoses similar to those of asymptomatic patients who have a similar disease stage.[27] Weight loss, tenesmus, and sciatic pain in a lower extremity are often ominous signs of late-stage rectal cancer.

Comorbidity

The surgeon should balance the risks and benefits of operation in patients with severe systemic diseases. Cardiovascular and pulmonary complications influence survival considerably.[30] Other factors that should be considered are prior pelvic radiation therapy for prostatic or gynecologic cancer, corticosteroid use, malnutrition, and an age older than 75 years.[28]

Other Conditions

Counseling by a stomal therapist is important before operation.[31] Patients who are blind,[32] have severe arthritis, or are mentally retarded may have a difficult time with a stoma. The use of a disposable plastic liner inside a colostomy appliance may facilitate adaptation in selected cases.[33] On occasion, because of religious, cultural, or personal reasons, patients may refuse conventional treatment.

Tumor-Related Factors

Stage

The depth of rectal wall invasion and lymph node metastasis are the most reliable prognostic predictors in rectal cancer.[34] The number[35] and the location[36] of positive lymph nodes also may be of prognostic value. The prognosis and treatment options for patients with rectal cancer are primarily determined by the TNM stage at diagnosis (Table 2).[37]

Differentiation

Rectal cancer is an adenocarcinoma in 98% of reported cases. Well-, moderately, and poorly differentiated and undifferentiated categories relate to the four histologic grades. Subgroups of colloid, mucinous, and signet ring cell types are indications of more aggressive disease.[27] Tumor differentiation is thought to be a reliable predictor of recurrence and survival.[38]

Table 2.—TNM Staging for Rectal Cancer*

Primary tumor (T)
  Tis Carcinoma in situ
  T1 Tumor invades submucosa
  T2 Tumor invades muscularis propria
  T3 Tumor invades through the muscularis propria into the subserosa or into nonperitonealized pericolic or perirectal tissues
  T4 Tumor perforates the visceral peritoneum; tumor is adherent to or directly invades other organs or structures (surgical or pathologic definition)
Regional lymph nodes (N)
  NX Unable to define nodes
  N0 No regional lymph node metastasis
  N1 Metastasis in 1 to 3 regional nodes
  N2 Metastasis in 4 or more regional nodes
Distant metastases (M)
  MX Distant metastasis cannot be assessed
  M0 No distant metastasis
  M1 Distant metastasis

Stage grouping

Stage	T	N	M
I	T1-T2	N0	M0
IIA	T3	N0	M0
IIB	T4	N0	M0
IIIA	T1-T2	N1	M0
IIIB	T3-T4	N1	M0
IIIC	Any T	N2	M0
IV	Any T	Any N	M1

*Additional descriptors: G (histologic grade), R 0-1 (residual tumor), L 0-1 (lymphatic invasion), V 0-1 (venous invasion), yTNM (during or after multimodality therapy), rTNM (recurrent tumor), aTNM (at autopsy).
Modified from the American Joint Committee on Cancer.[37] By permission of the American Joint Committee on Cancer.

Location
The distance of the cancer from the anal verge influences the treatment options available more than the prognosis.[27] In 1949, Kirklin et al.[39] showed that the location of the lesion with reference to the level of the peritoneal resection has no effect on prognosis. The anterior or posterior location of the cancer may influence prognosis.[40]

Size
In contrast to the depth of bowel wall penetration, tumor size does not correlate with disease stage, local recurrence, or lymphatic spread.[27]

DNA Ploidy
The DNA content or ploidy is a factor in the response to cytotoxic therapy in various malignancies. Cancers with DNA ploidies other than diploid are considered high-risk rectal cancers and are inversely correlated with survival.[41] Aneuploidy markedly increases the probability of positive lymph nodes and may have an implication for patient selection for local therapy.[42]

Obstruction and Perforation
Patients with obstruction or perforation usually have a poor prognosis.[27] Perforation that occurs during the operation causes seeding of cancer cells and should be documented in the operative report and be regarded as a locally advanced tumor regardless of the depth of bowel wall invasion.

Extension
Patients with extensive tumors adherent to other organs have a poor prognosis.[27] Direct extension to ovary, uterus, or small bowel does not affect prognosis in most cases if an en bloc resection is performed. When direct extension involves the bladder, prostate, or pelvic sidewall, the prognosis is poorer because complete resection for cure is often not possible.

Venous and Nerve Invasion
Tumors showing evidence of venous or nerve invasion have an increased rate of recurrence and distant metastasis.[43-45]

Response to Radiation
Tumor response to radiation is associated with improved tumor control and overall improved survival rate.[46] Tumor markers to predict radiosensitivity and prognosis are under investigation.[47] The presence of metastatic lymph nodes in the post-irradiated specimen is an ominous prognostic factor for survival.[48]

Surgeon-Related Factors
Among surgeons, both local recurrence and survival rates vary widely after curative resection for rectal cancer.[49,50] The dramatic differences in recurrence rates noted in the literature attest not only to stage of disease and differences in referral patterns but also to variance in the effectiveness of surgical techniques.[51] The Great Britain Large Bowel Cancer Project showed an unacceptable risk of local recurrence that seemed to be more surgeon-specific than disease-specific.[52]

Local recurrence rates of 25% to 35% have been reported in cooperative trials.[37] However, low recurrence rates of 8% with operation alone have been reported from Mayo Clinic.[25,53] Outcome is improved with both colorectal subspecialty training and the performance of a higher number of rectal cancer operations.[30,49,54] The surgeon has the responsibility to perform an oncologically appropriate dissection with adequate tumor-free margins and to prevent implantation of viable cancer cells in the suture line and surrounding tissues.

Distal Margins

The distal margin of resection should be measured in a fresh, unfixed state.[55] According to the observations of Quer et al.,[7] a 2-cm grossly tumor-free margin is acceptable because distal intramural and extramural lymphatic or vascular spreads rarely exceed 1.5 cm for a rectal tumor with the usual degree of differentiation in the absence of proximal obstruction. In the presence of poorly differentiated cancer, the need for a wider margin of resection is controversial.[56] The surgeon, when dealing with the individual case, must use his or her best judgment for determining that the resection is adequate and that the chance of cure is not decreased by doing a sphincter-saving operation.[57]

Lateral (Radial) Margins

The local recurrence rate correlates well with inadequate radial margins regardless of the type of resection, the stage of the tumor, or its degree of differentiation.[58] In patients with positive microscopic radial margins, whether additional radical operation is of more benefit than adjuvant chemoradiation is a basic question as yet unanswered in light of the limitations of the narrow confines of the true anatomical pelvis and the increased morbidity of extended lymphadenectomy.[59] R0, R1, R2 (R stands for residual tumor) have been added to the TNM classification for rectal cancer as additional prognostic indicators.[37]

Mesorectal Margins

Anatomically appropriate operations have been practiced by Mayo Clinic surgeons for 100 years. Adequate removal of the lymph-vascular pedicle within its fascial envelope allows radial and distal pelvic clearance and removal of regional lymph nodes.[51] The terms "total mesorectal excision,"[60] "sharp mesorectal excision,"[61] and "extrafascial excision"[62,63] are probably synonymous. For distal and mid-rectal cancers, the tissue within this envelope should be removed en bloc. The need to extend mesorectal excision more than 5 cm beyond a proximal rectal cancer has not been proved and may increase morbidity. We perform "tumor-specific"[25] mesorectal excision with similar local recurrence rates and less risk of anastomotic leak and usually no need for a temporary colostomy for cancer located in the upper portion of the rectum.

Implantation of Cancer Cells

We routinely irrigate the rectal stump with a tumoricidal solution to reduce the risk of implantation of cancer cells on the anastomosis. Iatrogenic perforation of the rectum and seepage of fragmented tumor particles during the dissection should be avoided at all costs, because they increase the risk of local recurrence.

PREOPERATIVE EVALUATION

Evaluation of the patient with rectal cancer necessitates a thorough understanding of the findings obtained through a history, physical examination, and pathologic and radiologic findings.

Preoperative staging is key to management.[64] Although the anticancer purpose of the operation is key, one must also strive to obtain optimal quality of life for the patient. The clinician must be able to determine whether the patient has disseminated disease, whether preoperative radiation therapy is indicated for a locally extensive lesion, whether a sphincter-saving operation is possible, or when a local treatment is appropriate. Knowledge of the pathologic findings and expert imaging of the pelvis are important to determine preoperatively the best approach for locoregional oncologic control of the tumor.

Histologic Documentation of Cancer

Before a patient is subjected to a radical operation, histologic confirmation of cancer is mandatory. Most rectal adenocarcinomas originate as in situ epithelial lesions from preexisting tubular adenomas. Rarely do they arise de novo. The in situ lesions are unlikely to metastasize and should be curable by simple, local measures.[65] Patients with large villous adenomas of the rectum require rectal ultrasonography, which can be useful for identification of an invasive portion to which a transanal biopsy can be guided.[66,67] On occasion, because of patient discomfort, an examination with the patient under anesthesia is necessary to obtain an adequate sample for the histologic documentation and to determine tumor resectability. Not all indurated or ulcerated rectal masses are cancers: solitary rectal ulcers[68] and pneumatosis cystoides intestinalis are not.[69] Nonetheless, histopathologically, a solitary rectal ulcer occasionally shows a mucosal reactive change to a deeper-seated malignancy.[70] Endometriosis can mimic rectal cancer on physical examination. Carcinoma can arise from an endometrial implant in the rectum.[71] Other malignant lesions such as melanomas,[72] lymphomas,[73] and neuroendocrine tumors[74] also can be found. Rarely, a cancer of the prostate may present as a rectal mass[75] or as a poorly differentiated carcinoma invading into the wall of the rectum.[28] Special staining for prostate-specific antigen may be needed to establish that the tumor is of prostatic origin. Carcinomas of the anal canal can be cured by combined treatment with external beam radiation and chemotherapy with fluorouracil and mitomycin. This approach is that used at Mayo Clinic and elsewhere.[76]

Disseminated Disease

The presence of distant metastasis must be ruled out before operation. In the presence of localized solitary liver metastases, a concomitant rectal resection and liver resection can be undertaken in good-risk patients providing both colorectal and hepatic surgical experts are present.[77]

Computed tomography of the abdomen and pelvis and chest radiography are routinely performed preoperatively. The preoperative computed tomography scan permanently stores information regarding the special distribution of tumor, which is valuable in the accurate planning of adjuvant therapy in patients with locally advanced tumors. Mid-rectal cancer may disseminate to the lung in the absence of liver metastasis. For patients with very distal rectal cancer, the inguinal and femoral nodes should be carefully palpated to rule out metastasis in those nodes.[78]

Synchronous Lesion

A complete evaluation of the colon is required in all patients to rule out a synchronous colonic lesion.[79,80] For this evaluation, colonoscopy is the procedure of choice. Barium enema and flexible sigmoidoscopy may be used as an alternative.

Locally Advanced or Nonresectable Lesion

Unfortunately, 5% to 10% of rectal cancers are not resectable at operation. Computed tomography accurately determines resectability for locally advanced rectal cancer in 85% of cases.[81] With regard to adjacent organ resection, computed tomography accurately determines the need for sacrectomy or hysterectomy, but it overestimates the need for urinary organ resection. In contrast to the adjuvant setting, in which the benefits of preoperative versus postoperative radiation therapy continue to be debated, for locally advanced rectal cancer preoperative chemoradiation is essential for tumor downstaging and increasing tumor resectability.[37,82,83]

Sphincter-Saving Operation

Traditionally, radical amputation has been the treatment of choice for distal and mid-rectal cancer. More recently, sphincter-saving procedures including low anterior resection, coloanal anastomosis, and local excision have been preferred.[65] These procedures allow preservation of anal sphincter function in patients who are carefully selected and when adequate oncologic treatment can be provided.

Patients present with various stages of rectal carcinoma. Sensitive and reliable staging techniques are needed to justify less-aggressive operation for early lesions and preoperative treatment for advanced rectal cancer. The accuracy of clinical staging by digital rectal examination is subjective and varies with the level of experience of the clinician. Its accuracy ranges from 44% to 83%.[84]

Digital rectal examination and rigid proctoscopy accurately measure the level of the tumor and document whether the lesion is ulcerated, necrotic, obstructive, or fixed. We have adopted the anal verge as point of reference and a distance of 12 cm from the anal verge as inclusion criteria for rectal cancer trials.[85]

Endoluminal rectal ultrasonography (Fig. 1) is the most widely used technique and has a T-staging accuracy of approximately 85% (range, 67%-93%).[55] With use of a high-frequency (5-7 MHz) transducer, sonography can resolve the rectal wall into five layers that correspond to the five histologic layers: mucosa, muscularis mucosa, submucosa, muscularis propria, and perirectal fat. There are some drawbacks that limit the clinical usefulness of the technique.[86] The technique is particularly operator-dependent. Interpretation of ultrasonograms is difficult, and the accuracy appears to be proportional to the experience of the observer. Assessment of a borderline situation (e.g., distinguishing between T2 and T3 tumors) can be difficult and of great clinical relevance. It is also generally accepted that accurate assessment of endosonographic findings is possible only during real-time examinations. Often, nodal metastases are not appreciated by endosonography because such nodes are not enlarged grossly. Because most lymph nodes involved by carcinoma of the rectum are less than 5 mm in diameter, nodal staging by rectal ultrasonography is of little predictive value unless ultrasound-guided biopsy can be used.[87]

Preoperative magnetic resonance imaging also can be used selectively.[88] With fluorodeoxyglucose-positron emission tomography, lymph node metastases may be detected that are not identified by other imaging techniques.[89] The major limitations of all imaging techniques are understaging as a result of microscopic invasion or overstaging caused by desmoplastic reaction. The choice of method is influenced by local expertise and availability.

A larger proportion of patients can benefit from sphincter-saving operations today than in the past. For many patients, the final decision for a sphincter-saving operation, however, can be made only at operation after full mobilization of the rectum.[11] A rectal amputation with a permanent colostomy should be performed in patients who have invasion of the sphincter apparatus, anal fistula, or inadequate sphincter function. Patients with large, poorly differentiated, locally advanced cancers necessitating

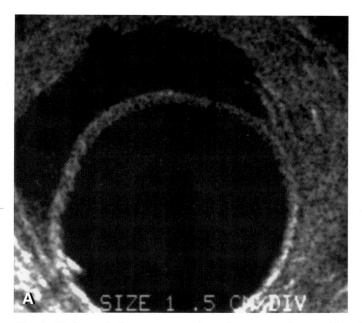 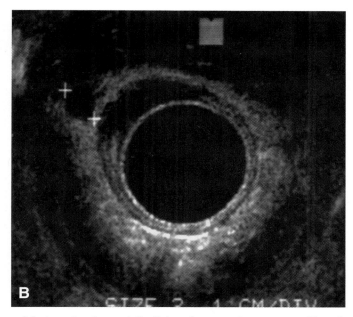

Fig. 1. Endorectal ultrasonograms of rectal cancer consistent with perirectal fat invasion (upper left of A*) and metastasis to a regional lymph node (between crosses in* B*).*

combined-method therapy and intraoperative radiation may be better served with colostomy than with a very low anastomosis because of impaired quality of life and poor functional outcome with an anastomosis.[90]

Local Treatment

The selection of patients who will benefit from wide local excision is always difficult.[91] The transanal treatment is commonly used in patients with small tumors and in physically compromised patients who are unable to tolerate transabdominal resection because of their extensive medical comorbid conditions, such as cardiac disease, pulmonary dysfunction, old age, or obesity. This treatment also is used in a small number of patients refusing colostomy or abdominal operation. For tumors that are mobile, T1 on ultrasonography, well- or moderately well-differentiated, less than 3 cm in size, and easily accessible, wide local excision seems to yield results comparable to those of more radical operation and with less postoperative morbidity.[8,92] The lesions should not invade blood vessel or lymphatic channels.[93] Immediate salvage radical operation is recommended if, in the specimen obtained at wide local excision, there are adverse pathologic findings, such as positive margins, vascular invasion, and invasion through muscularis propria.[94] Neoadjuvant therapy or radical operation should be considered for T2 lesions (i.e., invasion into the muscularis propria).[95-97] Local excision of rectal carcinoma can be curative only in the absence of vascular, lymphatic, and transmural spread.

The risk of lymph node metastasis increases to 17% when the tumor invades the muscularis propria (T2) and to 50% when it invades perirectal tissue (T3).[98] Additionally, poorly differentiated lesions metastasize to lymph nodes twice as frequently as well-differentiated lesions. Some tumors have "bad biology," and the prognosis is not good regardless of procedure. The tumor may be systemic and fatal at presentation. Further research is needed to identify accurately this subgroup of patients.[99]

Endocavitary radiotherapy is the delivery of low-energy (50 kV) x-rays through a specialized proctoscope. The tumor is identified within the viewing area of the treatment proctoscope, and radiation is delivered directly to the tumor. This technique does not require general anesthesia. Patients for whom curative treatment with endocavitary radiation is appropriate meet the following criteria. They have low-grade (grades 1 and 2) tumors that do not penetrate through the entire bowel wall. These tumors have a low risk of lymph node involvement. This technique is not appropriate for patients with involved lymph nodes, because little radiation penetrates through the bowel wall to the lymph node-bearing tissues. The tumors must be 10 cm or less from the dentate line, because this is as far as the treatment proctoscope can be inserted. The treatment proctoscope has a diameter of 3 cm. With the use of two adjacent overlapping fields, a tumor can be treated if it is no larger than 3 by 5 cm in greatest diameter. The tumor must be above the dentate line, because the squamous epithelium of the distal anal canal does not tolerate the high dose of radiation delivered with this technique. A commonly used treatment program includes the delivery of 120 Gy (12,000 rads) in four equal fractions. For 25 patients treated with curative intent at Mayo Clinic, the 5-year local control rate was 89% and the 5-year survival rate was 76%. The most substantial toxicity was ulceration, which occurred in 5 of the 25 patients.[100] In one of these five patients, a perforation developed after a biopsy of a radiation-induced ulcer. We urge caution during biopsy of radiation-induced lesions because serious complications can and do occur. A biopsy should not be performed to confirm the presence of a radiation-induced complication, but rather only when the lesion suggests the presence of cancer recurrence.

CONDUCT OF OPERATION

At Mayo Clinic, the most commonly performed operations for rectal cancer are the anterior resection, the low anterior resection with or without colonic pouch, the abdominoperineal resection, the wide local excision, and the Hartmann procedure for complicated carcinomas.[66,101] Over the years, a greater proportion of sphincter-saving operations have been performed. Factors that influence outcome of the operation have to be considered to select the appropriate operation for each patient. The operative technique performed at Mayo Clinic is well illustrated in two surgical atlases.[102,103] The use of a laparoscopic technique for rectal cancer has been described and may become more common in the future, depending on the results of clinical trials.[104,105]

Preparation

For most patients, preoperative bowel cleansing is performed on an outpatient basis. We favor orthograde lavage solutions for mechanical bowel preparation. Sodium phosphate-[106] or polyethylene glycol-based oral solutions[107] are used according to a patient's or surgeon's preference. Antibiotic prophylaxis with oral medication (neomycin and metronidazole) the day before operation or an intravenous preparation of a second-generation cephalosporin within 15 minutes of operation or both are given.

Thromboembolic complications are combated by the routine use of compression stockings, pneumatic compression devices, and subcutaneous heparin.[101,108] Adequate preoperative counseling[31] with a stomal therapist is beneficial for all patients in whom a permanent or temporary stoma is being considered. A stoma site is chosen and the skin is marked before the operation.[109]

Positioning

The modified Trendelenburg position is used to allow access to the perineum and to allow an assistant to stand between the patient's legs during operation. Allen stirrups are positioned to support the heels and calves, such that the lateral peroneal nerve is not subject to any pressure. The patient's arms are kept close to the body and are cushioned and protected. On occasion, the patient's right arm is extended to allow venous access by the anesthesiologist. A urinary catheter is inserted under sterile conditions. Ureteric stents are placed when invasion of the ureter is suspected in patients with large pelvic mass or in patients undergoing reoperation. The characteristics (level, size, mobility) of the tumor are assessed by digital rectal examination before irrigation of the rectum with 500 mL of diluted povidone-iodine solution. When an abdominoperineal resection is being done, the anus is first closed with a purse-string 0 silk suture to prevent soilage. A nasogastric decompression tube is not used routinely.[110]

Both the abdomen and the perineum are prepared and draped with a sterile technique. The instrument table (Mayo stand) is positioned above the patient's head. An exception to this positioning is for the transanal excision of a lesion located anteriorly, which necessitates a prone jackknife position for adequate exposure.

Incision

A lower midline incision skirting the umbilicus on the patient's right is the incision of choice for a rectal cancer operation. Extension of the incision until the stomach can be visualized is warranted when mobilization of the splenic flexure of the colon is required.

Intraoperative Staging

The liver is carefully palpated to rule out liver metastasis. Intraoperative liver ultrasonography is performed if suspicious lesions are present. The location of the rectal tumor above or below the peritoneal reflection should be determined, as should adherence of the tumor to surrounding structures such as the sacrum, iliac vessels, and pelvic floor muscles. Biopsy should be done for any suspicious para-aortic nodes or nodes near the inferior mesenteric artery. The most apical node should be tagged for the pathologist. Biopsy also should be performed for any suspicious liver, peritoneal, or omental metastasis.

Mobilization of Splenic Flexure, High or Low Ligation of Vessels

Often, the splenic flexure of the colon is mobilized as the first stage of the procedure when a low anterior resection or coloanal anastomosis is planned. The vessels to the tumor should be ligated before the tumor is manipulated. High ligation of the inferior mesenteric artery allows full mobilization of the descending and sigmoid colon, which continue to be vascularized by the middle colic artery through the marginal artery of Riolan. Division of the inferior mesenteric vein adjacent to the ligament of Treitz allows the descending colon to reach the deep pelvis in most patients, where a tension-free colonic pouch-anal anastomosis or low colorectal anastomosis can be performed.[61,111]

A narrowed sigmoid colon, containing diverticula and muscular hypertrophy or damaged by radiation, may not be suitable for a safe anastomosis. In these cases, the descending colon is preferable for the anastomosis. However, a healthy sigmoid colon can be used. For lesions located in the upper rectum, mobilization of the splenic flexure is usually unnecessary. High ligation of the inferior mesenteric artery does not improve 5-year survival rates in patients with cancer of the rectum or rectosigmoid.[112] If regional lymphadenopathy is present, the vessels should be taken to the origin of the inferior mesenteric artery.

Preservation of Autonomic Nerves
The sympathetic fibers of the superior hypogastric plexus arise from the aortic plexus and the two lateral lumbar splanchnic nerves. After incision of the peritoneum on the right and left sides at the level of the sacral promontory, the "shiny" appearance of the mesorectal envelope can be seen and the sympathetic nerves detected 1 cm lateral to the midline and 2 cm medial to each ureter. During mobilization of the posterior and lateral portion of the rectum, the hypogastric nerves along with the ureters should be carefully identified to avoid their injury, provided the approach does not compromise adequate tumor resection.

The branches of the pelvic plexus contain sympathetic and parasympathetic fibers that are important to sexual function. The plexus on each side is encased in the midportion of the lateral stalk posterolateral to the seminal vesicles and above the levator ani muscle. Dissection at this level can damage the neurovascular bundle that supplies the male genital organs.

The anterior mobilization starts in the avascular plane between the rectum and the seminal vesicles or vagina in the midline. The incision extends laterally and posteriorly to avoid injury to the neurovascular bundle. Injury to the neurovascular bundle may lead to retrograde ejaculation.[111] The hazards of pelvic dissection should be well known by the surgeon so as to preserve sexual function.[113-115] Documentation of the preoperative urinary and sexual function is advocated.

Rectal Excision
Avoidance of local recurrence depends on the adequacy of distal and lateral pelvic clearance and the excision of mesorectal fatty tissue within its fascial layer. With traction on the rectum in an anterior and cephalad direction, air is drawn in to dissect the natural plane between the rectum and sacrum (Fig. 2). A sharp dissection under direct vision in the avascular presacral space between the layer of the fascia of the rectum and Waldeyer's fascia with transection of the sacrorectal ligament facilitates full mobilization of the rectum beyond the tip of the coccyx posteriorly. Laterally, the peritoneum is incised just medial to the ureters. The lateral ligaments usually are divided with electrocautery. Occasionally, when the middle hemorrhoidal vessels are large, they need to be ligated.

The anterior plane of dissection includes Denonvilliers' fascia, particularly when the cancer is located anteriorly. In female patients, a combined total abdominal hysterectomy is indicated when the tumor is adherent to the vagina at the level of the posterior cervix. Excision of a portion of the posterior vagina is sometimes necessary.

After the rectum has been adequately mobilized, a noncrushing clamp is placed across the rectum distal to the tumor. A distal rectal washout is performed through the anus with a tumoricidal solution (sterile water or povidone-iodine) introduced with a 50-mL syringe. Patients who are candidates for adjuvant therapy should have metal clips placed in the tumor bed to demarcate the tumor location.

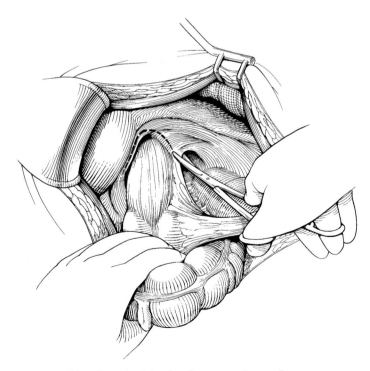

Fig. 2. "Air dissection" in the plane posterior to the mesorectum, caused by incising the peritoneum adjacent to the rectum with scissors and then manually pulling the sigmoid colon in an anterior and cephalad direction. (From Beahrs et al.[102] By permission of Mayo Foundation.)

Any close or positive margins also should be marked with clips. These clips can prevent geographic misses of adjuvant radiotherapy.

Type of Anastomosis

The technique of anastomosis may differ from one surgeon to another according to experience or preference. In general, we favor a double-stapled technique for low colorectal anastomosis, as described by Knight and Griffen.[10,11] Distal to a secure intestinal clamp (placed below the tumor to prevent spillage from the proximal open lumen), a 55- or 33-mm stapler (for very distal lesions) is placed. Pressure applied to the perineum by an assistant, elevating the region of the dissection a few centimeters, facilitates placement of the instrument. The rectum is then transected on the proximal edge of the stapler, after which the stapler is removed. At a previously selected site of proximal resection, the colon is divided proximally with a special purse-string instrument. The specimen is removed and sent to the pathologist to confirm that the margins of resection are adequate.

A suture is then placed at the cut end of the proximal colon by passing a 2-0 polypropylene suture on a Keith needle through the purse-string instrument. A bowel clamp is placed proximally to limit spillage as the purse-string sutures are loosened, and sizers are passed into the colonic lumen. The anvil of an end-to-end circular stapler with a diameter of 29 or 33 mm is then inserted proximally. The purse-string suture is tied. The circular stapler is introduced in the rectal segment. Its naked rod is directed to the previously placed staple line and centered immediately posterior to the staple row. After the anvil is fitted to the end of the rod, the proximal colon is advanced to the rectal segment. Great care is taken to avoid interposition of the vagina or seminal vesicle at the staple line. The circular stapler is closed and activated to effect a stapled anastomosis. The circular stapler is then opened, disengaged from the suture line, and removed. It is important to note that two complete rings of tissue have been removed by the instrument, ensuring that the staples have been properly placed. The anastomosis is then tested for a leak by insufflating air under pressure while the proximal colon is clamped and the pelvis filled with saline solution. If any leak is detected, it should be repaired. A no. 10 Jackson-Pratt drain is placed deep within the pelvis and exteriorized through a stab wound in the lower abdomen. The pelvic peritoneum is left open, and the well-vascularized omentum covers the anastomosis and limits the descent of the small bowel in the pelvis.

Colonic Pouch

Excision of the rectal reservoir can be detrimental to postoperative function. A straight distal colorectal and coloanal anastomosis often gives suboptimal functional results, especially in the first 6 to 18 months postoperatively. For patients with a limited life expectancy, any adaptation period may be too long.[64] Lazorthes et al.[116] and Parc et al.[117] described a technique of resection and coloanal anastomosis with a colon reservoir for rectal carcinoma. Disturbances in stool frequency and urgency appear to be a function of neorectal capacity and are inversely related to the length of the rectal stump.[118,119] The construction with a colonic J pouch has been reported to improve functional outcome in prospective randomized trials and physiologic studies comparing a colonic J pouch with straight reconstruction.[120-124] The construction of a colonic J pouch seems to be indicated when the distance of the anastomosis from the anal verge is less than 5 cm. After adequate colonic mobilization, a colonic pouch can be constructed with sutures or a surgical stapler (Fig. 3). The proximal colon is usually transected with a gastrointestinal anastomosis stapler. It is then folded into a J configuration with a length of 6 to 8 cm. The apex of the pouch is opened, and a single fire of a 75- or 90-mm linear cutting stapler should give adequate pouch length. A 2-0 polypropylene purse-string suture is placed around the opening at the pouch apex, and the anvil of the circular stapler is inserted. A double-stapled end-to-end anastomosis is performed after the very distal rectum has been closed with a 30-mm stapler. Alternatively, the pouch can be passed to the anus and a hand-sewn anastomosis performed. An endoanal anastomosis is often easier to perform in patients with physical limitation imposed by the pelvis. The use of a circular retractor with elastic hooks effaces the anal canal to facilitate creation of the anastomosis under direct vision. When a fatty colon is present, a straight coloanal anastomosis[125] or a coloplasty[126] can be used as an alternative to a colonic pouch.

Diverting Stoma

In patients undergoing proctectomy and colonic pouch-anal canal anastomosis, it is prudent to use a diverting stoma.[127] In addition, after preoperative chemoradiation, we routinely use such a diversion to reduce the risk of anastomotic leak leading to pelvic sepsis and subsequent fibrosis of the neorectum. If the anastomosis was technically difficult or when a small air leak cannot be repaired primarily, a diversion is mandatory. The use of a loop ileostomy allows adequate diversion without interference with the vascular supply of the colon.

Rectal Amputation With Permanent Colostomy

After completion of the abdominal mobilization of the rectum, a laparotomy pad is placed deep in the retrorectal space and the perineal phase of the operation begins. A

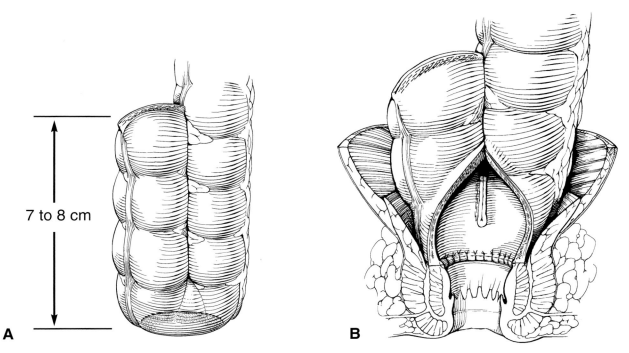

7 to 8 cm

A   **B**

Fig. 3. Colonic pouch after construction (A) *and after pouch-anal canal anastomosis* (B).

biconvex incision is made 3 to 4 cm from the anal verge, the anus having been closed with suture to prevent soilage. Rake retractors are used to expose the ischiorectal fat laterally. With cautery, the fat is incised until the anococcygeal ligament is palpated posteriorly and divided. With a curved Mayo scissors positioned on top of the coccyx, the posterior tissues are dissected until the laparotomy pad is detected. The levator muscles are palpated posteriorly and laterally and transected with electrocautery guided by the operating surgeon's index finger placed inside the pelvic cavity above the levators. When a large opening is created, the specimen is passed down by an assistant. This maneuver facilitates the dissection of the anterior attachments under direct vision, avoiding trauma to the prostate, urethra, and vagina. The perineal wound is closed primarily, approximating the ischiorectal fat, the subcutaneous fat, and the skin with resorbable suture. Two round suction drains are placed deep in the pelvis and exteriorized in the lower abdomen or on either side of the perineal incision.

An end colostomy is made in the left lower quadrant of the abdomen through the rectus abdominis muscle. The integrity of the vascular supply is verified before closure of the abdomen. Closure of the peritoneal space, lateral to the colostomy, is used by some but not all Mayo Clinic surgeons. A series of interrupted 2-0 chromic sutures are used to mature the colostomy, which should be slightly elevated and everted.

Wide Local Excision

The endoanal technique is our preferred approach.[8,92] Adequate muscle relaxation is provided by the anesthesiologist before insertion of the anal bivalved retractor. The tumor is visualized, and stay sutures are placed at 1 cm from the distal and lateral margins. A full-thickness incision is made by electrocautery at the lower part of the tumor just outside the stay sutures. The perirectal fat is seen in the deep portion. Hemostasis can be facilitated by the use of small hemostatic clips. The incision is gradually extended around the tumor. The tumor is progressively displaced distally by gentle traction on the stay sutures or Allis forceps until the upper margin is transected. The specimen is well oriented and sent to the pathologist. The rectal wound is irrigated with povidone-iodine solution and closed transversely with running 2-0 polyglactin 910 sutures.

En Bloc Excision of Adjacent Organs

Locally advanced rectal cancer[73] may involve the uterus, adnexa, and posterior vaginal wall in women or the seminal vesicles and prostate in men; the bladder may be invaded in both sexes. In the absence of distant or extrapelvic disease, an aggressive approach is indicated. A total pelvic exenteration with urinary diversion may be required to obtain tumor-free margins. Posterior rectal tumors fixed to the sacrum can be treated with abdominoperineal resection and sacrectomy in selected cases. The large perineal wounds that result require closure with a transpelvic musculocutaneous flap that uses the rectus abdominis muscle.[128] Immediate myocutaneous flap closure reduces the need for readmission and reoperation.[129] If tumor extends to an unresectable structure, we believe it is preferable to mark the tumor bed with clips, close the incision, and refer the patient for chemotherapy and radiotherapy. Consideration should also be given to specialized boost techniques such as intraoperative radiotherapy or brachytherapy.

Palliative Treatment

The goal of palliative treatment is to control symptoms caused by a rectal cancer thought to be unresectable for cure because of unresectable distant metastasis or extensive local growth. Palliation should be performed with acceptable morbidity and mortality. After a comprehensive assessment of the patient's overall medical condition, a decision is made to resect, to divert, or to use a transanal local procedure. In well-selected cases, we favor palliative abdominoperineal resection or anterior resection. These major resections are associated with fewer continued symptoms and improved quality of life than are nonresectional procedures.[130] However, not all patients are candidates for resection. A laparoscopic diversion is indicated in some cases. Various local procedures have been described as nonresectional palliative methods, such as endoscopic transanal resection,[131] electrocoagulation,[132] laser and photodynamic therapy,[133] argon endoscopic coagulation,[134] and other nonexcisional methods such as cryosurgery[135] and self-expanding mesh stent.[136] Results

of these procedures require further evaluation. Palliation also can be obtained with chemotherapy and radiotherapy in selected cases.

POSTOPERATIVE COMPLICATIONS

C. H. Mayo, M.D.,[2] stated in 1904 that "Statistics change from year to year with the ability of the operator, whose judgment increases through his mistakes and failures, and whose ability to select a justifiable operation for rectal cancer, according to the extent, location, fixation, glandular involvement, cachexia, and age, or invasion of the neighboring organs, such as vagina, uterus, prostate, or bladder, becomes more and more reliable." Although there has been a dramatic decline in the operative mortality rate after operation for rectal cancer, the morbidity rate remains surprisingly high. An operative mortality rate between 1% and 8% and morbidity rates between 21% and 76% have been reported.[137]

The profiles of intraoperative and early postoperative complications in 426 consecutive patients who underwent operations, excluding local excision, for rectal cancer at Mayo Clinic in Rochester, Minnesota, between 1984 and 1986 were analyzed (Table 3).[138] There were two deaths (0.5%). Both of the patients who died had liver metastasis. One patient had had an abdominoperineal resection and one had had a diverting colostomy only. There were no deaths among the patients who had low anterior resection, anterior resection, or resection with coloanal anastomosis. If potentially curative cases alone are considered, then

Table 3.—Rectal Cancer: Operative Procedures and Most Frequent Postoperative Complications

	Operative procedures											
	APR (n = 158)		LAR (n = 137)		AR (n = 71)		Coloanal (n = 25)		Hartmann's procedure (n = 24)		Colostomy only (n = 11)	
Complications	No.	%	No.	%	No.	%	No.	%	No.	%	No.	%
Urinary retention	50	32	25	18	12	17	5	20	1	4.2	1	9.1
Urinary tract infection	31	20	19	14	8	11	3	12	4	17	1	9.1
Perineal wound infection	25	16										
Atelectasis	16	10	4	2.9	6	8.4	2	8	2	8.3	2	18
Perineal wound breakdown	10	6.3										
Anastomotic leak			10	7.3	3	4.2	4	16				
Septicemia	8	5.1	3	2.2	2	2.8	1	4	1	4.2		
Small bowel obstruction	7	4.4	2	1.5	1	1.4	1	4	1	4.2	1	9.1
Abdominal wound infection	7	4.4	3	2.2	1	1.4			3	13	1	9.1

APR, abdominoperineal resection; AR, anterior resection; LAR, low anterior resection.
From Pollard et al.[138] By permission of the American Society of Colon and Rectal Surgeons.

there was no mortality. Intraoperative complications occurred in 34 patients (8%). The most common intraoperative complication was presacral bleeding, which occurred in 14 patients (3%), two of whom had hemorrhagic shock. A modified packing technique[139] and the use of thumbtacks[140] have been described to stop massive presacral hemorrhage. Splenic injury occurred in 2 patients (0.5%). There were no ureteral injuries. Intraoperative complications were not related to any particular operative procedure.

The overall postoperative complication rate was 50.2%, a high figure, but not different from that reported by other institutions. The most common complications were urologic. Urinary retention occurred in 94 patients (22.5%), and urinary tract infection in 66 patients (16%). Patients with obstructive airway disease and obesity had a significantly greater chance for development of postoperative atelectasis and pneumonia.

In the abdominoperineal resection group, the perineal wound was closed primarily in 151 patients (96%) and left open in 7 patients. Perineal infection occurred in 25 patients (16%) and perineal wound breakdown in 10 (6.6%) of the closed group. This resulted in a primary healing rate of 77%. Anastomotic leaks occurred in 17 patients (7.3%). Resection with coloanal anastomosis had the highest percentage of anastomotic leaks. For the patients undergoing low anterior resection and anterior resection, no difference in leak rate was noted when stapled anastomoses were compared with hand-sewn anastomoses. Although a complementary diversion of the fecal stream may not prevent an anastomotic leak, its use may make the leak less serious. An exploratory laparotomy may be avoided in some patients. When results with coloanal anastomosis from Mayo Clinic and Cleveland Clinic were combined,[125] major complications (leaks, stricture, failure) occurred in 39% of patients and minor complications in 23%. An anastomotic leak has serious consequences. Three of four patients with an anastomotic leak required reoperation and colostomy. Although there were no deaths, all patients required a prolonged hospitalization from 20 to 55 days.

Excluding anastomotic leaks, the other potentially life-threatening complications were infectious (pneumonia, septicemia) and cardiovascular (myocardial infarction, pulmonary embolus, pulmonary edema). Twenty-nine patients (6.8%) had serious infections or cardiovascular complications and survived. Less frequent postoperative complications were abdominal wound dehiscence (three patients), cholecystitis (three patients), cerebrovascular accident (two patients), peroneal nerve neurapraxia (two patients), renal failure (two patients), epileptic convulsion (two patients), epididymo-orchitis (one patient), hematemesis (one patient), ureteric edema (one patient),

transient ischemic episode (one patient), and perianastomotic abscess (one patient).

ADJUVANT CHEMOTHERAPY AND RADIOTHERAPY

Adjuvant therapy has been responsible for improving the survival rates of patients with high-risk rectal cancers. The first major randomized study to examine the role of adjuvant therapy was performed by the Gastrointestinal Tumor Study Group (GITSG).[16,141] Mayo Clinic participated in this study, which included patients with tumors that penetrated the rectal wall or involved lymph nodes. After complete resection, patients were randomized to one of four treatment arms. One group received no adjuvant therapy, the second group received chemotherapy alone (5-fluorouracil and methylchlorethyl-cyclohexylnitrosourea), the third group received postoperative pelvic radiotherapy alone (40-48 Gy in fractions of 1.8-2.0 Gy), and the fourth group received radiotherapy and chemotherapy. The 8-year survival rates were 28% in patients who had resection alone, 45% in those who received chemotherapy or radiotherapy alone postoperatively, and 58% in those who received radiotherapy and chemotherapy. The combination of postoperative radiotherapy and chemotherapy achieved significantly ($P = 0.005$) better survival than resection alone. This improvement led to a doubling of the 8-year survival rate.

Additionally, the Swedish Rectal Cancer Trial showed that preoperative radiotherapy also can improve the outcome of patients with rectal cancer.[142] In that trial, 1,168 patients with resectable rectal cancer were randomly assigned to preoperative pelvic radiotherapy (25 Gy in 5 fractions) followed by operation within 1 week or to operation alone. The radiotherapy did not increase postoperative mortality. After 5 years of follow-up, the rate of local recurrence was 11% in patients who had radiotherapy and operation and 27% in the operation-alone group ($P = 0.001$). The overall 5-year survival was 58% in the radiotherapy and operation group and 48% in the operation-alone group ($P = 0.002$). The conclusion was that a short-term regimen of high-dose preoperative radiotherapy reduced the rate of local recurrence and improved survival among patients with resectable rectal cancers.

The National Surgical Adjuvant Breast and Bowel Project (NSABP) performed three studies regarding postoperative adjuvant therapy of rectal cancers (NSABP R-01, R-02, R-03).[143-145] The first study (R-01) included 555 patients with Dukes' stages B and C tumors. After resection, patients were randomized to observation, chemotherapy (methotrexate, Oncovin [vincristine], 5-fluorouracil regimen), or pelvic radiotherapy alone. The chemotherapy provided better survival rates than resection alone or radiotherapy alone, and the radiotherapy improved local control but not survival. In the second study, R-02, 694 patients with Dukes' stages B and C tumors had resections and then were randomized to receive chemotherapy and radiotherapy or chemotherapy alone. The radiotherapy improved local rates but not survival compared with chemotherapy alone. This mirrored the results of the GITSG study. In the third study, R-03, patients were randomized to receive either preoperative or postoperative chemotherapy (5-fluorouracil and leucovorin) and radiotherapy. Approximately 130 patients were in each arm. In the preoperative group, 44% had a complete pathologic response. One year after randomization, 10% were dead in the preoperative arm and 6% in the postoperative arm. Sphincter sparing was 10% greater in the preoperative arm (Fig. 4), but toxicity was greater in the preoperative arm. Final results of this study will require more follow-up.

There are other adjuvant studies, but these are among the most important and influential. On the basis of the Swedish Rectal Cancer Trial, one can conclude that preoperative radiotherapy can improve both local control and survival of patients with resectable rectal cancers. For patients who have had resection performed but have tumors that have penetrated through the bowel wall or have spread to lymph nodes, the combination of postoperative radiotherapy and chemotherapy maximizes the chances of local control and survival, according to the findings of the GITSG and NSABP studies. Currently, it is unknown whether preoperative or postoperative adjuvant therapy is better.

There are special circumstances in which patients present with more advanced lesions and require special consideration. For patients with borderline resectable (tethered) or unresectable (fixed) tumors, the preoperative approach is favored because most tumors will be converted to resectable lesions, and this change leads to a lower probability of a positive margin. Our experience with postoperative external-beam radiation administered after subtotal resection was relatively unfavorable.[146] We achieved local control in 30% of patients with microscopically positive margins and in 17% of those with gross residual disease after subtotal resection. These results can improve with specialized boost techniques such as intraoperative radiotherapy. Preoperative administration of adjuvant therapy is preferable in these patients, thus avoiding most cases of subtotal resection. However, for patients who have subtotal resection or local failure, specialized boost techniques such as intraoperative electron irradiation or brachytherapy seem to provide better disease control than external-beam radiation alone.[147] Systemic therapy remains critical in patients with locally advanced or recurrent tumors, because it can reduce both local and distant failure rates.

FOLLOW-UP

The rationale for postoperative follow-up of rectal carcinoma is based on the assumption that detection of recurrence in asymptomatic patients at a stage more amenable to systemic and local salvage treatment can increase survival rates.[14] The majority of recurrences are detected within 2 years after surgical treatment. Follow-up programs are adjusted to the needs of an individual patient and must be cost-effective.[148,149] In the minimal follow-up plan, an appropriate investigation is instituted when a patient becomes symptomatic or signs are found on physical examination. Patients should, however, undergo surveillance for metachronous carcinoma and polyps for detection of other primary carcinomas.

For patients who participate in a colorectal carcinoma treatment protocol such as a multi-institutional adjuvant treatment study, the follow-up is intensive and includes a history and physical examination, a stool test for occult blood, endorectal ultrasonography for patients with low anterior resection, and a carcinoembryonic antigen test every 3 months for 2 years, every 6 months for 2 years, and then once a year. Chest radiography should be performed annually. Colonoscopy should be done at 1 year and every 3 to 5 years for detection of metachronous lesions. Other primary carcinomas also should be sought. An individual program can be outlined for patients with a high risk of recurrence not participating in a clinical trial, such as patients with Dukes' stage B and C carcinomas. The patient should be in good health and willing to have an additional operation as indicated.

Surgeons and patients should understand the limitations of follow-up to detect recurrences and metastases, no matter how extensive the follow-up. Given the infrequency of

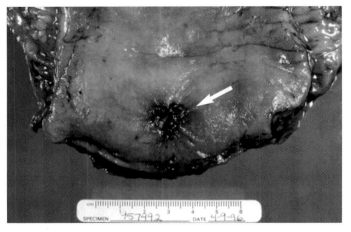

Fig. 4. A down-sized rectal cancer (arrow) *after preoperative chemoradiation that allowed a sphincter-saving operation to be done.*

isolated recurrence amenable to curative resection, a survival benefit of not more than 10% would be expected.[150] Patients should be encouraged to participate in the decision making of their follow-up plan or to participate in large randomized clinical trials that include more sensitive imaging tests capable of detecting treatable recurrences such as local, hepatic, and pulmonary metastasis.

The next step toward achieving a cost-effective plan consists of targeting the resources to the patients who are at highest risk for treatable recurrence.[151]

LOCALLY RECURRENT DISEASE

The value of operation in the management of local failure after curative resection of primary rectal cancer has been questioned, considering the amplitude and technical difficulties of these reoperations, their morbidity, and the limited survival after them. Treatment depends on the location and extent of recurrent disease and the previous therapy. Some patients with recurrence after local incision or anterior resection can be saved with abdominoperineal resection. Our results[152] with 65 patients who underwent operation for cure (i.e., with and without gross or microscopic residual disease at tumor margins) indicated that complete excision of locally recurrent rectal cancer can be accomplished safely and provide a long-term survival rate of 34% of patients at 5 years (Fig. 5). To obtain negative resection margins, en bloc resection of adherent surrounding organs, including vagina, uterus, bladder, prostate, and seminal vesicles anteriorly and sacrum posteriorly, is performed. Partial sacrectomy for posterior extension of recurrent tumor is safe and valuable. Lateral extension limits the surgeon's ability to achieve complete

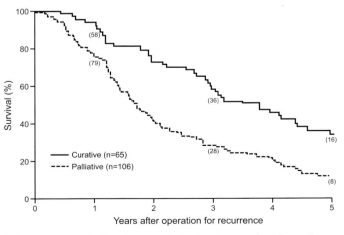

Fig. 5. Survival of patients with (palliative) and without (curative) cancer present at the margin of resection after operation for locally recurrent rectal cancer (P < 0.001). (From Suzuki et al.[152] By permission of the American Society of Colon and Rectal Surgeons.)

excision. The contraindications for an aggressive surgical approach are listed in Table 4. Adequate margins of resection and better local control of the tumor bed with a combination of external-beam radiation and 5-fluorouracil infusion and intraoperative radiation could conceivably improve these results.[19] In view of high systemic failure rates of more than 50% in patients with locally recurrent disease, routine use of systemic therapy is indicated as a component of the treatment regimen. Even with locally recurrent lesions, the aggressive multimethod approaches, including intraoperative radiotherapy, have resulted in improved local control and long-term survival rates of 20% compared with an expected 5% with conventional techniques.[19] The use of primary myocutaneous flap closure for large defects in patients treated with multimethod therapy and proctectomy (perineal wounds) or sacrectomy (posterior wounds) has resulted in complete wound healing in all patients.[121]

Proper selection of surgical candidates and the availability of a multidisciplinary experienced team consisting of a colorectal surgeon, an orthopedic surgeon, a urologist, a neurosurgeon, a plastic surgeon, and a radiation oncologist contribute to a more favorable outcome.[65]

FUTURE CONSIDERATIONS

Rectal cancer is a preventable disease. Every opportunity to promote screening of the general population should be encouraged to increase detection of early-stage lesions amenable to cure with less invasive procedures. Virtual colonoscopy,[153] molecular genetic markers,[154] video endoscopic resection,[155] endocavitary radiation therapy,[100] radioimmunoguided operation,[156] laparoscopic operation,[103,104] better-tolerated adjuvant therapy,[157] and immunotherapy[158,159] currently are being studied to improve the evaluation, treatment, and quality of life of patients with rectal cancer.

Table 4.—Contraindications to an Aggressive Surgical Approach in Locally Recurrent Rectal Cancer

Sciatic distribution of buttock and leg pain
Bilateral ureteral obstruction
Unilateral leg edema
Aortic node metastasis
Lateral deep pelvic sidewall extension
Direct tumor extension to multiple loops of small bowel
Extensive distant metastasis

Data from Suzuki et al.[152]

REFERENCES

1. Marquis R, Lasry JC, Heppell J, Potvin C, Falardeau M, Robidoux A: Quality of life of patients after restorative surgery for cancer of the rectum [French]. Ann Chir 46:830-838, 1992
2. Mayo CH: Cancer of the large bowel. Med Sentinel 12:466-473, 1904
3. Balfour DC: A method of anastomosis between sigmoid and rectum. Ann Surg Phila 51:239-241, 1910
4. Dixon CF: Surgical removal of lesions occurring in the sigmoid and rectosigmoid. Am J Surg 46:12-17, 1939
5. Waugh JM, Block MA, Gage RP: Three- and five-year survivals following combined abdominoperineal resection, abdominoperineal resection with sphincter preservation, and anterior resection for carcinoma of the rectum and lower part of the sigmoid colon. Ann Surg 142:752-757, 1955
6. Black BM: Combined abdominoendorectal resection: technical aspects and indications. Arch Surg 65:406-416, 1952
7. Quer EA, Dahlin DC, Mayo CW: Retrograde intramural spread of carcinoma of the rectum and rectosigmoid, a microscopic study. Surg Gynecol Obstet 96:24-30, 1953
8. Jackman RJ: Conservative management of selected patients with carcinoma of the rectum. Dis Colon Rectum 4:429-434, 1961
9. Hallenbeck GA, Judd ES, David C: An instrument for colorectal anastomosis without sutures. Dis Colon Rectum 6:98-101, 1963
10. Knight CD, Griffen FD: An improved technique for low anterior resection of the rectum using the EEA stapler. Surgery 88:710-714, 1980
11. Knight CD, Griffen FD: Techniques of low rectal reconstruction. Curr Probl Surg 20:387-456, 1983
12. Bess MA, Adson MA, Elveback LR, Moertel CG: Rectal cancer following colectomy for polyposis. Arch Surg 115:460-467, 1980
13. Beart RW Jr, Kelly KA: Randomized prospective evaluation of the EEA stapler for colorectal anastomoses. Am J Surg 141:143-147, 1981
14. Beart RW Jr, O'Connell MJ: Postoperative follow-up for patients with carcinoma of the colon. Mayo Clin Proc 58:361-363, 1983
15. Ahlquist DA, McGill DB, Schwartz S, Taylor WF, Owen RA: Fecal blood levels in health and disease: a study using Hemo-Quant. N Engl J Med 312:1422-1428, 1985
16. Gastrointestinal Tumor Study Group: Prolongation of the disease-free interval in surgically treated rectal carcinoma. N Engl J Med 312:1465-1472, 1985
17. Orkin BA, Dozois RR, Beart RW Jr, Patterson DE, Gunderson LL, Ilstrup DM: Extended resection for locally advanced primary adenocarcinoma of the rectum. Dis Colon Rectum 32:286-292, 1989
18. Kollmorgen CF, Meagher AP, Wolff BG, Pemberton JH, Martenson JA, Ilstrup DM: The long-term effect of adjuvant postoperative chemoradiotherapy for rectal carcinoma on bowel function. Ann Surg 220:676-682, 1994
19. Gunderson LL, Nelson H, Martenson JA, Cha S, Haddock M, Devine R, Fieck JM, Wolff B, Dozois R, O'Connell MJ: Intraoperative electron and external beam irradiation with or without 5-fluorouracil and maximum surgical resection for previously unirradiated, locally recurrent colorectal cancer. Dis Colon Rectum 39:1379-1395, 1996
20. Thibodeau SN, French AJ, Cunningham JM, Tester D, Burgart LJ, Roche PC, McDonnell SK, Schaid DJ, Vockley CW, Michels VV, Farr GH Jr, O'Connell MJ: Microsatellite instability in colorectal cancer: different mutator phenotypes and the principal involvement of hMLH1. Cancer Res 58:1713-1718, 1998
21. Landis SH, Murray T, Bolden S, Wingo PA: Cancer statistics, 1999. CA Cancer J Clin 49:8-31, 1999
22. Woolf SH: The best screening test for colorectal cancer—a personal choice (editorial). N Engl J Med 343:1641-1643, 2000
23. Winawer SJ, Fletcher RH, Miller L, Godlee F, Stolar MH, Mulrow CD, Woolf SH, Glick SN, Ganiats TG, Bond JH, Rosen L, Zapka JG, Olsen SJ, Giardiello FM, Sisk JE, Van Antwerp R, Brown-Davis C, Marciniak DA, Mayer RJ: Colorectal cancer screening: clinical guidelines and rationale. Gastroenterology 112:594-642, 1997
24. Ahlquist DA, Skoletsky JE, Boynton KA, Harrington JJ, Mahoney DW, Pierceall WE, Thibodeau SN, Shuber AP: Colorectal cancer screening by detection of altered human DNA in stool: feasibility of a multitarget assay panel. Gastroenterology 119:1219-1227, 2000
25. Zaheer S, Pemberton JH, Farouk R, Dozois RR, Wolff BG, Ilstrup D: Surgical treatment of adenocarcinoma of the rectum. Ann Surg 227:800-811, 1998
26. Sanfelippo PM, Beahrs OH: Carcinoma of the colon in patients under forty years of age. Surg Gynecol Obstet 138:169-170, 1974
27. American Society of Colon and Rectal Surgeons: Practical parameters for the treatment of rectal carcinoma—supporting documentation. Dis Colon Rectum 36:991-1006, 1993
28. Corman ML: Colon and Rectal Surgery. Fourth edition. Philadelphia, Lippincott-Raven, 1998, pp 738-744
29. Blumberg D, Paty PB, Picon AI, Guillem JG, Klimstra DS, Minsky BD, Quan SH, Cohen AM: Stage I rectal cancer: identification of high-risk patients. J Am Coll Surg 186:574-579, 1998
30. Bokey EL, Chapuis PH, Dent OF, Newland RC, Koorey SG, Zelas PJ, Stewart PJ: Factors affecting survival after excision of the rectum for cancer: a multivariate analysis. Dis Colon Rectum 40:3-10, 1997
31. Bryant RA: Ostomy patient management: care that engenders adaptation. Cancer Invest 11:565-577, 1993
32. Santiago E: Teaching a blind patient colostomy irrigation. Ostomy Wound Manage 46:18, 2000
33. Kelly AW, Nelson ML, Heppell J, Weaver A, Hentz J: Disposable plastic liners for a colostomy appliance: a controlled trial and follow-up survey of convenience, satisfaction, and costs. J Wound Ostomy Continence Nurs 27:272-278, 2000
34. Park YJ, Youk EG, Choi HS, Han SU, Park KJ, Lee KU, Choe KJ, Park JG: Experience of 1446 rectal cancer patients in Korea and analysis of prognostic factors. Int J Colorectal Dis 14:101-106, 1999
35. Pocard M, Panis Y, Malassagne B, Nemeth J, Hautefeuille P, Valleur P: Assessing the effectiveness of mesorectal excision in rectal cancer: prognostic value of the number of lymph nodes found in resected specimens. Dis Colon Rectum 41:839-845, 1998
36. Hojo K, Koyama Y, Moriya Y: Lymphatic spread and its prognostic value in patients with rectal cancer. Am J Surg 144:350-354, 1982
37. American Joint Committee on Cancer: Cancer Staging Manual. Sixth edition. Edited by FL Greene, DL Page, ID Fleming, AG Fritz, CM Balch, DG Haller, M Morrow. New York, Springer-Verlag, 2002, pp 113-123
38. Michelassi F, Vannucci L, Montag A, Goldberg R, Chappell R, Dytch H, Bibbo M, Block GE: Importance of tumor morphology for the long term prognosis of rectal adenocarcinoma. Am Surg 54:376-379, 1988

39. Kirklin JW, Dockerty MB, Waugh JM: The role of the peritoneal reflection in the prognosis of carcinoma of the rectum and sigmoid colon. Surg Gynecol Obstet 88:326-331, 1949

40. Emslie J, Beart R, Mohiuddin M, Marks G: Use of rectal cancer position as a prognostic indicator. Am Surg 64:958-961, 1998

41. Tang R, Ho YS, Chen HH, See LC, Wang JY: Different prognostic effect of postoperative chemoradiation therapy on diploid and nondiploid high-risk rectal cancers. Dis Colon Rectum 41:1494-1499, 1998

42. Zenni GC, Abraham K, Harford FJ, Potocki DM, Herman C, Dobrin PB: Characteristics of rectal carcinomas that predict the presence of lymph node metastases: implications for patient selection for local therapy. J Surg Oncol 67:99-103, 1998

43. Horn A, Dahl O, Morild I: Venous and neural invasion as predictors of recurrence in rectal adenocarcinoma. Dis Colon Rectum 34:798-804, 1991

44. Knudsen JB, Nilsson T, Sprechler M, Johansen A, Christensen N: Venous and nerve invasion as prognostic factors in postoperative survival of patients with resectable cancer of the rectum. Dis Colon Rectum 26:613-617, 1983

45. Moreira LF, Kenmotsu M, Gochi A, Tanaka N, Orita K: Lymphovascular and neural invasion in low-lying rectal carcinoma. Cancer Detect Prev 23:123-128, 1999

46. Wheeler JM, Warren BF, Jones AC, Mortensen NJ: Preoperative radiotherapy for rectal cancer: implications for surgeons, pathologists and radiologists. Br J Surg 86:1108-1120, 1999

47. Qiu H, Sirivongs P, Rothenberger M, Rothenberger DA, Garcia-Aguilar J: Molecular prognostic factors in rectal cancer treated by radiation and surgery. Dis Colon Rectum 43:451-459, 2000

48. Luna-Perez P, Trejo-Valdivia B, Labastida S, Garcia-Alvarado S, Rodriguez DF, Delgado S: Prognostic factors in patients with locally advanced rectal adenocarcinoma treated with preoperative radiotherapy and surgery. World J Surg 23:1069-1074, 1999

49. Hermanek P: Impact of surgeon's technique on outcome after treatment of rectal carcinoma. Dis Colon Rectum 42:559-562, 1999

50. Dahlberg M, Glimelius B, Pahlman L: Changing strategy for rectal cancer is associated with improved outcome. Br J Surg 86:379-384, 1999

51. Beart RW Jr: Mesorectal excision for rectal carcinoma: The new standard? Adv Surg 32:193-203, 1999

52. Phillips RK, Hittinger R, Blesovsky L, Fry JS, Fielding LP: Local recurrence following "curative" surgery for large bowel cancer. I. The overall picture. Br J Surg 71:12-16, 1984

53. Wilson SM, Beahrs OH: The curative treatment of carcinoma of the sigmoid, rectosigmoid, and rectum. Ann Surg 183:556-565, 1976

54. Frileux P, Parc R: Quality of surgical excision in cancer of the rectum: an important prognostic factor [French]. Gastroenterol Clin Biol 23:1355-1359, 1999

55. Wexner SD, Rotholtz NA: Surgeon influenced variables in resectional rectal cancer surgery. Dis Colon Rectum 43:1606-1627, 2000

56. Elliot MS, Todd IP, Nicholls RJ: Radical restorative surgery for poorly differentiated carcinoma of the mid-rectum. Br J Surg 69:273-274, 1982

57. Vandertoll DJ, Beahrs OH: Carcinoma of the rectum and low sigmoid: evaluation of anterior resection of 1,766 favorable lesions. Arch Surg 90:793-798, 1965

58. Quirke P, Durdey P, Dixon MF, Williams NS: Local recurrence of rectal adenocarcinoma due to inadequate surgical resection: histopathological study of lateral tumour spread and surgical excision. Lancet 2:996-999, 1986

59. Wolff BG: Lateral margins of resection in adenocarcinoma of the rectum. World J Surg 16:467-469, 1992

60. Heald RJ, Husband EM, Ryall RD: The mesorectum in rectal cancer surgery—the clue to pelvic recurrence? Br J Surg 69:613-616, 1982

61. Enker WE, Thaler HT, Cranor ML, Polyak T: Total mesorectal excision in the operative treatment of carcinoma of the rectum. J Am Coll Surg 181:335-346, 1995

62. Bissett IP, Hill GL: Extrafascial excision of the rectum for cancer: a technique for the avoidance of the complications of rectal mobilization. Semin Surg Oncol 18:207-215, 2000

63. Bissett IP, McKay GS, Parry BR, Hill GL: Results of extrafascial excision and conventional surgery for rectal cancer at Auckland Hospital. Aust N Z J Surg 70:704-709, 2000

64. Nicholls RJ: Surgery for rectal carcinoma. In Surgery of the Colon & Rectum. Edited by RJ Nicholls, RR Dozois. New York, Churchill Livingstone, 1997, pp 427-474

65. Dozois RR, Perry RE: Rectal cancer: current management. Curr Probl Surg 27:243-299, 1990

66. Nivatvongs S, Nicholson JD, Rothenberger DA, Balcos EG, Christenson CE, Nemer FD, Schottler JL, Goldberg SM: Villous adenomas of the rectum: the accuracy of clinical assessment. Surgery 87:549-551, 1980

67. Pikarsky A, Wexner S, Lebensart P, Efron J, Weiss E, Nogueras J, Reissman P: The use of rectal ultrasound for the correct diagnosis and treatment of rectal villous tumors. Am J Surg 179:261-265, 2000

68. Vaizey CJ, van den Bogaerde JB, Emmanuel AV, Talbot IC, Nicholls RJ, Kamm MA: Solitary rectal ulcer syndrome. Br J Surg 85:1617-1623, 1998

69. Soutter DI, Paloschi GB, Prentice RS: Pneumatosis cystoides intestinalis simulating malignant colonic obstruction. Can J Surg 28:272-273, 1985

70. Li SC, Hamilton SR: Malignant tumors in the rectum simulating solitary rectal ulcer syndrome in endoscopic biopsy specimens. Am J Surg Pathol 22:106-112, 1998

71. Lott JV, Rubin RJ, Salvati EP, Salazar GH: Endometrioid carcinoma of the rectum arising in endometriosis: report of a case. Dis Colon Rectum 21:56-60, 1978

72. Thibault C, Sagar P, Nivatvongs S, Ilstrup DM, Wolff BG: Anorectal melanoma—an incurable disease? Dis Colon Rectum 40:661-668, 1997

73. Devine RM, Beart RW Jr, Wolff BG: Malignant lymphoma of the rectum. Dis Colon Rectum 29:821-824, 1986

74. Robidoux A, Monte M, Heppell J, Schurch W: Small-cell carcinoma of the rectum. Dis Colon Rectum 28:594-596, 1985

75. Papa MZ, Koller M, Klein E, Bersuck D, Sarely M, Ben Arie G: Prostatic cancer presenting as a rectal mass: a surgical pitfall. Br J Surg 84:69-70, 1997

76. Ryan DP, Compton CC, Mayer RJ: Carcinoma of the anal canal. N Engl J Med 342:792-800, 2000

77. Chua HK, Wolff BG, Nagorney DM, Tsiotos GG, Munoz-Juarez M, Larson DR, Sondenaa K: Is combined colectomy and hepatectomy for synchronous metastatic colorectal cancer more efficient than staged? (Abstract.) Gastroenterology 118 Suppl 2:A1027, 2000

78. Tocchi A, Lepre L, Costa G, Liotta G, Mazzoni G, Agostini N, Miccini M: Rectal cancer and inguinal metastases: prognostic role and therapeutic indications. Dis Colon Rectum 42:1464-1466, 1999

79. Langevin JM, Nivatvongs S: The true incidence of synchronous cancer of the large bowel: a prospective study. Am J Surg 147:330-333, 1984

80. Isler JT, Brown PC, Lewis FG, Billingham RP: The role of pre-operative colonoscopy in colorectal cancer. Dis Colon Rectum 30:435-439, 1987

81. Farouk R, Nelson H, Radice E, Mercill S, Gunderson L: Accuracy of computed tomography in determining resectability for locally advanced primary or recurrent colorectal cancers. Am J Surg 175:283-287, 1998

82. Sentovich SM: Adjuvant therapy for colon and rectal cancer. Core subjects program. Am Soc Colon Rectal Surg 53-61, 1999

83. Farouk R, Nelson H, Gunderson LL: Aggressive multimodality treatment for locally advanced irresectable rectal cancer. Br J Surg 84:741-749, 1997

84. Nicholls RJ, Mason AY, Morson BC, Dixon AK, Fry IK: The clinical staging of rectal cancer. Br J Surg 69:404-409, 1982

85. Nelson H, Petrelli N, Carlin A, Couture J, Fleshman J, Guillem J, Miedema B, Ota D, Sargent D: Guidelines 2000 for colon and rectal cancer surgery. J Natl Cancer Inst 93:583-596, 2001

86. Stoker J, Rociu E, Wiersma TG, Lameris JS: Imaging of anorectal disease. Br J Surg 87:10-27, 2000

87. Herrera L, Villarreal JR: Incidence of metastases from rectal adenocarcinoma in small lymph nodes detected by a clearing technique. Dis Colon Rectum 35:783-788, 1992

88. Drew PJ, Farouk R, Turnbull LW, Ward SC, Hartley JE, Monson JR: Preoperative magnetic resonance staging of rectal cancer with an endorectal coil and dynamic gadolinium enhancement. Br J Surg 86:250-254, 1999

89. Whiteford MH, Whiteford HM, Yee LF, Ogunbiyi OA, Dehdashti F, Siegel BA, Birnbaum EH, Fleshman JW, Kodner IJ, Read TE: Usefulness of FDG-PET scan in the assessment of suspected metastatic or recurrent adenocarcinoma of the colon and rectum. Dis Colon Rectum 43:759-767, 2000

90. Shibata D, Guillem JG, Lanouette N, Paty P, Minsky B, Harrison L, Wong WD, Cohen A: Functional and quality-of-life outcomes in patients with rectal cancer after combined modality therapy, intraoperative radiation therapy, and sphincter preservation. Dis Colon Rectum 43:752-758, 2000

91. Temple LK, Naimark D, McLeod RS: Decision analysis as an aid to determining the management of early low rectal cancer for the individual patient. J Clin Oncol 17:312-318, 1999

92. Biggers OR, Beart RW Jr, Ilstrup DM: Local excision of rectal cancer. Dis Colon Rectum 29:374-377, 1986

93. Ruo L, Guillem JG: Major 20th-century advancements in the management of rectal cancer. Dis Colon Rectum 42:563-578, 1999

94. Baron PL, Enker WE, Zakowski MF, Urmacher C: Immediate vs. salvage resection after local treatment for early rectal cancer. Dis Colon Rectum 38:177-181, 1995

95. Wagman R, Minsky BD, Cohen AM, Saltz L, Paty PB, Guillem JG: Conservative management of rectal cancer with local excision and postoperative adjuvant therapy. Int J Radiat Oncol Biol Phys 44:841-846, 1999

96. Garcia-Aguilar J, Mellgren A, Sirivongs P, Buie D, Madoff RD, Rothenberger DA: Local excision of rectal cancer without adjuvant therapy: a word of caution. Ann Surg 231:345-351, 2000

97. Chakravarti A, Compton CC, Shellito PC, Wood WC, Landry J, Machuta SR, Kaufman D, Ancukiewicz M, Willett CG: Long-term follow-up of patients with rectal cancer managed by local excision with and without adjuvant irradiation. Ann Surg 230:49-54, 1999

98. Killingback M: Local excision of carcinoma of the rectum: indications. World J Surg 16:437-446, 1992

99. Bleday R, Breen E, Jessup JM, Burgess A, Sentovich SM, Steele G Jr: Prospective evaluation of local excision for small rectal cancers. Dis Colon Rectum 40:388-392, 1997

100. Schild SE, Martenson JA, Gunderson LL: Endocavitary radiotherapy of rectal cancer. Int J Radiat Oncol Biol Phys 34:677-682, 1996

101. Etchells E, McLeod RS, Geerts W, Barton P, Detsky AS: Economic analysis of low-dose heparin vs the low-molecular-weight heparin enoxaparin for prevention of venous thromboembolism after colorectal surgery. Arch Intern Med 159:1221-1228, 1999

102. Beahrs OH, Kiernan PD, Hubert JPJ: An Atlas of the Surgical Techniques of Oliver H. Beahrs. Philadelphia, WB Saunders Company, 1985

103. Keighley MRB, Pemberton JH, Fazio VW, Parc R: Atlas of Colorectal Surgery. New York, Churchill Livingstone, 1996

104. Nelson H: Laparoscopic surgery. In Surgery of the Colon & Rectum. Edited by RJ Nicholls, RR Dozois. New York, Churchill Livingstone, 1997, pp 865-878

105. Fleshman JW, Wexner SD, Anvari M, LaTulippe JF, Birnbaum EH, Kodner IJ, Read TE, Nogueras JJ, Weiss EG: Laparoscopic vs. open abdominoperineal resection for cancer. Dis Colon Rectum 42:930-939, 1999

106. Oliveira L, Wexner SD, Daniel N, DeMarta D, Weiss EG, Nogueras JJ, Bernstein M: Mechanical bowel preparation for elective colorectal surgery: a prospective randomized, surgeon-blinded trial comparing sodium phosphate and polyethylene glycol-based oral lavage solutions. Dis Colon Rectum 40:585-591, 1997

107. Wolff BG, Beart RW Jr, Dozois RR, Pemberton JH, Zinsmeister AR, Ready RL, Farnell MB, Washington JA II, Heppell J: A new bowel preparation for elective colon and rectal surgery: a prospective, randomized clinical trial. Arch Surg 123:895-900, 1988

108. McLeod RS: The risk of thromboembolism in patients undergoing colorectal surgery. Drugs 52 Suppl 7:38-41, 1996

109. Rozen BL: The value of a well-placed stoma. Cancer Pract 5:347-352, 1997

110. Wolff BG, Pemberton JH, van Heerden JA, Beart RW Jr, Nivatvongs S, Devine RM, Dozois RR, Ilstrup DM: Elective colon and rectal surgery without nasogastric decompression: a prospective, randomized trial. Ann Surg 209:670-673, 1989

111. Gordon PH, Nivatvongs S (editors): Principles and Practice of Surgery for the Colon, Rectum, and Anus. Second edition. St Louis, Quality Medical Publishing, 1999, pp 750-751

112. Pezim ME, Nicholls RJ: Survival after high or low ligation of the inferior mesenteric artery during curative surgery for rectal cancer. Ann Surg 200:729-733, 1984

113. Enker WE: Potency, cure, and local control in the operative treatment of rectal cancer. Arch Surg 127:1396-1401, 1992

114. Havenga K, Enker WE, McDermott K, Cohen AM, Minsky BD, Guillem J: Male and female sexual and urinary function after total mesorectal excision with autonomic nerve preservation for carcinoma of the rectum. J Am Coll Surg 182:495-502, 1996

115. Church JM, Raudkivi PJ, Hill GL: The surgical anatomy of the rectum—a review with particular relevance to the hazards of rectal mobilisation. Int J Colorectal Dis 2:158-166, 1987

116. Lazorthes F, Fages P, Chiotasso P, Lemozy J, Bloom E: Resection of the rectum with construction of a colonic reservoir and colo-anal anastomosis for carcinoma of the rectum. Br J Surg 73:136-138, 1986

117. Parc R, Tiret E, Frileux P, Moszkowski E, Loygue J: Resection and colo-anal anastomosis with colonic reservoir for rectal carcinoma. Br J Surg 73:139-141, 1986

118. Hallbook O, Nystrom PO, Sjodahl R: Physiologic characteristics of straight and colonic J-pouch anastomoses after rectal excision for cancer. Dis Colon Rectum 40:332-338, 1997

119. Hallbook O, Sjodahl R: Comparison between the colonic J pouch-anal anastomosis and healthy rectum: clinical and physiological function. Br J Surg 84:1437-1441, 1997

120. Hallbook O, Pahlman L, Krog M, Wexner SD, Sjodahl R: Randomized comparison of straight and colonic J pouch anastomosis after low anterior resection. Ann Surg 224:58-65, 1996

121. Hida J, Yasutomi M, Maruyama T, Fujimoto K, Nakajima A, Uchida T, Wakano T, Tokoro T, Kubo R, Shindo K: Indications for colonic J-pouch reconstruction after anterior resection for rectal cancer: determining the optimum level of anastomosis. Dis Colon Rectum 41:558-563, 1998

122. Lazorthes F, Chiotasso P, Gamagami RA, Istvan G, Chevreau P: Late clinical outcome in a randomized prospective comparison of colonic J pouch and straight coloanal anastomosis. Br J Surg 84:1449-1451, 1997

123. Hida J, Yasutomi M, Fujimoto K, Okuno K, Ieda S, Machidera N, Kubo R, Shindo K, Koh K: Functional outcome after low anterior resection with low anastomosis for rectal cancer using the colonic J-pouch: prospective randomized study for determination of optimum pouch size. Dis Colon Rectum 39:986-991, 1996

124. Williams N, Seow-Choen F: Physiological and functional outcome following ultra-low anterior resection with colon pouch-anal anastomosis. Br J Surg 85:1029-1035, 1998

125. Cavaliere F, Pemberton JH, Cosimelli M, Fazio VW, Beart RW Jr: Coloanal anastomosis for rectal cancer: long-term results at the Mayo and Cleveland Clinics. Dis Colon Rectum 38:807-812, 1995

126. Fazio VW, Mantyh CR, Hull TL: Colonic "coloplasty": novel technique to enhance low colorectal or coloanal anastomosis. Dis Colon Rectum 43:1448-1450, 2000

127. Dehni N, Schlegel RD, Cunningham C, Guiguet M, Tiret E, Parc R: Influence of a defunctioning stoma on leakage rates after low colorectal anastomosis and colonic J pouch-anal anastomosis. Br J Surg 85:1114-1117, 1998

128. Loessin SJ, Meland NB, Devine RM, Wolff BG, Nelson H, Zincke H: Management of sacral and perineal defects following abdominoperineal resection and radiation with transpelvic muscle flaps. Dis Colon Rectum 38:940-945, 1995

129. Radice E, Nelson H, Mercill S, Farouk R, Petty P, Gunderson L: Primary myocutaneous flap closure following resection of locally advanced pelvic malignancies. Br J Surg 86:349-354, 1999

130. Longo WE, Ballantyne GH, Bilchik AJ, Modlin IM: Advanced rectal cancer. What is the best palliation? Dis Colon Rectum 31:842-847, 1988

131. Irwin RJ: Resectoscopic transanal resection of extensive rectal adenomas. Aust N Z J Surg 54:375-377, 1984

132. Madden JL, Kandalaft S: Electrocoagulation: a primary and preferred method of treatment for cancer of the rectum. Ann Surg 166:413-419, 1967

133. Russin DJ, Kaplan SR, Goldberg RI, Barkin JS: Neodymium-YAG laser: a new palliative tool in the treatment of colorectal cancer. Arch Surg 121:1399-1403, 1986

134. Grund KE, Storek D, Farin G: Endoscopic argon plasma coagulation (APC): first clinical experiences in flexible endoscopy. Endosc Surg Allied Technol 2:42-46, 1994

135. Osborne DR, Higgins AF, Hobbs KE: Cryosurgery in the management of rectal tumours. Br J Surg 65:859-861, 1978

136. Spinelli P, Dal Fante M, Mancini A: Self-expanding mesh stent for endoscopic palliation of rectal obstructing tumors: a preliminary report. Surg Endosc 6:72-74, 1992

137. Rothenberger DA, Wong WD: Abdominoperineal resection for adenocarcinoma of the low rectum. World J Surg 16:478-485, 1992

138. Pollard CW, Nivatvongs S, Rojanasakul A, Ilstrup DM: Carcinoma of the rectum: profiles of intraoperative and early postoperative complications. Dis Colon Rectum 37:866-874, 1994

139. Metzger PP: Modified packing technique for control of presacral pelvic bleeding. Dis Colon Rectum 31:981-982, 1988

140. Nivatvongs S, Fang DT: The use of thumbtacks to stop massive presacral hemorrhage. Dis Colon Rectum 29:589-590, 1986

141. Douglass HO Jr, Moertel CG, Mayer RJ, Thomas PR, Lindblad AS, Mittleman A, Stablein DM, Bruckner HW: Survival after postoperative combination treatment of rectal cancer (letter). N Engl J Med 315:1294-1295, 1986

142. Swedish Rectal Cancer Trial: Improved survival with preoperative radiotherapy in resectable rectal cancer. N Engl J Med 336:980-987, 1997

143. Fisher B, Wolmark N, Rockette H, Redmond C, Deutsch M, Wickerham DL, Fisher ER, Caplan R, Jones J, Lerner H, Gordon P, Feldman M, Cruz A, Legault-Poisson S, Wexler M, Lawrence W, Robidoux A, and Other NSABP Investigators: Postoperative adjuvant chemotherapy or radiation therapy for rectal cancer: results from NSABP protocol R-01. J Natl Cancer Inst 80:21-29, 1988

144. Wolmark N, Wieand HS, Hyams DM, Colangelo L, Dimitrov NV, Romond EH, Wexler M, Prager D, Cruz AB Jr, Gordon PH, Petrelli NJ, Deutsch M, Mamounas E, Wickerham DL, Fisher ER, Rockette H, Fisher B: Randomized trial of postoperative adjuvant chemotherapy with or without radiotherapy for carcinoma of the rectum: National Surgical Adjuvant Breast and Bowel Project Protocol R-02. J Natl Cancer Inst 92:388-396, 2000

145. Hyams DM, Mamounas EP, Petrelli N, Rockette H, Jones J, Wieand HS, Deutsch M, Wickerham DL, Fisher B, Wolmark N: A clinical trial to evaluate the worth of preoperative multimodality therapy in patients with operable carcinoma of the rectum: a progress report of National Surgical Adjuvant Breast and Bowel Project Protocol R-03. Dis Colon Rectum 40:131-139, 1997

146. Schild SE, Martenson JA Jr, Gunderson LL, Dozois RR: Long-term survival and patterns of failure after postoperative radiation therapy for subtotally resected rectal adenocarcinoma. Int J Radiat Oncol Biol Phys 16:459-463, 1989

147. Gunderson LL, Wolff BG, Cha S, Haddock MG, Schild SE, Devine RM, Martenson JA: Intraoperative irradiation for locally advanced primary and recurrent rectal cancer. Probl Gen Surg 12:93-105, 1996

148. Galandiuk S, Wieand HS, Moertel CG, Cha SS, Fitzgibbons RJ Jr, Pemberton JH, Wolff BG: Patterns of recurrence after curative resection of carcinoma of the colon and rectum. Surg Gynecol Obstet 174:27-32, 1992

149. Schoemaker D, Black R, Giles L, Toouli J: Yearly colonoscopy, liver CT, and chest radiography do not influence 5-year survival of colorectal cancer patients. Gastroenterology 114:7-14, 1998

150. Richard CS, McLeod RS: Follow-up of patients after resection for colorectal cancer: a position paper of the Canadian Society of Surgical Oncology and the Canadian Society of Colon and Rectal Surgeons. Can J Surg 40:90-100, 1997

151. Rosen M, Chan L, Beart RW Jr, Vukasin P, Anthone G: Follow-up of colorectal cancer: a meta-analysis. Dis Colon Rectum 41:1116-1126, 1998

152. Suzuki K, Dozois RR, Devine RM, Nelson H, Weaver AL, Gunderson LL, Ilstrup DM: Curative reoperations for locally recurrent rectal cancer. Dis Colon Rectum 39:730-736, 1996

153. Johnson CD, Ahlquist DA: Computed tomography colonography (virtual colonoscopy): a new method for colorectal screening. Gut 44:301-305, 1999

154. Ahlquist DA, Thibodeau SN: Will molecular genetic markers help predict the clinical behavior of colorectal neoplasia? Gastroenterology 102:1419-1421, 1992

155. Winde G, Nottberg H, Keller R, Schmid KW, Bunte H: Surgical cure for early rectal carcinomas (T1): transanal endoscopic microsurgery vs. anterior resection. Dis Colon Rectum 39:969-976, 1996

156. Wolff BG, Bolton J, Baum R, Chetanneau A, Pecking A, Serafini AN, Fischman AJ, Hoover HC Jr, Klein JL, Wynant GE, Subramanian R, Goroff DK, Hanna MG Jr: Radioimmunoscintigraphy of recurrent, metastatic, or occult colorectal cancer with technetium Tc 99m 88BV59H21-2V67-66 (HumaSPECT-Tc), a totally human monoclonal antibody: patient management benefit from a phase III multicenter study. Dis Colon Rectum 41:953-962, 1998

157. O'Connell MJ, Martenson JA, Wieand HS, Krook JE, Macdonald JS, Haller DG, Mayer RJ, Gunderson LL, Rich TA: Improving adjuvant therapy for rectal cancer by combining protracted-infusion fluorouracil with radiation therapy after curative surgery. N Engl J Med 331:502-507, 1994

158. Stocchi L, Nelson H: Diagnostic and therapeutic applications of monoclonal antibodies in colorectal cancer. Dis Colon Rectum 41:232-250, 1998

159. Kugler A, Stuhler G, Walden P, Zoller G, Zobywalski A, Brossart P, Trefzer U, Ullrich S, Muller CA, Becker V, Gross AJ, Hemmerlein B, Kanz L, Muller GA, Ringert RH: Regression of human metastatic renal cell carcinoma after vaccination with tumor cell-dendritic cell hybrids. Nat Med 6:332-336, 2000

Chapter 42

COMMON ANORECTAL PROBLEMS

Santhat Nivatvongs, M.D.

This chapter presents Mayo Clinic's approach to four common anorectal problems: hemorrhoids, anal fissures, anorectal abscesses and anal fistulas, and pilonidal sinuses. The work of others is also cited.

HEMORRHOIDS

Hemorrhoids are not varicose veins, and not everyone has hemorrhoids. But, everyone has anal cushions. The anal cushions are composed of blood vessels, smooth muscle (Treitz's muscle), and elastic connective tissue in the submucosa (Fig. 1). They are located in the upper anal canal,

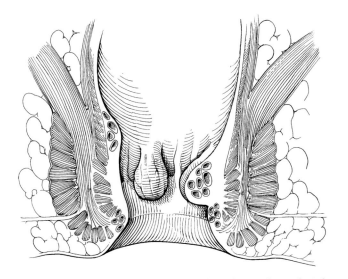

Fig. 1. The anal cushions are situated in the anal canal. They contain submucosal blood vessels, smooth muscle fibers, and connective tissue.

from the dentate line to the anorectal ring (puborectalis muscle). Three cushions lie in the following constant sites: left lateral, right anterolateral, and right posterolateral. Smaller discrete secondary cushions are usually present between these three main cushions. This anatomical arrangement is remarkably constant and bears no relationship to the terminal branching of the superior rectal artery, as previously thought. That this is the normal arrangement of anal cushions is borne out by their presence in children, the fetus, and even the embryo.[1]

The function of these cushions is to aid in anal continence. During defecation, when they become engorged with blood, they cushion the anal canal and support the anal canal lining. The anal cushions are supported by muscles that arise partly from the internal sphincter and partly from the conjoined longitudinal muscles. Hemorrhoid is the pathologic term used to describe the downward displacement of the anal cushions, causing dilatation of the contained venules.[1,2] Hence, hemorrhoids develop when the supporting tissues of the anal canal deteriorate.[3]

Nomenclature and Classification

External skin tags are discrete folds of skin arising from the anal verge. Such tags may be the result of thrombosed external hemorrhoids or may be a complication of inflammatory bowel disease independent of any hemorrhoid problem. External hemorrhoids comprise the dilated vascular plexus that is located below the dentate line and covered by squamous epithelium. Internal hemorrhoids are the symptomatic, exaggerated, submucosal vascular tissue located above the dentate line and covered by transitional and columnar epithelium. Internal hemorrhoids can be divided into categories. First-degree internal hemorrhoids bulge into the lumen of the anal canal and may produce painless bleeding. Second-degree internal hemorrhoids protrude at the time of a bowel movement but reduce spontaneously. Third-degree internal hemorrhoids protrude spontaneously or at the time of a bowel movement and require manual replacement. Fourth-degree internal hemorrhoids are permanently prolapsed and irreducible despite attempts at manual replacement. Mixed hemorrhoids have elements of internal and external hemorrhoids. Multiple skin tags often accompany and most frequently occur with external hemorrhoids but may, less frequently, be associated with internal hemorrhoids.

When the prolapse cannot be reduced because of swelling and spasm of the sphincter, strangulated hemorrhoids occur. Progression results in gangrenous hemorrhoids.

Prevalence

Using the data from the National Center for Health Statistics, Johanson and Sonnenberg[4] found that the prevalence rate was 4.4%. This figure could have been easily exaggerated because it is based on complaints. Obviously, not all the complaints are caused by true hemorrhoids. The diagnosis of hemorrhoids is not easy. It requires experienced physicians or surgeons to use a proper anoscope and, if necessary, to ask the patient to strain while sitting on the toilet bowl. A busy colon and rectal surgeon can hear a patient's complaint of "hemorrhoids" or see patients referred by other physicians for "hemorrhoids," only to find that many of these patients have other anal problems, ranging from pruritus ani to anal fissures, fistulas, and skin tags. Some do have true hemorrhoidal symptoms.

Assessing the true prevalence of hemorrhoids is virtually impossible. Not surprisingly, the reported prevalence rates have varied widely from 1% to 86%, depending on the method of ascertainment and the definition of "hemorrhoids."

Etiology and Pathogenesis

The sliding downward of anal cushions is the cause of hemorrhoids.[1] Hemorrhoids are associated with straining and with an irregular bowel habit, features compatible with the sliding anal lining theory. Hard, bulky stools causing straining and tenesmus from diarrhea are more likely to push the anal cushions out of the anal canal. Straining also causes engorgement of the cushions during defecation, making their displacement more likely. Repeated stretching disrupts the submucosal muscle of Treitz, resulting in prolapse. The anchoring and supporting connective tissue above the anal cushions has disintegrated and fragmented in patients with hemorrhoids.[3,5]

Many studies consistently show higher anal sphincter resting pressures in patients with hemorrhoids.[6-8] Another abnormality in many of these patients is the presence of ultraslow anal pressure waves (frequency, 0.9-1.6/minute) caused by contractions of the internal anal sphincter; the importance of this finding is not known.[9] Anal electrosensitivity and temperature sensation are reduced in patients with hemorrhoids, perhaps because the prolapse renders the rectal mucosa less sensitive. This change also may contribute to decreased continence. Rectal sensation to balloon distention is no different from that in control subjects.[2]

Predisposing and Associated Factors

Constipation aggravates symptoms of hemorrhoids. Tenesmus from diarrhea is another predisposing factor.[10] Pregnancy undoubtedly aggravates preexisting disease and, by mechanisms not well understood, predisposes to development of the disease in patients who were previously asymptomatic. In any patient with the combination of diarrhea and hemorrhoids, inflammatory bowel disease should be suspected and all attempts made to exclude it. Operative intervention in such patients may be fraught with greater complications.

Diagnosis

General assessment of the patient to ascertain the overall health status and to exclude associated disease, particularly bleeding disorders and liver disease with portal hypertension, should be the first phase of examination. Anemia from hemorrhoids is uncommon and can be corrected easily after treatment.[11] Inspection may reveal variable degrees of perianal skin abnormalities, protrusion of internal hemorrhoids, or normal appearance. Digital examination excludes distal rectal and anal canal neoplasms and enables assessment of the tone of the anal sphincter.

Anoscopy is performed to assess the extent of disease. With the anoscope in place, the patient is asked to strain as if having a bowel movement so the amount of prolapse can be assessed. During anoscopy, it is also important to look for and rule out a coexisting anal fissure, especially in patients complaining of pain or those in whom anal sphincter tone is deemed excessive.

Proctoscopy or flexible sigmoidoscopy must be performed in all patients to visualize the rectum and lower colon so that coexisting conditions can be excluded, particularly carcinoma, adenoma, and inflammatory bowel disease. Inflammatory bowel disease may produce symptoms similar to those from hemorrhoids and may potentiate any hemorrhoids present.

Colonoscopy should be performed in any patient with chronic diarrhea and a change in bowel habits. Screening colonoscopy should be considered in patients older than 50 years, especially those who have a family history of colorectal carcinoma.

Nonoperative Treatment

Diet and Bulk-Forming Agents
The rationale for adding bulk to the diet is to eliminate straining at defecation. In addition to consumption of fruits and vegetables, bulk in the diet can be supplemented easily with raw unprocessed oat bran (one-third to one-half cup per day). An alternative measure is to take psyllium seed (1 tablespoon per day). An adequate volume of fluids must be consumed each day. A high-fiber diet reduces symptoms of hemorrhoids and is ideal for the treatment of first-degree and some second-degree hemorrhoids.[12,13] It is important to impress on the patient that the urge to defecate should not be ignored.

Rubber Band Ligation
Rubber band ligation is a simple, quick, and effective nonoperative means of treating grades 1 and 2 and selected cases of grades 3 and 4 hemorrhoids.[14-17] The procedure is performed in the office, preferably after the patient has received a sodium biphosphate enema. Sedation is unnecessary. Although rubber band ligation has been used without resulting in problems in patients who have been taking aspirin, nonsteroidal anti-inflammatory drugs, and anticoagulants, it is advisable that use of these medications be stopped. Because most bleeding occurs 1 week to 10 days after rubber band ligation, one may proceed with the procedure and then have the patient discontinue use of the medications for about 2 weeks. Two rubber bands are placed on each drum in case one breaks. The procedure is performed through an anoscope with a rubber band ligator. The bands should be placed on the rectal mucosa and the top of the internal hemorrhoids[18,19] (Fig. 2). The external hemorrhoids must be left alone. Generally the ligation is performed at one site at a time. However, ligation of two or three sites at one time has had good results.[14,15] Subsequent ligation, if indicated, usually is performed 4 to 6 weeks later. Rubber band ligation is not without pain. Warm sitz baths help to relieve the pain from anal sphincter spasm, which occurs in some patients. An appropriate analgesic should be prescribed, and an increase in consumption of fruits and vegetables or a bulk-forming agent should be encouraged. Immediate severe or progressive pain is an indication of a misplaced rubber band ligation—one that is too close to the dentate line. Such bands require immediate removal.

There has been concern about the safety of rubber band ligation because of the rare reports of deaths resulting from acute perianal sepsis.[20] The clues to severe anal and perianal infection after rubber band ligation are a triad of symptoms: delayed anal pain, urinary retention, and fever.[21] Acute awareness of these rare but potentially life-threatening complications is essential, and immediate aggressive treatment is mandatory to prevent death.[22,23] Treatment should include administration of broad-spectrum antibiotics, drainage of an abscess (if present), and excision of necrotic tissues (if present). Because of possible severe complications, rubber band ligation is not advisable in patients with immunodeficiencies. This procedure also can be disastrous in patients who have tested positive for the human immunodeficiency virus.[24]

Other nonoperative procedures to treat hemorrhoids include infrared photocoagulation, electrocoagulation, sclerotherapy, cryotherapy, and anal stretch. None of these techniques are as effective as rubber band ligation.

Hemorrhoidectomy
Hemorrhoidectomy should be considered when 1) hemorrhoids are severely prolapsed and require manual replacement (grades 3 and 4), 2) patients fail to improve after multiple applications of nonoperative treatments, or 3) hemorrhoids are complicated by associated conditions

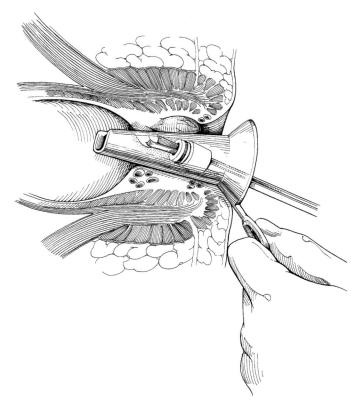

Fig. 2. Rubber band ligation. Note ligation of rectal mucosa at top of the internal hemorrhoid.

such as ulceration, fissure, fistula, large hypertrophied anal papilla, or extensive skin tags.

The choice of anesthesia should be individualized. In most cases, hemorrhoidectomy can be performed with the patient under local anesthesia in combination with mild sedation. However, in patients with deep "cheeks" of the buttocks, especially in muscular or obese men, a general or regional block anesthetic is preferable.[25] Even with general or regional anesthesia, the entire anal canal should be injected with 0.25% bupivacaine or 0.5% lidocaine containing 1:200,000 epinephrine, the epinephrine being used mainly for hemostatic purposes. The patient takes a bottle (45 mL) of sodium phosphate, mixing 1 tablespoon in a glass (8-ounce) of water the evening before. The advantage of cleansing the bowel preoperatively is that use of a laxative to stimulate bowel movement can be delayed to the fourth or fifth day postoperatively, when the maximal postoperative pain has started to subside.

Closed Hemorrhoidectomy

In 1931, Fansler[26] described the technique of hemorrhoidectomy in which the dissection was conducted in an anatomical method (intra-anal anatomical dissection). The key to this technique is use of the Fansler anal speculum (Fig. 3), which is 3 cm in diameter and 7 cm long. The entire hemorrhoidal tissues, along with the redundant skin, can be dissected easily in their normal anatomical location. There is no need to pull the hemorrhoidal pedicle toward the anus for suturing because the exposure is excellent all the way to the apex of the wound. Thus, prolapse of rectal mucosa or ectropion is almost unknown with this technique.

The procedure is performed with the patient in prone jackknife position with the cheeks of the buttocks taped apart (Fig. 4 A). With Lilly tonsil scissors (V. Mueller Co., McGaw Park, Illinois), an elliptical excision of external and internal hemorrhoids is begun at the perianal skin and is ended at the anorectal ring (Fig. 4 B). During the

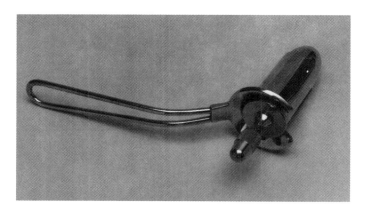

Fig. 3. Fansler anal speculum.

excision, the scissors is pressed firmly on the anal wall. This technique allows excision of a full thickness of mucosa and submucosa without injury to the underlying internal sphincter muscle. The strip of tissue excised should not be wider than 1.5 cm. It is important to use a three-point stitch at the apex of the wound to avoid a mass effect, which can cause tenesmus (Fig. 4 C). The entire wound is closed with running 3-0 chromic catgut sutures, 2 mm apart (Fig. 4 D). Chromic catgut closure results in excellent healing. If too much tissue has been inadvertently excised, the wound should be marsupialized and left open. The largest and most redundant hemorrhoid should be excised first. With this approach, the original plan to excise three quadrants may be modified, so that only a one- or two-quadrant hemorrhoidectomy is necessary. Some anal cushion should be preserved to maintain good anal continence,[27] particularly when patients approach the fifth and sixth decades of life. Ideally, the hemorrhoidectomy excision should not be performed in the posterior commissure unless plastic flap procedures are planned, because in this location the wound heals slowly and has a greater tendency to form a fissure (Fig. 4 E).

Circular Stapled Hemorrhoidectomy

Circular stapled hemorrhoidectomy is a new surgical technique. Its concept is to excise the redundant low rectal mucosa and submucosa with simultaneous stapling using a circular staple device. The internal hemorrhoids are not removed, and the external hemorrhoids are also left alone because they eventually regress.[28]

The kit consists of a 33-mm stapling gun with a nondetachable anvil, a purse-string speculum, a transparent anal dilator with an obturator, and a purse-string suture threader or a crochet hook (Fig. 5). The operation can be performed with the patient in the prone or lithotomy position, and the anesthesia can be local, general, or regional.

The anal dilator is inserted into the anal canal and secured in place with heavy sutures to the perianal skin (Fig. 6 A). The purse-string speculum is inserted through the anal dilator. A purse-string suture of 2-0 polypropylene is placed in the rectum 5 cm from the anal verge or 3 cm proximal to the dentate line (Fig. 6 B). It is important to place the suture in the submucosal layer. The stapler with the anvil fully extended is inserted through the purse-string suture and the purse-string suture is tied over the anvil. The purse-string suture tails are retrieved through the ports in the stapler gun with the crochet hook (Fig. 6 C). The stapler is then closed and fired. Compression on the gun is maintained for 20 to 30 seconds for hemostasis before the stapler is opened and removed. There is only one donut ring of removed tissue that should be checked for its completeness. The staple line should lie 1 to 2 cm above the top of

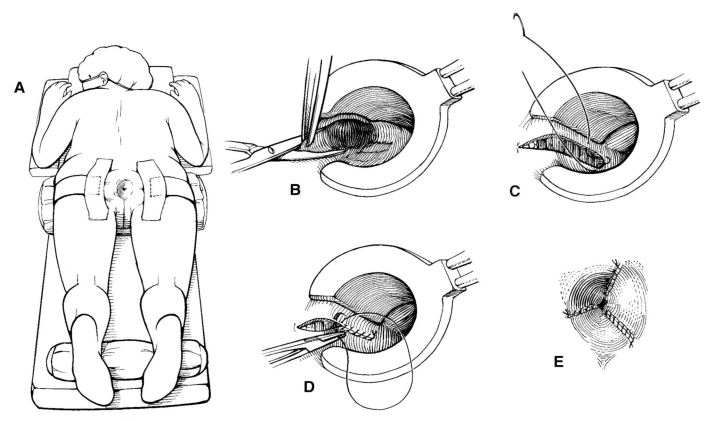

Fig. 4. Technique of closed hemorrhoidectomy. (A), Prone jackknife position with cheeks of buttock taped apart. (B), With Lilly tonsil scissors, an elliptical excision is begun at perianal skin and is ended at anorectal ring. (C), A three-point stitch at the apex of the wound. (D), A continuous suture with 3-0 chromic catgut. (E), At completion.

the internal hemorrhoids (Fig. 6 D). Stick ties should be placed for any active bleeding points.

This novel technique is associated with less pain and less disability than conventional hemorrhoidectomy. In a randomized controlled trial comparing the stapled hemorrhoidectomy with the Milligan-Morgan technique conducted by Mehigan et al.,[29] the stapled hemorrhoidectomy was associated with shorter anesthesia time, less pain, and shorter duration of disability. However, there was no statistical difference in patients' satisfaction at 4 months after operation (Table 1). The randomized controlled trial by Ho et al.[30] had a similar outcome (Table 2). However, the randomized controlled study by Cheetham et al.[31] comparing stapled hemorrhoidectomy with diathermy hemorrhoidectomy showed dismal results. Of 16 patients who had stapled hemorrhoidectomy and were followed for longer than 6 months, 5 (31%; 95% CI, 8.5%-54%) had symptoms of pain and fecal urgency that persisted for up to 15 months postoperatively. Because of these results, the randomized trial was suspended. In 64 patients studied by Beattie and Loudon,[32] results were promising 6 months after stapled hemorrhoidectomy. The median symptom score was 6 (range, 5-8) before the

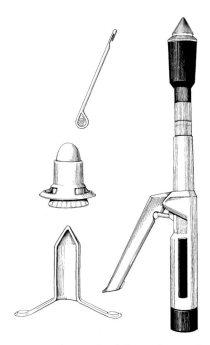

Fig. 5. A 33-mm hemorrhoidal circular stapler. From right to left, clockwise: stapler, purse-string speculum, anal dilator, suture threader. (Modified from Ethicon Endo-Surgery, Inc., Cincinnati, Ohio.)

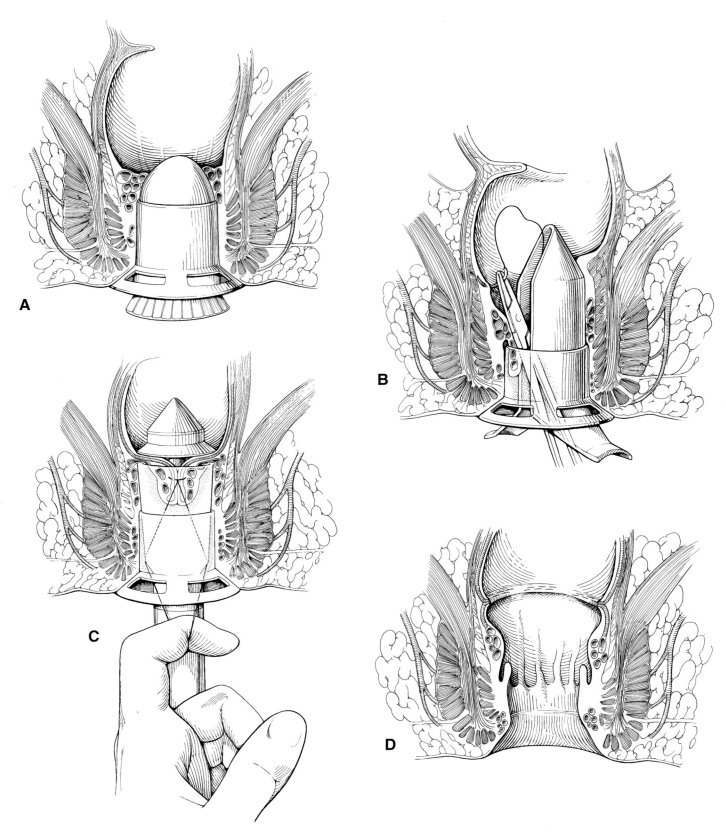

Fig. 6. Technique of stapled hemorrhoidectomy. (A), Anal dilator inserted into anal canal and secured with sutures. (B), Placement of purse-string suture 5 cm from anal verge with the purse-string speculum. (C), The purse-string suture is tied over the anvil, and the suture tails are retrieved through the ports in the stapler gun with the crochet hook. The stapler is then closed and fired. (D), The staple line at 1 to 2 cm above the internal hemorrhoids. (Modified from Ethicon Endo-Surgery, Inc., Cincinnati, Ohio.)

Table 1.—Hemorrhoidectomy: Results of a Randomized Controlled Trial

| | Technique | | |
	Stapled	Milligan-Morgan diathermy	P value
No. of patients	20	20	NS
Mean anesthesia time, min	18	22	0.007
Mean pain score on day 1	1.1	5.8	0.0007
Mean pain score on day 6	-4.4	1.2	0.0007
Mean time to return to work, d	17	34	0.002
Mean % satisfied at 4 mo	85	75	NS

NS, not significant.
Data from Mehigan et al.[29]

operation and 0 (range, 0-1) at 6 months after operation (P < 0.01). In addition, there were no recurrences, impaired continence, persistent anal pain, or urgency. Brown et al.[33] also found that stapled hemorrhoidectomy was feasible for acute thrombosed circumferential hemorrhoids. Although the pain was higher (P < 0.03) in the immediate postoperative period compared with pain after the Milligan-Morgan diathermy technique, the pain was lower at 6 weeks (P < 0.05). Patients in the stapled hemorrhoidectomy group also returned to work earlier, 14 days vs. 28 days (P < 0.05).

Although stapled hemorrhoidectomy has been shown to be safe, a life-threatening pelvic sepsis has been reported,[34] and a long-term result is not yet available.

Other Types of Hemorrhoidectomy

Excision and Ligation

This technique, described by Milligan et al.,[35] has been widely used in the United Kingdom and throughout the world.[36,37] The procedure is performed with the patient in the lithotomy position. The internal hemorrhoidal complexes are pulled down through the anus, producing the "triangle of exposure." The hemorrhoids are excised from the underlying sphincter muscle. The dissection is done proximally as far as the pedicles, where it is stick-tied with an absorbable suture. The wounds are left open.

Modified Whitehead Hemorrhoidectomy

In 1882, Whitehead,[38] of Manchester, England, described a technique for hemorrhoidectomy. A circular incision was made at the level of the dentate line. The submucosal and subdermal hemorrhoidal tissues then were dissected out. The redundant rectal mucosa was excised, and the remaining cut mucosal edge was sutured to the anoderm. Because of the high rate of complications, especially with ectropion, this technique soon fell out of favor. However, it has attracted the attention of some surgeons in the United States, where it has been revived with modifications.[39,40]

The Whitehead hemorrhoidectomy is performed with the patient in the prone position. The anal canal is exposed with the Buie self-retaining anal retractor. An incision is made at the level of the dentate line in one quadrant, and the flap of anoderm is raised. The submucosal and subdermal hemorrhoidal plexuses are excised, and the redundant rectal mucosa is excised transversely. The flap of anoderm is advanced proximally and sutured to the rectal mucosa. Hemorrhoids in other quadrants are removed similarly. The key to the success of this modified technique is suturing the flap of anoderm to the mucosa in the upper anal canal rather than pulling the mucosa down to the anoderm at the dentate line. In a long-term follow-up of 484 patients in the series reported by Wolff and Culp at Mayo Clinic,[40] there were no recurrences or ectropions. The cited advantage of this operation is for treatment of extensive circumferential hemorrhoids.

Laser Hemorrhoidectomy

Several years ago, the public demand for laser hemorrhoidectomy was great, because of hearsay and rumor that laser hemorrhoidectomy resulted in less pain and produced

Table 2.—Hemorrhoidectomy: Results of a Randomized Controlled Trial

| | Technique | | |
	Stapled	Milligan-Morgan diathermy	P value
No. of patients	62	57	NS
Mean anesthesia time, min	18	11	< 0.001
Mean pain score at 2 wk	3	5	< 0.005
% of patients with persistent pain at 3 mo	1	3	NS
No. of patients with incontinence at 6 wk	2	2	NS
Mean time to resume work, d	17	23	< 0.05
Mean cost, $	1,283	921	NS

Data from Ho et al.[30]

better results than conventional hemorrhoidectomy. Studies show no benefit of laser over conventional hemorrhoidectomy. Also, laser is more expensive and causes a greater degree of wound inflammation and dehiscence of the suture lines.[41,42]

Special Situations

Thrombosed External Hemorrhoids

The condition usually occurs without a known cause. Most patients give no history of straining or physical exertion and do not have a history of hemorrhoidal disease. The typical patient history is that of a painful mass in the perianal area. The pain usually is described as burning or throbbing, and its severity depends on the size of the thrombus. A thrombosed external hemorrhoid is an intravascular clot (Fig. 7). It is confined to the anoderm and does not cross proximally beyond the dentate line.

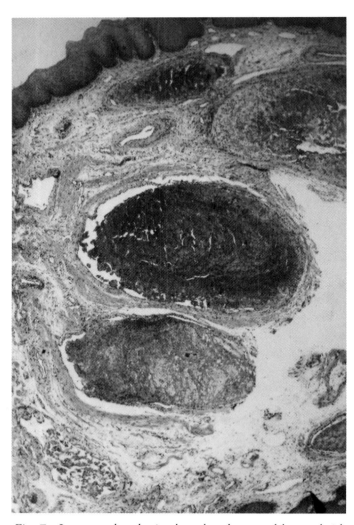

Fig. 7. Intravascular clot in thrombosed external hemorrhoid. (Hematoxylin-eosin; x40.)

The natural history of thrombosed external hemorrhoids is an abrupt onset of an anal mass and pain that peaks within 48 hours. The pain becomes minimal after the fourth day. If left alone, the thrombus shrinks and dissolves in a few weeks. Occasionally, the skin overlying the thrombus becomes necrotic, causing bleeding and discharge or infection, which may cause further necrosis and more pain. A large thrombus can result in a skin tag.

Because thrombosed external hemorrhoids are self-limited, the treatment is aimed at relief of severe pain and prevention of recurrent thromboses and residual skin tags. If the patient has intense pain, excision should be offered. However, if the pain already is subsiding and the thrombosed hemorrhoid has started to shrink, it is wise to manage it nonoperatively (Fig. 8). Management includes prescribing a nonconstipating analgesic drug, warm sitz baths for comfort, proper anal hygiene by hand washing, and bulk-producing agents such as bran or psyllium seed, if the patient is constipated. Suppositories have not proved helpful for treating this condition.

Proctoscopy or flexible sigmoidoscopy is performed to rule out associated anorectal disease. The procedure can be performed when the patient is evaluated initially if the examination can be done without undue pain, but usually it is postponed to a later date.

The thrombus can be excised in the office, clinic, or emergency department with proper equipment. A local anesthetic (0.25% bupivacaine containing 1:200,000 epinephrine) should be infiltrated to anesthetize the entire anal canal for accommodating a large Hill-Ferguson anal speculum for exposure. Excising the skin along with the mass is neither necessary nor desirable. Instead, an incision is made over the mass from the perianal skin to the level of the dentate line, and the thrombus can be easily dissected out with a scissors. Excessive skin is trimmed, and the

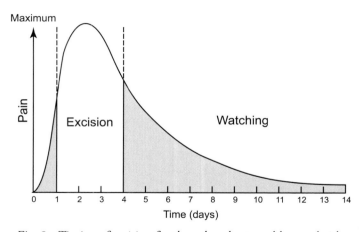

Fig. 8. Timing of excision for thrombosed external hemorrhoids.

wound is closed with running or interrupted 3-0 chromic catgut (Fig. 9). The relief of pain usually is immediate provided the wound is closed without tension. Postoperative care is aimed at keeping the wound clean by hand washing with soap and water. Warm sitz baths for 10 to 15 minutes three or four times daily are used for throbbing pain from spasm of the anal sphincter muscle. An analgesic drug is usually required during the first 24 hours.

Strangulated Hemorrhoids

Strangulated hemorrhoids arise from prolapsed third- or fourth-degree hemorrhoids that have become irreducible because of swelling (Fig. 10). The patient's history often reveals a long-standing hemorrhoidal prolapse on straining or at rest and marked edema of both external and internal hemorrhoids protruding through the anus. If untreated, the edema may progress to ulceration and necrosis. Pain is usually severe, and urinary retention may occur.

Proper treatment requires urgent or emergency hemorrhoidectomy. Because of the severe protrusion, it is usually easy to anesthetize the anal canal with the patient under local anesthesia. The operation should be performed in the operating room or in an ambulatory surgical center. Unless the tissues are necrotic, mucosa and skin can be closed as in elective hemorrhoidectomy. It is important to compress all the edema before starting the excision as a means to avoid taking too much normal tissue. Hemorrhoidectomy in the presence of strangulation and necrosis is a safe procedure provided all necrotic tissue is excised.[43-45]

Another approach to acute hemorrhoidal disease is to excise only the large blood clots of the external hemorrhoids and incise any large internal clots. All internal hemorrhoids that are prolapsed and reduced are ligated with rubber banding. This approach frequently requires three or more ligations. The procedure can be performed with the patient under local anesthesia. It is important to massage and squeeze the edematous anal tissues until collapsed before undertaking any excision, incision, and banding. When the procedure is properly performed, the relief is immediate, and a later hemorrhoidectomy is seldom necessary.[46,47]

While the patient is awaiting operation, temporary relief can be obtained by sprinkling the congested strangulated internal hemorrhoids with granulated sugar, as used in the treatment of strangulated rectal prolapse.[48]

Hemorrhoids in Pregnancy

During pregnancy, hemorrhoidectomy is indicated only if acute prolapse and thrombosis occur. It should be performed with the patient under local anesthesia. In the second and third trimesters, a left anterolateral position should be used.[49]

Prolapse and thrombosis of hemorrhoids occurring during delivery are indications for operation immediately postpartum. Similarly, operation is indicated for patients in whom hemorrhoidal disease was symptomatic before

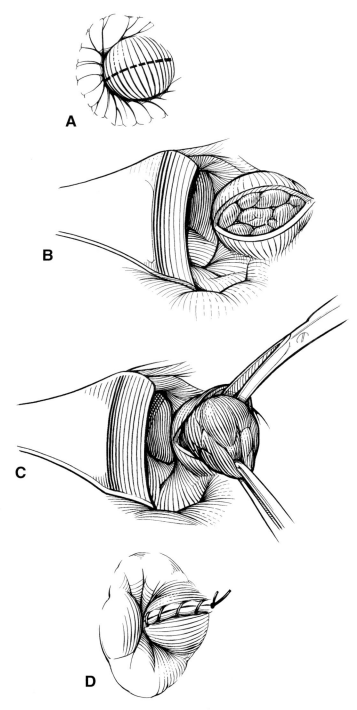

Fig. 9. Technique of evacuating blood clots in thrombosed external hemorrhoid. (A), Line of incision. (B), Hill-Ferguson retractor is used to expose the anal canal. (C), Evacuation of the blood clots. (D), Wound is closed without tension with continuous 3-0 chromic catgut.

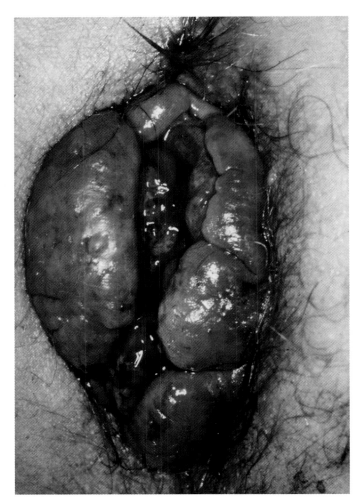

Fig. 10. Strangulated hemorrhoids.

pregnancy, is aggravated during pregnancy, and persists after delivery. In such patients, hemorrhoidectomy is best performed in the immediate postpartum period. Most patients have relief of symptoms the day after the operation.[50]

Hemorrhoids, Anorectal Varices, and Portal Hypertension

Anorectal varices in portal hypertension are common, observed in 78% of patients studied (89% in noncirrhotic patients and 56% in cirrhotic patients) ($P < 0.01$).[51] Patients with noncirrhotic portal hypertension or extrahepatic vein obstruction have large anorectal varices (> 5 mm) compared with cirrhotic patients (< 5 mm) ($P < 0.05$). Unlike esophageal varices, the risk of bleeding from anorectal varices is less than 2%.[51-53]

Despite the communication between systemic and portal systems in the anal canal, the incidence of hemorrhoidal disease in patients with portal hypertension is no greater than in the normal population.[3,52] Although

massive bleeding from prolapsed hemorrhoids in patients with portal hypertension is uncommon, it can be life-threatening. Treatment of encephalopathy, which includes administering nonabsorbable antibiotics and supplements of potassium, frequently causes severe diarrhea and breakdown of the anal canal lining, resulting in massive bleeding. Anoscopic examination is essential to identify the site of bleeding because proctoscopy or flexible sigmoidoscopy may miss the bleeding point entirely.

Once the bleeding site has been located, a stick-tie figure-of-eight suture of 2-0 synthetic absorbable material effectively stops the bleeding.[54] Coagulopathy and diarrhea must be corrected. Hemorrhoidectomy is reserved for the rare situation in which the stick-tie method fails to control the bleeding.[55]

Bleeding hemorrhoids in patients with portal hypertension must be distinguished from anorectal varices, a true consequence of portal hypertension. Anorectal varices occur in any of three specific zones: the perineal area, anal canal, and rectum.[56] The site of bleeding is usually in the squamous portion of the anal canal. Placement of running sutures of synthetic absorbable material starting as high as possible in the rectum and continuing to just outside the anus is the method of choice to control the bleeding.[52] A transjugular intrahepatic portosystemic shunt also has been successful.[57,58]

Hemorrhoids in Inflammatory Bowel Disease

Hemorrhoidal problems are uncommon in patients with inflammatory bowel disease.[59] Most anal problems result from perianal irritation and swelling caused by diarrhea rather than from hemorrhoids themselves. Hemorrhoids can be treated operatively or nonoperatively in patients with ulcerative colitis, but operation should be avoided in patients with active Crohn's disease.[59,60]

Hemorrhoids in Leukemia

Patients with leukemia or lymphoma or other conditions involving immunosuppression seldom present with hemorrhoidal disease.[61] The risks from operative intervention are great, and poor wound healing and postoperative abscesses are common. Operation is done as a last resort. *Escherichia coli* and *Pseudomonas aeruginosa* are the most common bacteria isolated from both blood and anorectal cultures.[61] Correction of any coexisting coagulation disorder and administration of appropriate antibiotics are important parts of the management of hemorrhoidal disease in this patient population. Anal infections in these patients lack classic signs of abscess formation. Fever, local pain, and local tenderness are the most common findings. The infected area usually has no pus but rather a cavity of necrotic tissue.

Hemorrhoids With Other Anorectal Diseases
If hemorrhoids are associated with other anorectal problems such as anal fissure or fistula in ano, hemorrhoidectomy in combination with sphincterotomy or fistulotomy can be done without added morbidity.

Recommendations for a Smooth Postoperative Course

The technical points for a smooth course after hemorrhoidectomy begin in the operating room. A well-performed hemorrhoidectomy with attention to detail, or "tricks," can make a difference. Most hemorrhoidectomies can be performed as outpatient procedures, or may require an overnight admission. Current recommendations are as follows:

1. Limit intravenous fluid to 250 mL during the operation.
2. When suitable, perform hemorrhoidectomy with the patient under local anesthesia. Buffer the anesthetic solution with sodium bicarbonate to minimize pain in cases of thrombosed external hemorrhoid.
3. Perform hemorrhoidectomy only to treat severe third- and fourth-degree hemorrhoids, including strangulated hemorrhoids. Do not operate on more than three quadrants. Frequently, only one or two quadrants require surgical treatment.
4. Avoid hemorrhoidectomy in the posterior quadrant. It does not heal well.
5. Do not excise a strip of mucosa more than 1.5 cm in width. The redundant anoderm and mucosa can be trimmed before closure. Close the wound with sutures 1 to 2 mm from the edges and 1 to 2 mm apart. Closure with tension is one of the sources of pain and wound separation.
6. Do not excise the hemorrhoids above the anorectal ring. Higher excision and suturing frequently cause urinary retention.
7. Inject the anesthetic agent into the internal sphincter at completion of the procedure, 2 to 3 mL in each quadrant. This will delay the pain for a few hours.
8. Provide a preemptive analgesia with ketorolac tromethamine, 30 mg intramuscularly, just before the patient leaves the operating room. Reduce the dosage to 15 mg in elderly patients. This agent is contraindicated in patients with impaired renal and hepatic function.
9. Prescribe an analgesic to be taken every 6 hours for 48 hours. Thereafter, it can be taken as needed.
10. Metronidazole, 500 mg orally 3 times a day for 5 days, has been shown to combat inflammation or infection and minimize pain.[62] This is generally unnecessary if the wounds are closed without tension.
11. For the first 3 days, have the patient take warm sitz baths to relieve the throbbing pain from the anal spasm. Baths should not exceed 10 to 15 minutes because water tends to macerate the skin, causing separation of the wounds. The anal area should be hand washed with soap and water and not with a washcloth. This cleansing should be done at least twice daily and after each bowel movement.
12. Encourage the patient to eat a high-fiber diet and drink plenty of fluid. Supplement the diet with a psyllium seed preparation or raw bran, as indicated. The first bowel movement can be delayed to the fourth or fifth day if a laxative was given preoperatively to empty the colon.

Summary

The current management of hemorrhoids at Mayo Clinic is summarized in Table 3.

ANAL FISSURES

Definition

Anal fissure is an ulcer in the distal portion of the anal canal which extends from the dentate line to the anal verge. Anal fissures can be classified as acute or chronic and further subdivided as either primary or secondary. A primary fissure occurs without association with other local or systemic diseases. A secondary fissure develops in association with other systemic diseases, such as Crohn's disease, leukemia, aplastic anemia, agranulocytosis, and infection with human immunodeficiency virus.

Etiology

It is generally agreed that the initiating factor in the development of a fissure is trauma to the anal canal, usually in the form of the passage of a hard and large fecal bolus or, less commonly, explosive diarrhea. One of the remarkable features of anal fissure is that it is nearly always located in the midline posteriorly, because of the elliptic arrangement of the external sphincter fibers in the posterior anal wall. This arrangement offers less support to the anal canal during the passage of a large fecal bolus and, thus, renders the posterior canal more prone to tear than elsewhere in the circumference of the anus.

Pathogenesis

Persistently hard bowel movements, in addition to initiating the process, may continuously aggravate the anal canal and result in failure of the fissure to heal. This factor must be considered when treatment is planned. Studies also have shown that after initiation of a tear in

Table 3. Summary of Management of Hemorrhoids at Mayo Clinic

Condition	Treatment
First-degree hemorrhoids	Exclusion of other causes of bleeding
	Diet, psyllium seed, or bran
	Rubber band ligation
	Electrocoagulation
Second-degree hemorrhoids	Rubber band ligation
	Electrocoagulation
Third-degree hemorrhoids	Rubber band ligation
	Closed hemorrhoidectomy
	Circular stapled hemorrhoidectomy
Fourth-degree hemorrhoids	Closed hemorrhoidectomy
	Circular stapled hemorrhoidectomy
Prolapsed strangulated hemorrhoids	Closed hemorrhoidectomy
	Circular stapled hemorrhoidectomy
	Multiple rubber band ligations
Thrombosed external hemorrhoids	If very painful, excision of clots
	If pain is resolving, conservative treatment
Perianal skin tags	If symptomatic, excision
Hypertrophied anal papillae	Asymptomatic: no treatment
	Symptomatic: excision

the anal canal, chronicity is perpetuated by persistent hypertonia of the internal sphincter.[63-67] The pain, tenderness, spasm, and fibrosis may be due to myositis of the internal sphincter.[68] Using laser Doppler flowmetry, Schouten et al.[69] found that the anodermal blood flow at the fissure site was substantially lower than at the posterior commissure of controls. Reduction of anal sphincter pressure by sphincterotomy improves anodermal blood flow at the posterior midline, resulting in healing of a fissure.

Clinical Manifestations

Anal pain, particularly during and after bowel movements, is the most prominent symptom. The pain is described as burning, throbbing, or dull aching. Bleeding is common and, as a rule, stains the toilet paper. If there is fever, a fissure may mimic an anorectal abscess, especially an intersphincteric abscess. In some patients with a painful fissure, dysuria or frequency of urination develops. Constipation is a common association, because the pain may cause patients to be reluctant to have a bowel movement.

Diagnosis

The diagnosis of an anal fissure is usually straightforward and can be made from the patient's history alone but needs to be confirmed by physical examination. The site of anal fissure differs between men and women. Anterior fissure is more common in women than in men—10% of all fissures in women and only 1% in men.[70] In men, the fissure is usually located in the midline posteriorly.

When performed gently, inspection of the anus by spreading the buttocks reveals the fissure in most cases (Fig. 11). Pain and apprehension may involuntarily draw the anus and the fissure upward, making it impossible to be seen. Coexisting large external hemorrhoids or skin folds may hide the fissure. Nonvisualization of the fissure does not rule out its presence. Digital examination is performed with a generous amount of 2% lidocaine jelly. The fissure can be appreciated as a small fibrotic defect that is tender. Digital examination also can detect tightness of the anal canal from spasm or fibrosis, another clue to the presence of a fissure. A small anoscope with a side view is useful to visualize the fissure. A small number of patients with chronic anal fissure have the classic triad: a sentinel pile (edematous adjacent skin), an anal ulcer, and a hypertrophied anal papilla. Proctoscopy or flexible sigmoidoscopy should be performed, if possible, to exclude any associated abnormalities of the anorectum and sigmoid colon, especially inflammatory bowel disease. In very painful fissure or in patients who cannot cooperate, the examination should be performed with the patient under general anesthesia.

Differential Diagnosis

Basically, all primary anal fissures occur in the posterior or anterior quadrants. Multiple fissures or fissures occurring

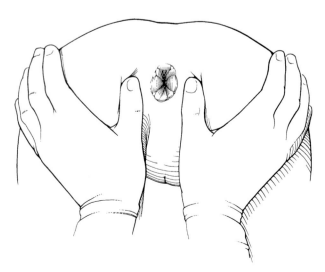

Fig. 11. Gentle spreading of the buttocks reveals an anal fissure.

in the lateral position arouse suspicion of other diseases such as Crohn's disease, ulcerative colitis, syphilis, tuberculosis, leukemia, and human immunodeficiency virus (Fig. 12). However, the majority of fissures in patients with Crohn's disease or ulcerative colitis occur in the posterior midline.

Management

Acute Fissure

Avoidance of constipation (or diarrhea) is the single most important nonoperative treatment. The aim of treatment of an acute anal fissure is to break the cycle of a hard stool (or diarrhea), pain, and reflex spasm. Warm sitz baths (40°C) substantially lower the anal resting pressure in patients with anal fissure.[71]

Conservative treatment of an acute anal fissure with bulk-forming agents and warm sitz baths is successful within 2 months in 40% to 50% of patients. For the 50% of patients who do not respond to the treatment, operation is recommended.[72-74] Unprocessed bran, 5 g three times a day, promotes healing in 84% of patients.[75]

Chronic Fissure

Nonoperative Treatment

Chronic anal fissures are usually deep, exposing the internal sphincter. Occasionally, chronic anal fissure has a triad of fissure, sentinel skin tag, and a hypertrophied anal papilla. Some patients with chronic anal fissure respond to warm sitz baths and bulk-forming agents, especially patients with associated constipation.

A relatively new medical treatment is the use of nitroglycerin or glyceryl trinitrate applied around the anus. The nitroglycerin paste (0.2%-0.3%) can be prepared at a hospital pharmacy by diluting commercial 2% nitroglycerin with petroleum. When organic nitrates are degraded, nitric oxide is released.[76] Nitric oxide is an inhibitory neurotransmitter in the internal sphincter.[77] Nitroglycerin reduces anal resting pressure and increases the anodermal blood flow.[78] The paste (an amount about the size of a peanut) is applied around the anal verge three times daily.

The success rate with nitroglycerin paste is 40% to 60%.[79-81] Although this result is less than ideal, the paste does not damage the sphincter muscle and thus fewer patients require a lateral sphincterotomy. Accordingly, nitroglycerin paste should be the first line of treatment. Patients should be warned of the temporary side effects of headache or light-headedness from the nitroglycerin. Nitroglycerin 0.3% is associated with a higher incidence of headache than 0.2%;[80] a higher concentration does not heal more fissures.[79] Thus, the 0.2% strength is recommended.

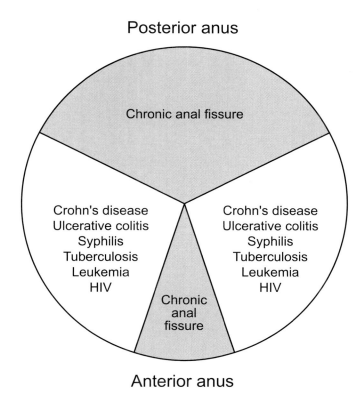

Fig. 12. Locations of chronic anal fissure and other anorectal conditions. HIV, human immunodeficiency virus. (Modified from Storer EH, Goldberg SM, Nivatvongs S: Colon, rectum, and anus. In Principles of Surgery. Third edition. Edited by SI Schwartz. New York, McGraw-Hill, 1979, p 1240. By permission of the publisher.)

Clostridium botulinum produces several toxins, of which types A, B, and E have been linked to cases of botulism in humans. Botulinum toxin type A is one of the most lethal biological toxins, but it is of therapeutic value in several muscle disorders such as strabismus, spasmodic torticollis, and achalasia.[82] Botulinum toxin exerts its effects on the peripheral nerve endings at the neuromuscular junction, resulting in flaccid paralysis due to irreversible and selective multiphasic blockade of acetylcholine. It also inhibits contractions in gastrointestinal smooth muscle.[83]

The success rate of botulinum toxin injection for healing anal fissure is between 60% and 83%.[82,84] The long-term outcome of this treatment remains to be determined. The effect of the toxin lasts for a few months, and the result after the resting anal pressure returns to the pretreatment level is still unknown. In the series reported by Maria et al.,[85] about a third of patients treated required a repeat treatment after 2 months of follow-up. Botulinum toxin is not inexpensive and is not convenient to use. It costs about $370 per vial (100 U) in the United States. It needs to be stored at −20°C and should be used within 4 hours after being diluted with a normal saline solution.

The dosage of botulinum toxin should be 20 U in two divided doses. The optimal sites for injection are the left and right lateral anal quadrants, and the injection is given into the internal sphincter muscle. Persistent fissures can be re-treated at a higher dose of 25 U. No adverse reactions or problems with fecal incontinence have been reported.

Anal Sphincter Stretch

The classic technique involves stretching the anal canal to a diameter that accommodates four fingers. The stretch also can be performed with a Park retractor, a Pratt anal speculum, or a rectosigmoid balloon. Surgeons have been attracted to the procedure by "its extreme simplicity." However, the technique is difficult to standardize and is criticized for causing uncontrolled tearing of the sphincter.[86] A proponent of this method cites the advantages of the absence of a wound and an early return to work for patients. Even though no incision is made, complications have been reported: bleeding from the fissure, perianal infection, Fournier's gangrene, rectal prolapse, and bacteremia.[86]

The results of anal stretch have been variable and are probably operator-dependent. Rates of fecal incontinence range from 0% to 27%.[87-89] Although the classic anal dilation has little place in current treatment, many investigators have reported excellent long-term results.[87-89] In a meta-analysis by Nelson,[90] anal stretch was more likely than sphincterotomy to result in persistence of fissure and incontinence to flatus.

In contrast to these poor results with anal dilation for anal fissure, Strugnell et al.[91] reported a success rate of 89% after the procedure with a median follow-up of 7.8 years. They emphasized the technique used:

> The procedure was performed with the patient under general anaesthesia and lying in the left lateral position. In addition patients were usually paralysed with suxamethonium (total neuromuscular blockade) during the procedure to prevent inadvertent contraction of the external sphincter and potential damage during dilation.
>
> Digital dilation was performed by controlled stretching evenly distributed around the anal circumference by rotating hands, and continued until it was perceived that no further reasonably achieved increase would occur. This required differing amounts of force according to the toughness of the internal sphincter.

Thus, with proper technique, some patients may benefit from a well-controlled anal stretch.

Lateral Internal Sphincterotomy

Lateral internal sphincterotomy has become the usual treatment of choice for an intractable anal fissure. Lessons learned include recognition that sphincterotomy through the posterior anal fissure was plagued with delayed or unhealed wounds and that internal sphincterotomy performed on the lateral anus healed the posterior or anterior fissure. A lateral internal sphincterotomy can be performed with local, regional, or general anesthesia. Local anesthesia is suitable in most patients, and the procedure is usually performed on an outpatient basis or in the office. The patient can be positioned in the prone, left antero-lateral, or lithotomy position. For surgeons less familiar with the anorectal anatomy or those just starting to perform lateral internal sphincterotomy, the procedure is best performed with an open approach.

For the closed technique, the anal canal is exposed with a Pratt bivalve anal speculum and gradually opened to its maximum. The stretched internal sphincter is easily felt and is bowstring-like. In the rare instance when the bowstring cannot be appreciated, it is essential to use the open technique. A small beaver blade (cataract knife) is stabbed through the skin at the palpable lateral border of the internal sphincter, in the intersphincteric space, with the blade in horizontal position. The knife blade is then advanced to the level of the dentate line. At this point, the blade is turned 90°, with the cutting edge of the knife behind the internal sphincter. Through shearing of the knife blade, the stretched muscle can be easily split apart as the knife is drawn back toward the anal verge. The stab wound is left open (Fig. 13).

With the open technique, a radial incision is less likely to separate than a transverse wound. A Pratt anal speculum exposes the lateral quadrant. A radial incision is made into the subcutaneous tissue, exposing the internal sphincter from its lateral edge to the level of the dentate line, after which the full thickness of the muscle is dissected and tented up with a hemostat. The muscle is incised in its full thickness from its lateral edge to the dentate line. The wound is closed with running 3-0 chromic catgut (Fig. 14). Closed internal sphincterotomy is preferable to open internal sphincterotomy. The stab wound heals rapidly. Lateral internal sphincterotomy is considered a minor operation. Garcia-Aguilar et al.[92] found that the closed technique was followed by less incontinence for gas and stool than the open technique ($P = 0.062$ for gas, $P < 0.001$ for soiling, $P < 0.001$ for stool). However, a meta-analysis by Nelson[90] showed no difference between the two techniques. The rates of incontinence and persistence of fissure varied from 0% to 20% and 3% to 29%, respectively. Review of all reports provided no insight to the wide variability. Nelson also found that the technique of sphincterotomy varies considerably, not only the length of incision but also the depth of incision. This may be a critical factor for the results.

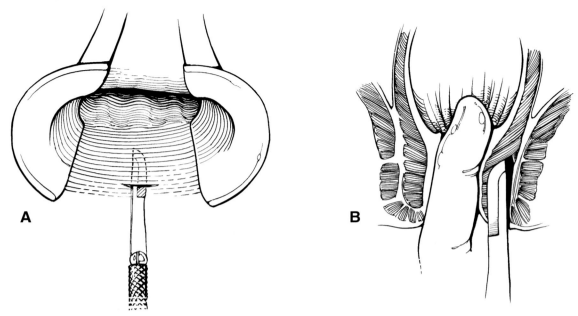

Fig. 13. Lateral internal sphincterotomy: closed technique. (A), Lateral anal canal is exposed with a Pratt anal speculum. A small beaver blade is stabbed into the intersphincteric groove with the cutting edge in a horizontal position. The knife is advanced behind the internal sphincter to the dentate line. (B), The cutting edge is turned toward the lumen and sawed through the internal sphincter with the index finger as a guide. It is important to stretch the anal canal while cutting.

In an anatomical and functional evaluation by Garcia-Aguilar et al.,[93] anal incontinence after lateral internal sphincterotomy was directly related to the length of the sphincterotomy. The series from Mayo Clinic[94] included 487 patients who were available for a long-term mean follow-up of 72 months (range, 6-145 months). Fissures healed by a median of 3 weeks in 96%. Fissures recurred in 8%, but two-thirds of these healed with conservative management alone. After more than 5 years, 6% of patients reported incontinence for flatus, 8% had minor fecal soiling, and 1% experienced incontinence for solid stool. Importantly, only 3% of patients stated that incontinence

had ever affected their quality of life. The outcome of operation was satisfactory for 98% of patients.

Unhealed or recurrent anal fissure after lateral internal sphincterotomy occurs in 1% to 3% of subjects.[94-96] Because a recurrence after lateral internal sphincterotomy usually is due to the technical failure of an inadequate internal sphincterotomy,[97] a second lateral internal sphincterotomy on the opposite side usually gives successful results.[63,98]

V-Y Advancement Flap
In a posterior anal fissure associated with marked redundant skin tags, a V-Y advancement flap works well. A triangular

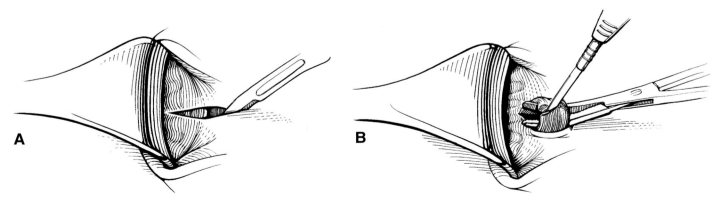

Fig. 14. Lateral internal sphincterotomy: open technique. (A), Lateral anal canal is exposed with a large Hill-Ferguson retractor. A radial incision is made from the dentate line to the anal verge, exposing the internal sphincter. (B), The internal sphincter is isolated with a curved clamp, and the muscle is cut with cautery. The wound is closed with continuous 3-0 chromic catgut.

skin flap, with the apex at the fissure and the wide base at the perianal skin, is created deep into the subcutaneous tissue. Internal sphincterotomy is performed in the bed of the fissure from the dentate line to its lateral border. If preferred, the fissure can be excised. The flap is then slid to cover the wound and closed with running 3-0 chromic catgut (Fig. 15).

Anal fissure may be associated with childbirth in 3% to 11% of patients who deliver vaginally. The fissure commonly occurs in the anterior midline. Shearing forces from the fetal head on the anal mucosa and mucosal tethering after childbirth rendering it more susceptible to trauma have both been incriminated but are difficult to substantiate. Postpartum anal fissure in primiparous women has been treated by reducing anal canal pressures, but most fissures heal with intensive medical management.[99]

When anal fissures occur in patients with weak sphincters, including those with a failed lateral internal sphincterotomy, previous obstetric trauma, or previous perianal operation, a flap can be used to cover the ulcer without performing an internal sphincterotomy. Nyam et al.[100] used island flaps in 21 patients and had a success rate of 100% after a median follow-up of 18 months (range, 2-28).

ANORECTAL ABSCESS AND FISTULA IN ANO

Anorectal Abscesses

Anorectal abscesses occur only in specific potential spaces around the anorectal region. It is essential to be familiar with and picture the anatomy of these spaces. The spaces are filled with fat, areolar tissues, and blood vessels. Their anatomical locations are self-explanatory (Fig. 16 and 17). Of note is the communication of these spaces on each side posteriorly (Fig. 18).

Pathogenesis and Avenue of Spread of Abscess

Current evidence suggests that infection in the anal glands is the origin of an anorectal abscess.[101] The average number of glands in a normal anal canal is 6 (range, 3-10).[102] Each gland is lined by stratified columnar epithelium with mucus-secreting or goblet cells interspersed within the glandular epithelial lining. These cells have a direct opening into an anal crypt at the dentate line. The anal glands are fairly evenly distributed around the anal canal. Eighty percent of the glands are submucosal in extent.[102] Intersphincteric or intramuscular glands cause the abscesses. The abscesses formed in the intersphincteric space can spread to the surrounding anorectal spaces (Fig. 18 and 19). The locations of abscesses, in order of frequency, are

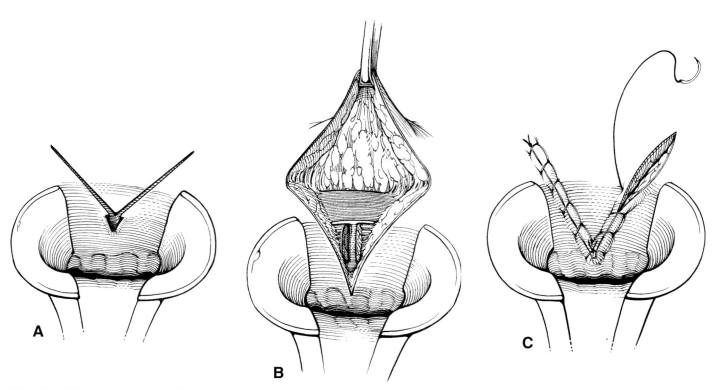

Fig. 15. V-Y advancement skin flap. (A), The posterior anal canal is exposed with a Pratt anal speculum. A triangular wide-base flap is outlined. (B), A full-thickness skin flap is raised. The internal sphincter is exposed to the dentate line and incised. (C), The flap is slid to cover the wound and the wound closed with continuous 3-0 chromic catgut.

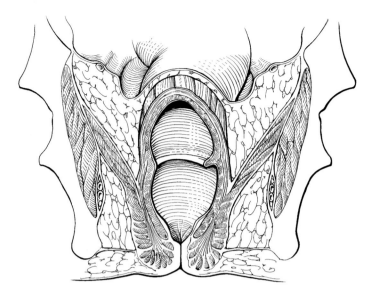

Fig. 16. Perianal and perirectal spaces (front view).

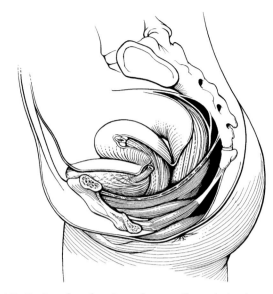

Fig. 17. Perianal and perirectal spaces (lateral view).

perianal, ischioanal (ischiorectal), intersphincteric, and supralevator. However, the incidence varies widely.[103,104]

Clinical Manifestations

The initial symptom of most anorectal abscesses is severe pain in the anal region. The pain is throbbing or dull aching, aggravated by walking, straining, coughing, and sneezing. Depending on the location of the abscess, a swollen mass may or may not be felt by the patient. Fever or even septicemia may be present. In some patients, urinary retention occurs.

Examination

Perianal and ischioanal (ischiorectal) abscesses cause an obvious swelling with marked tenderness. For an intersphincteric abscess, there is severe pain in the anal area with no sign of inflammation in the perianal region. However, the patient usually does not tolerate a digital examination unless a general anesthetic is given. Easily appreciated is an induration of the submucosal wall of the anal canal beginning at the dentate line and extending proximally for a variable distance. In a supralevator abscess, the severe pain usually is described as being in the coccyx. It can be an extension from an intersphincteric or an ischioanal abscess. The levator muscle is indurated. The supralevator abscess, as a rule, is difficult to diagnose, and intrarectal ultrasonography or magnetic resonance imaging is helpful. Further work-up with proctoscopy or flexible sigmoidoscopy should be postponed until the abscess has resolved.

Basic Principles in Management

Like an abscess in any part of the body, an anorectal abscess must be drained as soon as possible. When it is properly

treated, recovery is uncomplicated and morbidity is minimal, although some abscesses may progress to a fistula in ano. Delay in treatment or inadequate treatment occasionally causes extensive and life-threatening suppuration associated with massive tissue necrosis and septicemia and a risk of mortality.

In general, an antibiotic is not necessary after the abscess is adequately drained, but an antibiotic is advisable in certain groups of patients. In patients who have septicemia, immunodeficiency, severe diabetes mellitus, or agranulocytosis, a broad-spectrum antibiotic should be given. Patients with artificial heart valves or artificial joints also should have appropriate antibiotics.

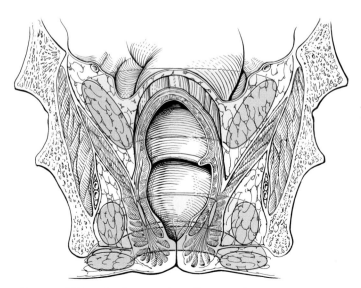

Fig. 18. "Horseshoe" connection of anorectal spaces.

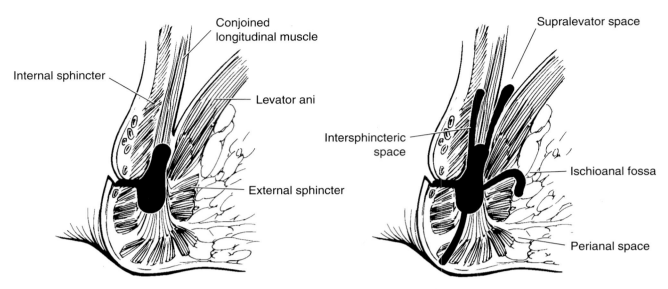

Fig. 19. *Avenues of extension of an intersphincteric abscess. (Modified from Parks.[101] By permission of BMJ Publishing Group.)*

Management

Perianal Abscess

This type is the most superficial and the easiest to treat. The abscess is usually small and can be drained with the patient under local anesthesia in the office, clinic, or emergency room. A cruciate incision is made on the most prominent part of the swelling, the skin edges being excised to prevent early closure of the incision. This is deepened down to the base of the abscess cavity (Fig. 20). It is essential to instill an adequate amount of anesthetic solution, deeply beyond the bottom of the abscess. The abscess cavity is thoroughly curetted and irrigated. Packing causes pain and is not necessary. Postoperatively, the wound is

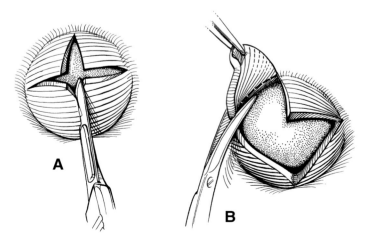

Fig. 20. *Incision and drainage of perianal abscess. (A), Cruciate incision. (B), Excision of dog ears.*

hand washed with soap and water, and a dry dressing is applied two or three times a day.

Ischioanal (Ischiorectal) Abscess

Small ischioanal abscesses on one side can be drained with the patient under local anesthesia, in the same manner as perianal abscess. A large ischioanal abscess usually has its origin in the deep postanal space and then spreads to the ischioanal space on one side or both sides as a "horseshoe" abscess. This type of abscess should be drained in the operating room with the patient under general or regional anesthesia.

The abscess should be drained through the deep postanal space. A longitudinal incision is made on the skin between the tip of the coccyx and the anus, exposing the anococcygeal ligament (superficial external sphincter). The anococcygeal ligament is then incised along its fibers; when the deep postanal space is entered, a pool of pus is found. A counterincision is made into the space at the ischioanal area on each side (Fig. 21). The abscess cavity is thoroughly curetted and irrigated. Postoperatively, the abscess cavity should be irrigated with diluted hydrogen peroxide (1:4 dilution) for 3 days. The openings are lightly packed. An alternative technique is to enter the deep postanal space through the anal canal by incising the internal sphincter in the posterior midline (Fig. 22).

Intersphincteric Abscess

Unlike perianal and ischioanal abscesses, an intersphincteric abscess has no apparent signs of swelling or induration in the perianal area. The diagnosis is made by having a strong suspicion, particularly when the anorectal pain

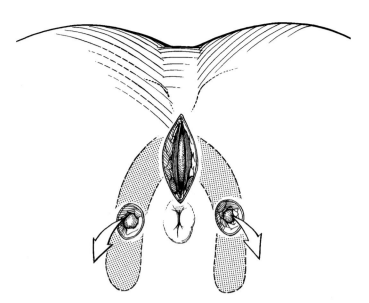

Fig. 21. Drainage of deep postanal space and counterdrainage of ischioanal spaces for horseshoe abscess.

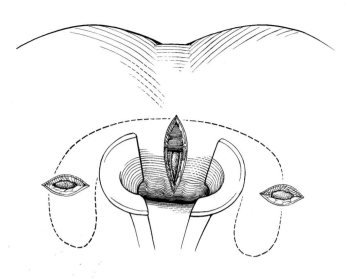

Fig. 22. Intra-anal drainage and counterdrainage of horseshoe abscess.

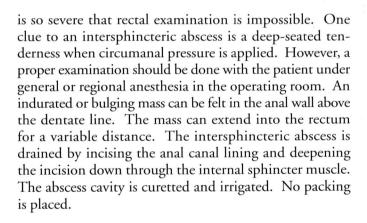

is so severe that rectal examination is impossible. One clue to an intersphincteric abscess is a deep-seated tenderness when circumanal pressure is applied. However, a proper examination should be done with the patient under general or regional anesthesia in the operating room. An indurated or bulging mass can be felt in the anal wall above the dentate line. The mass can extend into the rectum for a variable distance. The intersphincteric abscess is drained by incising the anal canal lining and deepening the incision down through the internal sphincter muscle. The abscess cavity is curetted and irrigated. No packing is placed.

Supralevator Abscess

This type of abscess is uncommon and can be difficult to diagnose. Because of its proximity to the abdominal cavity, a supralevator abscess can mimic acute intra-abdominal conditions. Digital examination reveals an indurated or bulging tender mass on either side of the lower rectum or posteriorly above the level of the anorectal ring. The supralevator abscess may arise in one of three ways. It may be due to an upward extension of an intersphincteric abscess, an upward extension of an ischioanal abscess, or an intra-abdominal disease, such as a diverticular abscess, an appendiceal abscess, or an abscess from Crohn's disease.

It is essential to determine the origin of the abscess before treatment. If the abscess is due to an upward extension of an intersphincteric abscess, it should be drained into the rectum. If it is drained through the ischioanal fossa, a complicated suprasphincteric fistula can be formed. If a supralevator abscess arises from an ischioanal abscess,

it should be drained through the ischioanal fossa; attempts at draining this kind of abscess into the rectum may result in an extrasphincteric fistula (Fig. 23). If the abscess is due to an intra-abdominal disease, the primary disease is treated, for example, by a colon resection, and the supralevator abscess is drained into the rectum through the ischioanal fossa or through the abdominal wall.

Bacteriology of Anorectal Abscesses

As a rule, bacteria in anorectal abscesses are fecal flora or cutaneous flora or both. Most surgeons do not send a specimen from the abscess for culture, with the belief that a culture is a waste of time, effort, and money.[105] Others,

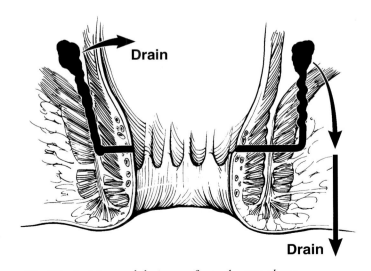

Fig. 23. Incision and drainage of supralevator abscess.

however, have suggested that a culture is worthwhile to determine the type of bacteria present in the abscess. There is strong evidence that patients whose abscesses grow gut organisms have a high incidence of anal fistulas after incision and drainage of the abscesses, whereas patients whose abscesses grow skin-derived organisms seldom have anal fistulas (*P* < 0.005).[106,107]

Although pus from anorectal abscesses contains large numbers of bacteria, chronic anal fistulas have much smaller numbers. The bacteria in chronic anal fistulas are normal commensals of the lower gastrointestinal tract.[108]

Recurrent Abscess and Fistula After Incision and Drainage

Theoretically, an anorectal abscess cavity will not heal completely unless the infected anal gland causing it is excised or self-destructs. Finding the internal opening or the infected gland is not easy. At the initial examination of anorectal abscesses, the internal opening is demonstrable in 14% to 35% of patients.[101-111] Abscess recurs after incision and drainage in 11% to 13% of patients,[103,112] whereas fistula in ano occurs in 16% to 41%.[103,110,112] Incision and drainage and primary fistulotomy has a recurrence or fistula in ano rate of 3% to 13%.[111,112] However, in 6.5% to 39% of patients, some degree of fecal incontinence develops.[111,112]

Because of the higher risk of fecal incontinence after a fistulotomy, most surgeons recommend an initial incision and drainage alone for anorectal abscesses. It is important to drain the abscess cavity completely and thoroughly curette and wash it. Most anorectal abscesses are drained with the patient under local anesthesia in the office, clinic, or emergency room.

Necrotizing Perianal and Perineal Infections (Fournier's Gangrene)

Fournier's gangrene is a synergistic necrotizing fasciitis, defined as a suppurative bacterial infection of the perirectal, perineal, or genital area, which leads to thrombosis of small subcutaneous vessels and often gangrene of the overlying skin. However, deeper extension to cause myonecrosis, which has sometimes been found in perineal infections, generally is not considered a feature of classic Fournier's gangrene. The bacterial synergism involves the production of exotoxins whose activities result in tissue necrosis and synthesis of gases that produce the repulsive stench and crepitus pathognomonic of anaerobic infections.[113] This is the most lethal form of infection in the anorectal area. Although some patients with neglected anorectal abscesses have progression to Fournier's gangrene, a considerable number of cases of overwhelming infection have no recognizable cause. Reported causes include genitourinary (24%),

anorectal (24%), intra-abdominal (10%), traumatic (2%), and undetermined (38%) causes.[114]

Clinical Manifestations

Necrotizing perianal and perirectal infections are usually the result of neglected or delayed treatment of the primary anorectal or perineal infection. Although patients with diabetes mellitus are more prone to this type of infection, this condition also can develop in patients who were previously healthy. Pain, tenderness, and swelling with crepitation of the perianal area, perineum, scrotum, or labia are characteristic. The swelling and crepitation may spread to the back, abdominal wall, and thigh. A distinct "black spot" on the skin is indicative of underlying tissue necrosis. Fever and a high leukocyte count are consistent findings.

Management

These infections are caused by synergistic, gram-negative, anaerobic or microaerophilic bacterial flora that cause considerable gas formation. Although *Clostridia perfringens* bacteria usually are present, they are not the major offending microorganisms. Therapy with multiple antibiotics is started as soon as possible. These antibiotics include penicillin for *Streptococcus* and *Clostridia*, metronidazole or clindamycin for anaerobes, especially *Bacteroides*, and a third-generation cephalosporin for coliform organisms and *Staphylococci*.[113] The antibiotic therapy should be adjusted according to the results of culture and sensitivity tests. Tetanus immunization also should be given.[114]

The most important aspect of treatment is immediate excision of all dead tissues, including the scrotal skin, if affected, irrespective of the size or site of the residual defect. Typically, the necrosis of underlying subcutaneous tissue is more extensive than is appreciated on physical examination. Hyperbaric oxygen treatment is not indicated unless myonecrosis caused by *Clostridia perfringens* is present.

Postoperatively, it is important to examine the patient several times a day. If the necrosis or infection is spreading, reoperation is indicated and has to be done as many times as necessary. Once the infection has been arrested, whirlpool treatment is helpful. The patient also should be evaluated for consideration of hyperalimentation, diverting colostomy, or cystostomy. Because of the extensive wound, skin grafting and creation of a new sac for the testes are usually necessary at a later date.

In the cumulative series of 1,726 cases reviewed by Eke[113] from 1950 to 1959, the mortality rate was 16%. Causes of death have included severe sepsis, coagulopathy, acute renal failure, diabetic ketoacidosis, and multiple organ failure.

Fistula in Ano

Fistula in ano is a chronic form of anorectal abscess that has spontaneously drained or been surgically drained but the abscess cavity does not heal completely. It becomes instead a fibrotic tract with a primary opening (internal opening) in the anal crypt at the dentate line and a secondary opening (external opening) in the perianal skin. Eisenhammer[115] stated that the anorectal abscess is the "parent of the fistula."

Classification

There are four main forms of fistula in ano, and they are based on the relationship of the fistula to the sphincter muscles[116] (Fig. 24).

Intersphincteric Fistula

The fistulous tract is in the intersphincteric plane. The external opening is usually in the perianal skin close to the anal verge.

Transsphincteric Fistula

The fistula starts in the intersphincteric plane or in the deep postanal space. The fistulous tract traverses the external sphincter, and the external opening is at the ischioanal fossa. Horseshoe fistulas are also in this category.

Suprasphincteric Fistula

The fistula starts in the intersphincteric plane in the mid anal canal and then passes upward to a point above the puborectal muscle. The fistula passes laterally over this muscle and downward between the puborectal and levator ani muscle into the ischioanal fossa.

Extrasphincteric Fistula

The fistula passes from the perineal skin through the ischioanal fossa and levator ani muscle and finally penetrates the rectal wall. Extrasphincteric fistulas may arise from cryptoglandular origin, trauma, a foreign body, or a pelvic abscess, such as diverticular or appendiceal abscess.

Clinical Manifestations

Most patients present with a previous history of anorectal abscess associated with intermittent drainage. Recurrence of an anorectal abscess suggests the presence of a fistula in ano. The external opening is usually visible as a red

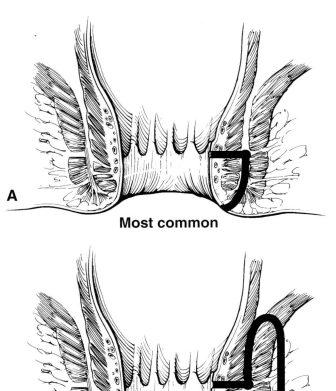

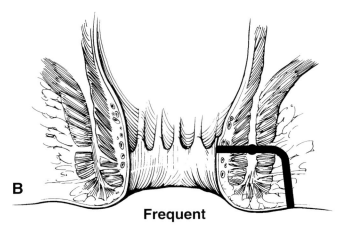

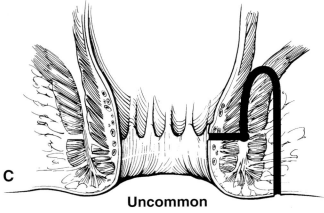

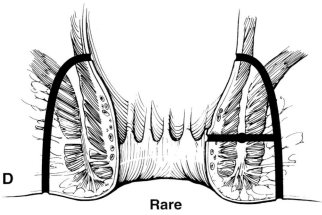

Fig. 24. A simplified classification of fistula in ano.

elevation of granulation tissue with purulent or serosanguineous discharge on compression. In a simple or superficial fistula the tract can be palpated as an indurated cord. Deep fistulas usually are not palpable.

Anoscopy should be done to identify the internal opening. Flexible sigmoidoscopy is performed to rule out other lesions and inflammatory bowel disease; if indicated, a full colonoscopy should be performed.

A fistula probe can be introduced into the fistulous tract to determine its direction, although it is not always possible to pass the probe through the internal opening. Most of the time this can be done with the patient under anesthesia in the operating room.

Several disorders must be considered in the differential diagnosis of a fistula in ano. Hidradenitis suppurativa is differentiated by the presence of multiple perianal openings with surrounding leatherlike hyperpigmented skin. A pilonidal sinus with perianal extensions and infected perianal sebaceous cysts must be considered. It is important to exclude fistulas associated with Crohn's disease and ulcerative colitis. Diverticulitis of the sigmoid colon, with perforation and fistulization to the perineum, rarely occurs. Low rectal and anal canal carcinomas may present as a fistula in the perineum.

Special Investigations

In the majority of patients who present with a fistula in ano, radiologic examination is of limited value. An experienced surgeon can find the complete fistulous tract in most patients. It, however, is helpful to investigate the course of the fistulous tracts in complicated cases.

Fistulography may help to delineate an extrasphincteric fistula of pelvic origin or may help in evaluation of patients with recurrent fistulas.[117] Reports of the usefulness of fistulography have been conflicting. For example, Kuijpers and Schulpen[118] found it accurate in only 16% of cases, whereas Weisman et al.[119] found that it revealed unsuspected conditions or directly altered surgical management in 48% of patients. Fistulography in properly selected patients may add useful information for definitive management of fistula in ano.

Intrarectal ultrasonography is unable to assess conditions outside the sphincters because of the limited focal range of the probe and lack of acoustic coupling when the probe is in the rectum. It is no more accurate than careful digital examination with the patient under anesthesia. Digital examination by an experienced operator can, however, lead to misdiagnosis of intersphincteric and extrasphincteric tracts and overlooking of supralevator extensions.[120] Magnetic resonance imaging is more accurate than intrarectal ultrasonography and is the method of choice when imaging is required for anal fistulas.[121,122]

Principles of Treatment

The presence of a symptomatic fistula in ano is an indication for operation because spontaneous healing of fistula in ano is very rare. Neglected fistulas may result in repeated abscesses and persistent drainage with its concomitant morbidity. Rarely, malignancy may supervene in a longstanding fistula. Because Crohn's disease is associated with anal fistulas, patients with any bowel symptoms suggestive of this condition should have their gastrointestinal tract investigated both endoscopically and radiographically. Control of active Crohn's disease must precede repair of any anal fistula associated with it.

The objective of fistula operation is simple: to cure the fistula with the lowest possible recurrence rate and with minimal, if any, alteration in continence and to do so in the shortest time. To approximate this ideal, a number of principles should be observed:[123] 1) the primary opening of a tract must be identified, 2) the relationship of the tract to the puborectalis muscle must be established, 3) division of the least amount of muscle in keeping with cure of the fistula should be practiced, 4) side tracts should be sought, and 5) the presence or absence of underlying disease should be determined.

The principles of fistula operation include unroofing the fistula, eliminating the primary opening (infective source), and establishing adequate drainage. Failure to open the entire tract may lead to recurrence. Fistulectomy, excision of the fistulous tract, has no advantages over fistulotomy, laying open the tract.

Technique

Before any operative treatment of fistula in ano, it is wise to ascertain whether the patient has normal continence. Fistula operation has an unenviable reputation because of the risks of recurrence and the possible impairment of anal continence. If the cryptoglandular origin of most fistulas is accepted, use of a lay-open technique is necessary and requires division of portions of both the internal and the external sphincters. The key landmark is the anorectal ring, because dividing this portion of the sphincter mechanism renders the patient incontinent.[123]

Simple Low Fistula

A prone jackknife position is preferred, but a lithotomy position with both legs in gynecologic stirrups also gives good exposure. An anal speculum such as the Pratt bivalve, Buie or Parks self-retaining retractor, or a Hill-Ferguson retractor can be used. A probe is introduced into the external opening and passed through the internal opening. The fistulous tract is then laid open with a knife or electrocautery (Fig. 25). Careful examination includes inspecting and probing to uncover the side or cephalad branches of the fistulous tracts. All the granulation tissues are curetted.

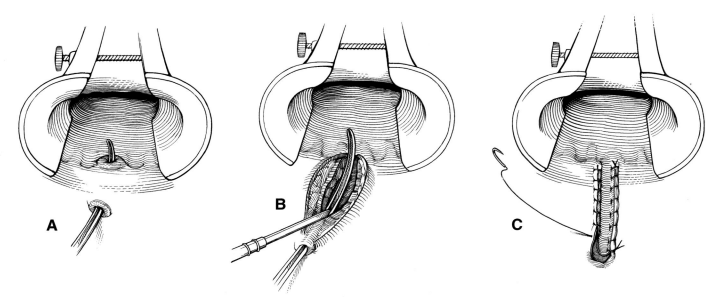

Fig. 25. Technique of fistulotomy for simple fistula. (A), The fistulous tract is probed. (B), The tract is laid open with cautery. (C), Marsupialization of wound.

To minimize the size of the wound, marsupialization is performed with 3-0 chromic catgut. No packing is inserted, but a mesh gauze is applied to catch the soiling. Postoperatively, the anal area is cleaned by hand washing with soap and water. Sitz baths do not clean, but they do macerate the wound and surrounding skin.

Horseshoe Fistula
The external openings are in the ischioanal area and curve posteriorly to join as a single tract to the internal opening in the posterior midline at the dentate line. This makes it impossible to probe the entire tract at once. The tract on each side is opened in a stepwise manner, with a probe used as a guide (Fig. 26). The granulation tissues are curetted, and marsupialization of the wound is done with 3-0 chromic catgut. No packing is required, and only dry cotton mesh gauze is applied. The wound is cleaned by hand washing with soap and water.

An alternative technique for horseshoe fistula was described by Hanley et al.[124] In that technique, the horseshoe-arms portion of the tracts are not laid open but are cored out. The T portion of the fistulous tract in the deep postanal space is identified and laid open (Fig. 27). The wounds are packed overnight for hemostasis. The wound is cleaned by hand washing. Hanley et al. reported that all 31 cases so treated had healing with a minimal defect and no problems with incontinence.

Advancement Rectal Flap
The rationale for advancing a rectal flap is to avoid laying open the fistulous tract, a procedure that inevitably necessitates cutting the overlying internal and external sphincter muscles. In the flap operation, the internal opening, the source of the fistula, is excised. This necessitates an en bloc excision of both the internal and the external sphincter muscles in a small area. The rest of the fistulous tract is cored out or curetted.

Mechanical bowel preparation and prophylactic antibiotics are used. The procedure is performed with the patient under general or regional anesthesia in a prone, jackknife position. An anorectal flap incorporating the internal sphincter muscle is raised starting at the internal opening and dissecting proximally. The internal opening is completely excised and the proximal tract is cored out. The flap is then patched over the defect and closed without tension. This operation is similar to the technique of repairing a rectovaginal fistula (Fig. 28). It should be used only in high transsphincteric or suprasphincteric chronic fistulas.

Many series have shown that preoperative resting or squeeze pressures do not change after the flap procedure.[125-127] The success rate for transsphincteric fistula repair ranges from 75% to 95%.[127-129] The success rate for repair of first-time fistulas (87%) is better than that for repair of recurrent fistulas (50%).[128] Hidaka et al.[127] reported a soiling frequency of 28% after repair in transsphincteric fistulas, but the preoperative condition was not stated. For suprasphincteric fistulas, they reported a recurrence rate of 9% and fecal soiling rate of 35%.

Advanced rectal flap procedures should be considered for the treatment of complex fistula in ano in properly selected patients.

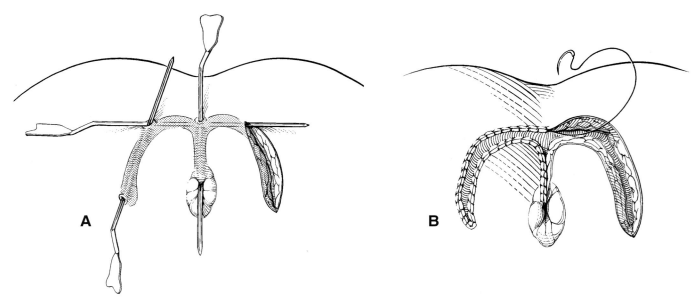

Fig. 26. Technique of fistulotomy for horseshoe fistula. (A), Laying open of the curved, fistulous tract in a straight-line manner, with a fistulous probe. (B), Marsupialization of wound.

Finding the Internal Opening

Even with a well-established fistulous tract that has a firm cord and an obvious external opening, the internal (primary) opening may not be apparent. The location of the external opening gives a hint to the site of the internal opening. The Goodsall rule is useful (Fig. 29). If the external opening is posterior to the imaginary transverse anal line, the fistulous tract curves posteriorly and opens to an internal opening in the posterior midline at the

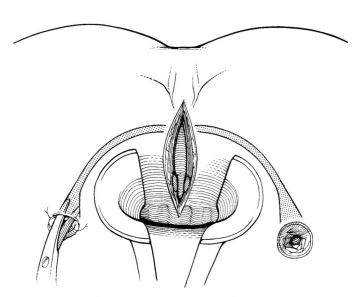

Fig. 27. Modification of Hanley's technique for horseshoe fistula. The side arms of the horseshoe fistulous tracts are cored out. The deep postanal space is opened, and the T portion of the fistulous tract is cored out into the anal canal.

dentate line. If the external opening is anterior to the transverse line, the fistulous tract usually runs directly into the anal canal at the dentate line. However, in an anterior external opening that is 3 cm or more from the anus, the tract is likely curving posteriorly to open to the midline posterior at the dentate line. The further the distance of the external opening from the anal margin, the greater the probability of a complicated upward extension.

Probing, when done, must be performed with care to prevent false channels and is best performed in the operating room. After the general introduction of a probe into the tract, a low fistula will pass straight toward the anus. Passage of a probe parallel to the anal canal indicates a high fistula, and it may be impossible to pass the probe into the internal opening.

Injection of diluted methylene blue is often helpful for finding the internal opening. When properly performed, this process is not messy, a trait for which it is notoriously known. The solution should be injected into the tract through a no. 18 intravenous catheter with a 3-mL syringe. A purse-string suture of 2-0 silk should be placed around the external opening and the gauze applied over it during the injection to minimize spillage. The dye drips through the internal opening. The fistulous tract stains blue and can be used as a guide for laying open the tract. Diluted hydrogen peroxide also can be used to identify the internal opening but not the tract.

Procedure When the Internal Opening Is Not Found

The fistulous tract should be cored out as far as possible and the rest of the tract curetted; reexploration is planned when

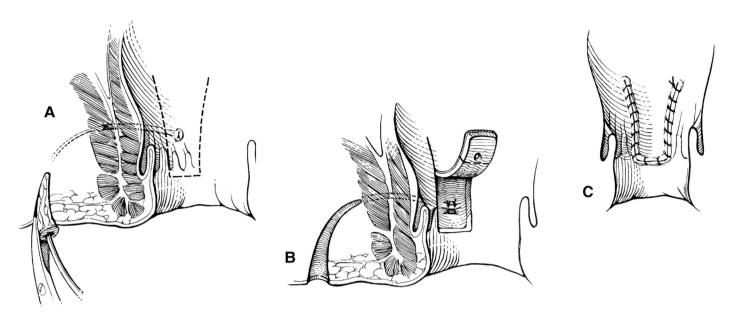

Fig. 28. Advancement rectal flap. (A), The fistulous tract is cored out, starting at the external opening. (B), A flap to include the internal sphincter is raised. The internal opening is excised and closed. (C), The flap is slid down to cover the wound.

it recurs. Recurrence is better than rendering the patient fecally incontinent.

Extent of Cutting of Sphincter Muscles

Division of only the lower half of the internal sphincter may result in minor alterations of continence in some patients, whereas in others division of the internal sphincter and a major portion of the external sphincter may cause no functional deficit. In elderly patients who already have a weakened sphincter mechanism, division of only the internal sphincter may result in partial incontinence. Thus, when there is doubt about the competence of the sphincter, it is wise to divide the muscle in stages.

When division of the sphincter muscle is considered, it must be remembered that there is no puborectalis muscle anteriorly. Division of muscle in this location is more hazardous than in other portions of the circumference. Therefore, appropriate care and attention must be exercised, especially in the female patient. Fistulotomy causes considerably lower anal sphincter resting and squeeze pressures and results in some degree of incontinence.[130-132]

The Use of Seton

Sushruta, a surgeon from India, is credited with describing the first use of a chemical seton in the *Treatise Sushruta Samhita* (600 B.C.). The operation involved insertion of a medicated thread into the fistulous tract.[133] The concept of using a seton (silk or other materials) to cut the anal sphincter muscle overlying the fistulous tract has been practiced since the time of Hippocrates (with horse hairs).

Before the 14th century, most surgeons avoided cutting the fistula with a knife for fear of massive fatal bleeding. Complicated fistulas were considered incurable at that time. With the teaching of John Arderne, cutting the anal sphincter with a knife to lay open the fistulous tract became the standard treatment and has largely replaced the use of seton as the primary treatment of fistula in ano.[134] During the past several years, seton has been revived for complicated and deep fistulas with the hope of avoiding or minimizing the risk of anal incontinence. Parks and Stitz[135] used a seton for 3 to 5 months in a high fistula

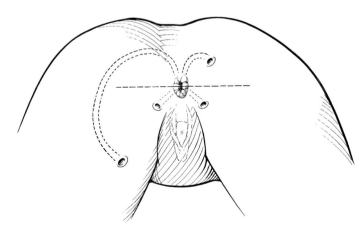

Fig. 29. Goodsall's rule: a straight tract when external opening is anterior; a curved tract to the posterior midline when external opening is posterior. When external opening is anterior but 3 cm or more away from anal verge, the tract curves to posterior midline.

before the fistulous tract was laid open. Hanley[136] advocated a rubber band seton, tying the seton loosely for 3 to 4 months to act as a drain and to create fibrosis. The rubber band was then tightened but not so tight that it caused pain or discomfort. The sphincter muscle was severed by the rubber band within 2 1/2 to 3 months. Culp[137] used a Penrose drain and tightened it to cut the muscle within 7 to 14 days. The rationale for using seton is threefold: 1) it stimulates fibrosis around the sphincter muscles and prevents them from gaping too far when the second-stage fistulotomy is performed, 2) it can be used to cut the sphincter muscle slowly, and 3) it acts as a drain.

It is essential to probe the entire fistulous tract. The limb of the tract lateral to the sphincter muscle is laid open and curetted. The skin overlying the sphincter is excised to at least 2 cm in width to prevent it from growing over. A 0 silk suture is then passed through the fistulous tract under the sphincter muscle. A few muscle fibers should be frayed before the silk is tied without any tension (Fig. 30). Silk is the best material for fibrotic reaction.

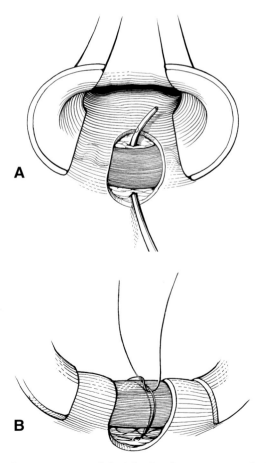

Fig. 30. Seton insertion. (A), The fistulous tract is probed and the surrounding skin excised. (B), A 0 silk suture is tied over the external sphincter.

In 4 to 6 weeks, when fibrosis has fully developed, the entire muscle encircled by the silk is incised, completing the second stage, the fistulotomy. This may require general or local anesthesia in the operating room. As a rule, the fibrotic muscle reverses itself within a few weeks.

For a cutting seton, it is best to use a rubber band and tie it around the sphincter without tension. It should be left for several weeks to allow fibrosis to form. The rubber band is then tightened and retightened with the aim of having it cut through the muscle in the next few weeks. The advantage of a cutting seton is that it avoids a second operation. Nonetheless, it is difficult to leave the rubber band in long enough. Cutting the muscle too soon before good fibrosis has developed defeats its purpose.

The success of the seton treatment of high or complex anal fistula varies from 5% to 62%.[138-142] These highly variable results probably reflect the different degree of complexity of the fistula and the amount of fibrosis developed at the time of cutting the muscle. Satisfaction with the outcome also varies between 63% and 96%.[138,140]

Fibrin Glue

Although fibrin sealant or glue has been used in Europe for more than 20 years, primarily as a hemostatic and adhesive agent, its application to anal fistula is relatively new. Early reports described use of autologous fibrinogen made by the blood bank from the patient's own donated blood.[143,144] The fibrinogen was injected into the fistula in an attempt to seal it and obliterate it. The technique has proved to be effective in selected cases of transsphincteric anal fistulas and rectovaginal fistulas.[145,146] Fibrin acts as a scaffold for fibroblast and blood vessels, thus promoting healing of the fistula. In 1998, the Food and Drug Administration approved a commercial fibrin sealant for use in patients. This has made a tremendous difference in further reducing costs, in addition to making the application quicker and easier. The fibrin sealant kit is easy to assemble, and fibrinogen within it is nearly 10 times the strength of the autologous version.[147]

The use of fibrin glue allows the fistulas to heal without the necessity to lay open the fistulous tract. Thus, all of the anal sphincter muscles are preserved. The fistulous tracts do require debridement before injection of the fibrin. The internal opening needs to be identified and is closed with chromic catgut before the fibrin glue is injected through the external opening. The fibrin sealant kit comes with a special syringe and needle for injection. The injected fibrinogen has a strong hemostatic quality; any oozing of blood from the fistulous tract created by debridement quickly stops after the injection. The glue sets immediately.[147] The patient is prepared in the same way as for a fistulotomy. This new treatment for anal fistulas is most appealing, but proper case selection and long-term results are not known yet.

Carcinoma in Chronic Anal Fistula

Carcinoma developing in long-standing anal fistula is rare. Fewer than 150 cases were reported in the literature up to 1981.[148] The most common form of carcinoma arising in a fistula in ano is colloid carcinoma (44%), followed by squamous cell carcinoma (34%) and adenocarcinoma (22%).[123] As for treatment, an abdominoperineal resection is required. The prognosis is poor.[123]

PILONIDAL DISEASE

Pilonidal sinus is a chronic subcutaneous abscess in the natal cleft that spontaneously drains through its cutaneous openings. It is not a "cyst," as it is called in many textbooks and articles.

Most authors now accept the acquired theory of causation. The exact mechanism of its origin, however, is not known. Bascom[149] believed the problem starts with folliculitis and the formation of an abscess that extends down into subcutaneous fat (Fig. 31). Karydakis,[150] however, believed that the loose hair, with its scales with chisel-like root ends, inserts into the depth of the natal cleft (Fig. 32). Once one hair inserts successfully, other hairs can insert more easily. The piercing of the skin and the foreign body (hair) lead to the abscess.

Observations from isolated reports point out that pilonidal sinus occurs in unusual locations, such as the umbilicus, a healed amputation stump, interdigital crypts, the penis, and a site of recurrent disease in an inadequately excised original area. All these reports support the acquired theory of this disease. Furthermore, pilonidal sinus is more likely to occur in a hirsute patient. It is an uncommon problem in the Chinese, who have relatively little hair in the sacral region.

Surgical Pathology

The main feature of a pilonidal sinus is the subcutaneous fibrous tract leading from the abscess to the skin surface. Most such tracts (93%) run cephalad; the rest (7%) run caudad and may be confused with a fistula in ano or with hidradenitis suppurativa.[151] Microscopic examination shows that the deeper abscess cavity and the tracts are lined by granulation tissue, not by the epithelium of the skin.[152]

Natural History

Pilonidal sinus is a chronic disease with a natural regression.[153] Usually, the disease does not manifest until puberty. It seldom occurs after the third decade of life. However, pilonidal sinus may occur at any age. When the disease commences in the third decade, it continues into the fourth decade in only 5% of patients, a suggestion that the disease has a natural tendency to "burn out" at about 30 years of age. The disease develops for the first time in the fourth decade in only a small group of patients.[153]

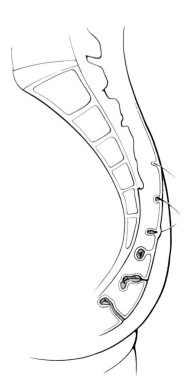

Fig. 31. Pathogenesis of pilonidal abscess and sinus.

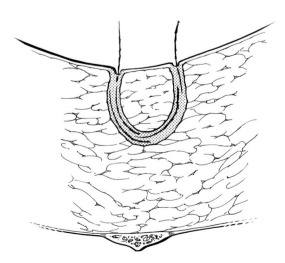

Fig. 32. Pathogenesis of pilonidal sinus. Insertion of hair into the central pit and extrusion through a sinus tract in chronic pilonidal sinus.

Predisposing Factors

Tiny skin dimples in the sacral coccygeal area are common in the normal population (9%), but most never develop into a pilonidal abscess.[154] Most pilonidal abscesses and their accompanying sinuses occur without known predisposing factors. A study by Akinci et al.[152] found four factors that favored pilonidal disease: familial tendency to pilonidal sinus, body weight more than 90 kg, driving a motor vehicle frequently or being a frequent passenger in one, and folliculitis or furuncle at any site of the body.

Clinical Manifestations

The average patient with pilonidal disease is a hirsute, moderately obese man in his second decade of life.[155] However, people of both sexes and any age can be affected. Pilonidal disease initially may be seen as an acute abscess in the sacral coccygeal area. It frequently ruptures spontaneously, leaving an unhealed sinus that drains chronically. Once a sinus "matures," pain is usually minimal. From 71% to 85% of patients with pilonidal infection are men.[156,157]

Diagnosis

The diagnosis of this condition is usually made easily. The patient's history suggests the problem. A painful, indurated swelling is the most common presentation of an acute sinus. In its earliest stage, only cellulitis may be present. In a chronic state, the diagnosis is confirmed by the sinus in the intergluteal fold approximately 5 cm above the anus. On careful examination, a pit or pits in the midline, which are the main source of the disease, almost always can be found (Fig. 33).

The differential diagnoses that must be considered include any furuncle in the skin, anal fistula, specific granulomas (e.g., syphilitic or tuberculous), and osteomyelitis with multiple draining sinuses in the skin. Actinomycosis in the sacral region has been described as virtually indistinguishable from pilonidal disease. When a fungus is suspected, the diagnosis should be confirmed from the presence of the fungus in smears of the discharge or in a culture of the discharge.

Treatment

Pilonidal Abscess

Although the infected epithelial sinus is in the midline, the abscess is usually lateral on either side of the midline and cephalad to the coccyx. Midline wounds in the intergluteal area heal poorly and slowly. Every attempt should be made to avoid a midline incision. If one is necessary, it should be made small. Drainage of a pilonidal abscess almost always can be performed with the patient under local anesthesia in the clinic, office, or emergency room. A longitudinal incision is made lateral to the midline in the coccygeal area (Fig. 34). The incision is deepened into the subcutaneous tissue, entering the abscess cavity. Hair, usually present in the abscess cavity, must be removed. All infected granulation tissue and necrotic debris are thoroughly curetted. The skin edges are trimmed to make the abscess cavity an open wound. It is important to look for the midline pit, which, as a rule, is tiny. It may not be apparent because of the swelling; if this is the case, the

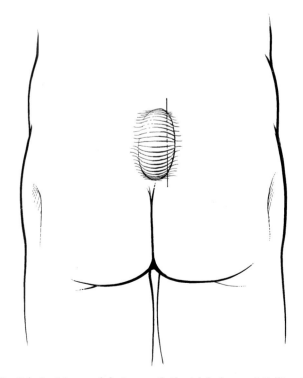

Fig. 34. *Incision and drainage of pilonidal abscess. Midline incision should be avoided.*

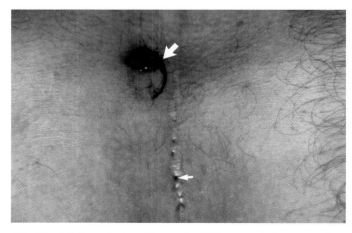

Fig. 33. *Midline pits* (small arrow). *Hairs extrude from secondary sinus* (large arrow).

patient should return a few days later for another look. A probe should be introduced into it and the tract laid open to meet the lateral incision. The wound is lightly packed with fine mesh gauze. An antibiotic is not indicated. The patient is instructed to irrigate the wound with diluted hydrogen peroxide (1:4 dilution) twice a day for 2 or 3 days. This effectively removes the residual debris. Thereafter, the wound should be washed with soap and water twice a day. The hairs around the wound should be shaved or plucked until the wound has completely healed.

Pilonidal Sinus
Pilonidal sinus can be treated several ways: nonoperative treatment, lateral incision and laying open of midline pits, incision and marsupialization, wide local excision with or without primary closure, excision and Z-plasty, and advancing flap operation (Karydakis procedure).

Nonoperative Treatment
The immediate cause of the infection in pilonidal sinus is a collection of loose hairs and debris in the internatal cleft. These hairs must be removed.

The most important conservative treatment was developed at the Tripler Army Medical Center, Hawaii. Armstrong and Barcia[158] treated pilonidal disease mainly by shaving all hairs within the natal cleft, 5 cm from the anus to the presacrum. Visible hairs within the sinus were removed, but no attempt was made to extract the hairs within the sinus. A lateral incision for drainage was made only if there was an abscess. This conservative method was applied to 101 consecutive patients during a 1-year period. The wounds healed in all patients. Unfortunately, the duration of follow-up and recurrence rates were not stated in the study.

Injecting phenol into the sinus tract has been advocated by some authors. Most surgeons have abandoned this method because of a low rate of success.[159]

Lateral Incision and Laying Open of Midline Sinuses
Lord[160] advocated the congenital theory and Bascom[149] was a strong advocate of the acquired cause, but their concepts of treatment were remarkably similar. Both advocated excision of the midline pits or sinuses and thorough cleansing of hair and debris from the sinus tract. Bascom[161] emphasized avoiding midline wounds by using a longitudinal incision lateral to the midline to enter the chronic abscess cavity. Of the 149 patients, with a mean follow-up of 3 1/2 years (longest, 9 years), the cure rate was 84%. The advantages of this technique are minimal operations and small wounds. The operations can be done on an outpatient basis. The healing is rapid and usually complete within 3 weeks. This is the technique of choice for most primary pilonidal sinuses, with or without abscess. Using this technique, Senapati et al.[162] reported a success rate of 90% in 218 patients at a mean follow-up of 12.1 months (range, 1-60 months). Excision of the midline pits, despite the small wound, is sometimes slow to heal. A better way is to lay open the midline pits toward the lateral incision (Fig. 35). This is an important point to minimize a recurrence.

Incision and Marsupialization
An open type of operation with marsupialization of the wound was advocated at Mayo Clinic by Buie[163] and later by Culp.[164] The technique consists of opening the sinus tract in the midline. The debris and granulation tissue in the tract are scraped with a curette. The fibrous tissue in the tract is saved and is sutured to the edges of the wound. This technique minimizes the size and depth of the wound and prevents the wound from premature closure.[164] In addition, it is easy to pack and clean the wound (Fig. 36). The average healing time is 4 to 6 weeks, with prolonged healing (12 to 20 weeks) in 2% to 4% and recurrence in 8%.[157,165] Although this technique is simple, the problem is that the wound is in the midline, which delays or causes incomplete healing.

Wide Local Excision With or Without Primary Closure
En bloc excision is made around a midline pilonidal sinus, deep down to the presacral fascia. The wound takes a long time to heal, and incomplete healing is frequent because of its midline location.[166-169] This radical technique has no advantages over marsupialization and should be abandoned.

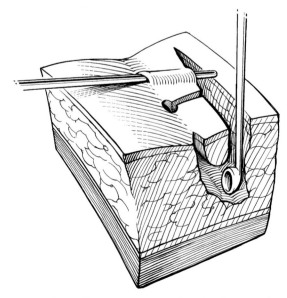

Fig. 35. Lateral incision to enter chronic abscess cavity. The sinus tract from the midline pit is laid open. The granulation tissues are curetted.

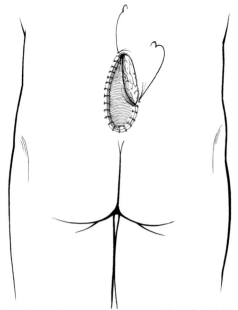

Fig. 36. Incision and marsupialization. The edge of skin is sutured to the fibrotic tissue at the base of the wound.

Excision and Z-plasty

Excision of pilonidal sinuses with primary closure of the wound is simple but has a high recurrence rate. The use of primary closure, however, is appealing because successful wound healing can be accomplished within 7 to 10 days. To avoid recurrence or breakdown of the midline wound, the anatomy of the natal crease must be altered. Z-plasty can be done to achieve this goal (Fig. 37). Primary excision of pilonidal sinuses with a Z-plasty closure fills out and flattens the natal crease, directs the hair points away from

the midline, prevents maceration, reduces the suction effect of the soft tissue of the buttocks, and minimizes friction between the adjacent surfaces of the buttocks.[170,171] The main disadvantage of this procedure is that it is rather extensive for a noncomplicated pilonidal sinus. Moreover, it is not suitable for performance on an outpatient basis.

Advancing Flap Operation (Karydakis Procedure)

According to Karydakis,[150] recurrent pilonidal sinuses occur because of the reentry of hair into the intergluteal fold. The individual hairs are then forced by friction into the depths of the fold. He designed an operative technique to avoid these problems. A "semilateral" incision is made over the sinuses all the way down to the presacral fascia (Fig. 38). Mobilization is carried to the opposite side so that the entire flap can be advanced toward the other side on closure. A closed suction drain is placed. This technique avoids the midline wound. In a series of 7,471 patients who received the advancing flap procedure, the complication rate was 8.5%, mainly infection and fluid collection. The mean hospital stay was 3 days, but many patients required only a 1-day hospitalization. Less commonly, the procedure was performed on an outpatient basis. The recurrence rate was 1%, and follow-up ranged from 2 to 20 years. With each recurrence, reentry of hair through skin defects was observed. The Karydakis flap procedure has proved to be an effective operation for pilonidal sinuses,[150,172] but it is a moderately extensive procedure.

Summary of Treatment

Many operations for pilonidal disease are worse than the disease itself. The treatment for pilonidal disease should

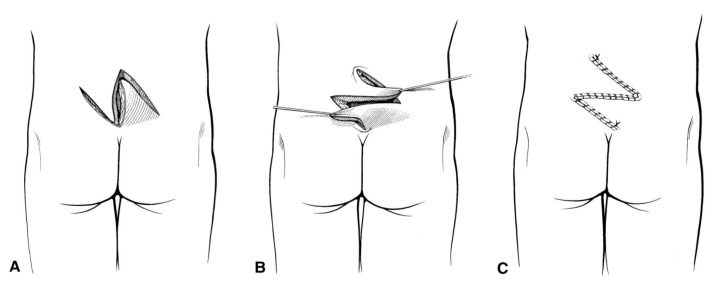

Fig. 37. Technique of excision and Z-plasty. (A), The midline pilonidal sinuses are excised. The limbs of the Z are created. (B), Subcutaneous skin flaps are raised and interposed. (C), Closure of the skin.

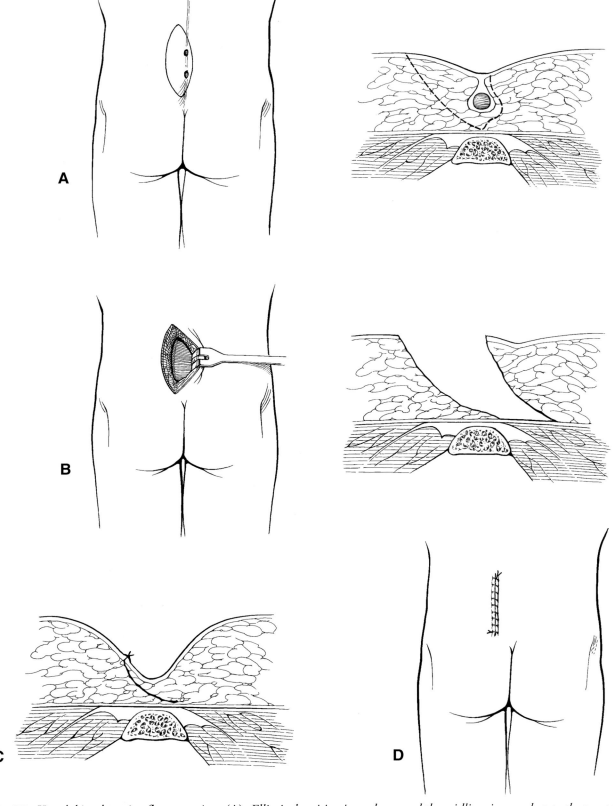

Fig. 38. Karydakis advancing flap operation. (A), Elliptical excision is made around the midline sinuses, deep to the presacral fascia and off the midline to one side. (B), Wound on side is undermined, creating a full-thickness flap. (C), The flap is closed to the edge of the wound on the opposite side. (D), Closed wound is off the midline. (Modified from Karydakis GE: New approach to the problem of pilonidal sinus. Lancet 2:1414-1415, 1973. By permission of The Lancet Publishing Group.)

be simple. Most operations, if not all, can be performed on an outpatient basis, with minimal loss of work time.

A simple incision and drainage of the abscess lateral to the midline, with vigorous removal of all the hairs and debris, shaving hairs around the wound, and laying open of midline pits, is all that is necessary for an acute pilonidal abscess. For a chronic pilonidal sinus, the method of choice is a lateral incision into the chronic abscess cavity, with removal of all hair and granulation tissues. This is to be done along with laying open of the midline pit with its tract to the lateral wound.

The surgeon must make it clear to the patients and their families that they are responsible for the second half of the treatment. The wounds must be irrigated or cleaned in the shower with soap and water to remove hair and debris. The skin around the wound should be shaved to remove all hair, or the hair should be plucked every 10 to 14 days.

Role of Hair

During the initial operation, all hair lying free in the pilonidal sinus must be removed. The wound will not heal if even a single hair is present or enters the wound. Hair can enter the wound in three ways. First, hair from the edges of the wound often can be misdirected and can grow into the wound. The best way to avoid this problem is to pluck these hairs every 10 to 14 days until the wound is healed completely. Second, hair in the adjacent area, particularly from the perianal area, can grow to considerable length, and tips of the hair can get into the wound. Shaving or trimming with scissors is required. Third, loose hair is the most common offender. Motion in the intergluteal cleft has been shown to attract loose hair, which then sticks in the area. Washing with soap is an easy way to loosen these sticky hairs.

Recurrent Disease

The time needed for healing of a pilonidal wound depends on the type of operation and the extent of the disease. The recurrence rate varies widely from series to series (0%-37%).[150,157,167] Recurrence is caused by the spontaneous reinsertion of the loose hair into the natal cleft. The mechanism is the same for primary pilonidal disease, and the treatment is also the same.

Unhealed Wound

Not uncommonly, the wound does not heal after operation for a pilonidal sinus. Most often, the base of the wound is filled with gelatinous granulation tissue, which is often the result of improper postoperative wound care. Hair may grow into the edges of the wound, preventing complete healing. Some wounds are kept clean and yet do not heal. Almost all unhealed wounds are in the midline natal cleft area. The lateral incision technique usually avoids this problem.

For a *curettage*, *reexcision*, and *saucerization* procedure, the hair around the unhealed wound must be shaved and plucked, after which a complete curettage of the granulation tissue is done. If the shape of the wound appears to fold together causing "pocketing," it should be refashioned and saucerization performed to avoid accumulation of discharge. If the wound is infected with anaerobic bacteria, administering an antibiotic can improve healing. The wound should be washed with soap and water, followed by light packing with mesh gauze twice a day.

Some pilonidal wounds heal well initially but fail to form epithelium. The problem is mainly mechanical, especially in obese patients and those with a narrow intergluteal cleft. The motion of the buttocks traumatizes the wound constantly. For *reverse bandaging*, a wide piece of adhesive tape is placed on each side of the wound, stretching it outward (Fig. 39). The tapes are tied in front of the abdomen. The net effect is to flatten the wound and remove most of the angle of the intergluteal cleft.[173] This technique may be useful in some cases.

If the wound is extensive and conservative management fails, the wound should be excised. In this situation, a *gluteus maximus myocutaneous flap* offers a secure repair.[174] However, the procedure is rather extensive for a simple disease (Fig. 40).

The unique method of *excision and flap closure* for treating the unhealed wound was devised by Bascom.[175] The basic approach is to excise the unhealed skin and the underlying subcutaneous tissue. The natal cleft is flattened by replacing the defect at the depth of the cleft with a skin flap over the wound. This operation is easier than it appears

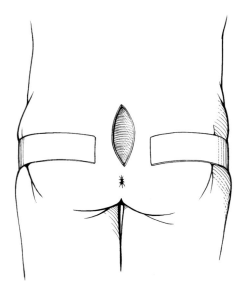

Fig. 39. Reverse bandaging technique for unhealed pilonidal wound. Patient's buttocks are strapped with tape in a reverse direction, spreading the wound open.

and is less extensive than the gluteus maximus myocutaneous and other types of flaps. The fat is not mobilized. The flap is a full-thickness skin flap. It is the operation of choice for extensive recurrent pilonidal disease. The procedure is performed with the patient under general or spinal anesthesia. A broad-spectrum antibiotic is administered when the patient is called to the operating room, and this treatment is continued until the drain is removed 4 or 5 days later. The patient is placed in the prone jackknife position.

With the patient's buttocks pressed together, the lines of contact of the cheeks of the buttocks are marked with a felt-tipped pen (Fig. 41 *A*). The cheeks of the buttocks are then taped apart, and the skin is prepared and draped (Fig. 41 *B*). The skin in this region is infiltrated with 0.25 bupivacaine containing 1:200,000 epinephrine to decrease bleeding. A triangle-shaped section of skin overlying the unhealed wound is excised, extending above and lateral to the apex in the cleft. The lower end of the incision is

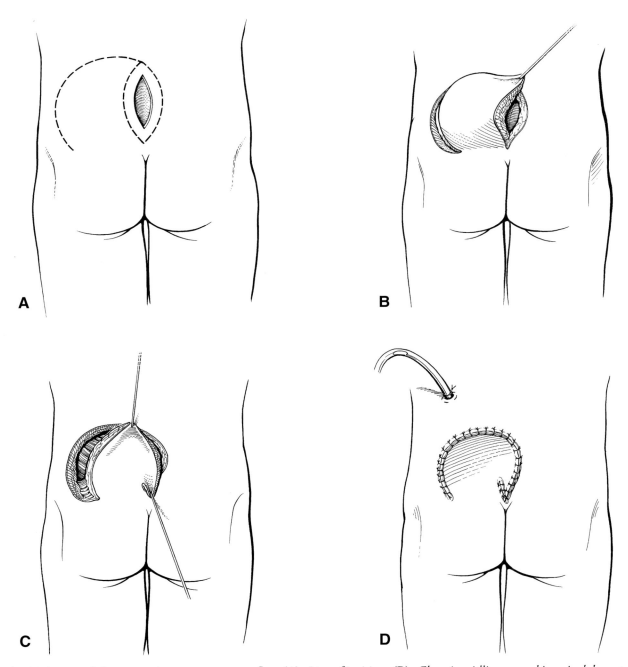

Fig. 40. Technique of gluteus maximus myocutaneous flap. (A), Line of incision. (B), Chronic midline wound is excised down to presacral fascia, and the myocutaneous flap created. (C), Rotation of flap to cover the presacral defect. (D), Closure of wound, with a suction drain.

curved medially toward the anus to avoid "dog ear" on closure (Fig. 41 C). The granulation tissue and hairs are removed. No fat or muscle is mobilized.

After the skin flap (dissected only into the dermis) is raised out to the previously marked line on the left side, the tapes are released. The skin flap is positioned to overlap the edges of the wound on the right side. The excess skin is excised. A closed suction drain is placed in the subcutaneous tissue. The subcutaneous tissue is closed with 3-0 chromic catgut, and the skin is closed with subcuticular 3-0 synthetic monofilament absorbable suture (Fig. 41 D and E). The suture line can be reinforced with a running suture or tape strips can be applied. When properly performed, this line of skin closure is off the midline.

Pilonidal Sinus and Carcinoma

Carcinoma arising in a chronic pilonidal sinus is rare. In a review of the world literature from 1900 to 1994, only 44 patients were described: 39 had squamous cell carcinomas, 3 had basal cell carcinomas, 1 had an adenocarcinoma (sweat gland type), and 1 had an unspecified carcinoma.[176] The cause of pilonidal carcinoma seems to be the same as that by which other chronic inflamed wounds, such as scars, skin ulcers, and chronic fistulas, undergo malignant degeneration. The average duration of pilonidal disease is 23 years. Pilonidal carcinoma has a distinctive appearance, and the diagnosis usually can be made on inspection of the patient. A central ulceration is often present with a friable, indurated, erythematous, and fungating margin. Biopsy confirms the diagnosis. The cancers are usually well-differentiated squamous cell carcinomas, frequently with focal areas of keratinization and rare mitotic figures. The carcinomas grow locally before metastasizing to inguinal lymph nodes. Preoperative evaluation of patients with pilonidal carcinoma should include examination of the inguinal areas, the perineum, and the anorectum. Treatment involves wide local excision to include the presacral fascia. According to a review of the literature, the recurrence rate is 34%, and death from the disease occurs in 18% of patients on follow-up of 29 months.[176]

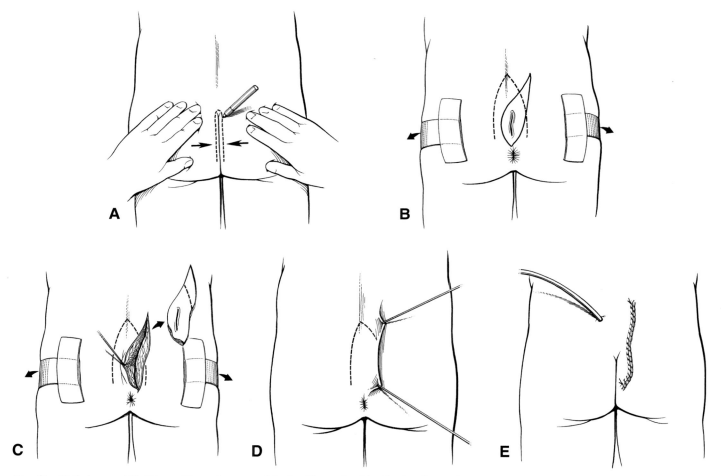

Fig. 41. Cleft closure. (A), Natural lines of contact of cheeks of buttock. (B), Cheeks of buttock are taped apart, and line of excision of the unhealed wound is outlined. (C), Excision of wound. Note triangular shape. (D), Dermal flap is raised to the marked line on the opposite side. (E), The flap is closed and suction drain is placed. Note that suture line is off the midline. (Modified from Bascom.[175] By permission of Excerpta Medica.)

REFERENCES

1. Thomson WH: The nature of haemorrhoids. Br J Surg 62:542-552, 1975
2. Loder PB, Kamm MA, Nicholls RJ, Phillips RK: Haemorrhoids: pathology, pathophysiology and aetiology. Br J Surg 81:946-954, 1994
3. Bernstein WC: What are hemorrhoids and what is their relationship to the portal venous system? Dis Colon Rectum 26:829-834, 1983
4. Johanson JF, Sonnenberg A: Temporal changes in the occurrence of hemorrhoids in the United States and England. Dis Colon Rectum 34:585-591, 1991
5. Haas PA, Fox TA Jr, Haas GP: The pathogenesis of hemorrhoids. Dis Colon Rectum 27:442-450, 1984
6. Hiltunen KM, Matikainen M: Anal manometric findings in symptomatic hemorrhoids. Dis Colon Rectum 28:807-809, 1985
7. Sun WM, Peck RJ, Shorthouse AJ, Read NW: Haemorrhoids are associated not with hypertrophy of the internal anal sphincter, but with hypertension of the anal cushions. Br J Surg 79:592-594, 1992
8. Lin JK: Anal manometric studies in hemorrhoids and anal fissures. Dis Colon Rectum 32:839-842, 1989
9. Waldron DJ, Kumar D, Hallan RI, Williams NS: Prolonged ambulant assessment of anorectal function in patients with prolapsing hemorrhoids. Dis Colon Rectum 32:968-974, 1989
10. Johanson JF, Sonnenberg A: Constipation is not a risk factor for hemorrhoids: a case-control study of potential etiological agents. Am J Gastroenterol 89:1981-1986, 1994
11. Kluiber RM, Wolff BG: Evaluation of anemia caused by hemorrhoidal bleeding. Dis Colon Rectum 37:1006-1007, 1994
12. Moesgaard F, Nielsen ML, Hansen JB, Knudsen JT: High-fiber diet reduces bleeding and pain in patients with hemorrhoids: a double-blind trial of Vi-Siblin. Dis Colon Rectum 25:454-456, 1982
13. Senapati A, Nicholls RJ: A randomised trial to compare the results of injection sclerotherapy with a bulk laxative alone in the treatment of bleeding haemorrhoids. Int J Colorectal Dis 3:124-126, 1988
14. Wrobleski DE, Corman ML, Veidenheimer MC, Coller JA: Long-term evaluation of rubber ring ligation in hemorrhoidal disease. Dis Colon Rectum 23:478-482, 1980
15. Lee HH, Spencer RJ, Beart RW Jr: Multiple hemorrhoidal bandings in a single session. Dis Colon Rectum 37:37-41, 1994
16. MacRae HM, McLeod RS: Comparison of hemorrhoidal treatment modalities: a meta-analysis. Dis Colon Rectum 38:687-694, 1995
17. Jensen SL, Harling H, Arseth-hansen P, Tange G: The natural history of symptomatic haemorrhoids. Int J Colorectal Dis 4:41-44, 1989
18. Alexander-Williams J, Crapp AR: Conservative management of haemorrhoids. Part I: injection, freezing and ligation. Clin Gastroenterol 4:595-618, 1975
19. Nivatvongs S, Goldberg SM: An improved technique of rubber band ligation of hemorrhoids. Am J Surg 144:378-380, 1982
20. Russell TR, Donohue JH: Hemorrhoidal banding: a warning. Dis Colon Rectum 28:291-293, 1985
21. Shemesh EI, Kodner IJ, Fry RD, Neufeld DM: Severe complication of rubber band ligation of internal hemorrhoids. Dis Colon Rectum 30:199-200, 1987
22. Scarpa FJ, Hillis W, Sabetta JR: Pelvic cellulitis: a life-threatening complication of hemorrhoidal banding. Surgery 103:383-385, 1988

23. Quevedo-Bonilla G, Farkas AM, Abcarian H, Hambrick E, Orsay CP: Septic complications of hemorrhoidal banding. Arch Surg 123:650-651, 1988
24. Buchmann P, Seefeld U: Rubber band ligation for piles can be disastrous in HIV-positive patients. Int J Colorectal Dis 4:57-58, 1989
25. Nivatvongs S, Fang DT, Kennedy HL: The shape of the buttocks: a useful guide for selection of anesthesia and patient position in anorectal surgery. Dis Colon Rectum 26:85-86, 1983
26. Fansler WA: Hemorrhoidectomy—anatomical method. Lancet 51:529-531, 1931
27. Gibbons CP, Trowbridge EA, Bannister JJ, Read NW: Role of anal cushions in maintaining continence. Lancet 1:886-888, 1986
28. Beattie GC, Loudon MA: Circumferential stapled anoplasty in the management of haemorrhoids and mucosal prolapse. Colorectal Dis 2:170-175, 2000
29. Mehigan BJ, Monson JR, Hartley JE: Stapling procedure for haemorrhoids versus Milligan-Morgan haemorrhoidectomy: randomised controlled trial. Lancet 355:782-785, 2000
30. Ho YH, Cheong WK, Tsang C, Ho J, Eu KW, Tang CL, Seow-Choen F: Stapled hemorrhoidectomy—cost and effectiveness: randomized, controlled trial including incontinence scoring, anorectal manometry, and endoanal ultrasound assessments at up to three months. Dis Colon Rectum 43:1666-1675, 2000
31. Cheetham MJ, Mortensen NJ, Nystrom PO, Kamm MA, Phillips RK: Persistent pain and faecal urgency after stapled haemorrhoidectomy. Lancet 356:730-733, 2000
32. Beattie GC, Loudon MA: Follow-up confirms sustained benefit of circumferential stapled anoplasty in the management of prolapsing haemorrhoids. Br J Surg 88:850-852, 2001
33. Brown SR, Ballan K, Ho E, Ho Fams YH, Seow-Choen F: Stapled mucosectomy for acute thrombosed circumferentially prolapsed piles: a prospective randomized comparison with conventional haemorrhoidectomy. Colorect Dis 3:175-178, 2001
34. Molloy RG, Kingsmore D: Life threatening pelvic sepsis after stapled haemorrhoidectomy (letter). Lancet 355:810, 2000
35. Milligan ETC, Morgan CN, Jones LE, Officer R: Surgical anatomy of the anal canal, and operative treatment of haemorrhoids. Lancet 2:1119-1124, 1937
36. Andrews BT, Layer GT, Jackson BT, Nicholls RJ: Randomized trial comparing diathermy hemorrhoidectomy with the scissor dissection Milligan-Morgan operation. Dis Colon Rectum 36:580-583, 1993
37. Seow-Choen F, Ho YH, Ang HG, Goh HS: Prospective, randomized trial comparing pain and clinical function after conventional scissors excision/ligation vs. diathermy excision without ligation for symptomatic prolapsed hemorrhoids. Dis Colon Rectum 35:1165-1169, 1992
38. Whitehead W: The surgical treatment of haemorrhoids. Br Med J 1:148-150, 1882
39. Bonello JC: Who's afraid of the dentate line? The Whitehead hemorrhoidectomy. Am J Surg 156:182-186, 1988
40. Wolff BG, Culp CE: The Whitehead hemorrhoidectomy: an unjustly maligned procedure. Dis Colon Rectum 31:587-590, 1988
41. Senagore A, Mazier WP, Luchtefeld MA, MacKeigan JM, Wengert T: Treatment of advanced hemorrhoidal disease: a prospective, randomized comparison of cold scalpel vs. contact Nd:YAG laser. Dis Colon Rectum 36:1042-1049, 1993
42. Leff EI: Hemorrhoidectomy—laser vs. nonlaser: outpatient surgical experience. Dis Colon Rectum 35:743-746, 1992

43. Eu KW, Seow-Choen F, Goh HS: Comparison of emergency and elective haemorrhoidectomy. Br J Surg 81:308-310, 1994

44. Sacco S, Mortilla MG, Tonielli E, Morganti I, Cola B: Emergency hemorrhoidectomy for complicated hemorrhoids. Coloproctology 9:157-159, 1987

45. Allen PIM, Goldman M: Prolapsed thrombosed piles: a reappraisal. Coloproctology 9:210-212, 1987

46. Salvati EP: Management of acute hemorrhoidal disease. Perspect Colon Rectal Surg 3:309-314, 1990

47. Rasmussen OO, Larsen KG, Naver L, Christiansen J: Emergency haemorrhoidectomy compared with incision and banding for the treatment of acute strangulated haemorrhoids: a prospective randomised study. Eur J Surg 157:613-614, 1991

48. Myers JO, Rothenberger DA: Sugar in the reduction of incarcerated prolapsed bowel: report of two cases. Dis Colon Rectum 34:416-418, 1991

49. Nivatvongs S: Alternative positioning of patients for hemorrhoidectomy. Dis Colon Rectum 23:308-309, 1980

50. Saleeby RG Jr, Rosen L, Stasik JJ, Riether RD, Sheets J, Khubchandani IT: Hemorrhoidectomy during pregnancy: Risk or relief? Dis Colon Rectum 34:260-261, 1991

51. Chawla Y, Dilawari JB: Anorectal varices—their frequency in cirrhotic and non-cirrhotic portal hypertension. Gut 32:309-311, 1991

52. Hosking SW, Smart HL, Johnson AG, Triger DR: Anorectal varices, haemorrhoids, and portal hypertension. Lancet 1:349-352, 1989

53. Johansen K, Bardin J, Orloff MJ: Massive bleeding from hemorrhoidal varices in portal hypertension. JAMA 244:2084-2085, 1980

54. Nivatvongs S: Suture of massive hemorrhoidal bleeding in portal hypertension. Dis Colon Rectum 28:878-879, 1985

55. Jacobs DM, Bubrick MP, Onstad GR, Hitchcock CR: The relationship of hemorrhoids to portal hypertension. Dis Colon Rectum 23:567-569, 1980

56. Hosking SW, Johnson AG: Bleeding anorectal varices—a misunderstood condition. Surgery 104:70-73, 1988

57. Katz JA, Rubin RA, Cope C, Holland G, Brass CA: Recurrent bleeding from anorectal varices: successful treatment with a transjugular intrahepatic portosystemic shunt. Am J Gastroenterol 88:1104-1107, 1993

58. Shibata D, Brophy DP, Gordon FD, Anastopoulos HT, Sentovich SM, Bleday R: Transjugular intrahepatic portosystemic shunt for treatment of bleeding ectopic varices with portal hypertension. Dis Colon Rectum 42:1581-1585, 1999

59. Jeffery PJ, Parks AG, Ritchie JK: Treatment of haemorrhoids in patients with inflammatory bowel disease. Lancet 1:1084-1085, 1977

60. Wolkomir AF, Luchtefeld MA: Surgery for symptomatic hemorrhoids and anal fissures in Crohn's disease. Dis Colon Rectum 36:545-547, 1993

61. Grewal H, Guillem JG, Quan SH, Enker WE, Cohen AM: Anorectal disease in neutropenic leukemic patients: operative vs. nonoperative management. Dis Colon Rectum 37:1095-1099, 1994

62. Carapeti EA, Kamm MA, McDonald PJ, Phillips RK: Double-blind randomised controlled trial of effect of metronidazole on pain after day-case haemorrhoidectomy. Lancet 351:169-172, 1998

63. Xynos E, Tzortzinis A, Chrysos E, Tzovaras G, Vassilakis JS: Anal manometry in patients with fissure-in-ano before and after internal sphincterotomy. Int J Colorectal Dis 8:125-128, 1993

64. Farouk R, Duthie GS, MacGregor AB, Bartolo DC: Sustained internal sphincter hypertonia in patients with chronic anal fissure. Dis Colon Rectum 37:424-429, 1994

65. Keck JO, Staniunas RJ, Coller JA, Barrett RC, Oster ME: Computer-generated profiles of the anal canal in patients with anal fissure. Dis Colon Rectum 38:72-79, 1995

66. Williams N, Scott NA, Irving MH: Effect of lateral sphincterotomy on internal anal sphincter function: a computerized vector manometry study. Dis Colon Rectum 38:700-704, 1995

67. Prohm P, Bonner C: Is manometry essential for surgery of chronic fissure-in-ano? Dis Colon Rectum 38:735-738, 1995

68. Brown AC, Sumfest JM, Rozwadowski JV: Histopathology of the internal anal sphincter in chronic anal fissure. Dis Colon Rectum 32:680-683, 1989

69. Schouten WR, Briel JW, Auwerda JJ, De Graaf EJ: Ischaemic nature of anal fissure. Br J Surg 83:63-65, 1996

70. Goligher JC: Surgery of the Anus, Rectum and Colon. Fifth edition. London, Baillière Tindall, 1984, pp 170-191

71. Dodi G, Bogoni F, Infantino A, Pianon P, Mortellaro LM, Lise M: Hot or cold in anal pain? A study of the changes in internal anal sphincter pressure profiles. Dis Colon Rectum 29:248-251, 1986

72. Hananel N, Gordon PH: Re-examination of clinical manifestations and response to therapy of fissure-in-ano. Dis Colon Rectum 40:229-233, 1997

73. Shub HA, Salvati EP, Rubin RJ: Conservative treatment of anal fissure: an unselected, retrospective and continuous study. Dis Colon Rectum 21:582-583, 1978

74. Lock MR, Thomson JP: Fissure-in-ano: the initial management and prognosis. Br J Surg 64:355-358, 1977

75. Jensen SL: Treatment of first episodes of acute anal fissure: prospective randomised study of lignocaine ointment versus hydrocortisone ointment or warm sitz baths plus bran. Br Med J (Clin Res Ed) 292:1167-1169, 1986

76. Parker JD, Parker JO: Nitrate therapy for stable angina pectoris. N Engl J Med 338:520-531, 1998

77. O'Kelly T, Brading A, Mortensen N: Nerve mediated relaxation of the human internal anal sphincter: the role of nitric oxide. Gut 34:689-693, 1993

78. Loder PB, Kamm MA, Nicholls RJ, Phillips RK: 'Reversible chemical sphincterotomy' by local application of glyceryl trinitrate. Br J Surg 81:1386-1389, 1994

79. Carapeti EA, Kamm MA, McDonald PJ, Chadwick SJ, Melville D, Phillips RK: Randomised controlled trial shows that glyceryl trinitrate heals anal fissures, higher doses are not more effective, and there is a high recurrence rate. Gut 44:727-730, 1999

80. Kennedy ML, Sowter S, Nguyen H, Lubowski DZ: Glyceryl trinitrate ointment for the treatment of chronic anal fissure: results of a placebo-controlled trial and long-term follow-up. Dis Colon Rectum 42:1000-1006, 1999

81. Hyman NH, Cataldo PA: Nitroglycerin ointment for anal fissures: effective treatment or just a headache? Dis Colon Rectum 42:383-385, 1999

82. Pitt J, Boulos PB: Chemical sphincterotomy for anal fissure: review. Colorect Dis 1:2-8, 1999

83. Maria G, Brisinda G, Bentivoglio AR, Cassetta E, Gui D, Albanese A: Influence of botulinum toxin site of injections on healing rate in patients with chronic anal fissure. Am J Surg 179:46-50, 2000

84. Maria G, Cassetta E, Gui D, Brisinda G, Bentivoglio AR, Albanese A: A comparison of botulinum toxin and saline for the treatment of chronic anal fissure. N Engl J Med 338:217-220, 1998

85. Maria G, Brisinda G, Bentivoglio AR, Cassetta E, Gui D, Albanese A: Botulinum toxin injections in the internal anal sphincter for the treatment of chronic anal fissure: long-term results after two different dosage regimens. Ann Surg 228:664-669, 1998

86. Lund JN, Scholefield JH: Aetiology and treatment of anal fissure. Br J Surg 83:1335-1344, 1996

87. Isbister WH, Prasad J: Fissure in ano. Aust N Z J Surg 65:107-108, 1995

88. Nielsen MB, Rasmussen OO, Pedersen JF, Christiansen J: Risk of sphincter damage and anal incontinence after anal dilatation for fissure-in-ano: an endosonographic study. Dis Colon Rectum 36:677-680, 1993

89. Sohn N, Weinstein MA: Anal dilatation for anal fissures. Semin Colon Rectum Surg 8:17-23, 1997

90. Nelson RL: Meta-analysis of operative techniques for fissure-in-ano. Dis Colon Rectum 42:1424-1428, 1999

91. Strugnell NA, Cooke SG, Lucarotti ME, Thomson WH: Controlled digital anal dilatation under total neuromuscular blockade for chronic anal fissure: a justifiable procedure. Br J Surg 86:651-655, 1999

92. Garcia-Aguilar J, Belmonte C, Wong WD, Lowry AC, Madoff RD: Open vs. closed sphincterotomy for chronic anal fissure: long-term results. Dis Colon Rectum 39:440-443, 1996

93. Garcia-Aguilar J, Belmonte Montes C, Perez JJ, Jensen L, Madoff RD, Wong WD: Incontinence after lateral internal sphincterotomy: anatomic and functional evaluation. Dis Colon Rectum 41:423-427, 1998

94. Nyam DC, Pemberton JH: Long-term results of lateral internal sphincterotomy for chronic anal fissure with particular reference to incidence of fecal incontinence. Dis Colon Rectum 42:1306-1310, 1999

95. Usatoff V, Polglase AL: The longer term results of internal anal sphincterotomy for anal fissure. Aust N Z J Surg 65:576-578, 1995

96. Hananel N, Gordon PH: Lateral internal sphincterotomy for fissure-in-ano—revisited. Dis Colon Rectum 40:597-602, 1997

97. Farouk R, Gunn J, Lee PWR, Monson JRT: Failure of lateral internal sphincterotomy for the treatment of chronic anal fissure is due to technical failure (abstract). Br J Surg 83 Suppl 1:60, 1996

98. Gordon PH, Vasilevsky CA: Symposium on outpatient anorectal procedures. Lateral internal sphincterotomy: rationale, technique and anesthesia. Can J Surg 28:228-230, 1985

99. Corby H, Donnelly VS, O'Herlihy C, O'Connell PR: Anal canal pressures are low in women with postpartum anal fissure. Br J Surg 84:86-88, 1997

100. Nyam DC, Wilson RG, Stewart KJ, Farouk R, Bartolo DC: Island advancement flaps in the management of anal fissures. Br J Surg 82:326-328, 1995

101. Parks AG: Pathogenesis and treatment of fistula-in-ano. Br Med J 1:463-469, 1961

102. Seow-Choen F, Ho JM: Histoanatomy of anal glands. Dis Colon Rectum 37:1215-1218, 1994

103. Vasilevsky CA, Gordon PH: The incidence of recurrent abscesses or fistula-in-ano following anorectal suppuration. Dis Colon Rectum 27:126-130, 1984

104. Prasad ML, Read DR, Abcarian H: Supralevator abscess: diagnosis and treatment. Dis Colon Rectum 24:456-461, 1981

105. Nicholls G, Heaton ND, Lewis AM: Use of bacteriology in anorectal sepsis as an indicator of anal fistula: experience in a distinct general hospital. J R Soc Med 83:625-626, 1990

106. Grace RH, Harper IA, Thompson RG: Anorectal sepsis: microbiology in relation to fistula-in-ano. Br J Surg 69:401-403, 1982

107. Eykyn SJ, Grace RH: The relevance of microbiology in the management of anorectal sepsis. Ann R Coll Surg Engl 68:237-239, 1986

108. Seow-Choen F, Hay AJ, Heard S, Phillips RK: Bacteriology of anal fistulae. Br J Surg 79:27-28, 1992

109. Ramanujam PS, Prasad ML, Abcarian H, Tan AB: Perianal abscesses and fistulas: a study of 1023 patients. Dis Colon Rectum 27:593-597, 1984

110. Henrichsen S, Christiansen J: Incidence of fistula-in-ano complicating anorectal sepsis: a prospective study. Br J Surg 73:371-372, 1986

111. Seow-Choen F, Leong AF, Goh HS: Results of a policy of selective immediate fistulotomy for primary anal abscess. Aust N Z J Surg 63:485-489, 1993

112. Schouten WR, van Vroonhoven TJ: Treatment of anorectal abscess with or without primary fistulectomy: results of a prospective randomized trial. Dis Colon Rectum 34:60-63, 1991

113. Eke N: Fournier's gangrene: a review of 1726 cases. Br J Surg 87:718-728, 2000

114. Heppell J, Benard F: Life-threatening perineal sepsis. Perspect Colorect Surg 4:1-18, 1991

115. Eisenhammer S: The internal anal sphincter and the anorectal abscess. Surg Gynecol Obstet 103:501-506, 1956

116. Parks AG, Gordon PH, Hardcastle JD: A classification of fistula-in-ano. Br J Surg 63:1-12, 1976

117. Parks AG, Gordon PH: Fistula-in-ano: perineal fistula of intra-abdominal or intrapelvic origin simulating fistula-in-ano—report of seven cases. Dis Colon Rectum 19:500-506, 1976

118. Kuijpers HC, Schulpen T: Fistulography for fistula-in-ano: Is it useful? Dis Colon Rectum 28:103-104, 1985

119. Weisman RI, Orsay CP, Pearl RK, Abcarian H: The role of fistulography in fistula-in-ano: report of five cases. Dis Colon Rectum 34:181-184, 1991

120. Choen S, Burnett S, Bartram CI, Nicholls RJ: Comparison between anal endosonography and digital examination in the evaluation of anal fistulae. Br J Surg 78:445-447, 1991

121. Lunniss PJ, Barker PG, Sultan AH, Armstrong P, Reznek RH, Bartram CI, Cottam KS, Phillips RK: Magnetic resonance imaging of fistula-in-ano. Dis Colon Rectum 37:708-718, 1994

122. Beckingham IJ, Spencer JA, Ward J, Dyke GW, Adams C, Ambrose NS: Prospective evaluation of dynamic contrast enhanced magnetic resonance imaging in the evaluation of fistula in ano. Br J Surg 83:1396-1398, 1996

123. Gordon PH: Anorectal abscesses and fistula-in-ano. In Principles and Practice of Surgery for the Colon, Rectum, and Anus. Second edition. Edited by PH Gordon, S Nivatvongs. St Louis, Quality Medical Publishing, 1999, pp 241-286

124. Hanley PH, Ray JE, Pennington EE, Grablowsky OM: Fistula-in-ano: a ten-year follow-up study of horseshoe-abscess fistula-in-ano. Dis Colon Rectum 19:507-515, 1976

125. Kreis ME, Jehle EC, Ohlemann M, Becker HD, Starlinger MJ: Functional results after transanal rectal advancement flap repair of trans-sphincteric fistula. Br J Surg 85:240-242, 1998

126. Lewis WG, Finan PJ, Holdsworth PJ, Sagar PM, Stephenson BM: Clinical results and manometric studies after rectal flap advancement for infra-levator trans-sphincteric fistula-in-ano. Int J Colorect Dis 10:189-192, 1995

127. Hidaka H, Kuroki M, Hirokuni T, Toyama Y, Nagata Y, Takano M, Tsuji Y: Follow-up studies of sphincter-preserving

operations for anal fistulas. Dis Colon Rectum 40 Suppl:S107-S111, 1997

128. Schouten WR, Zimmerman DD, Briel JW: Transanal advancement flap repair of transsphincteric fistulas. Dis Colon Rectum 42:1419-1422, 1999

129. Miller GV, Finan PJ: Flap advancement and core fistulectomy for complex rectal fistula. Br J Surg 85:108-110, 1998

130. Pescatori M, Maria G, Anastasio G, Rinallo L: Anal manometry improves the outcome of surgery for fistula-in-ano. Dis Colon Rectum 32:588-592, 1989

131. Sainio P, Husa A: A prospective manometric study of the effect of anal fistula surgery on anorectal function. Acta Chir Scand 151:279-288, 1985

132. Belliveau P, Thomson JP, Parks AG: Fistula-in-ano: a manometric study. Dis Colon Rectum 26:152-154, 1983

133. McCourtney JS, Finlay IG: Setons in the surgical management of fistula in ano. Br J Surg 82:448-452, 1995

134. Perrin WS: President's address: some landmarks in the history of rectal surgery. Proc R Soc Med 25:338-346, 1932

135. Parks AG, Stitz RW: The treatment of high fistula-in-ano. Dis Colon Rectum 19:487-499, 1976

136. Hanley PH: Rubber band seton in the management of abscess-anal fistula. Ann Surg 187:435-437, 1978

137. Culp CE: Use of Penrose drains to treat certain anal fistulas: a primary operative seton. Mayo Clin Proc 59:613-617, 1984

138. Hamalainen KP, Sainio AP: Cutting seton for anal fistulas: high risk of minor control defects. Dis Colon Rectum 40:1443-1446, 1997

139. Williams JG, MacLeod CA, Rothenberger DA, Goldberg SM: Seton treatment of high anal fistulae. Br J Surg 78:1159-1161, 1991

140. Lunniss PJ, Kamm MA, Phillips RK: Factors affecting continence after surgery for anal fistula. Br J Surg 81:1382-1385, 1994

141. Christensen A, Nilas L, Christiansen J: Treatment of transsphincteric anal fistulas by the seton technique. Dis Colon Rectum 29:454-455, 1986

142. Pearl RK, Andrews JR, Orsay CP, Weisman RI, Prasad ML, Nelson RL, Cintron JR, Abcarian H: Role of the seton in the management of anorectal fistulas. Dis Colon Rectum 36:573-577, 1993

143. Park JJ, Cintron JR, Siedentop KH, Orsay CP, Pearl RK, Nelson RL, Abcarian H: Technical manual for manufacturing autologous fibrin tissue adhesive. Dis Colon Rectum 42:1334-1338, 1999

144. Abel ME, Chiu YS, Russell TR, Volpe PA: Autologous fibrin glue in the treatment of rectovaginal and complex fistulas. Dis Colon Rectum 36:447-449, 1993

145. Cintron JR, Park JJ, Orsay CP, Pearl RK, Nelson RL, Abcarian H: Repair of fistulas-in-ano using autologous fibrin tissue adhesive. Dis Colon Rectum 42:607-613, 1999

146. Venkatesh KS, Ramanujam P: Fibrin glue application in the treatment of recurrent anorectal fistulas. Dis Colon Rectum 42:1136-1139, 1999

147. Chiu YSY: Repair of fistulas-in-ano using autologous fibrin tissue adhesive. Dis Colon Rectum 42:613, 1999

148. Getz SB Jr, Ough YD, Patterson RB, Kovalcik PJ: Mucinous adenocarcinoma developing in chronic anal fistula: report of two cases and review of the literature. Dis Colon Rectum 24:562-566, 1981

149. Bascom J: Pilonidal disease: origin from follicles of hairs and results of follicle removal as treatment. Surgery 87:567-572, 1980

150. Karydakis GE: Easy and successful treatment of pilonidal sinus after explanation of its causative process. Aust N Z J Surg 62:385-389, 1992

151. Notaras MJ: A review of three popular methods of treatment of postanal (pilonidal) sinus disease. Br J Surg 57:886-890, 1970

152. Akinci OF, Bozer M, Uzunkoy A, Duzgun SA, Coskun A: Incidence and aetiological factors in pilonidal sinus among Turkish soldiers. Eur J Surg 165:339-342, 1999

153. Clothier PR, Haywood IR: The natural history of the post anal (pilonidal) sinus. Ann R Coll Surg Engl 66:201-203, 1984

154. Klass AA: The so-called pilo-nidal sinus. Can Med Assoc J 75:737-742, 1956

155. Sondenaa K, Andersen E, Nesvik I, Soreide JA: Patient characteristics and symptoms in chronic pilonidal sinus disease. Int J Colorectal Dis 10:39-42, 1995

156. Kooistra HP: Pilonidal sinuses: review of literature and report of 350 cases. Am J Surg 55:3-17, 1942

157. Solla JA, Rothenberger DA: Chronic pilonidal disease: an assessment of 150 cases. Dis Colon Rectum 33:758-761, 1990

158. Armstrong JH, Barcia PJ: Pilonidal sinus disease: the conservative approach. Arch Surg 129:914-917, 1994

159. Schneider IH, Thaler K, Kockerling F: Treatment of pilonidal sinuses by phenol injections. Int J Colorectal Dis 9:200-202, 1994

160. Lord PH: Anorectal problems: etiology of pilonidal sinus. Dis Colon Rectum 18:661-664, 1975

161. Bascom J: Pilonidal disease: long-term results of follicle removal. Dis Colon Rectum 26:800-807, 1983

162. Senapati A, Cripps NP, Thompson MR: Bascom's operation in the day-surgical management of symptomatic pilonidal sinus. Br J Surg 87:1067-1070, 2000

163. Buie LA: Jeep disease (pilonidal disease of mechanized warfare). South Med J 37:103-109, 1944

164. Culp CE: Pilonidal disease and its treatment. Surg Clin North Am 47:1007-1014, 1967

165. Bissett IP, Isbister WH: The management of patients with pilonidal disease—a comparative study. Aust N Z J Surg 57:939-942, 1987

166. Isbister WH, Prasad J: Pilonidal disease. Aust N Z J Surg 65:561-563, 1995

167. Allen-Mersh TG: Pilonidal sinus: finding the right track for treatment. Br J Surg 77:123-132, 1990

168. Kronborg O, Christensen K, Zimmermann-Nielsen C: Chronic pilonidal disease: a randomized trial with a complete 3-year follow-up. Br J Surg 72:303-304, 1985

169. Duchateau J, De Mol J, Bostoen H, Allegaert W: Pilonidal sinus: Excision–marsupialization–phenolization? Acta Chir Belg 85:325-328, 1985

170. Toubanakis G: Treatment of pilonidal sinus disease with the Z-plasty procedure (modified). Am Surg 52:611-612, 1986

171. Mansoory A, Dickson D: Z-plasty for treatment of disease of the pilonidal sinus. Surg Gynecol Obstet 155:409-411, 1982

172. Kitchen PR: Pilonidal sinus: experience with the Karydakis flap. Br J Surg 83:1452-1455, 1996

173. Rosenberg I: The dilemma of pilonidal disease: reverse bandaging for cure of the reluctant pilonidal wound. Dis Colon Rectum 20:290-291, 1977

174. Perez-Gurri JA, Temple WJ, Ketcham AS: Gluteus maximus myocutaneous flap for the treatment of recalcitrant pilonidal disease. Dis Colon Rectum 27:262-264, 1984

175. Bascom JU: Repeat pilonidal operations. Am J Surg 154:118-122, 1987

176. Davis KA, Mock CN, Versaci A, Lentrichia P: Malignant degeneration of pilonidal cysts. Am Surg 60:200-204, 1994

Chapter 43

RECTAL PROLAPSE AND SOLITARY RECTAL ULCER SYNDROME

Santhat Nivatvongs, M.D.

RECTAL PROLAPSE

Rectal prolapse is a protrusion of the full thickness of the rectal wall caused by an infolding of the wall into or through the anus (Fig. 1). The folds on the rectal wall are circular. The condition must not be confused with a rectal mucosal prolapse or prolapsed hemorrhoids, both of which have radial folds of redundant mucosa extruding through the anus (Fig. 2).

The three grades of rectal prolapse[1] are grade 1 (hidden prolapse), the intussusception is in the rectum and does not come into the anal canal; grade 2, the prolapse comes to but not through the anus; and grade 3 (overt prolapse), the prolapse protrudes through the anus.

Etiology and Pathophysiology

Cineradiographic studies show that rectal prolapse is the result of intussusception or infolding of the rectum, usually beginning 6 to 8 cm from the anal verge.[2] However, the cause of a spontaneous intussusception is still unknown. It was once thought that weakness of the pelvic floor muscle was the main cause of rectal prolapse. However, electromyography shows normal pelvic floor muscle in some patients[3] and weakness in others.[4] Excessive straining at defecation seems to be an important factor in the pathogenesis of rectal prolapse. The anatomical abnormalities commonly found in patients with this condition are the result of prolonged rectal prolapse and not the cause. These are a deep pelvic cul-de-sac, an elongated mesorectum, diastasis of the levator ani muscle, perineal descent, a patulous anus, and loss of support to the uterus and bladder. Fecal incontinence in rectal prolapse is the result of a neuropathy of the pudendal nerves due to

stretching caused by the prolapse. The incontinence is not caused by a mechanical stretching of the anal sphincter by the prolapse, as previously believed.[5]

Clinical Features and Diagnosis

The diagnosis of rectal prolapse is easy if the prolapse has come through the anus. Pain is not the typical symptom, although most patients complain of pressure in the perineum or mild, dull aching. Constipation due to difficulty defecating is common. In many patients, the main complaint is leaking of mucus. Worsening of the prolapse is gradual. When the prolapse comes to but not through the anus, the diagnosis can be difficult and must

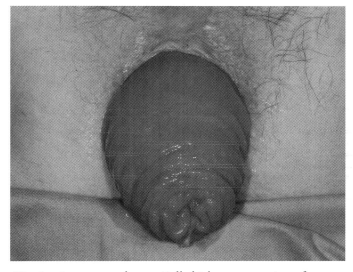

Fig. 1. An overt prolapse. Full-thickness protrusion of rectum through anus.

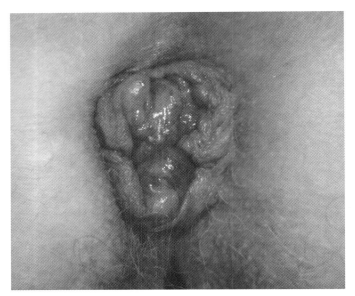

Fig. 2. Rectal mucosal prolapse. Note radial protrusion of anorectal mucosa.

be differentiated from rectal mucosal prolapse or prolapsed hemorrhoids. In grade 2 rectal prolapse, there is some degree of descending perineum, with bulging of perineum and a prominent ring of external sphincter, forming a "donut" sign (Fig. 3). Patients with grade 1 (hidden) prolapse or rectal intussusception may have as their only complaint difficult defecation or bleeding from

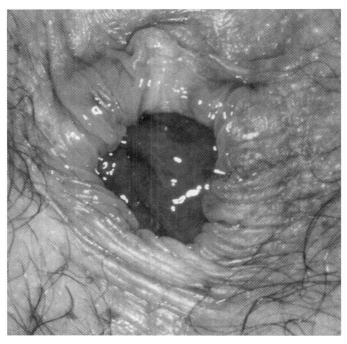

Fig. 3. Grade 2 rectal prolapse. The rectum protrudes to but not through the anus, forming a "donut" sign.

an associated rectal ulcer. Cinedefecography must be used to confirm the diagnosis.

Examination should always include straining in the toilet. Frequently, the patient cannot produce the prolapse in a lateral or prone jackknife position. The examiner should observe the movement of the perineum and the degree of descending perineum on straining. Digital examination gives a good clue to the status of the resting anal tone and the anal squeeze pressure.

Flexible sigmoidoscopy or proctoscopy and anoscopy are useful to confirm the diagnosis. In rectal prolapse, the lower rectal mucosa is red and hyperemic from the trauma. The changes may be circumferential or patchy. The patient may have areas of ulceration typical for a "solitary rectal ulcer." Colonoscopy is advised as a cancer screening examination for patients older than 50 years. A barium enema should be avoided because many patients have difficulty evacuating the barium. The straining may result in strangulation of the prolapse.

Women predominate, the female:male ratio being 9:1.[6] The mean age at presentation for this disorder is 65 years in women and 44 years in men.[6] About 40% of women with rectal prolapse have not had children,[7] refuting childbirth as a cause.[8] By the time patients seek medical help, about 50% already have fecal incontinence. Patients with a long-standing rectal prolapse frequently also have urinary incontinence.

Investigation
Anal manometry will not change the surgical approach and is not helpful for predicting postoperative functional results. Electromyography and measurement of the terminal motor latency of the pudendal nerve are useful for confirming damage to the innervation of the external anal sphincter and the pelvic floor muscles. Patients with damage to the pudendal nerve usually continue to have fecal incontinence after successful repair of the rectal prolapse. Cinedefecography is used to confirm the diagnosis of rectal intussusception, especially in patients with hidden prolapse (Fig. 4).

Complications
Complications from rectal prolapse are uncommon.

Bleeding
Severe bleeding may occur in patients with associated rectal ulceration. A repair of rectal prolapse to stop the intussusception may be needed if local management, including electrocoagulation and injection of diluted epinephrine solution, fails to stop the bleeding. Preventing recurring intussusception of the rectum usually partially heals the rectal ulcer.

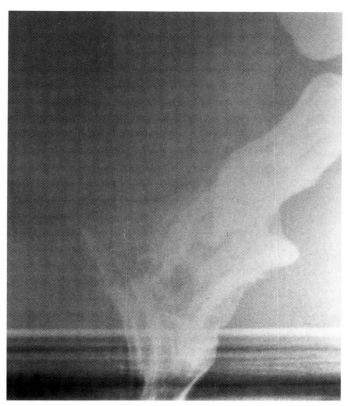

Fig. 4. Grade 1 (hidden) rectal prolapse. The rectum intussuscepts into the upper anal canal.

Incarceration
When the prolapse remains out for prolonged periods, it may become congested and eventually incarcerated, strangulated, or even gangrenous. This condition, however, is not common. The edematous prolapse can be treated effectively by sprinkling granulated sugar on the edematous mucosa to reduce the edema and, thus, aid in reduction.[9] Incarcerated, strangulated, or gangrenous prolapse that cannot be reduced requires a transperineal rectosigmoidectomy.[10]

Small Intestinal Evisceration
This exceedingly rare complication may occur during straining at defecation, resulting in rupture of the lining of the pelvic cul-de-sac. Until 1994, 57 cases had been reported.[11] An urgent exploratory celiotomy is indicated. The eviscerated small intestine usually can be reduced, the cul-de-sac sutured, and a rectosigmoid resection with rectopexy performed. In the presence of generalized peritonitis, however, an anastomosis should be avoided and Hartmann's procedure performed.

Operative Repair
There are more than 100 techniques for repair of rectal prolapse, and none of them are perfect. Repair of rectal prolapse can remove the protrusion or intussusception of the rectum but not the underlying cause of the problem. Each patient may have a unique, underlying difficulty different from that of others. For example, some patients have constipation because of pelvic floor problems, whereas others have colonic inertia. Some patients have mild fecal incontinence, whereas others have severe fecal incontinence from pudendal neuropathy. Some patients have urgent bowel movements, others do not. The repair should fit the clinical situation of each patient, taking into account the patient's general health and life expectancy.

The two general approaches are abdominal and perineal. The abdominal approach is recognized as having a smaller recurrence rate, although a prospective, randomized, controlled study has never been conducted to compare the two approaches. However, the abdominal approach is a major operation. It should not be performed in many patients. The perineal approach has a higher recurrence rate, but it is impressively well tolerated by patients.

Abdominal Approach

Rectosigmoid Resection and Rectopexy
This technique, originally described by Frykman in 1955,[12] had not caught on until recently, when it was found that the results of this procedure (with some modification) are as good as or better than the popular technique of rectal suspension with use of a mesh to anchor the rectum.[13,14]

A mechanical bowel preparation and prophylactic antibiotics are indicated. The important part of the operation must include a full mobilization of the rectum down to the pelvic floor. Lateral ligaments to the rectum should be preserved, because their division may cause problems with defecation and decrease rectal compliance.[15,16] The redundant rectum and sigmoid colon are transected at a convenient site to remove the slack, and an anastomosis is made between the proximal rectum and the distal sigmoid colon. The superior rectal artery also should be preserved to ensure a good blood supply to the entire rectum. The lateral peritoneum and the endopelvic fascia on each side are sutured to the presacral fascia with 2-0 polypropylene below the promontory of the sacrum (Fig. 5). The rectum should lie comfortably along the curve of the sacrum. Unless there is oozing of blood, a pelvic drain is not used. Some surgeons perform suture rectopexy without rectosigmoid resection.[17] Others perform rectosigmoid resection without rectopexy.[18] Both groups report satisfactory results. The mortality rate with this approach is 0% to 6.7%, morbidity 0% to 20%, and recurrence 0% to 9% with 2 to 4 years of follow-up.[11]

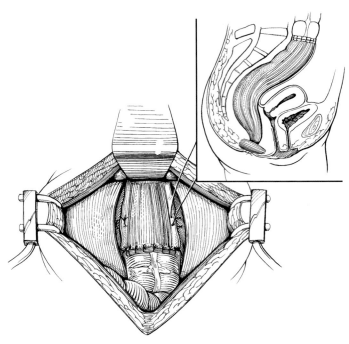

Fig. 5. Rectopexy. The lateral peritoneum and the endopelvic fascia on each side of rectum are sutured to presacral fascia below promontory of sacrum.

Suspension of Rectum With Prosthetic Mesh (Ripstein or Wells Procedure)

The anterior mesh sling (Ripstein repair) has long been the most popular repair for rectal prolapse in the United States. This technique has been plagued with rectal obstruction. In 1987, Ripstein abandoned this technique in favor of the posterior sling as described by Wells in 1959.[19]

Polypropylene (Marlex) and polytef (Teflon) are the most common materials used; polypropylene is the easier to sew because it is stiffer. Other materials such as poly-tetrafluoroethylene (Gortex), another polypropylene (Prolene), and polyglycolic acid (Vicryl) also have been used. Polyvinyl alcohol (Ivalon sponge), a popular material used in the United Kingdom, is not approved by the Food and Drug Administration for use in the United States. In this technique, the rectum is fully mobilized to the pelvic floor muscle. A rectangular sheet of mesh about 6 x 4 cm is sutured in the midline to the presacral fascia at the level of the second and third sacral vertebrae with three interrupted 2-0 polypropylene sutures. The mesh is then folded around the rectum to reach about three-quarters of its circumference. Excess mesh is excised. The edges of the mesh are then sutured to the anterior rectal wall with interrupted 2-0 polypropylene (Fig. 6). Because of the foreign body in the pelvis, a rectosigmoid colon resection is not advised. The results of anterior and posterior rectopexy are

comparable. The mortality rate is 0% to 4%, and the morbidity rate ranges widely from 3% to 52%, depending on whether minor complications are included. The recurrence rate is between 0% and 16%, depending on the duration of follow-up.[11]

Laparoscopic Approach

Laparoscopic repair has become a favorite approach for some surgeons who are well trained in laparoscopic techniques. The laparoscopic approach is used to mobilize the rectum and sigmoid colon. A suprapubic or Pfannenstiel incision is then made, and the mobilized bowel is delivered to the exterior. The proximal rectum and distal sigmoid colon are then resected and anastomosed. Rectopexy is next accomplished laparoscopically in the same manner as in the open technique. For an intracorporeal technique, the rectum is divided with a laparoscopic linear stapler at a convenient area that allows easy circular stapled anastomosis by way of the anus. The divided rectum, along with the sigmoid colon, is then exteriorized by way of a 4- to 5-cm periumbilical or suprapubic midline incision. The redundant rectum and sigmoid colon are then resected. A purse-string suture is used to secure the anvil of the circular stapler in the proximal cut end of sigmoid colon, which is then returned to the abdominal cavity. After closure of the abdominal incision, the pneumoperitoneum is reestablished and the two ends of the bowel are anastomosed with a circular stapler passed by way of the anal canal into the distal rectum. If rectopexy is to be done, intracorporeal suturing skills are needed for placement of the rectopexy sutures.

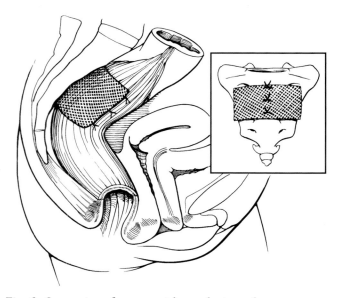

Fig. 6. Suspension of rectum with prosthetic mesh.

The laparoscopic approach to rectal prolapse that includes rectopexy with or without rectosigmoid colon resection is effective. It has low morbidity and mortality rates and is well tolerated by elderly patients.[20,21] The long-term follow-up data are not yet available, but short-term follow-up results show an acceptable recurrence of 0% to 6% at a median follow-up of 18 to 30 months.[20,22,23]

Perineal Approach

Although numerous varieties of perineal procedures for rectal prolapse have been described, two techniques are practical and provide satisfactory outcome. These are perineal rectosigmoidectomy (Altemeier procedure) and rectal "mucosectomy" with anorectal wall plication (Delorme procedure).

Mechanical bowel preparation should be used before operation and prophylactic antibiotics during operation, as with a transabdominal approach.

Perineal Rectosigmoidectomy (Altemeier Procedure)

In 1882, Auffret[24] recognized that a complete rectal prolapse was an intussusception, although he could not explain its cause or mechanism. He was the first to perform a transperineal rectosigmoidectomy in a patient with rectal prolapse that had progressed to strangulation. The prolapse was 70 cm in length. Auffret removed a total of 90 cm of the bowel transperineally, through the prolapse itself. This was performed with the patient under general anesthesia with ether. The patient died the next day. In 1933, Miles[25] reported his experience with transperineal rectosigmoidectomy in 31 cases. One postoperative death occurred, and one recurrence developed 5 years after the operation. This operation subsequently gained popularity, particularly at St. Mark's Hospital in London. However, enthusiasm faded when subsequent studies showed a recurrence rate of 27% in the first year and as high as 50% after 3 years of follow-up evaluation.[26] It was the excellent results of Altemeier et al.[27] in 1971 that stimulated the enthusiasm for this procedure, especially in the United States. They reported a 19-year experience with a series of 106 consecutive cases of rectal prolapse with only three recurrences (duration of follow-up was not specified).

This technique is suitable for an overt rectal prolapse (grade 3) that protrudes at least 3 cm from the anal verge. A lithotomy or a prone jackknife position can be used. A Foley catheter is placed into the bladder before the operation. The patient is placed in lithotomy position on hanging (gynecologic) stirrups. A general endotracheal anesthetic is preferred, but a spinal, caudal, or, if necessary, local anesthetic also can be used. A self-retaining retractor or a Gelpi retractor gives an excellent exposure.

After the anorectum is thoroughly irrigated with diluted povidone-iodine solution, the prolapse is pulled down to its maximum with Babcock clamps. The dentate line can be easily recognized with its distinct anoderm. A circular incision is made 2 cm proximal to the dentate line (Fig. 7 A) with electrocautery. The incision cuts through the mucosa, submucosa, muscle, and serosa of the everting rectum. The serosal layer of the inner rectal tube is exposed. It is dissected free from the surrounding tissues. At this point, the anterior peritoneal attachments of the rectum are dissected free and an opening is made into the peritoneal cavity (Fig. 7 B). With the patient in slight Trendelenburg position, the small bowel falls back into the abdominal cavity. The rectum remains attached by its mesorectum and the sigmoid colon by its mesentery laterally and posteriorly. The attachments are clamped, divided, and tied with 2-0 or 3-0 chromic catgut (Fig. 7 C). Other flimsy attachments can be cut with scissors or electrocautery. The dissection is carried further proximally until the rectum and sigmoid colon no longer come down. It is important not to cut the mesorectum or mesosigmoid too far proximal from the anal verge, otherwise the anastomotic line will be on tension and not have sufficient blood supply. The previously cut anterior peritoneum is now sutured to the anterior wall of the rectum or sigmoid colon, or it can be left open (Fig. 7 D).

If the patient has good anal continence, a sphincter repair is unnecessary. Alternatively, if the patient has severe fecal incontinence, it is reasonable to approximate the levator ani, puborectalis, and the external anal sphincter muscles with 2-0 polyglactin 910. These sutures can be placed anterior or posterior to the anal canal and rectum or both (Fig. 7 E). The rectal tube, or the sigmoid colon, is transected at the level of the anal verge and redundant bowel is removed (Fig. 7 F). The proximal cut end of the anal canal is then anastomosed to the distal cut end of the sigmoid colon with interrupted or running 3-0 polyglactin 910. No drain or packing is placed (Fig. 7 G and H).

The morbidity rate associated with this operation is between 5% and 24%, and the mortality rate is 0% to 6%.[11] The recurrence rate is 0% to 60%.[11,28] The largest series with long-term follow-up was reported by Kim et al.[6] A total of 183 patients, median age 75 years (range, 14-100 years), underwent perineal rectosigmoidectomy. The recurrence rate was 16% after a mean follow-up of 47 months (range, 12-165 months). The overall complication rate was 14%. Despite very low anastomosis, the leak rate was only 2%, and stricture at the anastomosis occurred in only 2%. There was only one death in the 183 patients. Seventy-six percent of patients were satisfied with the outcome of their operation.

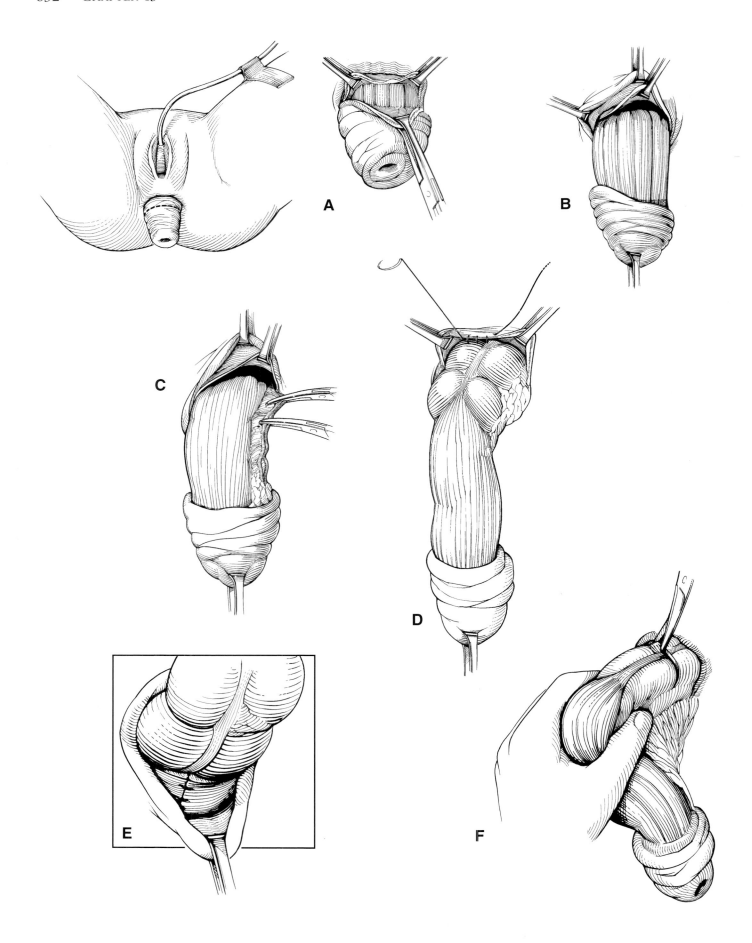

A

B

C

D

E

F

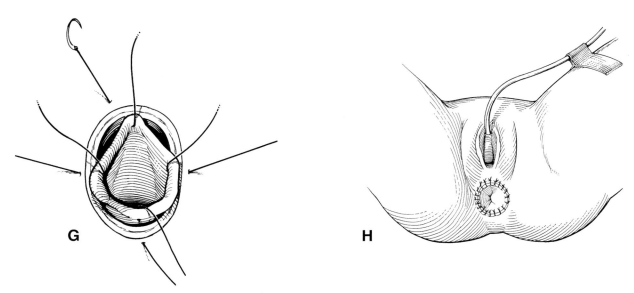

Fig. 7. Perineal rectosigmoidectomy (Altemeier procedure). (A), A circumferential incision is made on the prolapsed rectum, 2 cm proximal to the dentate line. (B), The peritoneal attachment on anterior rectal wall is opened. (C), Division of the mesorectum or mesosigmoid to fully mobilize the rectum and sigmoid colon. (D), The previously opened peritoneum is sutured to the rectal or colonic wall. (E), Approximation of puborectalis. (F), Excision of prolapsing rectal tube and sigmoid colon. (G), Stay sutures of 3-0 polyglactin 910 are placed at four quadrants. (H), At completion.

Anorectal "Mucosectomy" and Plication of Anorectum (Modified Delorme Procedure)

In 1900, Delorme[29] described a technique of repair of rectal prolapse by peeling the mucosa of the prolapsed rectum all around, starting just proximal to the dentate line and continuing to the proximal end of the prolapse. The denuded rectal wall then was plicated to shorten the anorectum, resulting in reduction of the prolapse into the anal canal. This operation never became popular or widely used. However, during the past 2 decades, there have been sporadic reports of the use of the Delorme procedure (with some modifications) as a primary treatment for complete rectal prolapse. Uhlig and Sullivan[30] and Berman et al.[31] applied Delorme's concept of shortening the rectum with "mucosectomy" and plication but modified the technique from extra-anal mucosectomy to intra-anal mucosectomy. This modified technique is suitable for a prolapse that protrudes less than 3 cm from the anus, in which case the perineal rectosigmoidectomy cannot be performed.

This operation should be performed with the patient in prone jackknife position. A self-retaining retractor or a Gelpi retractor gives an excellent exposure. The anorectum is irrigated thoroughly with diluted povidone-iodine solution. The anal canal is injected submucosally all around with 0.25% bupivacaine containing 1:200,000 epinephrine to decrease bleeding. A Pratt anal speculum is inserted into the anal canal for exposure. With electrocautery or scissors, the mucosa and submucosa 1 cm above the dentate line are cut circumferentially (Fig. 8 *A*). The mucosal-submucosal tube is dissected from the underlying internal sphincter and carried up to the anorectal ring (Fig. 8 *B*). A small Richardson or a right-angle retractor should be available to aid the exposure. The tube is pulled down for traction, and the right-angle retractor is appropriately placed for the exposure. Gauze can be inserted into the tube for better traction and identification. The dissection is carried proximally until the rectum no longer comes down and feels tight on traction. At this point, the tube is transected at its upper part (Fig. 8 *C*). Usually the dissection can go up to 10 to 15 cm from the anal verge. A Pratt anal speculum again is inserted into the anal canal to expose the upper cut end of the mucosa. A stitch of 3-0 polyglactin 910 suture is placed at the upper end as the first bite. In the subsequent bites, the denuded muscle wall of the rectum is taken in a left-right fashion (Fig. 8 *D*) in a distally progressing series until the last bite takes the distal cut end just above the dentate line. Eight such stitches are placed and tied, resulting in an anastomosis between the upper end and the lower cut ends. Additional sutures are placed to complete the anastomosis. At completion, the prolapsed rectum is shortened by its pleated wall (Fig. 8 *E*). No packing is placed in the anorectum.

The clear advantage of the Delorme procedure over the Altemeier procedure is that it is less extensive. The prolapsed rectum is shortened by plication of the muscular wall instead of resection. There are wide ranges in the results of the Delorme procedure. The mortality rate is low, 0% to 2.5%.[11] The morbidity rate ranges between 0% and 62.5%, depending on inclusion or exclusion of minor complications. The functional results have varied, but

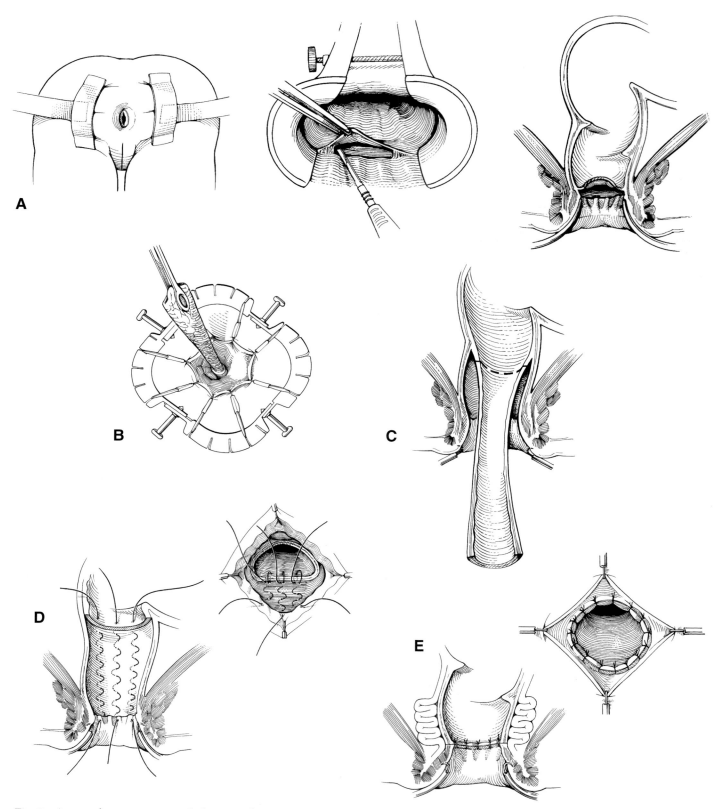

Fig. 8. Anorectal mucosectomy and plication of anorectum (modified Delorme procecdure). (A), Patient is placed in prone position. With use of a Pratt anal speculum for exposure, a circumferential incision is made 1 cm proximal to the dentate line. (B), The mucosa-submucosa layer is dissected from the underlying internal sphincter and tunica muscularis. The dissection is carried proximally until it is taut. (C), The mucosal-submucosal tube is divided. (D), The upper cut end of mucosa-submucosa is brought down to the mucosa-submucosa of the anal canal, taking along the denuded anorectal wall. We use 3-0 polyglactin 910. (E), At completion of the approximation, the anorectum is plicated.

reported results are somewhat better than might be expected for a perineal procedure. The satisfactory results have been reported to be between 74% and 93%.[11] Recurrence ranges widely between 5% and 35%, largely depending on the method and the duration of follow-up.[11,28]

Summary

The surgeon must tailor the operation to fit the patient. Abdominal rectopexy with or without resection is a major operation with potentially high morbidity and mortality rates and possible problems with defecation, but this approach has a low recurrence rate. The perineal approach (perineal rectosigmoidectomy and the Delorme procedure) provides lower morbidity and mortality rates, less pain, and a shorter duration of hospital stay, but recurrence rates are much higher in the long term. Despite this, the perineal approach has appeal in elderly patients or in patients in the high surgical risk category because it causes less morbidity. For younger patients, the benefits of the perineal approach, being a lesser procedure, must be weighed against a higher recurrence rate. The functional results between the two approaches are comparable.[6,28]

SOLITARY RECTAL ULCER SYNDROME

Solitary rectal ulcer syndrome is an uncommon one in which a chronic ulcer appears in the rectum. The most common site is at 7 to 10 cm from the anal verge. The term "solitary rectal ulcer" is misleading because there may be more than one ulcer and there is a stage of the disease when no gross ulcer is present. Moreover, the lesion can occur in areas of the large bowel other than the rectum.

The cause of solitary rectal ulcer syndrome is unknown. The syndrome is strongly associated with abnormal perineal descent.[32] More than half of patients have an obvious associated rectal prolapse of variable degree,[4,33,34] and many of the rest have an occult type or rectal intussusception.[35]

The ulcer is shallow and has a sharply demarcated hyperemic edge. It is characteristically covered with a white, gray, or yellowish slough. The gross appearance of the lesion may be misinterpreted as proctitis, Crohn's ulceration, or carcinoma. Microscopic features are characterized by thickening of the muscularis mucosa with extension of collagen fibers into the lamina propria and absence of a large number of inflammatory cells in the lamina propria. Rectal bleeding, passage of mucus through the rectum, and tenesmus are almost invariably present. Difficulty in defecation is frequently the main problem and an incapacitating one for which patients seek help. They describe difficulty in initiation of defecation and excessive straining at stool.

Proctoscopy or flexible sigmoidoscopy is the mainstay in diagnosis, allowing direct visualization of the lesions. The procedures allow a biopsy specimen to be taken. Defecography is the radiologic investigation of choice. It may show an internal or occult rectal intussusception. Electromyography of pelvic floor muscles may show hyperactivity of puborectalis muscle at rest and during straining.[34] Single-fiber electromyography shows evidence of pudendal nerve damage in 60% of patients. The degree of damage correlates with the degree of descent of perineum.[36]

There may be an association between colitis cystica profunda and solitary rectal ulcer. Colitis cystica profunda is a rare condition in which normal mucosal glands are found in the submucosa of the colon and rectum. Its cause is unclear, but the condition seems to be the result of epithelial displacement during the course of a disease, such as infectious diarrhea, colitis, trauma from instrumentation or other injuries, biopsy, polypectomy, digital trauma, radiation, and rectal prolapse. Because of its similarity in clinical presentation and association with rectal trauma and rectal prolapse, some authors regard colitis cystica profunda of the rectum as part of the same disease as solitary rectal ulcer syndrome.[2,37]

Management

Conservative Treatment

Because the principal complaint in the majority of cases of solitary rectal ulcer syndrome is difficult defecation, the aim of treatment is to resolve this problem. Bulk-forming agents, avoidance of purgative laxatives, and the use of suppositories all may help to reduce the need to strain at bowel movements. In patients who have hyperactivity of the puborectalis muscle on straining, biofeedback should be tried.

Surgical Treatment

Excision of the rectal ulcer is, as a rule, ineffective; the rectal ulcer returns. In patients with evidence of rectal prolapse and a rectal ulcer, repair of the prolapse should be considered. This can be performed with an abdominal or a transperineal approach. The difficulty occurs in patients with solitary rectal ulcer syndrome who do not seem to have an overt rectal prolapse. In them, it is impossible to offer any rational form of treatment. Nonetheless, operations for rectal prolapse can improve or cure many of these patients.[38-41] The surgeon should make clear to patients, however, that there is a considerable chance of failure if a rectal prolapse repair is done.

REFERENCES

1. Beahrs OH, Theuerkauf FJ Jr, Hill JR: Procidentia: surgical treatment. Dis Colon Rectum 15:337-346, 1972

2. Broden B, Snellman B: Procidentia of the rectum studied with cineradiography: a contribution to the discussion of causative mechanism. Dis Colon Rectum 11:330-347, 1968

3. Neill ME, Parks AG, Swash M: Physiological studies of the anal sphincter musculature in faecal incontinence and rectal prolapse. Br J Surg 68:531-536, 1981

4. Sun WM, Read NW, Donnelly TC, Bannister JJ, Shorthouse AJ: A common pathophysiology for full thickness rectal prolapse, anterior mucosal prolapse and solitary rectal ulcer. Br J Surg 76:290-295, 1989

5. Parks AG, Swash M, Urich H: Sphincter denervation in anorectal incontinence and rectal prolapse. Gut 18:656-665, 1977

6. Kim DS, Tsang CB, Wong WD, Lowry AC, Goldberg SM, Madoff RD: Complete rectal prolapse: evolution of management and results. Dis Colon Rectum 42:460-466, 1999

7. Jurgeleit HC, Corman ML, Coller JA, Veidenheimer MC: Symposium: procidentia of the rectum: teflon sling repair of rectal prolapse, Lahey Clinic experience. Dis Colon Rectum 18:464-467, 1975

8. Karasick S, Spettell CM: Defecography: Does parity play a role in the development of rectal prolapse? Eur Radiol 9:450-453, 1999

9. Myers JO, Rothenberger DA: Sugar in the reduction of incarcerated prolapsed bowel: report of two cases. Dis Colon Rectum 34:416-418, 1991

10. Ramanujam PS, Venkatesh KS: Management of acute incarcerated rectal prolapse. Dis Colon Rectum 35:1154-1156, 1992

11. Gordon PH: Rectal procidentia. In Principles and Practice of Surgery for the Colon, Rectum, and Anus. Second edition. Edited by PH Gordon, S Nivatvongs. St Louis, Quality Medical Publishing, 1999, pp 503-540

12. Frykman HM: Abdominal proctopexy and primary sigmoid resection for rectal procidentia. Am J Surg 90:780-787, 1955

13. Graf W, Karlbom U, Pahlman L, Nilsson S, Ejerblad S: Functional results after abdominal suture rectopexy for rectal prolapse or intussusception. Eur J Surg 162:905-911, 1996

14. Duthie GS, Bartolo DC: Abdominal rectopexy for rectal prolapse: a comparison of techniques. Br J Surg 79:107-113, 1992

15. Mollen RM, Kuijpers JH, van Hoek F: Effects of rectal mobilization and lateral ligaments division on colonic and anorectal function. Dis Colon Rectum 43:1283-1287, 2000

16. Speakman CT, Madden MV, Nicholls RJ, Kamm MA: Lateral ligament division during rectopexy causes constipation but prevents recurrence: results of a prospective randomized study. Br J Surg 78:1431-1433, 1991

17. Blatchford GJ, Perry RE, Thorson AG, Christensen MA: Rectopexy without resection for rectal prolapse. Am J Surg 158:574-576, 1989

18. Wolff BG, Dietzen CD: Abdominal resectional procedures for rectal prolapse. Semin Colon Rectal Surg 2:184-186, 1991

19. McMahan JD, Ripstein CB: Rectal prolapse: an update on the rectal sling procedure. Am Surg 53:37-40, 1987

20. Heah SM, Hartley JE, Hurley J, Duthie GS, Monson JR: Laparoscopic suture rectopexy without resection is effective treatment for full-thickness rectal prolapse. Dis Colon Rectum 43:638-643, 2000

21. Stewart BT, Stitz RW, Lumley JW: Laparoscopically assisted colorectal surgery in the elderly. Br J Surg 86:938-941, 1999

22. Kessler H, Jerby BL, Milsom JW: Successful treatment of rectal prolapse by laparoscopic suture rectopexy. Surg Endosc 13:858-861, 1999

23. Stevenson AR, Stitz RW, Lumley JW: Laparoscopic-assisted resection-rectopexy for rectal prolapse: early and medium follow-up. Dis Colon Rectum 41:46-54, 1998

24. Auffret M: Un cas de procidence du gros intestin d'une longueur de 90 centimètres; opération par excision; double rangée de suture; mort. Progr Méd Par Med Chir Pharm 10:650-652, 1882

25. Miles WE: Recto-sigmoidectomy as a method of treatment for procidentia recti. Proc R Soc Med 26:1445-1448, 1933

26. Porter N: Collective results of operations for rectal prolapse. Proc R Soc Med 55:1087-1091, 1962

27. Altemeier WA, Culbertson WR, Schowengerdt C, Hunt J: Nineteen years' experience with the one-stage perineal repair of rectal prolapse. Ann Surg 173:993-1006, 1971

28. Madoff RD, Mellgren A: One hundred years of rectal prolapse surgery. Dis Colon Rectum 42:441-450, 1999

29. Delorme M: Communication: sur le traitement des prolapsus du rectum totaux, par l'excision de la muqueuse rectale ou rectocolique. Bull et mém Soc Chirurgiens de Paris 26:499-518, 1900

30. Uhlig BE, Sullivan ES: The modified Delorme operation: its place in surgical treatment for massive rectal prolapse. Dis Colon Rectum 22:513-521, 1979

31. Berman IR, Harris MS, Rabeler MB: Delorme's transrectal excision for internal rectal prolapse: patient selection, technique, and three-year follow-up. Dis Colon Rectum 33:573-580, 1990

32. Snooks SJ, Nicholls RJ, Henry MM, Swash M: Electrophysiological and manometric assessment of the pelvic floor in the solitary rectal ulcer syndrome. Br J Surg 72:131-133, 1985

33. Kuijpers HC, Schreve RH, ten Cate Hoedemakers H: Diagnosis of functional disorders of defecation causing the solitary rectal ulcer syndrome. Dis Colon Rectum 29:126-129, 1986

34. Martin CJ, Parks TG, Biggart JD: Solitary rectal ulcer syndrome in Northern Ireland: 1971-1980. Br J Surg 68:744-747, 1981

35. Johansson C, Ihre T, Ahlback SO: Disturbances in the defecation mechanism with special reference to intussusception of the rectum (internal procidentia). Dis Colon Rectum 28:920-924, 1985

36. Mackle EJ, Parks TG: Solitary rectal ulcer syndrome: aetiology, investigation and management. Dig Dis 8:294-304, 1990

37. Ford MJ, Anderson JR, Gilmour HM, Holt S, Sircus W, Heading RC: Clinical spectrum of "solitary ulcer" of the rectum. Gastroenterology 84:1533-1540, 1983

38. Lowry AC, Goldberg SM: Internal and overt rectal procidentia. Gastroenterol Clin North Am 16:47-70, 1987

39. Nicholls RJ, Simson JN: Anteroposterior rectopexy in the treatment of solitary rectal ulcer syndrome without overt rectal prolapse. Br J Surg 73:222-224, 1986

40. Berman IR, Manning DH, Dudley-Wright K: Anatomic specificity in the diagnosis and treatment of internal rectal prolapse. Dis Colon Rectum 28:816-826, 1985

41. Keighley MR, Shouler P: Clinical and manometric features of the solitary rectal ulcer syndrome. Dis Colon Rectum 27:507-512, 1984

Chapter 44

ABDOMINAL TRAUMA

Daniel J. Johnson, M.D.
Daniel C. Cullinane, M.D.

The historical roots of surgery can be found in the management of traumatic wounds. The traditional focus of treatment was limited to surface and extremity injuries. Abdominal trauma was managed expectantly during wartime, and surgical intervention was uncommon. The opening of major body cavities to treat injury began in earnest during World War I.[1] However, the diagnosis and management of abdominal injuries have changed dramatically since then, as have the patterns of injury. Steady advances have occurred in diagnosis, treatment, antibiotics, and operating room asepsis. These improvements, in combination with the prompt evacuation and rapid surgical treatment of the wounded soldier, have carried over into the management of trauma in civilians.

Trauma surgery is the science of missed injuries. The abdominal cavity regularly conceals life-threatening injuries and hemorrhage. Ongoing improvements in diagnosis and treatment can limit the number of missed injuries substantially, resulting in reduced treatment failures and improved outcomes. Changes in surgical methods and techniques do not come as rapidly as changes in technology in the information age. New treatments are proposed many years before they become the standard of care, if they ever reach that level.

This chapter highlights some recent advances in diagnosis and treatment that have streamlined the care of abdominal trauma.

ANATOMICAL CONSIDERATIONS

The abdomen includes all the contents of the peritoneal cavity and the retroperitoneal structures. The bony thorax and pelvis provide protection for certain abdominal organs (Fig. 1). However, this shield of protection can confound the diagnosis and management of injuries to these organs. The major solid organs (liver, spleen, and kidneys) reside within the thoracic abdomen and so are vulnerable only to major blunt force trauma, but they are easily injured with all types of penetrating objects. The bony pelvis contains fewer vital structures. Nonetheless, the pelvic organs are well protected against all except the extremes of blunt force.

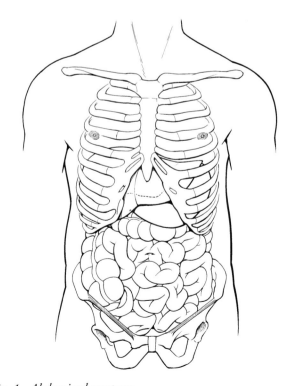

Fig. 1. Abdominal anatomy.

The rich blood supply of the pelvic region, however, presents a different set of challenges for the trauma surgeon when blunt forces prevail.

The retroperitoneal abdomen is divided into three zones. Zone 1 includes midline retroperitoneal structures such as the duodenum, pancreas, aorta, and vena cava. Zone 2 encompasses the lateral retroperitoneum and includes the kidneys, ureters, and parts of the ascending and descending colon. Zone 3 is the pelvic retroperitoneum. These distinct regions have treatment implications when decisions need to be made about the exploration of retroperitoneal hematomas.

EPIDEMIOLOGY

Blunt trauma predominates. The distribution of blunt and penetrating trauma depends on the locale, in that major urban areas have a higher proportion of penetrating trauma. Fabian and Croce[2] reported that, in Memphis, 27% of trauma admissions in 1996 were due to penetrating injuries and 73% to blunt injuries. Among these admissions, laparotomy was done in 36% of the penetrating traumas and only 7.6% of the blunt traumas. These rates are similar to those in other reports.[3] At Mayo Clinic in Rochester, Minnesota, 90% of trauma admissions during the same period were due to blunt forces. Nationally, penetrating trauma declined during the 1990s. Favorable economic factors are thought to be responsible.

The liver and spleen are the most frequently injured organs in blunt trauma. Hollow visceral injuries are more infrequent and can be difficult to diagnose. In penetrating trauma, the most frequently injured organs, in decreasing order of frequency, are small bowel, liver, and colon.[2] Multiple organ injuries are typical in penetrating trauma.

DIAGNOSIS

An organized and systematic approach to the trauma victim must be undertaken to reduce the risk of missed injury and to prevent death. The Advanced Trauma Life Support course for physicians describes this approach.[4] Unrecognized injuries to intra-abdominal organs have historically been a major source of preventable deaths, and considerable work has been devoted to development of the right tools for determining the need for surgical intervention.[5] Figures 2 and 3 depict management schemes that might be

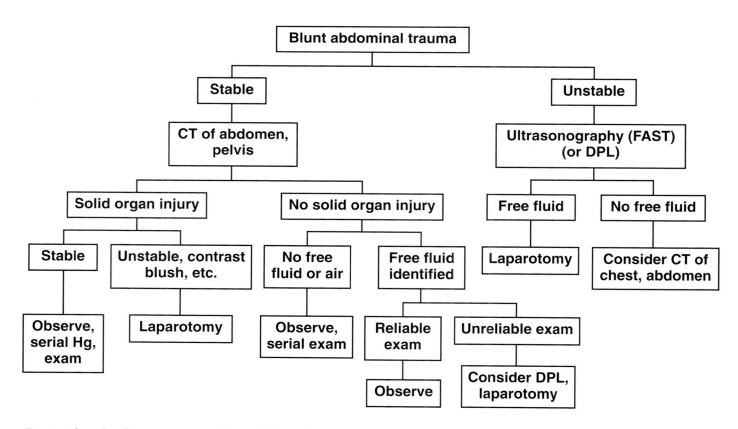

Fig. 2. Algorithm for management of blunt abdominal trauma. CT, computed tomography; DPL, diagnostic peritoneal lavage; FAST, focused abdominal sonography for trauma; Hg, hemoglobin.

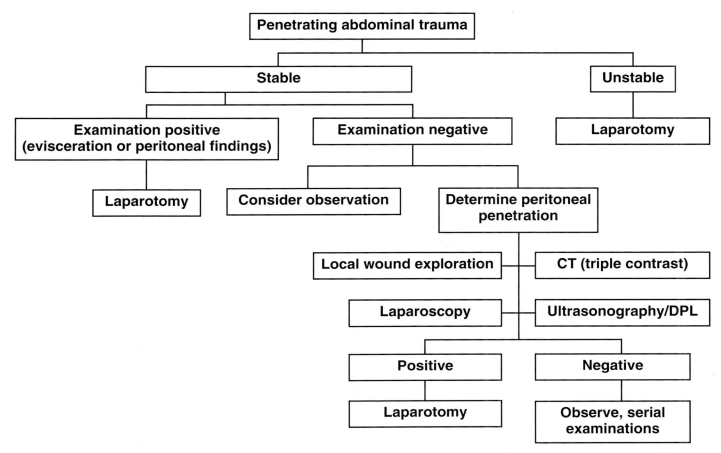

Fig. 3. Algorithm for management of penetrating abdominal trauma. CT, computed tomography; DPL, diagnostic peritoneal lavage.

helpful for blunt and penetrating abdominal trauma. These are sample algorithms that can be used in the decision-making and diagnostic process. The various diagnostic methods available are described below and range from the very simple to the more technologically complex.

History and Physical Examination

The importance of the history and physical examination cannot be overstated. These basic elements of the trauma evaluation are often overlooked in favor of more definitive diagnostic tests. Not every patient with trauma can provide an accurate history because of, for example, superimposed head injury, intoxication, severe pain, or shock. The traumatic event, therefore, is reconstructed with the help of eyewitnesses and police, fire, and emergency medical service personnel in lieu of an alert and cooperative victim.

Key elements in the history can determine the mechanism of trauma and will yield clues to the pattern of organ injury, whether due to blunt or to penetrating forces. In vehicle collisions, the speed and direction of impact, whether safety restraints or airbags were in use, intrusion into the passenger compartment of the vehicle, deaths of other victims at the scene, and ejection from the vehicle are important details. For example, in front-impact collisions where change in velocity is 35 mph or more, the risk of thoracic aortic transection is considerable. Much less force, however, can injure the spleen or liver. In other types of injury, the wounding mechanism should be determined, including the type and length of an impaling object, height of the fall, type of assaulting weapon, and the proximity of the assailant. Drug and alcohol intake can alter mental status. Knowledge of such ingestions is important in the evaluation of head injury and abdominal trauma.

Physical examination has historically been the mainstay of diagnosis in abdominal trauma. This is still true for penetrating trauma, in which the decision for operative intervention is often based solely on physical findings and signs and symptoms. The physical examination in blunt trauma is notoriously unreliable for both negative and positive findings.[3,6] Nonetheless, this component of the evaluation should not be overlooked. Certain physical signs such as bruising over the left upper quadrant or a seat belt mark over the mid abdomen can yield valuable clues about the type of underlying abdominal injury.

Physical signs of abdominal injury and hemodynamic compromise typically are the best indications of the need for urgent laparotomy in blunt trauma. Alternatively, in penetrating trauma, the mere presence of a wound over the torso, even in the absence of other physical signs, might be sufficient grounds for laparotomy. The physical examination can be compromised by neurologic injury (found in up to 25% of patients) and substance use (up to 50% of trauma victims).[2] Remote painful injuries also confound evaluation of the injured abdomen.

Laboratory Tests

Blood samples are routinely obtained during evaluation of trauma. Complete blood count and electrolyte, amylase, and blood alcohol determinations are performed on the sample. In addition, at Mayo Clinic, blood is also obtained for typing and screening or, depending on the extent of known injuries, crossmatching for transfusion. Liver function tests also may be a part of the routine panel at certain institutions. Routine blood work is usually more helpful in evaluation of blunt trauma than of penetrating trauma. However, in both types of trauma, these tests are usually adjunctive and rarely helpful for determining the need for surgical intervention.

The hemoglobin value is of little use before resuscitation of the patient with trauma, unless it is exceptionally low. The leukocyte count can be increased in response to stress and is, therefore, not specific. However, a value more than $12,000/mm^3$ may point to an occult intestinal injury in patients with no other obvious injury and no other reason to evaluate the abdomen.[7] The serum amylase value seems to be randomly increased in patients with known or suspected abdominal trauma. The low specificity and accuracy of this value limit its clinical usefulness in evaluating abdominal trauma.[8] Lipase levels seem to offer no advantage and, along with amylase, are an unnecessary part of routine evaluation of blunt trauma.[9]

Increased liver transaminase values may point to the presence of an occult hepatic injury or ischemia in the absence of any other reason to evaluate the abdomen in blunt trauma. These are sensitive but nonspecific indicators. They may have more usefulness in pediatric patients with trauma, in whom nonoperative management is a more zealously held standard.

Plain Radiography

The use of plain radiography in the modern management of trauma is limited. This is especially true of abdominal trauma. Supine chest radiography is standard in evaluation of the victim of blunt and penetrating abdominal trauma according to the Advanced Trauma Life Support protocol.[4] Aside from possible evidence of thoracic trauma,

however, few findings reveal the presence of abdominal injuries. Lower rib fractures (5-12) support the need for diagnostic evaluation of the abdomen because the underlying solid visceral organs could be involved. Injuries to the diaphragm may be apparent on chest radiography, but radiographs may be normal and findings nonspecific in such injuries also.[10] Free intra-abdominal air is virtually never seen on a supine radiograph, and its presence would likely lead to more definitive diagnostic tests.

Abdominal radiography is also of very limited diagnostic use, unless a foreign body or projectile missile needs to be located. This is not a routine component of the evaluation of blunt abdominal trauma, even though occasionally there may be some useful findings. Retroperitoneal air can be seen and may indicate an injury to the duodenum or colon. This extraluminal air is a nonspecific finding, however, and can be related to bronchopulmonary barotrauma. Other possibly important findings include displacement of viscera by fluid or hematoma, gastric distention by air or food, and free intraperitoneal air (which may require a cross-table lateral view to identify).

Pelvic radiography, another test that is considered standard in the evaluation of blunt trauma, can reveal an injury to the bony pelvis. The amount of force required to crack bones in the pelvic ring also can disrupt intra-abdominal organs and vascular structures. An evaluation of the abdomen with any of the accepted methods described below is probably warranted even when relatively minor pelvic fractures are discovered on plain radiography. Computed tomography of the abdomen and pelvis, however, is the preferable method because of the added advantage of defining the precise anatomy of the bony injuries. Also, because of the presence of considerable lower abdominal and pelvic pain with pelvic fractures, we have adopted a liberal policy of using abdominal computed tomography when a pelvic fracture is found on plain radiography.

Diagnostic Peritoneal Lavage

Byrne described the peritoneal tap in 1956.[11] This was a four-quadrant dry tap, and it had a false-negative rate of about 36%. The modern peritoneal lavage was developed by Root in 1965 and involved the instillation of fluid into the abdominal cavity to test the effluent for blood cells.[12] Three techniques have been used for diagnostic peritoneal lavage: open, closed, and semi-open. The open technique, as described originally, involves a skin incision with direct visualization and opening of the fascia and peritoneum for insertion of the lavage catheter. The closed technique, as described by Lazarus and Nelson in 1979, uses an over-the-guidewire Seldinger method for insertion of the catheter into the peritoneum.[13] The semi-open method uses a cut-down followed by exposure of the fascia and puncture by a needle or trochar blindly through the fascia into the peritoneum. Because of the speed and safety of the closed technique, we use this method for the rare patient who cannot undergo a reliable ultrasonographic examination. We currently use a kit that has an 8F, 24-cm catheter with multiple perforations oriented along the catheter in a spiral fashion.

After placement of the catheter, the peritoneal cavity is aspirated. The aspiration of 10 mL of blood or any enteric contents indicates a positive result. Typically, if there is minimal or no aspirate, 1,000 mL of saline is instilled and allowed to drain out by gravity. This fluid is examined with a cell count and a determination of amylase level. An erythrocyte value of more than $100,000/mm^3$ or a leukocyte value more than $500/mm^3$ is considered a positive result. Because these results are extremely sensitive but are not very specific, the nontherapeutic laparotomy rate can be as high as 30%. The complication rate is low (< 1% of 10,358 cases), but there is the risk of bowel, bladder, and vascular perforation.[14]

With the closed technique, a peritoneal lavage catheter can be placed by one operator in less than 5 minutes. If the results are equivocal, however, waiting for the cell counts can seem like an eternity. Peritoneal lavage is a legitimate screening tool for abdominal injury, but positive results do not mandate laparotomy in stable patients. This method recently was replaced by ultrasonography, a noninvasive method that provides similar information. Current indications for peritoneal lavage include the lack of ultrasonography capability in the trauma room and the finding of indeterminate free fluid on computed tomography.

The practice at Mayo Clinic is to perform FAST ultrasonography (described below) to determine whether free intraperitoneal fluid is present in patients who present in shock. If the result of ultrasonography is equivocal or of poor quality, then a closed diagnostic peritoneal lavage is performed. We consider this test result positive if 10 mL of blood or fluid containing bile or particulate matter is withdrawn. If the lavage result is not grossly positive, other sources of hemorrhage are sought. Saline is not instilled unless the procedure is being done to diagnose a hollow viscus injury. Abdominal computed tomography then can be performed without the confusion caused by the residual free saline from the lavage. We believe that if enough free blood cannot be withdrawn from the abdominal cavity through the catheter, the shock is likely due to an extra-abdominal source of hemorrhage.

Ultrasonography

Ultrasonography of the injured abdomen was first described by Aufschnaiter and Kofler in 1983,[15] but it did not become popular in the United States until the early 1990s.

This examination is rapid, hence the acronym FAST (focused abdominal sonography for trauma), inexpensive (after the initial capital outlay), and highly sensitive (comparable to the diagnostic peritoneal lavage that it replaces). The learning curve is steep, and 200 examinations are necessary for maximal proficiency.[16]

This examination is performed with a portable unit in the trauma resuscitation room. Only one operator is required, and results are obtained instantly. The examination does not require a radiologist because this tool has proven effectiveness in the hands of surgeons and emergency medicine physicians specifically trained in its use.[16,17] The ultrasound probe is used to evaluate the subphrenic spaces, the subhepatic space, the paracolic gutters, the pelvis, the pericardium, and possibly even the pleural spaces. Limitations to effective examination include obesity, subcutaneous air, and bowel gas. This test is probably no more useful for determining the need for laparotomy than diagnostic peritoneal lavage, but it does have the advantages of safety and immediate results. Therefore, it is an excellent screening tool.

Ultrasonography has a limited ability to detect specific organ injuries within the abdomen. We have noticed considerable difficulty with splenic injuries that have not bled freely into the peritoneal cavity. Approximately 20% of splenic injuries will have contained hemorrhage with little or no substantial free intraperitoneal blood.[18] Patients are at risk for delayed hemorrhage if the diagnosis is not ascertained by other means. In our experience, ultrasonography is most useful in the hypotensive patient to determine the need for immediate laparotomy.

Computed Tomography

Computed tomography (CT) has revolutionized the care of abdominal trauma, for the management of both the initial injuries and subsequent complications. Federle et al.,[19] in 1981, were the first to describe the use of this tool for abdominal injuries. Since that time, advances in technology have led to improved image quality and speed of imaging. Time constraints traditionally have limited use of the test to only the most stable of patients. In early reports, an abdominal CT evaluation took an average of 55 minutes, and an extra 20 minutes was necessary if a head scan was added.[20] Helical CT scanning has decreased the scanning time to 6 to 10 minutes and has provided better quality to assist in the management of complex combined injuries of the head, chest, abdomen, and pelvis.[21,22] Three-dimensional reconstruction is an added tool that enhances the evaluation of bony pelvic, abdominal vascular, and facial injuries.

A complete evaluation of the traumatized abdomen includes images of the lower chest and pelvis. Typically, oral and intravenous contrast agents should be used if not precluded by allergy or other complicating circumstances. However, because of the lack of added sensitivity for diagnosing blunt hollow visceral injuries, we have eliminated the use of an oral contrast agent for abdominal CT. Mesenteric and intestinal injuries are suggested by other features, such as the presence of free fluid without solid organ injury or mesenteric streaking. The contrast agent takes time to pass through the intestines and often does not leave the stomach. These factors, along with the risk of aspiration, negate the increased yield that an oral contrast agent might afford.

Sensitivity, specificity, and accuracy with CT are more than 97% in some series and compare favorably with other diagnostic methods such as diagnostic peritoneal lavage.[23] CT scanning has not usually measured up to diagnostic peritoneal lavage or ultrasonography if time and cost are considered the most important factors. These comparisons, however, are not appropriate, because CT stands alone in its ability to identify specific organ injuries, determine the extent of the injury, and quantify the amount of blood present within the abdomen. Other advantages include the detection of retroperitoneal injuries and bony injuries of the pelvis. CT not only identifies the injured organs but also aids in determining which injuries can be managed nonsurgically.[18]

There are, however, certain limitations to CT in addition to the time and cost factors. Identification of injuries to the bowel, pancreas, and diaphragm has been elusive because their CT findings can be subtle and nonspecific. These particular injuries and their diagnoses are discussed subsequently in this chapter. Complications also can occur with the use of oral contrast agents, and controversy remains regarding their necessity.[24] There is a perceived risk of aspiration, but proponents of oral contrast use have reported a low incidence of this complication.[25] The incidence of vomiting without actual aspiration is not known.

CT has its greatest use in the evaluation of blunt trauma. However, CT can be very helpful in some cases of penetrating trauma to the lower chest, flank, or pelvic or perineal regions. Peritoneal penetration is often difficult to determine in these cases, especially in the absence of physical findings. Subtle findings on CT may indicate the need for laparotomy, whereas negative results might avoid an unnecessary operation. Rectal contrast study is sometimes recommended, particularly in the evaluation of penetrating back, flank, or perineal injuries. We have found CT to be very useful in these circumstances. Often, the path of the projectile or knife can be followed on serial images, and if it is determined to be away from the abdominal cavity, the patient can be dismissed after a brief period of observation.

Laparoscopy

Laparoscopic, or minimally invasive, operation has revolutionized general surgery since the late 1980s. In addition to cholecystectomy, laparoscopy provides certain advantages in elective splenectomy, antireflux procedures, hernia repair, and colon resection. In trauma, however, laparoscopy is still a technology searching for an application. Laparoscopy was first proposed as a diagnostic tool for abdominal trauma in 1976, and its current use remains in the diagnostic realm.[26]

As an adjunctive method for assessing the need for therapeutic laparotomy, laparoscopy has been reasonably successful for blunt and penetrating trauma.[27-30] Several studies have touted its value for avoiding unnecessary or nontherapeutic laparotomy, but because of the push toward observation in many types of abdominal injuries, proper comparisons between observation and laparoscopy have not yet been made.[31] Laparoscopy should more appropriately be compared with CT because they might have a similar role in determining the need for therapeutic laparotomy. As with CT, hemodynamic stability is a necessity before any laparoscopic undertaking.

There are numerous drawbacks to the use of laparoscopy in abdominal trauma. Some of the theoretic or historical disadvantages include the need for general anesthesia, the risk of tension pneumothorax with diaphragmatic injuries, gas embolism with major venous injuries, and increased intracranial pressure in patients with closed head injury. None of these risks have proved to be major limitations, however. Cost and time issues are considerable compared with other diagnostic means. As many as 57% of known injuries have been missed by laparoscopic examination because visualization of the spleen, small bowel, duodenum, pancreas, and retroperitoneal structures is difficult.[32]

Therapeutic indications for laparoscopy in abdominal trauma are still being developed. Treatment of injuries to the liver, spleen, stomach, gallbladder, and diaphragm has been reported.[28,33] The small bowel can now be "run" from the ligament of Treitz to the ileocecal junction with available technology and expertise. A gasless laparoscopic evaluation also has been developed in which strategically placed struts are used to maintain exposure. In time, more and more procedures will be attempted given the zeal that many laparoscopic surgeons have for advancing their field.

Laparoscopy has one clear indication in the evaluation of penetrating trauma to the flank or thoracic abdomen when other diagnostic methods might fail to clearly determine the presence of peritoneal or diaphragmatic perforation.[28,29] In these situations, we have used laparoscopy when the surgeon considered the risk of observation to be too high. Treatment algorithms have been established which show the role of laparoscopy in avoiding laparotomy when there is no other clear reason to operate besides the existence of a proximity wound. The exact role of laparoscopy in blunt trauma has yet to be developed.

NONOPERATIVE MANAGEMENT

The use of nonoperative management strategies has always been difficult for the trauma surgeon. This approach has been embraced with fervor in pediatric trauma, whereas specialists in adult trauma have been converted only gradually, especially for many types of blunt injury. Some advantages of nonsurgical management include less cost, fewer postoperative complications, and less pain for the patient. Advances in CT technology have greatly enhanced our ability to detect and conservatively manage abdominal trauma. Although these methods are often preferred in solid organ blunt injuries, there are also indications for nonsurgical management of penetrating injuries.

Blunt Trauma

Nonoperative management should be considered only in hemodynamically stable patients, although the definition of "stable" remains elusive. Very select criteria should be used to determine the suitability for nonoperative management of patients with trauma. Between 60% and 70% of blunt solid organ injuries can be managed nonoperatively, and the success rate is typically more than 90%.[34,35] In these cases, CT has been used as a screening and scoring tool. The value of follow-up CT remains questionable, however.

Blunt splenic injuries are managed conservatively in 61% to 77% of cases, and the failure rate is about 10%.[18,36] Failure is associated with several factors, including age older than 55 years, Injury Severity Score, Glasgow Coma Score, injury grade, and quantity of hemoperitoneum. These factors are all relative, and there seem to be no absolute contraindications in adult patients except for hemodynamic instability. Grading of splenic injuries on the basis of CT findings traditionally has been a pitfall in considering nonoperative management. Considerable hemoperitoneum and the presence of contrast blush indicating active hemorrhage are more reliable CT findings that point to the need for operative intervention.

Blunt liver injuries are more suited than splenic injuries to nonoperative management, possibly because bleeding is more often venous. The same requirement of hemodynamic stability applies to observation without surgical intervention in patients with blunt liver injuries. CT and arteriography are important adjuncts in the management of such injuries. Large series of liver injuries have shown that higher rates of nonoperative management and lower failure rates can be achieved compared with splenic injuries.[37] Conservative management of liver trauma is associated with reduced mortality, lower rate of infection, decreased numbers of transfusions, and decreased durations of hospital stay.[38] As with operative management, complications can include "biloma," abscess, and vascular-biliary fistula.

Penetrating Trauma

There are three important questions to ask when evaluating the victim of penetrating abdominal trauma: 1) does the patient need immediate operation? 2) has the peritoneal cavity been penetrated? 3) has a visceral injury resulted from that penetration? With the use of clinical examination and select imaging studies, this algorithm determines which patients can be managed successfully without operation. With regard to the first question, if the patient is hemodynamically stable and does not have obvious peritoneal irritation or evisceration, immediate operation is not necessary, and the evaluation can proceed to the second question in the algorithm.

Peritoneal penetration can often be difficult to determine, especially when other factors make the examination difficult. Penetrating wounds, especially stab wounds, to the abdomen can be managed selectively.[39] Serial physical examination alone can be used to screen patients who may be suitable candidates for observation.[40,41]

Low rates of false-negative examinations can be achieved, and unnecessary and nontherapeutic laparotomies can be avoided. Other diagnostic methods, such as local wound exploration, diagnostic peritoneal lavage, and laparoscopy, can be used to supplement the physical examination and determine whether peritoneal penetration has occurred.[42] These diagnostic tools were discussed above.

If the abdomen has been penetrated, laparotomy can still be avoided if the patient's condition remains stable and there are no other signs of intraperitoneal injury. Serial physical examination and laparoscopy can be used to rule out visceral injury in penetration of the anterior abdomen. Triple-contrast CT also can be used to evaluate penetrating injuries to any portion of the torso, including wounds to the anterior abdomen, flank, back, and perineum.[43,44] At Mayo Clinic, we have limited the use of CT to stable patients with penetrating injuries to the back or posterior flank. CT, however, may not provide much additional benefit over physical examination in determining which patients need laparotomy for treatment of a visceral wound. More attention has been given to the selective management of abdominal stab wounds, but gunshot wounds can be managed similarly. The risk of visceral injury is somewhat higher, though, because direct penetration of the organ is not always necessary to produce injury.

OPERATIVE MANAGEMENT

Indications

The presence of hemorrhagic shock and physical findings consistent with abdominal injury are the historical standards by which operative indications are judged. Most trauma surgeons still hold this combination of findings at the top of their list of reasons for surgical intervention. Clinical presentations cover a wide range in abdominal trauma, however, and the role of nonoperative management continues to expand, as discussed above. Therefore, after clinical indications, the second major indication for laparotomy is failed conservative management. This rather broad category exposes the need for various thresholds to determine when conservative treatment has failed. Many trauma centers have established unambiguous criteria to decide when patients with abdominal trauma need operative management. We consider any failure of nonoperative management within the first 6 hours to be a failure of triage or an error in judgment; thus, adherence to protocol is vitally important. The indications for surgical intervention therefore can be based on physical findings, hemodynamic stability, findings on imaging studies, or prior clinical experience. These apply to either blunt or penetrating abdominal trauma.

Conduct of the Operation

After the decision to operate on the abdomen, the patient is placed on the operating table in the supine position and preparation for operation proceeds from the chin to the knees. This wide area allows access to the neck, chest, abdomen, and groin for either surgical exposure or venous cannulation (neck or groin) in the event of rapid or unexplained blood loss. The operating room is kept at 80°F to prevent the accelerated hypothermia that can occur in patients with trauma. The abdominal incision typically extends from the xiphoid process to the pubis, although there is a role for more limited incisions when the exact nature of the injury has been established preoperatively. In penetrating trauma, especially stab wounds, a much smaller incision can be made to ascertain whether peritoneal penetration has occurred, if this was not previously determined. Laparoscopy seems to be a viable diagnostic substitute in these types of penetrating wounds, however. Inadequate exposure and visualization of the peritoneal contents because of an undersized incision is an unacceptable reason for missed injuries.

Large amounts of blood may be encountered on first entering the abdomen. Until the blood is completely evacuated, ongoing active hemorrhage must be suspected. In this case, the abdomen must be packed with either laparoscopy sponges or sterile towels to reproduce the tamponade afforded by the closed abdomen. All four quadrants should be rapidly packed while as much blood and clot as possible are evacuated manually. Every region of the abdomen then should be systematically examined until the source or sources of bleeding have been identified. Therapeutic maneuvers for these sites can then be undertaken.

Hemorrhage control is the first priority in managing abdominal trauma. It should, therefore, be accomplished before any other definitive therapy. This may require the temporary placement of clamps or packs until a more thorough assessment can be made. The next priority is control of gastrointestinal spillage. Again, temporary clamps can be placed, and definitive closure of the injuries can be deferred until later in the operation or, if necessary, another day. After these two initial goals are achieved, the abdomen can be explored systematically. This typically involves the sequential examination of all four quadrants, liver, and spleen; inspection of the entire gastrointestinal tract from esophagus to rectum (including the duodenum, mesentery, and lesser sac); and visualization of the pelvis and retroperitoneum. The retroperitoneum should be explored in select circumstances. Hematoma or soilage in zone 1 requires a careful exploration, and exploration of zone 2 or 3 should be limited to patients with obvious gastrointestinal soilage or rapidly expanding hematoma.

"Damage Control" Laparotomy

In a small subset of trauma patients (about 10%), abdominal injuries are of such severity that definitive repair cannot be accomplished during the original laparotomy. In these patients, efforts are directed toward control of surgical bleeding and gastrointestinal leakage, followed by temporary closure and planned reoperation after the patient's condition has been stabilized. The decision to pursue this course of action must be made early in the procedure, preferably within the first few minutes.[45] If hypothermia, coagulopathy, and acidosis are present, the surgeon must decide whether to "bail out" or continue with the operation. This decision is primarily based on experience and judgment because there are few hard data to support any clear criteria. Blood loss of 4 to 5 liters, temperature less than 34°C, and pH less than 7.25 have been proposed as cutoff values, but the experience has been largely anecdotal in small series of patients.[46]

This method was recently called the "damage control" laparotomy, but the use of temporary abdominal packs can be traced back to the treatment of battlefield wounds during World War II.[47] Subsequent to this, packing and planned reoperation were abandoned in favor of definitive treatment of all injuries at the initial operation. In 1979, Calne et al.[48] described four patients with severe hepatic trauma who underwent packing and treatment at a second operation. These salvage measures gained popularity for liver injuries in the early 1980s, but the indications have expanded to include other types of severe abdominal injuries.[49,50] Trauma to the liver, pancreas, duodenum, small bowel, retroperitoneum, and pelvis has been treated with temporizing measures and planned reoperation. The mortality rates have ranged from 40% to 60%, largely due to the severity of injuries and the loss of physiologic reserve, but select series report somewhat better results.[45]

The "damage control" procedure should follow a carefully scripted sequence based on the condition of the patient and the nature of the injuries. Bleeding is the first priority and can be controlled with direct repair or ligation of certain vessels. Temporary shunting also can be considered, but there is little experience with this method in abdominal vascular injury.[45] Packing should be used to control nonsurgical bleeding from solid organs and the retroperitoneum. Overpacking and underpacking need to be avoided, and the packs should be strategically placed to provide the right amount of tamponade.[51] The next priority is gastrointestinal spillage, which can be controlled temporarily with bowel clamps, staples, umbilical tape ligation, or external tube drainage. At Mayo Clinic, we use a gastrointestinal stapler to resect and seal the injured intestines. This temporary iatrogenic intestinal obstruction has not affected morbidity or mortality rates. Definitive repair then can be undertaken at the subsequent operation. The abdomen should then be closed temporarily with one of the methods described in Chapter 45. The patient is then transferred to the intensive care unit, where all hemodynamic, acid-base, temperature, and coagulation abnormalities are corrected.

The timing of reoperation is often based on clinical judgment because there are no clear guidelines. In some reports, 48 to 72 hours has usually been the timeframe within which the second laparotomy is performed. During this period, bowel edema should have resolved substantially enough to allow for definitive gastrointestinal repairs and fascial closure of the abdomen. Subsequent procedures for abdominal closure or irrigation and debridement are often necessary for patients who survive. Patients who can be returned to the operating room earlier seem to have a better outcome, but this result may be a function of the severity of their underlying injuries.[47,50] Patients undergoing "damage control" laparotomy experience various complications, including abdominal compartment syndrome, multisystem organ failure, gastrointestinal fistula, and abdominal abscess. Again, these problems are often based on the nature and severity of the underlying injuries.

Temporary Closure

Primary closure of the trauma laparotomy is ideal, but occasionally it is not possible because of the risk of abdominal compartment syndrome, the presence of damaged abdominal wall tissue, or the need to reexplore for definitive treatment. Various temporary closures and materials have been used with different degrees of success. The choice of methods depends on the surgeon's preference and the risks associated with the various prosthetics.

The simplest method involves closing the skin with either heavy nylon suture or towel clips.[52] The fascia is left open with this method, and the expansible qualities of the skin allow for bowel edema and fluid accumulation within the abdomen. Closure with towel clips is quick and easy but very disturbing to the count-compulsive operating room personnel. We largely have abandoned this type of closure because of the skin necrosis that often results. Other methods involve the use of absorbable and nonabsorbable prosthetics, which can be temporarily sewn to either the skin or the fascia. Absorbable materials include polyglactin acid and polyglycolic acid meshes, and the nonabsorbable materials include plastic irrigation bags (Bogota bags), polypropylene mesh, reinforced silicone, and polytetrafluoroethylene.[53,54] These range from inexpensive to very expensive, and the choice depends on the ability of the material to provide strength and dependability with few complications.[53]

Mesh materials, although strong and easy to use, have a high risk of fistula formation when they have direct contact with the bowel.[55] Other substances such as irrigation bags, polytetrafluoroethylene, and silicone are smooth and do not permit the adherence or ingrowth of tissue. At some point, all nondegradable substances have to be removed to allow for definitive closure, skin grafting of the open wound, or secondary healing if the wound is small. A broader discussion of the techniques of temporary closure are discussed in Chapter 45.

Splenic Injury

Surgical management of splenic injuries becomes necessary when conservative management fails or when the injury is discovered at the time of laparotomy for hemorrhagic shock or separate organ injuries. Every attempt should be made to salvage the injured spleen unless uncontrollable hemorrhage or severe destruction of the tissue necessitates splenectomy. The decision to save or sacrifice the spleen should be made early and depends on the condition of both the patient and the other organs within the abdomen.

Splenic salvage can be accomplished by splenorrhaphy, partial splenectomy, or splenic wrap with an absorbable mesh material.[56] Splenorrhaphy is used for simple lacerations and is best accomplished with permanent monofilament suture. Some type of pledget material is often necessary because of the friable nature of the splenic capsule. Partial splenectomy is used when portions of the organ are crushed or devitalized. What percentage of the organ needs to remain to preserve normal splenic function is unknown, however. Splenic wrap has been used for binding a fragmented spleen that is not amenable to other types of repair. Absorbable mesh material is used for this purpose. The long-term effects on splenic function are unknown, and there is a risk of infection, especially when there are associated injuries of the bowel.

Hepatobiliary Injury

The operative treatment of liver injury depends on the severity and depth of the wound and the associated blood loss. Most liver injuries can be treated nonoperatively, but when conservative management fails or these injuries are discovered during laparotomy for other reasons, a systematic management approach needs to be undertaken. Hemorrhage control is the primary goal of treatment, followed by debridement of devitalized tissue and control of bile leakage. The actual suture closure of liver defects or lacerations should not be a primary goal of therapy.

Hemorrhage control usually begins with temporary packing of the laceration to allow complete mobilization of both lobes of the liver. After this step, the exact sources of bleeding can be assessed more thoroughly. The temporary packing sometimes can produce adequate hemostasis, but the use of cautery, sutures, or clips on the exact bleeding points is often necessary. Massive or uncontrollable hemorrhage may necessitate vascular isolation or inflow occlusion of the liver to allow identification of specific sites, including the hepatic veins or vena cava.[57] Other measures to control bleeding include temporary packing and reexploration, as described above, hepatorraphy with mattress sutures, or placement of a mesh wrap.[58]

Crush injury or vascular embarrassment often can devitalize large areas of the liver. Resectional debridement is a surgical technique that allows for removal of devitalized tissue without performing a specific anatomical resection.[38,59] This technique also can be used to control hemorrhage when a segment of the liver has been partially detached by the trauma. If large areas of ischemic or devitalized liver are present, we do not perform resectional debridement at the initial operation. This usually is performed at a subsequent operation after the patient has been resuscitated and hypothermia or coagulopathy has been corrected. Anatomical or segmental lobar resection can be used if the injury occurs along specific anatomical lines, which is rarely the case.

Injuries of the intrahepatic bile ducts commonly are associated with major disruptions of liver parenchyma and usually are treated with clips or ligation when recognized at the time of operation. In nonoperative management of liver injuries, intrahepatic bile duct injuries usually present as bilomas, and conservative management with drainage is usually successful. Extrahepatic biliary injuries are rare because the ducts are small and they are relatively flexible within the porta hepatis. Techniques that can be used to manage these injuries include suture repair, T-tube drainage, hepaticojejunostomy, and late reconstruction after damage control measures.[60,61] Penetrating injuries, especially gunshot wounds, present a greater challenge because of the major loss of duct tissue that can result.

Gallbladder injuries are also rare, occurring in about 2% of both blunt and penetrating trauma.[62] Aside from discovery at laparotomy, gallbladder injuries can be difficult to diagnose without a high degree of suspicion and the liberal use of sophisticated imaging such as CT and nuclear radiography. Management ranges from observation for hematomas to suture repair for minor lacerations to cholecystopexy for avulsions to cholecystectomy.[63] Cholecystectomy seems to be the safest approach, however.

Stomach Injury

Injuries to the stomach are rare and are most commonly the result of penetrating trauma. Blunt rupture of the stomach is exceedingly rare, and only small numbers of cases have been reported in the world's literature. The reported rate in blunt trauma admissions is 0.025%.[64] The stomach is protected by its thick wall, rich blood supply, and safe location in the thoracic abdomen. The stomach seems to be most vulnerable to blunt injury when it is full of food and relatively thin-walled. The anterior wall and greater curvature are the areas most often affected by injury.

Gastric injuries can be diagnosed with CT and peritoneal lavage and on the basis of clinical presentation. Shock from hemorrhage is rare in the absence of associated injuries. Peritoneal findings from spillage may lead to the discovery of this injury at laparotomy. Most gastric injuries can be treated with simple suture repair. Complex injuries require debridement before repair. Gastric resection has been reported for the most severe blunt gastric rupture.[65] Morbidity and mortality result from the severity of the associated injuries.

Pancreatic and Duodenal Injury

Pancreatic and duodenal injuries are often discussed together because of their shared blood supply and protected location in the retroperitoneum. These structures are more commonly injured by penetrating trauma; blunt injuries are somewhat rare. Treatment depends on the severity of the damage and individual surgeon's judgment based on experience and well-established management principles. Considerable morbidity and mortality can result from these injuries; early mortality is most often due to hemorrhage from associated vascular or solid organ injuries.

Pancreatic injuries are due to penetrating forces in two-thirds of cases. Associated injuries are present in 90% of cases, and the overall mortality has been reported to be as high as 26%, due to associated major vascular injury.[66] Most penetrating pancreatic injuries are discovered at laparotomy, and the diagnosis of blunt injury relies on CT scanning or a high degree of suspicion. Late diagnosis remains a problem and usually results from false-negative interpretation of CT scan or misinterpretation of clinical findings. Conservative (nonoperative) management of blunt injuries is an option if major ductal disruption can be ruled out. There is a role for endoscopic retrograde cholangiopancreatography in this management scheme when other diagnostic tools cannot determine whether a ductal injury has occurred.[67,68] Magnetic resonance cholangiopancreatography also has been described as a possible adjunct to the diagnosis and management of pancreatic injuries.[69]

Operative treatment of pancreatic injuries ranges from exploration and drainage to pancreatic-duodenal resection (the Whipple operation). Most authors advocate conservative treatment, especially if ductal injury is not suspected or cannot be proved. All hematomas surrounding the pancreas should be explored to determine whether the gland has been injured. Intraoperative transduodenal pancreatography has been advocated by some authors. The complication rate from the duodenotomy is apparently low.[70] The presence of ductal injury, however, does not mandate more aggressive surgical therapy or resection in every case. Debridement and drainage are sufficient in the majority of both blunt and penetrating injuries. Transection of the body and tail is best managed with distal pancreatectomy and drainage. Injuries to the pancreatic head can be challenging, and treatment choices range from drainage alone to resection, depending on the severity of injury (resection for grade 3 or 4) or the presence of an associated duodenal injury. Drainage of the disrupted gland into a Roux loop of bowel is not recommended unless the pancreatic head has been removed.

Complications from pancreatic injuries are difficult to manage. These include fistula, pseudocyst, abscess, pancreatitis, and anastomotic leak. The fistula rate is about 5%, but the abscess rate can be as high as 60% in penetrating trauma, especially when an associated colonic or duodenal injury is present.[66] The late mortality rate from these complications can be as high as 30%.[71]

Avoiding complications, therefore, is a primary goal of surgical management.

Postoperative drainage is an important adjunct in the management of pancreatic injuries. The type of drain used may influence the postoperative abscess rate. Traditionally, large sump catheters and Penrose drains were used to control pancreatic leakage, but the bacterial contamination and abscess rates were unacceptable. Closed suction drains have shown an advantage for reducing these rates of infection.[72] Also, the use of octreotide, a synthetic somatostatin analogue, may be beneficial in pancreatic injuries. In a retrospective study, Amirata et al.[73] reported no pancreatic complications in pancreatic injuries treated with octreotide postoperatively and a 29% rate in injuries not treated. This matter requires further investigation.

Duodenal injuries present similar diagnostic and therapeutic conundrums. Associated pancreatic injuries are present in 25% of cases.[74] Because approximately 85% of these injuries are due to penetrating forces, diagnosis is usually made at the time of laparotomy.[75] That assumes a thorough exploration of the abdomen and retroperitoneum. Any staining of blood or bile around the duodenum should prompt complete mobilization and inspection of all four of its parts.

Diagnosis of blunt injuries requires a high degree of suspicion aided by clinical examination and CT. When peritoneal lavage was used more widely, bile staining or particulate debris in the fluid might result from an intraperitoneal perforation of the duodenum, but these findings are not specific for duodenal injury. Injuries confined to the retroperitoneum, however, are difficult to diagnose with methods other than CT.

Duodenal hematomas, induced by blunt trauma, usually can be detected on CT and are amenable to conservative management.[76] Distinguishing hematoma from perforation on imaging studies can be difficult; thus, clinical judgment is important in the decision to operate. Conservative treatment for 5 days is usually sufficient to allow resolution of the hematoma and associated symptoms.[77] Nasogastric decompression and total parenteral nutrition have long been considered standard therapy, but these should be applied on an individual basis.

Surgical treatment of duodenal perforations depends on the nature of the injury and the amount of tissue damage. The varied and creative surgical options for managing these injuries are listed in Table 1. Simple repair is successful in 70% to 85% of the injuries.[75] More extensive surgical treatment such as a Whipple procedure may be necessary in 3% of cases.[78] Pyloric exclusion is a surgical maneuver proposed by Vaughan et al. in 1977.[79] This procedure closes the pylorus to the passage of food and secretions in

Table 1.—Surgical Options for Duodenal Injuries

Simple closure
Jejunal serosal patch
Resection and duodenojejunostomy
Duodenal exclusion
Duodenal diverticulization
Pancreatoduodenectomy (Whipple operation)

order to give the duodenum an opportunity to heal. Taking this concept one step further, Berne et al.[80] proposed the "duodenal diverticulization" procedure, which excludes the pylorus by removing it along with the gastric antrum. In effect, an end-duodenal diverticulum is created in case a fistula occurs. This method is aggressive and not currently recommended. We continue to use pyloric exclusion for the most extensive duodenal injuries. A purse-string closure of the pylorus is performed through a separate gastrotomy. A loop of jejunum is then brought up the gastrotomy, and a hand-sewn anastomosis is created. No other luminal tubes are placed when this method is used.

Tube decompression of the duodenum can be added to any repair, but its actual usefulness is questionable.[78] Stone and Fabian[81] suggested a three-tube method of treatment, placing a gastrostomy, retrograde duodenostomy, and a feeding jejunostomy (Fig. 4). This method is a safe and conservative approach, but it may not be necessary in the management of low-grade injuries requiring only simple repair. Closed suction drainage is an important adjunct of treatment, as it is with pancreatic trauma.

Complications from duodenal injuries include fistula, suture line leak, and abscess. The fistula rate ranges from 2% to 14%, and most fistulas can be managed conservatively.[75] The overall mortality rate from duodenal trauma ranges from 13% to 28%, and late mortality from 6% to 12%. Sound surgical judgment and aggressive early management help to limit complications from these injuries.

Small Bowel Injury

Small bowel injury is relatively infrequent in blunt abdominal trauma, occurring in 5% to 15% of cases.[82] In penetrating trauma, small bowel injury is more common. One series reported the overall frequency to be 1.1% in all patients with trauma admitted during a 12-year period.[83] The diagnosis of small bowel injury can be difficult, particularly in blunt injury, and the delays in diagnosis and treatment cause considerable morbidity.[84]

Each method of evaluation has potentially important pitfalls, but CT is emerging as the diagnostic tool of choice in blunt intestinal trauma.[85] The overall accuracy was reported to be as high as 94% in one series.[86] The CT findings range from small amounts of free fluid to free air to contrast extravasation. Rizzo et al.[87] found that all surgically proven small bowel injuries had free fluid on CT. Although this finding is very nonspecific, it should raise suspicion, especially when no other organ injury explains this fluid. Free air, however, was found in only half of the patients with bowel lacerations in that study. We generally perform either a diagnostic peritoneal lavage or immediate laparotomy, depending on the condition of the patient, if free fluid is seen on CT without an associated solid organ injury.

Injuries to the small bowel range from hematoma to serosal tears to complete transection and include mesenteric lacerations with compromised circulation and bowel ischemia. The treatment varies accordingly, and simple repair is the most widely used management technique. Resection and anastomosis also may be necessary, especially if there is devitalized or marginally perfused bowel.

The debate over stapled or hand-sewn anastomosis continues; recent literature has questioned which method of anastomosis is better in the patient with trauma. Brundage et al.[88] reported a higher rate of complication and leak in stapled anastomoses, although their study included injuries along the entire abdominal gastrointestinal tract. Conversely, Witzke et al.[83] examined small bowel injuries only and found a slightly higher rate of abscess in stapled bowel but no difference in the rates of

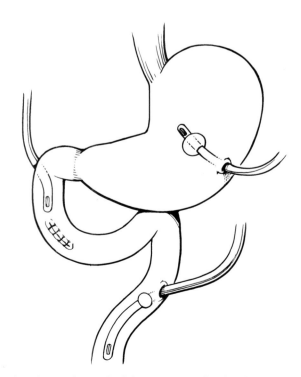

Fig. 4. Three-tube method for managing duodenal injuries.

small bowel obstruction, fistula, or leak compared with hand-sewn connections. Hand-sewing may be the safest approach, especially when the bowel is edematous, because the staples cannot accommodate the differences in the thickness of the bowel.

Colon Injury

The management of colon injuries has evolved since World War II, but controversy still remains as to which method of treatment best suits the needs of the patient. Colostomy was considered the standard of care for all types of colon injury during World War II and was thought to be responsible for a dramatic decline in the mortality rate from colon injury compared with that during World War I.[89] Performing a colostomy proximal to the area of injury was once considered a standard accessory to the repair or resection of colon injuries. Exteriorization of minor colon repairs was also an acceptable method of treatment. Either choice required considerable follow-up care and a second surgical procedure to return the colon to the abdominal cavity.

In 1979, Stone and Fabian[90] published results of a prospective randomized trial that advocated primary repair of colon injuries. They found decreased complication and infection rates compared with rates in patients treated with diverting colostomy. Colostomy was still reserved for a subset of severely injured patients who were not included in the data analysis. Other reports have confirmed these findings and extended the role of primary repair to all types and severity of colon injury.[91,92] Leak and abscess rates are low to nonexistent in these series. Most of the published reports concern penetrating injuries, but many of the management principles can be applied to blunt injury.

During the past 20 years, colon injuries have come to be treated either with debridement and primary repair or with resection and anastomosis. These methods have been rendered without concern for associated factors such as shock and fecal contamination. Some reports, however, continue to advocate colostomy for more severe injuries.[93] Durham et al.[94] advocated that patients with a high abdominal trauma index and high colon injury score should be considered for colostomy, even though they could not show a difference in outcome in this subset of severe injuries. Rectal injuries have been conspicuously absent from all of these series, and the principles of repair or resection, drainage, and diverting colostomy should be considered the standard treatment of these injuries.

CONCLUSION

The management of abdominal trauma has developed steadily since World War I. Improvements in diagnosis and treatment have standardized care, facilitated detection of injury, reduced morbidity, and increased survival. Standard guidelines continue to be developed and refined for a wide range of abdominal injuries.

Ultrasonography has become an effective screening tool and has nearly replaced peritoneal lavage in this capacity. Considerable improvements in CT technology have enhanced the speed and quality of the imaging, making it the standard of care in injury diagnosis and management. These tools have helped the surgeon decide which patients are the most suitable candidates for non-surgical management.

When surgical management is deemed necessary, however, the most important tools are still the surgeon's judgment, skill, and experience. Appropriate application of these qualities becomes the key to success. "Damage control" laparotomy, although not necessarily new, has received considerable attention in recent years. Application of this treatment has improved the care of patients with the most severely injured abdomens. New methods of handling old problems will continue to be developed.

REFERENCES

1. Davis JH: History of trauma. *In* Trauma. Second edition. Edited by EE Moore, KL Mattox, DV Feliciano. Norwalk, CT, Appleton & Lange, 1991, pp 3-14
2. Fabian TC, Croce MA: Abdominal trauma, including indications for celiotomy. *In* Trauma. Fourth edition. Edited by KL Mattox, DV Feliciano, EE Moore. New York, McGraw-Hill, 2000, pp 583-602
3. Mackersie RC, Tiwary AD, Shackford SR, Hoyt DB: Intra-abdominal injury following blunt trauma: identifying the high-risk patient using objective risk factors. Arch Surg 124:809-813, 1989
4. Advanced Trauma Life Support Program for Doctors: ATLS. Sixth edition. Chicago, American College of Surgeons, 1997
5. West JG, Trunkey DD, Lim RC: Systems of trauma care: a study of two counties. Arch Surg 114:455-460, 1979
6. Davis JJ, Cohn I Jr, Nance FC: Diagnosis and management of blunt abdominal trauma. Ann Surg 183:672-678, 1976
7. Harris HW, Morabito DJ, Mackersie RC, Halvorsen RA, Schecter WP: Leukocytosis and free fluid are important indicators of isolated intestinal injury after blunt trauma. J Trauma 46:656-659, 1999
8. Mure AJ, Josloff R, Rothberg J, O'Malley KF, Ross SE: Serum amylase determination and blunt abdominal trauma. Am Surg 57:210-213, 1991
9. Buechter KJ, Arnold M, Steele B, Martin L, Byers P, Gomez G, Zeppa R, Augenstein J: The use of serum amylase and lipase in evaluating and managing blunt abdominal trauma. Am Surg 56:204-208, 1990
10. Gelman R, Mirvis SE, Gens D: Diaphragmatic rupture due to blunt trauma: sensitivity of plain chest radiographs. AJR Am J Roentgenol 156:51-57, 1991
11. Byrne RV: Diagnostic abdominal tap. West J Surg 64:369-373, 1956
12. Root HD, Hauser CW, McKinley CR, LaFave JW, Mendiola RP Jr: Diagnostic peritoneal lavage. Surgery 57:633-637, 1965
13. Lazarus HM, Nelson JA: A technique for peritoneal lavage without risk or complication. Surg Gynecol Obstet 149:889-892, 1979
14. Powell DC, Bivins BA, Bell RM: Diagnostic peritoneal lavage. Surg Gynecol Obstet 155:257-264, 1982
15. Aufschnaiter M, Kofler H: Sonographic acute diagnosis in polytrauma [German]. Aktuelle Traumatologie 13:55-57, 1983
16. Rozycki GS, Ochsner MG, Jaffin JH, Champion HR: Prospective evaluation of surgeons' use of ultrasound in the evaluation of trauma patients. J Trauma 34:516-526, 1993
17. Schlager D, Lazzareschi G, Whitten D, Sanders AB: A prospective study of ultrasonography in the ED by emergency physicians. Am J Emerg Med 12:185-189, 1994
18. Peitzman AB, Heil B, Rivera L, Federle MB, Harbrecht BG, Clancy KD, Croce M, Enderson BL, Morris JA, Shatz D, Meredith JW, Ochoa JB, Fakhry SM, Cushman JG, Minei JP, McCarthy M, Luchette FA, Townsend R, Tinkoff G, Block EF, Ross S, Frykberg ER, Bell RM, Davis F III, Weireter L, Shapiro MB: Blunt splenic injury in adults: Multi-institutional Study of the Eastern Association for the Surgery of Trauma. J Trauma 49:177-187, 2000
19. Federle MP, Goldberg HI, Kaiser JA, Moss AA, Jeffrey RB Jr, Mall JC: Evaluation of abdominal trauma by computed tomography. Radiology 138:637-644, 1981
20. Pevec WC, Peitzman AB, Udekwu AO, McCoy B, Straub W: Computed tomography in the evaluation of blunt abdominal trauma. Surg Gynecol Obstet 173:262-267, 1991
21. Novelline RA, Rhea JT, Bell T: Helical CT of abdominal trauma. Radiol Clin North Am 37:591-612, 1999
22. Shuman WP: CT of blunt abdominal trauma in adults. Radiology 205:297-306, 1997
23. Blow O, Bassam D, Butler K, Cephas GA, Brady W, Young JS: Speed and efficiency in the resuscitation of blunt trauma patients with multiple injuries: the advantage of diagnostic peritoneal lavage over abdominal computerized tomography. J Trauma 44:287-290, 1998
24. Stafford RE, McGonigal MD, Weigelt JA, Johnson TJ: Oral contrast solution and computed tomography for blunt abdominal trauma: a randomized study. Arch Surg 134:622-626, 1999
25. Federle MP, Yagan N, Peitzman AB, Krugh J: Abdominal trauma: use of oral contrast material for CT is safe. Radiology 205:91-93, 1997
26. Gazzaniga AB, Stanton WW, Bartlett RH: Laparoscopy in the diagnosis of blunt and penetrating injuries to the abdomen. Am J Surg 131:315-318, 1976
27. Rossi P, Mullins D, Thal E: Role of laparoscopy in the evaluation of abdominal trauma. Am J Surg 166:707-710, 1993
28. Zantut LF, Ivatury RR, Smith RS, Kawahara NT, Porter JM, Fry WR, Poggetti R, Birolini D, Organ CH Jr: Diagnostic and therapeutic laparoscopy for penetrating abdominal trauma: a multicenter experience. J Trauma 42:825-829, 1997
29. Ivatury RR, Simon RJ, Weksler B, Bayard V, Stahl WM: Laparoscopy in the evaluation of the intrathoracic abdomen after penetrating injury. J Trauma 33:101-108, 1992
30. Livingston DH, Tortella BJ, Blackwood J, Machiedo GW, Rush BF Jr: The role of laparoscopy in abdominal trauma. J Trauma 33:471-475, 1992
31. Townsend MC, Flancbaum L, Choban PS, Cloutier CT: Diagnostic laparoscopy as an adjunct to selective conservative management of solid organ injuries after blunt abdominal trauma. J Trauma 35:647-651, 1993
32. Elliott DC, Rodriguez A, Moncure M, Myers RA, Shillinglaw W, Davis F, Goldberg A, Mitchell K, McRitchie D: The accuracy of diagnostic laparoscopy in trauma patients: a prospective, controlled study. Int Surg 83:294-298, 1998
33. Smith RS, Fry WR, Morabito DJ, Koehler RH, Organ CH Jr: Therapeutic laparoscopy in trauma. Am J Surg 170:632-636, 1995
34. Allins A, Ho T, Nguyen TH, Cohen M, Waxman K, Hiatt JR: Limited value of routine follow-up CT scans in nonoperative management of blunt liver and splenic injuries. Am Surg 62:883-886, 1996
35. Sartorelli KH, Frumiento C, Rogers FB, Osler TM: Nonoperative management of hepatic, splenic, and renal injuries in adults with multiple injuries. J Trauma 49:56-61, 2000
36. Bee TK, Croce MA, Miller PR, Pritchard FE, Fabian TC: Failures of splenic nonoperative management: Is the glass half empy or half full? J Trauma 50:230-236, 2001
37. Malhotra AK, Fabian TC, Croce MA, Gavin TJ, Kudsk KA, Minard G, Pritchard FE: Blunt hepatic injury: a paradigm shift from operative to nonoperative management in the 1990s. Ann Surg 231:804-813, 2000
38. David Richardson J, Franklin GA, Lukan JK, Carrillo EH, Spain DA, Miller FB, Wilson MA, Polk HC Jr, Flint LM: Evolution in the management of hepatic trauma: a 25-year perspective. Ann Surg 232:324-330, 2000
39. Nance FC, Cohn I Jr: Surgical judgment in the management of stab wounds of the abdomen: a retrospective and prospective

analysis based on a study of 600 stabbed patients. Ann Surg 170:569-580, 1969

40. Demetriades D, Rabinowitz B: Indications for operation in abdominal stab wounds: a prospective study of 651 patients. Ann Surg 205:129-132, 1987

41. Zubowski R, Nallathambi M, Ivatury R, Stahl W: Selective conservatism in abdominal stab wounds: the efficacy of serial physical examination. J Trauma 28:1665-1668, 1988

42. Feliciano DV, Bitondo CG, Steed G, Mattox KL, Burch JM, Jordan GL Jr: Five hundred open taps or lavages in patients with abdominal stab wounds. Am J Surg 148:772-777, 1984

43. Phillips T, Sclafani SJ, Goldstein A, Scalea T, Panetta T, Shaftan G: Use of the contrast-enhanced CT enema in the management of penetrating trauma to the flank and back. J Trauma 26:593-601, 1986

44. Himmelman RG, Martin M, Gilkey S, Barrett JA: Triple-contrast CT scans in penetrating back and flank trauma. J Trauma 31:852-855, 1991

45. Hirshberg A, Mattox KL: Planned reoperation for severe trauma. Ann Surg 222:3-8, 1995

46. Carrillo C, Fogler RJ, Shaftan GW: Delayed gastrointestinal reconstruction following massive abdominal trauma. J Trauma 34:233-235, 1993

47. Abikhaled JA, Granchi TS, Wall MJ, Hirshberg A, Mattox KL: Prolonged abdominal packing for trauma is associated with increased morbidity and mortality. Am Surg 63:1109-1112, 1997

48. Calne RY, McMaster P, Pentlow BD: The treatment of major liver trauma by primary packing with transfer of the patient for definitive treatment. Br J Surg 66:338-339, 1979

49. Stone HH, Strom PR, Mullins RJ: Management of the major coagulopathy with onset during laparotomy. Ann Surg 197:532-535, 1983

50. Talberg S, Trooskin SZ, Scalea T, Vieux E, Atweh N, Duncan A, Sclafani S: Packing and re-exploration for patients with non-hepatic injuries. J Trauma 33:121-124, 1992

51. Hirshberg A, Walden R: Damage control for abdominal trauma. Surg Clin North Am 77:813-820, 1997

52. Smith PC, Tweddell JS, Bessey PQ: Alternative approaches to abdominal wound closure in severely injured patients with massive visceral edema. J Trauma 32:16-20, 1992

53. Mayberry JC, Mullins RJ, Trunkey DD: Absorbable mesh prosthesis closure for abdominal trauma and other catastrophies. Adv Surg 33:217-241, 1999

54. Fernandez L, Norwood S, Roettger R, Wilkins HE III: Temporary intravenous bag silo closure in severe abdominal trauma. J Trauma 40:258-260, 1996

55. Nagy KK, Fildes JJ, Mahr C, Roberts RR, Krosner SM, Joseph KT, Barrett J: Experience with three prosthetic materials in temporary abdominal wall closure. Am Surg 62:331-335, 1996

56. Fingerhut A, Oberlin P, Cotte JL, Aziz L, Etienne JC, Vinson-Bonnet B, Aubert JD, Rea S: Splenic salvage using an absorbable mesh: feasibility, reliability, and safety. Br J Surg 79:325-327, 1992

57. Buckman RF Jr, Miraliakbari R, Badellino MM: Juxtahepatic venous injuries: a critical review of reported management strategies. J Trauma 48:978-984, 2000

58. Jacobson LE, Kirton OC, Gomez GA: The use of an absorbable mesh wrap in the management of major liver injuries. Surgery 111:455-461, 1992

59. Pachter HL, Feliciano DV: Complex hepatic injuries. Surg Clin North Am 76:763-782, 1996

60. Dawson DL, Jurkovich GJ: Hepatic duct disruption from blunt abdominal trauma: case report and literature review. J Trauma 31:1698-1702, 1991

61. Feliciano DV: Biliary injuries as a result of blunt and penetrating trauma. Surg Clin North Am 74:897-907, 1994

62. Penn I: Injuries of the gall-bladder. Br J Surg 49:636-641, 1962

63. Sharma O: Blunt gallbladder injuries: presentation of twenty-two cases with review of the literature. J Trauma 39:576-580, 1995

64. Allen GS, Moore FA, Cox CS Jr, Wilson JT, Cohn JM, Duke JH: Hollow visceral injury and blunt trauma. J Trauma 45:69-75, 1998

65. Nanji SA, Mock C: Gastric rupture resulting from blunt abdominal trauma and requiring gastric resection. J Trauma 47:410-412, 1999

66. Ivatury RR, Nallathambi M, Rao P, Stahl WM: Penetrating pancreatic injuries: analysis of 103 consecutive cases. Am Surg 56:90-95, 1990

67. Hayward SR, Lucas CE, Sugawa C, Ledgerwood AM: Emergent endoscopic retrograde cholangiopancreatography: a highly specific test for acute pancreatic trauma. Arch Surg 124:745-746, 1989

68. Wright MJ, Stanski C: Blunt pancreatic trauma: a difficult injury. South Med J 93:383-385, 2000

69. Nirula R, Velmahos GC, Demetriades D: Magnetic resonance cholangiopancreatography in pancreatic trauma: a new diagnostic modality? J Trauma 47:585-587, 1999

70. Berni GA, Bandyk DF, Oreskovich MR, Carrico CJ: Role of intraoperative pancreatography in patients with injury to the pancreas. Am J Surg 143:602-605, 1982

71. Jones RC: Management of pancreatic trauma. Am J Surg 150:698-704, 1985

72. Fabian TC, Kudsk KA, Croce MA, Payne LW, Mangiante EC, Voeller GR, Britt LG: Superiority of closed suction drainage for pancreatic trauma: a randomized, prospective study. Ann Surg 211:724-728, 1990

73. Amirata E, Livingston DH, Elcavage J: Octreotide acetate decreases pancreatic complications after pancreatic trauma. Am J Surg 168:345-347, 1994

74. Nassoura ZE, Ivatury RR, Simon RJ, Kihtir T, Stahl WM: A prospective reappraisal of primary repair of penetrating duodenal injuries. Am Surg 60:35-39, 1994

75. Weigelt JA: Duodenal injuries. Surg Clin North Am 70:529-539, 1990

76. Kunin JR, Korobkin M, Ellis JH, Francis IR, Kane NM, Siegel SE: Duodenal injuries caused by blunt abdominal trauma: value of CT in differentiating perforation from hematoma. AJR Am J Roentgenol 160:1221-1223, 1993

77. Jones WR, Hardin WJ, Davis JT, Hardy JD: Intramural hematoma of the duodenum: a review of the literature and case report. Ann Surg 173:534-544, 1971

78. Snyder WH III, Weigelt JA, Watkins WL, Bietz DS: The surgical management of duodenal trauma: precepts based on a review of 247 cases. Arch Surg 115:422-429, 1980

79. Vaughan GD III, Frazier OH, Graham DY, Mattox KL, Petmecky FF, Jordan GL Jr: The use of pyloric exclusion in the management of severe duodenal injuries. Am J Surg 134:785-790, 1977

80. Berne CJ, Donovan AJ, White EJ, Yellin AE: Duodenal "diverticulization" for duodenal and pancreatic injury. Am J Surg 127:503-507, 1974

81. Stone HH, Fabian TC: Management of duodenal wounds. J Trauma 19:334-339, 1979

82. Dauterive AH, Flancbaum L, Cox EF: Blunt intestinal trauma: a modern-day review. Ann Surg 201:198-203, 1985

83. Witzke JD, Kraatz JJ, Morken JM, Ney AL, West MA, Van Camp JM, Zera RT, Rodriguez JL: Stapled versus hand sewn anastomoses in patients with small bowel injury: a changing perspective. J Trauma 49:660-665, 2000

84. Schenk WG III, Lonchyna V, Moylan JA: Perforation of the jejunum from blunt abdominal trauma. J Trauma 23:54-56, 1983

85. Brownstein MR, Bunting T, Meyer AA, Fakhry SM: Diagnosis and management of blunt small bowel injury: a survey of the membership of the American Association for the Surgery of Trauma. J Trauma 48:402-407, 2000

86. Sherck J, Shatney C, Sensaki K, Selivanov V: The accuracy of computed tomography in the diagnosis of blunt small-bowel perforation. Am J Surg 168:670-675, 1994

87. Rizzo MJ, Federle MP, Griffiths BG: Bowel and mesenteric injury following blunt abdominal trauma: evaluation with CT. Radiology 173:143-148, 1989

88. Brundage SI, Jurkovich GJ, Grossman DC, Tong WC, Mack CD, Maier RV: Stapled versus sutured gastrointestinal anastomoses in the trauma patient. J Trauma 47:500-507, 1999

89. Ogilvie WH: Abdominal wounds in the Western Desert. Surg Gynecol Obstet 78:225-238, 1944

90. Stone HH, Fabian TC: Management of perforating colon trauma: randomization between primary closure and exteriorization. Ann Surg 190:430-436, 1979

91. Sasaki LS, Allaben RD, Golwala R, Mittal VK: Primary repair of colon injuries: a prospective randomized study. J Trauma 39:895-901, 1995

92. Jacobson LE, Gomez GA, Broadie TA: Primary repair of 58 consecutive penetrating injuries of the colon: Should colostomy be abandoned? Am Surg 63:170-177, 1997

93. Cornwell EE III, Velmahos GC, Berne TV, Murray JA, Chahwan S, Asensio J, Demetriades D: The fate of colonic suture lines in high-risk trauma patients: a prospective analysis. J Am Coll Surg 187:58-63, 1998

94. Durham RM, Pruitt C, Moran J, Longo WE: Civilian colon trauma: factors that predict success by primary repair. Dis Colon Rectum 40:685-692, 1997

Chapter 45

THE UNCLOSABLE ABDOMEN AND THE DEHISCED WOUND

Daniel C. Cullinane, M.D.
Michael P. Bannon, M.D.

Today, advances in surgery and critical care allow patients who otherwise would have died to survive. Nonetheless, physicians treating these surviving patients face new clinical problems. One of the most challenging problems is the unclosable abdomen. Closure of the abdominal incision may not be possible in patients being operated on for severe abdominal tissue destruction, infection, inflammation, or ischemia. If closure is attempted, the abdominal compartment syndrome (ACS) may result. In addition, postoperative fascial dehiscence and wound disruption are likely to occur.

We present the Mayo Clinic approach to critically ill patients with intensive abdominal tissue damage due to trauma, vascular compromise, or infection. In particular, we address the management of the unclosable abdomen, ACS, fascial dehiscence, and delayed abdominal wall reconstruction.

THE UNCLOSABLE ABDOMEN

Elective laparotomy in stabilized surgical patients is preceded by a complete preoperative work-up that addresses and optimizes the patient's condition. The operation itself is conducted with optimal exposure, optimal resources, and minimal tissue injury. The wound is closed primarily.

In contrast, operations for traumatic injuries and emergency abdominal catastrophes generally are done without benefit of such advantages. The patients are often in shock, have poorly controlled comorbid conditions, and have tissue injury that is often several hours or days old. Although most of these patients are reasonable candidates for a completed operation, about 10% have an unclosable abdomen.

To survive, they require an abbreviated procedure with only a temporary closure of the abdominal wound (Table 1).[1]

Attempts to close an abdomen are futile in the patient who has reached physiologic exhaustion and is requiring active resuscitation.[2-4] Even if the abdominal fascia is closed, ACS may develop due to postoperative intra-abdominal hypertension (IAH) that can result in fascial dehiscence. Management of these critically ill patients requires knowledge and experience with ACS. The initial focus is on accomplishing decompressive laparotomy, temporary abdominal closure, and prevention of fascial dehiscence. Techniques of abdominal wall reconstruction are used later.

ABDOMINAL COMPARTMENT SYNDROME

Compartment syndromes that occur in the extremities are well known. The soft tissue swelling subsequent to

Table 1.—Indications for Temporary Abdominal Closure

Clinical condition of patient
    Hemodynamic instability precludes definitive repair
    Excessive peritoneal edema precludes abdominal wall closure without resultant abdominal compartment syndrome
    Uncontrolled bleeding or coagulopathy
    Massive abdominal wall loss due to infection
Treatment dilemma
    Inability to eliminate or control source of intra-abdominal infection
    Incomplete debridement of necrotic tissue
    Uncertainty about viability of remaining bowel

ischemia or reperfusion, fractures, crush injury, or infection results in venous hypertension, followed by arterial insufficiency and tissue infarction. Prompt recognition and urgent decompression often aid limb salvage. Increased intra-abdominal pressure (IAP) has been recognized as a cause of cardiopulmonary and renal insufficiency in critically ill surgical patients for 20 years.[5,6] Before ACS was identified, many patients succumbed to respiratory failure because of the associated increase in ventilatory pressure.

ACS can be described broadly as an organ dysfunction attributable to increased IAP. Oliguria is often evident and is accompanied by markedly increased peak inspiratory airway pressures on controlled mechanical ventilation. Hypotension and poor cardiac output also often develop due to impaired venous return resulting from compression of the inferior vena cava. If not recognized and treated promptly, ACS is uniformly fatal.[7-9]

Clinically significant increases in IAP and ACS have been reported in various conditions (Table 2). The common presentation is that of a severe systemic inflammatory response syndrome in an underperfused patient. With ongoing resuscitation and tissue edema, the patient has an acute increase in the volume of abdominal contents. Tissue edema causes decreased compliance of the abdominal wall. The resulting increased IAP leads to pressure-related end-organ dysfunction.

Pathogenesis

One of the most consistent findings in animal studies of ACS is decreased cardiac output associated with increased IAP.[10,11] Although intravenous fluids can improve cardiac output and hypotension transiently, a vicious cycle eventually ensues with continuing fluid administration further increasing edema and IAP.[7] The clinical deterioration does not improve until IAP is relieved with a decompressive laparotomy.

Table 2.—Risk Factors for Development of Abdominal Compartment Syndrome

Blunt and penetrating abdominal trauma
Ruptured abdominal aortic aneurysm
Retroperitoneal hemorrhage
Pneumoperitoneum
Neoplasm
Pancreatitis
Ascites
Liver transplantation
Burns
Abdominal sepsis

With increasing IAP, the arterial partial pressure of oxygen (PO_2) begins to decrease, and the arterial partial pressure of carbon dioxide (PCO_2) increases. The intrathoracic pressure also increases in proportion to the IAP. When IAP exceeds 25 mm Hg, greatly increased end-inspiratory pressure is required to achieve a fixed tidal volume.[8] Because increased intrathoracic pressure may artificially increase the readings of central venous pressure and pulmonary capillary wedge pressure, intravascular volume may be low despite normal or increased filling pressure. The mechanism of IAP that affects pulmonary function is largely mechanical. As IAP increases, the diaphragm is forced higher into the chest, compressing the lungs. Adequate ventilation then requires increasing airway pressure to maintain a constant tidal volume. Poor compliance and loss of functional reserve capacity impair oxygenation and ventilation, mimicking the acute respiratory distress syndrome. Although the pulmonary manifestations of ACS are similar to those of the acute respiratory distress syndrome, its pathophysiology resembles that of an extraparenchymal restrictive lung disease.[9]

Renal failure and renal insufficiency are observed often in ACS. Reversible renal failure due to IAP has been documented in animal studies and in the clinical setting.[5-7] In animals, an IAP greater than 20 mm Hg is associated with anuria. The renal failure with ACS is likely due to a combination of renal vein and inferior vena cava compression caused by the increased IAP. This condition will not improve spontaneously and can lead to permanent organ dysfunction if the abdomen is not decompressed.[12,13]

Diagnosis

The diagnosis of ACS is almost entirely clinical. In our experience, common signs are a tensely distended abdomen, increased peak airway pressure, and hypercapnia. Oliguria, described by many authors as a hallmark of the problem, is inconsistent; about 50% of patients with ACS nevertheless maintain adequate urine output.[8] This is likely due to the large volume of intravenous crystalloid these patients receive for resuscitation. The level at which IAP causes ACS is not known, because different patients do not respond uniformly to the same level of IAP. Although physiologic changes are evident with an IAP of 10 mm Hg to 15 mm Hg, decompressive laparotomy may not be indicated at this level (Table 3). At an IAP of more than 25 mm Hg, many patients will ultimately require decompression to survive.[13,14]

Generally, IAP is measured indirectly. Previously, IAP was assessed by inserting a catheter into the inferior vena cava. Mechanical and infectious complications have led to the abandonment of this technique.

The urinary bladder, which is an extraperitoneal intra-abdominal structure, is commonly used as a conduit to

Table 3.—Grades of Abdominal Compartment Syndrome and Likely Treatments

Grade	Intra-abdominal pressure, mm Hg	Treatment
I	< 10	Observation
II	10-19	Observation and limitation of intravenous fluids, if possible
III	20-29	Decompressive laparotomy possibly indicated
IV	> 30	Decompressive laparotomy indicated

assess IAP. The compliant wall of the bladder acts as a diaphragm, allowing changes in IAP to be reflected as changes in pressure in the intravesicular lumen. Bladder pressure can be monitored intermittently or continuously. The technique (Fig. 1) is to first clamp the bladder catheter distal to the aspiration port, then clean the port with a povidone-iodine topical solution. Seventy milliliters of saline is injected into the aspiration port. An 18-gauge needle is inserted into the aspiration port and connected to the bedside monitor to transduce the column of fluid.[15]

Another less commonly used indirect measure of IAP is intragastric pressure. This technique involves filling the stomach with saline and using a nasogastric tube connected to a pressure transducer. However, because there is some risk of aspiration with this technique and because measuring intravesicular pressure is simpler and more reproducible, the intragastric pressure technique is not used at Mayo Clinic.

Intra-abdominal Hypertension

Development of IAH and ACS are not synonymous. Although it is impossible to have ACS without IAH, the reverse is not true. Normal IAP is less than 10 cm H_2O. Postoperatively, many surgical patients will have an IAP in the range of 10 to 20 cm H_2O. Clearly, these patients do not all have ACS. When the physiologic consequences of IAP begin to have an impact on the cardiopulmonary system and renal function, the IAP causes ACS regardless of the absolute pressure. Most trauma or critical care surgeons would agree, however, that an IAP of more than 25 cm H_2O may cause at least subclinical organ dysfunction and thus warrants decompressive laparotomy.[9,13] Measuring IAP in patients who are not sedated and on control mode ventilation is likely to result in an artificially high abdominal pressure reading. For intravesicular pressure to be of clinical value, the patient must be on control mode ventilation with heavy sedation and chemical paralysis.

Decompressive Laparotomy

After a diagnosis of ACS is made, an abdominal decompression should be done as quickly as possible. The decompressive laparotomy can be performed either in the intensive care unit or in the operating room. Deciding where to perform the decompressive laparotomy depends on several factors, of which the patient's physiology is the most important. Many patients are too sick to be transported safely. A calculated decision must be made about the cause of the ACS. If it is primarily due to edema, the procedure can be done safely and efficiently at the bedside in the intensive care unit.[16] The typical supplies for a bedside procedure are listed in Table 4. If there are strong indications of ongoing hemorrhage, the procedure should be done in the operating room where there is adequate instrumentation, lighting, and suture material readily available.

Most anesthetic machines in operating rooms cannot sustain the high level of ventilatory support typically required in ACS. If the operating room is required, the patient should be transported with a portable ventilator capable of maintaining high ventilatory pressure and positive end-expiratory pressure. A respiratory therapist should accompany the patient to the operating room and use the same ventilator from the intensive care unit until the patient's abdomen is decompressed and the patient's ventilatory function is stabilized. Then, ventilation through the anesthesia machine may be appropriate. The rapid change in physiology that accompanies abdominal decompression mandates that two experienced clinicians attend the patient. One surgeon is the designated operator, and the other is a critical care physician who manages the cardiorespiratory changes that occur with decompression.

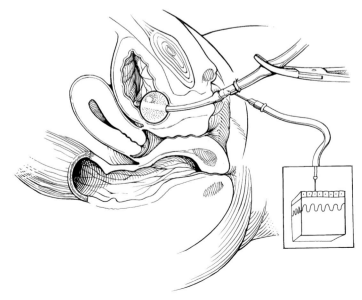

Fig. 1. Measurement of intravesicular pressure.

Table 4.—Supplies Required for Bedside Decompressive Laparotomy

23 x 33-inch iodine-impregnated adhesive plastic surgical drape	Sterile gloves (assorted sizes)
100 mL evacuators with antireflux valve (2)	Surgical masks
	Sterile water (2 liters)
10 mm x 20 cm flat silicone drains (2)	Sterile scissors
	Sterile hemostats (2)
Y connectors for suction lines (2)	Needle driver
18 x 24-inch plastic surgical drape	Shall-Cross clamps (2)
Sterile Yankauer suction device (2)	Suture material
Povidone-iodine (1 bottle)	Sterile towels (2 packs)
Scalpel #10 (disposable)	Sterile laparotomy pads (10)
Cautery (disposable)	Surgical drape spray adhesive (2 cans)
Surgical gowns	

The abdomen is prepped with a povidone-iodine topical solution, and sterile laparotomy drapes are applied. The previous fascial closure is slowly undone, allowing the critical care physician to compensate for changes in ventilation and hemodynamics. After the previous closure is taken down, the cause of the ACS is sought. Generally, bowel edema and "third-spaced" fluid is found. If bleeding is encountered or a considerable amount of clotted blood is present, the source of the hemorrhage must be addressed. After the abdomen has been explored, any existing omentum is used to cover exposed viscera. Then a temporary closure technique is used to cover the abdomen.

Physiologic Changes After Relief of Abdominal Compartment Syndrome

The accurate assessment of intravascular volume is essential in the management of critically ill patients. This is especially true in patients with IAH, who frequently have clinically significant third-spaced fluid losses and decreased venous return. Traditionally, intracardiac filling pressures, such as pulmonary capillary wedge pressure and central venous pressure, have been used to assess preload status. Their use is based on the assumption that when ventricular compliance remains constant, intracardiac pressures accurately reflect ventricular end-diastolic volumes. The poor correlation between cardiac index and pulmonary capillary wedge pressure or central venous pressure in critically ill surgical patients has been reported.[17-20] This poor correlation is due, in part, to changing ventricular compliance in the critically ill patient, which causes a variable relationship between pressure and volume. Increased IAP and intrathoracic pressure, which occur in IAH,

unpredictably increase intracardiac pressure measurements. Dependence on pulmonary capillary wedge pressure or central venous pressure to guide fluid resuscitation in these patients may lead to inappropriate therapy.[17,18]

Right ventricular volume measurements are independent of pressure or volume relationships, and, unlike intracardiac filling pressures, increased IAP or intrathoracic pressure does not confound their interpretation. Several studies have identified a better correlation between right ventricular end-diastolic volume index and cardiac index than between pulmonary capillary wedge pressure and cardiac index in trauma patients undergoing shock resuscitation.[17-19]

Relieving IAP associated with ACS causes dramatic changes in cardiac and ventilatory variables. Sudden, severe hypotension may occur during or immediately after abdominal decompression. Sudden cardiac arrest also has been reported and may be mediated by a sudden reperfusion syndrome.[16] Release of pressure on the vena cava allows the sudden washout of anaerobic metabolic products. In the underperfused, acidotic host, the addition of these metabolic acids can cause sudden cardiac arrest. Depending on the acid-base status of the patient, sodium bicarbonate is sometimes used empirically before abdominal decompression to aid in buffering the washout of metabolic acids.

During decompression, the increased airway pressure associated with ACS suddenly decreases. Most patients are kept on pressure-controlled ventilation to limit their peak airway pressure. The physician who is managing the critical care of the patient during a decompressive laparotomy should monitor tidal volumes and maintain reasonable ventilatory settings to prevent hyperinflation and barotrauma. The positive end-expiratory pressure and the concentration of inspired oxygen also can be decreased as oxygenation improves rapidly after decompression.

FASCIAL DEHISCENCE

Incidence

The published incidence of fascial dehiscence is 0% to 3% in patients at risk, although the latter figure is considered extremely high.[21,22] Most surgeons believe that the true incidence of dehiscence in all laparotomies is less than 1% and that it is about 6% in emergency laparotomies.[21-23]

Etiology

Many factors predispose patients to the development of fascial dehiscence (Table 5). Both technical and host factors determine the incidence. Although the incidence is low, the mortality is 15% to 30%, because of the factors that predispose the patient to evisceration. Although a broken suture or failed knot is occasionally observed, wound dehiscence is caused more often by the suture cutting through the tissue. The suture may be placed too close to the wound edge, which allows the fascia to tear. More commonly, however, infection or increased IAP cause weakening and fascial necrosis. Thus, the cause of fascial dehiscence is often multifactorial. A typical patient may be a nutritionally depleted host who has wound infection and increased IAP due to coughing or straining.

Host Factors

Host factors are influential in the development of wound dehiscence and evisceration. Advanced age, poor vascularity, male sex, pulmonary disease, malnutrition, and immunosuppression impede the healing process and predispose the patient to wound complications.[21,22,24-32]

Advanced age is thought to impair wound healing. Several studies have found the incidence of wound disruption in patients older than 45 to be 5 times greater than that of a younger cohort.[27,33] The increased incidence of wound complications may be due to diminished cell proliferation in the healing wounds of elderly surgical patients.[29]

The indications for operation also may influence the development of wound complications. Operations for acute abdominal catastrophes and trauma predispose the patient to dehiscence and evisceration.[21,22,26,28] Whether these complications are due to the effects of the operation or a breakdown in technique is not known. Abdominal sepsis and wound infection also impair healing and disrupt the fascial muscle layer. Operations on the gastrointestinal tract are followed by the greatest incidence of wound dehiscence. All of these situations share the common thread of peritoneal contamination, which increases the incidence of infection, dehiscence, and evisceration when present to any extent.[27]

Male sex also may lead to a higher rate of dehiscence. Most studies report a wound dehiscence rate in men that is at least double that in women.[21,29] Although the reason for the difference has not been established, it may be because women, in general, have a more relaxed abdominal wall, do more vigorous postoperative activity, or have a genetic difference in collagen formation.

Pulmonary dysfunction and chronic cough also are thought to lead to a higher rate of dehiscence and hernia. The cessation of smoking may minimize but not eliminate this risk. Chronic lung disease and chronic cough have long been implicated, but findings are contradictory.[26,27]

Obesity has consistently been cited as causing wound failure. A body weight that is more than 130% of ideal weight or a body mass index of more than 28 is predictive of dehiscence and hernia formation.[33,34] One theory about the cause of obesity-related wound failure cites the increased IAP observed in morbidly obese patients. Other authors suggest that the cause may be tension from an obese abdominal wall or technical difficulties in closing an obese abdominal wall.[21,28]

Local Wound Factors

Postoperative wound infection predisposes patients both to fascial dehiscence and to postoperative incisional hernia. Wound infection remains the most consistent factor in wound dehiscence.[35] The prevention of infection or its early recognition and treatment are key to minimizing the effects of this serious complication.

Tension on the suture line is the second leading cause of fascial dehiscence and necrosis. Poor surgical technique can strangulate tissue and allow overly tight sutures to cut through the fascia. Abdominal distention and IAH cause increased tension and ischemia of the abdominal wall. In theory, local wound circulation and healing are best supported by an interrupted suture 1 cm apart that incorporates 1 cm of tissue on each side of the wound. However, dehiscence has not been found to occur more frequently with a continuous suture technique.[24,35]

Most large series show little difference in outcome or a slight advantage to continuous methods of closure, particularly an en masse closure.[30] More important than the type of suture material is the use of a properly performed, wide-spaced en masse closure. Closure of the peritoneum offers minimal strength and can be omitted. The abdominal fascia heals by forming a dense fibrous scar at the opposing fascial edges. The purpose of the suture is to approximate the fascial edges while the fibrous scar matures. Wide bites at 1-cm intervals should be taken from the edge of the fascia to a minimum depth of 1 cm. Shorter intervals between sutures may weaken the fascia with multiple perforations. Before closure, the omentum is drawn under the fascia wherever possible to cover the viscera and minimize bowel adhesion to the overlying abdominal wall.

Table 5.—Risk Factors for Fascial Dehiscence and Subsequent Ventral Hernia

Wound infection	Advanced age
Intra-abdominal hypertension	Obesity
Male sex	Early reoperation
Abdominal distention	Comorbid disease
Pulmonary infection	

Type of Incision

The type of abdominal incision has long been debated by surgeons. The most frequent abdominal incision in adults is the midline incision. This incision offers the advantages of speed, versatility, and ease for entering and closing the abdomen. Although the choice of abdominal incision (vertical vs. transverse) is often cited when discussing fascial dehiscence, the data suggesting that vertical incisions are inherently weaker than transverse incisions are flawed, and available studies are often not comparable.[28,36-38] Typically, vertical incisions are used in the emergency setting for trauma, hemorrhage, sepsis, or reoperation. The higher incidence of fascial dehiscence and incisional hernia in such patients is to be expected. Most controlled studies have not demonstrated an inherent strength advantage to transverse abdominal incisions.[28]

Prevention

Although fascial repair with nonabsorbable or long-term absorbable suture and proper surgical technique minimize the incidence of dehiscence, no technique offers absolute prevention. The time to consider the technical factors for minimizing the possibility of a wound separation is during the initial operation, not when evisceration has occurred. A rapid, technically perfect operation done with minimal contamination gives the patient the best opportunity to heal properly and thus to avoid a catastrophic wound complication. Postoperatively, the risk can be minimized by attending promptly and carefully to the avoidance of abdominal distention, the prevention of ACS, good pulmonary hygiene, and wound infections.

Retention Sutures

Retention sutures, which are often used along with a tenuous primary fascial closure, are often inappropriate. Instead, patients are best served with a temporary abdominal closure or a planned ventral hernia created by placement of absorbable mesh. Closing an already impaired abdominal wall under tension is an invitation for further dehiscence or ACS.

As mentioned above, most wound dehiscence occurs when sutures tear through soft fascia rather than because of suture or knot failure.[31,32] Conventional retention sutures may reduce the lateral distracting forces on a midline wound, thereby lessening tension on the suture in the midline. Such thinking leads the surgeon to tie the retention sutures tightly to reduce tension on the midline. This approach causes bow-stringing of the sutures across the curved peritoneal cavity and allows them to saw into the bowel. Tightly tied sutures also may predispose to abdominal wall ischemia.[28,31,32] The result is a dehisced abdominal wall and exposed small bowel with fistulous openings, an extremely difficult condition to manage.

Retention sutures will not prevent a dehiscence or hernia formation, but they will prevent evisceration.[39] To avoid the complications noted earlier, the surgeon should place retention sutures loosely, if they are used. The correctly placed suture must enter the skin at a more medial position than it traverses the fascia (Fig. 2). This placement minimizes cutting and subsequent necrosis of the skin. Retention sutures can be safely removed 14 to 21 days postoperatively.

When placed traditionally through all layers of the abdominal wall, retention sutures can cause bowel obstruction, enterocutaneous fistula, or adhesions. Retention sutures can be horizontal mattress sutures (Fig. 2) that are kept extraperitoneal to avoid interference with wound care and complications from erosion into the underlying bowel. Nonetheless, the ischemic and skin-cutting effects of retention sutures often outweigh their limited prophylactic value.[40,41]

Diagnosis

Mortality from abdominal wound dehiscence is 15% to 30% in patients at risk.[35] To promptly diagnose and treat dehiscence, surgeons must recognize both host and technical risk factors. Few patients will present with an abdominal dehiscence in the first 4 to 5 days postoperatively. In those who do, a technical factor is often responsible for the problem. Certainly, poor wound healing cannot be the cause of such early postoperative wound failure.

Frequently, dehiscence occurs 6 to 8 days after an operation. The abdominal wound begins leaking serosanguineous, salmon-pink drainage.[32] In patients with more

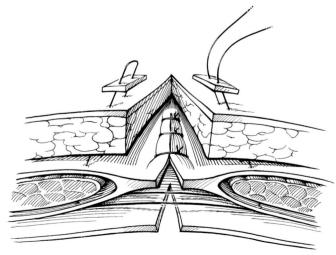

Fig. 2. Cross section of a horizontal mattress retention suture. Note extraperitoneal placement.

risk factors or paroxysmal coughing, the problems should be addressed immediately. When dehiscence is suspected, the patient should be brought to the operating room for wound exploration and possible fascial closure. If the patient has already had an evisceration, the exposed intestine should first be covered with sterile gauze soaked in warm saline. The stomach is then decompressed with a nasogastric tube, and the patient is taken to the operating room for exploration.

Operative Management
The cause of the dehiscence will determine the operating technique. The basic tenet of reoperation for wound dehiscence or evisceration is to avoid the repetition of any technical errors of the first operation. If IAH was the cause of fascial failure, then a temporary closure will certainly be required. If local wound sepsis was the cause, skin closure usually is contraindicated.

At Mayo Clinic, we reopen the wound along its entire length and carefully do an exploratory laparotomy. We search thoroughly for intra-abdominal abscesses and anastomotic integrity. If an abscess is found, we irrigate the cavity locally and remove any devitalized tissue or foreign material. We drain through a separate incision in the fascia away from the primary wound or any stomas. Because local infection and excessive tension often result in ischemic, soft fascia, we thoroughly debride any areas of devitalized fascia before closure of any type.

When the fascia is of good quality and the wound requires only minimal debridement, reclosure of the fascia is appropriate. Generally, we use an interrupted closure after reoperation. Sometimes we also use retention sutures. These are placed extraperitoneally (Fig. 2) to decrease the possibility of enterocutaneous fistulas. The sutures also should not be tied tightly, because doing so will lead to more fascial ischemia or necrosis. When the fascia is under tension, no attempt should be made at primary closure.

When extensive debridement is required or there is IAH, we create a temporary fascial bridge. We generally use an absorbable mesh such as polyglactin 910 or an absorbable polyglycolic acid mesh (Fig. 3). We allow the wound to granulate through the mesh, then apply a skin graft later (see below). The resulting hernia from using absorbable mesh can be treated later, whereas the complications of permanent mesh in this situation can be devastating.

Techniques of Temporary Closure
When a temporary abdominal closure is necessary, several techniques can be used. Two techniques routinely used at Mayo Clinic are the vacuum-packed dressing and the Esmarch bandage, both of which offer rapid secure closure of the abdomen. The temporary abdominal closure requires

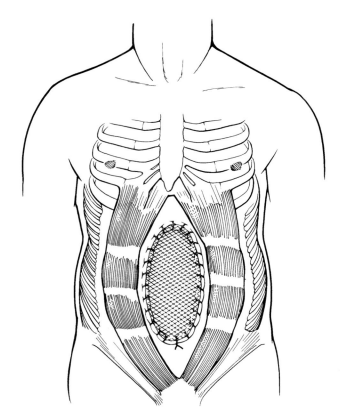

Fig. 3. Polyglactin 910 absorbable mesh coverage of viscera for patient with unclosable abdomen.

ease and speed of application, minimal damage to existing tissue, and adequate containment of the abdominal viscera. In addition, the cost of materials and the time needed to apply them should be low. In both of these techniques, an occlusive adhesive plastic drape is applied as an outer layer. This allows continuous suction to be applied through intra-abdominal drains that remove third-spaced fluid. Both techniques provide reasonably secure abdominal coverage. Patients are sedated and mechanically ventilated until they can be returned to the operating room. Neuromuscular blocking agents are used occasionally.

We have not used many of the other techniques of temporary abdominal closure because they require more time to apply and have more wound complications associated with them. We have abandoned the routine use of towel clips as a skin closure, because they lead to increased skin necrosis. We also no longer use techniques involving the suture of prosthetic material to either the skin or the fascia, because they require extra time and may cause tissue destruction from the massive edema that occurs with resuscitation.

The Vacuum-Packed Technique
The vacuum-packed technique is a three-layer temporary closure that does not require suturing. First, any available

omentum is placed over the intestine. Then an 18 x 18-inch bowel isolation bag is placed over the edematous intestine to provide protection from potential trauma. Next, a sterile blue surgical towel is placed on top of the isolation bag under the fascia laterally to the anterior axillary line. The surgical towel provides a temporary fascial bridge along the length of the wound (Fig. 4). One or two 10-mm flat, fluted, closed suction drains are placed along the fascia and covered by another folded blue surgical towel. The surgical drapes are removed and Benzoin spray is applied to the skin of the abdomen. After the spray is dry, two large iodine-impregnated adhesive plastic surgical drapes are applied to the entire abdomen. After the patient is moved to the surgical intensive care unit, low, continuous wall suction is applied to the surgical drains. These abdominal drains effectively remove third-spaced abdominal fluid that accumulates under the occlusive dressing.

The Esmarch Technique

The Esmarch technique[42] is a slightly less complicated, albeit more expensive, method for rapid, temporary abdominal closure. Two strips of 4-inch–wide sterile latex Esmarch bandage are cut to span the length of the incision, rinsed in saline, and stapled longitudinally, one to each cutaneous edge. To minimize fluid leakage, staples are spaced about 5 mm apart. The two strips of bandage are held side by side vertically, then the edges are turned in and stapled to form a silo (Fig. 5). The bandage is placed directly over the intestine. Then two flat, fluted Blake surgical drainage tubes made of polymeric silicone are placed on top of it, and the surgical drapes are removed. Benzoin spray is applied to the entire abdominal skin, and after it is dry, two large iodine-impregnated adhesive plastic surgical drapes are used to cover the entire abdomen. The patient is then transported to the intensive care unit for further resuscitation. The drains are placed on low continuous suction to remove accumulated third-spaced fluid.

Postoperative Care

The patient who has an open abdomen presents a complex clinical challenge. Because fluid loss can be considerable, 10 L to 20 L of intravenous fluid is typically required for the first 24 hours after decompression. The drains placed during the temporary closure capture much of the third-spaced abdominal fluid. This not only makes nursing care easier by minimizing fluid leakage but also may prevent recurrent ACS caused by intra-abdominal fluid retention.

The patient's clinical response to resuscitation determines the appropriate time to return to the operating room for further management. This generally occurs 24 to 48 hours after the initial procedure. Temporary closure can be kept in place for a longer period if the patient's condition does not improve sufficiently. After the patient has met the goals of resuscitation, any intra-abdominal packing is removed. If gastrointestinal tract continuity needs to be reestablished after a damage control procedure, it can be done at this time. In most cases, the patient will have met resuscitative goals 48 hours after injury, at which time all packing is removed. Because abdominal packing is done under stressful conditions and surgical counts are either unreliable or impossible because of time constraints, we obtain an abdominal

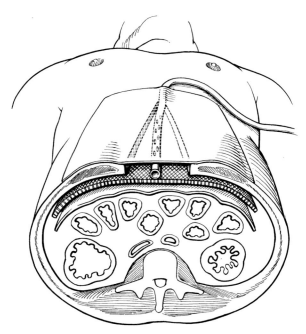

Fig. 4. Vacuum-packed technique using a blue surgical towel (hatched area) as a temporary fascial bridge.

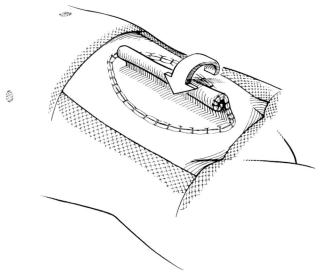

Fig. 5. Temporary abdominal closure using an Esmarch bandage.

radiograph in the operating room to ensure the removal of all intra-abdominal packing.

In most patients, the large-volume resuscitation will have left the patient with a positive fluid balance, and the abdominal wall will not close primarily after the second laparotomy. After an extensive washout with the pulse irrigator, a second temporary closure is fashioned. When the patient shows signs of recovery and begins spontaneous diuresis, about 5 days postoperatively, fascial closure can be attempted with reasonable success. Our practice is to leave the skin open and allow the wound to heal by secondary intention because of the likelihood of wound infections associated with skin closure after multiple laparotomies.

When a patient remains critically ill and continues to be edematous, a primary fascial closure often cannot be performed. An absorbable mesh such as polyglactin 910 or an absorbable polyglycolic acid mesh is sewn to the fascia to provide a temporary fascial bridge. Wet-dry wound dressings are applied, and after a few days, granulation tissue begins to grow through the mesh. We allow the abdomen to granulate and contract for 2 to 4 weeks, depending on the patient's clinical condition. When a clean bed of granulation tissue is present, we use a partial-thickness skin graft to provide coverage. The patient is then left with a large ventral hernia that can be repaired several months later.

ABDOMINAL WALL RECONSTRUCTION

Deciding whether to do abdominal wall reconstruction to repair the ventral hernia depends on the individual patient. Some patients, particularly those who are elderly, morbidly obese, or otherwise debilitated, are not good surgical candidates. Younger patients who have returned to full activity often can have reconstruction 6 to 12 months after they are dismissed. Regardless, no patient should have major abdominal wall reconstruction without maximization of nutritional and functional status. Reconstructive abdominal surgery is a major undertaking with substantial morbidity. Operating on a nutritionally depleted host who has extensive adhesions can lead to enterocutaneous fistula, infection, or a recurrence of hernia.

Reconstruction of the muscular abdominal wall should be done after the patient has recovered from the critical illness. The patient must be anabolic and must have reached maximal rehabilitative goals. Several techniques enable the surgeon to avoid or minimize placement of prosthetic materials, two of which are commonly used at Mayo Clinic. Some patients will have stomas left from the initial hospitalization. As long as the reconstruction can be done without the use of prosthetic material, stoma closure can

be done at the same time without additional clinical morbidity. Skin grafts over the abdominal viscera must be allowed sufficient time, generally 6 to 12 months, to mature and separate from the viscera. If a skin graft can be grasped by the examiner and pinched away from the underlying viscera as a separate layer, it can be excised safely with minimal risk of creating an enterotomy or other abdominal organ injury during dissection of the hernia margins. Because of the loss of abdominal domain in many of these patients, the anesthesiologist should constantly assess the peak airway pressure during closure of the midline fascia. If peak airway pressure consistently exceeds 30 cm H_2O to 40 cm H_2O despite maximal relaxation, a primary closure is unlikely to be possible and prosthetic mesh will be needed.

Fascial or Release Technique

With sharp dissection, the previous skin graft is carefully separated from the contents of the abdomen. Initially, the graft is taken off laterally, then dissection continues circumferentially. Next, large, bilateral, subcutaneous skin flaps are created by sharply separating the subcutaneous tissue from the fascia of the abdominal wall to the level of the anterior axillary line. The junction of the rectus abdominis muscle and the fascia of the external oblique muscle are identified. The fascia of the external oblique muscle is incised longitudinally from the costal margin to an area inferior to the umbilicus. This incision is curved medially at the superior aspect of the incision (Fig. 6). Then, the external oblique muscle is carefully divided with cautery, taking care not to divide the underlying areas. About 8 cm to 10 cm of fascial advancement can be obtained on each side.[43] Doing so allows reliable, tension-free midline abdominal closure for fascial gaps of 16 cm to 20 cm. After the lateral fascial release is complete, the midline incision is closed (Fig. 7), either with interrupted sutures or with running heavy monofilament absorbable suture. Bilateral, 10-mm, flat, fluted, closed suction drains are placed under the subcutaneous flaps to prevent the formation of a "seroma." The skin is then closed with running 3-0 absorbable subcutaneous sutures. Drains are removed after 3 to 4 days.

Tissue Expander Technique

An alternative to lateral fascial release is the use of tissue expanders to stretch the abdominal musculature and allow tension-free midline closure.[44] Using tissue expanders allows adequate fascial stretching without disrupting the inherent strength of the abdominal wall or the neurovascular supply.

The tissue expander is placed lateral to the rectus abdominus muscle between the fascia of the external and internal oblique muscles. Transverse incisions 5 cm long

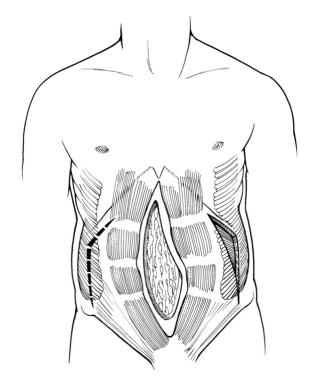

Fig. 6. Fascial release technique: incision of external oblique fascia and muscle.

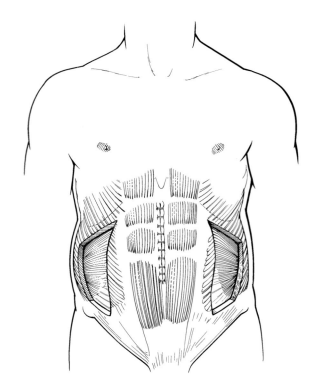

Fig. 7. Fascial release technique: closure of midline incision. Note expansion laterally to accomodate oblique muscle separation incisions.

are created below the costal margin. Dissection is made through the subcutaneous tissue, and the incision is made in the fascia of the external oblique muscle in the downward and medial direction of its fibers. Blunt dissection separates the areolar tissue beneath the fascia of the external

oblique muscle. The tissue expander is placed in the natural pocket beneath the fascia of the external oblique muscle (Fig. 8 and 9). The expander is then properly oriented and filled with 50 to 100 mL of saline. The fascia and skin are then closed. After 3 weeks of healing, the

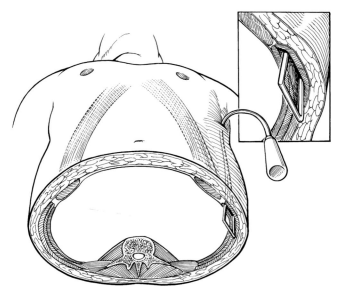

Fig. 8. Creation of fascial space between the external and internal oblique abdominal muscles for insertion of tissue expander.

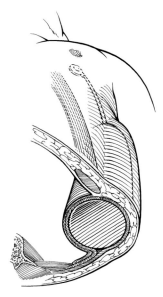

Fig. 9. Tissue expander in place beneath external oblique fascia.

expanders are filled with 50 to 125 mL of saline every 2 weeks as tolerated. After six to eight filling cycles, the patient is prepared for abdominal wall reconstruction. In the subsequent definitive operation, the skin graft over the bowel is excised and the fascial borders are identified. The tissue expanders are deflated and removed immediately before fascial closure. In most patients, the midline fascia can be closed without substantial tension. For other patients, a panel of permanent prosthetic material is used to repair the abdominal wall defect.

CONCLUSION

During the past decade, surgeons have increasingly recognized the consequences of IAH and ACS. High-volume fluid resuscitation and advanced ventilation strategies have enabled patients to survive critical illnesses that would have been fatal a decade ago. Along with these advances, however, come new clinical challenges, such as ACS. With better understanding of ACS and increasing experience in its managament, surgeons can continue to advance the treatment of these critically ill patients. As treatment for ACS becomes more sophisticated, we find that temporary closure techniques may be useful in patients who have operation for gastrointestinal or vascular conditions and in trauma or burn emergencies. We believe that more liberal use of damage control procedures could ultimately save more lives.

Fascial dehiscence and evisceration are vexing problems for abdominal surgeons. In most cases, the outcome is certain even before the scalpel touches the skin. Many of the known risk factors cannot be controlled, and even a technically perfect operation cannot prevent the occurrence of dehiscence. Improved outcomes require prompt recognition and treatment. A delay to diagnosis or a repetition of previous technical errors often leads to an unfavorable outcome.

REFERENCES

1. Morris JA Jr, Eddy VA, Rutherford EJ: The trauma celiotomy: the evolving concepts of damage control. Curr Probl Surg 33:609, 1996
2. Wittmann DH, Schein M, Condon RE: Management of secondary peritonitis. Ann Surg 224:10-18, 1996
3. Moore EE, Burch JM, Franciose RJ, Offner PJ, Biffl WL: Staged physiologic restoration and damage control surgery. World J Surg 22:1184-1190, 1998
4. Brasel KJ, Ku J, Baker CC, Rutherford EJ: Damage control in the critically ill and injured patient. New Horizons 7:73-86, 1999
5. Richards WO, Scovill W, Shin B, Reed W: Acute renal failure associated with increased intra-abdominal pressure. Ann Surg 197:183-187, 1983
6. Doty JM, Saggi BH, Sugerman HJ, Blocher CR, Pin R, Fakhry I, Gehr TW, Sica DA: Effect of increased renal venous pressure on renal function. J Trauma 47:1000-1003, 1999
7. Schein M, Ivatury R: Intra-abdominal hypertension and the abdominal compartment syndrome. Br J Surg 85:1027-1028, 1998
8. Eddy V, Nunn C, Morris JA Jr: Abdominal compartment syndrome: the Nashville experience. Surg Clin North Am 77:801-812, 1997
9. Burch JM, Moore EE, Moore FA, Franciose R: The abdominal compartment syndrome. Surg Clin North Am 76:833-842, 1996
10. Barnes GE, Laine GA, Giam PY, Smith EE, Granger HJ: Cardiovascular responses to elevation of intra-abdominal hydrostatic pressure. Am J Physiol 248:R208-R213, 1985
11. Kashtan J, Green JF, Parsons EQ, Holcroft JW: Hemodynamic effect of increased abdominal pressure. J Surg Res 30:249-255, 1981
12. Ivatury R, Porter J, Simon R, Islam S, John R, Stahl W: Intra-abdominal hypertension after life threatening penetrating abdominal trauma: incidence, prophylaxis, and clinical relevance to gastric mucosa pH and abdominal compartment syndrome (abstract). J Trauma 43:194, 1997
13. Ivatury RR, Diebel L, Porter JM, Simon RJ: Intra-abdominal hypertension and the abdominal compartment syndrome. Surg Clin North Am 77:783-800, 1997
14. Schein M, Wittmann DH, Aprahamian CC, Condon RE: The abdominal compartment syndrome: the physiological and clinical consequences of elevated intra-abdominal pressure. J Am Coll Surg 180:745-753, 1995
15. Cheatham ML, Safcsak K: Intraabdominal pressure: a revised method for measurement. J Am Coll Surg 186:594-595, 1998

16. Morris JA Jr, Eddy VA, Blinman TA, Rutherford EJ, Sharp KW: The staged celiotomy for trauma: issues in unpacking and reconstruction. Ann Surg 217:576-584, 1993

17. Cheatham ML, Safcsak K, Block EF, Nelson LD: Preload assessment in patients with an open abdomen. J Trauma 46:16-22, 1999

18. Chang MC, Blinman TA, Rutherford EJ, Nelson LD, Morris JA Jr: Preload assessment in trauma patients during large-volume shock resuscitation. Arch Surg 131:728-731, 1996

19. Diebel LN, Myers T, Dulchavsky S: Effects of increasing airway pressure and PEEP on the assessment of cardiac preload. J Trauma 42:585-590, 1997

20. Eddy VA, Morris JA Jr, Cullinane DC: Hypothermia, coagulopathy, and acidosis. Surg Clin North Am 80:845-854, 2000

21. Keill RH, Keitzer WF, Nichols WK, Henzel J, DeWeese MS: Abdominal wound dehiscence. Arch Surg 106:573-577, 1973

22. Bucknall TE, Cox PJ, Ellis H: Burst abdomen and incisional hernia: a prospective study of 1129 major laparotomies. Br Med J (Clin Res Ed) 284:931-933, 1982

23. Webster C, Neumayer L, Smout R, Horn S, Daley J, Henderson W, Khuri S, National Veterans Affairs Surgical Quality Improvement Program: Prognostic models of abdominal wound dehiscence after laparotomy. J Surg Res 109:130-137, 2003

24. Richards PC, Balch CM, Aldrete JS: Abdominal wound closure: a randomized prospective study of 571 patients comparing continuous vs. interrupted suture techniques. Ann Surg 197:238-243, 1983

25. Seid MH, McDaniel-Owens LM, Poole GV Jr, Meeks GR: A randomized trial of abdominal incision suture technique and wound strength in rats. Arch Surg 130:394-397, 1995

26. Greenburg AG, Saik RP, Peskin GW: Wound dehiscence: pathophysiology and prevention. Arch Surg 114:143-146, 1979

27. Penninckx FM, Poelmans SV, Kerremans RP, Beckers JP: Abdominal wound dehiscence in gastroenterological surgery. Ann Surg 189:345-352, 1979

28. Poole GV Jr: Mechanical factors in abdominal wound closure: the prevention of fascial dehiscence. Surgery 97:631-640, 1985

29. White H, Cook J, Ward M: Abdominal wound dehiscence: a 10-year survey from a district general hospital. Ann R Coll Surg Engl 59:337-341, 1977

30. Brolin RE: Prospective, randomized evaluation of midline fascial closure in gastric bariatric operations. Am J Surg 172:328-331, 1996

31. Gislason H, Gronbech JE, Soreide O: Burst abdomen and incisional hernia after major gastrointestinal operations—comparison of three closure techniques. Eur J Surg 161:349-354, 1995

32. Grace RH, Cox S: Incidence of incisional hernia after dehiscence of the abdominal wound. Am J Surg 131:210-212, 1976

33. Riou JP, Cohen JR, Johnson H Jr: Factors influencing wound dehiscence. Am J Surg 163:324-330, 1992

34. Wolf AM, Kortner B, Kuhlmann HW: Results of bariatric surgery. Int J Obes Relat Metab Disord 25 Suppl 1:S113-S114, 2001

35. Hunt TK: Diagnosis and treatment of wound failure. Adv Surg 8:287-309, 1974

36. Greenall MJ, Evans M, Pollock AV: Midline or transverse laparotomy? A random controlled clinical trial. Part I. Influence on healing. Br J Surg 67:188-190, 1980

37. Makela JT, Kiviniemi H, Juvonen T, Laitinen S: Factors influencing wound dehiscence after midline laparotomy. Am J Surg 170:387-390, 1995

38. Hendrix SL, Schimp V, Martin J, Singh A, Kruger M, McNeeley SG: The legendary superior strength of the Pfannenstiel incision: A myth? Am J Obstet Gynecol 182:1446-1451, 2000

39. Gislason H, Soreide O, Viste A: Wound complications after major gastrointestinal operations: the surgeon as a risk factor. Dig Surg 16:512-514, 1999

40. Rink AD, Goldschmidt D, Dietrich J, Nagelschmidt M, Vestweber KH: Negative side-effects of retention sutures for abdominal wound closure. A prospective randomised study. Eur J Surg 166:932-937, 2000

41. Gislason H, Viste A: Closure of burst abdomen after major gastrointestinal operations—comparison of different surgical techniques and later development of incisional hernia. Eur J Surg 165:958-961, 1999

42. Cohn SM, Burns GA, Sawyer MD, Tolomeo C, Milner KA, Spector S: Esmarch closure of laparotomy incisions in unstable trauma patients. J Trauma 39:978-979, 1995

43. Lucas CE, Ledgerwood AM: Autologous closure of giant abdominal wall defects. Am Surg 64:607-610, 1998

44. Jacobsen WM, Petty PM, Bite U, Johnson CH: Massive abdominal-wall hernia reconstruction with expanded external/internal oblique and transversalis musculofascia. Plast Reconstr Surg 100:326-335, 1997

Ventral and Incisional Hernias

David R. Farley, M.D.
Mark D. Sawyer, M.D.
Michael G. Sarr, M.D.

Ever since the Mayo brothers described their "Mayo repair" of umbilical and ventral hernias using the so-called pants-over-vest technique, Mayo Clinic has had an interest in and referral practice addressing repair of both straightforward and complex abdominal wall hernias. Over the years, techniques have come and gone, incorporable mesh repairs have become popular, and the original "Mayo repair" is no longer promoted. Moreover, minimally invasive techniques have been introduced into many different gastrointestinal procedures, including repair of selected ventral and incisional hernias. However, one thing that has not changed is the presence of these hernias. Although we may have learned how to prevent their occurrence in selected situations by maximizing nutrition, avoiding undue tension, selecting more durable suture, and adopting a minimal access approach to certain common disorders previously necessitating a long celiotomy (e.g., cholecystectomy, Nissen fundoplication), open celiotomies are still necessary, and operations for incisional hernias continue to be common for the general surgeon.

This chapter addresses the physiology, clinical presentation, and diagnosis of both primary and secondary ventral abdominal wall hernias exclusive of groin hernias. Much of the chapter focuses on our preferred approaches for individual situations. No one approach is best for all patients, and surgeons should be skilled in a broad spectrum of operative techniques to meet the needs of each patient.

THE PROBLEM

More than 1 million celiotomies are performed annually in the United States for, for example, colectomy, aortic aneurysm repair, bariatric procedures, gynecologic disorders, and kidney and prostate disease. As many as 11%[1-3] of all celiotomies eventually lead to an abdominal wall defect or incisional hernia. In addition to these "iatrogenic" hernias, primary umbilical, epigastric, and the more unusual spigelian and lumbar hernias also require repair. In the United States alone, more than 90,000 ventral and incisional hernias are repaired annually.[4] Although many patients live with and tolerate such defects, most enlarging or symptomatic incisional hernias probably should be repaired. Nearly half of such repairs become necessary within 1 year of the primary procedure, but a third of patients present with hernia or hernia develops at least 5 years later.[5] The appropriate surgical reintervention for symptoms can be painful, expensive, and time-consuming. Productivity and job hours are lost, and the threat of subsequent adhesions or bowel obstruction and the possibility of re-recurrence often make incisional and ventral hernia repairs fraught with disappointment for patient and surgeon alike. The failure rate for primary direct repair of incisional hernias is realistically as high as 49% to 58%.[6-8]

PHYSIOLOGY

The cause of incisional hernia early postoperatively may be directly related either to poor surgical technique or to inordinate tension at the time of primary closure, but other factors that are not correctable by the surgeon are also important. Deep wound infection, obesity, pulmonary difficulties, and malnutrition are all well-known factors that greatly increase the risk of a subsequent incisional hernia. Patients with an extensive history of smoking, constipation, chronic obstructive pulmonary disease or asthma, ascites, and other conditions also have a higher risk for development of ventral hernia, both in the short term and over time (sometimes decades later). The premature return to heavy lifting, maneuvers that put undue stress on the healing fascia, and other such inappropriate physical activities often have been blamed (possibly unduly so) as factors contributing to an increased incidence of incisional hernia. Aside from the obvious audible "popping" of sutures that occasionally occurs when a patient is emerging from anesthesia, it is unclear whether strenuous activities need to be strictly avoided. Avoidance may be a surgical dictum that should be revisited. For instance, daily activities such as getting out of bed or a chair, coughing, having a bowel movement, or bending over to put on one's shoes are unavoidable, yet clearly they increase the strain on an abdominal wall closure. We need only remember our previous approach to inguinal herniorrhaphy in the pre-1950 era, when patients were kept bedridden for 1 to 2 weeks to "allow the incision to heal." No one would consider this approach today. Similarly, the periumbilical closure site for the 10-mm laparoscope used for laparoscopic cholecystectomy formally is a mini-celiotomy with a direct primary fascial "closure," but we doubt that many surgeons urge their patients to avoid heavy lifting for the requisite 6 to 12 weeks that most suggest as dictum for a routine midline celiotomy done for some other intra-abdominal disorder.

More current thought about healing of a surgically created or congenital fascial defect involves the physiologic process of wound healing, and several general concepts are important. Fascial healing depends on a complex interplay of inflammation, neovascularization, and the laying down and subsequent remodeling of the collagen fibers. The remodeling of collagen fibers depends intimately on collagen synthesis, proteolytic degradation with reorganization and restructuring not only of the physical orientation of the "scar" but also a change in the types of collagen deposited dependent on physicomechanical forces exerted on the wound. An analogy can be drawn to bony healing, which is maximized and highly dependent on stress and strain forces. Some investigators have suggested that the relative types of collagen laid down vary between patients, possibly explaining the increased incidence of incisional hernia in certain subjects. For instance, patients undergoing abdominal aortic aneurysmectomy have a well-recognized increased incidence of incisional hernia after transabdominal repair. An apparent biochemical defect in them may be related to the incisional hernia and the aneurysmal dilatation of the aortic wall, again being a disruption of modeling of the structural wall of the aorta and of the abdominal fascia. A similar abnormality in collagen deposition occurs in patients with direct inguinal hernias.

CLINICAL PRESENTATION AND DIAGNOSIS

Ventral herniorrhaphy is best detected by obtaining a complete history and performing a thorough physical examination. Symptoms often involve past sensations of "ripping" or "tearing." Pain is an infrequent complaint unless the hernia defect is small and the herniated contents become transiently incarcerated. A classic example is the patient with an epigastric (congenital) hernia in which the preperitoneal fat becomes acutely incarcerated and strangulated; the presentation then becomes that of a small, tender, mid epigastric midline mass. More commonly, an abdominal or flank bulge that comes with exertion and goes with relaxation is virtually pathognomonic of a hernia. Patients often feel the bulge reduce intra-abdominally, surprisingly most often without any notable pain or discomfort. With very large hernias, the patient often complains of feelings of "falling out" with loss of the abdominal domain. Less commonly, the patient may describe intermittent symptoms of partial small bowel obstruction. Bloating, constipation, or nonspecific gastrointestinal complaints, although often attributed to the hernia, usually are unrelated.

Even though the defect is usually obvious on evaluation, some examinations can be extremely difficult if the patient is obese, the hernia is incarcerated, or there is a great deal of scarring in the area from previous operations or from secondary healing after a previous deep wound infection. Other disorders may elicit referral for a ventral hernia. Simple rectus diastasis may mimic a ventral hernia. This harmless anomaly of acquired laxity, widening, and thinning of an otherwise intact linea alba extends from the xiphoid to the umbilicus but is obviously not a hernia. A large lipoma may confuse the unwary clinician (Fig. 1). A previous mesh repair with abdominal wall laxity (but no defect as such) may look every bit like a surgical problem, when in fact it is not (Fig. 2). Similarly, diffuse bulges in the region of previous flank incisions are not uncommon and usually are not true hernias (i.e., defects in the abdominal wall). The absence of a palpable fascial "edge" or no prior operative intervention in the region should tip off the astute clinician to some disorder that probably will not improve with operative intervention (e.g., rectus diastasis, mesh laxity).[3]

However, other complicated hernias may not be evident as a reducible bulge. For instance, small fascial defects may become "plugged" with incarcerated preperitoneal fat, omentum, or bowel. This situation is most common with epigastric, umbilical, or laparoscopic port-site hernias. This situation is similar to that of a femoral hernia that presents as a mass below the inguinal ligament. A more unusual defect that can be extremely difficult to appreciate is the intraparietal (intramural) hernia that may

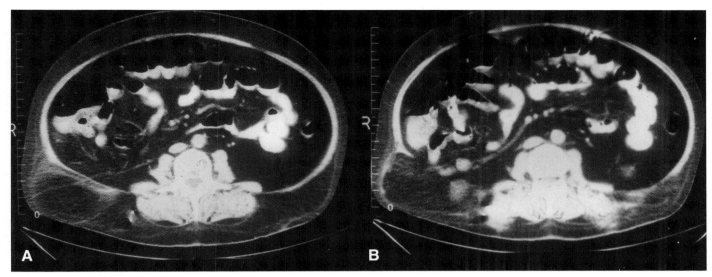

Fig. 1. (A), *Computed tomogram of a right-sided flank hernia, which may look like a large lipoma.* (B), *Scrutiny of another image from the same scan clearly identifies the right flank bulge as a hernia.*

complicate a spigelian hernia. These hernias involve abdominal wall defects that lie beneath an intact anterior fascia; the hernia sac thus dissects under the intact anterior fascia, extending laterally within the abdominal wall but not presenting as an anterior bulge.

When it is difficult to delineate the presence or the extent of a ventral hernia by palpation, computed tomography can be helpful. This imaging technique is most helpful for very obese patients in whom the physical examination is unreliable or in patients suspected of having a lumbar or intramural hernia (e.g., nonpalpable spigelian

hernia). The suspected diagnosis should be communicated to the radiologist before the test is performed such that a detailed examination can be performed in the anatomical region of interest. It is often surprising how large a hernia sac can be that remains "hidden" within the abdominal wall. Computed tomography often shows a disruption of the fascial continuity, provided thin cuts are taken; this potential problem points out the importance of direct communication with the radiologist. The presence of abdominal viscera outside the fascial confines of the peritoneal cavity is diagnostic, but the absence of this

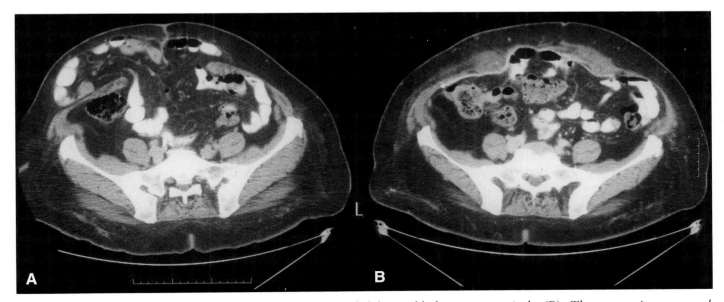

Fig. 2. (A), *Computed tomogram from a patient complaining of abdominal bulging preoperatively.* (B), *The same patient presented postoperatively with minor bulging. Scan highlights good coverage of the fascial defect with mesh and no evidence of recurrent hernia.*

specific finding is not necessarily helpful. Computed tomography is performed with the patient supine. The herniated contents may have reduced into the abdominal cavity.

We have found ultrasonography to be less reliable for the diagnosis of a suspected abdominal wall hernia, for many reasons: marked operator dependence, unclear tissue images of incarcerated nonhollow tissue, inability of the surgeon to interpret the images, and less precise characterization of fascial incontinence. We have no experience with the use of peritoneography with intraperitoneal administration of contrast agent and see little, if any, indication for such an invasive procedure. We can envision the potential use of laparoscopy for a difficult-to-diagnose hernia, provided the patient is markedly symptomatic, other noninvasive imaging techniques have been tried, and the surgeon plans to repair the hernia, if it is present, at the time of laparoscopy.

INDICATIONS FOR OPERATION

The indication for ventral hernia repair is the secure diagnosis of an abdominal wall defect that causes symptoms, usually pain or specific gastrointestinal alterations. Repair for cosmesis is also a recognized indication in selected patients. Abdominal hernia defects enlarge with time and eventually become symptomatic; most asymptomatic hernias, therefore, should be repaired electively. However, operative intervention is not mandated in asymptomatic, elderly patients with seemingly stable defects or in high-risk patients with minimally symptomatic or asymptomatic defects, especially those with a limited life expectancy.

Contraindications for ventral hernia repair include considerable uncorrectable comorbid conditions or the inability to tolerate general or controlled regional anesthesia. Long-standing defects with loss of the abdominal domain may contraindicate repair in patients with severe pulmonary compromise—placing the abdominal contents back into the abdomen and elevating the diaphragm may be more than the patient with chronic obstructive pulmonary disease, bronchiectasis, or severe asthma can tolerate. Some of these huge defects, especially those associated with loss of the anterior abdominal wall due to trauma or infection, may not be repairable. Others that have become so large that the abdominal domain is essentially gone with herniation of most of the intra-abdominal viscera also may not be repairable.

A frequent clinical situation is the extremely obese patient with a ventral hernia. In this case, repair of the ventral hernia ideally is postponed until the patient has lost weight both to decrease the operative morbidity and to increase the possibility of a successful long-term repair.

Obesity is a well-recognized factor predisposing to recurrence. However, in many obese patients the ventral herniorrhaphy is put off indefinitely until the patient loses weight. All too commonly, the weight is not lost, the ventral herniorrhaphy is not done, and the hernia becomes progressively larger. The clinical situation then becomes a vicious circle of enlarging hernia with a contraindication to repair (i.e., obesity). These patients require an aggressive approach. Initially, when the hernia is small, a multidisciplinary program of aggressive weight loss should be instituted; if unsuccessful after a defined time, operative repair (probably a mesh-based technique, see below) should be undertaken despite the lack of weight loss. In a patient with morbid obesity, a primary bariatric surgical approach is indicated initially in an attempt to treat the underlying problem (i.e., the obesity) and to treat the hernia secondarily provided a primary repair is possible. A patient with severe obesity may have a huge ventral hernia, either a primary umbilical hernia (the repair of which has been delayed) or an incisional hernia. In this situation, an aggressive surgical approach to weight loss (and not the hernia) is indicated. The hernia can be fixed after the bariatric procedure when the patient's weight is less; the repair will be easier, and the chances of success will be far better. This approach treats the entire patient and the cause of the hernia and not just the hernia itself.

Historically, the standard of care at Mayo Clinic has been to repair first-time ventral or incisional hernias in a primary fashion with permanent suture. Primary reapproximation usually is accomplished in small hernia defects when it is possible without tension and with good fascial edges. The original Mayo repair, or so-called pants-over-vest technique, in which the edge of one side of the defect is brought to overlap the other edge, theoretically offers many advantages for preventing recurrence. However, clearly it increases tension of the fascial closure. Surgeons have long argued whether a running suture technique or multiple interrupted sutures are best. There are no compelling data to select one technique over the other. A running suture is designed to distribute the tension along the entire length of the wound, yet if the suture breaks the entire closure is jeopardized. In contrast, an interrupted suture closure maximizes tension at the site of each individual suture, yet if one suture breaks the entire wound is not threatened. Theoretic argument supports both techniques. Similarly, the type of suture material (e.g., absorbable, braided, synthetic) is also hotly debated among surgeons without solid objective data to define the superiority of one type of suture material over the other. Even the authors of this chapter differ in the technique and suture material used for a primary reapproximation-type repair.

For hernias that are large, would lead to undue tension, or involve weak, attenuated, or absent fascia, use of some form of prosthetic material is indicated. Many surgeons either cut a piece of polypropylene mesh or polytetrafluoroethylene to match the defect and then sew the prosthesis to the edges of the fascia, but other approaches are an onlay technique or a sandwich-type repair with two sheets of prosthetic material, one sheet anterior to the anterior rectus sheath and the other posterior to the undersurface of the abdominal wall. This sandwich technique reinforces fascial closure in some, but not all, patients. All prosthetic mesh closures rely on the sutures used to hold the prosthetic mesh in place.

As our referral practice has developed, patients with morbid obesity, severe abdominal infection or trauma, advancing age, a history of multiple failed hernia repairs (up to 12 attempts), fistulas, and bowel obstruction have altered our approach. Primary closure may work well in healthy, thin patients with a small first-time recurrence, but more detailed repairs that use a different approach have been adopted to deal with these more complex incisional hernia defects. In such clinical situations, a laparoscopic approach, the Rives-Stoppa technique, and the rectus sheath rollover have great advantages.

LAPAROSCOPIC REPAIR OF INCISIONAL HERNIA

Laparoscopic repair, in contrast to an open procedure, typically is not advisable for a strangulated viscus. Chronically incarcerated bowel may be challenging to reduce laparoscopically without injury of the bowel with spillage of luminal content, but clearly it is not an absolute contraindication unless the abdomen is markedly distended or the patient has signs of local sepsis. A fascial defect more than 6 inches wide may be difficult to repair endoscopically, and hernias associated closely with the symphysis pubis can be troublesome to fix no matter the access (laparoscopic or open).

Conduct of Operation

A peripheral venous catheter is placed, and a general anesthetic is administered. A urinary catheter is inserted, and the arms are tucked at the patient's side. Abduction of the arms to 90° allows the surgeon more room to access the abdomen with large midline defects, with defects well off the midline, and in obese patients. Wide skin preparation of the entire abdomen from the nipples to the knees is prudent. The initial incision should be placed as far away as possible from the actual abdominal wall hernia; the vicinity of the anterior axillary line is ideal. Our preference is to place the 12-mm incision

somewhere cephalad to the level of the umbilicus on either the right or the left side—whichever allows the greatest distance from the hernia defect. The fascia is exposed and divided, and a muscle-splitting technique used. The peritoneum is incised, and a 12-mm trocar is placed under direct vision. A pneumoperitoneum is created with pressures from 10 to 15 mm Hg. The abdomen is explored. Two 5-mm trocars are placed on either side of the working camera port (Fig. 3). Ideally, both 5-mm trocars are placed at a distance sufficient to allow the graspers to be at 45° angles to the camera while the defect is repaired. Sometimes this positioning is not possible with larger defects.

Adhesions and omentum are released with sharp dissection and electrocautery. The entire posterior intraperitoneal surface of the anterior abdominal wall is exposed, and attachments to the small bowel, colon, and liver are released. With a fully exposed abdominal wall, the defect becomes obvious (Fig. 4). The defect is measured on the outside of the abdomen, and a large piece of mesh is tailored to be at least 6 cm greater in total diameter (allowing a 3-cm overlap circumferentially). A total of at least 4 permanent sutures (generally we use 8 to 12 for larger defects) are placed into a two-sided mesh and tied, the tails left 8 inches long and opposite the slippery side of the mesh

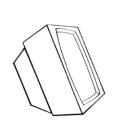
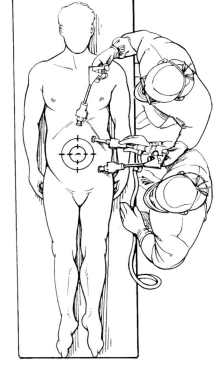

Fig. 3. Two 5-mm working ports flank a 12-mm trocar site used for the camera.

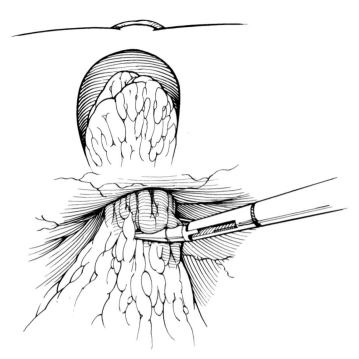

Fig. 4. Intraperitoneal look of a typical periumbilical defect.

(Fig. 5). The fashioned mesh and suture combination is rolled tightly and placed directly into the abdomen through the largest trocar. For larger pieces of mesh, the 12-mm port must be removed, and the mesh is inserted as the pneumoperitoneum releases. Thereafter, the 12-mm trocar is reinserted and the abdomen is reinsufflated.

With the use of graspers through the 5-mm trocars, the mesh is unrolled. A no. 11 blade is used to create 2-mm incisions (the number of incisions equals the number of sutures tied to the mesh), which allow an endoscopic grabbing device to be inserted into the abdomen. The graspers, working internally, pass each suture through the separate fascial punctures made by the suturing device. One-centimeter fascial bites are carefully obtained through each solitary 2-mm incision. Sequentially, the 4 to 12 separate stitches are passed through the abdominal wall to allow secure, circumferential fascial bites (Fig. 6). Our preference is to place the sutures farthest away from the camera first. The sutures are pulled anteriorly, and mesh placement is assessed. A wrinkled mesh, or one under too much tension, is easily adjusted by replacing the sutures through a different fascial site. With accurate placement, the sutures are tied and cut. The mesh is fixed circumferentially with a tacking device (Fig. 7). Additional clips are placed within the middle of the mesh to coapt it to the abdominal wall and help minimize seroma formation.

Hemostasis is secured, and the pneumoperitoneum is released. The trocars are removed, and the 12-mm fascial defect is closed primarily in layers with interrupted absorbable suture. The 5- and 12-mm skin incisions are closed with a subcuticular absorbable suture, and the 2-mm incisions are simply dressed. An abdominal binder is placed, and the patient is extubated and admitted to the hospital. A patient-controlled anesthesia pump is offered.

Advantages and Disadvantages

The advantages of a laparoscopic approach to ventral herniorrhaphy are primarily those of a minimal access technique. Smaller incisions usually are associated with less pain and possibly both a shorter hospitalization and a quicker return to normal activity. Other potential advantages are that the incisions used are distant to the prosthetic material placed; wound infections thus would not be contiguous with the prosthetic material.

The disadvantages of a laparoscopic repair are primarily threefold. First, the prosthetic material used in the repair is placed intraperitoneally. Thus, at least one side of the graft is in direct contact with the intraperitoneal viscera. Most surgeons, including us, use a polytetrafluoroethylene material that leads to formation of a pseudocapsule between the graft and the viscera.

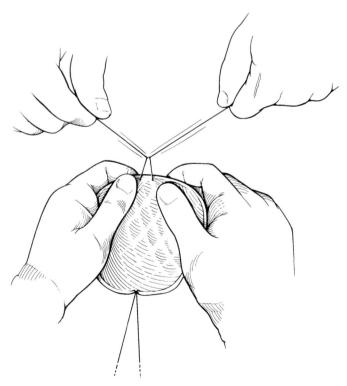

Fig. 5. A two-sided panel is created with at least four (8-inch) permanent sutures tied near the edges circumferentially. Knots lie on the "roughened side," allowing only the "slippery side" access to contact with omentum, bowel, and liver.

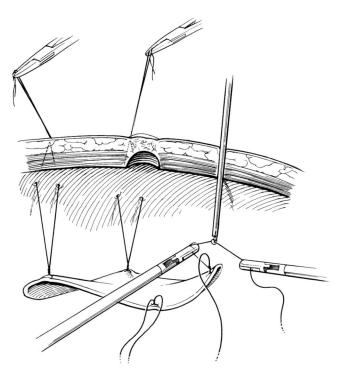

Fig. 6. Sequential passage of sutures through separate fascial sites (but the same skin incision) allows 1-cm fascial bites to hold the mesh securely.

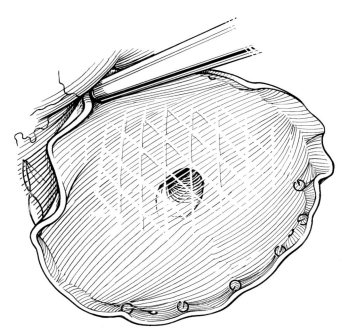

Fig. 7. A tacking device is used to fix the panel circumferentially.

Second, currently the graft of choice does not have a latticework that allows good, solid tissue ingrowth and thereby tissue fixation. The anterior surface of the polytetrafluoroethylene graft either has holes through the graft or has a roughened texture; nevertheless, tissue fixation is poor. Possibly some of the newer prosthetic materials with polytetrafluoroethylene on the visceral side and a woven polypropylene layer bonded to the parietal side will prove applicable.

Third, a laparoscopic approach may not be possible. Multiple adhesions intraperitoneally or dense fixation of intraperitoneal structures to the hernia sac may prevent adequate visualization and freeing up of all the edges of the defect. Without this clearance, safe and effective prosthetic fixation is not possible.

Surgical Outcomes

Decade-long follow-up does not yet exist for laparoscopic repairs of incisional hernia. We have performed more than 120 such laparoscopic ventral hernioplasties at Mayo Clinic in Rochester, Minnesota. Repairs are painful, and most patients require 1 to 4 days of hospitalization. Conversion to an open approach was necessary in one patient with severe adhesions after 7 previous celiotomies. Patient satisfaction has been high and greatest in patients with three or more previous attempts at herniorrhaphy.

The mean duration of follow-up in our patients is now more than 3 years. Hernia recurrence was suspected in five patients. In two patients, hernias developed within the former primary incision: adjacent to, but outside the confines of the previous mesh repair (i.e., the new defect was located cephalad or caudad to the previous repair of smaller midline hernias). We repaired both hernias secondarily with mesh. We now tend to place mesh under the entire midline incision even though the actual hernia defect may be much smaller. Previous incisions seem to act like a "zipper" in that the entire incision line remains the area of the abdominal wall with the greatest weakness and under the greatest stress or tension. One patient, status post a Hartmann procedure and two failed midline hernia repairs, was delighted with the laparoscopic procedure, but a hernia later developed in the old stoma site. It, too, was fixed safely with a laparoscopic approach. Two other patients reported a recurrent bulge, but computed tomography showed contained abdominal contents behind a tension-free mesh repair. The abdominal wall was lax (as candidly described to each patient preoperatively), but the hernia defect remained well covered.

COMPONENT SEPARATION OF ABDOMINAL WALL

One of the prime tenets of herniorrhaphy is the absence of tension in the closure. Several approaches are available: substitution of prosthesis for tissue, augmentation of the patient's tissues, and various methods of "component separation" of the abdominal wall to relax the parietes to allow a tension-free closure.[9] Other considerations include the location of the fascial defect, the availability of natural tissue, the adverse effects of prosthetic material, and, perhaps most important, the size of the defect. An ideal repair of ventral hernias includes closure of the wound without tension, use of the patient's own tissues rather than prosthetic material, and restoration of normal parietal anatomy with an acceptable rate of recurrence of a fascial defect (≤ 10%).

For ventral hernias resulting from midline incisional fascial defects, the patient's tissues are often adequate for repair, provided the defect is not excessively wide (< 30 cm). Ventral incisional hernias that do not involve any loss of the components of the abdominal wall (e.g., fascia, muscle, fat, skin) are often self-limited because the abdominal wall retracts laterally to a certain extent but cannot progress farther than the upper and lower limits of the incision permit. For most midline abdominal incisions, the lateral regression of the fascial margin does not often expand the defect beyond 25 to 30 cm. This limitation of the lateral extent of many ventral incisional hernias may allow herniorrhaphy with the patient's own tissues, minimal tension, and the restoration of normal anatomy.

The technique described below, under the appropriate conditions, may be used in solitary fashion as the herniorrhaphy or they may be used in combination with other techniques to provide a satisfactory result. The decision, as always, is left to the surgeon's best judgment.

Conduct of Operation

These techniques involve modification of the anterolateral parietes and necessitate substantial exposure of the anterior abdominal wall. The patient is positioned supine with wide skin preparation to the posterior axillary line. Because of the wide mobilization and potential need for prosthetic material, use of a broad-spectrum prophylactic antibiotic is prudent. The first step, therefore, is to dissect the abdominal pannus off the parietes, the skin and subcutaneous fat complex being taken directly off the fascia. Although this plane is fairly straightforward, care must be taken to ensure a clean removal of fat from the fascia yet avoid inadvertent incision of the fascia itself. The blood supply to this skin and fat complex comes from laterally within the complex; previous lateral transmural incisions, especially vertical ones (e.g., paramedian incisions), may jeopardize viability of the flap. We prefer to use electrocautery, turning the blade slightly upward from the direction of the dissection. This maneuver presents a more diffuse surface to the cutting edge, allowing downward pressure to permit close apposition of the blade to the

fascia without incision and resultant exposure of the underlying muscle. Perforating vessels encountered from the parietes to the pannus may be electrocauterized in most instances, especially on the pannus. Bleeding vessels from the parietes are easily controlled with suture ligatures of absorbable suture material into the musculoaponeurotic layers. This method may in fact be preferable, because there is less disruption of the fascia.

The dissection is carried laterally 2 or 3 cm beyond the lateral border of the rectus sheath. Of note, most of the sensation of the abdominal wall progresses circumferentially from the sensory roots of the spinal cord; even extensive separation of the pannus from the aponeuroses usually does not result in a substantial or permanent sensory deficit. If the rectus muscle is not easily visible, simultaneous palpation above and below the abdominal wall usually clearly demarcates the limits of the rectus sheath. Once the anterior parietes are sufficiently exposed, we prefer use of two techniques of component separation of the abdominal wall to allow the patient's tissues to appose in the midline without undue tension: release and rollover of the rectus sheath and release of the external oblique musculoaponeurosis. These techniques may be used separately or in concert, depending on the size of the defect.

The first technique, the rectus sheath rollover, rotates the anterior rectus sheath medially and anteriorly. The anterior rectus sheath is incised vertically along its length, beginning at the middle of the defect approximately 1 cm medial to the lateral border of the rectus sheath. The incision is carried rostrally and caudally from this point, progressing medially as it travels toward the apices of the wound. The rationale for this lateral medial drift is the oblong shape of hernial defects; the defect is usually widest at the center and narrows toward the superior and inferior aspects. Thus, the amount of rectus sheath rotation necessary is maximal at the midpoint of the wound and becomes progressively less toward the rostral and caudal extents of the hernia. After the anterior rectus sheath is incised laterally, the anterior rectus sheath is freed from the underlying rectus muscle, proceeding medially. Care must be taken to avoid creating defects in the anterior rectus sheath at this point; the tendinous insertions of the rectus muscle are far more adherent to the sheath than the remainder of the rectus muscle. Kocher clamps applied to the anterior rectus fascia just medial to the relaxing incision can provide traction to rotate the anterior rectus sheath medially and anteriorly, thereby allowing gain of as much as 5 to 10 cm of medial approximation of the parietes. This technique may be enough to close defects of less than 10 to 15 cm in width without undue tension. For larger defects, the external oblique release (described below) may be necessary.

The second technique of component separation involves release of the external oblique fascia accomplished by vertical incision of the external oblique musculoaponeurotic layer just lateral to the lateral border of the rectus sheath. The incision functions as a relaxing incision, allowing the rectus sheath to slide medially and the internal oblique and transverse abdominus layers to slide laterally. For this maneuver to be successful, the incision must completely transect the external oblique fascia. Usually, the incision itself is satisfactory; on occasion it may be necessary to free the external oblique muscle from the internal oblique muscle to obtain adequate release to allow a tension-free closure. In contrast to the rectus rollover incision, this release is made roughly 1 cm lateral to the lateral border of the rectus sheath throughout its entire length.

Suturing of the fascia may, of course, be accomplished in many ways. We prefer a running closure, progressing from both apices of the wound and meeting in the center. A running horizontal suture provides theoretical benefits in terms of distribution of tension. A simple suture, interrupted or running, presents the tissue with a point of contact only as wide as the suture itself, and a running horizontal mattress suture spreads the tension over a length of suture between the fascial entrance points. The sutures are started just inside the cut edge of the rectus sheath, passed through rectus muscle, and brought out again through the anterior sheath more medially, and a mirror-image bite is taken through the contralateral sheath. The suture is reversed with bites taken back to the first side, 1.5 to 2.0 cm from the previous suture. The running suture has the additional benefit of gradually pulling the fascia together where tension is least, lessening the tension toward the center of the wound. We prefer no. 1 loop polydioxanone suture with a knot tied at the beginning rather than the technique of passing the suture through the loop; use of a doubled suture anchored with a weak link of a single strand makes little sense. Although polydioxanone suture is absorbable, its strength lasts well beyond the time most fascial healing takes place.

Because of the rather extensive dissection in the suprafascial plane, fluid accumulation above the repair is the rule. We routinely place closed suction drains for 3 to 5 days postoperatively to avoid the accumulation of clinically significant "seromas." The drains are removed when drainage is less than 50 mL in 24 hours. The surgeon may want to remove the drains sooner when prosthetic material has been placed (see below) in order to minimize the risk of bacterial contamination. Prophylactic antibiotics are not used beyond the effective perioperative time frame, microbial antibiotic resistance being a global concern.

These techniques may allow tension-free apposition of the fascia in the midline, but the surgeon may want to augment the closure with application of prosthetic material. Most simply, an appropriately sized portion of prosthetic material may be sutured to the anterior aspect of the fascia at the lateral cut edge of the rectus sheath incision. This has the salutary effect of replacing the rotated anterior rectus sheath, which theoretically may be more important below the linea semicircularis, where there is no posterior rectus sheath. Alternatively, the above-described techniques may be used after a Rives-Stoppa–type repair (see below) with placement of prosthetic material posterior to the rectus muscle.

In summary, these techniques provide a means of restoring nearly normal musculoaponeurotic anatomy and may be used alone or in conjunction with prosthetic materials to provide a satisfactory closure. Variations of component separation of the abdominal wall parietes substantially reduce tissue tension and may avoid the need for prosthetic material if desired (e.g., clean-contaminated, contaminated, or dirty wounds). Use of these techniques does not preclude simultaneous creation of enteric stomas. Given the overall utility of these techniques, every general surgeon who repairs large ventral hernias should be skilled in their use.

Advantages and Disadvantages

The major advantages of these techniques are twofold: restoration of a nearly normal tension-free musculoaponeurotic anatomy and avoidance of prosthetic material. By releasing parts of just the anterior fasciae of the lateral aspects of the abdominal wall, autogenous anterior rectus fascia (or rectus muscle) is released to allow a tension-free primary fascial closure in the midline with primary coverage by the mobilized skin or fat components. The second advantage, avoidance of the need for prosthetic material, is especially important in clean-contaminated, contaminated, or even grossly contaminated wounds. Use of this technique should be closely questioned in grossly contaminated wounds because a large extent of the anterior fascia is jeopardized if a deep wound space infection occurs. Use of this technique does not preclude simultaneous creation of enteric stomas.

A disadvantage of component separation techniques is a higher rate of recurrent hernias, usually about 15%. Although this is arguably greater than with some of the radical repairs that use prosthetic material (recurrence rates about 5%), the advantage of avoiding infected mesh may make the somewhat higher rate of recurrence acceptable. Another potential disadvantage is the need for a very wide lateral dissection with the possibility of devascularization of the skin and subcutaneous fat complex at the medial edge. Also, the lateral relaxing incisions weaken the abdominal wall laterally, especially in the lower abdomen.

Surgical Outcomes

An in-house hospital stay of 3 to 7 days is the rule after the component separation technique, depending on three main factors: pain control, wound serum drainage, and ileus. We routinely administer diazepam in the first few postoperative days to alleviate the muscle spasms, which are common. Other than this, the postoperative pain control regimen is standard: patient-controlled analgesia with a narcotic (usually morphine) followed by an oral medication such as oxycodone when parenteral narcotics are no longer necessary. Use of an abdominal binder is routine; it aids in patient comfort and may diminish trauma to the fresh closure by limiting stresses such as coughing.

Drains are left in place until their output is less than 50 mL in 24 hours. This usually occurs within 3 days, although it may take up to a week. Beyond this time frame, the risk of infection becomes prohibitory, and drains are removed, accepting the possibility of a seroma that may require percutaneous drainage. Development of a wound infection obviously prolongs convalescence, because the extent of the flaps may preclude successful wound dressing changes at home (at least at first), even if a visiting nurse is employed. In the case of infection, the wound is opened, and wet-to-dry dressings are changed three times daily until granulation tissue has formed. If the wound is clean and well granulated, the flaps may be allowed to seal down, resulting in a more manageable wound.

Long-term problems are chiefly those of recurrence. Hernia may recur in up to 10% to 15% of patients, in both our experience and that of others (Russell Postier, M.D., University of Nebraska, personal communication). Most recurrences are in small areas where suture has pulled through weak fascia; the authors have not yet seen a full dehiscence of the wound.

More minor difficulties are areas of anesthesia or dysesthesia associated with the extensive dissection of the abdominal wall. A few patients may have areas of numbness or occasional pangs of pain; most of these are minor according to the patients' subjective assessment and may be alleviated or resolved entirely with time. In one particularly thin patient in whom polypropylene mesh was used to replace the anterior fascial layer after a rectus rollover, a turned-up corner of mesh irritated the dermis and necessitated a local trimming.

RIVES-STOPPA TECHNIQUE OF VENTRAL HERNIORRHAPHY

After having noted an unacceptably high recurrence rate of incisional hernias with the standard primary reapproximation repairs and after the typical onlay type of prosthetic material repairs, we have been pleased with our modification[10,11] of the Rives-Stoppa intramural prosthetic mesh repair of large ventral and incisional hernias.[12,13] This operative repair was developed because of the importance of a tension-free approach in which the final strength of the repair derives not from sutures holding the prosthetic material to the edge of the fascial defect but rather from ingrowth of fibrous tissue into the prosthesis with solid fixation of the prosthesis in place to "patch" the defect, if not reapproximate the edges. Several concepts are important. First, the prosthesis should allow tissue ingrowth and incorporation of the permanent prosthesis as an integral part of the reconstructed abdominal wall. Thus, a mesh prosthesis (as opposed to a sheet of polytetrafluoroethylene, which does not allow substantial tissue ingrowth) is highly preferable. Second, because the strength of the repair is not in the suture fixation but rather in tissue ingrowth, the larger the surface area for tissue ingrowth, the stronger the repair (Fig. 8). Although we do not suggest this more aggressive repair for all ventral or incisional hernias, we do favor this "radical" hernioplasty for most recurrent incisional hernias or for large primary ventral hernias in patients with one or more risk factors for recurrence.

Conduct of Operation

The basic concept of the Rives-Stoppa technique is to patch the hernia defect "from behind" with a large sheet of permanent prosthetic mesh and to place the mesh intramurally within the abdominal wall (intraparietally). This intramural location is designed so the prosthesis does not come in direct contact with the intraperitoneal contents but rather has at least one layer of autogenous tissue interposed between the mesh and the intraperitoneal organs.[11] To do this, a plane should be developed behind (posterior to) the rectus muscles but anterior to the posterior rectus fascia. This space is created 5 to 10 cm wider than the perimeter of the fascial defect.

After supine placement of the patient and a very wide antiseptic skin preparation, laterally to the mid axillary lines bilaterally, usually the previous incision is reopened if it is an incisional hernia or an incision is made centered over the defect. Perioperative intravenous antibiotic prophylaxis usually directed at skin flora is used routinely. All attempts should be made to dissect the hernia sac from the subcutaneous tissues but to stay extraperitoneal. At this point, the redundant hernia sac is not excised "back to good, healthy fascia," as in the classic primary approximation repair. Instead, the hernia sac is maintained intact to serve as a barrier of autogenous tissue between the mesh and the intraperitoneal content (Fig. 9). If tears or defects in the peritoneal hernia sac are created

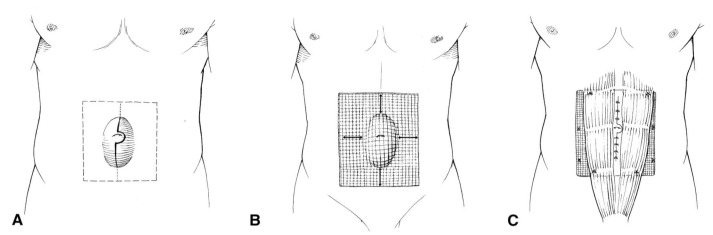

Fig. 8. *Basic concept of modified Rives-Stoppa technique. The hernia defect (central elliptical area, A) is "patched" with a large sheet of prosthetic mesh (B) placed posterior to the rectus abdominis muscles (C). Note extension of the mesh 5 to 10 cm beyond the lateral superior and inferior extent of the defect. This large surface area maximizes tissue ingrowth into and through mesh, fixing it in place. (A and B from Sakorafas and Sarr.[11] By permission of Mayo Foundation.)*

during mobilization of the hernia sac or if the peritoneum is entered consciously to facilitate mobilization of the hernia sac in patients with multiply recurrent or very caudal hernias, then the peritoneal defects are closed with a running absorbable suture material.

Next the retrorectus plane is developed. This maneuver is most easily accomplished by palpating the medial edge of the rectus sheath and creating an anterior fasciotomy to expose the medial edge of the rectus muscle. With blunt (and, if necessary, sharp) dissection, the rectus muscle is retracted anteriorly while the posterior rectus sheath is mobilized off the posterior aspect of the rectus muscle. This space usually has not been transgressed and is readily developed laterally to the lateral margin of the rectus muscles unless

the patient has had a previous subcostal or paramedian incision or unless the patient has had a previous ileostomy or colostomy. In cases of previous ileostomy or colostomy, care should be taken to avoid injuring a knuckle of bowel caught up in a persistent fascial defect in the posterior rectus or endoabdominal fascia. This retrorectus plane is developed at least 5 to 10 cm rostral and caudal to the extent of the defect or to the pubis inferiorly or the xiphoid rostrally if the defect involves all the infraumbilical or epigastric region. Note that the rectus muscles do not arise from the costal margin but rather from the ribs one or more interspaces rostral to the costal margin. This is important because the mesh can be placed up and over the costal margin and, if necessary, can be sewn to the edge of the costal margin.

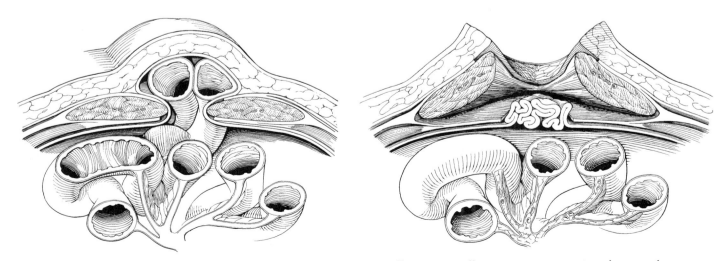

Fig. 9. *Basic concept of modified Rives-Stoppa technique. Maintenance of hernia sac will serve as autogenous tissue between the prosthetic mesh and the intraperitoneal content.*

While this retrorectus space is developed, several concepts should be kept in mind. First, the space should be considerably larger than the fascial defect, extending at least 5 to 10 cm beyond the circumference of the defect. Second, there must be a fascial layer anterior to the mesh lateral to the fascial defect to which the mesh will be anchored during the early postoperative phase of tissue ingrowth.

Once the retrorectus space is developed, the mesh is anchored in place to secure its location over the next 3 to 6 weeks when tissue incorporation occurs. This anchoring suture is placed by making a short 0.5-cm stab through the skin of the anterior abdominal wall at the lateral extent of the retrorectus space. With use of a heavy absorbable suture (1-0 polydioxanone) and a long needle that has been straightened into a ski shape, the needle is passed through the stab wound into the subcutaneous space, through the rectus fascia and lateral rectus muscle into the mobilized retrorectus space, through the mesh in horizontal mattress fashion, then back out the abdominal wall through the same stab wound, with care taken to leave at least 1 cm between the ends of the suture where the needle passed through the anterior fascia (Fig. 10). When the suture is tied, the knot will lie in the subcutaneous space, and the mesh will be anchored to the anterior rectus fascia. Usually about 12 such anchoring sutures are placed, in a fashion similar to the numbers on a clock, around the mesh. Rostrally, the mesh can be sewn to the xiphoid or costal margin if necessary and caudally to the pubis or Cooper's ligaments bilaterally; we use a permanent suture for these areas of fixation.

After the mesh is secured in place without any wrinkling and under only slight tension, one should attempt to reapproximate the medial edges of the anterior rectus sheath

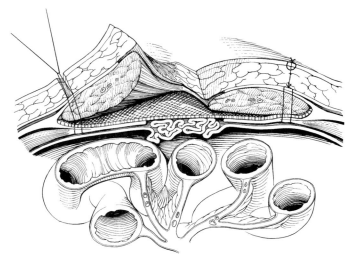

Fig. 10. Anchoring of mesh in place. Note transmural placement of sutures through skin stab wound.

over the mesh, even if this results in tension at this suture line. This reapproximation is done not for strength (because the defect has already been "patched" with the mesh) but rather to place another layer of autogenous tissue between the mesh and the skin in an attempt to minimize the risk of infection. We also place one or two closed suction drains anterior to the mesh for several days postoperatively.

This technique can be used for many types of abdominal wall incisional hernias, including midline, subcostal, paramedian, transverse, and flank. The variations of where the "intramural" space is created depend on the site of the hernia. One need only keep at least one good fascial layer anterior to the mesh to allow a stable anchoring of the mesh until tissue incorporation can occur.

Several special situations may occur. On occasion, not enough autogenous tissue (omentum or hernia sac) is present to intersperse between the mesh and the bowel in the middle of the defect. In this situation, we have used a composite-type prosthesis. Several composite approaches are possible, either sewing a sheet of polytetrafluoroethylene to the polypropylene mesh in the area exposed to the intraperitoneal content (with a commercially available prosthesis with polypropylene bonded to a thin layer of polytetrafluoroethylene) or placing a sheet of absorbable polyglycolic mesh between the bowel and the polypropylene mesh.

In another special situation, the skin or subcutaneous complex overlying the hernia is very thin and attenuated and the hernia defect is very large. In this case the lateral fascial edge cannot be approximated over the mesh and there is inadequate skin or subcutaneous tissue laterally to mobilize over the mesh. In this case, we tend to make the incision directly into the peritoneum, find the medial edge of the rectus from its posterior (intraperitoneal) aspect, incise the medial edge of the posterior rectus sheath, and then mobilize the space posterior to the rectus muscle but anterior to the posterior rectus sheath. When the mesh is in position, the mesh situated between the medial edges of the posterior rectus sheath will be exposed to the intraperitoneal content; usually, a polytetrafluoroethylene surface is used. However, the mesh laterally is still placed intramurally, and the tissue incorporation still occurs intramurally.

Advantages and Disadvantages

The advantages of a Reves-Stoppa repair depend primarily on patient selection. This radical hernioplasty is not indicated for all patients, especially those with small primary hernias. However, for multiple recurrent, complex abdominal wall hernias, especially with very large or multiple "Swiss cheese" defects and multiple intra-abdominal adhesions, this technique has the lowest reported long-term recurrence rate (see below) and can effectively patch the entire hernia defect without tension and without reliance on suture fixation to the fascial edge for long-term repair.

Another major advantage is that if another celiotomy is required in the future, the abdomen can be entered directly through the mesh prosthesis. Indeed, subsequent closure should be a very secure one without concern about incisional hernia because the repair involves reapproximation of the mesh-to-mesh, which should not break down provided a permanent suture is used.

This technique does, however, have several potential disadvantages. First, this procedure is a "big" operation, takes 1 1/2 to 3 hours, and necessitates a 3- to 5-day hospitalization. Second, because it uses a large sheet of prosthetic material, infection is always a major concern. If the bowel is inadvertently entered during the dissection, some consideration should be given to abandoning the use of prosthetic material. Similarly, if a clean-contaminated procedure (e.g., colectomy, small bowel resection, gastrectomy, appendectomy) is conducted at the same time of planned Rives-Stoppa herniorrhaphy, placement of the mesh prosthesis also should be strongly questioned. Third, because a large surface area is mobilized, seroma formation is not uncommon. We routinely place closed suction drains in an attempt to control the tissue fluid transudation; however, the drain itself is a two-way street for bacteria, and the surgeon always must weigh the risk:benefit ratio of maintaining the drain for more than a few days postoperatively. No data exist concerning the efficacy of "prophylactic" antibiotics while the drains are in place. Finally, patients often complain of a pulling or tearing sensation, usually in the lower abdomen in the areas of the anchoring sutures. We warn all our patients about this possibility, but it remains a substantial complaint for 2 to 4 months.

Surgical Outcomes

Because of the extensive dissection needed, this operative repair is not done as an outpatient procedure, and convalescence is long. Average hospital stay is about 3 to 5 days, but if an extensive intraperitoneal adhesiolysis is needed, postoperative ileus may occur and delay dismissal. In most instances, dismissal is dictated by pain control.

Wound problems involve primarily wound infections, skin or subcutaneous necrosis or breakdown, and seromas or hematomas. Because this is a clean operation, primary wound infections should be uncommon. However, if the skin or subcutaneous complex covering the hernia is attenuated or consists of scar, every attempt should be made to excise the attenuated areas and reapproximate healthy fat and epidermis, but under no tension. We close the wound with a running absorbable dermal closure (polyglycolic acid) with reinforcing skin staples that are left in place for 3 weeks. A real problem is development of wound hematomas and seromas. If large, they can drain through the incision, thereby increasing the incidence of wound and mesh infection. Should a stable hematoma or seroma form without concern of spontaneous rupture, we follow it noninterventionally. If pending rupture appears evident, we place a drain percutaneously. On occasion, late chronic seromas represent a pseudobursa with a secretory, mesothelial lining and necessitate formal excision of the wall of the bursa. We have had to excise three such chronic seromas in about 250 patients.

We have been using this technique since 1991. Our initial experience with 50 patients was reported in 1996.[10] Recurrent hernias developed in two patients (4%). Since then, our total experience has grown by about 200 patients. There have been four other recurrent hernias (total recurrence rate 6/250, 3%). Two recurrent hernias developed at the edge of the mesh repair in a previous incision; our interpretation is that we did not extend the mesh far enough to include those incisions. Now we tend to expect all previous abdominal wall incisions to be at risk and try to include all abdominal wall incisions in our patch repair whenever possible. Two other "recurrent" hernias were in patients who had mesh infections necessitating excision of the mesh, which left a recurrent hernia.

Mesh infections are the major concern to the surgeon and the patient. Early in our experience, we placed prosthetic material with this technique at the time of other clean-contaminated gastrointestinal procedures. Of our eight mesh infections (total infection rate, 4%), three occurred in this situation. Currently, we do not use this technique if the gut is to be opened. Instead, we use an absorbable polyglycolic acid prosthesis sewn to the fascia edges (without mobilizing the retrorectus space) or some of the newer tissue matrix products for temporary closure and plan the permanent repair for 3 to 6 months later. One of the other five mesh infections occurred during the initial hospitalization because a knuckle of small bowel stuck in a previous colostomy site was injured (and not recognized intraoperatively). The other mesh infections occurred in patients who had a prior onlay-type prosthetic mesh repair. We excised the previous prosthetic mesh, waited 6 months, and then performed the modified Rives-Stoppa technique. Despite high-dose perioperative antibiotics, mesh infections occurred about 1 to 3 months postoperatively and mesh removal was necessary. Although anecdotal, we believe that a previous mesh infection places patients at a much higher risk of mesh infection at a later date. Probably some other type of herniorrhaphy, if possible, should be considered in these patients (e.g., component separation techniques).

CONCLUSION

The laparoscopic, component separation, and Rives-Stoppa techniques for incisional abdominal hernia defects bolster the techniques of general surgeons who are attempting to rid patients of symptomatic hernias. With primary repair, recurrence rates are as high as 58% or more, and the documented low recurrence rate of these more radical techniques is a welcome change for patients and surgeons. The key to herniorrhaphy is to repair the hernia with a tension-free technique and, if mesh is used, with wide coverage beyond the extent of the defect. Whether by minimally invasive or open approach, all three techniques are painful and typically necessitate several days of hospitalization with temporary need for intravenous narcotics.

REFERENCES

1. Santora TA, Roslyn JJ: Incisional hernia. Surg Clin North Am 73:557-570, 1993
2. Carlson MA, Ludwig KA, Condon RE: Ventral hernia and other complications of 1,000 midline incisions. South Med J 88:450-453, 1995
3. Israelsson LA, Jonsson T, Knutsson A: Suture technique and wound healing in midline laparotomy incisions. Eur J Surg 162:605-609, 1996
4. Toy FK, Bailey RW, Carey S, Chappuis CW, Gagner M, Josephs LG, Mangiante EC, Park AE, Pomp A, Smoot RT Jr, Uddo JF Jr, Voeller GR: Prospective, multicenter study of laparoscopic ventral hernioplasty: preliminary results. Surg Endosc 12:955-959, 1998
5. Mudge M, Hughes LE: Incisional hernia: a 10 year prospective study of incidence and attitudes. Br J Surg 72:70-71, 1985
6. van der Linden FT, van Vroonhoven TJ: Long-term results after surgical correction of incisional hernia. Neth J Surg 40:127-129, 1988
7. Koller R, Miholic J, Jakl RJ: Repair of incisional hernias with expanded polytetrafluoroethylene. Eur J Surg 163:261-266, 1997
8. Paul A, Korenkov M, Peters S, Kohler L, Fischer S, Troidl H: Unacceptable results of the Mayo procedure for repair of abdominal incisional hernias. Eur J Surg 164:361-367, 1998
9. Ramirez OM, Ruas E, Dellon AL: "Components separation" method for closure of abdominal-wall defects: an anatomic and clinical study. Plast Reconstr Surg 86:519-526, 1990
10. Temudom T, Siadati M, Sarr MG: Repair of complex giant or recurrent ventral hernias by using tension-free intraparietal prosthetic mesh (Stoppa technique): lessons learned from our initial experience (fifty patients). Surgery 120:738-743, 1996
11. Sakorafas GH, Sarr MG: Intraparietal retrorectus tension-free prosthetic mesh: a simple and effective method of repair of complex ventral hernias via a modified Stoppa technique: surgical technique. Acta Chir Belg 99:109-112, 1999
12. Rives J: Major incisional hernia. In Surgery of the Abdominal Wall. Edited by JP Chevrel. Berlin, Springer-Verlag, 1987, pp 116-144
13. Stoppa RE: The treatment of complicated groin and incisional hernias. World J Surg 13:545-554, 1989

Chapter 47

INGUINAL HERNIA: OPEN REPAIR

Mark E. Freeman, M.D.
Stephen L. Smith, M.D.

It may be true that no two general surgeons repair an inguinal hernia exactly alike. It also may be true that every general surgeon thinks his or her particular repair is the best. It is certainly true that open inguinal hernia repair techniques continue to evolve and remain controversial.

No single inguinal hernia repair is accepted by all 21 general surgeons who perform this procedure at the three Mayo Clinic sites. In a poll of these 21 surgeons, 8 (38%) most frequently use an anterior, tension-free Lichtenstein repair, 5 (24%) prefer a Bassini repair, 4 (19%) most commonly perform a mesh plug procedure, and 4 (19%) perform preperitoneal laparoscopic repairs most often. In the previous 5 years, these surgeons had performed 10 different repairs. In addition to the operations listed above, these repairs included, in decreasing order of frequency, transperitoneal laparoscopic, McVay, Nyhus preperitoneal, Stoppa, Shouldice, and Marcy. The number of repairs used by each surgeon ranged from 2 to 7 (mean, 3.6).

The current techniques of open inguinal hernia repair and the changes in recent years at Mayo Clinic mirror the techniques and changes across the United States and around the world. This chapter reviews our past open inguinal hernia repairs, discusses the current repairs, and speculates on future trends.

HISTORY OF HERNIA REPAIR

The word "hernia" is derived from Latin, meaning "rupture or tear." The earliest recorded reference to the diagnosis of a hernia is in the Egyptian Papyrus of Ebers, about 1550 B.C.[1] These observations included "a swelling on the surface of a belly" and "caused by coughing."[1]

About 50 A.D., Celsus published an explicit description of the contemporary hernia operation of his day. He highlighted hemostasis by vessel ligature and efforts to save the testicle.[2] Galen of Pergamum, the most prominent and influential physician of the Greco-Roman period, later recommended ligature of the cord and sac with amputation of the testicle.[3] He proposed that the cause of herniation was a rupture of the peritoneum and stretching of the muscles and fascia.

Galen's recommendation for routinely sacrificing the testicle during hernia repair went unchallenged for the next 1,000 years. It was not until the 13th century that William of Salicet broke ranks and proposed that surgeons "...permit the testicle to redescend to its place, and do not dream...of extirpating it."[4] Further important advancements were not made until the 19th century.

In 1814, Antonia Scarpa published a treatise on hernia surgery, entitled *Sull'ernia Memorie Anatomico-Chirurgiche*. He introduced the term "sliding hernia" and stressed the importance of studying inguinal anatomy. Several decades later, Astley Paston Cooper authored a major contribution to the hernia literature entitled "The Anatomy and Surgical Treatment of Abdominal Hernias." He defined the transversalis fascia and established it as the main barrier to abdominal herniation. In 1804, Cooper wrote, "No disease of the human body...requires in its treatment a greater combination of accurate anatomical knowledge, with surgical skill, than hernia in all its varieties."

Surgical repair of hernia was revolutionized in 1889 by the Italian surgeon Eduardo Bassini. Bassini described a technique designed to "restore those conditions in the area of the hernial orifice which exist under normal circumstances."[5] He proposed suturing of the transversalis fascia and conjoined tendon to the inguinal ligament. One year later in the United States, William Halsted published a report describing a similar repair, which included a relaxing incision.[6,7]

Shortly thereafter, Georg Lotheissen described another tissue repair that involved anchoring the transversalis fascia to Cooper's ligament.[8] This method was later refined and popularized by McVay in the 1950s.[9] A third major tissue repair was developed by Shouldice, Obney, and Ryan in the 1950s.[10] Their multilayered repair stressed the use of local anesthesia, early ambulation, and one continuous suture line.

The next major milestone in hernia surgery was introduction of the tension-free repair by Lichtenstein in 1986.[11] He reported that reconstruction of the floor of the inguinal canal with a synthetic mesh had very low rates of complication and recurrence. This work established the safety and effectiveness of routine use of mesh in the repair of inguinal hernia and paved the way for introduction of other mesh prosthesis hernioplasties.

More recently, laparoscopic surgery has been added to the types of inguinal herniorrhaphy, and it is discussed in Chapter 48.

ANATOMY OF THE INGUINAL REGION

Crucial to the successful repair of an inguinal hernia is an understanding of the regional anatomy. The abdominal wall may most simply be broken down into anterior and posterior laminar aspects. The anterior wall primarily is made up of the internal and external abdominal oblique muscles and aponeuroses. The posterior abdominal wall consists of the transversus abdominis muscle and the transversalis fascia. It is this posterior wall that contains the defect through which the herniated contents can protrude. The anterior structures are simply displaced by the herniated contents coming through the posterior wall.

The inferior margin of the transversus abdominis muscle joins with the internal abdominal oblique muscle at the internal inguinal ring to form an aponeurotic arch. The aponeurotic arch fuses with the internal oblique aponeurosis to form the conjoined tendon. Although commonly discussed, a true conjoined tendon occurs in less than 10% of patients, according to anatomical studies.[12,13]

The aponeurosis of the external abdominal oblique muscle has both a superficial and a deep layer. This most anterior aponeurotic layer fuses with the internal oblique and the transversus abdominis aponeuroses to form the anterior rectus sheath in the groin. The external oblique aponeurosis acts as the superficial border of the inguinal canal and is reflected posteriorly to form the inguinal (Poupart's) ligament. The inguinal ligament is an inferior thickened portion of the external abdominal aponeurosis as it rolls posteriorly under the most medial fibers. It attaches laterally to the anterior iliac spine and medially to the superior pubic ramus and pubic tubercle.

The inguinal canal exists as a potential space between the fibers of the external oblique aponeurosis, the transversus abdominis muscle, and the transversalis fascia. It is approximately 4 cm in length and travels from the internal inguinal ring laterally to the external inguinal ring medially. The spermatic cord (in males) and round ligament (in females) are the major structures that travel through this canal. The deep layer (or floor) of the inguinal canal is formed by the transversus abdominis aponeurosis and the transversalis fascia. This relatively weak posterior wall is the most important structure from a surgical perspective. The posterior wall contains an area referred to as Hesselbach's triangle, which is bounded laterally by the deep inferior epigastric vessels, medially by the lateral edge of the rectus abdominis muscle, and inferiorly by the inguinal ligament. Hernia defects through the posterior wall in this region are classified as direct hernias. Hernias lateral to Hesselbach's triangle or through a slack internal inguinal ring are classified as indirect hernias.[14]

Cooper's ligament is simply the posterior periosteum of the superior pubic ramus as it joins with fascial condensations of the transversalis fascia. This structure is extremely constant in form and is known for its dense fibrous tissue. This layer, which is often 2 to 3 mm thick, is used as an anchor for suture in several repairs.

The iliopubic tract is of considerable strength in most humans and thus is useful in inguinal hernia repair. It consists of a thick fascial band originating from the iliopectineal ligament. It runs from the anterior iliac spine to the iliopectineal eminence and inserts into Cooper's ligament. The iliopubic tract lies just adjacent and deep to the middle portion of the inguinal ligament; however, they are easily separable and distinct layers. The inguinal ligament arises from the external oblique aponeurosis and the iliopubic tract from part of the transversus abdominis muscle and the transversalis fascia.

ETIOLOGY OF HERNIA FORMATION

Inguinal hernia formation is thought to have several basic causes, including a patent processus vaginalis, a defective shutter or "sphincter" mechanism at the internal inguinal ring, weakened abdominal fascia, and increased abdominal pressure.

Direct inguinal hernias are formed by the mechanical breakdown of the transversalis fascia of the posterior inguinal wall over time. Causes of increased intra-abdominal pressure, such as cough, constipation, pregnancy, obesity, exertion, prostate hypertrophy, and peritoneal dialysis, increase the risk of direct hernia formation. However, many people have these conditions and never have an inguinal hernia, and hernias develop in people who do not have these conditions. This can be explained by the inguinal canal laminar structure or by the shutter and sphincter mechanisms.

The "shutter mechanism" is described as a movement of the transversus abdominis aponeurotic arch. The arch remains convex until the transversus abdominis and internal abdominal oblique muscles are tensed, at which point the arch flattens out. This action supports the floor of the inguinal canal by moving the arch toward the iliopubic tract so that it covers the internal inguinal ring. One theory of direct hernia formation is that a defective aponeurotic arch structure will not support the floor of the inguinal canal on exertion.[15,16] This exposes a single, thin layer of transversalis fascia in Hesselbach's triangle to increased intra-abdominal pressure.

The "sphincter mechanism" describes the movement of the transversalis fascia sling as it is pulled superiorly and laterally to close the internal inguinal ring during transversus abdominis contraction. This allows for tightening of the internal inguinal ring around the spermatic cord structures during episodes of increased intra-abdominal pressure. For both the shutter and the sphincter mechanisms to function properly, the anterior and posterior laminar layers must be allowed to slide past one another.[17]

Hernia repairs that suture posterior structures to the anterior inguinal ligament are thought to disrupt these two delicate mechanisms. The so-called tension-free inguinal hernia repair attempts to support these mechanisms with prosthetic mesh.

The indirect hernia can be the result of a congenital process, unlike the direct inguinal hernia, which is acquired. During development, the testes normally descend from a retroperitoneal location into the scrotum along a tubular processus vaginalis. If the processus vaginalis remains patent, it may exist as a preformed or potential indirect hernia sac. A patent processus vaginalis does not indicate that an indirect hernia will occur. Numerous studies have shown that although a large percentage of cadavers have a patent processus vaginalis, few of the patients actually had ever reported symptoms or signs of an indirect hernia.[18,19] This is due to the fact that the cause of indirect hernias is not only a patent processus vaginalis but also the weakening of the fibers of the transversalis fascia at the internal inguinal ring.

DIAGNOSIS AND IMAGING

Presentation
Hernia formation usually occurs slowly over a long time. The most common initial symptom of an inguinal hernia is the presence of a small bulge in the groin, with or without mild discomfort on exertion or long periods of standing. Discomfort most often occurs early in the course of hernia formation as the tissues are stretched and dilated. With time, patients often notice that the bulge increases in size and at times no longer disappears when they lie supine. If there is no associated discomfort, patients can become adept at manually reducing the hernia. Pain, if present, is usually described as sharp, localized, worse with straining, and improved at rest.

Some hernias occur acutely. Acute-onset inguinal hernias are usually indirect and are due to sudden excessive exertion. Patients often report pain or discomfort before they notice a small bulge above the inguinal ligament.

The most common cause of presentation for emergency surgical repair is an episode of incarceration. Incarceration occurs when the contents of the hernia are extruded beyond the peritoneal cavity and are no longer reducible. This is due to edema and adhesion formation between the hernia sac and its contents or even between the contents alone. Hernia strangulation, interruption of the blood supply to the hernia content, is less common. Clues to the diagnosis of strangulation include acute-onset pain associated with fever and tachycardia. Erythema of the skin over the hernia and extreme tenderness also may occur. Nausea, vomiting, and septic symptoms may develop later in the course of the disease.

Interview
During the initial consultation with the patient, it is important to elicit a thorough history. Specific information regarding a possible inciting event and the factors predisposing to increased abdominal pressure is gathered.

Examination
Examination of an inguinal hernia begins with visual inspection of the groin and genitals while the patient is standing. Often a reducible bulge is present which expands with coughing or the Valsalva maneuver. Other, less obvious hernias may be visualized only with straining. An indirect hernia often travels from a lateral to medial position and may extend into the scrotum along the path of the inguinal ligament. Alternatively, a direct hernia usually begins medially and protrudes forward toward the examiner. The exact type of hernia is not always obvious on physical examination.

The examiner's finger is used to invaginate the scrotum, with the tip of the finger placed in or through the external inguinal ring. On coughing, an indirect hernia is usually felt protruding through the internal inguinal ring at the tip of the finger, whereas a direct hernia is usually felt lateral to the external ring. After examination of the external ring, the floor of the inguinal canal and the internal ring must be palpated thoroughly. In women, the entire length of the inguinal region is palpated externally.

An attempt should always be made to reduce the content of the hernia into its proper location. Beginning at the most distal aspect, gentle yet firm pressure is used to reposition the hernial content into the abdominal cavity. An incarcerated hernia will not reduce. A strangulated hernia also is not reducible, but often it is extremely tender, firm, and erythematous.

An inguinal hernia can almost always be diagnosed on the basis of the physical examination. On rare occasions, such as the obese patient with a recurrent hernia, computed tomography or ultrasonography may be useful.

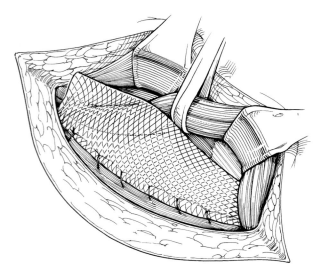

Fig. 1. Lichtenstein repair: placement of mesh over posterior wall of canal.

TYPES OF OPERATIONS

Lichtenstein Repair

Irving Lichtenstein was one of the first surgeons to recognize suture-line tension as the primary cause of most recurrent hernias. In 1974, he described a method of plugging femoral and recurrent inguinal hernias with rolled cylindrical mesh. In 1986, he described a procedure using prosthetic mesh that had been performed in more than 300 patients. No attempt was made to approximate the transversus abdominis or internal oblique to the inguinal ligament, and no stitches were placed in the internal inguinal ring. In 1989, he described 1,000 cases in which this technique had been used. There were few complications and no recurrences during 1 to 5 years of follow-up. He broke ranks from the surgical establishment by proposing the use of prosthetic mesh in routine hernia operations.[11]

Technique

After a standard inguinal incision is made, the external oblique is incised to reveal the inguinal canal, and the cord is mobilized. Indirect hernia sacs are invaginated into the abdomen after being dissected free. Inguinoscrotal sacs are divided in the canal. The distal portion is left wide open and undissected. A direct hernia sac may be imbricated posteriorly with an absorbable suture.

The posterior wall of the canal is covered with an appropriately tailored size and shape of polypropylene mesh (Fig. 1). The mesh must be wide enough to cover the entire canal floor. It should be able to lie over the inguinal ligament, reach underneath the superior aspect of the external abdominal oblique, and overlap the pubic tubercle by 2 to 3 cm. The mesh is sutured to the pubic tubercle and inguinal ligament beyond the internal ring with a continuous polypropylene suture. The superior aspect is similarly sutured to the internal oblique muscle or aponeurosis. The lateral "tails" are passed around the spermatic cord at the internal ring, are crossed, and then are sutured down to each other and the inguinal ligament (Fig. 2). This creates a new internal ring and preserves the "shutter mechanism." The external oblique is then closed with a continuous suture over the cord. The remainder of the wound is closed routinely.

This technique was revolutionary in that no definitive suturing of fascial tissues is used, unlike all previously described repairs.

Bassini Repair

In 1887, Eduardo Bassini introduced a hernia operation that would become one of the most common to be performed during the next century. He reported considerably lower morbidity, mortality, and recurrence rates than the best herniologists of his day. This rather obscure surgeon from Padua caused a sensation, and contemporary surgeons flocked to observe his techniques. During the many years since this first description, innumerable variations of Bassini's original technique have been performed. The original Bassini repair is described here.[20,21]

Technique

The incision was made 5 to 7 cm in length from the pubic tubercle toward the iliac spine. The external oblique was opened. The cord was surrounded. Apparently, according to illustrations, Bassini excised cremaster muscle, genital

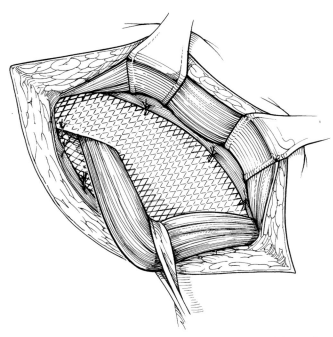

Fig. 2. Lichtenstein repair: mesh "tails" secured lateral to spermatic cord.

nerve, and "lipomata" of the cord. The sac was dissected free and opened. It is believed that Bassini then cut open the inguinal floor and separated off the underlying preperitoneal fat with his thumb for 3 cm in all directions and exposed the iliopectineal ligament. The musculature lateral to the internal ring was incised for 2 to 3 cm to allow lateral

displacement of the cord with the repair. The sac was dissected for 2 cm into the iliac fossa to ensure high ligation. It was twisted, ligated, transfixed, and divided (Fig. 3). Repair of the floor included 6 to 8 interrupted silk sutures spaced 4 mm apart. Each suture was placed like a purse string, passing into and out of the fascial layers exposed. No sutures were placed lateral to the cord (Fig. 4). At closure, the external oblique was addressed first, being closed over the transplanted cord.

Clearly, this operation is not the one that most current surgeons were taught, and it is not the same procedure currently referred to as a Bassini repair.[22,23]

Mesh Plug Repair

In the early 19th century, C. W. Wutzer, a professor of surgery in Bonn, was one of the first to propose use of an external wooden plug for the treatment of inguinal hernias. In 1886, William Macewen reported use of an internal plug for the inguinal canal which was made from a portion of the hernia sac itself. However, after the advent of the Bassini repair in 1887, this method never became popular. Irving Lichtenstein, in 1974, was one of the first modern surgeons to report on the use of plugs from rolled synthetic mesh. In the late 1980s, Arthur Gilbert improved the design of the cylindrical plugs into a cone or umbrella shape, which allowed for more circumferential coverage, although these plugs were never popular. In 1998, Robbins and Rutkow resurrected the mesh plug idea and developed a preformed umbrella-shaped plug

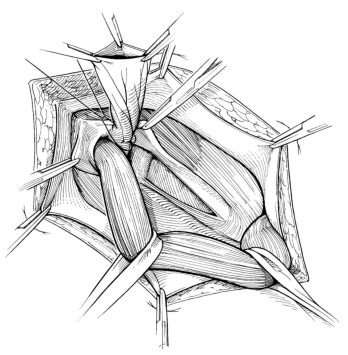

Fig. 3. Bassini repair: high ligation of indirect inguinal hernia sac.

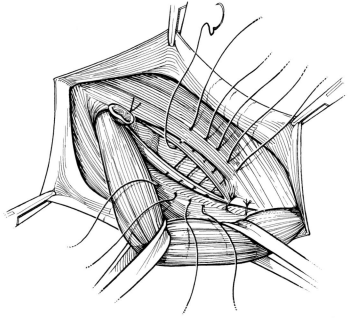

Fig. 4. Bassini repair: placement of interrupted sutures in the inguinal floor.

made from polyethylene mesh. This is often used in conjunction with a mesh patch. The so-called mesh plug technique is rapidly gaining in popularity.[24]

Technique

A 4- to 5-cm incision is made over the internal inguinal ring. The external oblique aponeurosis is incised to reveal the inguinal canal, and a self-retaining retractor is inserted into the wound. The ilioinguinal and genitofemoral nerves are preserved if identified, although no calculated effort is made to identify them. The spermatic cord is then mobilized at the level of the pubic tubercle, and a Penrose drain is passed underneath for manipulation.

A high dissection of the spermatic cord is performed, separating the sac from the cremasteric fibers (Fig. 5). The free sac and any lipomas then are simply invaginated into the abdominal cavity. An umbrella-shaped plug is inserted into the opening of the internal ring just below the crura, tapered end first (Fig. 6). In small indirect hernias, several small stitches suffice to keep the plug in place. For large indirect hernias, the plug is sutured to the internal ring with multiple interrupted sutures. If the preformed plug appears too large for the defect or the patient's habitus, the distal wide portion may be tailored to fit appropriately.

Direct hernias are treated somewhat differently. The transversalis fascia defect is elevated and the midportion is incised to reveal the preperitoneal fat. The sac, the overlying transversalis, and the transversus abdominis are then invaginated into the abdominal cavity, and a mesh plug is

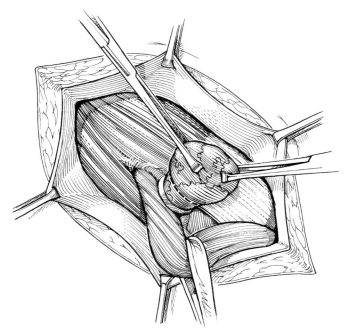

Fig. 5. Mesh plug repair: separation of indirect inguinal hernia sac from the spermatic cord.

inserted into the newly created defect. The plug is then sutured into place with multiple interrupted sutures to any surrounding tissue (Fig. 7). The use of two or more mesh plugs has been advocated for pantaloon hernias or hernias with multiple defects.

All repairs are reinforced with a flat piece of polyethylene mesh. This may be placed with a sutureless technique or absorbable tacking sutures from the pubic tubercle to an area lateral to the internal inguinal ring. The lateral portion of the patch has two limbs, which are sutured snugly around the spermatic cord. This mesh layer serves only as protection from future herniation by increased tissue ingrowth into the inguinal canal.

The cord is replaced anterior to the mesh, and the external oblique aponeurosis is approximated over the cord with a continuous absorbable suture. Standard closure is then completed.

McVay Cooper's Ligament Repair

Astley Cooper was the first to identify the thick band of superior rami periosteum and transversalis fascia reflection that now bears his name. Interestingly, although he described the structure, he never used Cooper's ligament in his repair and prescribed a truss for all but incarcerated hernias. Georg Lotheissen, in 1897, was the first surgeon to report suturing the conjoined tendon to Cooper's ligament. He performed this operation in a female patient with a twice recurrent inguinal hernia in whom the inguinal ligament was destroyed. In 1942, Chester McVay described a variation of the Cooper ligament repair. His work emphasized the ability to repair direct, large indirect, and femoral hernias. He also championed the use of a relaxing incision in the anterior rectus sheath. The McVay Cooper's ligament repair is the only anterior suture repair that may repair all three types of groin hernias.[9]

Technique

As in the Bassini repair, an inguinal incision is made, the cord is mobilized, and the inguinal floor is opened. Cooper's ligament is identified and cleared. The anterior femoral fascia is identified and dissected free in a medial direction, with care taken to avoid the femoral artery and vein. If a femoral hernia is present, the sac is brought up to an inguinal location. Next, the transversus abdominis arch is mobilized superiorly. A 4- to 5-cm relaxing incision is then made superiorly along the line where aponeurosis of the internal abdominal oblique joins the anterior rectus sheath.

The spermatic cord is then incised, and any adipose tissue or "lipomas" are dissected free. The cremaster muscle fibers are divided at the level of the internal inguinal ring, and the external spermatic artery is divided near the inferior epigastric artery.

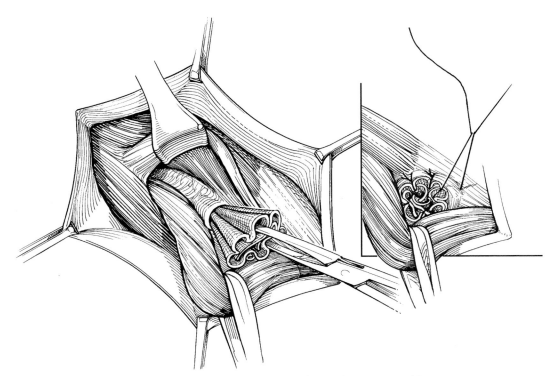

Fig. 6. Mesh plug repair: placement of plug into internal ring opening of an indirect inguinal hernia.

The spermatic cord is then inspected for the presence of an indirect hernia sac. If an indirect hernia sac is located, it is incised and explored. Direct hernia sacs can simply be inverted. However, excision is reasonable for those that are extremely large.

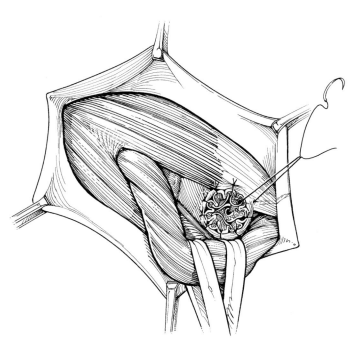

Fig. 7. Mesh plug repair: circumferential suturing of a plug in a direct inguinal hernia.

The first step in the repair is careful imbrication of the preperitoneal tissue, with avoidance of any injury to underlying bowel or bladder. A running absorbable suture is used to retract this tissue from the operating field. Interrupted sutures are then placed between the transversus abdominis arch, the transversalis fascia, and Cooper's ligament, beginning at the pubic tubercle and moving laterally to the edge of the femoral vein. It is vital to the success of the repair that thick bites of both Cooper's ligament and the transversus abdominis arch are taken, and not simply the internal oblique.

The next step is repair of the femoral canal. Four transition sutures are used to approximate the anterior femoral fascia to Cooper's ligament. It is imperative to place the first transition stitch just lateral to the last stitch of the previous suture line. The remainder of the transition stitches also may be placed more lateral to the previous Cooper's ligament sutures.

After placement of the transition stitches, the transversus abdominis arch is approximated to the anterior femoral fascia. This suture line is continued medial to lateral, but not beyond the spermatic cord, so that it will exit the newly created internal ring tangentially. An instrument then may be inserted into the newly created inguinal ring to ensure proper closure. The cord is allowed to return to its native position.

The defect created by the relaxing incision may be secured with several interrupted sutures or covered with a piece of mesh. The external oblique is then reapproximated over the cord, and the remainder of the closure is completed.

Nyhus (Preperitoneal) Repair

Beginning in 1959, Nyhus and associates advocated use of a preperitoneal approach. It has been understood for some time that the most important structures in the cause of hernia formation are the transversus abdominis muscle and its aponeurosis and the transversalis fascia. The Nyhus posterior preperitoneal approach emphasizes the benefits of a posterior repair using the iliopubic tract. These benefits include direct exposure of the posterior structures, avoiding scar tissue present in recurrent hernia, and the relative safety of releasing incarcerated or strangulated hernias.[25]

Technique

A transverse abdominal incision is made 3 cm above the inguinal ligament, slightly superior to the conventional inguinal hernia incision. The subcutaneous tissue is dissected to reveal the anterior rectus sheath. An incision is then made through the anterior rectus sheath at a level superior to the internal inguinal ring. The rectus muscle is retracted medially, and the incision is carried out laterally through the entire external oblique, internal oblique, and transversus abdominis muscles to expose the transversalis fascia.

The transversalis fascia is then incised carefully, and the preperitoneal space is entered without disturbing the underlying peritoneum. With minimal blunt dissection, the posterior inguinal wall and any herniation can be visualized.

A direct hernia can be reduced easily with blunt dissection of the preperitoneal space. The margins of the hernia sac should be identified as the hernia is reduced. There is usually no need to excise the direct hernia sac, although severely redundant tissue may be invaginated and excised. Care should be taken to avoid bladder injury at this level. The direct defect is closed with interrupted permanent sutures. The medial Cooper's ligament located inferiorly is sutured to the thickened transversalis fascia and the transversus abdominis aponeurotic arch located superiorly. Occasionally, the iliopubic tract is damaged from direct herniation; in this case, the transversus abdominis aponeurotic arch is the lone superior fascial structure.

If an indirect hernia sac is present, it may be reduced with gentle traction. As opposed to a direct sac, the indirect sac is ligated and the excess sac is removed.

Small indirect defects can be repaired by approximating the anterior crus to the iliopubic tract and posterior crus of the internal inguinal ring with interrupted suture. Larger defects are repaired differently. The anterior crus of the transversalis sling and the iliopubic tract medial to the spermatic cord are approximated with interrupted suture.

Two or three sutures are used to create an artificial internal ring so that the spermatic cord lies superior and lateral to the femoral artery. Two or three more sutures are used to close the defect laterally.

If a large indirect hernia is present which destroys the posterior wall near Hesselbach's triangle, the medial aspect is repaired as a direct hernia. A new internal inguinal ring is created laterally, as described previously.

The posterior wall is inspected for further hernia defects. Once all the defects have been identified and repaired, a layered closure is accomplished.

Stoppa Repair

The Stoppa, or giant, prosthetic reinforcement of the visceral sac was introduced in 1987 and has since become an invaluable tool for dealing with problematic bilateral or recurrent groin hernias. Stoppa's procedure was an interesting innovation because it is nearly sutureless, it is tension-free, and the hernia defect is almost entirely ignored. The repair involves reinforcing the transversalis fascia with a large sheet of polyester mesh placed in the preperitoneal space. Postoperatively, increasing abdominal pressure actually assists with holding the mesh in place.[26]

Technique

A transverse abdominal incision is placed 2 to 3 cm below the level of the anterior superior iliac spine, but superior to any hernia defects that may be present. The rectus sheath and external and internal oblique musculature are also divided. The abdominal wall is retracted as the rectus muscle is bluntly dissected from the rectus sheath. The lateral edge of the rectus is then inspected for the transversalis fascia. This layer is incised, the preperitoneal space then being revealed. The inferior epigastric vessels are visualized and bluntly dissected free.

A prosthetic mesh sheet is tailored to fit the abdominal wall. The mesh is usually diamond-shaped with the bottom wider than the top and the lateral edge longer than the medial aspect. The length of the superior edge of the mesh should equal the distance from the midline to the anterior superior iliac spine minus 1 cm. The medial distance should be 14 cm with the inferior-lateral corner extended approximately 2 to 4 cm.

The mesh is sutured into place with 2 or 3 interrupted absorbable stitches along the superior border 2 to 3 cm above the incision. Three long clamps are used to slide the mesh inferiorly into the preperitoneal space. The medial aspect is placed into the space of Retzius, behind the pubic symphysis and superficial to the bladder. The clamp at the middle of the inferior border of the mesh is placed over the obturator foramen, superior ramus of the pubis, and the iliac vessels. The clamp at the inferior lateral border is positioned into the iliac fossa, over the internal inguinal ring and "parietalized" spermatic cord.

The retractors and clamps are removed cautiously. Care must be taken to avoid any wrinkling or shifting of the mesh during withdrawal of the instruments before closure.

Shouldice Repair

The Shouldice repair was first reported in the 1950s. The operation consists of a four-layer repair with tissue imbrication that uses two single stainless steel wires. The proposed advantage of the repair is the ability to use only local anesthesia to allow for early ambulation. It has been described as a multilayered Bassini repair.[10]

Technique

After standard incision and exposure, cremaster muscle fibers are incised at the level of the internal inguinal ring and are separated from the spermatic cord, the result being medial and lateral muscle flaps. An indirect hernia sac should be identified and dissected free from the cord at the level of the internal ring and below. Essential to the repair is that all of the attachments to the internal ring are freed at this point.

The transversalis fascia is incised at the level of the internal ring, and the incision is carried down inferomedially to the level of the pubic tubercle. The cribriform fascia of the thigh is incised below the level of the inguinal ligament. The femoral ring may be examined from both above the inguinal ligament and below from the femoral orifice. The internal oblique, transversus abdominis, and transversalis fascia are identified medially. The iliopubic tract is then identified laterally adjacent to the cremasteric stump.

The posterior wall of the inguinal canal is then reapproximated with a stainless steel wire. The suture is passed through the iliopubic tract and then through the transversalis fascia, rectus, transversus abdominis, and internal oblique. The suture is tied, but the free end is used as a continuous suture. The running suture line travels down toward the internal ring, incorporating the cremasteric stump laterally. The suture is reversed and is used to approximate the free border of the transversus arch to the inguinal ligament all the way to the pubic crest, where the wire is tied.

The second wire suture is used to create an artificial inguinal ligament by suturing the internal abdominal oblique and transversus abdominis to the external oblique aponeurosis. This suture line begins at the internal inguinal ring and travels to the pubic crest, where it reverses itself. A 2-cm bite of the medial external abdominal oblique is used to cover the medial edge of the floor of the inguinal canal. A continuous suture line is carried laterally, parallel to the inguinal ligament. This creates a second artificial inguinal ligament just superficial to the previous suture line. The wire is sutured into position at the internal ring.

The medial cremasteric stump is sutured near the pubic tubercle to prevent descent of the testicle. The spermatic cord is allowed to return to its position, and the external abdominal oblique is closed with a continuous absorbable suture. Standard closure may be undertaken.

COMPLICATIONS OF HERNIA OPERATION

Infection

The risk for development of a postoperative wound infection is 1% to 2%, regardless of which type of procedure is performed.[27] Risk factors for development of wound infection after open hernia repair include sex, age, drain placement, and duration of operation, among others.[28] Women and patients older than 70 years have a substantially higher risk of infection.[29] Multiple studies have shown that routine perioperative antibiotics have no effect on infection rates.[30,31]

The use of monofilament biomaterial is also recommended over the use of the braided material because the latter harbors small spaces or pores, which preclude entry and surveillance by macrophages.[32] Although earlier reports claimed increased risk of infection, recent studies have shown no substantial difference in the infection rates of patients with or without prosthetic materials.[31,33]

Bleeding

Bleeding is one of the most common complications of an inguinal hernia repair. Considerable postoperative bleeding or hematoma formation occurs in approximately 1.3% of patients.[34] To decrease the risk, one should avoid blind clamping and suture placement and instead control bleeding through direct vision at all times.

Injuries to the femoral vein have been reported as a result of inaccurate suture placement through the anterior wall or a lateral stitch placed in Cooper's ligament causing compression. The femoral artery is also at risk because it lies just deep to the transversalis fascia and lateral to the deep inguinal ring and femoral vein.

Neuralgia

Neuralgia is an unfortunate complication of hernia operation which can be difficult to explain. Neuralgia with neurapraxia and hyperesthesia is reported in 1.5% of patients after open hernia repair,[34] but the incidence may be much higher. The nerves most commonly involved are the ilioinguinal, iliohypogastric, and genitofemoral nerves because of their distinct anatomical variation and proximity.

The most common type of neuralgia is due to the formation of a neuroma. A neuroma is formed by the proliferation of fibers around the nerve after partial or complete transection. The pain can be intense at the site, often imitating an electric shock. A distinct hyperesthesia is also noted along the corresponding dermatome. Projected pain, or that caused by a suture encasing an intact nerve, is often elicited by light touch.

Testicular Complications
Ischemic orchitis and testicular atrophy are the two most common complications involving the testicle. Ischemic orchitis is usually noted within the first 24 to 72 hours postoperatively as a painful enlargement of the testicle, often associated with fever. In a fraction of these patients, testicular atrophy ultimately develops over time; however, it is impossible to predict which patients will be affected. The ischemia is thought to be due to venous congestion from thrombosis of veins in the spermatic cord. The frequency of testicular atrophy has been reported to be 0.036% with primary repairs and 0.46% with recurrent repairs.[35]

Femoral Venous Thrombosis and Pulmonary Embolus
Femoral venous thrombosis and pulmonary embolus are infrequent complications of inguinal hernia repair, but when they occur they can be deadly. Wantz[36] found thrombosis leading to pulmonary embolus after hernioplasty in 3 (0.07%) of 4,114 patients. However, thrombophlebitis is much more common, occurring in 1.4% of inguinal hernia repairs.

Recurrent Hernia
Recurrence is the single most common complication of open inguinal hernia repair, ranging from 1% to 20% in indirect hernias and 3.5% to 20.9% in direct hernias.[37] The single most common cause of hernia recurrence is a technical failure and is usually due to excess tension. Also, many recurrent hernias are not truly recurrent but were present as a second, or missed, hernia at the time of initial operation. In the hands of the average general surgeon, studies reveal that prosthetic or mesh repairs have considerably lower recurrence rates (Table 1).

CONCLUSION
There are many accepted ways to repair an inguinal hernia. The inguinal hernia repair techniques used at Mayo Clinic are varied and reflect the numerous techniques performed nationally and internationally.

The trends in inguinal hernia repair at Mayo Clinic were assessed in a comparison of statistics from 1989 and 1999 at all three Mayo Clinic sites. These results showed a considerable transition. In 1989, no Mayo Clinic surgeon was performing laparoscopic repairs, and 97% of repairs done were with suture alone. By 1999, only 29% of repairs were performed with only suture and 71% involved mesh; 12% of the repairs were laparoscopic and 59% were anterior tension-free repairs.

The preferred procedures have changed in the past 30 years. The most recent trends toward the use of prosthetic materials and tension-free repairs have been mirrored in the Mayo Clinic system, and these will continue to evolve.

Table 1.—Frequency of Recurrent Hernia After Inguinal Hernia Repair

Type of repair	Subsequent recurrence, % of patients
Suture repair	
Bassini	2.9-25
Shouldice	0.2-2.7
McVay	1.5-15.5
Nyhus	3.2-32.2
Prosthetic repair	
Tension-free	0-1.7
Mesh plug	0-1.6
Stoppa	0-7

REFERENCES

1. Lyons AS, Petrucelli RJI: Medicine: An Illustrated History. New York, Abradale Press/Abrams, 1987
2. Celsus: De medicina (English translation by WG Spencer). Cambridge, Harvard University Press, 1938
3. Read RC: The development of inguinal herniorrhaphy. Surg Clin North Am 64:185-196, 1984
4. Pifteau P: Chirurgie de Guillaume de Salicet. Toulouse, Imprimerie Saint-Cyprien, 1898
5. Bassini E: Nuovo metodo operativo per la cura dell'ernia inguinale. Padova, Italy, Prosperini, 1889
6. Halsted WS: The radical cure of inguinal hernia in the male. Johns Hopkins Hosp Bull 4:17-24, 1893
7. Halsted WS: Surgical Papers. Vol 1. Baltimore, Johns Hopkins Press, 1924
8. Lotheissen G: Zur radikol Operation der Schlenkelhernien. Zentralbl Chir 25:548, 1898
9. McVay CB, Anson BJ: Inguinal and femoral hernioplasty. Surg Gynecol Obstet 88:473-485, 1949
10. Shouldice EE: The treatment of hernia. Ontario Med Rev 20:670-684, 1953
11. Lichtenstein IL: Hernia Repair Without Disability. Second edition. St Louis, Ishiyaku Euroamerica, 1986
12. Sorg J, Skandalakis JE, Gray SW: The emperor's new clothes or the myth of the conjoined tendon. Am Surg 45:588-589, 1979
13. Nyhus LM, Condon RE: Hernia. Fourth edition. Philadelphia, JB Lippincott, 1995
14. Nyhus LM, Klein MS, Rogers FB: Inguinal hernia. Curr Probl Surg 28:401-450, 1991
15. Spangen L, Anderson R, Ohlsson L: Nonpalpable inguinal hernia in women. In Hernia. Third edition. Edited by LM Nyhus, RE Condon. Philadelphia, JB Lippincott, 1989, pp 74-77
16. Lytle WJ: Internal inguinal ring. Br J Surg 32:441-446, 1945
17. Zimmerman LM: Essential problems in surgical treatment of inguinal hernia. Surg Gynecol Obstet 71:654-663, 1940
18. Hughson W: Persistent or preformed sac in relation to oblique inguinal hernia. Surg Gynecol Obstet 41:610-614, 1925
19. Keith A: Origin and nature of hernia. Br J Surg 11:455-475, 1924
20. Bassini E: Sulla cura radicale dell'ernia inguinale. Arch Soc Ital Chir 4:380, 1887
21. Bassini E: Nuovo metodo per la cura radicale dell'ernia inguinale. Atti Congr Assoc Med Ital 2:179-182, 1887
22. Catterina A: Bassini's operation for the radical treatment of inguinal hernia (translated by R Vicchi-Borghesi, L Secchi). London, Lewis, 1934
23. Wantz GE: The operation of Bassini as described by Attilio Catterina. Surg Gynecol Obstet 168:67-80, 1989
24. Robbins AW, Rutkow IM: Mesh plug repair and groin hernia surgery. Surg Clin North Am 78:1007-1023, 1998
25. Nyhus LM: Iliopubic tract repair of inguinal and femoral hernia: the posterior (preperitoneal) approach. Surg Clin North Am 73:487-499, 1993
26. Wantz GE: Giant prosthetic reinforcement of the visceral sac: the Stoppa groin hernia repair. Surg Clin North Am 78:1075-1087, 1998
27. Amid PK: Classification of biomaterials and their related complications in abdominal wall hernia surgery. Hernia 1:15-21, 1997
28. Olson M, O'Connor M, Schwartz ML: Surgical wound infections: a 5-year prospective study of 20,193 wounds at the Minneapolis VA Medical Center. Ann Surg 199:253-259, 1984
29. Simchen E, Rozin R, Wax Y: The Israeli Study of Surgical Infection of drains and the risk of wound infection in operations for hernia. Surg Gynecol Obstet 170:331-337, 1990
30. Lazorthes F, Chiotasso P, Massip P, Materre JP, Sarkissian M: Local antibiotic prophylaxis in inguinal hernia repair. Surg Gynecol Obstet 175:569-570, 1992
31. Gilbert AI, Felton LL: Infection in inguinal hernia repair considering biomaterials and antibiotics. Surg Gynecol Obstet 177:126-130, 1993
32. Bendavid R: Complications of groin hernia surgery. Surg Clin North Am 78:1089-1103, 1998
33. Martin RE, Sureih S, Classen JN: Polypropylene mesh in 450 hernia repairs: evaluation of wound infections. Contemp Surg 20:46-48, 1982
34. Rydell WB: Inguinal and femoral hernioplasties. Arch Surg 87:493, 1963
35. Bendavid R, Andrews DF, Gilbert AI: Testicular atrophy: incidence and relationship to the type of hernia and to multiple recurrent hernias. Probl Gen Surg 12:225-227, 1995
36. Wantz GE: The Canadian repair of inguinal hernia. In Hernia. Third edition. Edited by LM Nyhus, RE Condon. Philadelphia, JB Lippincott, 1989, pp 236-248
37. Bendavid R: Expectations of hernia surgery (inguinal and femoral). In Principles and Practice of Surgical Laparoscopy. Edited by S Paterson-Brown, J Garden. Philadelphia, WB Saunders, 1994, pp 387-414

Chapter 48

ENDOSCOPIC INGUINAL HERNIA REPAIR

David R. Farley, M.D.
John H. Donohue, M.D.

About 700,000 inguinal hernias are repaired each year in the United States.[1] Various techniques are available to treat the nagging and sometimes dangerous problem of groin hernia. Millions of job hours are lost because of the associated lack of productivity after repair in the typically healthy, young male patient (> 90% of all patients with inguinal hernia are men[2]). Even though various operative techniques are useful for repair of hernias, the endoscopic approaches, totally extraperitoneal (TEP) and transabdominal preperitoneal (TAPP), have definite advantages in selected patients.

PHYSIOLOGY

Although "hernia" is the Latin word for "rupture," modern definitions typically generalize a hernia as the protrusion of an organ or tissue through or beyond the structure that normally confines it.[3] By definition, an inguinal hernia exists when the processus vaginalis remains patent in childhood (an "indirect" defect occurs at the internal ring) or whenever intra-abdominal tissue breaks through the transversalis fascia in the Hesselbach triangle (a "direct" defect). Although most hernias are indirect, or congenital, clinical symptoms typically are delayed into the middle years of life (most hernia repairs are done in 45- to 64-year-old men[2]) as the effects of the aging process, tissue breakdown, and repetitive exertion or factors increasing abdominal pressure become prominent. Increased intra-abdominal pressure can be generated from excessive coughing (e.g., chronic obstructive pulmonary disease, bronchitis, smoking), obesity, constipation, sneezing, asthma, benign prostatic hypertrophy, and ascites.[4]

DIAGNOSIS AND IMAGING

Most inguinal hernias are diagnosed on the basis of a thorough history that reveals groin discomfort, pain, or aching, with or without a visible bulge. Most commonly, symptoms occur as the day progresses and are not appreciated on awakening. Physical examination invariably reveals a reducible mass in the inguinal canal or a clear impulse with straining or coughing. In patients with characteristic groin symptoms who lack obvious physical findings, computed tomography, magnetic resonance imaging, or ultrasonography may be of benefit, but our preference has been to explore the groin for a presumed inguinal hernia if the history is consistent with this diagnosis. If the symptoms are atypical and the examination does not reveal a hernia, we favor observation and subsequent reexamination. An imaging study should be considered if the patient has substantial complaints. A diagnostic laparoscopy also may be considered in such cases, but it is not currently a routine part of our practice.

INDICATIONS FOR OPERATION

The vast majority of inguinal herniorrhaphies are performed for symptomatic inguinal hernias. We do offer elective repair for asymptomatic defects in fit patients, but we are careful to stress the elective nature of operative intervention in this patient population. Asymptomatic but enlarging inguinal hernias should be repaired.

Although hospital charges are higher for the TEP and TAPP approaches than for open mesh herniorrhaphy, their advantages make both options viable procedures in appropriately selected patients.

Both TEP and TAPP repairs are excellent methods of fixing virtually all groin hernias. The indications for use of TEP or TAPP repair include 1) a recurrent hernia previously repaired with an open anterior technique (especially if a mesh prosthesis was used), 2) bilateral hernias, 3) unilateral defects in patients wanting prompt return to activities with heavy exertion, and 4) patients wanting maximal cosmesis. A previous lower midline incision makes TAPP or TEP repair more difficult, but it is not a contraindication to this type of procedure. There are few absolute contraindications for endoscopic repairs in patients able to tolerate general anesthesia. Patients who have had an open prostatectomy, bladder operation, or placement of an aortofemoral vascular prosthesis are usually not considered candidates for laparoscopic inguinal hernia repair. Strangulated hernias invariably should not be fixed through a totally extraperitoneal approach because it can be difficult to ensure that adequate and safe reduction of the hernia has been achieved. Large scrotal or chronically incarcerated hernias can be difficult and problematic to fix by either the TEP or TAPP technique. Although groin hernias in female patients are easily repaired with either technique, we believe that most women are better served by an open herniorrhaphy, usually without a mesh prosthesis and with local anesthesia. Patients requiring immediate return to anticoagulation are encouraged to forgo the TEP or TAPP technique to avoid potential retroperitoneal bleeding that can be difficult to detect.

OPERATIVE TECHNIQUE

TEP

The patient is asked to empty the bladder immediately before entering the operating room. An intravenous catheter is placed and a general anesthetic is administered. Nasogastric and urinary catheters are unnecessary. The lower abdomen is prepared with a soap or iodine-type solution. A 1.5-cm incision is created within the inferior portion of the umbilicus. Blunt dissection is carried down to the rectus sheath, and the rectus fascia is exposed on one side of the midline (opposite the side of the planned inguinal hernia repair). A 1-cm vertical fasciotomy of the anterior rectus sheath allows identification of the underlying rectus muscle. The rectus muscle is retracted laterally and elevated with S-shaped retractors. The posterior rectus fascia is visualized and protected. A balloon dilator is inserted through the anterior fasciotomy and placed behind the rectus muscle. The lubricated balloon dilator slides easily to the pubic symphysis.

The endoscope is placed within the instrument, and dilation of the balloon with pneumatic compression is begun. Approximately 40 compressions of the plastic bulb

generate a working space the size of a grapefruit. This expansion is accomplished in a controlled fashion, and visualization of the symphysis pubis, rectus muscles, bladder, and inferior epigastric vessels is clear. Direct hernias typically are seen to reduce from this vantage point. The balloon subsequently is deflated and the dilator is removed. A 10-mm port is placed through the off-center fasciotomy and secured in place. Carbon dioxide insufflation creates a pneumopelvis at 10 mm Hg, and a 30° laparoscope is inserted and the pelvis is explored.

The symphysis pubis, Cooper's ligaments, bladder, rectus muscles, and both sets of inferior epigastric vessels typically are visualized before dissection. Two horizontal 5-mm incisions are created directly in the midline (the first lies 1 cm cephalad to the symphysis pubis and the second lies an additional 3 to 5 cm further cephalad). Two 5-mm trocars are inserted safely under direct vision into the previously created space. Two graspers are used through the 5-mm working ports (Fig. 1). The symphysis pubis is noted, Cooper's ligaments are cleared of fatty tissue, and the epigastric vessels are left attached to the underside of the rectus muscle. Importantly, dissection is carried out laterally but posterior to the inferior epigastric vessels and extended as far laterally as possible. This potential space is created with blunt dissection. Cautery is unnecessary for the TEP repair.

The abdominal musculature and fascia are tented anteriorly and the peritoneal reflection is displaced posteriorly (Fig. 2). With full mobilization, pulsations of the iliac vessels are seen and the spermatic cord is identified. Both

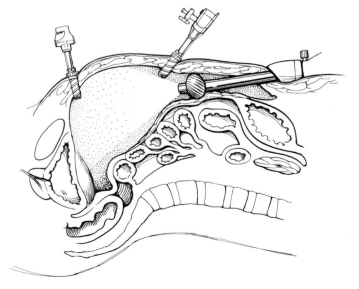

Fig. 1. Sagittal view of a totally extraperitoneal procedure after balloon insufflation in the preperitoneal space. The camera, working through a 10-mm umbilical port site, allows visualization of dissection by graspers working from midline 5-mm ports.

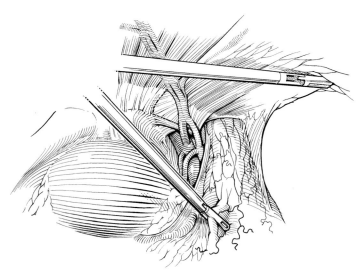

Fig. 2. Caudad view. From the umbilical camera port, a right indirect inguinal hernia is identified. Graspers tease the hernia sac cephalad, with great care taken to avoid injury to the urinary bladder or regional vessels (iliac artery and vein, epigastric artery and vein).

the vas deferens and gonadal vessels are easily appreciated. In thin patients devoid of adipose tissue, the genitofemoral nerve is readily identifiable on the underlying psoas muscle. The peritoneal sac is mobilized and released from the spermatic cord. The medial umbilical ligament is released, care being taken to protect the underlying iliac artery and vein.

With the entire retroperitoneum of a unilateral lower quadrant mobilized and skeletonized, the peritoneal sac is reflected cephalad, and a nylon mesh is placed to cover the defect (Fig. 3). For most groin defects, a 10- by 12-cm piece of mesh is sufficient. Larger pieces of mesh are appropriate for larger hernias or large patients. The mesh is inserted blindly through the 10-mm trocar. With use of the two 5-mm working ports, the mesh is rotated in place to widely cover the indirect, direct, and femoral hernia regions. A tacking device is used to secure the mesh to Cooper's ligament, and the medial, cephalad, and lateral aspects of the mesh are coapted with the abdominal wall. One must refrain from placing tacks on the inferior edge of the mesh and lateral to Cooper's ligament (the "triangle of doom" houses the iliac vessels and the "quadrilateral of pain" hides the ilioinguinal, iliohypogastric, lateral femoral cutaneous, and genitofemoral nerves[4]). The mesh is placed in a tension-free manner and the hernia sac is positioned rostral to the mesh so as to minimize the chance that the peritoneal contents will slide posterior and underneath the just-placed mesh.

The contralateral side is always explored and assessed for potential repair. Under full visualization, the pneumopelvis is released, and the working space is obliterated as

graspers hold the lower, lateral corner of the mesh in place. The 5-mm trocars are removed, followed by the 10-mm camera port. The anterior rectus sheath fasciotomy is closed with a single interrupted 2-0 absorbable suture. All skin incisions are closed with a 4-0 subcuticular absorbable stitch, and a local anesthetic is used to anesthetize all three incisions. The patient is extubated in the operating room and is dismissed later the same day. Oral analgesics are prescribed.

TAPP

The operation is performed with the patient under general anesthesia and positioned supine. Intraoperative decompression of the bladder and stomach is not necessary. Only a limited shave of the mid abdomen at the level of the umbilicus is performed. The lower half of the abdomen and pubic area are prepared in the standard fashion.

A vertical incision is made at the caudal aspect of the umbilicus. Pneumoperitoneum may be induced with a Veress needle or Hasson cannula, followed by placement of a 10-mm cannula. A 30°-angled 10-mm laparoscope is used for the procedure. The surgeon usually stands on the contralateral side with the camera operator for unilateral hernias. For the right-handed surgeon, bilateral or left-sided hernias can be easily repaired standing on the patient's left side.

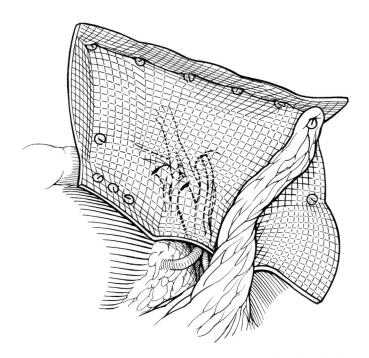

Fig. 3. A 4- by 5-inch panel of mesh is placed and tacked to widely cover the regions of groin hernia: direct, indirect, and femoral. The peritoneal sac must not be allowed access posterior to the inferior or deep portion of the mesh. It is tacked to the right rostral corner of the mesh

With the patient in 10°-Trendelenburg position, the lower abdomen and pelvis can be readily inspected. Both groins should be evaluated for clinically undetected hernias. In some patients with inguinal hernia, no peritoneal protrusion is apparent (only preperitoneal fat is herniated). In this case, repair of the inguinal defect is still required. Two additional ports are placed for TAPP laparoscopic hernia repair, each in the semilunar line at the level of the umbilicus or slightly caudad to this level. For unilateral hernias, 12-mm contralateral and 5-mm ipsilateral ports are placed. For bilateral hernias, two 12-mm ports are inserted (Fig. 4). If a 5-mm tacker is used, both working ports may be 5 mm.

With cautery or scissors, a transverse peritoneal incision is made 5 cm cephalad to the symphysis pubis from near the midline to a point cephalad to the anterior superior iliac spine. The preperitoneal space is dissected bluntly, and the peritoneum is retracted posteriorly with a grasper in the left hand and structures are pushed anteriorly with a grasper in the right hand. If an indirect hernia is present, the peritoneal sac should be grasped with the left hand instrument and pulled cephalad, and small bits of the spermatic cord structures are gently grasped and pushed caudally (Fig. 4). Large indirect hernias can be fully reduced without injury. Small amounts of herniated preperitoneal fat also should be reduced fully within the abdominal cavity. The hernia sac should be separated from the spermatic cord far enough proximally to ensure that the peritoneum does not retract back through the internal ring once the tissues are released from traction. Direct hernias are more readily reduced and usually consist of small, sharply defined defects in the transversalis fascia.

Medially, the bladder is bluntly pushed away from the pubic rami and symphysis pubis. Cooper's ligament is clearly seen near the caudal end of the medial dissection. In the central zone of the operative field, the inferior epigastric vessels are visualized cephalad, the spermatic cord and internal inguinal ring centrally, and the external iliac artery and vein caudally. If a slit piece of mesh is placed, the spermatic cord structures must be cleared circumferentially. Laterally, the abdominal muscular tissue is seen cephalad and the iliopsoas muscle is visualized posterior to the inguinal ligament.

A 15- by 10-cm piece of polypropylene mesh with rounded corners is used, a slit being made to accommodate the spermatic cord. The prosthesis is back-loaded into the 12-mm cannula, pushed out of the cannula with a grasper, and opened. Once the prosthesis has been positioned properly with the tail wrapped around the spermatic cord (Fig. 5), staples are used to fix the mesh into position. Most are placed in the cephalad portion of the mesh. The staples placed near the caudad edge of the mesh are fixed to Cooper's ligament medially, but staples are not placed posterior to the inguinal ligament in the central or lateral portions of the mesh so as to avoid injury to the external iliac vessels and the femoral and femorocutaneous nerves (Fig. 6). For this reason, when the sides of the mesh are approximated around the slit, it is important that the underlying tissues are not included.

After a final inspection of the preperitoneal space for hemorrhage, the peritoneal incision is reapproximated

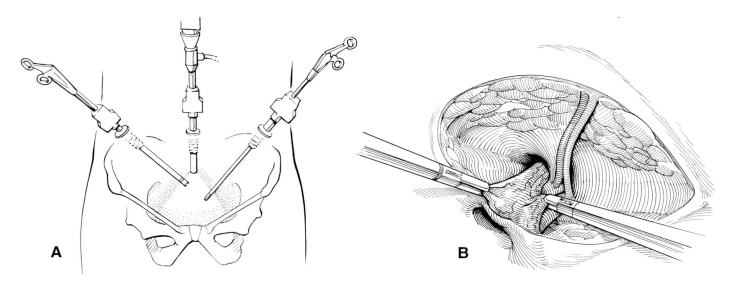

Fig. 4. (A), *Placement of laparoscopic ports for a transabdominal preperitoneal repair of a left indirect inguinal hernia.* (B), *After completion of the preperitoneal dissection, the hernia sac is held in the left-hand grasper and the skeletonized spermatic cord in the right-hand instrument.*

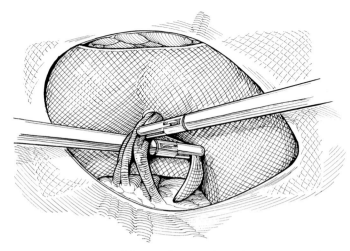

Fig. 5. Positioning of the prosthetic mesh in the preperitoneal space with placement of the lateral tail around the spermatic cord.

with staples. The caudad edge usually can be pulled cephalad; this creates an overlap of the two edges and lessens the risk of herniation and postoperative adhesions (Fig. 7). If the peritoneal incision cannot be closed completely, a sheet of oxidized cellulose is used to cover the peritoneal defect.

The lateral cannulas are removed under direct vision, followed by the umbilical port. The fascial defects at the 10-mm and 12-mm cannula sites are closed with figure-of-eight sutures of 0-polyglactin. The skin edges of all three incisions are approximated with 3-0 subcuticular polyglactin. The wounds are dressed with quarter-inch butterfly strips and adhesive dressings. The patient is extubated in the operating room and is allowed to return home on the same day. Oral analgesics are prescribed.

SURGICAL OUTCOME

TEP

We have performed more than 1,200 TEP procedures at Mayo Clinic in Rochester, Minnesota. With a mean follow-up of more than 3 years, eight hernia recurrences have been identified (0.7%). Six of the eight recurrences occurred within our first 40 surgical repairs. Urinary retention developed in some 70 men, and one superficial wound infection was noted. Patients were unequivocally satisfied with this procedure, reporting that soreness lasted a few days to 2 weeks. Interestingly, all 137 patients undergoing the TEP repair for a recurrent hernia commented that this technique was less painful and less taxing than their previous repair(s). Most patients are fully ambulatory the day of operation and most are back to work within 1 week. Full exertional activities are allowed when they can be performed pain-free.

TAPP

Our results with 206 TAPP hernia repairs in 173 patients (including 31 simultaneous bilateral and 2 delayed

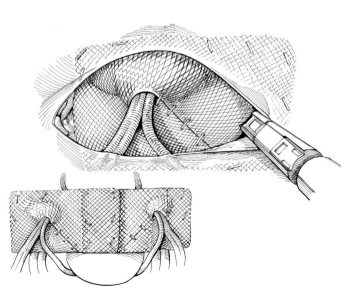

Fig. 6. The staples along the cephalad edge of the prosthesis and those to approximate the slit in the mesh have been placed. The staple gun secures the mesh medially to Cooper's ligament. No staples should be placed in the lateral shaded region.

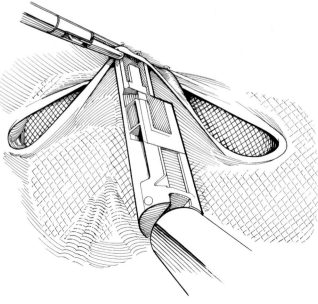

Fig. 7. Closure of the peritoneal incision with overlapping of the peritoneum to minimize adhesions and the risk of herniation through the incision.

contralateral TAPP herniorrhaphies) performed during a 3-year period (1992-1995) were published previously.[5] With a mean follow-up of 29 months, there were six recurrent hernias (2.8%), half of them due to technical problems involving inadequate mesh coverage. Nearly 70% of patients were treated as outpatients. Urinary retention (56%), pain (22%), and nausea or emesis (9%) were the most common causes for overnight admission. One patient with a history of partial cystectomy required conversion to laparotomy for a bladder injury. Four patients required later reoperation for the following complications: trocar site hernias (two), hematoma (one), and genitofemoral nerve entrapment (one). Minor complications, including postoperative discomfort, "seromas," and small hematomas, occurred in 25% of patients and were treated conservatively. The median time to full activity or employment was 7 days for unilateral and 12 days for bilateral TAPP herniorrhaphy.

LONG-TERM FOLLOW-UP

TEP

Numerous studies document low morbidity rates, low recurrence rates, excellent cosmesis, and prompt return to normal activities with the TEP repair.[6-9] Although the cost of repair is initially slightly greater, early return to work or activity is cost-effective.[1] Long-term follow-up showing recurrence rates of less than 3% highlight the advantages of TEP versus older-type open repairs (e.g., Bassini, McVay, Marcy). Advantages of the TEP repair over common, modern open mesh techniques are the ability to repair bilateral defects through the same small incisions, mesh coverage prevents subsequent defects in the femoral region, recurrent hernias are repaired through virginal planes, and cosmesis is superb. Our current rate of recurrence is less than 1%, and the TEP approach is offered to all patients considering general anesthesia.

TAPP

Large single-institution studies[10,11] show low complication rates (4.6%-7.6%) and a recurrence rate of just over 1%. In several randomized, prospective trials comparing open and laparoscopic inguinal herniorrhaphy,[12] costs were greater for the laparoscopic procedure, the overall complication and recurrence rates were comparable, but less narcotic use and recovery time were needed in the patients who had laparoscopy. In uncontrolled comparisons,[13,14] hernia recurrences and the incidence of postoperative complications were higher with TAPP than TEP repairs. Because TAPP repair was the initial laparoscopic procedure performed and TEP repair was adopted only later in these experiences, it is unknown whether these differences are related to surgeon experience or advantages of the TEP technique. The routine creation of a peritoneal incision does create the potential for postoperative adhesions and possible bowel obstruction in the TAPP repair. This is a rare complication when an experienced surgeon performs the operation. However, because of this difficulty and increased experience with TEP repair, many laparoscopic surgeons now prefer the totally extraperitoneal approach.

CONCLUSION

The TEP and TAPP procedures for inguinal hernia are straightforward, viable options in this era of tension-free herniorrhaphy. The recurrence rate is less than 2% for each repair, and patient acceptance has been uniform and complete. Morbidity with these outpatient procedures has been minimal. Although general surgeons at Mayo Clinic retain their own operative preferences, patients with inguinal hernia generally have open repair with an anterior approach with mesh if they want local or attended local anesthesia or have large, incarcerated hernias. Patients with bilateral or recurrent inguinal hernia or with serious cosmetic concerns who prefer general anesthesia are encouraged to undergo TEP or TAPP repairs.

REFERENCES

1. Becker SM, Curcillo PG, Goodyear J, LeBlanc K: The hernia debate: current perspectives on repair techniques. Medical Crossfire: General Surgery Edition. Vol 1. No. 2, 1999
2. Rutkow IM, Robbins AW: Demographic, classificatory, and socioeconomic aspects of hernia repair in the United States. Surg Clin North Am 73:413-426, 1993
3. Oakes D: Hernias. In Fundamentals of Surgery. Edited by JE Niederhuber. Stamford, CT, Appleton & Lange, 1998, pp 390-401
4. Scott DJ, Jones DB: Hernias and abdominal wall defects. In Surgery: Basic Science and Clinical Evidence. Edited by JA Norton, RR Bollinger, AE Chang, SF Lowry, SJ Mulvihill, HI Pass, RW Thompson. New York, Springer-Verlag, 2001, pp 787-823
5. Barry MK, Donohue JH, Harmsen WS, Ilstrup DM: Transabdominal preperitoneal laparoscopic inguinal herniorrhaphy: assessment of initial experience. Mayo Clin Proc 73:717-723, 1998
6. Liem MS, van der Graaf Y, van Steensel CJ, Boelhouwer RU, Clevers GJ, Meijer WS, Stassen LP, Vente JP, Weidema WF, Schrijvers AJ, van Vroonhoven TJ: Comparison of conventional anterior surgery and laparoscopic surgery for inguinal-hernia repair. N Engl J Med 336:1541-1547, 1997
7. Champault G, Rizk N, Catheline J-M, Barrat C, Turner R, Boutelier P: Inguinal hernia repair. Totally pre-peritoneal laparoscopic approach versus Stoppa operation. Randomized trial: 100 cases. Hernia 1:31-36, 1997
8. Bessell JR, Baxter P, Riddell P, Watkin S, Maddern GJ: A randomized controlled trial of laparoscopic extraperitoneal hernia repair as a day surgical procedure. Surg Endosc 10:495-500, 1996
9. Smith CD: Laparoscopic totally extraperitoneal inguinal hernia repair. Operative Tech Gen Surg 1:185-196, 1999
10. Leibl BJ, Schmedt CG, Schwarz J, Daubler P, Kraft K, Schlossnickel B, Bittner R: A single institution's experience with transperitoneal laparoscopic hernia repair. Am J Surg 175:446-451, 1998
11. Birth M, Friedman RL, Melullis M, Weiser HF: Laparoscopic transabdominal preperitoneal hernioplasty: results of 1000 consecutive cases. J Laparoendosc Surg 6:293-300, 1996
12. Memon MA, Rice D, Donohue JH: Laparoscopic herniorrhaphy. J Am Coll Surg 184:325-335, 1997
13. Ramshaw BJ, Tucker JG, Conner T, Mason EM, Duncan TD, Lucas GW: A comparison of the approaches to laparoscopic herniorrhaphy. Surg Endosc 10:29-32, 1996
14. Kald A, Anderberg B, Smedh K, Karlsson M: Transperitoneal or totally extraperitoneal approach in laparoscopic hernia repair: results of 491 consecutive herniorrhaphies. Surg Laparosc Endosc 7:86-89, 1997

Chapter 49

COMMON PEDIATRIC GASTROINTESTINAL DISORDERS

David A. Rodeberg, M.D.
Christopher R. Moir, M.D.

With the exception of appendicitis, most pediatric surgical gastrointestinal disorders are uncommon and diverse. The challenge with children who have abdominal pain is to arrive at a diagnosis in a timely fashion yet use the least invasive and most efficient means of investigation. A simplified diagnostic algorithm that concentrates on the age of the patient and the symptoms of abdominal pain and emesis can be used. Age groups are created by a "rule of threes" that is not only reasonably accurate but also simple and direct for categorizing patients into different risk groups suggesting certain surgical disorders.

This chapter describes the common gastrointestinal disorders by age and provides a systematic description of pediatric surgical gastrointestinal disorders and their treatment. The most common pediatric surgical diseases and procedures are discussed, and some rare conditions are included for completeness and to illustrate recent major advances in surgical therapy.

AGE GROUPS

Infants 0 to 3 Months
The most common presenting symptom in this age group is emesis. Affected infants may be irritable, fussy, or colicky, but the onset of emesis and its character may lead to the correct diagnosis.

Nonbilious Emesis
The two most common causes of nonbilious emesis in infants up to 3 months old are gastroesophageal reflux and hypertrophic pyloric stenosis. The history of the vomiting generally differentiates these two conditions. Gastroesophageal reflux is often described as "spitting up," whereas pyloric stenosis is associated with the three Ps: persistent, progressive, and projectile.

Bilious Emesis
This chapter, and almost all others dealing with bilious emesis in the neonate, advises that "bilious emesis in the neonate is a surgical emergency." Surgical conditions are not necessarily always found, but the possibility of missing a malrotation and volvulus mandates such an approach. Nonsurgical conditions usually involve sepsis or metabolic derangements due to inborn errors of metabolism.

Children 3 Months to 3 Years
In this age group, intussusception is most likely to be diagnosed. Malrotation, Hirschsprung's disease, and incarcerated hernias also may occur in this age group, but with decreasing frequency as the child ages. Bilious emesis loses its significance with increasing age.

Children Older Than 3 Years
In this age group, appendicitis is so common that any other diagnosis should be viewed with some skepticism.

MALROTATION
Abnormalities of rotation and fixation are important conditions that present during infancy and early childhood and are frequently life-threatening. The incidence of malrotation is approximately 1 in 6,000 live births. In autopsy studies, the frequency is approximately 0.5%. This

discrepancy suggests that many patients are asymptomatic throughout life. However, more than half of patients who become symptomatic present within the first month of life and the vast majority within the first year.[1]

The cause of malrotation is best understood by first understanding the developmental transformation of the embryonic midgut. During development, the midgut grows more rapidly than the peritoneal cavity. To accommodate this discrepancy, the midgut herniates into the amnionic cavity during the 4th week of gestation. The superior mesenteric artery (SMA) is the stalk on which this herniation occurs. The bowel then returns to the peritoneal cavity during the 10th week of gestation, and this process is completed by the 11th week. During the return to the peritoneal cavity, the bowel undergoes a 270° counterclockwise rotation around the SMA axis. After the bowel has completely returned to the peritoneal cavity, and until birth, the duodenum and the ascending and descending colon all undergo fixation to the posterior peritoneum. If rotation has occurred normally, the ligament of Treitz should be to the left of the vertebral column, level with the antrum of the stomach, and the duodenum should pass behind the SMA. If rotation is complete for the colon, the cecum should be in the right lower quadrant with the transverse colon anterior to the SMA. If rotation of either the duodenum or colon is arrested, fixation cannot occur.

The most common malrotation anomaly clinically observed is malrotation of the entire midgut in which the ligament of Treitz is located to the right of the vertebral column and the duodenum has a corkscrew configuration (Fig. 1). Duodenal obstruction is a frequent problem and is caused by an intrinsic component due to the corkscrew configuration and an extrinsic component due to Ladd bands. Ladd bands are adhesions that connect the right colon to the right pericolic gutter and extend across the anterior duodenum, causing external compression. These adhesions are remnants of the retroperitoneal attachments that normally secure the ascending colon. Complete malrotation results in the majority of the small bowel being located in the right side of the abdomen. Also, the colon is not rotated, and thus the cecum lies in the mid abdomen. In complete malrotation, the duodenum and colon typically are fused, one on each side of the SMA, and thus the base of the small bowel mesentery is narrowed. This narrow pedicle around the SMA is the axis about which a midgut volvulus revolves.

Among patients with malrotation and fixation abnormalities, 30% to 62% have associated anomalies, usually related to the gastrointestinal tract.[2] The most frequent anomalies include duodenal and other small bowel atresias. Patients with congenital diaphragmatic hernia and abdominal wall defects such as omphalocele and gastroschisis have malrotation caused by an inability to complete

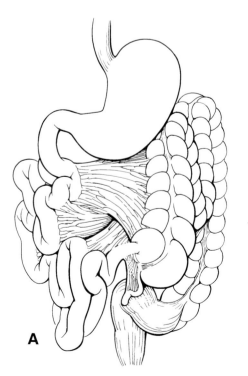
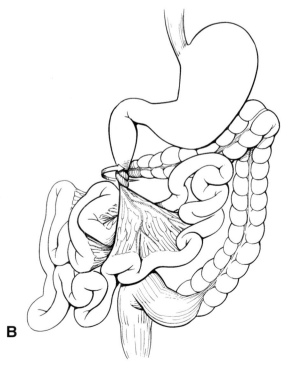

Fig. 1. (A), *Complete malrotation.* (B), *Volvulus. The small bowel has twisted around the superior mesenteric artery axis, wrapping the colon about its base.*

rotation and fixation, with bowel remaining outside the abdominal cavity.

Malrotation can manifest in several ways. Some patients remain asymptomatic throughout life and the malrotation is discovered incidentally during an unrelated work-up. However, most symptomatic patients present before the first year of life. The usual presentations for children with malrotation can be grouped as any combination of volvulus (intestinal ischemia and obstruction), duodenal obstruction, or abdominal pain. Midgut volvulus is a surgical emergency. Delay in treatment can result in intestinal ischemia and necrosis leading to short-gut syndrome or death. Because the obstruction is beyond the ampulla of Vater, these children have bilious emesis. In children, the sudden appearance of bilious emesis is the predominant symptom, initiating the adage that "bilious emesis means malrotation until proven otherwise."[3] Bilious vomiting requires an immediate evaluation to rule out a midgut volvulus. Other signs and symptoms that develop with volvulus include abdominal distention, dehydration, and irritability. Subsequently, as the bowel becomes ischemic, patients become lethargic and septic shock develops. This is manifested by abdominal wall erythema, peritoneal irritation, metabolic acidosis, thrombocytopenia, leukopenia, hemodynamic instability, respiratory compromise, and, with mucosal necrosis, hematemesis or melena. Waiting for signs of intestinal compromise is dangerous, because the ability to salvage ischemic small bowel is greatly diminished and a delay in therapy increases morbidity and mortality. Affected children do not always present with a fulminant course because the volvulus may be incomplete or segmental or may occur intermittently. This presentation usually occurs in older children who have intermittent emesis (which may or may not be bilious), chronic abdominal pain, early satiety, failure to thrive, malabsorption, and weight loss.

There are many causes for the abdominal pain associated with malrotation. Obstruction may lead to crampy abdominal pain and bilious emesis. Occlusion of the mesenteric venous and lymphatic systems leads to edema of the bowel wall, mesentery, and lymph nodes, all of which may cause some discomfort. Chronic arterial insufficiency caused by a partial volvulus may result in intestinal angina, chronic pain, and diarrhea.

As stated previously, duodenal obstruction occurs in patients with malrotation for two reasons: the corkscrew configuration of the nonrotated duodenum and the presence of Ladd bands.[4] These lesions lead to the "double bubble" sign: the presence of bowel gas in the stomach and in the proximal duodenum on abdominal radiography.

The standard for diagnosis of malrotation is an upper gastrointestinal series.[5] If the ligament of Treitz is identified to the left of the vertebral column at a level parallel to the gastric antrum or duodenal bulb, malrotation is not present. If this criterion is not met, the patient has abnormal rotation. Typically with malrotation, the ligament of Treitz is found to the right of the vertebral column and inferior to the duodenal bulb (Fig. 2 A). In patients with volvulus, an obstruction is present in the third portion of the duodenum, classically having the appearance of a bird's beak on an upper gastrointestinal contrast radiograph. If the duodenum is only partially obstructed, a spiral- or corkscrew-type abnormality may be observed (Fig. 2 B). In the past, a barium enema examination frequently was used to diagnose malrotation. However, an abnormally positioned cecum is present in approximately 15% of patients with normal rotation of the small intestine. More importantly, patients with malrotation and duodenal obstruction may have a normally positioned cecum. Ultrasonography has been used to evaluate patients for malrotation. Normally, the superior mesenteric vein (SMV) lies to the right of the SMA. If the SMV lies either anterior or to the left of the SMA, malrotation may be present. However, this study should not be relied on as the definitive test for malrotation.

The preoperative management of malrotation is straightforward. Children who are acutely ill with midgut volvulus or obstruction require urgent operative intervention. Operative therapy should not be delayed. Resuscitation can be performed in the operating room. These patients need aggressive fluid resuscitation, broad-spectrum antibiotics, nasogastric decompression, and placement of a urinary catheter. Blood tests, including a type and cross-match for possible transfusion, should be done. In contrast, children who are clinically asymptomatic should have operation delayed pending further evaluation.

The correction of malrotation involves seven surgical steps: 1) incision and evisceration, 2) correction of malrotation, 3) mobilization of the duodenum, 4) lysis of Ladd bands and widening of the mesenteric base, 5) search for intrinsic obstruction, 6) appendectomy, and 7) placement of the small bowel to the right side of the abdomen and colon to the left. The incision is usually transverse in the right upper quadrant. When the peritoneal cavity is entered, the small bowel is found to be anterior and is visualized before the transverse colon. The small bowel should be completely eviscerated to determine whether midgut volvulus is present. After the small bowel is eviscerated, the next step is to reduce the bowel if a volvulus is present. Usually the volvulus occurs in a clockwise direction; therefore, the bowel should be turned counterclockwise to correct the volvulus. Reduction of a volvulus usually necessitates turning the bowel counterclockwise more than 360°. After reduction of the volvulus associated with bowel ischemia or necrosis, restoration of blood flow may cause the release of toxic substances from the bowel, inducing hypotension. Therefore, before reduction occurs, the anesthetist should be alerted and a fluid bolus given. Once the small bowel has been turned counterclockwise sufficiently to flatten the mesentery, warm sponges should be placed on the bowel and the bowel observed for a time. If a single area of necrosis is present, it should be resected and either a primary anastomosis or end-ostomies created, depending on peritoneal contamination and the patient's condition. If multiple areas of bowel are necrotic, they should be resected and a proximal stoma created. One of the goals is to retain as much bowel length as possible; thus, if segments of bowel are of questionable viability, they should be left in continuity and a second-look procedure performed within 24 to 36 hours. After the midgut volvulus is corrected, attention should be turned to division of the Ladd bands. These bands extend from the right pericolic gutter, across the duodenum to the right colon. These bands should be completely divided on both the lateral and the medial aspects of the duodenum until the duodenum appears to be grossly normal with no evidence of external compression. A Kocher maneuver is required to lyse the Ladd bands fully.

The next step in operative management is to widen the mesenteric base. As previously stated, if the base is narrow, the patient is predisposed to the development of volvulus. Dividing the adhesions that connect the duodenum to the cecum and right colon widens the mesenteric base. To ensure that the base of the mesentery is widened, the peritoneal covering over the mesentery surrounding the SMA also should be divided.

Next, attention should be turned to the duodenum. The duodenum should be mobilized fully with the Kocher maneuver and mobilization of the ligament of Treitz. In doing so, the entire duodenum and proximal jejunum should be easily visualized and areas of obstruction identified. Areas of small intestinal atresia should be sought and corrected. An appendectomy should be performed because the cecum will no longer be in the right lower quadrant after the Ladd procedure. A subsequent bout of appendicitis might then present atypically and not be recognized, putting the patient at increased risk. This risk can be abolished by appendectomy. Once all these procedures have been completed, the small bowel should be returned to the abdominal cavity by placing the third and fourth portions of the duodenum straight down the right lateral aspect of the peritoneal cavity and then placing the rest of the small bowel in the right side of the peritoneal cavity. Finally, the entire colon should be distributed in the left side of the peritoneal cavity with the cecum positioned in the left upper quadrant.

Postoperatively, patients frequently require continued intravenous fluid hydration and nasogastric decompres-

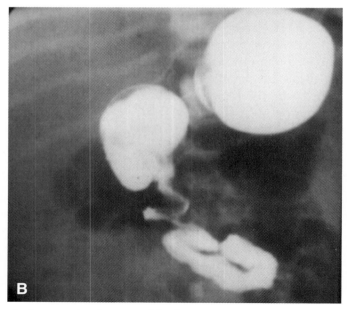

Fig. 2. Upper gastrointestinal contrast studies. (A), Malrotation without volvulus, typical malposition of duodenojejunal juncture. Small bowel is to right of midline, and the colon and cecum are to the left. (B), Malrotation with volvulus. Duodenum has corkscrew configuration.

sion for several days before bowel function returns and enteral nutrition can be initiated. Postoperative complications include recurrent volvulus in 0% to 10% of patients.[6] Predisposing factors for recurrent volvulus include an unrecognized narrow mesenteric base and lack of peritoneal adhesions. Gastrointestinal motility disturbances are common.[7] Small bowel obstruction due to adhesions, prolonged ileus, or bleeding caused by aggressive operative dissection are all possible complications. The most devastating postoperative complication is short-gut syndrome. Approximately 18% of cases of short-gut syndrome are due to midgut volvulus.[8]

The operative mortality rate for this procedure ranges from 3% to 9% and is usually attributed to volvulus, intestinal gangrene, prematurity, or other associated congenital abnormalities.[2]

PYLORIC STENOSIS

Pyloric stenosis is common in pediatric patients, occurring in approximately 1 in 300 live births. There is a familial association in approximately 5% of cases. It occurs most commonly in children 2 to 6 weeks old. It also seems to be more common in white first-born males. The obstruction is due to hypertrophy of the circular smooth muscle at the pylorus causing an obstruction of the gastric outlet. The classic clinical presentation is projectile, nonbilious vomiting. Patients usually have intermittent emesis that progressively becomes worse. After emesis, the children usually continue to be hungry and are willing to eat again. Because these children have prolonged episodes of emesis, it is not uncommon for them to be dehydrated and have electrolyte abnormalities.

The physical examination is facilitated by placing a nasogastric tube to decompress the stomach, which allows for easier palpation of the pyloric area. A palpable pyloric "olive" should be present in 70% to 80% of patients. If an olive is palpated, no radiographic work-up is required. However, if the olive cannot be palpated, the patient should undergo radiographic imaging. Ultrasonography frequently shows the pylorus to be more than 15 mm long or more than 3.5 mm wide (Fig. 3). An upper gastrointestinal study shows an elongated pylorus with a narrow string sign of contrast passing through the pylorus. Frequently, the stomach is dilated and gastric emptying is delayed. We favor use of an upper gastrointestinal series to also obtain information about gastroesophageal reflux disease, pyloric atresia, duodenal web, or malrotation.

Once the diagnosis has been made, the child should be prepared for the operating room. The orogastric tube should be on suction to keep the stomach decompressed. Patients are frequently dehydrated and have hypochloremic,

hypokalemic metabolic alkalosis. For correction of these conditions, the patient should be given multiple boluses of 0.45% NaCl with 20 mEq KCl. For severe hypochloremia, 0.9% NaCl with 20 mEq KCl is used. If the patient has no electrolyte abnormalities and is not severely dehydrated, the operation can take place. However, if the child has electrolyte abnormalities, then fluid resuscitation and electrolyte correction should be accomplished first.

There are two operative procedures for pyloric stenosis: the classic Ramstedt pyloromyotomy and laparoscopic pyloromyotomy. For the Ramstedt procedure, a right upper quadrant transverse abdominal incision is made through the rectus abdominis muscle into the peritoneal cavity. The pylorus is brought through the incision to the surface, and a longitudinal incision is made through the serosa over the length of the hypertrophied pyloric musculature. The knife is then rotated and the knife handle is used to break apart the hypertrophied musculature further until the mucosa can be seen. A Benson spreader is used to distance the muscular edges from each other so that the pylorus is widely patent. Once this has been completed, some saline should be placed over the mucosa and air instilled into the gastric lumen to ensure that there has been no mucosal perforation. If a mucosal injury is found, two options are available. If the injury to the mucosa is small, a primary repair of the mucosa can be performed with interrupted polyglactin 910 sutures. If the mucosal defect is large, the pyloromyotomy should be completely closed, the bowel rotated, and a new pyloromyotomy attempted elsewhere on the pylorus.

Recently, laparoscopic pyloromyotomy has become feasible. For this procedure, a laparoscope is inserted through the umbilicus and 5-mm trocars are placed, one in the right upper quadrant and one in the left upper quadrant. The pylorus is secured with a Babcock clamp through one of the trocars and a beaver-blade scalpel is inserted through the other. With the scalpel, the pyloromyotomy is achieved in the same fashion as the open procedure.

Regardless of which procedure is used to perform the pyloromyotomy, the patient continues to receive fluids intravenously and enteral nutrition is begun 6 hours postoperatively. In the past, a protocol of progressive increases in feeding volume and concentration was used. However, currently patients are fed ad libitum by 6 hours after operation. Patients tolerate this feeding without difficulty, and it has decreased the duration of hospitalization. It is not uncommon for children to have one or two more episodes of emesis as they are being fed during the first 24 hours. However, if the emesis continues beyond 48 hours, the pyloromyotomy may be incomplete. Reoperation then is needed for completion of the pyloromyotomy.

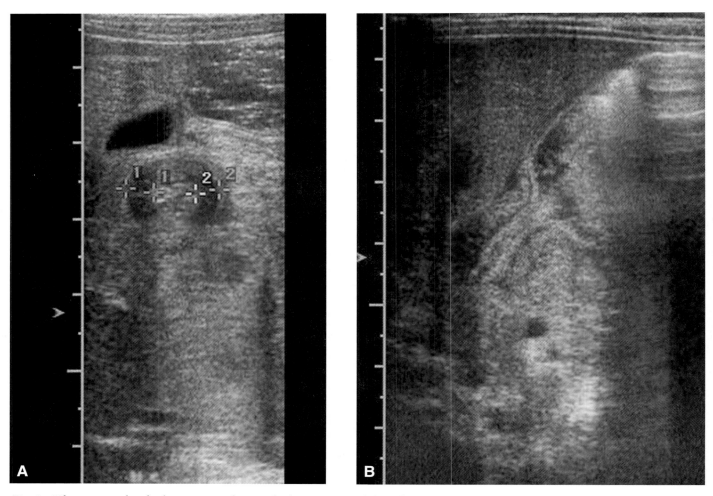

Fig. 3. Ultrasonographs of pyloric stenosis showing both cross-section (A) and transverse (B) views.

ATRESIA

Small bowel atresia or stenosis is a common cause of small bowel obstruction in the newborn. The incidence has been estimated to be 1 in 300 to 1,500 live births.[9] The cause of these lesions is hypothesized to be an ischemic event during gestation.

Several functional gastrointestinal abnormalities are associated with these lesions. The proximal dilated intestine frequently has abnormal motility.[10] The dysmotility usually resolves after the mechanical obstruction has been corrected. However, the more dilated the bowel, the longer the dysmotility persists. Patients also have a transient impairment of intestinal absorption and mucosal transport.

A classification system developed by Grosfeld divides these abnormalities into four major groups (Fig. 4). It is hypothesized that type 1 atresias result from incomplete recanalization of the embryonic intestine. However, the other types (II-IV) seem to be more consistent with intrauterine ischemia or interruptions of mesenteric blood flow during gestation.

Atresias frequently are diagnosed during routine prenatal ultrasonography. Intestinal atresia or bowel obstruction is suspected in women with maternal polyhydramnios because a proximal obstruction results in diminished intestinal absorption of amniotic fluid.[11] Frequently, prenatal ultrasonography also reveals multiple dilated loops of intestine. After delivery, abdominal distention and bilious vomiting are the major findings.[12] As expected, the magnitude of abdominal distention is related to the point of obstruction; distal lesions produce greater amounts of abdominal distention. Many children also fail to pass meconium.

The diagnosis of intestinal atresia is confirmed from plain abdominal radiographs that show distended, air-filled bowel loops and an absence of distal bowel gas. A diatrizoate meglumine-diatrizoate sodium enema should be performed to rule out meconium ileus or large bowel atresia and to confirm the diagnosis of small bowel obstruction. The enema study in small bowel atresia should show a microcolon and a small, unused ileum. An upper gastrointestinal contrast study is not routinely necessary.

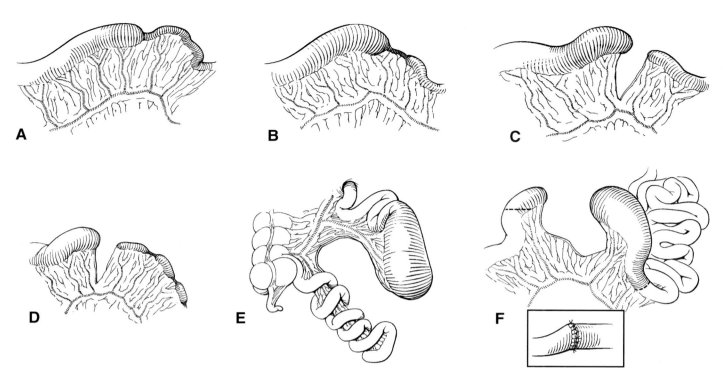

Fig. 4. Classification of intestinal atresia: (A), *type 1, membranous atresia with intact bowel and mesentery;* (B), *type II, blind ends separated by a fibrous cord;* (C), *type IIIa, blind ends separated by a V-shaped mesenteric defect;* (D), *type IV, multiple atresias ("string of sausages");* (E), *type IIIb, "apple peel" or "Christmas tree" atresia;* (F), *operative strategies for dealing with size discrepancies of bowel ends include resection of dilated portion with a primary anastomosis or, if this requires too much bowel to be removed, the distal end can be opened at an oblique angle to widen the distal bowel.*

The treatment of affected newborns is straightforward. They should receive intravenous fluid resuscitation, nasogastric tube decompression, and antibiotics. A right upper quadrant transverse abdominal incision is performed, and the small bowel is eviscerated. The entire small bowel should be inspected. A classic transition point is frequently observed. Atresias are equally distributed between the jejunum and ileum. Because more than 20% of patients have more than one site of atresia, the entire small bowel and colon must be evaluated.[13] Evaluation includes injection of saline distal to the obvious transition point and the milking of the saline through the small bowel and colon to ensure that there are no other obstructions. The goals of this operative procedure are to resect the stricture(s), restore gastrointestinal tract continuity, and maintain intestinal length. Frequently, the proximal segment of the bowel is very dilated and may appear ischemic. All nonviable tissue should be excised. If bowel length permits, the dilated segment also should be resected. The resection of the dilated bowel is thought to hasten the return of normal bowel motility. The distal unused small bowel is opened along the antimesenteric border so that an end-to-oblique single-layer anastomosis can be performed.

When small bowel atresias occur in association with gastroschisis, they are frequently difficult to identify during the initial operation because of the peritoneal inflammation. Affected children should be managed by returning the bowel to the peritoneal cavity and repairing the gastroschisis defect. After 6 to 8 weeks, the children should be re-explored. The peritoneal and intestinal inflammation will have resolved enough to allow adequate exploration and repair of any atresias that may be present. If the peritoneal inflammation is minimal, a primary resection and anastomosis may be performed.

The outcome for management of atresias in children is excellent in that survival rates are 90%.[14] The most common complications are anastomotic problems, such as leak or stricture, which may occur in 10% to 15% of children. Necrotizing enterocolitis and adhesions causing small bowel obstruction also are frequent complications. Short-gut syndrome occurs if less than 20 to 30 cm of small bowel remains after repair of the atresias.[15] Patients with short-gut syndrome frequently require prolonged parenteral nutrition with concurrent enteral nutrition until the small bowel has adapted. The dysmotility of the dilated proximal segment of bowel may persist for several months.

TRACHEOESOPHAGEAL FISTULA

Tracheoesophageal fistula (TEF) is present in approximately 1 of 1,500 to 4,000 live births. The cause of TEF is uncertain; however, it is probably related to a defect during fetal development. The trachea and esophagus start as a single bud off the primitive foregut. During the 4th week of gestation, lateral invaginations occur that divide the trachea from the esophagus. Some defect is thought to occur during this period which causes the development of the TEF. A genetic component also seems to be present; however, the exact mechanism is unknown.

There are many variants of TEF (Fig. 5). The most common is type C, a proximal esophageal atresia and a distal TEF. It occurs in 85% of all patients. Type A, the next most common (8%), is an isolated esophageal atresia. The type E fistula is the classically described H-type fistula with an intact trachea and esophagus but a small communication in the cervical region. This variant occurs in 4% of patients. Type B is a distal esophageal atresia and proximal TEF. Type D is an esophageal atresia with both distal and proximal fistulas. Both types B and D occur in 1% of patients.

All types of TEF, other than the H type, are usually diagnosed within the first days of life. It is also becoming more common for TEF to be detected prenatally during routine ultrasonography. Typical findings on prenatal ultrasonography include a dilated proximal esophageal pouch and polyhydramnios. At birth, patients experience considerable respiratory distress, related to the preferential streaming of inhaled air into the stomach rather than the lungs. Excessive salivation can be present with secretions collecting in the proximal esophageal pouch and subsequently spilling over into the lungs. Also, feeding problems are common, including choking, coughing, and cyanosis. Because gas can preferentially flow into the stomach, patients can present with acute gastric dilatation. This exacerbates gastroesophageal reflux, forcing gastric contents through the fistula into the trachea. This, in turn, causes a chemical pneumonitis.

The diagnosis of TEF can be confirmed by placement of a nasogastric tube into the proximal esophageal pouch. Chest and abdominal radiography can confirm that the nasogastric tube was not passed and may show the tube curled within the esophagus (Fig. 6). If there is a communication between the trachea and the distal esophagus, air will be present within the gastrointestinal tract. If, however, there is no communication between the gastrointestinal tract and the trachea distally, then the patient will have a gasless abdomen. Occasionally, it is necessary to instill a very small volume of barium into the proximal esophageal pouch to confirm the diagnosis.

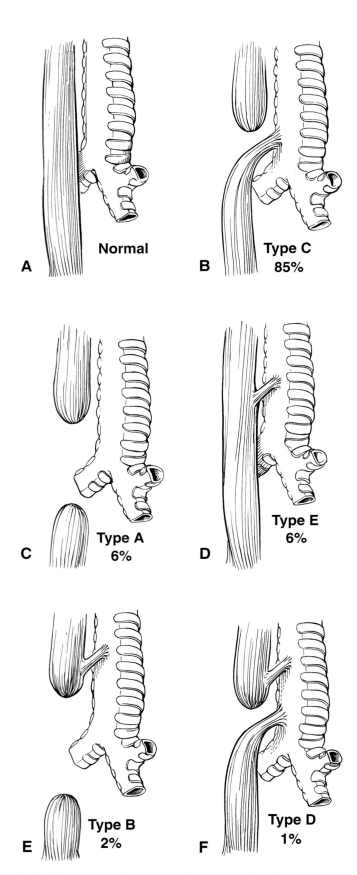

Fig. 5. The gross classification and frequencies of tracheoesophageal fistula.

If TEF is suspected, it is important to evaluate the patient for other associated anomalies. Anomalies are found in 50% to 70% of patients, the most common being cardiac lesions, found in 30% of patients. The most common cardiac anomalies include patent ductus arteriosus and septal defects. Other gastrointestinal tract abnormalities occur in 12% of patients and include imperforate anus, duodenal atresia, and pyloric stenosis. Trisomy 21 and trisomy 18 are also associated with TEF. VACTERL syndrome (vertebral body, anal, cardiac, tracheoesophageal fistulas, renal, and limb anomalies) is found in 30% of patients. For evaluation of these anomalies, cardiac echocardiography should be performed. During the test, the aorta should be evaluated to determine whether there is a left-sided or right-sided arch. This information can affect the approach that is used to repair the TEF. The patient should also undergo ultrasonography to evaluate the kidneys, ureters, and bladder. Radiography of the vertebral column and upper extremities should be done. Physical examination is sufficient to evaluate the anus.

Once the diagnosis of TEF has been made, a sump suction catheter should be placed into the proximal esophageal pouch to prevent the collection of secretions and minimize the risk of aspiration. For prevention of reflux of gastric contents into the distal esophagus and then into the trachea, the patient should be maintained in a reverse Trendelenburg position. Patients who are stable from a cardiac and respiratory point of view may undergo repair of their TEF at 24 to 48 hours after birth.

In the operating room, the patients are placed in left lateral decubitus position for a right thoracic incision. The dissection is done in an extrapleural approach through the fourth intercostal space. The azygos vein is divided, and the fistula is usually found behind the azygos vein. The fistula is divided, leaving a small cuff of the fistula tract on the trachea. The trachea is closed with interrupted 5-0 sutures. Once the proximal esophageal pouch is identified, a primary end-to-end esophageal anastomosis is performed. A chest tube is placed to provide drainage and is brought out extrapleurally.

If the distance between the ends of the esophagus is large enough to prevent primary closure without undue tension, several maneuvers can be performed. First, both the proximal and the distal esophagus should be dissected for maximal mobilization. If this is unsuccessful, then a circular myotomy can be performed in the proximal pouch, the mucosa being left intact. The myotomy allows the proximal pouch to be lengthened. If the circular myotomy would not create enough length, then a spiral myotomy can be performed along the length of the proximal pouch; this gives more length to the proximal esophagus than the circular myotomy. A second option is to bring the ends of the esophagus as close as possible to each other and then secure them to the periosteum of the vertebral column with a nonabsorbable suture. After the patient has had a chance to grow, a delayed repair can be performed. In pure esophageal atresia, patients with type A are more likely to have a large distance between the esophageal ends. In this instance, three options are available. The first is to do a gastric pull-up and create a thoracic or cervical esophageal-gastric anastomosis. This requires a combined abdominal and thoracic or abdominal and cervical approach. The second option necessitates a colonic interposition, in which either the right or the left colon, based on a vascular pedicle, is brought up through a retrogastric position into the chest and anastomosed to the esophagus and stomach. The third option is similar to the second, except that an isolated small bowel segment is used as the conduit instead of colon.

Patients who are unstable and not candidates for immediate repair may undergo a delayed repair after their cardiac

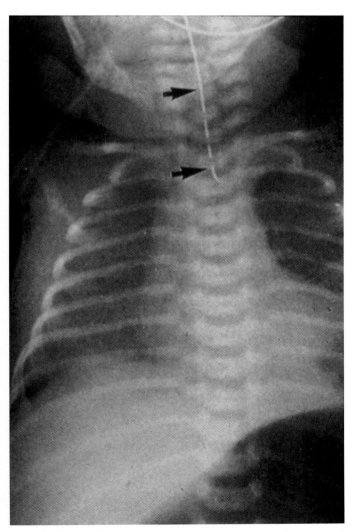

Fig. 6. Chest radiograph showing a nasogastric tube in proximal pouch of a tracheoesophageal fistula (arrows).

or pulmonary disease has been corrected. These children are managed by nasogastric decompression of the proximal pouch. Total parenteral nutrition is provided, and these patients frequently also require a gastrostomy tube to provide gastric decompression. If the patient is having difficulty ventilating because of the preferential gas flow into the stomach, then a Fogarty catheter can be used to occlude the fistula. If this is not successful at stopping the gas flow, the patient may require immediate division of the fistula without any attempts being made to reconstruct the esophagus. The esophageal reconstruction can be delayed until the patient is more stable.

Patients with an H-type tracheoesophageal fistula do not require a thoracic approach. The fistula occurs in the cervical area and therefore is approached through a right cervical incision. Preoperatively, patients should have a catheter placed through the fistula during bronchoscopy. This aids in identification of the fistula during operation. The fistula is divided and the openings oversewn.

Postoperatively, patients with TEF continue to require nasogastric decompression. The end of the tube frequently is placed superior to the anastomosis. However, some surgeons prefer placing it through the anastomosis and into the stomach. This allows access for subsequent enteral nutrition. The patient is not fed by mouth for approximately 7 days and then undergoes a radiologic contrast study of the esophagus. If there is no evidence of any leak, the patient is fed, and after 24 hours the chest tube is removed. A leak occurs in 10% to 20% of patients. If there is no distal obstruction, this should close spontaneously within several weeks. While this is awaited, the patient should receive nothing by mouth, the chest tube should be left in place, and nutrition should be provided either parenterally or enterally distal to the stomach.

The overall survival rate for patients with TEF is approximately 80% to 90%. The mortality rate is usually related to the presence of other anomalies, the most important of which are the cardiac lesions. The distal esophagus in patients with TEF frequently has decreased motility, resulting in 25% to 30% of patients having problems with gastroesophageal reflux disease. The reflux often first becomes apparent postoperatively. Many patients will require therapy with histamine$_2$-receptor blockers or proton pump inhibitors. Unfortunately, a lower esophageal stricture will develop in some of these patients. These patients should be treated initially with dilation. However, the stricture may re-form. These patients should then undergo a loose Nissen or a Thal fundoplication. In 15% to 30% of patients, a stricture will develop at the esophageal anastomosis. This usually can be corrected with dilations, either intraoperatively or with fluoroscopy. Strictures may necessitate repetitive dilations 3 or 4 times over several

months. However, if this nonoperative therapy is unsuccessful, then an operation with excision of the stricture and primary anastomosis is necessary. A recurrent TEF can occur in 10% of patients and is usually the result of a leak at the anastomotic site. A recurrent TEF will not spontaneously close and immediate operative repair is needed. Tracheomalacia occurs in 25% of patients and is related to dilation of the proximal esophageal pouch, causing compression of the tracheal rings.

NECROTIZING ENTEROCOLITIS

Necrotizing enterocolitis (NEC) is the most common surgical emergency in the neonatal intensive care unit, affecting from 1% to 7% of all admissions to the unit. The mortality rate is 20% to 40%.[16] NEC may occur in up to 10% of premature infants weighing less than 1,500 g.[17] In more than 90% of cases the patient is premature, has low birth weight, and is physiologically stressed. As the neonate matures, both within and outside the uterus, the susceptibility to NEC decreases. NEC can involve any segment of the gastrointestinal tract but seems to involve commonly the distal ileum and cecum. These are watershed areas of the SMA. NEC involves the distal small bowel and colon in 44% of affected infants, only the small bowel in 30%, and only the colon in 26%.[18] In approximately 20% of patients, the entire small bowel and colon are involved (pannecrosis), a condition incompatible with survival. In more than 50% of patients, multiple segments of bowel are involved, and the disease occurs in a patchy distribution.

An episode of NEC is frequently first detected from signs of physiologic instability such as lethargy, temperature instability, apnea or bradycardia, hypoglycemia, and hemodynamic instability.[19] Patients recently may have begun formula feeds and have sudden development of signs of gastrointestinal distress, including increased gastric residuals or bilious aspirate from the orogastric tube, abdominal distention, vomiting, blood per rectum, and decreased stool and urine output. These initial findings are consistent with and often difficult to distinguish from neonatal septicemia. With disease progression, bloody stools may develop. Patients with bowel necrosis and perforation will have evidence of peritonitis with abdominal wall erythema, edema, tenderness, or a palpable inflammatory mass. Systemic inflammatory response syndrome is evidenced by lethargy, oliguria, hypotension, and tachycardia. Temperature instability and episodes of apnea and bradycardia also frequently occur. Occasionally, the leukocyte count is increased, there is a left shift, or, more commonly, neutropenia is present, which may denote a worse prognosis. A decreasing platelet count indicates intestinal ischemia and necrosis and may be related to the systemic inflammatory response syndrome associated with disease progression. A metabolic acidosis frequently occurs as a result of the intravascular hypovolemia and the septic response.

Abdominal radiographs show several findings. The most common finding is gas-filled dilated loops of bowel. Evidence of pneumatosis intestinalis is the hallmark of NEC (Fig. 7). This finding, however, may be absent in up to 20% of patients with NEC. Pneumatosis is usually seen early and transiently in the course of NEC. Portal vein gas also may be seen in the area of the liver shadow. Sequential radiographs may show the presence of persistent and fixed dilated loops of the small intestine. These fixed loops are suggestive of, but not diagnostic of, intestinal necrosis; in approximately 43% of patients, the condition resolves with medical management.[20] Plain abdominal radiographs also may show ascites that can be associated with intestinal necrosis. Extensive ascites mandates that paracentesis be performed to determine whether necrosis or perforation has occurred. The only absolute indication for operation is perforation, which usually results in free intraperitoneal air. This finding is best visualized with a left lateral decubitus view, in which a liver-air interface can be easily seen next to the abdominal wall. Perforation may occur in up to 30% of patients without any free intraperitoneal air demonstrable by radiographic studies.[21] As a general rule, contrast studies are to be avoided in the diagnosis of NEC.

Once the diagnosis of NEC has been established, medical therapy is initiated unless there is a clear indication for laparotomy, such as intestinal perforation. The initial management of NEC involves discontinuing any oral intake and decompressing the stomach with an orogastric tube. Because of continued third-space fluid losses into the bowel lumen, the bowel wall, and the peritoneal cavity, the patient usually requires intravenous fluid therapy at 1.5 to 2 times maintenance volume. Boluses of additional fluid may be required to maintain urine output at more than 1 mL/kg per hour. Serial physical examinations, abdominal radiography, and determination of leukocyte counts, platelet counts, and electrolyte values are performed every 6 hours. Blood cultures are obtained and broad-spectrum antibiotic therapy is initiated. Fortunately, with aggressive medical management and support, 60% to 70% of patients will improve and a laparotomy will be avoided.

There are several key indicators for the conversion from medical management to operative care. The three best indicators for operative intervention are pneumoperitoneum, portal vein gas, or positive results on paracentesis.[21] Several other indications for operative intervention

qualify as markers for intestinal gangrene. Optimally, an operation should be performed when gangrene is present but before perforation occurs. This scenario is associated with a lower mortality rate (30%) than when the disease has progressed to perforation (64%). The markers of intestinal gangrene are less sensitive and specific and thus are not, by themselves, absolute indications for operation. Examples include erythema of the abdominal wall, a palpable mass, portal vein gas, or a persistently dilated loop of bowel on plain radiography. In addition, patients who do not respond to maximal medical management and continue to have clinical deterioration (worsening thrombocytopenia, acidosis, and hemodynamic instability) usually have necrotic bowel and require surgical resection. Pneumatosis intestinalis alone should not be used as an indication for operation, because more than half of patients will improve and not require operative intervention.

The main goals of laparotomy are to remove gangrenous bowel, to create an ostomy and a mucous fistula,

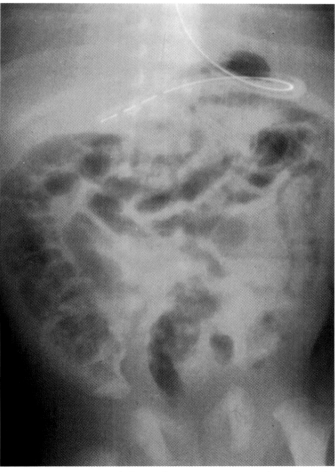

Fig. 7. Pneumatosis coli form of necrotizing enterocolitis. In right lower quadrant, cystic form of pneumatosis is shown. Loops of bowel and the rectum are outlined by the linear form of pneumatosis.

and to preserve as much bowel length as possible. With the patient under general endotracheal anesthesia, a supraumbilical or infraumbilical transverse incision is made. The entire gastrointestinal tract from the gastroesophageal junction to the distal rectosigmoid should be inspected. All areas of frankly necrotic or compromised bowel are identified during this exploration. The extent of involvement then is assessed, with the knowledge that approximately 30 cm of small bowel is needed to prevent the complication of short-gut syndrome. If a single area, such as the ileum and right colon, is involved, necrotic bowel can be resected utilizing a diverting end ileostomy and mucous fistula. Unlike adult patients, the ostomy and mucous fistula may be brought out through the incision in proximity without concern for the development of a wound infection or increased morbidity.[22] If multiple areas needing resection are discovered, primary reanastomosis of the distal bowel segments with a proximal stoma at the first point of resection is the procedure of choice. Patients with multiple areas of bowel ischemia but not frank necrosis may benefit from a high diverting jejunostomy with bowel rest. If the patient remains unstable, reexploration can be performed 24 to 48 hours later. The stomas are secured to the fascia with a few interrupted absorbable sutures with 1 to 2 cm of bowel protruding. No attempt is made to mature the ostomies because maturation will occur spontaneously during the next several days. The skin is left open or approximated with a few adhesive tapes, and the ostomies are covered with nonadherent gauze containing bismuth tribromophenate and petrolatum.

Before intestinal continuity is reestablished, a barium enema study or distal (mucous fistula) colostography should be performed to ensure that there are no areas of stricture in the remaining distal bowel. In 12% to 45% of patients, a stricture develops after a severe NEC episode. The strictures usually appear 4 to 6 weeks after injury.[23] They occur as a result of submucosal fibrosis in areas that previously had been ischemic. Colonic strictures typically are seen, but strictures of the small intestine occasionally are present. All strictures should be resected at the time of stoma takedown.

The mortality rate for these critically ill infants has improved steadily during the past decade as a result of early medical or surgical intervention and improved neonatal critical care. Overall, approximately 50% of patients who weigh less than 1,000 g survive an episode of severe NEC. In larger preterm infants (>1,500 g), approximately 75% survive.[24] Among those who survive, a considerable number will have short-gut syndrome, necessitating long-term management and support. Patients at risk for short-gut syndrome that necessitates prolonged parenteral nutrition have less than 20 to 30 cm of small bowel with an ileocecal valve or 40 to 50 cm without an ileocecal valve. Approximately 6% of patients will have a recurrence of their NEC within 1 month of their first episode, often requiring reinstitution of medical management and possibly operation. Another major long-term complication in patients with NEC is neurologic injury as a result of prematurity and perinatal stress. It occurs at rates similar to those in premature infants in general.

MECONIUM SYNDROMES

Meconium ileus is a form of small bowel obstruction that presents in the first few days of life. It is often the earliest manifestation of cystic fibrosis and occurs in 10% to 20% of patients with cystic fibrosis.[25] Thickened meconium adheres to the mucosal surface of the bowel, causing an obstruction in the terminal ileum. All patients who have meconium ileus should be tested for cystic fibrosis with a sweat chloride test. There is no correlation between the development of meconium ileus and the severity of future pancreatic exocrine insufficiency. However, a disease called "meconium ileus equivalent," which occurs later in childhood or in adults, results in partial or complete small bowel obstruction due to abnormally thick fecal material. Meconium ileus equivalent results from diminished exocrine pancreatic secretion or inadequate pancreatic enzyme replacement, abnormal intestinal mucus, and decreased intestinal motility. The treatment of this condition is the same as that of meconium ileus.

Meconium ileus is an accumulation of inspissated meconium in the terminal ileum. The disease usually presents in an otherwise healthy-appearing neonate in whom, during the first few days of life, abdominal distention develops in association with bilious vomiting and an inability to pass meconium. Abdominal radiographs show multiple dilated intestinal loops consistent with intestinal obstruction. Air bubbles are often identified within the meconium in the right lower quadrant and are referred to as a soap-bubble sign or a ground-glass sign.[26]

The initial management of patients with meconium ileus includes intravenous fluid resuscitation, nasogastric tube decompression, and the administration of broad-spectrum antibiotics. Patients with uncomplicated meconium ileus should undergo a meglumine diatrizoate enema, which can be both diagnostic and therapeutic. The enema should not be attempted in patients with evidence of a complicated meconium ileus, volvulus, necrotic bowel, atresia, perforation, or peritonitis. On infusion of the meglumine diatrizoate into the bowel, the contrast is refluxed up around the meconium in the terminal ileum and proximal to the obstruction. The hyperosmolar fluid then draws free water into the bowel lumen, liquefying the meconium pellets and allowing them to be passed spontaneously. Because the preparation draws free water into the lumen of the bowel, the patient must be adequately hydrated before and during the enema. If the first attempt to reflux contrast material above the level of the obstruction is unsuccessful, the enema can be repeated 2 or 3 times. This treatment of meconium ileus has a success rate of more than 50%.[27] However, if the enema is unsuccessful after several attempts, then the patient should undergo laparotomy.

The operative strategy for meconium ileus is to create an enterotomy proximal to the area of obstruction and irrigate with either a dilute meglumine diatrizoate solution or 4% acetylcysteine solution. If this is unsuccessful, attempts can be made to milk the pellets of inspissated meconium out through the enterotomy. Rarely is resection and primary anastomosis required. Patients with complicated meconium ileus have volvulus, intestinal necrosis, atresia, or a meconium pseudocyst necessitating resection of nonviable segments of bowel, distal irrigation, and exteriorization. The operative survival rate for these children is more than 90%.[28]

Meconium plug syndrome also presents in the neonatal period as a distal intestinal obstruction. The meconium plug syndrome results in the deposition of thickened meconium in the distal colon and is thought to result from decreased intestinal motility. Meconium plug syndrome frequently occurs in association with maternal diabetes mellitus, hypothyroidism, or childbirth. The hypoglycemia that occurs in infants of diabetic mothers is hypothesized to induce glucagon secretion that subsequently causes decreased intestinal motility. Patients with meconium plug frequently are premature infants who otherwise appear healthy but present with a distal intestinal obstruction. This obstruction results in substantial abdominal distention with little or no meconium being passed. Plain abdominal radiography frequently shows multiple dilated loops of small bowel and the soap-bubble or ground-glass appearance of meconium in the rectum. As with the meconium ileus, a water-soluble contrast enema is frequently diagnostic and therapeutic. Patients should undergo suction rectal biopsy to rule out Hirschsprung's disease. In the absence of Hirschsprung's disease, there are no long-term sequelae from meconium plug syndrome.

INTESTINAL DUPLICATIONS AND CYSTS

Enteric duplications are rare congenital anomalies. Although these lesions may present at any age, more than 80% of patients present within the first 2 years of life.[29] The duplications present as cystic abnormalities of the gastrointestinal tract found anywhere from the esophagus to the anus. The lesions often contain many different types of mucosa, including acid-secreting gastric mucosa.

The small intestine is the most common location for enteric duplications, accounting for approximately 50% of these anomalies.[30] Within the small intestine the most common location is the ileum. Small bowel duplications are usually found within the mesentery. They share a common blood supply and a common muscular wall with the adjacent normal bowel. There are two types of intestinal duplications: cystic and tubular. Two-thirds of all lesions are cystic. Communication between the lumen of the duplication and the adjacent bowel is rare, but it is diagnostic when present. The communication may occur anywhere along the common wall. If it is present distally, the duplication often drains spontaneously into the small bowel and may remain asymptomatic. However, a proximal fistula results in the accumulation of secretions in the distal blind end of the duplication, causing adjacent bowel obstruction, perforation, or volvulus.

Duplications usually present as an acute intestinal obstruction. However, small bowel lesions may present with indolent, vague abdominal pain or intermittent gastrointestinal bleeding. Gastric mucosa can be present within duplications, causing ulceration of adjacent bowel.[31] Peptic ulceration or hemorrhage occurs most commonly in patients with jejunal duplications, because a higher percentage of jejunal lesions contain gastric mucosa. Therefore, patients with proximal lesions more commonly present with acute gastrointestinal bleeding, melena, perforation, or fistulization. In contrast, ileal duplications are more likely to present with acute intestinal obstruction resulting from the enlarged duplication compressing the adjacent bowel. Also, bowel obstruction may result from a duplication causing torsion, volvulus, or intussusception of the involved bowel.

During physical examination, an abdominal mass is infrequently palpable. Because many children present with operative indications, such as acute bowel obstruction or a complication of peptic ulcer disease, imaging and other confirmatory studies are often not performed. However, ultrasonography has been shown to be an excellent diagnostic method for detecting enteric duplications and differentiating solid from cystic lesions. Ultrasonography shows a classic triple-layer effect. Computed tomography and magnetic resonance imaging also can visualize duplications as a large cystic lesion of unclear cause. When gastric mucosa is present, technetium scanning will show the lesion.

The treatment of intestinal duplications depends on the amount of bowel involved. Complete excision of the duplication and attached bowel followed by primary anastomosis is performed if the involved segment is short.

However, excision of long tubular duplications could result in short-gut syndrome. Therefore, other operative strategies are performed for long tubular duplications. If no gastric mucosa is present in the duplication, a communication can be created at the distal end of the common wall, allowing drainage of the duplication into the small intestine. However, if gastric mucosa is present, this could result in peptic ulcer disease. In patients whose duplication contains gastric mucosa, a counterincision should be performed away from the common wall and the mucosa stripped from the entire duplication.[32] Once the mucosa has been stripped, the muscular walls are left in place. These muscular walls subsequently collapse, obliterating the duplication space.

The outcome for patients with intestinal duplications is excellent and depends upon the presence of associated congenital anomalies. If these lesions are not diagnosed and persist into adulthood, malignancy can arise within the duplication.[33] However, these lesions are uniformly benign in the pediatric patient. Any mortality associated with the lesions is usually due to bleeding or sepsis from perforation and is related to a delay in diagnosis and definitive treatment.

INTUSSUSCEPTION

Intussusception is the invagination of a segment of intestine into an adjoining intestinal segment. Intussusception is one of the most common causes of acute abdominal pain in children younger than 5 years. Most cases (80%-90%) occur in children between the ages of 3 months and 3 years.[34]

The most common cause of intussusception is idiopathic. Only 2% to 12% of all pediatric patients have an identifiable anatomical lead point.[35] Anatomical lead points are more common in neonates (60%-75%) and patients older than 5 years (57% in older children and 97% in adults). The most common lead point is thought to be an enlarged Peyer's patch after a viral illness.[36] However, a Meckel diverticulum is the most common anatomical lead point identified on pathologic specimens. Other lead points include polyps, benign hamartomas associated with Peutz-Jeghers syndrome, submucosal hematomas due to Schönlein-Henoch purpura, cysts, or malignancies. With each contraction during peristalsis, the length of the intussusceptum increases, drawing it further and further into the lumen of the adjacent bowel. Intussusception results in a cycle of lymphatic obstruction, venous congestion, arterial compromise, and eventual necrosis of the intussusceptum.

The typical history for intussusception is a young infant with sudden abdominal pain, crying, and drawing up of the knees. The abdominal pain is short-lived and occurs in 15- to 30-minute intervals. Between episodes of pain, the child is comfortable and quiet. As time passes, systemic toxicity and other symptoms of intestinal obstruction, such as abdominal distention and bilious emesis, develop. As the mucosal blood supply is compromised, the patient sloughs mucosa, resulting in the classic red currant jelly stool. If the disease process continues to evolve, sepsis and hemodynamic instability and shock develop. Frequently, on physical examination, the mass of the intussusception is palpable in the right upper quadrant, and the right lower quadrant may feel "empty" (25%-60% of patients). On rectal examination, 60% to 90% of patients have either gross or occult blood. Abdominal radiography frequently shows a pattern of small bowel obstruction with dilated proximal loops and the absence of distal bowel gas.[37] Ultrasonography has become the noninvasive diagnostic procedure of choice.[38]

Contrast enemas done by a radiologist are both diagnostic and therapeutic.[39] Patients with evidence of clinical peritonitis or perforation should not undergo a contrast enema but instead should proceed directly to laparotomy. Frequently, a clinical history of longer than 48 hours or radiographic evidence of a complete bowel obstruction is associated with intestinal gangrene. Therefore, successful contrast enema reduction is unlikely and operative intervention is more probable for these patients. For uncomplicated cases, the success rate for contrast enema reduction of the intussusception ranges from 50% to 90%. Contrast enema allows visualization and reduction of the intussusception under fluoroscopic observation. As the intussusception is reduced through the ileocecal valve, the contrast should reflux freely into the small intestine. This finding is essential to document a successful reduction. Another method that is gaining popularity is an ultrasound-guided hydrostatic reduction. Ultrasonography shows the intussuscepted segment of bowel as either a bull's-eye (transverse view) or a kidney-shaped mass (longitudinal view). Saline or air introduced into the colon may be used to provide the pressure necessary for reduction.[40] The reduction process is observed with real-time ultrasonography. Greater rates of reduction are reported with air insufflation (up to 95%) than with saline enemas.[41] After successful reduction, perioperative antibiotic therapy should be continued for 24 hours, with subsequent initiation of feedings.

Children with peritonitis or perforation and children in whom pressure reduction is unsuccessful should undergo laparotomy. These patients should initially receive fluid resuscitation, nasogastric tube decompression, and broad-spectrum antibiotics. A right transverse supraumbilical incision is made. The bowel should be gently compressed with warm saline-soaked pads in an attempt to reduce tissue edema and facilitate reduction. The intussusceptum is expressed from the intussuscipiens by placing gentle pressure at the apex of the intussusceptum and milking it proximally (Fig. 8). This action is similar to that used in squeezing a tube of toothpaste from the bottom. The intussusceptum should never be pulled, because traction may disrupt this fragile and compromised bowel. Manual reduction of the intussusception should be successful in approximately 90% of children. After the intestine is reduced, the bowel is examined for any surgical lead points, and bowel viability is assessed. If a lead point is identified, this should be resected and a primary anastomosis performed. An intussusception that cannot be reduced suggests that the intestine is gangrenous. In this case, the intussusception should be resected and a primary anastomosis performed. Once the intussusception has been corrected, an appendectomy should be performed.

Complications associated with intussusception include perforation during or after nonoperative reduction (< 0.2% of patients).[42] After successful hydrostatic reduction of the intussusception, intussusception may recur (5%-10%).[43] The recurrence rate after surgical reduction is lower, but it still may be 1% to 4%. Recurrences most commonly present within 2 to 3 days. Recurrences are treated with hydrostatic or pneumatic reduction unless operative indications are present. If patients have several episodes of intussusception, colonoscopy and subsequent laparotomy are warranted to look for an anatomical lead point.

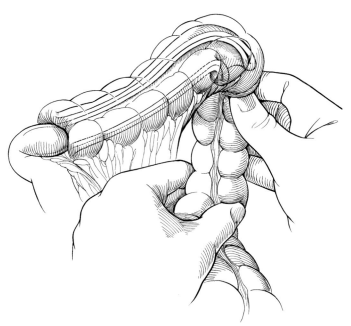

Fig. 8. Manual reduction of intussusception. If a barium enema fails or intussusception is encountered during a laparotomy for intestinal obstruction, manual reduction is required. The intestine is occluded immediately distal to the intussusception with the fingers of one hand and stripped proximally with the fingers of the other. In effect, this maneuver increases intraluminal pressure just as an enema does. The intestine should not be pulled. If reduction is not readily achieved, resection and anastomosis should be performed.

OMPHALOMESENTERIC DUCT REMNANTS (MECKEL'S DIVERTICULUM)

Meckel's diverticulum is discussed in Chapter 26, and, therefore, only pediatric concerns are addressed in this section. As a reminder, Meckel's diverticulum frequently follows the rule of two's: found in 2% of the population, contains two types of ectopic mucosa in 60% of patients (gastric or pancreatic), commonly presents in patients younger than 2 years old, is found approximately 2 feet from the ileocecal valve, and is about 2 inches long.[44]

Among patients with Meckel's diverticulum, 65% to 95% remain asymptomatic throughout life. The symptoms at presentation depend on the patient's age. Infants most commonly present with bowel obstruction due either to intussusception of the Meckel diverticulum or to volvulus of the small bowel around a fibrous remnant of omphalomesenteric duct. Hydrostatic reduction of the intussusception is seldom successful. If a volvulus has occurred, patients present with evidence of small bowel obstruction associated with sudden and severe abdominal pain and abdominal findings characteristic of intestinal

ischemia. Signs of intestinal ischemia, including acidosis, peritonitis, and shock, may occur before any evidence of intestinal obstruction.

Hemorrhage is more often found in older patients and is the most common presentation for Meckel's diverticulum. Hemorrhage from a Meckel diverticulum is the most common cause of substantial gastrointestinal bleeding in pediatric patients. The bleeding classically presents as bright red blood from the rectum, usually painless and often massive. The bleeding is a result of peptic ulceration in adjacent normal ileum due to ectopic gastric mucosa within the diverticulum. Because bleeding from a Meckel diverticulum is the most common cause of hematochezia in pediatric patients, the initial diagnostic study should be pentagastrin-stimulated technetium isotope scanning. This detects the ectopic gastric mucosa within the diverticulum with a sensitivity of more than 90%.[45]

There are many other, less common, ways for Meckel's diverticula to present. They may become inflamed, presenting clinically like appendicitis. Perforated diverticulitis is more likely to result in pneumoperitoneum and diffuse peritonitis compared with appendicitis. Because these diverticula are large, it is more difficult for a perforation to be walled off. A patent omphalomesenteric duct acts as a conduit connecting the umbilicus to the terminal ileum and manifests as feculent drainage from the umbilicus. An omphalomesenteric sinus frequently presents as umbilical granuloma or a persistently draining sinus at the umbilicus. Initial treatment for the granuloma is cauterization with silver nitrate. If this is unsuccessful, operative resection may be required. If a sinus is identified, it should be evaluated with preoperative imaging. Water-soluble contrast sinography frequently shows a fistulous communication to the bladder or gastrointestinal tract. Ultrasonography also may be diagnostic. An omphalomesenteric cyst most frequently presents in an infraumbilical midline position as either a mass or an infected cyst.

In patients with an omphalomesenteric sinus or patent omphalomesenteric duct, exploration may be done through a relatively small infra-umbilical incision. The omphalomesenteric remnant is dissected free distally and is completely resected. Any connection to the bowel is divided and oversewn. In patients with evidence of a bleeding Meckel diverticulum, obstruction, or diverticulitis, exploration should be done through a right lower quadrant transverse incision. For patients with Meckel's diverticulum, a V-shaped incision excising the anomaly and a segment of the antimesenteric border of the small bowel should result in complete excision of the lesion and any damaged adjacent tissue. The resultant defect in the bowel usually can be closed transversely. Some diverticula with a narrow base and no evidence of ectopic tissue can be treated with a GIA stapler fired across the base of the diverticulum. If a large area of small bowel is involved by the diverticulum, a primary resection of the lesion and its associated small bowel may be appropriate. A primary anastomosis in a hemodynamically stable patient with minimal peritoneal soiling is appropriate. For unstable patients with gross peritoneal contamination, exteriorization is preferable.

The approach to a Meckel diverticulum that is incidentally discovered at laparotomy is currently controversial. The controversy centers around the 5% of Meckel's diverticula that become symptomatic.[46] Lesions that have palpable ectopic mucosa, a prominent arterial supply, a fibrous omphalomesenteric duct remnant, evidence of inflammation, or a narrow base are all more likely to become symptomatic with bleeding, obstruction, or diverticulitis. Therefore, all of these lesions should undergo resection. Any lesions with attachments to the umbilicus also should be resected or detached to prevent volvulus and internal hernias. Finally, any patient who presents with complaints of abdominal pain and who, at laparotomy, has no other identifiable cause for the symptoms should have the diverticulum resected. However, some studies suggest that all incidentally discovered Meckel's diverticula should be resected, especially in the pediatric population.[46,47]

GASTROINTESTINAL BLEEDING

Although concerning to parents, gastrointestinal tract bleeding in children is usually a limited process without physiologic sequelae.[48] The common causes for such bleeding in children are age-dependent.

The initial steps in evaluating a child with gastrointestinal bleeding are identical throughout the different age ranges and include identifying the source of the bleeding, assessing the volume and significance of the bleeding, and initiating resuscitation. As in adults, the initial diagnostic maneuver is to place a nasogastric tube. This will give an indication of whether the source is the upper or lower gastrointestinal tract. Initial resuscitation should proceed with maintenance intravenous fluid and lactated Ringer boluses until normal hemodynamic values and good urinary output have been achieved. Patients who do not respond after two boluses of 20 mL/kg may require a transfusion. Patients can lose 30% to 40% of their intravascular volume without having any clinical findings of hypotension. Thus it is easy to underestimate both the magnitude of blood loss and the adequacy of resuscitation. During resuscitation, all patients should have laboratory studies performed, including a complete blood count, platelet count, liver function tests, and coagulation studies.

The most common cause of gastrointestinal bleeding in neonates occurs in those who have had some form of neonatal distress resulting in stress gastritis. These patients frequently have a coffee-ground gastric aspirate or melena. Another common cause is vitamin K deficiency that results in hemorrhagic diseases of the newborn. This condition should be treated with 1 mg of vitamin K given intramuscularly. Swallowed maternal blood also results in a large volume of blood-tinged nasogastric aspirate and can be evaluated with the Apt test. Nasogastric decompression, intravenous fluids, and histamine$_2$-receptor blockers are often sufficient treatment. Further evaluation is not warranted unless the bleeding continues or worsens. If the bleeding does worsen or continues despite adequate conservative therapy, endoscopy should be performed. Rarely is surgical intervention required.

For lower gastrointestinal tract bleeding, anal fissures are the most common cause in newborns through preschoolers. Fissures result in bright-red blood that streaks the stool or in small bright-red spots on the diaper. Anal speculum examination is usually sufficient to confirm the diagnosis of an anal fissure. In almost all patients, treatment with stool softeners and warm sitz baths is successful, but occasionally anal dilations are needed.[49] The next most common causes of lower gastrointestinal tract bleeding in neonates are NEC and malrotation with volvulus. Even with an aggressive evaluation, the cause of gastrointestinal bleeding in newborns remains undiagnosed in approximately 50% of cases. This uncertainty is acceptable. The vast majority of patients never require an operation.

During infancy, the most common causes of upper gastrointestinal bleeding include esophagitis and gastritis due to gastroesophageal reflux disease and peptic ulcer disease. These diagnoses are often confirmed with both endoscopy and intraluminal pH monitoring. Both peptic ulcer disease and gastroesophageal reflux disease usually respond to conservative therapy with histamine$_2$-receptor blockers or proton pump inhibitors, and prokinetic agents also are used for gastroesophageal reflux disease. Anal fissure continues to be the most common cause of lower gastrointestinal tract bleeding in infants. However, in this age group, intussusception and gangrenous bowel, most likely due to volvulus, become more prevalent and require consideration and evaluation.

In preschool children older than 1 year, peptic ulcer disease with its comorbid conditions of esophagitis and gastritis is the most common cause of upper gastrointestinal bleeding. These patients should be evaluated endoscopically and, as in adults, treated with an initial trial of medical therapy. Intestinal obstruction or continued bleeding indicates the need for surgical intervention. The most common sources of lower gastrointestinal bleeding in preschool children are colonic polyps and Meckel's diverticulum.

In school-aged and adolescent children, the most common cause of upper gastrointestinal bleeding is peptic ulcer disease, but bleeding from esophageal varices, due either to portal vein thrombosis or hepatic cirrhosis, has become more prevalent. Esophageal varices commonly present with massive hematemesis. Endoscopy is usually diagnostic and therapeutic with banding or sclerotherapy of the visualized varices. Frequently, replacement of coagulation factors and transfusions of packed red blood cells are also needed. A common cause of lower gastrointestinal tract bleeding in school-age and adolescent children is polyps. Also, inflammatory bowel disease becomes more prevalent in adolescent children and is discussed extensively elsewhere in this book.

As expected, the diagnostic work-up for each age group varies with the probable causes (Fig. 9). However, if the bleeding has stopped and all of the study results are negative, observation is warranted in anticipation that these same evaluations will be performed again if the patient has another bleed and may yield a definitive diagnostic answer.

POLYPOID DISEASE

The four major polypoid diseases in pediatric patients include juvenile polyps, Peutz-Jeghers syndrome, familial adenomatous polyposis, and Gardner's syndrome. In children, 80% of all polyps are juvenile polyps.[50] The cause of these polyps is uncertain. Juvenile polyps are benign hamartomas found throughout the colon, but not in the small bowel. Usually they are solitary lesions. Juvenile polyps occur in approximately 1% of children between the ages of 3 and 5 years and are rarely present beyond adolescence.[51] The clinical presentation for these lesions is most commonly intermittent small-volume bleeding due to ulceration. Juvenile polyps in the sigmoid or rectum also may prolapse out of the anus or cause intussusception. Diagnosis of these lesions is easily accomplished with either sigmoidoscopy in combination with barium enema or colonoscopy. Treatment for juvenile polyps is primarily snare removal during endoscopy. Approximately 80% of these lesions spontaneously regress.[52] This regression is thought to be due to twisting of the polyp on the vascular pedicle leading to infarction of the polyp and sloughing. These lesions must be differentiated from the juvenile polyposis syndromes, which are much less common but do have the potential for malignant degeneration. The polyposis syndromes are characterized by more than five polyps in the colon, polyps throughout the gastrointestinal tract, and any number of polyps associated with a family history of juvenile polyposis.[53]

Peutz-Jeghers syndrome consists of multiple benign hamartoma polyps that occur most frequently in the small bowel (55%), although they may occur anywhere from stomach to rectum.[54] Patients also have excessive melanotic pigmentation on the buccal mucosa and lips and around the mouth. These areas of increased pigmentation are present at birth and fade by puberty. There is a family history of Peutz-Jeghers syndrome in approximately 50% of patients. The disease is transmitted as an autosomal dominant disorder. The mean age at clinical presentation is 30 years, although a range of 2 to 82 years has been described. Frequently, patients present with abdominal pain and obstruction caused by intussusception. The intussusception may be transient with partial obstruction that can resolve spontaneously. However, the intussusception also may present as a lesion that cannot be radiographically reduced. The diagnosis of Peutz-Jeghers syndrome should be suspected in patients with melanotic lesions who present with abdominal pain, obstruction, or anemia or melena. The diagnosis can be made with upper and lower endoscopy and small bowel contrast study.

Patients with Peutz-Jeghers syndrome have an increased lifelong risk for cancer, both intestinal and extraintestinal, and the cancer mortality rate is 50% by 60 years of age.[54]

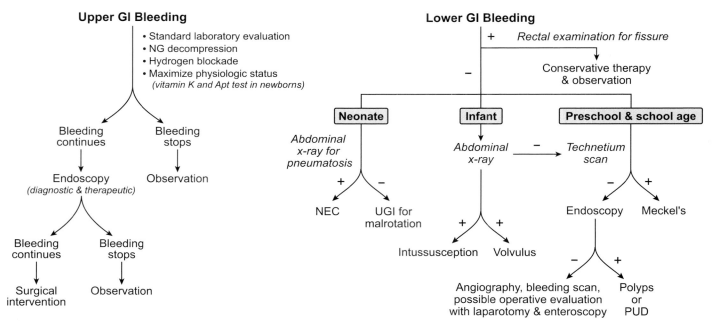

Fig. 9. Algorithm for the diagnostic work-up of upper and lower gastrointestinal (GI) bleeding. NEC, necrotizing enterocolitis; NG, nasogastric; PUD, peptic ulcer disease; UGI, upper gastrointestinal radiography.

Malignant degeneration of the hamartomatous polyps has been reported. Extraintestinal tumors in patients with Peutz-Jeghers syndrome include pancreatic, testicular, ovarian, cervical, and breast. Because of this malignant potential, recommendations for the treatment of Peutz-Jeghers syndrome have changed. All polyps more than 5 mm in diameter should be removed. Small bowel polyps may be removed during laparotomy with intraoperative enteroscopy. Any tumors detected need aggressive surgical therapy. The current recommendations for follow-up include annual 1) breast and pelvic examinations with cervical smears and pelvic ultrasonography, 2) testicular ultrasonography, and 3) pancreatic ultrasonography. Esophagogastroduodenoscopy and colonoscopy, in conjunction with a small bowel contrast radiographic study, should be performed biannually. Finally, mammography is recommended at ages 25, 30, 33, 35, biannually until 50, and then annually.[54]

Familial adenomatous polyposis and Gardner's syndrome[55-57] are discussed in Chapter 40.

HIRSCHSPRUNG'S DISEASE

Hirschsprung's disease is a neurogenic form of intestinal obstruction in which there is an absence of ganglion cells in the myenteric and submucosal plexus. This lack of an intact intrinsic nervous system results in failure of relaxation of the internal anal sphincter and bowel wall due to an increased contractile adrenergic response in the aganglionic segment. Hirschsprung's disease is thought to occur as a result of incomplete caudal migration of the myenteric nervous system; however, a discrete pathogenic mechanism for this arrest of caudal migration is undetermined. Invariably, the aganglionosis begins at the anorectal line, involving the submucosal and myenteric plexuses and the internal sphincter. The aganglionosis then extends proximally to the level of the rectosigmoid area in approximately 80% of patients, to the splenic flexure in 10%, and to the cecum or a segment of small bowel in 10%.[58] On histologic examination, the aganglionosis is associated with hypertrophy of nerve fibers and an increase of staining for acetylcholine esterase activity. The small bowel proximal to the level of aganglionosis shows muscle hypertrophy.

Patients with Hirschsprung's disease present with symptoms consistent with colonic obstruction. The incidence is 1:4,000 to 7,000, and there is a male preponderance of 4:1.[59] The vast majority of children have delayed passage of meconium beyond 24 hours after birth.[60] They also may have considerable abdominal distention and bilious emesis. Ten percent of patients may present with enterocolitis due to stasis and bacterial overgrowth in the bowel proximal to the level of obstruction. The enterocolitis may be severe and can progress to sepsis. Other associated anomalies are rare; however, Down syndrome (trisomy 21) is present in about 13% of patients and is associated with a worse prognosis.[61]

The diagnosis of Hirschsprung's disease is established with a combination of radiologic and pathologic studies. Abdominal radiography will show dilated loops of small bowel consistent with a distal intestinal obstruction. A barium enema study may show a dilated colon proximal to an area of aganglionosis with a visible transition point; however, this is usually not present until 3 to 6 weeks of age. Time is required for the proximal bowel to become dilated (Fig. 10). Another criterion is failure to evacuate barium within 24 hours after a barium radiographic study.[62] The absence of ganglion cells within the submucosal Meissner plexus on rectal biopsy is the standard for diagnosis of Hirschsprung's disease. In a newborn patient, a suction rectal biopsy is sufficient to demonstrate this lesion. In older children, suction rectal biopsy is frequently inadequate; therefore, a full-thickness biopsy specimen from the posterior rectal wall should be obtained during examination with the patient under anesthesia. Rectal biopsy in which both acetylcholine esterase staining and ganglion cells are evaluated is accurate in 99% of patients.[63] Anorectal manometry also can be performed in children older than 40 weeks gestation and more than 3 kg in weight. It will show absence of the rectoanal inhibitory reflex in patients with Hirschprung's disease.[64]

The traditional treatment of Hirschsprung's disease has been a left lower quadrant transverse incision and visualization of the rectosigmoid colon. Multiple partial-thickness biopsy specimens are obtained, and the transition point from aganglionosis to normal bowel is determined pathologically. Just proximal to this transition zone, a diverting loop colostomy is performed. Definitive repair is delayed 3 to 4 months to allow the patient to grow and the dilated bowel to return to normal caliber.

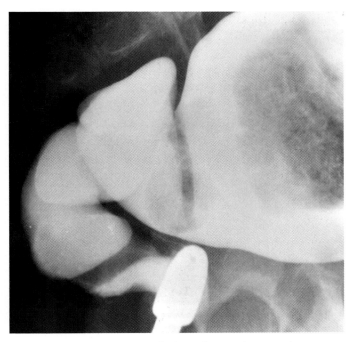

Fig. 10. Barium enema study, lateral view, showing classic transition point of dilated rectum in Hirschsprung's disease.

There has been a recent trend to perform the definitive procedure within the first week of life.[65] In this case, the diagnosis is made and the colon is kept decompressed with daily enemas. This technique obviates a two-stage procedure. The definitive procedure then may be performed by the traditional transabdominal approach or by the more recently described laparoscopy-assisted or transanal approaches.[66] Three different definitive operations can be performed: the Soave, the Duhamel, and the Swenson procedures. The two most commonly performed are the Soave and the Duhamel. The Soave, or endorectal pull-through, includes resection of the aganglionic portion of bowel and a rectal "mucosectomy" to the level of the dentate line.[67] The normal bowel is then passed through the rectal muscular cuff and sewn to the mucosal edge at the dentate line. In the Duhamel procedure, approximately 9 cm of aganglionic rectum is left in place. Normal bowel is tunneled posteriorly behind the rectum and is brought through a posterior incision at the dentate line. The normal bowel is then sutured to the posterior half of the dentate line, and a common channel is created between the aganglionic and normal bowel with a GIA stapler fired along their shared wall.[68] Care should be taken not to leave a blind-ended stump at the end of the aganglionic bowel. Because this area is unable to contract, gastrointestinal contents can accumulate within the stump, causing problems with stasis, obstruction, and infection. Some investigators consider a Duhamel procedure to be the procedure of choice for total colonic aganglionosis because it provides some colonic absorptive capacity from the aganglionic rectum that is preserved.

There are some long-term complications associated with Hirschsprung's disease and its treatment. In 10% of patients, constipation remains a considerable problem after operation. A similar percentage of patients have problems with incontinence.[69] Patients in whom enterocolitis develops should be treated with rectal and colonic irrigations and intravenous antibiotics. If there is no response to these measures or toxicity develops, a colostomy should be performed to provide decompression.

IMPERFORATE ANUS

Imperforate anus involves a spectrum of anatomical abnormalities characterized by the anus not being located within the middle of the anal sphincteric complex. It is usually classified as either low or high. In low lesions, there is a fistulous tract connecting the rectum to the midline of the perineum. Higher lesions are characterized by either rectal agenesis with no fistulous opening or a fistulous communication to either the vagina or uterus in the female or the urethra or bladder in the male.

The incidence of imperforate anus is 1:5,000.[70] High lesions are two times more common in males than females. The embryology of these defects is hypothesized to be due to maldevelopment of cloacal separation between the rectum and the genitourinary system or an abnormality of the dorsal cloacal membrane. Higher lesions are thought to occur early in gestation, at 4 to 6 weeks, and lower lesions occur at 10 to 12 weeks' gestation. Not uncommonly, imperforate anus is an isolated malformation. However, it can be associated with small bowel atresias, the VACTERL syndrome (vertebral, anal, cardiac, tracheoesophageal fistula, renal, limb anomalies), Down syndrome, and cardiac defects. The most common problem is genitourinary anomalies. They occur in 20% of patients who have low lesions and 60% of patients with high lesions.[71] These anomalies most commonly include renal agenesis or vesicular-ureteral reflux.

Imperforate anus usually is detected during the initial physical examination when an anus cannot be identified or the anus is not located in its proper anatomical position at the mid point between the tip of the coccyx and the most inferior portion of the vestibule or scrotum. If a fistulous tract is not identified along the midline of the perineum, then the child should be observed for 24 to 48 hours for meconium to be expelled either from the vagina of girls or in the urine of boys. Children with high lesions frequently have a diminished gluteal fold and sphincter contraction and have an abnormal sacrum. The poor gluteal fold and diminished sphincter contraction probably are due to improper formation of the sphincter complex in the absence of the rectum.

The diagnostic work-up should include chest radiography with a nasogastric tube in position to rule out a tracheoesophageal fistula. Abdominal and pelvic radiographs should be obtained to look for vertebral and sacral anomalies. Sacral anomalies are associated with poor long-term functional outcome because affected patients frequently have fecal and urinary incontinence after operation. Abdominal and pelvic ultrasonography should be performed to look for the rectal stump, to evaluate the kidneys, to rule out genitourinary obstruction, and to evaluate for a tethered spinal cord.[72] Urinalysis should be done to look for meconium and large intestinal cells in the urine, which indicate a fistulous tract from the rectum. Voiding cystourethrography should be done before dismissal from the hospital to rule out vesicular-ureteral reflux.

Patients initially are treated with intravenous fluids and nasogastric decompression until their work-up is complete. Any patient with a high lesion who does not have a perineal fistula should undergo an initial diverting colostomy. The purposes of the diverting colostomy are to protect the genitourinary system from continued fecal contamination and to allow time for the patient to grow before operative correction. The definitive procedure is performed when the patient is approximately 6 months old. At the time of ostomy formation, it is important to irrigate the meconium from the distal bowel so that it does not become inspissated or cause infection of the genitourinary tract. Low lesions may be treated one of two ways. If the child is of adequate size, a definitive procedure is performed shortly after birth. If the child is small, the fistulous tract may undergo progressive dilations to allow easy passage of meconium and colonic decompression. This conservative therapy may continue until the child increases in size, after which a definitive operative procedure can be performed.

The definitive operative procedure for low lesions is a limited posterior sagittal anorectoplasty.[73] This involves placing the patient in a prone jackknife position and determining the center of the sphincter complex with electrical stimulation of the skin. A midline incision is made from the middle of the sphincter complex down to and around the fistulous opening. The fistula is then mobilized from its surrounding soft tissue structures back into the middle of the sphincter complex. The sphincter complex is then reapproximated with absorbable sutures anterior to the fistula. Then the mucosal lining of the fistulous tract is sutured into its new position in the middle of the sphincter complex. On completion of the procedure, electrostimulation of the sphincter complex should demonstrate circumferential contraction around the new anal opening.

In high lesions that have previously required a colostomy, the child should undergo distal colostography to determine the anatomy of the distal fistula and rectal stump. Once this information has been obtained, a posterior sagittal anorectoplasty can be performed, usually at 3 to 6 months of age. A midline incision is started at the tip of the sacrum and carried down through the middle of the sphincter complex until the fistula or rectal stump is identified. If a fistula is present, the fistula is divided and suture ligated. The rectal stump is then mobilized from surrounding soft tissue structures and brought down into position through the middle of the sphincter complex. The sphincter complex is closed both anteriorly and posteriorly around the newly positioned rectum, and exit of the new rectum through the middle of the sphincter complex is ensured. The mucosa of the fistula or rectum is then sutured to the skin, and the rest of the perineal incision is closed. On completion of the procedure, there should be circumferential contracture of the sphincter complex around the newly positioned anus.

Once the definitive procedure has been performed, a 3-week interval should pass to allow healing of the anastomosis. Subsequently, daily dilations should be performed to prevent stricture of the anastomosis, and these should be continued for 3 months. The diverting colostomy may be closed 6 to 8 weeks after the sagittal anorectoplasty has been performed.

Complications are not uncommon. The most common complication is constipation, which occurs in the majority of patients. It usually can be managed with minimal medical therapy. Intractable constipation may occur in 25% of patients.[74] The patients are also at risk for the development of rectal prolapse and anal stenosis, each of which occurs in approximately 30% of patients. Incontinence is the most distressing complication and is related to the level of the anomaly. Incontinence is present after operation in 10% of patients with low lesions and in 25% to 50% of patients with high lesions.[75] The other major determinant of incontinence is central nervous system or spinal anomalies.

REFERENCES

1. Seashore JH, Touloukian RJ: Midgut volvulus: an ever-present threat. Arch Pediatr Adolesc Med 148:43-46, 1994
2. Messineo A, MacMillan JH, Palder SB, Filler RM: Clinical factors affecting mortality in children with malrotation of the intestine. J Pediatr Surg 27:1343-1345, 1992
3. Powell DM, Othersen HB, Smith CD: Malrotation of the intestines in children: the effect of age on presentation and therapy. J Pediatr Surg 24:777-780, 1989
4. Lewis JE Jr: Partial duodenal obstruction with incomplete duodenal rotation. J Pediatr Surg 1:47-53, 1966
5. Schey WL, Donaldson JS, Sty JR: Malrotation of bowel: variable patterns with different surgical considerations. J Pediatr Surg 28:96-101, 1993
6. Stauffer UG, Herrmann P: Comparison of late results in patients with corrected intestinal malrotation with and without fixation of the mesentery. J Pediatr Surg 15:9-12, 1980
7. Coombs RC, Buick RG, Gornall PG, Corkery JJ, Booth IW: Intestinal malrotation: the role of small intestinal dysmotility in the cause of persistent symptoms. J Pediatr Surg 26:553-556, 1991
8. Warner BW, Ziegler MM: Management of the short bowel syndrome in the pediatric population. Pediatr Clin North Am 40:1335-1350, 1993
9. Hays DM: Intestinal atresia and stenosis. Curr Probl Surg October 1969, pp 1-48
10. Doolin EJ, Ormsbee HS, Hill JL: Motility abnormality in intestinal atresia. J Pediatr Surg 22:320-324, 1987
11. Phelps S, Fisher R, Partington A, Dykes E: Prenatal ultrasound diagnosis of gastrointestinal malformations. J Pediatr Surg 32:438-440, 1997
12. Grosfeld JL: Alimentary tract obstruction in the newborn. Curr Probl Pediatr 5:3-47, 1975
13. Grosfeld JL, Ballantine TV, Shoemaker R: Operative management of intestinal atresia and stenosis based on pathologic findings. J Pediatr Surg 14:368-375, 1979
14. Rescorla FJ, Grosfeld JL: Intestinal atresia and stenosis: analysis of survival in 120 cases. Surgery 98:668-676, 1985
15. Kurkchubasche AG, Rowe MI, Smith SD: Adaptation in short-bowel syndrome: reassessing old limits. J Pediatr Surg 28:1069-1071, 1993
16. Holman RC, Stehr-Green JK, Zelasky MT: Necrotizing enterocolitis mortality in the United States, 1979-85. Am J Public Health 79:987-989, 1989
17. Uauy RD, Fanaroff AA, Korones SB, Phillips EA, Phillips JB, Wright LL: Necrotizing enterocolitis in very low birth weight infants: biodemographic and clinical correlates. National Institute of Child Health and Human Development Neonatal Research Network. J Pediatr 119:630-638, 1991
18. Ballance WA, Dahms BB, Shenker N, Kliegman RM: Pathology of neonatal necrotizing enterocolitis: a ten-year experience. J Pediatr 117:S6-S13, 1990
19. Kanto WP Jr, Hunter JE, Stoll BJ: Recognition and medical management of necrotizing enterocolitis. Clin Perinatol 21:335-346, 1994
20. Leonard T Jr, Johnson JF, Pettett PG: Critical evaluation of the persistent loop sign in necrotizing enterocolitis. Radiology 142:385-386, 1982
21. Kosloske AM: Indications for operation in necrotizing enterocolitis revisited. J Pediatr Surg 29:663-666, 1994
22. Musemeche CA, Kosloske AM, Ricketts RR: Enterostomy in necrotizing enterocolitis: an analysis of techniques and timing of closure. J Pediatr Surg 22:479-483, 1987
23. Janik JS, Ein SH, Mancer K: Intestinal stricture after necrotizing enterocolitis. J Pediatr Surg 16:438-443, 1981
24. Ricketts RR, Jerles ML: Neonatal necrotizing enterocolitis: experience with 100 consecutive surgical patients. World J Surg 14:600-605, 1990
25. Welsh MJ, Tsui L-C, Boat TF, Beaudet AL: Cystic fibrosis. In The Metabolic and Molecular Bases of Inherited Disease. Vol III. Seventh edition. Edited by CR Scriver, AL Beaudet, WS Sly, D Valle. New York, McGraw-Hill, 1995, pp 3799-3876
26. Neuhauser EBD: Roentgen changes associated with pancreatic insufficiency in early life. Radiology 46:319-328, 1946
27. Kao SC, Franken EA Jr: Nonoperative treatment of simple meconium ileus: a survey of the Society for Pediatric Radiology. Pediatr Radiol 25:97-100, 1995
28. Del Pin CA, Czyrko C, Ziegler MM, Scanlin TF, Bishop HC: Management and survival of meconium ileus: a 30-year review. Ann Surg 215:179-185, 1992
29. Bower RJ, Sieber WK, Kiesewetter WB: Alimentary tract duplications in children. Ann Surg 188:669-674, 1978
30. Holcomb GW III, Gheissari A, O'Neill JA Jr, Shorter NA, Bishop HC: Surgical management of alimentary tract duplications. Ann Surg 209:167-174, 1989
31. Wardell S, Vidican DE: Ileal duplication cyst causing massive bleeding in a child. J Clin Gastroenterol 12:681-684, 1990
32. Bar-Maor JA, Shoshany G, Israel O, Halpern M, Etzioni A: Tubular duplication of the jejunum and ileum lined entirely by gastric mucosa. J Pediatr Gastroenterol Nutr 4:303-306, 1985
33. Orr MM, Edwards AJ: Neoplastic change in duplications of the alimentary tract. Br J Surg 62:269-274, 1975
34. Doody DP: Intussusception. In Surgery of Infants and Children: Scientific Principles and Practice. Edited by KT Oldham, PM Colombani, RP Foglia. Philadelphia, Lippincott Raven Publishers, 1997, pp 1241-1248
35. Young DG: Intussusception. In Pediatric Surgery. Vol 2. Fifth edition. Edited by A O'Neill Jr, MI Rowe, JL Grosfeld, EW Fonkalsrud, AG Coran. St Louis, Mosby, 1998, pp 1185-1198
36. Bell TM, Steyn JH: Viruses in lymph nodes of children with mesenteric adenitis and intussusception. Br Med J 2:700-702, 1962
37. Lazar L, Rathaus V, Erez I, Katz S: Interrupted air column in the large bowel on plain abdominal film: a new radiological sign of intussusception. J Pediatr Surg 30:1551-1553, 1995
38. Barr LL: Sonography in the infant with acute abdominal symptoms. Semin Ultrasound CT MR 15:275-289, 1994
39. Eklof OA, Johanson L, Lohr G: Childhood intussusception: hydrostatic reducibility and incidence of leading points in different age groups. Pediatr Radiol 10:83-86, 1980
40. Kirks DR: Air intussusception reduction: "the winds of change." Pediatr Radiol 25:89-91, 1995
41. Guo JZ, Ma XY, Zhou QH: Results of air pressure enema reduction of intussusception: 6,396 cases in 13 years. J Pediatr Surg 21:1201-1203, 1986
42. Katz ME, Kolm P: Intussusception reduction 1991: an international survey of pediatric radiologists. Pediatr Radiol 22:318-322, 1992
43. Stringer MD, Pablot SM, Brereton RJ: Paediatric intussusception. Br J Surg 79:867-876, 1992
44. Amoury RA, Snyder CL: Meckel's diverticulum. In Pediatric Surgery. Fifth edition. Edited by JA O'Neill Jr, MI Rowe, JL

Grosfeld, EW Fonkalsrud, AG Coran. St Louis, Mosby, 1998, pp 1173-1184

45. Sfakianakis GN, Conway JJ: Detection of ectopic gastric mucosa in Meckel's diverticulum and in other aberrations by scintigraphy: II. Indications and methods: a 10-year experience. J Nucl Med 22:732-738, 1981

46. Cullen JJ, Kelly KA, Moir CR, Hodge DO, Zinsmeister AR, Melton LJ III: Surgical management of Meckel's diverticulum: an epidemiologic, population-based study. Ann Surg 220:564-568, 1994

47. Mackey WC, Dineen P: A fifty year experience with Meckel's diverticulum. Surg Gynecol Obstet 156:56-64, 1983

48. Sherman NJ, Clatworthy HW Jr: Gastrointestinal bleeding in neonates: a study of 94 cases. Surgery 62:614-619, 1967

49. Berman WF, Holtzapple PG: Gastrointestinal hemorrhage. Pediatr Clin North Am 22:885-895, 1975

50. Louw JH: Polypoid lesions of the large bowel in children with particular reference to benign lymphoid polyposis. J Pediatr Surg 3:195-209, 1968

51. Mestre JR: The changing pattern of juvenile polyps. Am J Gastroenterol 81:312-314, 1986

52. Nelson EW Jr, Rodgers BM, Zawatzky L: Endoscopic appearance of auto-amputated polyps in juvenile polyposis coli. J Pediatr Surg 12:773-776, 1977

53. Jass JR: Juvenile polyposis. In Familial Adenomatous Polyposis and Other Polyposis Syndromes. Edited by R Phillips, AD Spigelman, JPS Thomson. London, E. Arnold, 1994, pp 203-214

54. Spigelman AD, Phillips RKS: Peutz-Jeghers syndrome. In Familial Adenomatous Polyposis and Other Polyposis Syndromes. Edited by R Phillips, AD Spigelman, JPS Thomson. London, E. Arnold, 1994, pp 188-202

55. Gardner EJ, Richards RC: Multiple cutaneous and subcutaneous lesions occurring simultaneously with hereditary polyposis and osteomatosis. Am J Hum Genet 5:139-147, 1953

56. Farmer KCR, Hawley PR, Phillips RKS: Desmoid disease. In Familial Adenomatous Polyposis and Other Polyposis Syndromes. Edited by R Phillips, AD Spigelman, JPS Thomson. London, E. Arnold, 1994, pp 128-142

57. Eagel BA, Zentler-Munro P, Smith IE: Mesenteric desmoid tumours in Gardner's syndrome—review of medical treatments. Postgrad Med J 65:497-501, 1989

58. Ikeda K, Goto S: Diagnosis and treatment of Hirschsprung's disease in Japan: an analysis of 1628 patients. Ann Surg 199:400-405, 1984

59. Russell MB, Russell CA, Niebuhr E: An epidemiological study of Hirschsprung's disease and additional anomalies. Acta Paediatr 83:68-71, 1994

60. Klein MD, Philippart AI: Hirschsprung's disease: three decades' experience at a single institution. J Pediatr Surg 28:1291-1293, 1993

61. Quinn FM, Surana R, Puri P: The influence of trisomy 21 on outcome in children with Hirschsprung's disease. J Pediatr Surg 29:781-783, 1994

62. Rosenfield NS, Ablow RC, Markowitz RI, DiPietro M, Seashore JH, Touloukian RJ, Cicchetti DV: Hirschsprung disease: accuracy of the barium enema examination. Radiology 150:393-400, 1984

63. Andrassy RJ, Isaacs H, Weitzman JJ: Rectal suction biopsy for the diagnosis of Hirschsprung's disease. Ann Surg 193:419-424, 1981

64. Ito Y, Donahoe PK, Hendren WH: Maturation of the rectoanal response in premature and perinatal infants. J Pediatr Surg 12:477-482, 1977

65. Cilley RE, Statter MB, Hirschl RB, Coran AG: Definitive treatment of Hirschsprung's disease in the newborn with a one-stage procedure. Surgery 115:551-556, 1994

66. Smith BM, Steiner RB, Lobe TE: Laparoscopic Duhamel pullthrough procedure for Hirschsprung's disease in childhood. J Laparoendosc Surg 4:273-276, 1994

67. Boley SJ: An endorectal pull-through operation with primary anastomosis for Hirchsprung's disease. Surg Gynecol Obstet 127:353-357, 1968

68. Talbert JL, Seashore JH, Ravitch MM: Evaluation of a modified Duhamel operation for correction of Hirschsprung's disease. Ann Surg 179:671-675, 1974

69. Teitelbaum DH, Coran AG, Weitzman JJ, Ziegler MM, Kane T: Hirschsprung's disease and related neuromuscular disorders of the intestine. In Pediatric Surgery. Vol 2. Fifth edition. Edited by JA O'Neill Jr, MI Rowe, JL Grosfeld, EW Fonkalsrud, AG Coran. St Louis, Mosby, 1998, pp 1381-1424

70. Stephens FD, Smith ED: Ano-rectal Malformations in Children. Chicago, Year Book Medical Publishers, 1971

71. McLorie GA, Sheldon CA, Fleisher M, Churchill BM: The genitourinary system in patients with imperforate anus. J Pediatr Surg 22:1100-1104, 1987

72. Willital GH: Advances in the diagnosis of anal and rectal atresia by ultrasonic-echo examination. J Pediatr Surg 6:454-457, 1971

73. Kiely EM, Peña A: Anorectal malformations. In Pediatric Surgery. Vol 2. Fifth edition. Edited by JA O'Neill Jr, MI Rowe, JL Grosfeld, EW Fonkalsrud, AG Coran. St Louis, Mosby, 1998, pp 1425-1448

74. Yeung CK, Kiely EM: Low anorectal anomalies: a critical appraisal. Pediatr Surg Int 6:333-335, 1991

75. Nixon HH, Puri P: The results of treatment of anorectal anomalies: a thirteen to twenty year follow-up. J Pediatr Surg 12:27-37, 1977

INDEX

Note: Page numbers followed by f indicate figures; those followed by t indicate tables.

Abdomen, unclosable, 653, 653t
Abdominal aortic reconstruction, ischemic colitis
    after, 521
Abdominal compartment syndrome, 653–656,
    654t
    decompressive laparotomy for, 655–656, 656t
    diagnosis of, 654–655, 655f, 655t
    intra-abdominal hypertension and, 655
    pathogenesis of, 654
    physiologic changes after relief of, 656
Abdominal decompression, for abdominal com-
    partment syndrome, 655–656, 656t
Abdominal exploration
    for mesenteric venous thrombosis, 451, 451f
    water-soluble, for small bowel obstruction, 433
Abdominal trauma, 637–652
    anatomy and, 637f, 637–638
    blunt, nonoperative management of, 643
    diagnosis of, 638f, 638–643, 639f
        computed tomography in, 641–642
        diagnostic peritoneal lavage in, 640–641
        history and physical examination in,
            639–640
        laboratory tests in, 640
        laparoscopy in, 642–643
        plain radiography in, 640
        ultrasonography in, 641
    epidemiology of, 638
    nonoperative management of, 643
    operative management of, 644–649
        for colon injury, 649
        "damage control" laparotomy for, 644–645
        for hepatobiliary injury, 646
        indications for, 644
        operative procedure for, 644
        for pancreatic and duodenal injury,
            646–648, 648f, 648t
        for small bowel injury, 648–649
        for splenic injury, 645–646
        for stomach injury, 646
        temporary closure for, 645
    penetrating, nonoperative management of, 643
Abdominal wall, component separation of, for
    ventral hernias, 671–674
Abdominal wall reconstruction, 661–663
    fascial or release technique for, 661, 662f
    tissue expander technique for, 661–663, 662f
Abdominoperineal resection, for rectal cancer,
    576
Ablation
    alcohol, for hepatic cysts, 201, 202
    hepatic, for hepatic colorectal metastases, 182
    for hepatocellular carcinoma, 167–168
    nerve, for chronic pancreatitis, 337–338
    radiofrequency, for neuroendocrine hepatic
        metastases, 185
Abscesses
    anorectal. See Anorectal abscesses
    appendiceal, 530, 531
    intra-abdominal, after pancreatoduodenec-
        tomy, 288
    pilonidal, treatment of, 616f, 616–617
    splenic, 367
Accidents, with morbid obesity, 141

Achalasia, 37–45
    epidemiology and pathophysiology of, 37, 38f
    patient evaluation in, 37–39, 39f
    treatment of, 39–44
        botulinum toxin in, 39–40
        esophageal resection for, 45
        esophagomyotomy for, 41–42
        laparoscopic myotomy for, 43–44, 44f
        pharmacologic, 39
        pneumatic dilation for, 40f, 40–41
        surgical myotomy for, 41
        surgical outcome in, 44
        thoracoscopic myotomy for, 43
        transabdominal cardiomyotomy for, 42, 42f
        transthoracic cardiomyotomy for, 42–43, 43f
Acidosis, metabolic, following pancreas transplan-
    tation, 349
Adenocarcinoma. See specific sites
Adenoma
    bile duct, 195–196
    hepatocellular, 193–195, 195f, 196f
    of upper gastrointestinal tract, associated with
        familial adenomatous polyposis, 565–566
        surveillance for, 566
        treatment of, 565–566
Adhesions, small bowel obstruction due to, 435
Adrenal rest tumor, hepatic, 199
Adson, Martin A., 14, 15f
    hepatic surgery and, 159
    islet cell tumors and, 299
Advancing flap operation, for pilonidal sinus,
    618, 619f
Aflatoxins, hepatocellular carcinoma and, 160
Air embolus, with hepatic resection, 180
Alcohol ablation, for hepatic cysts, 201, 202
Alkaline reflux gastritis, after gastric operations,
    132
    medical and dietary interventions for, 133
    operative treatment of, 136
Altemeier procedure, 631, 632f–633f
Ampicillin, for colonic diverticula, 493
Ampullectomy, for pancreatic and periampullary
    carcinoma, 284
Amputation, rectal, for rectal cancer, 578–579
Anal canal anastomoses. See Ileal pouch-anal
    canal anastomosis; Jejunal pouch-anal canal
    anastomosis
Anal cancer, following proctocolectomy and ileal
    pouch-anal canal anastomosis, 541
Anal fissures, 599–604
    clinical manifestations of, 600
    definition of, 599
    diagnosis of, 600, 600f
    differential diagnosis of, 600–601, 601f
    etiology of, 599
    management of, 601–604
        for acute fissures, 601
        anal sphincter stretch for, 602
        for chronic fissures, 601–604
        lateral internal sphincterotomy for,
            602–603, 603f
        nonoperative, 601–602
        V-Y advancement flap for, 603–604, 604f
    pathogenesis of, 599–600

Anal fistulas. See Fistula in ano
Anal sphincter stretch, for anal fissures, 602
Anemia
    with glucagonoma, 312
    hemolytic, congenital, 366–367
Aneurysms. See Visceral artery aneurysms; specific
    arteries
Angiomyolipoma, hepatic, 198
Angioplasty, for chronic mesenteric ischemia,
    464t, 464–465
Annandale, Thomas, 421–422
Anorectal abscesses, 604f, 604–608, 605f
    bacteriology of, 607–608
    clinical manifestations of, 605
    examination of, 605
    fistula after incision and drainage of, 608
    management of, 605–607
        for intersphincteric abscesses, 606–607
        for ischioanal abscesses, 606, 607f
        for perianal abscesses, 606, 606f
        for supralevator abscesses, 607, 607f
    pathogenesis and avenue of spread of,
        604–605, 605f, 606f
    recurrent, 608
Anorectal manometry, 477–478, 479f
Anorectal "mucosectomy," with plication of
    anorectum, for rectal prolapse, 633, 634f,
    635
Anorectal necrotizing fasciitis, 608
Anorectal plication, anorectal "mucosectomy"
    with, for rectal prolapse, 633, 634f, 635
Anorectal varices, in portal hypertension, 598
Anorectoplasty, sagittal, posterior, for imperforate
    anus, 718
Antacids, for peptic ulcers, 109, 109t
Antibiotics. See also specific antibiotics
    for appendicitis, 528
Anticholinergic agents, for peptic ulcers, 109t,
    109–110
Anticoagulation, for mesenteric venous thrombo-
    sis, 450
Antireflux surgery. See Gastroesophageal reflux
    disease
Anus. See also Anorectal entries
    Crohn's disease involving, surgical treatment
        of, 416–418, 417f, 418f
    imperforate, in pediatric patients, 717–719
Appendicitis, 525–532
    antibiotics for, 528
    complicated, 530
    diagnosis of, 525–526, 526f
    imaging studies in, 526–527, 527f, 528f
    laparoscopic appendectomy for, 529f,
        529–530, 530f
        open appendectomy versus, 531
    open appendectomy for, 528–529
        laparoscopic appendectomy versus, 531
    with perforation, 530
    postoperative complications with, 530–531
    supportive care for, 528
Appendix, Crohn's disease involving, 415
Aspiration, percutaneous, for hepatic cysts,
    201
Atresia, in pediatric patients, 704–705, 705f

Balfour, Donald C., 6, 6f, 14, 570
Balloon expulsion test, 478
Bariatric surgery. *See also specific procedures*
    historical background of, 142–149
    indications for, 141t, 141–142
    at Mayo Clinic, 149–156, 151f
        current approach to, 150–151, 151t
        gastric bypass technique for, 151–153, 152f
        reoperation and, 155–156
        results of, 153–154
        in special situations, 154–155
Barium enema, for colon cancer detection, 508
Barium esophagography, in gastroesophageal reflux
    disease, 25
Barrett's esophagus, 58
    in gastroesophageal reflux disease, 25–26
Bassini repair, 682–683, 683f
Beahrs, Oliver H., 10, 12, 12f, 14
    islet cell tumors and, 299
Bench-work procedure, for pancreas transplanta-
    tion, 344–345, 345f, 346f
Bile acid therapy, for gallstones, 236–237, 237t
Bile duct adenoma, 195–196
Bile duct stones, of common bile duct. *See* Chole-
    docholithiasis
Bile duct strictures, benign, classification of, 249,
    250f
Bile duct trauma, operative management of, 646
Biliary "colic," 227, 228f
Biliary cystadenoma, 201
Biliary-enteric anastomosis
    double, for biliary strictures, 257
    single, for biliary strictures, 256
Biliary hamartoma, 196
Biliary leak, after pancreatoduodenectomy, 288
Biliary lithotripsy, 237–238
Biliary pancreatitis, in choledocholithiasis, 239,
    239t
Biliary reconstruction, in liver transplantation
    recipients, 217, 217f, 218f
Biliary sludge, 227
Biliary stents, for pancreatic and periampullary car-
    cinoma, 287
Biliary stone disease. *See* Choledocholithiasis; Gall-
    stone(s)
Biliary strictures, benign, 247–260
    anatomy and vascular supply of biliary tree and,
        247–248, 248f
    causes of, 250–253
    diagnosis of, 253
    iatrogenic, 251–253
    operative treatment of, 253–257
        for Bismuth type I injuries, 254–255,
            255f–257f
        for Bismuth type II and III injuries, 255–256,
            257f, 258f
        for Bismuth type IV injuries, 256–257
        for Bismuth type V injuries, 257
        gallbladder use for, 257
        outcome of, 257–259, 259t
    pathophysiology of, 248–249
Biliary tree, anatomy and vascular supply of,
    247–428, 248f
Biliopancreatic bypass, partial, historical back-
    ground of, 148–149, 149f
Bilious drainage, following hepatic resection, 180
Bismuth, for peptic ulcers, 109, 109t
Black, B. Marden, 14, 16f
Bladder anastomosis
    for drainage of pancreatic exocrine secretions,
        346, 347f
    for pancreatic exocrine secretion drainage,
        breakdown of, 349
Blue days, 10
Bobbs, John S., cholecystectomy and, 225

Botulinum toxin
    for achalasia, 39–40
    for anal fissures, 601–602
Bowel. *See* Colon *entries;* Colonic *entries;* Small
    intestinal *entries;* Small intestine; *specific
    regions of bowel*
Bowel resection. *See also* Colon resection
    for Crohn's disease, 411–412, 415, 416f
    for mesenteric venous thrombosis, 451–452
    for small bowel obstruction, 434
Braasch, William F., 4–5, 5f, 12, 14
Branches of Mayo Clinic, 10, 14
Breast carcinoma, hepatic metastases from, hepatic
    resection for, 186
Brinton, William, 422
Brooke ileostomy
    for Crohn's disease, 415, 417f
    proctocolectomy and. *See* Proctocolectomy,
        Brooke ileostomy and
Buie, Louis A., 14
Bulk-forming agents, for hemorrhoids, 591
Bypass grafting, for chronic mesenteric ischemia,
    459–465
        operative technique for, 460–463, 461f–463f
        results of, 463–464, 464t

CA 19-9, in pancreatic and periampullary carci-
    noma, 274–275
Cancer. *See* Malignancies; *specific types and sites*
Carcinoid tumor
    in Meckel's diverticula, 405
    small intestinal, 379–380, 380f
Carcinoma. *See specific sites*
Cardiomyotomy
    transabdominal, for achalasia, 42, 42f
    transthoracic, for achalasia, 42–43, 43f
Cecal volvulus, 554–556
    cecal, treatment of, 555–556
    diagnosis of, 554–555, 555f
Cecopexy, for volvulus, 555–556
Cecorectal anastomosis, for functional constipa-
    tion, 481
Cecostomy, for volvulus, 555–556
Celiac artery aneurysms, 471–472, 472f, 473f
Celiotomy, abdominal wall defects following,
    665
Celsus, 679
Chemical ablation, for hepatocellular carcinoma,
    167–168
Chemoprotection, for hepatocellular carcinoma,
    169
Chemoradiation therapy
    for esophageal carcinoma
        with surgery, 69, 70
        without operation, 70
    with pancreatoduodenectomy, 288–289
Chemotherapy. *See also* Chemoradiation therapy
    adjuvant
        for hepatocellular carcinoma, 168–169
        for pancreatic cystic neoplasms, 358–359
        with pancreatoduodenectomy, 288
        preoperative, for esophageal carcinoma, 68
        for rectal cancer, 581–582, 582f
        with surgery for gastric cancer, 84–85
    infusional, hepatic arterial, for hepatic colorectal
        metastases, 182–183
Chest radiography, in gastroesophageal reflux dis-
    ease, 25
Children. *See also* Pediatric gastrointestinal disor-
    ders
    bariatric surgery in, 154
Cholangiocarcinoma
    intrahepatic, 170–171
    liver transplantation for, 211

Cholangiocellular tumors, benign, 195–196
Cholangiography, intraoperative, choledocholithi-
    asis discovered during, management of,
    240–241, 241f
Cholecystectomy, 14
    laparoscopic, 233–235, 234f, 236t, 237t
        choledocholithiasis discovered during, man-
            agement of, 240–241, 241f
        for gallbladder carcinoma, 267
    open, 232–233
    radical, for gallbladder carcinoma, 266f,
        266–267, 267f
    timing of, 236
Cholecystitis
    acute calculus, 227–229, 228f
    chronic, 227, 228f
    emphysematous, 229
Cholecystojejunostomy, for pancreatic and peri-
    ampullary carcinoma, 284–285
Cholecystostomy, 231–232, 232f
    open, 231, 232f
    percutaneous, 231, 232f
Choledochoduodenostomy
    for biliary strictures, 254–255, 256f
    for pancreatic and periampullary carcinoma,
        284–285
Choledochojejunostomy, for biliary strictures, 255,
    257f
Choledocholithiasis, 228f, 238–243
    asymptomatic, 238
    biliary anatomy and, 225–226
    with biliary pancreatitis, 239, 239t
    classification of, 238
    diagnosis of, 240, 240f
    historical background of, 225
    with intermittent jaundice, 238
    management of, 240–243, 241f
        for choledocholithiasis discovered during
            laparoscopic cholecystectomy and intra-
            operative cholangiography, 240–241,
            241f
        laparoscopic common bile duct exploration
            for, 242–243
        open common bile duct exploration for, 242,
            242f
        with retained stones, 241–242
        for suspected choledocholithiasis, 240
    pathogenesis of, 238
    suspected, management of, 240
Cholesterol gallstones, 226, 226f
Ciprofloxacin, for colonic diverticula, 492
Cirrhosis, hepatocellular carcinoma and, 160
Clagett, Oscar T. (Jim), 3, 3f, 4, 6, 9
Clapesattle, Helen, 12, 19
Clostridium botulinum toxin
    for achalasia, 39–40
    for anal fissures, 601–602
Cole, Warren, cholecystography and, 225
Colectomy
    abdominal, ileorectal anastomosis and,
        548–549
        advantages and disadvantages of, 548
        procedure for, 548–549, 549f
        results with, 549
    for Crohn's disease, 415, 417f
    with ileorectal anastomosis, for familial adeno-
        matous polyposis, 560–561, 561f
    with ileorectostomy, for functional constipation,
        480–481, 482f
    segmental, for functional constipation, 481
Colic artery aneurysms, 473
Colitis. *See also* Ischemic colitis; Ulcerative colitis
    necrotizing enterocolitis as, in pediatric patients,
        708–710, 709f
Collis esophageal lengthening procedure, 30, 31f

Colon
  Crohn's disease involving, surgical treatment of, 415, 416f, 417f
  injury of, operative management of, 649
  motor disorders of. See Constipation, functional
  vascular anatomy of, 519f, 519–520
Colon cancer, 507–518. See also Colorectal cancer
  diagnosis of, 508
  physiology, biochemistry, molecular biology, and pathology of, 507–508
  surgical treatment of
    with bleeding, 517
    controversies regarding, 515–517
    general oncologic principles and, 509, 509t
    indications for, 508–509
    laparoscopic left hemicolectomy, sigmoid colonic resection, and low anterior resection for, 512–514, 513f, 514f
    laparoscopic right hemicolectomy for, 511–512
    laparoscopy in, 515–516
    left hemicolectomy for, 511
    long-term follow-up of, 515, 516t
    for obstructing tumors, 516
    outcomes with, 514–515
    with perforated viscus, 516–517
    prophylactic oophorectomy in, 516
    right hemicolectomy for, 509, 510f, 511f
    sigmoid colonic anterior resection and low anterior resection for, 511
    in special circumstances, 514
    transverse colon resection for, 510
  with ulcerative colitis, 535
Colon cutoff sign, in acute pancreatitis, 323
Colon resection. See also Bowel resection
  for diverticula, 493–499
    elective, 496
    emergency, 494–496, 495f
    laparoscopic, 496–499, 498f–500f
  for ischemic colitis, 522–523
    conduct of, 522, 522f
    indications for, 522
    long-term follow-up of, 523
    outcomes with, 522–523
  segmental, for functional constipation, 481
  of sigmoid colon, for colon cancer, 511, 512–514, 513f, 514f
  of transverse colon, for colon cancer, 510
  for volvulus, 555, 556, 557
Colon screening, for cancer, 508
Colon surveillance, for cancer, 508
Colonic decompression, for volvulus, 555, 556–557
Colonic diverticula, 489–505
  bleeding due to, 500–502
    clinical presentation of, 500
    management of, 500–502
    natural history of, 500
    pathophysiology of, 500
  clinical presentation of, 490–491
  diagnosis and imaging of, 491–492
  medical therapy for, 492
  pathology and pathophysiology of, 489–490, 490f
  surgical treatment of, 493–500
    elective, laparotomy for, 496
    emergency, laparotomy for, 494–496, 495t
    indications for, 493–494
    laparoscopic resection for, 496–499, 498f–500f
    outcomes and long-term follow-up of, 499–500
  terminology for, 489
Colonic lavage, on-table, for diverticula, 496

Colonic necrosis, in acute pancreatitis, treatment of, 331
Colonic obstruction
  cancer causing, 516
  in ulcerative colitis, 535
  volvulus and. See Colonic volvulus
Colonic perforation, in ulcerative colitis, 535
Colonic pouch, for rectal cancer, 578, 579f
Colonic transit, evaluation of, 476–477, 477f, 478f
Colonic volvulus, 553–558
  age of patients and, 553
  cecal, 554–556
    diagnosis of, 554–555, 555f
    treatment of, 555–556
  etiology of, 553–554, 554f
  incidence of, 553
  of sigmoid colon, 556–557
    diagnosis of, 556, 556f
    treatment of, 556–557
  of transverse colon, 557
Colonoscopy
  for colon cancer detection, 508
  for ischemic colitis detection, 521
Colorectal cancer. See also Colon cancer; Rectal cancer
  familial adenomatous polyposis and, 559–560
  hepatic metastases from, hepatic resection for, 181f, 181t, 181–182, 182f
  screening for, 570–571
Colostomy
  for rectal cancer, 578–579
  transverse, with drainage, for diverticula, 495, 495t
Common bile duct exploration
  laparoscopic, for choledocholithiasis, 242–243
  open, for choledocholithiasis, 242, 242f
Common bile duct stones. See Choledocholithiasis
Component separation of abdominal wall, for ventral hernias, 671–674
Constipation, functional, 475–487
  diagnosis of, 476–479
    anorectal function evaluation in, 477–479, 479f
    approach for, in tertiary referral practice, 479, 480f
    colonic transit evaluation in, 476–477, 477f, 478f
    history and physical examination in, 476
    psychologic evaluation in, 476
  etiology and pathogenesis of, 475–476
  surgical treatment of, 480–484
    long-term follow-up of, 482–484, 484t
    operations for, 480–481, 482f
    outcomes with, 482, 483t
Continent ileostomy, proctocolectomy and, 545–548
  background and rationale for, 545
  indications for and contraindications to, 545–546
  posthospital care with, 546–547
  procedure for, 546, 546f
  results with, 547–548
Contrast agents, water-soluble, for small bowel obstruction, 432–533
Cooper, Astley Paston, 421, 679, 684
Cooper's ligament, 680
Coronary artery disease, with morbid obesity, 140–141
Cost-effectiveness, 14, 16
Courvoisier, Ludwig, cholecystectomy and, 225
Crohn's disease, 409–420
  diagnosis of, 410
  etiology of, 409

Crohn's disease (Continued)
  hemorrhoids in, 598
  incidence of, 409
  natural history of, 409–410, 410t
  surgical treatment of
    for anus and rectum, 416–418, 417f, 418f
    for colon, 415, 416f, 417f
    for esophagus, duodenum, and stomach, 412, 412f, 413f
    indications for, 411, 411t
    laparoscopic, 415, 418
    outcome of, 418–419
    preoperative preparation for, 411
    for small bowel, 412–415, 413f–415f
    surgical principles and, 411–412
Cryoablation
  hepatic, for hepatic colorectal metastases, 182
  for hepatocellular carcinoma, 168
Cullen sign, in acute pancreatitis, 322
Curettage, for pilonidal sinus, 620
Cyst(s). See also Pseudocysts
  hepatic. See Liver, cystic lesions of
  intestinal, in pediatric patients, 711–712
  pancreatic. See Pancreatic cystic tumors
  splenic, 367
Cystadenocarcinoma, 201
Cystadenoma
  biliary, 201
  serous, 352, 352f
    operative treatment of, 357, 359
Cyst excision, for hepatic cysts, 201
Cyst fenestration, for hepatic cysts, 202, 201
Cystitis, following pancreas transplantation, 349–350
Cystoduodenostomy, for pancreatic pseudocysts, Roux-en-Y, 331
Cystogastrostomy, for pancreatic pseudocysts, 330–331, 331
Cystojejunostomy, Roux-en-Y, for pancreatic pseudocysts, 331
Cytokines, manipulation of, for acute pancreatitis, 324
Cytoreductive hepatic surgery, for neuroendocrine hepatic metastases, 183–185, 184t

"Damage control" laparotomy, for abdominal trauma, 644–645
Defecography, 478
Degenerative joint disease
  with bariatric surgery, 154
  premature, with morbid obesity, 140
Dehiscence, fascial. See Fascial dehiscence
Delivery, following proctocolectomy and ileal pouch-anal canal anastomosis, 540
Delorme procedure, modified, 633, 634f, 635
Desmoid tumors, associated with familial adenomatous polyposis, 563–565, 564f
  surveillance for, 565
  treatment of, 564–565
Detorsion, for volvulus, 555–556, 557
Diabetes mellitus
  complications of
    end-stage renal disease as, 342
    pancreas transplantation after, 341–360
  with morbid obesity, 140
Diagnostic peritoneal lavage, in abdominal trauma, 640–641
Diarrhea
  following continent ileostomy and proctocolectomy, 548
  after gastric operations, 131, 132
  operative treatment of, 135
Dickson, Claude F., 14

Diet
  gastric cancer and, 76
  for hemorrhoids, 591
Dieulafoy lesions, 122–123
  etiology of, 122
  management of, 123
  presentation and diagnosis of, 122
Diffuse esophageal spasm, 45–46
Dilation, for esophageal carcinoma, 70
Discrimination, with morbid obesity, 141
Dissolution, of gallstones
  contact, 237, 238f
  medical, 236–237, 237t
Diverticula. See Diverticulitis; Diverticulosis; specific sites, e.g., Colonic diverticula
Diverticulectomy
  incidental, 405–406
  laparoscopic, with myotomy and fundoplication, for epiphrenic esophageal diverticula, 50–52, 51f–53f
  therapeutic, 405
  thoracoscopic, with myotomy and fundoplication, for epiphrenic esophageal diverticula, 50–52, 51f–53f
Diverticulitis, 491
  complicated, 489
  definition of, 489
  simple, 489
Diverticulosis, 490–491
  definition of, 489
Dixon, C. F., 570
Dor partial anterior fundoplication, 30
Drainage
  bilious, following hepatic resection, 180
  external, for pancreatic pseudocysts, 330
  internal, for pancreatic pseudocysts, 330–331
  of pancreatic exocrine secretions, with pancreatic transplantation, 346, 347f, 348f, 349
  percutaneous, for pancreatic pseudocysts, 330
  serosanguineous, following hepatic resection, 180
Drug therapy. See also specific drugs and drug types
  for peptic ulcers, 109t, 109–110
Duhamel procedure, 717
Dumping syndrome
  with bariatric surgery, 153
  after gastric operations, 131–132
  operative treatment of, 135
Duodenal diverticula, 397–398
  bile duct strictures with, 250
  diagnosis of, 398
  location, incidence, and cause of, 397
  signs and symptoms of, 397–398
  treatment of, 398
Duodenal injury, operative management of, 646–648, 648f, 648t
Duodenal switch, with distal bypass, historical background of, 149, 149f
Duodenal ulcers. See also Peptic ulcers
  bile duct strictures with, 250–251
Duodenum
  anatomy of, 375
  Crohn's disease involving, surgical treatment of, 412, 412f, 413f
  villous tumors of. See Villous tumors of duodenum

Edis, A. J., islet cell tumors and, 299
Education, continuing, 13
Educational programs, 8
Elderly persons
  bariatric surgery in, 154
  ischemic colitis in, 520
Electromyography, in functional constipation, 479

Ellis, F. Henry (Bunky), 14, 15f
Embolism
  mesenteric, surgical treatment of, 444, 445f
  pulmonary, following hernia repair, for inguinal hernias, 688
Emesis, nonbilious and bilious, in infants, 699
Emphysematous cholecystitis, 229
En bloc excision, for rectal cancer, 579–580
Endorectal pull-through, 717
End-stage renal disease, in diabetes, 342
End-to-end anastomosis, for biliary strictures, 254, 255f
Enteric anastomosis
  for pancreatic exocrine secretion drainage, 346, 348f
  for pancreatic exocrine secretion drainage, breakdown of, 349
Enterocolitis, necrotizing, in pediatric patients, 708–710, 709f
Enteroliths, within jejunoileal diverticula, 401
E sign, in acute pancreatitis, 323
Esmarch technique, for fascial dehiscence, 660, 660f
Esophageal bypass, for esophageal carcinoma, 70
Esophageal carcinoma, 57–73
  choice of treatment for, 60–61
  combined treatment for, 67–70, 68t
    chemoradiation without operation as, 70
    preoperative chemotherapy in, 68, 69
    preoperative external beam radiation in, 68–70
  diagnosis of, 58–59, 58f–60f, 59t
  dilation and stents for, 70
  endoscopic laser therapy for, 71
  etiology and epidemiology of, 57
  intraoperative electron irradiation for, 71
  palliative therapy for, 70
  pathology and pathogenesis of, 57–58, 58f
  photodynamic therapy for, 70
  prevention of, 71
  signs and symptoms of, 58
  staging of, 59–60, 61t
  surgical outcome with, 67
  surgical therapy for, 61–67
    esophagectomy and bypass as, 70
    Ivor Lewis esophagogastrectomy as, 62–66, 63f–65f
    transhiatal esophagogastrectomy as, 66–67, 67f
  thoracoscopic operations for, 71
Esophageal diverticula, epiphrenic, 49f, 49–55, 50f
  etiology and pathophysiology of, 49
  operative treatment of, 50–53
    laparoscopic esophageal myotomy, diverticulectomy, and fundoplication for, 50–52, 51f–53f
    thoracoscopic esophageal myotomy, diverticulectomy, and fundoplication for, 52–53, 53f, 54f
  surgical outcome with, 53–54
  symptoms and diagnosis of, 49–50
Esophageal lengthening procedure, Collis, 30, 31f
Esophageal manometry, in gastroesophageal reflux disease, 24
Esophageal motility disorders, 37–47. See also specific disorders
  nonspecific, 46
  secondary, 46
Esophageal myotomy, diverticulectomy, and fundoplication
  laparoscopic, 50–52, 51f–53f
  thoracoscopic, 52–53, 53f, 54f
Esophageal pH monitoring, 24-hour, in gastroesophageal reflux disease, 24–25
Esophageal resection, for achalasia, 45

Esophageal sphincter, lower
  in gastroesophageal reflux disease, 23–24
  pneumatic dilation of, for achalasia, 40f, 40–41
Esophagectomy, with bypass, for esophageal carcinoma, 70
Esophagoduodenoscopy, with biopsies, in gastroesophageal reflux disease, 24
Esophagogastrectomy
  Ivor Lewis, 62–63
  transhiatal, 66–67, 67f
Esophagography, barium, in gastroesophageal reflux disease, 25
Esophagomyotomy, for achalasia, 41–42
Esophagus
  Crohn's disease involving, surgical treatment of, 412
  nutcracker, 46
Ethanol injection, percutaneous, for hepatocellular carcinoma, 167–168
Evacuation proctography, 478
Excision and flap closure, for pilonidal sinus, 620–622, 622f
External beam radiation therapy
  intraoperative, for esophageal carcinoma, 71
  postoperative, for esophageal carcinoma, 69–70
  preoperative, for esophageal carcinoma, 68–69
    with chemotherapy, 69
Extracorporeal shock-wave lithotripsy, 237–238
Extraperitonealization, for volvulus, 557

Familial adenomatous polyposis, 559–563
  colorectal, 559–563
    clinical course of, 559–560
    natural history of, 559–560
    surgical treatment of, 560–563, 561t, 562t, 563f
  desmoid tumors associated with, 563–565, 564f
    surveillance for, 565
    treatment of, 564–565
  upper gastrointestinal disease associated with, 565–566
    surveillance for, 566
    treatment of, 565–566
  villous tumors of duodenum associated with, 391
Fascial dehiscence, 656–661
  diagnosis of, 658–659
  etiology of, 656–658, 657t
    host factors in, 657
    incision type in, 658
    local wound factors in, 657
  incidence of, 656
  operative management of, 659f, 659–661
    postoperative care and, 660–661
    temporary closure techniques for, 659–660, 660f
  prevention of, 658
  retention sutures for, 658, 658f
Fascial technique, for abdominal wall reconstruction, 661, 662f
Fatty change, focal, hepatic, 200
Fecal occult blood testing, 508
Femoral venous thrombosis, following hernia repair, for inguinal hernias, 688
Fibrin glue, for fistula in ano surgery, 614–615
Fibrolamellar hepatocellular carcinoma, 169f, 169–170, 170f
Fissures, anal. See Anal fissures
Fistula(s)
  anorectal, after incision and drainage of anorectal abscesses, 608
  in Crohn's disease, 414–415, 415f, 417–418
  following proctocolectomy and ileal pouch-anal canal anastomosis, 541

Fistula(s) *(Continued)*
  pancreatic, in acute pancreatitis, treatment of, 331
  tracheoesophageal, in pediatric patients, 706f, 706–708, 707f
Fistula in ano, 609–615
  assessment of, 610
  chronic, carcinoma in, 615
  classification of, 609, 609f
  clinical manifestations of, 609–610
  extrasphincteric, 609
  horseshoe, treatment of, 611, 612f
  intersphincteric, 609
  suprasphincteric, 609
  transsphincteric, 609
  treatment of, 610–615
    advancement rectal flap for, 611, 613f
    extent of cutting sphincter muscles and, 613
    fibrin glue in, 614–615
    for horseshoe fistula, 611, 612f
    locating internal opening in, 612, 613f
    seton use in, 613–614, 614f
    for simple low fistula, 610–611, 611f
    when internal opening is not found, 612–613
Fistulography, in fistula in ano, 610
Fistulotomy, for fistula in ano. *See* Fistula in ano, treatment of
Focal fatty change, hepatic, 200
Focal nodular hyperplasia, 192–193, 193f, 194f
Fournier's gangrene, 608
Franco, Pierre, 421
Frey procedure, for chronic pancreatitis, 337, 338f
Fundoplication
  laparoscopic, with myotomy and diverticulectomy, for epiphrenic esophageal diverticula, 50–52, 51f–53f
  Nissen, laparoscopic, 26–29, 27f–29f
  partial anterior, Dor, 30
  thoracoscopic, with myotomy and diverticulectomy, for epiphrenic esophageal diverticula, 50–52, 51f–53f
  Toupet, partial posterior, laparoscopic, 29, 29f

Galen of Pergamum, 679
Gallbladder, as conduit, double, for biliary strictures, 257
Gallbladder carcinoma, 261–270
  clinical presentation of, 263
  etiology of, 261–262
  imaging of, 264
  laboratory evaluation of, 264
  natural history of, 262
  operative treatment of
    conduct of, 265–268, 265f–268f
    diagnostic laparoscopy for, 265
    indications for, 264–265
    outcome of, 268, 269t
    preoperative preparation for, 265
  pathology of, 262
  prognostic factors for, 262, 262f, 263t
Gallbladder trauma, operative management of, 646
Gallstone(s), 225–238
  acute calculus cholecystitis and, 227–229, 228f
  asymptomatic, 227
  biliary anatomy and, 225–226
  biliary "colic" with, 227, 228f
  biliary sludge and, 227
  cholesterol, 226, 226f
  chronic cholecystitis and, 227, 228f
  contact dissolution as, 237, 238f
  diagnosis of, 230, 230f, 231f
  emphysematous cholecystitis and, 229
  gallstone ileus and, 229
  historical background of, 225

Gallstone(s) *(Continued)*
  medical management of, 236–238
    biliary lithotripsy as, 237–238
    contact dissolution as, 237, 238f
    medical dissolution as, 236–237, 237t
  Mirizzi syndrome and, 228f, 229
  with morbid obesity, 141
  pancreatitis due to, 332, 333t
  pigmented, 226–227
  surgical management of, 231–236
    cholecystostomy for, 231–232, 232f
    laparoscopic cholecystectomy for, 233–235, 234f, 236t, 237t
    open cholecystectomy for, 232–233
    timing of cholecystectomy for, 236
Gallstone ileus, 229
Gallstone pancreatitis, treatment of, 332
Gangrene
  appendicitis with, 530
  Fournier's, 608
Gastrectomy
  distal, gastric emptying after, 129
  for gastric adenocarcinoma, 79f–81f, 79–83, 80t, 81t
    Mayo Clinic approach for, 83f, 83–84, 84f
  for gastric lymphoma, 96, 97–98
  proximal, gastric emptying after, 131
Gastric acid, peptic ulcer and, 104–105
Gastric adenocarcinoma, 75–90
  diagnosis and preoperative evaluation of, 78–79
  epidemiology and risk factors for, 75–77
  following gastrectomy, distal, 121
  hepatic metastases from, hepatic resection for, 187
  pathology of, 77t, 77–78
  surgical management of, 79f–81f, 79–83, 80t, 81t
    adjuvant and neoadjuvant therapy and, 84–85
    long-term follow-up of, 85–86
    Mayo Clinic operative approach for, 83f, 83–84, 84f
Gastric artery aneurysms, 472–473
Gastric bypass
  distal, historical background of, 149, 149f
  for esophageal carcinoma, 70
  historical background of, 147f, 147–148, 148t
  Roux-en-Y
    vertical, 150, 151f
    vertical disconnected, 150, 151f
    vertical disconnected very, very long-limb, 150–154, 151f
      results of, 153–154
      technique of, 151–153, 152f
Gastric emptying
  disorders of, after gastric operations, 131–137
    diagnosis of, 132–133
    medical and dietary interventions for, 133
    operative treatment of, 134t, 134–137, 136f
    preoperative considerations for, 133–134
    prevention of, 137
  after gastric operations, 128–131
  physiology of, 127–128, 128f
Gastric lymphoma, 91–101
  primary
    B-cell
      large, diffuse, 94, 97
      marginal zone, of MALT type, 93–94, 94f, 96–97
    clinical features of, 92
    clinical staging of, 92–93
    definition of, 91
    diagnosis of, 92
    epidemiology of, 92
    pathology of, 93t, 93–94, 94f

Gastric lymphoma *(Continued)*
    staging of, 95, 95f, 95t
    treatment of, 95–98
      general, 95–96
      recommendations for, 98, 98t
      surgical, 96–98
Gastric motility, physiology of, 127–128, 128f
Gastric motor disorders. *See also* Gastroparesis
  following gastrectomy, 121
Gastric outlet obstruction, peptic ulcers with, 108
Gastric polyps, 76
Gastric remnant, care of, 132
Gastric remnant cancer, after gastric operations, 136–137
Gastric resection, distal, for peptic ulcers, 114, 114f
Gastric ulcers. *See* Peptic ulcers
Gastric vagotomy, proximal, for peptic ulcers, 113, 113f, 115
Gastrinoma, 306–310
  diagnosis of, 307, 307t
  localization and treatment of, 307–309, 308f, 308t, 309f
  in multiple endocrine neoplasia I, 309–310, 310f
Gastritis, alkaline reflux, after gastric operations, 132
  medical and dietary interventions for, 133
  operative treatment of, 136
Gastroduodenal artery aneurysms, 473–474
Gastroenterostomy, 14, 14f
Gastroepiploic artery aneurysms, 472–473
Gastroesophageal reflux disease, 23–35
  diagnosis and imaging of, 24–25
  indications for operation in, 25–26, 26f
  operative procedures for, 26–30
    Collis esophageal lengthening procedure as, 30, 31f
    Dor partial anterior fundoplication as, 30
    Hill repair as, 30
    laparoscopic Nissen fundoplication as, 26–29, 27f–29f
    laparoscopic paraesophageal hernia repair as, 29–30, 30f
    laparoscopic Toupet partial posterior fundoplication as, 29, 29f
    redo laparoscopic antireflux procedures as, 30
  physiology and pathology of, 23–24
  surgical failures in, 26, 26f
  surgical outcome with, 30–35
    long-term, 32–33, 34f
    perioperative complications and, 31–32
    postoperative complications and short-term outcome and, 32, 33f
Gastrointestinal surgery, Mayo Clinic contributions to, 13–14
Gastrointestinal tract hemorrhage, after pancreatoduodenectomy, 288
Gastrojejunostomy
  for Crohn's disease, 412, 412f
  retrocolic, for duodenal obstruction with pancreatic and periampullary carcinoma, 285
  Roux-en-Y, gastric emptying after, 129–130, 130f
Gastroparesis
  after gastric operations, 131
    medical and dietary interventions for, 133
    operative treatment of, 134t, 134–135, 136f
  after pancreatoduodenectomy, 287
Gastroplasty
  historical background of, 144–147, 145f, 146f, 146t
  vertical banded, 150, 151f
Gastrostomy
  anterior, for pancreatic pseudocysts, 331
  endoscopic, percutaneous, for pancreatic and periampullary carcinoma, 287

Genetic testing, for familial adenomatous polyposis, 560
  surgical decision making based on, 562–563
Genitourinary cancer, hepatic metastases from, hepatic resection for, 185–186
Gentamicin, for colonic diverticula, 493
Gilbert, Arthur, 683
Glucagonoma, 310–313, 311f, 311t
  VIPoma syndrome and, 312–313, 313t
Gluteus maximus myocutaneous flaps, for pilonidal sinus, 620, 621f
Glyceryl trinitrate, for anal fissures, 601
Governance of Mayo Clinic, 8–9
Graft pancreatitis, following pancreas transplantation, 349
Graft rejection, following pancreas transplantation, 348–349
  monitoring for, 347–348
Graham, Ewarts, cholecystography and, 225
Graham, Roscoe, islet cell tumors and, 299
Grant, C. S., islet cell tumors and, 299
Grey Turner sign, in acute pancreatitis, 322
Group practice, integration of, 3–4

Hair, in pilonidal sinus, 620
Halsted, William, 680
Hamartoma, biliary, 196
Harrington, Stuart W. (Tack), 14, 16f
Hartmann's procedure, for diverticula, 495, 495t
Harwick, Harry J., 7, 7f, 9, 16
Heat ablation, for hepatocellular carcinoma, 168
Helicobacter pylori
  eradication of, 96, 97, 98
  gastric lymphoma associated with, 91, 93–94
  peptic ulcer and, 107
    medical therapy for, 110
    pathogenesis of, 105, 106
Heller, Ernst, 41
Hemangioma, 196–197, 197f, 198f, 367
Hematologic disorders, 365–373
  chronic myeloid disorders as, 367
  congenital hemolytic anemias as, 366
  diagnosis of, 368
  hemangiomas as, 368
  historical background of, 365
  imaging studies in, 368
  lymphomas as, 367
  platelet disorders as, 366
  primary splenic malignancies as, 368
  sinistral portal hypertension as, 368
  splenectomy for, 368–373, 369f–373f
  splenic abscesses and cysts as, 367
  splenic anatomy and physiology and, 365–366
  splenic torsion as, 367–368
Hemicolectomy
  left
    for colon cancer, 511
    laparoscopic, for colon cancer, 512–514, 513f, 514f
  right
    for colon cancer, 509, 510f, 511f
    laparoscopic, for colon cancer, 511–512
Hemolytic anemias, congenital, 366–367
Hemorrhage
  with colon cancer, 517
  from colonic diverticula, 500–502
    clinical presentation of, 500
    management of, 500–502
    natural history of, 500
    pathophysiology of, 500
  following hernia repair, for inguinal hernias, 687
  following pancreas transplantation, 349
  with hepatic resection, 180

Hemorrhage (*Continued*)
  with jejunoileal diverticula, 401
  with Meckel's diverticula, 403
  after pancreatoduodenectomy, 288
  in pediatric patients, 714–715, 716f
  peptic ulcers with, 107–108
    duodenal, 116–117
    operation for, 119–120
  with rectal prolapse, 628
  in ulcerative colitis, 535
Hemorrhoids, 589f, 589–599
  diagnosis of, 590–591
  etiology and pathogenesis of, 590
  external, thrombosed, 596f, 596–597, 597f
  in inflammatory bowel disease, 598
  in leukemia, 598
  nomenclature and classification of, 589–590
  nonoperative treatment of, 591
  with other anorectal diseases, 599
  in portal hypertension, 598
  predisposing and associated factors for, 590
  in pregnancy, 597–598
  prevalence of, 590
  strangulated, 597, 598f
  surgical treatment of, 591–596
    circular stapled hemorrhoidectomy for, 592–593, 593f, 594f, 595, 595t
    closed hemorrhoidectomy for, 592, 592f, 593f
    excision and ligation for, 595
    laser hemorrhoidectomy for, 595–596
    modified Whitehead hemorrhoidectomy for, 595
    recommendations for smooth postoperative course with, 599
Hench, Philip S., 8, 8f
Hepatectomy
  in liver transplantation recipient, 214–215, 215f
  partial, for hepatocellular carcinoma, operative technique for, 171, 171f–174f
Hepatic artery aneurysms, 470–471
Hepatic cancer. *See* Hepatocellular carcinoma; Intrahepatic cholangiocarcinoma
Hepatic failure, following hepatic resection, 180–181
Hepatic insufficiency, following hepatic resection, 180–181
Hepatic metastases, 177–189
  colorectal, nonresectional, 182–183
  hepatic resection for. *See* Hepatic resection, for hepatic metastases
  from neuroendocrine tumors, hepatic resection for, 183–185
  from noncolorectal, nonneuroendocrine tumors, hepatic resection for, 185–187
Hepaticojejunostomy
  for biliary strictures, 255
  Roux-en-Y, for pancreatic and periampullary carcinoma, 284
Hepatic resection
  for gallbladder carcinoma, 266, 266f
  for hepatic metastases
    colorectal, results of, 181f, 181t, 181–182, 182f
    complications of, 180–181
    neuroendocrine, 183–185
    for neuroendocrine metastases, 183–185
    noncolorectal, nonneuroendocrine, 185–187
    operative technique for, 178–179, 179f
    patient selection for, 177–178
    postoperative care for, 179–180
    preoperative care for, 178
  for hepatocellular carcinoma, 165–166
  repeat, for hepatocellular carcinoma, 167
Hepatic splenosis, 200

Hepatitis B virus, hepatocellular carcinoma and, 159–160
Hepatitis C virus, hepatocellular carcinoma and, 160
Hepatobiliary injury, operative management of, 646
Hepatocellular adenoma, 193–195, 195f, 196f
Hepatocellular carcinoma, 159–170, 171–176
  clinical features of, 161
  epidemiology of, 159
  etiology of, 159–160
  fibrolamellar, 169f, 169–170, 170f
  laboratory findings in, 161
  liver biopsy in, 164, 165f
  liver transplantation for, 210–211
  natural history of, 162
  pathology of, 160–161, 161f
  patient selection in, 162f, 162–164, 163f
  prevention of, 169
  staging of, 164, 166t
  surveillance for, 164–165
  treatment of, 165–169
    ablation as, 167–168
    adjuvant therapy in, 168–169
    operative technique for, 171, 171f–174f
    orthotopic liver transplantation as, 166–167
    for recurrent disease, repeat hepatic resection as, 167
Hepatocellular tumors, benign, 192–195, 193f–196f
Hepp-Couinaud approach, for biliary strictures, 257
Hernia(s)
  incisional, with bariatric surgery, 153
  very large, 155
  inguinal. *See* Inguinal hernias
  ventral. *See* Ventral hernias
Hernia repair
  for inguinal hernias. *See* Inguinal hernias
  for paraesophageal hernias, laparoscopic, 29–30, 30f
  for ventral hernias
    component separation of abdominal wall and, 671–674
    indications for, 668–669
    laparoscopic, 669–671, 669f–671f
    Rives-Stoppa technique of, 674–677, 675f, 676f
Hill repair, 30
Hirschsprung's disease, in pediatric patients, 716–717, 717f
Hodgkin's disease, 367
H_2-receptor antagonists, for peptic ulcers, 109t, 110
Hydrochloric acid, peptic ulcer and, 104–105
Hyperlipidemia, with morbid obesity, 141
Hypertension
  intra-abdominal, 655–656
  with morbid obesity, 140
  portal
    hemorrhoids and anorectal varices in, 597–598
    liver transplantation for, 211
  sinistral, 367

Ileal artery aneurysms, 473
Ileal pouch-anal canal anastomosis
  for familial adenomatous polyposis, ileorectal anastomosis versus, 562
  for functional constipation, 481
  proctocolectomy with, 536–542
    clinical results with, 538–542
    for familial adenomatous polyposis, 560, 561–562, 562t

Ileal pouch-anal canal anastomosis (Continued)
    physiologic results with, 542
    preparation for, 536
    procedure for, 536–538, 537f
    rationale for, 536
Ileal pouch-distal rectal anastomosis, proctocolectomy with, 542–543, 543f
Ileorectal anastomosis
    abdominal colectomy and, 548–549
        advantages and disadvantages of, 548
        procedure for, 548–549, 549f
        results with, 549
    colectomy with, for familial adenomatous polyposis, 560–561, 561f
    for functional constipation, 481
    ileal pouch-anal canal anastomosis versus, for familial adenomatous polyposis, 562
Ileorectostomy
    colectomy with, for functional constipation, 480–481, 482f
    for Crohn's disease, 415, 417f
Ileostomy
    Brooke
        for Crohn's disease, 415, 417f
        proctocolectomy and. See Proctocolectomy, Brooke ileostomy and
    continent, proctocolectomy and, 545–548
        background and rationale for, 545
        indications for and contraindications to, 545–546
        posthospital care with, 546–547
        procedure for, 546, 546f
        results with, 547–548
    for functional constipation, 481
    proctocolectomy with, for familial adenomatous polyposis, 563, 563f
    for volvulus, 555
Ileum, anatomy of, 375–376
Ileus, gallstone, 229
Iliopubic tract, 680
Imipenem-cilastin, for colonic diverticula, 493
Immune thrombocytopenic purpura, 366
Immunosuppression, following pancreas transplantation, 347, 348f
Imperforate anus, in pediatric patients, 717–719
Incisional hernias, with bariatric surgery, 153
    very large, 155
Infants. See Pediatric gastrointestinal disorders
Infection. See also specific infections
    in acute pancreatitis, 326–327, 327f
        treatment of, 328–329, 329t
    following hernia repair, for inguinal hernias, 687
Inflammation
    bile duct strictures with, 250–251
    with Meckel's diverticula, 404, 405f
Inflammatory bowel disease. See Crohn's disease; Ulcerative colitis
Inflammatory pseudotumor, hepatic, 199–200
Inguinal hernias, 679–689, 691–697
    diagnosis and imaging of, 681–682, 691
    endoscopic repair of, 691–697
        indications for, 691–692
        long-term follow-up of, 696
        outcome with, 695–696
        totally extraperitoneal, 692f, 692–693, 693f, 695, 696
        transabdominal preperitoneal, 693–695, 694f, 695f, 695–696
    etiology of, 680–681
    inguinal region anatomy of and, 680
    physiology of, 691
    recurrent, 688, 688t
    surgical repair of, 682–688
        Bassini method for, 682–683, 683f

Inguinal hernias (Continued)
    complications of, 687–688
    historical background of, 679–680
    Lichtenstein method for, 682, 682f, 683f
    McVay Cooper's ligament repair for, 684–686
    mesh plug repair for, 683–684, 684f, 685f
    Nyhus repair for, 686
    Shouldice repair for, 687
    Stoppa repair for, 686–687
Instrument design at Mayo Clinic, 11–12
Insulinoma, 300–306
    adult nesidioblastosis and, 305–306, 306f
    clinical evaluation of, 301, 301t
    clinical presentation of, 300–301, 301t
    historical background of, 299, 300
    localization of, 301–303, 302f, 303t
    malignant, 306
    MEN I with hyperinsulinism and, 305, 306f
    operative treatment of, 303–305, 304f, 305f
Integrated group practice, 3–4
Intestinal cysts, in pediatric patients, 711–712
Intestinal duplications, in pediatric patients, 711–712
Intestinal viability, assessment of
    with mesenteric ischemia, acute, 445
    with small bowel obstruction, 433
Intestine. See Bowel entries; Colon entries; Colonic entries; Small intestinal entries; Small intestine entries
Intra-abdominal abscess, after pancreatoduodenectomy, 288
Intra-abdominal hemorrhage
    in acute pancreatitis, treatment of, 331
    after pancreatoduodenectomy, 288
Intra-abdominal hypertension, 655–656
Intrahepatic cholangiocarcinoma, 170–171
Intrarectal ultrasonography, in fistula in ano, 610
Intussusception
    with Meckel's diverticula, 404–405
        diagnosis of, 405–406
    in pediatric patients, 712–713, 713f
Ischemic colitis, 519–524
    after abdominal aortic reconstruction, 521
    colonic vascular anatomy and, 519f, 519–520
    colonoscopy in, 521
    etiology of, 520t, 520–521
    nonischemic, in elderly patients, 520
    occlusive, acute, 521
    pathology of, 520
    patient groups and, 520–521
    physical examination in, 521
    radiographic diagnosis of, 522
    surgical treatment of, 22–523
        indications for, 522
        long-term follow-up of, 522–523
        outcomes with, 522–523
        procedure for, 522, 522f
    in young adults, 520
Islet cell tumors, 299–319, 300f. See also Insulinoma
    carcinoma as, 314f, 314–315
    gastrinoma as, 306–310
        diagnosis of, 307, 307t
        localization and treatment of, 307–309, 308f, 308t, 309f
        in multiple endocrine neoplasia I, 309–310, 310f
    glucagonoma as, 310–313, 311f, 311t
        VIPoma syndrome and, 312–313, 313t
    historical background of, 299–300
    in multiple endocrine neoplasia I, 315f, 315–316
    somatostatinoma syndrome and, 313–314, 314t
    very rare, 316

Islet transplantation, 343
Ivor Lewis esophagogastrectomy, 62–63, 63f–65f

Jaundice, intermittent, choledocholithiasis with, 238
Jejunal artery aneurysms, 473
Jejunal pouch-anal canal anastomosis, proctocolectomy and, 549–550
    advantages of, 549
    procedure for, 549, 550f
    results with, 550
Jejunoileal bypass, historical background of, 142–144, 144t
Jejunoileal diverticula, 399–402
    diagnosis of, 400–401
    location, incidence, and cause of, 399, 399f
    signs and symptoms of, 399–400, 400f
    treatment of, 401–402
Jejunum, anatomy of, 375
Judd, E. Starr, 14, 15f
Juvenile polyps, 715

Karydakis procedure, 618, 619f
Kendall, Edward C., 8, 8f
Kidney transplantation, with pancreas transplantation, 341–342, 342t
Kirklin, John W., 6–7, 7f, 17, 19, 20
Kocher maneuver, for duodenal diverticula, 398
Kock pouch, proctocolectomy and, 545–548
    background and rationale for, 545
    indications for and contraindications to, 545–546
    posthospital care with, 546–547
    procedure for, 546, 546f
    results with, 547–548

Langenbuch, Carl, cholecystectomy and, 225
Langerhans, Paul, 299
Laparoscopic procedures. See specific procedures
Laparotomy, for diverticula
    elective, 496
    emergency, 494–496, 495f
Large intestine. See Bowel entries; Colon entries; Colonic entries
Laser therapy, endoscopic, for esophageal carcinoma, 71
Laxatives
    bulk-forming, for hemorrhoids, 591
    for hemorrhoids, 591
Leiomyoma, hepatic, 198–199
Leiomyosarcoma, small intestinal, 381–382, 382f
Leukemia, hemorrhoids in, 598
Lichtenstein, Irving, 682, 683
Lichtenstein repair, 682, 682f, 683f
Lifestyle modifications, for peptic ulcers, 109
Ligamentum teres approach, for biliary strictures, 255–256
Linkage analysis testing, for familial adenomatous polyposis, 560
Lipoma, hepatic, 198
Lipomatous tumors, hepatic, 198
Lithotripsy, biliary, 237–238
Liver. See also Hepatic entries
    benign tumors of, 191–200
        cholangiocellular, 195–196
        classification of, 191, 192t
        diagnosis and imaging of, 191–192
        hepatocellular, 192–195, 193f–196f
        mesenchymal, 198–199
        neural, 199
        newer operative approaches for, 203
        vascular, 196–197, 197f, 198f

Liver *(Continued)*
cystic lesions of, 191–192
classification of, 191, 192t
congenital, 200–202
diagnosis and imaging of, 191–192
neoplastic, 202
newer operative approaches for, 203
traumatic, 202–203
polycystic disease of, 201–202
Liver biopsy, for hepatocellular carcinoma, 164, 165f
Liver cancer. *See* Hepatic metastases; Hepatocellular carcinoma; Intrahepatic cholangiocarcinoma
Liver resection. *See* Hepatic resection
Liver transplantation, 209–223
for benign hepatic neoplasms and cysts, 203
for cholangiocarcinoma, 211
for hepatocellular carcinoma, 210–211
indications for, 210
liver diseases necessitating, 209–210, 210f
living-donor, 219–222, 220f
donor evaluation for, 220–221
donor operation for, 221
need for, 220
postoperative management for, 222
recipient operation for, 221–222
organ allocation and acceptance for, 212
organ procurement in cadaver donors and, 212–214, 213f
orthotopic, for hepatocellular carcinoma, 166–167
patient evaluation for, 211–212
for portal hypertension, 211
recipient operation for, 214–218
biliary reconstruction and, 217, 217f, 218f
caval replacement and venous bypass and, 216
hepatectomy as, 214–215, 215f
implantation and reperfusion and, 215–216, 216f
portal vein thrombosis and, 216–217
postoperative and long-term care for, 217–218, 218f, 219f
split liver, 218–219
Living-donor liver transplantation, 219–222, 220f
donor evaluation for, 220–221
donor operation for, 221
need for, 220
postoperative management for, 222
recipient operation for, 221–222
Longmire procedure, for biliary strictures, 256
Lotheissen, Georg, 680, 684
Lower esophageal sphincter
in gastroesophageal reflux disease, 23–24
pneumatic dilation of, for achalasia, 40f, 40–41
Lymphadenectomy
extended, for pancreatic and periampullary carcinoma, 283–284
for gastric cancer, 80f, 80t, 80–83, 81f, 81t
regional, for gallbladder carcinoma, 266–267, 267f
Lymphangioma, hepatic, 197–198
Lymphedema, with morbid obesity, 141
Lymphoma, 367
gastric. *See* Gastric lymphoma
Hodgkin's, 367
non-Hodgkin, 367
small intestinal, 380–381, 381f, 381t

Macewen, William, 683
Malabsorption, with jejunoileal diverticula, 399–400
treatment of, 401
Malabsorptive procedures, historical background of, 148–149, 149f

Malignancies. *See also specific malignancies*
with morbid obesity, 141
Malrotation, in pediatric patients, 699–703, 700f, 702f
Manometry, anorectal, 477–478, 479f
Marsupialization, for pilonidal sinus, 617
Mayo, Charles Horace, 1–3, 3f, 4, 5, 19
rectal cancer and, 569–570, 580
small bowel carcinoma and, 382
small bowel obstruction and, 422
Mayo, Louise Abigail Wright, 1, 2f
Mayo Properties Association, 4
Mayo, William James, 1–3, 2f, 4, 5, 9, 16–17, 19, 20, 21
biliary strictures and, 247
colonic diverticula and, 489
gastric adenocarcinoma and, 75
islet cell tumors and, 299
small bowel obstruction and, 422
spleen and, 365
splenectomy and, 371, 372
Mayo, William Worrall, 1, 2f, 19, 21
Mayo Clinic
branches of, 10, 14
commitment to ideals and standards at, 16–17
cost-effectiveness at, 14, 16
daily life of surgeons at, 10–13
expanding role of philanthropy for, 16
governance of, 8–9
historical background of, 1–10
instrument design at, 11–12
relationship focus at, 6–7
research at, 8, 13
surgical technique development at, 11
surgical technique standardization at, 12
teamwork at, 12–13, 16
Mayo Foundation, 4, 9, 10
McIlrath, D. C., islet cell tumors and, 299
McVay, Chester, 684
McVay Cooper's ligament repair, 684–686
Meckel, Johann Friederich, 402
Meckel's diverticula, 402–406
diagnosis of, 404–405
embryology and anatomy and, 402–403, 403f
signs and symptoms of, 403–404, 404f, 405f
surgical therapy for, 405–406
Meconium ileus, 710–711
Meconium plug syndrome, 711
Medical records system, 4–6
Megacolon, toxic, in ulcerative colitis, 535
Melanoma, hepatic metastases from, hepatic resection for, 186
Mesenchymal hamartoma, hepatic, 199
Mesenchymal tumors, hepatic, benign, 198–199
Mesenteric artery aneurysms, superior, 471
Mesenteric ischemia
acute, 441–446
diagnosis of, 442–443
mortality rates associated with, 441, 441t
pathophysiology and etiology of, 441–442, 442f
surgical treatment of
assessment of intestinal viability and, 445
for embolic occlusive disease, 444, 445f
indications for, 443
for nonocclusive disease, 445
outcomes of, 445
preoperative preparation for, 443
for thrombotic occlusive disease, 444–445
chronic, 457–466
clinical presentation of, 457–458, 458t
diagnosis of, 458–459, 460f
prevalence of, 457
surgical treatment of, 459–465, 464t

Mesenteric ischemia *(Continued)*
choice of operation for, 459
operative technique for, 460–463, 461f–463f
results of, 463–464, 464t
Mesenteric venous thrombosis, acute, 447–455
clinical classification of, 448
clinical presentation of, 448–449, 449t
diagnostic tests for, 449f, 449–450, 450f
etiology of, 447–448, 448t
incidence of, 447
treatment of, 450–453, 453f
clinical outcome of, 452, 452f, 452t, 453f
nonsurgical, 450–451
surgical, 451f, 451–452
Mesh plug repair, for inguinal hernias, 683–684, 684f, 685f
Mesosigmoidoplasty, for volvulus, 557
Mesothelioma, hepatic, benign, 199
Metabolic acidosis, following pancreas transplantation, 349
Metabolic disorders, following gastric operations, 121
Metastatic disease
hepatic. *See* Hepatic metastases
small intestinal, 382, 383f
Methyl-*tert*-butyl ether, for gallstones, 237, 238f
Metronidazole, for colonic diverticula, 492, 493
Mirizzi syndrome, 228f, 229
bile duct strictures in, 250–251
Mono-octanoin, for gallstones, 237
Morbidity, in hospital, with bariatric surgery, 153
Morbid obesity, 139–157
bariatric surgery for. *See* Bariatric surgery
medical complications of, 140t, 140–142, 141t
Mortality
in hospital, with bariatric surgery, 153
with mesenteric ischemia, acute, 441, 441t
after pancreatoduodenectomy, 288
Mucinous cystic neoplasm, pancreatic, 352–353, 353f
operative treatment of, 357–358, 359f, 359–361, 360f
Mucosa-associated lymphoid tissue, gastric lymphoma associated with, 91, 93–94, 94f
Mucosal defense, against gastric acid and pepsin, 105
Multiple endocrine neoplasia, type I
historical background of, 299–300
with hyperinsulinism, 305, 306f
pancreas in, 315f, 315–316, 316f
Zollinger-Ellison syndrome in, 309–310, 310f
Myeloid disorders, chronic, 367
Myotomy
laparoscopic
for achalasia, 43–44, 44f
with diverticulectomy and fundoplication, for epiphrenic esophageal diverticula, 50–52, 51f–53f
surgical
for achalasia, 41
for diffuse esophageal spasm, 46
thoracoscopic
for achalasia, 43
with diverticulectomy and fundoplication, for epiphrenic esophageal diverticula, 52–53, 53f, 54f

Nagorney, D. M., islet cell tumors and, 299
Nasogastric suction, for small bowel obstruction, 432
Necrolytic migratory erythema, with glucagonoma, 311f, 311–312
Necrosectomy, technique for, 328–329, 329t

Necrosis
    colonic, in acute pancreatitis, treatment of, 331
    pancreatic, in acute pancreatitis, 326, 326f, 327f
        treatment of, 328–329, 329t
Necrotizing enterocolitis, in pediatric patients,
    708–710, 709f
Necrotizing fasciitis, anorectal, 608
Neoplasms. See Malignancies; *specific types and sites*
Nerve ablation, for chronic pancreatitis, 337–338
Nesidioblastosis, adult, 305–306, 306f
Neuralgia, following hernia repair, for inguinal
    hernias, 687–688
Neural tumors, hepatic, 199
Neuroendocrine tumors, hepatic metastases from,
    hepatic resection for, 183–185
Nipple valve, malfunction of, following continent
    ileostomy and proctocolectomy, 547–548
Nissen fundoplication, laparoscopic, 26–29,
    27f–29f
Nitroglycerin, for anal fissures, 601
Nodular regenerative hyperplasia, 195
Non-Hodgkin lymphoma, 367
Nonsteroidal anti-inflammatory drugs, peptic
    ulcers and, 105
    prophylaxis for, 111
Nutcracker esophagus, 46
Nutritional support, for acute pancreatitis, 324
Nyhus repair, 686

Obesity, morbid, 139–157
    bariatric surgery for. See Bariatric surgery
    medical complications of, 140t, 140–142, 141t
Omphalomesenteric duct remnants, 713–714
Oophorectomy, prophylactic, with colon cancer,
    516
Orange days, 10
Orthotopic liver transplantation, for hepatocellular
    carcinoma, 166–167
Ostracism, with morbid obesity, 141

Pancreas. See also Pancreatic *entries*
    exocrine secretions of, pancreatic transplantation
        and, 346
    injury of, operative management of, 646–647
Pancreatectomy
    for chronic pancreatitis, 336
    historical background of, 299
Pancreatic anastomotic leak, after pancreatoduo-
    denectomy, 287–288
Pancreatic and periampullary carcinoma, 271–297,
    272f
    biomolecular markers for, 274–275
    diagnosis of, 275–278
        angiography in, 277–278
        clinical evaluation in, 275
        computed tomography in, 275–277, 276f
        endoscopic retrograde cholangiopancreatogra-
            phy in, 277
        endoscopic ultrasonography in, 278
        laboratory evaluation in, 275
        laparoscopy in, 278
        magnetic resonance imaging and magnetic
            resonance spectroscopy in, 277
        perioperative or intraoperative biopsy in, 278
        positron-emission tomography in, 277
    lymph node metastases of, 273, 274f
    operative treatment of
        conduct of, 279–285, 287–288
            adjuvant therapy with, 288–289
            ampullectomy for, 284
            extended lymphadenectomy in, 283–284
            long-term follow-up of, 289t, 289–291,
                290f, 290t, 291f

Pancreatic and periampullary carcinoma
    (*Continued*)
        outcome of, 287–288
        for palliative surgery, 284–285
        postoperative management and, 287
        for potentially curative resection, 279–283,
            280f–286f
        indication for, 279
    pathology of, 272
    perineural invasion of, 273–274
    staging of, 273t, 273–274
Pancreatic artery aneurysms, 473–474
Pancreatic cancer. See also Pancreatic and peri-
    ampullary carcinoma
    hepatic metastases from, hepatic resection for,
        187
Pancreatic cystic tumors, 351–363
    adjuvant therapy for, 358–359
    diagnosis and imaging of, 354–357, 355t
        angiography for, 356
        computed tomography and ultrasonography
            for, 355–356, 356f
        endoscopic retrograde cholangiopancreatogra-
            phy for, 356, 357f
        laparoscopy for, 356–357
        magnetic resonance pancreatography for,
            356, 357f
    histopathologic classification of, 351t,
        351–354
    operative treatment of, 357–358
        for intraductal papillary mucinous tumor,
            358
        for mucinous cystic neoplasm, 357–358,
            359f, 359–361, 360f
        for neoplasms discovered incidentally at oper-
            ation, 358
        for serous cystadenoma, 357, 359
        surgical outcomes and long-term follow-up
            of, 359–361
Pancreatic fistulas, in acute pancreatitis, treatment
    of, 331
Pancreatic heterotopia, 199
Pancreatic necrosis, in acute pancreatitis, 326,
    326f, 327f
    treatment of, 328–329, 329t
Pancreaticoduodenal artery aneurysms, 473–474
Pancreaticoduodenectomy, for chronic pancreati-
    tis, 335, 336f, 336–337, 337f
Pancreatic pseudocysts
    in acute pancreatitis, 325f, 325–326
    surgical treatment of, 329–331
Pancreatic resection
    for chronic pancreatitis, 336–337, 337f, 338f
    for pseudocysts, 330
Pancreatic transplantation, 341–350
    alone, 341, 342, 342t
    benefits of, 343–344
    indications for, 341
    islet transplantation as, 343
    after kidney transplantation, 341, 342, 342t
    for nonuremic diabetic patients, 342–343
    postoperative complications of, 348–350
    postoperative management for, 346–350
        immunosuppression in, 347, 348f
        monitoring for rejection and, 347–348
    preoperative evaluation and preparation for,
        342
    simultaneous with kidney transplantation, 341,
        342, 342t
    surgical technique for, 344–346
        for bench-work procedure, 344–345, 345f,
            346f
        exocrine secretions and, 346, 347f, 348f
        for pancreas recovery, 344
        for pancreatic transplant, 345, 346f

Pancreatitis, 321–340
    acute, 321–332
        complications of, 325–327, 325f–327f
        diagnosis of, 322–323
        etiology of, 321, 322t
        management of, 323t, 323–324, 324t
        outcomes of, 332, 332t
        pathogenesis of, 321–322
        severity scoring of, 325
        surgery for, 327–332
            with colonic necrosis, 331
            with infected necrosis, 328
            with intra-abdominal hemorrhage, 331
            necrosectomy as, 328–329, 329t
            with nonresolving sterile necrosis, 328
            with pancreatic fistulas, 331
            with pancreatic pseudocysts, 329–331
            with severe gallstone pancreatitis, 332
    biliary, in choledocholithiasis, 239, 239t
    chronic, 332–338
        bile duct strictures with, 251
        clinical presentation of, 333
        diagnosis of, 333–334, 334f
        etiology of, 332, 333t
        management of, 334–338
            medical therapy in, 334–335
            surgical, 335–338, 336f–338f
        pathogenesis of, 333
    graft, following pancreas transplantation, 349
Pancreatoduodenectomy
    for pancreatic and periampullary carcinoma,
        279–283, 280f–286f
        adjuvant therapy with, 288–289
        alternatives to, 284
        extended lymphadenectomy with, 283–284
        long-term follow-up of, 289t, 289–291, 290f,
            290t, 291f
        outcome of, 287–288
        postoperative management and, 287
    for villous tumors of duodenum, 391, 393–394
Papaverine, for mesenteric ischemia, acute, 445
Papillary mucinous tumor, pancreatic, intraductal,
    353f, 353–354, 354f
    operative treatment of, 358
Paraesophageal hernia repair, laparoscopic, 29–30,
    30f
Pathologists, 13
Patient consultations, 10–12
Patient focus, 4–6
Pearse, A. G. E., islet cell tumors and, 299
Pediatric gastrointestinal disorders, 699–721
    atresia as, 704–705, 705f
    bleeding as, 714–715, 716f
    in children 3 months to 3 years, 699
    in children older than 3 years, 699
    Hirschsprung's disease as, 716–717, 717f
    imperforate anus as, 717–719
    in infants 0 to 3 months of age, 699
    intestinal duplications and cysts as, 711–712
    intussusception as, 712–713, 713f
    malrotation as, 699–703, 700f, 702f
    meconium syndromes as, 710–711
    necrotizing enterocolitis as, 708–710, 709f
    omphalomesenteric duct remnants as, 713–714
    polypoid disease as, 715–716
    pyloric stenosis as, 703, 704f
    tracheoesophageal fistula as, 706f, 706–708,
        707f
Peliosis hepatis, 200
Peptic ulcers, 103–126
    anastomotic (stomal), 120–121
    Dieulafoy lesion as, 122–123
        etiology of, 122
        management of, 123
        presentation and diagnosis of, 122

Peptic ulcers (Continued)
duodenal, bile duct strictures with, 250–251
epidemiology of, 104
hemorrhage with, 107–108
historical background of, 103–104
medical therapy for, 108–111
for duodenal ulcers, 110
for gastric ulcers, 110–111
for Helicobacter pylori, 110
lifestyle modifications as, 109
pharmacologic, 109t, 109–110
prophylactic, for NSAID-associated ulcers, 111
obstruction with, 108
pathogenesis of, 104–106
acid secretion and mucosal defense and, 104–105
Helicobacter pylori in, 105, 106
nonsteroidal anti-inflammatory drugs in, 105
smoking in, 105
Zollinger-Ellison syndrome and, 105–106
perforation of, 108
stress
acute, 121–122
management of, 122
pathogenesis of, 121
surgical therapy for, 111–121
adverse outcomes of, 120–121
for duodenal ulcer, 115–118
with complications, 116–118
elective operations for, 115–116, 116t
for gastric ulcer, 118–120
with complications, 119–120
elective, 119
indications for, 119
types of ulcers and, 118f, 118–119
operative techniques for, 111–114, 112t, 112f–114f
operative trends and, 111
physiologic effects of operation and, 114–115
uncomplicated, 106–107
Periampullary carcinoma. See Pancreatic and peri-ampullary carcinoma
Peripancreatic fluid collections, in acute pancreatitis, 325f, 325–326
treatment of, 329–331
Peutz-Jeghers syndrome, 715–716
pH monitoring, esophageal, 24-hour, in gastro-esophageal reflux disease, 24–25
Philanthropy, expanding role of, 16
Photodynamic therapy, for esophageal carcinoma, 70
Pigmented gallstones, 226–227
Pilonidal carcinoma, 622
Pilonidal sinus, 615f, 615–632
carcinoma and, 622
clinical manifestations of, 616
diagnosis of, 616, 616f
natural history of, 615
predisposing factors for, 616
surgical pathology of, 615
treatment of, 616–622
for abscess, 616f, 616–617
for sinus, 617–622, 617f–622f
Piperacillin-tazobactam, for colonic diverticula, 493
Plastic surgical reconstruction, following bariatric surgery, 155
Platelet disorders, 366–368
Plummer, Henry S., 4, 4f
Pneumatic dilation, for achalasia, 40f, 40–41
Polycystic liver disease, 201–202
Polyp(s). See also Familial adenomatous polyposis
gastric, 76
in pediatric patients, 715–716
villous tumors of duodenum associated with, 391

Polypectomy, prior, excision of site of, 514
Portal hypertension
hemorrhoids and anorectal varices in, 598
liver transplantation for, 211
sinistral, 367
Portal vein thrombosis, in liver transplantation recipients, 216–217
Pouchitis
following proctocolectomy and continent ileostomy, 548
following proctocolectomy and ileal pouch-anal canal anastomosis, 540
Praxagoras, 421
Pregnancy
following proctocolectomy and ileal pouch-anal canal anastomosis, 539–540
hemorrhoids in, 597–598
Priestley, James T., 9, 9f
islet cell tumors and, 299
Proctectomy
completion, for functional constipation, 481
for Crohn's disease, 416
Proctocolectomy
Brooke ileostomy and, 543–545
advantages and disadvantages of, 543
indications for, 543
operative technique for, 544, 544f
postoperative care with, 544–545
preoperative preparation for, 543–544
results with, 545
continent ileostomy and, 545–548
background and rationale for, 545
indications for and contraindications to, 545–546
posthospital care with, 546–547
procedure for, 546, 546f
results with, 547–548
for Crohn's disease, 415, 417f
with ileal pouch-anal anastomosis, for familial adenomatous polyposis, 560, 561–562, 562t
ileal pouch-anal canal anastomosis and, 536–542
clinical results with, 538–542
physiologic results with, 542
preparation for, 536
procedure for, 536–538, 537f
rationale for, 536
ileal pouch-distal rectal anastomosis and, 542–543, 543f
with ileostomy, for familial adenomatous polyposis, 563, 563f
jejunal pouch-anal canal anastomosis and, 549–550
advantages of, 549
procedure for, 549, 550f
results with, 550
prophylactic, for familial adenomatous polyposis, 560
Proctography, evacuation, 478
Prostaglandin analogues, for peptic ulcers, 109, 109t
Proton pump inhibitors, for peptic ulcers, 109t, 110
Pseudoachalasia, 39
Pseudocysts
in acute pancreatitis, 325f, 325–326
pancreatic
in acute pancreatitis, 325f, 325–326
surgical treatment of, 329–331
Pseudolipoma, hepatic, 198
Pseudotumor, inflammatory, hepatic, 199–200
Pulmonary embolism, following hernia repair, for inguinal hernias, 688
Pyloric stenosis, in pediatric patients, 703, 704f

Pyloromyotomy
laparoscopic, 703
Ramstedt, 703
Pyloroplasty, gastric emptying after, 129

Radiation therapy. See also Chemoradiation therapy
adjuvant
for pancreatic cystic neoplasms, 358–359
with pancreatoduodenectomy, 288
for rectal cancer, 581–582
endocavitary, for rectal cancer, 575–576
Radiofrequency ablation, for neuroendocrine hepatic metastases, 185
Radiopaque markers, for colonic transit evaluation, 476–477, 477f
Ramstedt pyloromyotomy, 703
Rankin, Fred W., 3
small bowel carcinoma and, 382
Rectal amputation, for rectal cancer, 578–579
Rectal cancer, 569–588. See also Colorectal cancer
factors influencing treatment of, 571–573
patient-related, 571
surgeon-related, 572–573
tumor-related, 571–572, 572t
following proctocolectomy and ileal pouch-anal canal anastomosis, 541
future directions for, 583
landmarks in treatment at Mayo Clinic and, 569–570, 570t
preoperative evaluation and, 573–574
disseminated disease and, 574
histological, 573–574
locally advanced or nonresectable lesions and, 574
synchronous lesions and, 574
screening for, 570–571
surgical treatment of
adjuvant chemotherapy and radiotherapy with, 581–582, 582f
follow-up of, 582–583
locally recurrent disease and, 583, 583f, 583t
local treatment for, 575–576
operative procedure for, 576–580, 577f, 579f
postoperative complications and, 580t, 580–581
preparation for, 576
sphincter-saving operation for, 574–575, 575f
Rectal excision
local, for rectal cancer, 577f, 577–578
wide local, for rectal cancer, 579
Rectal flaps, advancement, for fistula in ano, 611, 613f
Rectal prolapse, 627f, 627–635, 628f
clinical features and diagnosis of, 627–628, 628f
complications of, 628–629
etiology of, 627
incarcerated, 629
investigation of, 628, 629f
operative repair of, 629–635
abdominal approach for, 629–631, 630f
laparoscopic, 630–631
perineal approach for, 631–635, 632f–634f
pathophysiology of, 627
Rectal resection, anterior
low, for rectal cancer, 576
for rectal cancer, 576
Rectal ulcer, solitary, 635
Rectopexy, for rectal prolapse, 629, 630f
Rectosigmoidectomy, perineal, 631, 632f–633f
Rectosigmoid resection, for rectal prolapse, 629
Rectum. See Anorectal entries; Colorectal entries; Rectal entries
Redo procedures, antireflux, laparoscopic, 30

Reexcision, for pilonidal sinus, 620
Reflux gastritis, alkaline, after gastric operations, 132
    medical and dietary interventions for, 133
    operative treatment of, 136
Relationship focus at Mayo Clinic, 6–7
Release technique, for abdominal wall reconstruction, 661, 662f
ReMine, W. H., islet cell tumors and, 299
Renal injury, bile duct strictures due to, 249
Reoperation
    bariatric, 155–156
    following proctocolectomy and ileal pouch-anal canal anastomosis, 541–542
Research, 8, 13
Reverse bandaging, for pilonidal sinus, 620, 620f
Ripstein procedure, 630, 630f
Rives-Stoppa technique, 674–677, 675f, 676f
Root, Mabel C., 4, 5f
Rubber band ligation, for hemorrhoids, 591, 591f

Sarcoma, hepatic metastases from, hepatic resection for, 186
Saucerization, for pilonidal sinus, 620
Scarpa, Antonia, 679
Schedules, 10
Schwannoma, hepatic, 199
Scintigraphy, for colonic transit evaluation, 477, 478f
Selective vagotomy, for peptic ulcers, 113
Sentinel loop sign, in acute pancreatitis, 323
Sepsis, after pancreatoduodenectomy, 288
Serosanguineous drainage, following hepatic resection, 180
Seton, for fistula in ano surgery, 613–614, 614f
Sexual function, following proctocolectomy and ileal pouch-anal canal anastomosis, 539
Shouldice repair, 687
Sigmoidopexy
    endoscopic, for volvulus, 557
    for volvulus, 557
Sigmoidoscopy, flexible, for colon cancer detection, 508
Sleep apnea, with morbid obesity, 141
Sleeve resection, for Crohn's disease, 412, 413f
Small intestinal anastomosis
    for pancreatic exocrine secretion drainage, breakdown of, 349
    for pancreatic exocrine secretion drainage, 346, 348f
Small intestinal atresia, in pediatric patients, 704–705, 705f
Small intestinal bypass, historical background of, 142, 143f
Small intestinal diverticula, 397–408
    duodenal, 397–398
        bile duct strictures with, 250
        diagnosis of, 398
        location, incidence, and cause of, 397
        signs and symptoms of, 397–398
        treatment of, 398
    jejunoileal, 399–402
        diagnosis of, 400–401
        location, incidence, and cause of, 399, 399f
        signs and symptoms of, 399–400, 400f
        treatment of, 401–402
    Meckel's, 402–406
        diagnosis of, 404–405
        embryology and anatomy and, 402–403, 403f
        signs and symptoms of, 403–404, 404f, 405f
        surgical therapy for, 405–406

Small intestinal obstruction, 421–439
    with bariatric surgery, 154
    classification of, 422, 423t
    complete, 422
    diagnosis and imaging of, 423–425, 426f–430f, 427
    etiopathogenesis of, 422–423, 423t, 424f, 425f
    functional, 422
    historical background of, 421–422
    incomplete, 422
    with jejunoileal diverticula, 401
    management of, 428–436
        conservative therapy in, 432–433
        during early postoperative period, 434–435
        initial steps in, 428–432, 431f
        laparoscopy in, 435–436, 436t
        operative therapy in, 433–434
        prevention and, 435
    mechanical, 422
    with Meckel's diverticula, 403–404, 404f
    outcome with, 436–437
    simple, 422
    strangulated, 422
Small intestinal resection. See also Bowel resection
    for jejunoileal diverticula, 401, 402
    for small bowel obstruction, 434
Small intestinal tumors
    malignant, 375–385
        adenocarcinoma as, 377–379, 378f, 379t
        anatomy and, 375–376
        carcinoid tumor as, 379–380, 380f
        diagnosis and imaging of, 376–377, 377f
        incidence of, 376
        leiomyosarcoma as, 381–382, 382f
        lymphoma as, 380–381, 381f, 381t
        metastatic, 382, 383f
        pathophysiology of, 376
        surgical approach for, 382–384
    villous, of duodenum. See Villous tumors of duodenum
Small intestine
    Crohn's disease involving, surgical treatment of, 412–415, 413f–415f
    injury of, operative management of, 648–649
Smoking, peptic ulcer and, 105
Soave procedure, 717
Social ostracism and discrimination, with morbid obesity, 141
Solitary rectal ulcer syndrome, 635
Somatostatinoma syndrome, 313–314, 314t
Sphincterotomy
    for Crohn's disease, 417
    endoscopic, for acute pancreatitis, 332
    lateral internal, for anal fissures, 602–603, 603f
Spleen
    abscesses of, 367
    anatomy and physiology of, 365–366
    cysts of, 367
    historical background of, 365
    injury of, operative management of, 645–646
    torsion of, 367–368
Splenectomy, 368–373
    laparoscopic, 368–371, 369f–371f
    open, 371
    partial, for splenic trauma, 646
    preoperative preparation for, 368
    results with, 371–372, 372f, 373f
Splenic artery aneurysms, 468t, 468–470, 469f
Splenic malignancies, primary, 367
Splenorrhaphy, for splenic trauma, 645–646
Splenosis, hepatic, 200
Split liver transplantation, 218–219
Stapling, hand sewing versus, for small bowel anastomoses, 648–649

Stenting
    biliary, for pancreatic and periampullary carcinoma, 287
    for esophageal carcinoma, 70
    of visceral arteries, for chronic mesenteric ischemia, 464t, 464–465
Stomach. See also Gastric entries
    Crohn's disease involving, surgical treatment of, 412, 412f
    injury of, operative management of, 646
Stoppa repair, 686–687
Stress ulcers, 121–122
    hemorrhage of, management of, 122
    prophylaxis for, 121–122
Strictureplasty, for Crohn's disease, 412, 412f, 413f, 413–414
    Finney-type, 413, 414f
    Heineke-Mikulicz-type, 413, 413f
Strictures
    biliary. See Biliary strictures
    following proctocolectomy and ileal pouch-anal canal anastomosis, 540
Sucralfate, for peptic ulcers, 109, 109t
Surgeons, daily life at Mayo Clinic, 10–13
Surgical techniques
    development at Mayo Clinic, 11
    standardization at Mayo Clinic, 12
Swenson procedure, 717

Tait, Lawson, 422
Teamwork at Mayo Clinic, 12–13, 16
Teratoma, hepatic, benign, 199
Testicular complications, following hernia repair, for inguinal hernias, 688
Thermal ablation, for hepatocellular carcinoma, 168
Thoracoscopic operations. See specific procedures
Thoracotomy, right, 64, 64f
Thrombectomy, for mesenteric venous thrombosis, 451–452
Thrombolytic therapy, for mesenteric venous thrombosis, 450–451
Thrombosis
    acute mesenteric ischemia due to, surgical treatment of, 444–445
    femoral vein, following hernia repair, for inguinal hernias, 688
    following pancreas transplantation, 349
    mesenteric artery, superior, surgical treatment of, 444–445
    mesenteric vein. See Mesenteric venous thrombosis, acute
    portal vein, recipient operation for liver transplantation and, 216–217
Tissue expander technique, for abdominal wall reconstruction, 661–663, 662f
Toupet partial posterior fundoplication, laparoscopic, 29, 29f
Toxic megacolon, in ulcerative colitis, 535
Tracheoesophageal fistula, in pediatric patients, 706f, 706–708, 707f
Transhiatal esophagogastrectomy, 66–67, 67f
Traumatic cysts, hepatic, 202
Treves, Frederick, 422
Truncal vagotomy, for peptic ulcers, 111–112, 112f, 115
Tube decompression, for duodenal trauma, 648, 648f
Tumors. See Malignancies; specific types and sites

Ulcer(s), peptic. See Peptic ulcers
Ulcerative colitis, 533–552
    diagnosis of, 533–534
    fulminant, 534–535

Ulcerative colitis (Continued)
hemorrhoids in, 598
medical treatment of, 534, 534t
signs and symptoms of, 533, 533t
surgical treatment of, 534–550
abdominal colectomy and ileorectal anastomosis for, 548–549, 549f
alternatives for, 536, 536t
indications for, 534t, 534–536
proctocolectomy and Brooke ileostomy for,
543–545, 544f
proctocolectomy and continent ileostomy for,
545–548, 546f
proctocolectomy and ileal pouch anal canal
anastomosis for. See Proctocolectomy,
ileal pouch-anal canal anastomosis and
proctocolectomy and ileal pouch-distal rectal
anastomosis for, 542–543, 543f
proctocolectomy and jejunal pouch-anal canal
anastomosis for, 549–550, 550f
rationale for, 536
Unclosable abdomen, 653, 653t
Urethritis, following pancreas transplantation,
349–350

Vacuum-packed technique, for fascial dehiscence,
659–660, 660f
Vagotomy
gastric
proximal
gastric emptying after, 128–129, 129t
for peptic ulcers, 113, 113f, 115
truncal, gastric emptying after, 129
physiologic effects of, 114
selective, for peptic ulcers, 113
truncal, for peptic ulcers, 111–112, 112f, 115
van Heerden, J. A., islet cell tumors and, 299
Varices, anorectal, in portal hypertension, 598

Vascular tumors, hepatic, benign, 196–198, 197f,
198f
Venous stasis disease, with morbid obesity, 141
Venous thrombosis, femoral, following hernia
repair, for inguinal hernias, 688
Ventral hernias, 665–671
clinical presentation and diagnosis of, 666–668,
667f
physiology of, 665–666
surgical treatment of
component separation of abdominal wall in,
671–674
indications for, 668–669
laparoscopic, 669–671, 669f–671f
Rives-Stoppa technique of, 674–677, 675f,
676f
ventral. See Incisional hernias
Verner-Morrison syndrome, 312–313, 313t
Villous tumors of duodenum, 387–396
distribution of, 388
historical background of, 387
operation for, 389–391
conduct of, 391–393, 391f–393f
long-term follow-up of, 394f, 394–395, 395f
Mayo Clinic experience with, 393–394
morbidity and mortality with, 394
with polyposis syndromes, 391
for sporadic VTD, 390–391
size and histology of, 387–388, 388t
symptoms, signs, and diagnosis of, 388–389,
389f
VIPoma syndrome, 312–313, 313t
Visceral artery aneurysms, 467t, 467–474
of celiac artery, 471–472, 472f, 473f
of colic artery, 473
of gastric artery, 472–473
of gastroduodenal artery, 473–474
of gastroepiploic artery, 472–473
of hepatic artery, 470–471

Visceral artery aneurysms (Continued)
of ileal artery, 473
of jejunal artery, 473
of pancreatic artery, 473–474
of pancreaticoduodenal artery, 473–474
of splenic artery, 468t, 468–470, 469f
of superior mesenteric artery, 471
Viscus perforation, with colon cancer, 516–517
Volvulus
colonic. See Colonic volvulus
with Meckel's diverticula, 404, 404f
in pediatric patients, 700f, 701, 703
V-Y advancement flap, for anal fissures, 603–604,
604f

Walters, H. Waltman, 14, 15f
Warfarin, for mesenteric venous thrombosis, 450
Water-soluble contrast agents, for small bowel
obstruction, 432–533
Waugh, John M., 14
hepatic surgery and, 159
Weight loss, with bariatric surgery, 153
Wells procedure, 630, 630f
Whipple procedure. See Pancreatoduodenectomy
"Whirl sign," in cecal volvulus, 554, 555f
Whitehead hemorrhoidectomy, modified, 595
William of Salicet, 679
Work-related ostracism and discrimination, with
morbid obesity, 141
Wutzer, C. W., 683

Zollinger-Ellison syndrome, 105–106, 306–310
diagnosis of, 307, 307t
localization and treatment of gastrinomas in,
307–309, 308f, 308t, 309f
in multiple endocrine neoplasia I, 309–310, 310f
Z-plasty, for pilonidal sinus, 618, 618f